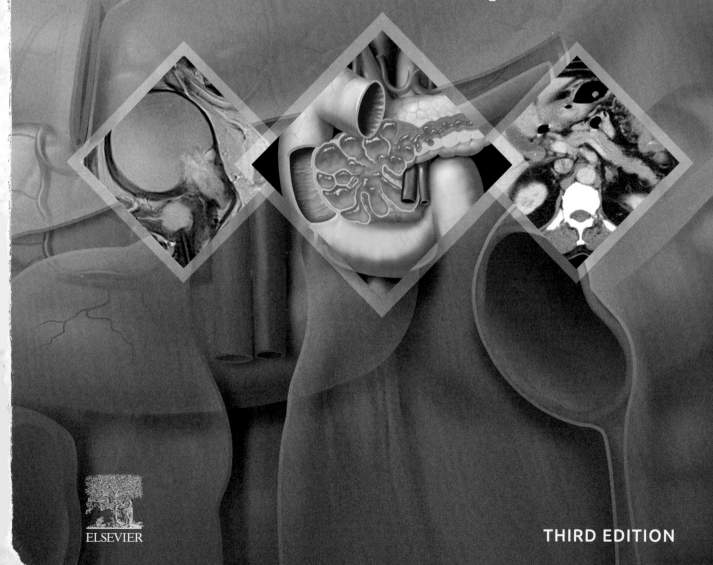

ExpertDDX

Abdomen and Pelvis

Zaheer | Raman
Foster | Fananapazir

ELSEVIER

THIRD EDITION

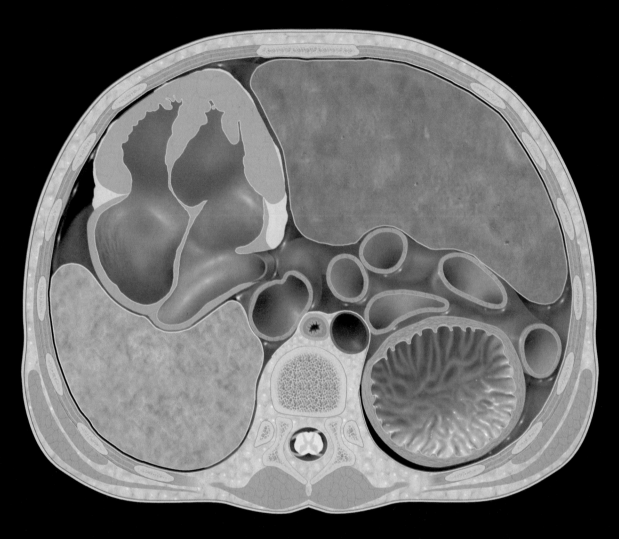

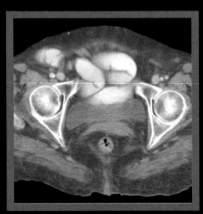

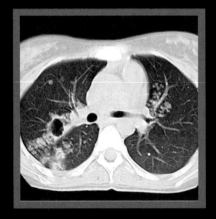

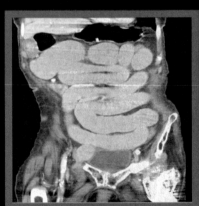

ExpertDDX
Abdomen and Pelvis

THIRD EDITION

Atif Zaheer, MD
Professor of Radiology, Oncology and Medicine
The Johns Hopkins University School of Medicine
Baltimore, Maryland

Siva P. Raman, MD
Bay Imaging Consultants
Walnut Creek, California

Bryan R. Foster, MD
Professor
Department of Radiology
Oregon Health & Science University
Portland, Oregon

Ghaneh Fananapazir, MD, FSAR, FSRU, FSABI
Professor of Radiology
University of California, Davis
Davis, California

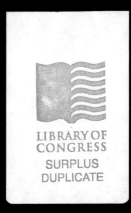

Elsevier
1600 John F. Kennedy Blvd.
Ste 1800
Philadelphia, PA 19103-2899

EXPERTDDX: ABDOMEN AND PELVIS, THIRD EDITION

ISBN: 978-0-323-87866-1

Notices

Practitioners and researchers must always rely on their own experience and knowledge in evaluating and using any information, methods, compounds or experiments described herein. Because of rapid advances in the medical sciences, in particular, independent verification of diagnoses and drug dosages should be made. To the fullest extent of the law, no responsibility is assumed by Elsevier, authors, editors or contributors for any injury and/or damage to persons or property as a matter of products liability, negligence or otherwise, or from any use or operation of any methods, products, instructions, or ideas contained in the material herein.

Previous edition copyrighted 2017.

Library of Congress Control Number: 2022942209

Printed in Canada by Friesens, Altona, Manitoba, Canada

Last digit is the print number: 9 8 7 6 5 4 3 2 1

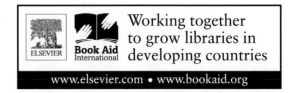

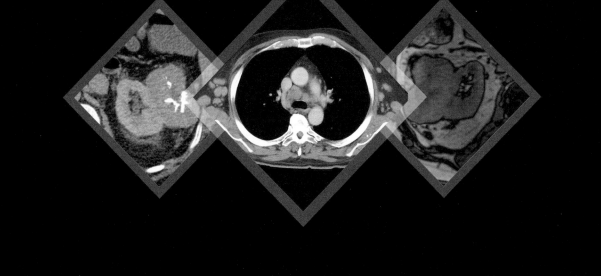

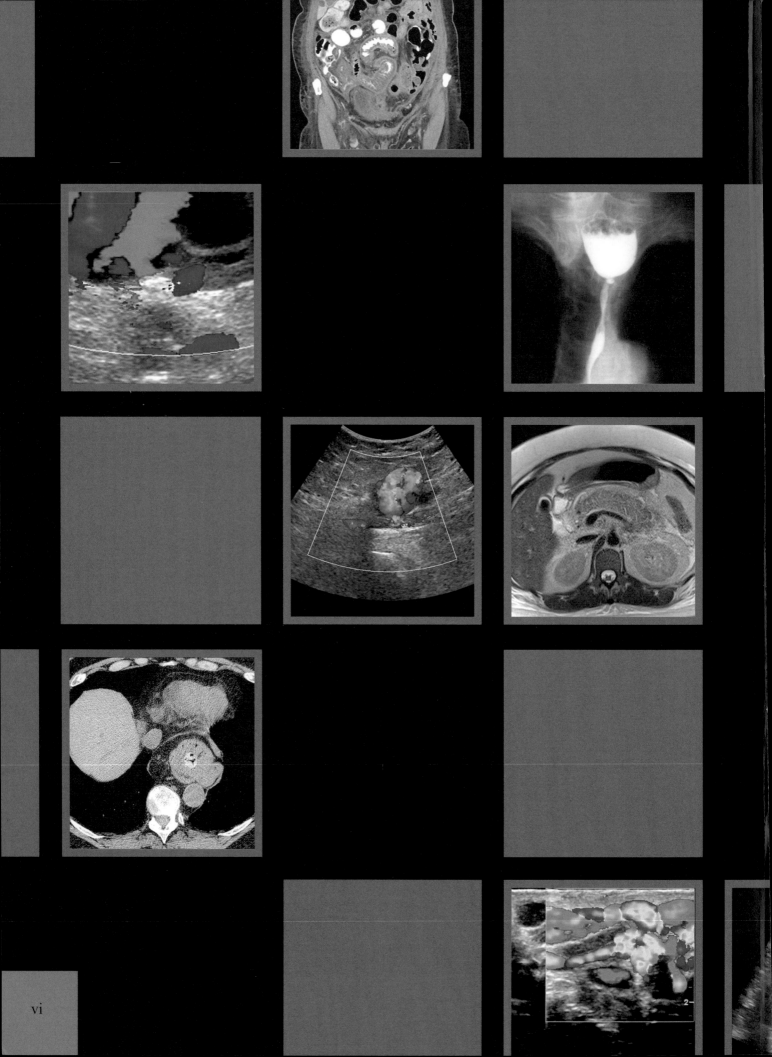

Contributing Authors

Akram M. Shaaban, MBBCh
Professor
Department of Radiology and Imaging Sciences
University of Utah
Salt Lake City, Utah

Jacqueline K. Anderson, BS
Medical Student
Mayo Clinic Alix School of Medicine
Scottsdale, Arizona

Molly B. Carnahan, MD
Fellow
Department of Radiology
Mayo Clinic
Phoenix, Arizona

Additional Contributors

Gregory E. Antonio, MD, DRANZCR, FHKCR
Shweta Bhatt, MD
Amir A. Borhani, MD
Michael P. Federle, MD, FACR
Alessandro Furlan, MD
Matthew T. Heller, MD, FSAR

Aya Kamaya, MD, FSRU, FSAR
Eric K. H. Liu, PhD, RDMS
L. Nayeli Morimoto, MD
Hee Sun Park, MD, PhD
Maryam Rezvani, MD
Narendra Shet, MD
Katherine To'o, MD

Mitchell Tublin, MD
Fauzia Vandermeer, MD
Ashish P. Wasnik, MD, FSAR
Jade Wong-You-Cheong, MBChB, MRCP, FRCR, FSRU, FSAR

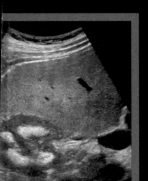

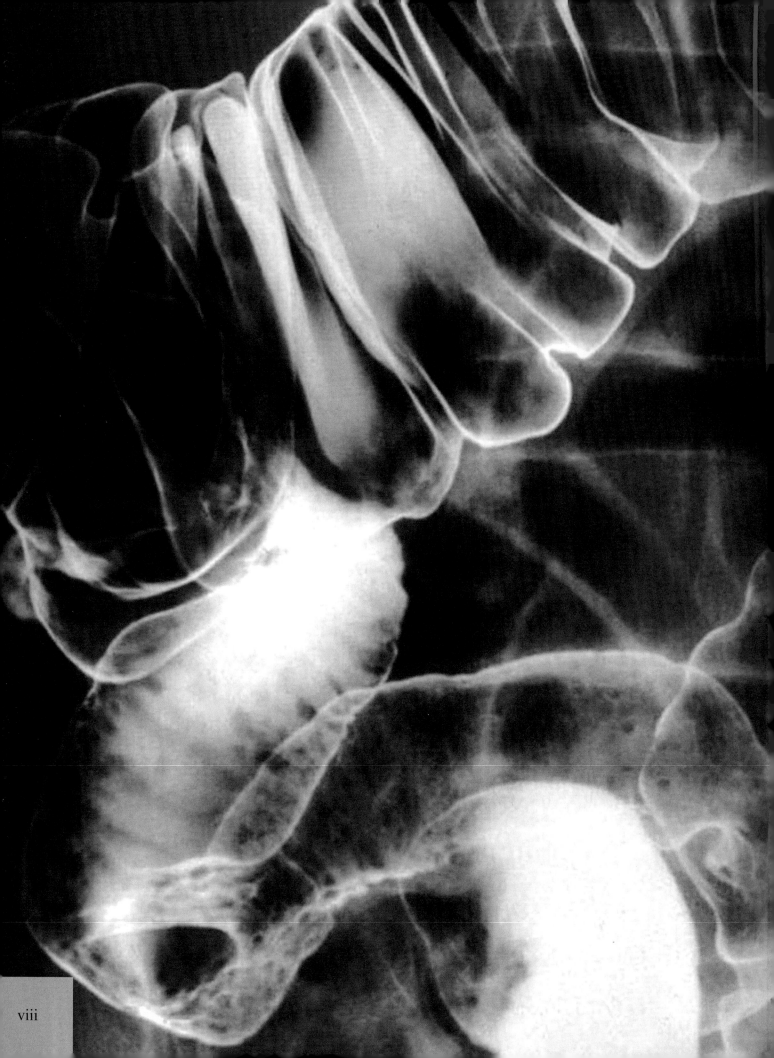

Preface

Radiologists play an important role in deciphering complex clinical scenarios and require skills to tackle cases based on the patient's clinical presentation, such as pain in a particular location or a specific radiographic appearance, e.g., a T2-hypointense liver mass. In order to provide a helpful differential diagnosis, the radiologist will attempt to recall information learned during their training, past experiences, or, in more recent venues, CME meetings. Standard radiology texts may serve as another helpful source, but these run the problem of not being organized by specific diseases or clinical presentation and may not be helpful or efficient in quickly generating a useful differential diagnosis. Internet searches are usually a knee-jerk reaction for most in search of an expedient result, yet these searches only lead the clinician into a maze of countless unvetted and unreliable sources.

Our series of *Expert Differential Diagnosis* ("ExpertDDx") books draw on the accumulated experience and expertise of our Elsevier authors, many of whom have authored and helped edit the encyclopedic *Diagnostic Imaging* books. Our goal is to identify the most common and important clinical and imaging challenges and to organize the differential diagnoses into common, less common, and rare groups for such scenarios. Information on characteristic imaging studies, along with the key clinical and imaging features that allow one to distinguish among the possible etiologies, is provided. For this third edition of *ExpertDDx: Abdomen and Pelvis*, we have significantly added and widened MR findings-based differential diagnoses. Furthermore, we have added and broadened sections on organ transplant-related abnormalities and symptom-based differential considerations, such as flank and abdominal pain. The differential considerations for multiple disorders are modified in the light of several classifications, including LI-RADS for liver, O-RADS for ovarian masses, and the updated Tanaka classification for pancreatic cysts, as the parameters of all these have changed since the previous edition of *ExpertDDx: Abdomen and Pelvis* was published in 2017.

We hope you find this to be a valuable resource that helps you provide the best medical care in your everyday practice.

Atif Zaheer, MD
Professor of Radiology, Oncology and Medicine
The Johns Hopkins University School of Medicine
Baltimore, Maryland

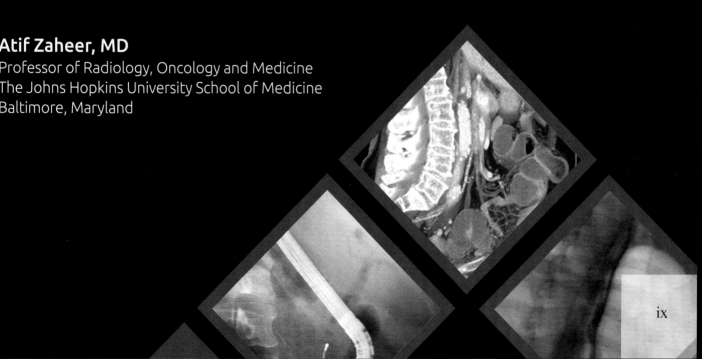

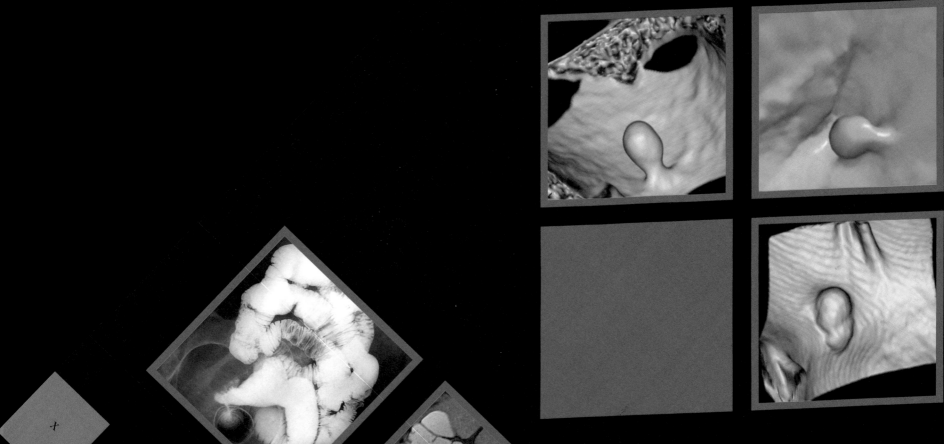

Acknowledgments

LEAD EDITOR
Arthur G. Gelsinger, MA

LEAD ILLUSTRATOR
Laura C. Wissler, MA

TEXT EDITORS
Rebecca L. Bluth, BA
Nina Themann, BA
Terry W. Ferrell, MS
Megg Morin, BA
Kathryn Watkins, BA
Shannon Kelly, MA

ILLUSTRATIONS
Lane R. Bennion, MS
Richard Coombs, MS

IMAGE EDITORS
Jeffrey J. Marmorstone, BS
Lisa A. M. Steadman, BS

ART DIRECTION AND DESIGN
Cindy Lin, BFA

PRODUCTION EDITORS
Emily C. Fassett, BA
John Pecorelli, BS

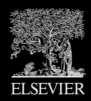

ELSEVIER

Sections

SECTION 1: **Peritoneum and Mesentery**

SECTION 2: **Abdominal Wall**

SECTION 3: **Esophagus**

SECTION 4: **Stomach**

SECTION 5: **Duodenum**

SECTION 6: **Small Intestine**

SECTION 7: **Colon**

SECTION 8: **Spleen**

SECTION 9: **Liver**

SECTION 10: **Gallbladder**

SECTION 11: **Biliary Tract**

SECTION 12: **Pancreas**

SECTION 13: **Retroperitoneum**

SECTION 14: **Adrenal**

SECTION 15: **Kidney**

SECTION 16: **Collecting System**

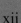

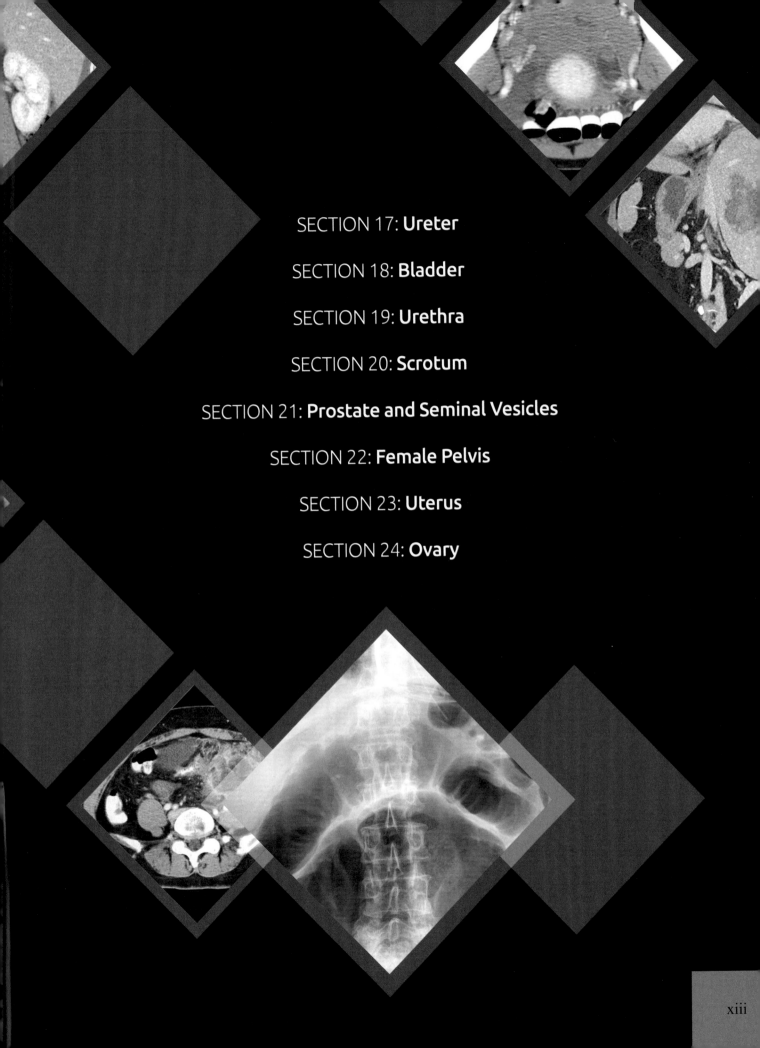

SECTION 17: **Ureter**

SECTION 18: **Bladder**

SECTION 19: **Urethra**

SECTION 20: **Scrotum**

SECTION 21: **Prostate and Seminal Vesicles**

SECTION 22: **Female Pelvis**

SECTION 23: **Uterus**

SECTION 24: **Ovary**

TABLE OF CONTENTS

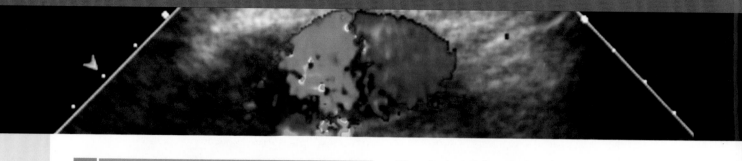

SECTION 1: PERITONEUM AND MESENTERY

GENERIC IMAGING PATTERNS

4   Mesenteric or Omental Mass (Solid)
    Siva P. Raman, MD
10 Mesenteric or Omental Mass (Cystic)
    Siva P. Raman, MD
14 Fat-Containing Lesion, Peritoneal Cavity
    Siva P. Raman, MD
18 Mesenteric Lymphadenopathy
    Siva P. Raman, MD
22 Abdominal Calcifications
    Siva P. Raman, MD
28 Pneumoperitoneum
    Siva P. Raman, MD
32 Hemoperitoneum
    Siva P. Raman, MD
36 Misty (Infiltrated) Mesentery
    Siva P. Raman, MD

MODALITY-SPECIFIC IMAGING FINDINGS

COMPUTED TOMOGRAPHY

42 High-Attenuation (Hyperdense) Ascites
    Siva P. Raman, MD

SECTION 2: ABDOMINAL WALL

ANATOMICALLY BASED DIFFERENTIALS

48 Abdominal Wall Mass
    Siva P. Raman, MD
52 Mass in Iliopsoas Compartment
    Siva P. Raman, MD
54 Groin Mass
    Siva P. Raman, MD
58 Elevated or Deformed Hemidiaphragm
    Siva P. Raman, MD
60 Defect in Abdominal Wall (Hernia)
    Siva P. Raman, MD

SECTION 3: ESOPHAGUS

GENERIC IMAGING PATTERNS

66 Intraluminal Mass, Esophagus
    Atif Zaheer, MD and Michael P. Federle, MD, FACR
68 Extrinsic Mass, Esophagus
    Atif Zaheer, MD and Michael P. Federle, MD, FACR
72 Lesion at Pharyngoesophageal Junction
    Atif Zaheer, MD and Michael P. Federle, MD, FACR
74 Esophageal Ulceration
    Atif Zaheer, MD and Michael P. Federle, MD, FACR
76 Mucosal Nodularity, Esophagus
    Atif Zaheer, MD and Michael P. Federle, MD, FACR
78 Esophageal Strictures
    Atif Zaheer, MD and Michael P. Federle, MD, FACR
80 Dilated Esophagus
    Atif Zaheer, MD and Michael P. Federle, MD, FACR
82 Esophageal Outpouchings (Diverticula)
    Atif Zaheer, MD and Michael P. Federle, MD, FACR
84 Esophageal Dysmotility
    Atif Zaheer, MD and Michael P. Federle, MD, FACR

CLINICALLY BASED DIFFERENTIALS

86 Odynophagia
    Atif Zaheer, MD and Michael P. Federle, MD, FACR

SECTION 4: STOMACH

GENERIC IMAGING PATTERNS

90 Gastric Mass Lesions
    Atif Zaheer, MD and Michael P. Federle, MD, FACR
96 Intramural Mass, Stomach
    Atif Zaheer, MD and Michael P. Federle, MD, FACR
98 Target or Bull's-Eye Lesions, Stomach
    Atif Zaheer, MD and Michael P. Federle, MD, FACR
100 Gastric Ulceration (Without Mass)
    Atif Zaheer, MD and Michael P. Federle, MD, FACR
102 Intrathoracic Stomach
    Atif Zaheer, MD and Michael P. Federle, MD, FACR
104 Thickened Gastric Folds
    Atif Zaheer, MD and Michael P. Federle, MD, FACR
110 Gastric Dilation or Outlet Obstruction
    Atif Zaheer, MD and Michael P. Federle, MD, FACR
114 Linitis Plastica, Limited Distensibility
    Atif Zaheer, MD and Michael P. Federle, MD, FACR

CLINICALLY BASED DIFFERENTIALS

118 Epigastric Pain
    Atif Zaheer, MD and Michael P. Federle, MD, FACR
124 Left Upper Quadrant Mass
    Atif Zaheer, MD and Michael P. Federle, MD, FACR

SECTION 5: DUODENUM

GENERIC IMAGING PATTERNS

130 Duodenal Mass
    Atif Zaheer, MD and Michael P. Federle, MD, FACR

TABLE OF CONTENTS

136 Dilated Duodenum
Atif Zaheer, MD and Michael P. Federle, MD, FACR
138 Thickened Duodenal Folds
Atif Zaheer, MD and Michael P. Federle, MD, FACR

SECTION 6: SMALL INTESTINE

GENERIC IMAGING PATTERNS

142 Multiple Masses or Filling Defects, Small Bowel
Atif Zaheer, MD and Michael P. Federle, MD, FACR
144 Cluster of Dilated Small Bowel
Atif Zaheer, MD and Michael P. Federle, MD, FACR
146 Aneurysmal Dilation of Small Bowel Lumen
Atif Zaheer, MD and Michael P. Federle, MD, FACR
148 Stenosis, Terminal Ileum
Atif Zaheer, MD and Michael P. Federle, MD, FACR
150 Segmental or Diffuse Small Bowel Wall Thickening
Atif Zaheer, MD and Michael P. Federle, MD, FACR
156 Pneumatosis of Small Intestine or Colon
Atif Zaheer, MD and Michael P. Federle, MD, FACR

CLINICALLY BASED DIFFERENTIALS

160 Occult GI Bleeding
Atif Zaheer, MD and Michael P. Federle, MD, FACR
164 Small Bowel Obstruction
Atif Zaheer, MD and Michael P. Federle, MD, FACR

SECTION 7: COLON

GENERIC IMAGING PATTERNS

172 Solitary Colonic Filling Defect
Atif Zaheer, MD and Michael P. Federle, MD, FACR
174 Multiple Colonic Filling Defects
Atif Zaheer, MD and Michael P. Federle, MD, FACR
176 Mass or Inflammation of Ileocecal Area
Atif Zaheer, MD and Michael P. Federle, MD, FACR
182 Colonic Ileus or Dilation
Atif Zaheer, MD and Michael P. Federle, MD, FACR
186 Toxic Megacolon
Atif Zaheer, MD and Michael P. Federle, MD, FACR
188 Rectal or Colonic Fistula
Atif Zaheer, MD and Michael P. Federle, MD, FACR
194 Segmental Colonic Narrowing
Atif Zaheer, MD and Michael P. Federle, MD, FACR
198 Colonic Thumbprinting
Atif Zaheer, MD and Michael P. Federle, MD, FACR
200 Colonic Wall Thickening
Atif Zaheer, MD and Michael P. Federle, MD, FACR
206 Smooth Ahaustral Colon
Atif Zaheer, MD and Michael P. Federle, MD, FACR

CLINICALLY BASED DIFFERENTIALS

208 Acute Right Lower Quadrant Pain
Atif Zaheer, MD and Michael P. Federle, MD, FACR
214 Acute Left Abdominal Pain
Atif Zaheer, MD and Michael P. Federle, MD, FACR

SECTION 8: SPLEEN

GENERIC IMAGING PATTERNS

222 Splenomegaly
Siva P. Raman, MD
226 Multiple Splenic Calcifications
Siva P. Raman, MD
228 Solid Splenic Mass or Masses
Siva P. Raman, MD
230 Cystic Splenic Mass
Siva P. Raman, MD

MODALITY-SPECIFIC IMAGING FINDINGS

COMPUTED TOMOGRAPHY

232 Diffuse Increased Attenuation, Spleen
Siva P. Raman, MD

SECTION 9: LIVER

GENERIC IMAGING PATTERNS

236 Liver Mass With Central or Eccentric Scar
Atif Zaheer, MD and Michael P. Federle, MD, FACR
240 Focal Liver Lesion With Hemorrhage
Atif Zaheer, MD and Michael P. Federle, MD, FACR
244 Liver "Mass" With Capsular Retraction
Atif Zaheer, MD and Michael P. Federle, MD, FACR
246 Fat-Containing Liver Mass
Atif Zaheer, MD and Michael P. Federle, MD, FACR
248 Cystic Hepatic Mass
Atif Zaheer, MD and Michael P. Federle, MD, FACR
252 Focal Hypervascular Liver Lesion
Atif Zaheer, MD and Michael P. Federle, MD, FACR
258 Liver Mass With Mosaic Enhancement
Atif Zaheer, MD
262 Mosaic or Patchy Hepatogram
Atif Zaheer, MD and Michael P. Federle, MD, FACR
266 Hepatic Calcifications
Atif Zaheer, MD and Michael P. Federle, MD, FACR
270 Liver Lesion Containing Gas
Atif Zaheer, MD and Michael P. Federle, MD, FACR
274 Portal Venous Gas
Atif Zaheer, MD and Michael P. Federle, MD, FACR
276 Widened Hepatic Fissures
Atif Zaheer, MD and Michael P. Federle, MD, FACR
278 Dysmorphic Liver With Abnormal Bile Ducts
Atif Zaheer, MD and Michael P. Federle, MD, FACR
282 Focal Hyperperfusion Abnormality (THAD or THID)
Atif Zaheer, MD and Michael P. Federle, MD, FACR
288 Periportal Lucency or Edema
Atif Zaheer, MD and Michael P. Federle, MD, FACR

MODALITY-SPECIFIC IMAGING FINDINGS

MAGNETIC RESONANCE IMAGING

294 Multiple Hypointense Liver Lesions (T2WI)
Atif Zaheer, MD and Michael P. Federle, MD, FACR

TABLE OF CONTENTS

298 **Hyperintense Liver Lesions (T1WI)**
Atif Zaheer, MD and Michael P. Federle, MD, FACR
304 **Liver Lesion With Capsule or Halo on MR**
Atif Zaheer, MD and Michael P. Federle, MD, FACR

COMPUTED TOMOGRAPHY

308 **Multiple Hypodense Liver Lesions**
Atif Zaheer, MD and Michael P. Federle, MD, FACR
314 **Focal Hyperdense Hepatic Mass on Nonenhanced CT**
Atif Zaheer, MD and Michael P. Federle, MD, FACR
318 **Widespread Low Attenuation Within Liver**
Atif Zaheer, MD and Michael P. Federle, MD, FACR

ULTRASOUND

322 **Focal Hepatic Echogenic Lesion ± Acoustic Shadowing**
Atif Zaheer, MD, Gregory E. Antonio, MD, DRANZCR, FHKCR, and Eric K. H. Liu, PhD, RDMS
328 **Hyperechoic Liver, Diffuse**
Atif Zaheer, MD, Gregory E. Antonio, MD, DRANZCR, FHKCR, and Eric K. H. Liu, PhD, RDMS
330 **Hepatomegaly**
Hee Sun Park, MD, PhD, Aya Kamaya, MD, FSRU, FSAR, and Siva P. Raman, MD
334 **Diffusely Abnormal Liver Echogenicity**
Hee Sun Park, MD, PhD, Aya Kamaya, MD, FSRU, FSAR, and Atif Zaheer, MD
336 **Anechoic Liver Lesion**
Hee Sun Park, MD, PhD, Aya Kamaya, MD, FSRU, FSAR, and Atif Zaheer, MD
340 **Hypoechoic Liver Mass**
Hee Sun Park, MD, PhD, Aya Kamaya, MD, FSRU, FSAR, and Atif Zaheer, MD
344 **Echogenic Liver Mass**
Hee Sun Park, MD, PhD, Aya Kamaya, MD, FSRU, FSAR, and Atif Zaheer, MD
348 **Target Lesions in Liver**
Hee Sun Park, MD, PhD, Aya Kamaya, MD, FSRU, FSAR, and Atif Zaheer, MD
350 **Multiple Hypo-, Hyper- or Anechoic Liver Lesions**
Hee Sun Park, MD, PhD, Aya Kamaya, MD, FSRU, FSAR, and Atif Zaheer, MD
354 **Hepatic Mass With Central Scar**
Hee Sun Park, MD, PhD, Aya Kamaya, MD, FSRU, FSAR, and Siva P. Raman, MD
356 **Periportal Lesion**
Hee Sun Park, MD, PhD, Aya Kamaya, MD, FSRU, FSAR, and Siva P. Raman, MD
360 **Irregular Hepatic Surface**
Aya Kamaya, MD, FSRU, FSAR and Siva P. Raman, MD
362 **Portal Vein Abnormality**
Hee Sun Park, MD, PhD, Aya Kamaya, MD, FSRU, FSAR, and Siva P. Raman, MD

SECTION 10: GALLBLADDER

GENERIC IMAGING PATTERNS

366 **Distended Gallbladder**
Siva P. Raman, MD

368 **Gas in Bile Ducts or Gallbladder**
Siva P. Raman, MD
372 **Focal Gallbladder Wall Thickening**
Siva P. Raman, MD
374 **Diffuse Gallbladder Wall Thickening**
Jade Wong-You-Cheong, MBChB, MRCP, FRCR, FSRU, FSAR and Atif Zaheer, MD

MODALITY-SPECIFIC IMAGING FINDINGS

COMPUTED TOMOGRAPHY

378 **High-Attenuation (Hyperdense) Bile in Gallbladder**
Siva P. Raman, MD

ULTRASOUND

380 **Hyperechoic Gallbladder Wall**
Jade Wong-You-Cheong, MBChB, MRCP, FRCR, FSRU, FSAR and Atif Zaheer, MD
382 **Echogenic Material in Gallbladder**
Jade Wong-You-Cheong, MBChB, MRCP, FRCR, FSRU, FSAR and Atif Zaheer, MD
384 **Dilated Gallbladder**
Jade Wong-You-Cheong, MBChB, MRCP, FRCR, FSRU, FSAR and Atif Zaheer, MD
388 **Intrahepatic and Extrahepatic Duct Dilatation**
L. Nayeli Morimoto, MD, Aya Kamaya, MD, FSRU, FSAR, and Siva P. Raman, MD

CLINICALLY BASED DIFFERENTIALS

390 **Right Upper Quadrant Pain**
Siva P. Raman, MD

SECTION 11: BILIARY TRACT

GENERIC IMAGING PATTERNS

398 **Dilated Common Bile Duct**
Siva P. Raman, MD
404 **Asymmetric Dilation of Intrahepatic Bile Ducts**
Siva P. Raman, MD
408 **Biliary Strictures, Multiple**
Siva P. Raman, MD

MODALITY-SPECIFIC IMAGING FINDINGS

MAGNETIC RESONANCE IMAGING

412 **Hypointense Lesion in Biliary Tree (MRCP)**
Siva P. Raman, MD

SECTION 12: PANCREAS

GENERIC IMAGING PATTERNS

416 **Hypovascular Pancreatic Mass**
Siva P. Raman, MD
422 **Hypervascular Pancreatic Mass**
Siva P. Raman, MD
426 **Cystic Pancreatic Mass**
Siva P. Raman, MD

TABLE OF CONTENTS

432 **Atrophy or Fatty Replacement of Pancreas**
Siva P. Raman, MD

434 **Dilated Pancreatic Duct**
Siva P. Raman, MD

438 **Infiltration of Peripancreatic Fat Planes**
Siva P. Raman, MD

444 **Pancreatic Calcifications**
Siva P. Raman, MD

MODALITY-SPECIFIC IMAGING FINDINGS

ULTRASOUND

448 **Cystic Pancreatic Lesion**
Fauzia Vandermeer, MD and Siva P. Raman, MD

452 **Solid Pancreatic Lesion**
Fauzia Vandermeer, MD and Siva P. Raman, MD

456 **Pancreatic Duct Dilatation**
Fauzia Vandermeer, MD and Siva P. Raman, MD

SECTION 13: RETROPERITONEUM

GENERIC IMAGING PATTERNS

460 **Retroperitoneal Mass, Cystic**
Matthew T. Heller, MD, FSAR and Bryan R. Foster, MD

466 **Retroperitoneal Mass, Soft Tissue Density**
Bryan R. Foster, MD

472 **Retroperitoneal Mass, Fat Containing**
Matthew T. Heller, MD, FSAR and Bryan R. Foster, MD

476 **Retroperitoneal Hemorrhage**
Matthew T. Heller, MD, FSAR and Bryan R. Foster, MD

SECTION 14: ADRENAL

GENERIC IMAGING PATTERNS

480 **Adrenal Mass**
Mitchell Tublin, MD and Ghaneh Fananapazir, MD, FSAR, FSRU, FSABI

SECTION 15: KIDNEY

GENERIC IMAGING PATTERNS

488 **Calcifications Within Kidney**
Ghaneh Fananapazir, MD, FSAR, FSRU, FSABI

492 **Congenital Renal Anomalies**
Ghaneh Fananapazir, MD, FSAR, FSRU, FSABI and Jacqueline K. Anderson, BS

496 **Kidney Transplant Dysfunction**
Ghaneh Fananapazir, MD, FSAR, FSRU, FSABI

500 **Solid Renal Mass**
Ghaneh Fananapazir, MD, FSAR, FSRU, FSABI

504 **Cystic Renal Mass**
Ghaneh Fananapazir, MD, FSAR, FSRU, FSABI and Jacqueline K. Anderson, BS

508 **Bilateral Renal Cysts**
Ghaneh Fananapazir, MD, FSAR, FSRU, FSABI and Alessandro Furlan, MD

512 **Infiltrative Renal Lesions**
Ghaneh Fananapazir, MD, FSAR, FSRU, FSABI

516 **Perirenal and Subcapsular Mass Lesions**
Ghaneh Fananapazir, MD, FSAR, FSRU, FSABI

520 **Fat-Containing Renal Mass**
Ghaneh Fananapazir, MD, FSAR, FSRU, FSABI

524 **Renal Sinus Lesion**
Ghaneh Fananapazir, MD, FSAR, FSRU, FSABI and Jacqueline K. Anderson, BS

528 **Gas in or Around Kidney**
Ghaneh Fananapazir, MD, FSAR, FSRU, FSABI, Molly B. Carnahan, MD, and Alessandro Furlan, MD

530 **Delayed or Persistent Nephrogram**
Ghaneh Fananapazir, MD, FSAR, FSRU, FSABI and Amir A. Borhani, MD

534 **Wedge-Shaped or Striated Nephrogram**
Ghaneh Fananapazir, MD, FSAR, FSRU, FSABI and Alessandro Furlan, MD

538 **Acute Flank Pain**
Bryan R. Foster, MD

MODALITY-SPECIFIC IMAGING FINDINGS

ULTRASOUND

544 **Enlarged Kidney**
Ghaneh Fananapazir, MD, FSAR, FSRU, FSABI, Jacqueline K. Anderson, BS, and Jade Wong-You-Cheong, MBChB, MRCP, FRCR, FSRU, FSAR

548 **Small Kidney**
Jade Wong-You-Cheong, MBChB, MRCP, FRCR, FSRU, FSAR

552 **Hyperechoic Kidney**
Ghaneh Fananapazir, MD, FSAR, FSRU, FSABI

556 **Dilated Renal Pelvis**
Narendra Shet, MD

560 **Hyperechoic Renal Mass**
Ghaneh Fananapazir, MD, FSAR, FSRU, FSABI and Mitchell Tublin, MD

SECTION 16: COLLECTING SYSTEM

566 **Dilated Renal Calyces**
Bryan R. Foster, MD and Alessandro Furlan, MD

570 **Filling Defect, Renal Pelvis**
Amir A. Borhani, MD and Bryan R. Foster, MD

SECTION 17: URETER

GENERIC IMAGING PATTERNS

576 **Ureteral Filling Defect or Stricture**
Amir A. Borhani, MD and Bryan R. Foster, MD

580 **Cystic Dilation of Distal Ureter**
Amir A. Borhani, MD and Bryan R. Foster, MD

SECTION 18: BLADDER

GENERIC IMAGING PATTERNS

584 **Filling Defect in Urinary Bladder**
Bryan R. Foster, MD and Amir A. Borhani, MD

590 **Urinary Bladder Outpouching**
Amir A. Borhani, MD and Bryan R. Foster, MD

TABLE OF CONTENTS

592   **Gas Within Urinary Bladder**
Amir A. Borhani, MD and Bryan R. Foster, MD

594   **Abnormal Bladder Wall**
Bryan R. Foster, MD and Ashish P. Wasnik, MD, FSAR

SECTION 19: URETHRA

GENERIC IMAGING PATTERNS

600   **Urethral Stricture**
Matthew T. Heller, MD, FSAR and Bryan R. Foster, MD

SECTION 20: SCROTUM

GENERIC IMAGING PATTERNS

604   **Intratesticular Mass**
Bryan R. Foster, MD and Mitchell Tublin, MD

608   **Testicular Cystic Lesions**
Bryan R. Foster, MD and Mitchell Tublin, MD

610   **Extratesticular Cystic Mass**
Mitchell Tublin, MD and Bryan R. Foster, MD

612   **Extratesticular Solid Mass**
Bryan R. Foster, MD and Mitchell Tublin, MD

616   **Diffuse Testicular Enlargement**
Shweta Bhatt, MD and Bryan R. Foster, MD

618   **Decreased Testicular Size**
Shweta Bhatt, MD and Bryan R. Foster, MD

620   **Testicular Calcifications**
Shweta Bhatt, MD and Bryan R. Foster, MD

SECTION 21: PROSTATE AND SEMINAL VESICLES

GENERIC IMAGING PATTERNS

624   **Focal Lesion in Prostate**
Bryan R. Foster, MD and Alessandro Furlan, MD

630   **Enlarged Prostate**
Katherine To'o, MD and Bryan R. Foster, MD

SECTION 22: FEMALE PELVIS

GENERIC IMAGING PATTERNS

634   **Pelvic Fluid**
Akram M. Shaaban, MBBCh

638   **Female Lower Genital Cysts**
Akram M. Shaaban, MBBCh

644   **Extraovarian Adnexal Mass**
Maryam Rezvani, MD and Akram M. Shaaban, MBBCh

CLINICALLY BASED DIFFERENTIALS

650   **Acute Pelvic Pain in Nonpregnant Women**
Akram M. Shaaban, MBBCh

SECTION 23: UTERUS

GENERIC IMAGING PATTERNS

658   **Enlarged Uterus**
Maryam Rezvani, MD and Akram M. Shaaban, MBBCh

662   **Thickened Endometrium**
Maryam Rezvani, MD and Akram M. Shaaban, MBBCh

CLINICALLY BASED DIFFERENTIALS

668   **Abnormal Uterine Bleeding**
Maryam Rezvani, MD and Akram M. Shaaban, MBBCh

SECTION 24: OVARY

GENERIC IMAGING PATTERNS

676   **Multilocular Ovarian Cysts**
Akram M. Shaaban, MBBCh

682   **Unilocular Ovarian Cysts**
Akram M. Shaaban, MBBCh

688   **Solid Ovarian Masses**
Akram M. Shaaban, MBBCh

692   **Calcified Ovarian Masses**
Akram M. Shaaban, MBBCh

MODALITY-SPECIFIC IMAGING FINDINGS

MAGNETIC RESONANCE IMAGING

696   **Ovarian Lesions With Low T2 Signal Intensity**
Akram M. Shaaban, MBBCh

ExpertDDX

Abdomen and Pelvis

Zaheer | Raman
Foster | Fananapazir

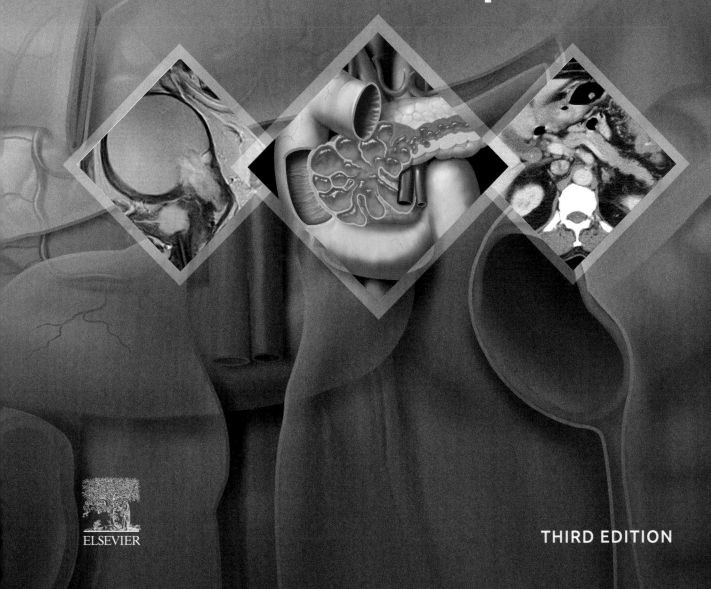

ELSEVIER

THIRD EDITION

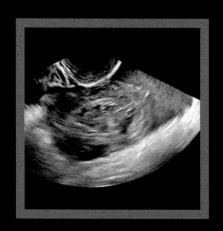
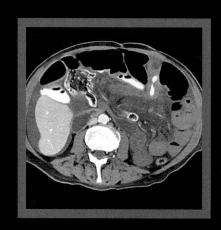
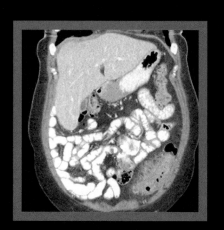
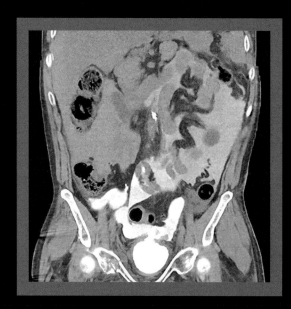
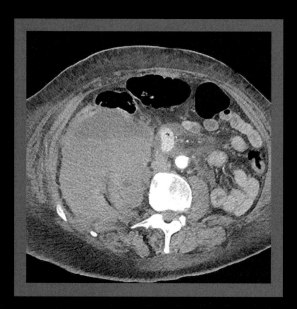
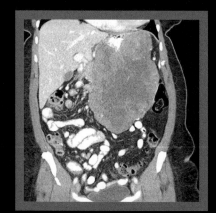
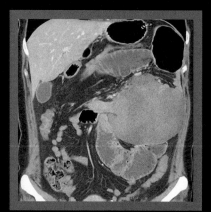
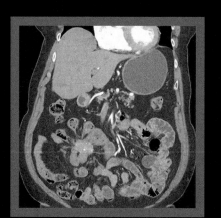

SECTION 1
Peritoneum and Mesentery

Generic Imaging Patterns

Mesenteric or Omental Mass (Solid)   4
Mesenteric or Omental Mass (Cystic)   10
Fat-Containing Lesion, Peritoneal Cavity   14
Mesenteric Lymphadenopathy   18
Abdominal Calcifications   22
Pneumoperitoneum   28
Hemoperitoneum   32
Misty (Infiltrated) Mesentery   36

Modality-Specific Imaging Findings

Computed Tomography
    High-Attenuation (Hyperdense) Ascites   42

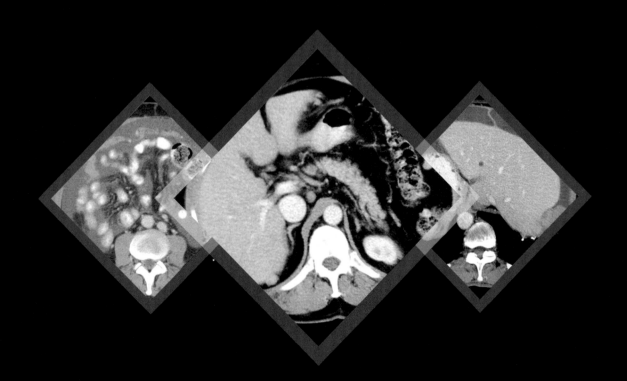

DIFFERENTIAL DIAGNOSIS

Common

- Peritoneal Metastases
- Lymphoma
- Mesenteric Lymphadenopathy
- Acute Pancreatitis
- Diaphragmatic Insertions (Mimic)
- Mesenteric Hematoma (Mimic)

Less Common

- Mesothelioma
- Desmoid
- Sclerosing Mesenteritis
- Tuberculous Peritonitis
- Carcinoid Tumor
- Splenosis
- Gastrointestinal Stromal Tumor
- Fat Necrosis
- Primary Papillary Serous Carcinoma

Rare but Important

- Sarcoma of Mesentery or Retroperitoneum
- Leukemia
- Benign Mesenchymal Tumors
- Leiomyomatosis Peritonealis Disseminata
- Other Systemic Diseases

ESSENTIAL INFORMATION

Key Differential Diagnosis Issues

- Peritoneal metastases are, by far, most common cause of solid mass in omentum
- Lymphadenopathy is, by far, most common etiology for solid mesenteric mass

Helpful Clues for Common Diagnoses

- **Peritoneal Metastases**
  - Most common with primary gynecologic (ovary, uterus) and GI malignancies
  - May result in discrete soft tissue masses in omentum and mesentery, usually in conjunction with ascites and peritoneal thickening, nodularity, and enhancement
- **Lymphoma**
  - Very common cause of mesenteric lymphadenopathy, usually in conjunction with lymphadenopathy elsewhere
  - Lymphoma can rarely involve omentum (i.e., peritoneal lymphomatosis), producing confluent soft tissue infiltration that is virtually indistinguishable from carcinomatosis
    - Usually in association with significant lymphadenopathy or extranodal disease elsewhere
    - May be associated with ascites but less commonly than carcinomatosis
    - Uncommon and most often seen with immunocompromised patients or aggressive forms of lymphoma (such as Burkitt lymphoma)
- **Mesenteric Lymphadenopathy**
  - Many potential infectious, inflammatory, and neoplastic causes (which can manifest as discrete nodes or confluent nodal masses)
  - Substantial lymphadenopathy should raise concern for malignancy but can also be seen with infections or be reactive to inflammatory processes in abdomen
- **Acute Pancreatitis**
  - May produce extrapancreatic necrosis due to leakage of pancreatic enzymes into adjacent mesenteric fat with resultant fat necrosis
    - Can appear very nodular and mass-like, potentially mimicking tumor spread or carcinomatosis
  - Inflammation from pancreatitis may extend into mesentery, creating phlegmon that mimics solid mass
- **Diaphragmatic Insertions (Mimic)**
  - Slips of diaphragm may insert on ribs and costal cartilages, potentially mimicking peritoneal or omental nodularity on axial images
  - Key is to visualize elongated shape of these "masses" and their contiguity with rest of diaphragm
    - Diagnosis easily confirmed on multiplanar reformats
- **Mesenteric Hematoma (Mimic)**
  - Usually seen in patients with history of trauma or coagulopathy and could mimic hyperdense "mass"

Helpful Clues for Less Common Diagnoses

- **Mesothelioma**
  - May rarely arise from peritoneum, accounting for 20% of all mesotheliomas
  - Appearance similar to carcinomatosis, including omental/mesenteric nodularity and masses, peritoneal thickening/enhancement, and pleated appearance of mesentery
    - May be associated with ascites but usually less than is seen with carcinomatosis
    - Can be localized (solitary dominant mass) or diffuse (extensive peritoneal involvement)
  - Presence of pleural plaques can be important clue given relationship between mesothelioma and asbestos
- **Desmoid**
  - Benign, aggressive mesenchymal neoplasm that can involve abdominal wall or mesentery
  - Predisposing risk factors include prior surgery, trauma, Gardner syndrome, or familial polyposis
  - Appears as locally aggressive soft tissue mass, which can compress and invade adjacent structures
  - Variable appearance but typically hypoenhancing with low signal on T1WI and high signal on T2WI MR
    - Can appear well circumscribed or infiltrative
- **Sclerosing Mesenteritis**
  - Idiopathic inflammatory and fibrotic disorder of mesentery that ranges in appearance from subtle "misty mesentery" to discrete fibrotic mass
  - End-stage disease may result in discrete fibrotic mass (with frequent coarse calcification) that occludes vasculature and produces bowel obstructions
  - Usually located in left upper quadrant, but appearance may be difficult to differentiate from carcinoid tumor
- **Tuberculous Peritonitis**
  - Involvement of peritoneum can result in thickening and nodularity that appears similar to carcinomatosis
  - Results in peritoneal thickening, nodularity, and ascites
  - Frequently associated with tuberculous lymphadenitis, which manifests as necrotic lymphadenopathy

- **Carcinoid Tumor**
  - Spiculated mesenteric mass in right left quadrant, often with calcification, which is frequently associated with desmoplastic reaction and tethering of adjacent bowel/vasculature
  - Mesenteric mass represents metastasis, with primary tumor most commonly present in terminal ileum
    - Primary ileal tumor may not always be visible on CT but often is hypervascular on arterial-phase images
- **Splenosis**
  - Traumatic rupture of spleen resulting in implantation of splenic tissue throughout peritoneal cavity
  - Enhancing nodules should have identical enhancement on all phases of imaging to normal spleen
  - Absence of spleen is important clue to diagnosis, but confirmation can be obtained with Tc-99m heat-denatured RBC scan
- **Gastrointestinal Stromal Tumor**
  - Commonly arises from stomach or small bowel but can be exophytic with extensive mesenteric component
  - Can be massive in size, occupying much of abdomen, making it very difficult to ascertain exact site of origin
    - Should always be strongly considered when confronted by solitary dominant mass occupying sizable portion of abdomen
  - Variable enhancement (can be hypodense or relatively vascular) with frequent internal heterogeneity, ulceration, and necrosis
- **Fat Necrosis**
  - Includes postsurgical fat necrosis, epiploic appendagitis, and omental infarcts; can appear very mass-like and simulate malignancy
  - Diagnosis contingent on presence of internal fat and clinical history, although internal fat can be quite insubstantial in some cases
- **Primary Papillary Serous Carcinoma**
  - Rare malignancy seen primarily in postmenopausal women with evidence of diffuse peritoneal tumor spread (e.g., ascites, tumor implants, etc.)

- Identical in appearance and histology to peritoneal carcinomatosis secondary to ovarian cancer but without evidence of primary ovarian mass

Helpful Clues for Rare Diagnoses

- **Sarcoma of Mesentery or Retroperitoneum**
  - Primary peritoneal sarcomas are uncommon, although large retroperitoneal sarcomas can grow into peritoneal space
  - Most common primary peritoneal sarcoma is malignant fibrous histiocytoma
  - Usually no specific imaging features for different sarcomas, which appear as nonspecific, large mass
- **Leukemia**
  - Can rarely infiltrate peritoneum with imaging findings similar to carcinomatosis or lymphomatosis
  - Most often seen with acute myeloid leukemia (AML)
- **Benign Mesenchymal Tumors**
  - Encompass wide variety of benign masses, including hemangiomas, lipomas, and nerve sheath tumors
  - Hemangiomas appear as low-density, poorly marginated masses with characteristic internal phleboliths
  - Lipoma demonstrates uniform fat density without internal complexity to suggest liposarcoma
  - Mesenteric plexiform neurofibromas are most commonly seen in neurofibromatosis type 1
    - Mesenteric low-density mass with branching appearance
- **Leiomyomatosis Peritonealis Disseminata**
  - Dissemination of multiple smooth muscle nodules throughout peritoneum, usually in premenopausal patients with history of uterine fibroids
  - Imaging demonstrates multiple peritoneal soft tissue nodules with CT attenuation and MR signal characteristics (usually hypointense on T2WI) similar to uterine fibroids
- **Other Systemic Diseases**
  - Amyloidosis, extramedullary hematopoiesis, Erdheim-Chester, and sarcoidosis have reported cases of mass-like omental/mesenteric involvement

Peritoneal Metastases

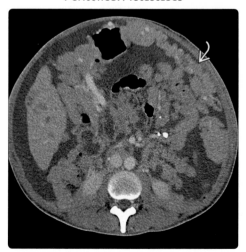

Peritoneal Metastases

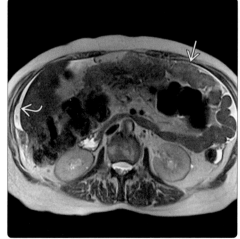

(Left) Axial CECT in a patient with melanoma shows extensive peritoneal carcinomatosis with omental caking ➡ and ascites. (Right) Axial T2 MR shows extensive omental caking ➡ throughout the anterior omentum, along with a small amount of ascites ➡, compatible with peritoneal carcinomatosis.

Peritoneal Metastases

Peritoneal Metastases

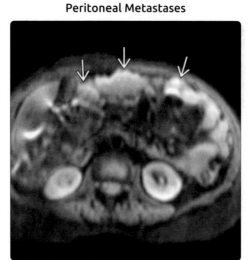

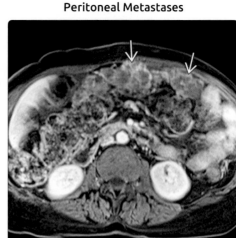

(Left) *Axial DWI MR in a patient with cholangiocarcinoma shows abnormal restricted diffusion ➡ throughout the anterior omentum.* (Right) *Axial T1 C+ FS MR in the same patient shows that the restricted diffusion corresponds to multiple hypoenhancing peritoneal metastases ➡ throughout the omentum.*

Lymphoma

Lymphoma

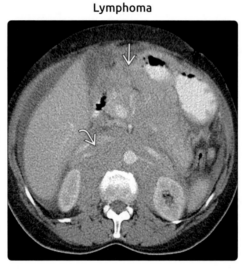

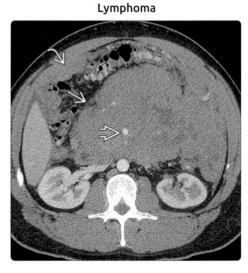

(Left) *Axial CECT shows extensive confluent retroperitoneal ➡ and mesenteric ➡ lymphadenopathy secondary to non-Hodgkin lymphoma.* (Right) *Axial CECT shows a large, confluent mesenteric mass ➡ in a patient with non-Hodgkin lymphoma. Note how the mass surrounds vessels ➡ without any appreciable narrowing or attenuation, a classic feature. Also note the presence of infiltrating soft tissue throughout the omentum ➡, compatible with lymphomatosis.*

Lymphoma

Lymphoma

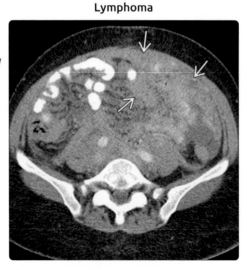

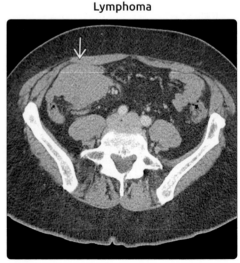

(Left) *Axial CECT in an AIDS patient shows extensive soft tissue infiltration ➡ throughout the mesentery and omentum, reflecting lymphomatous involvement (i.e., lymphomatosis).* (Right) *Axial CECT shows a solid mass ➡ in the right lower quadrant intimately associated with loops of bowel, ultimately found to represent non-Hodgkin lymphoma.*

Mesenteric Lymphadenopathy

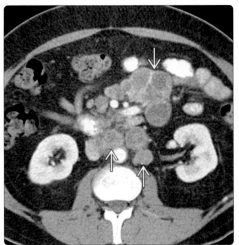

Acute Pancreatitis

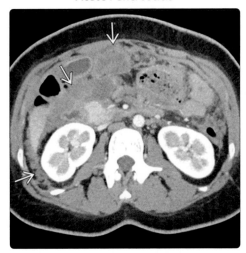

(Left) *Axial CECT shows extensive necrotic lymphadenopathy* ➡ *in the mesentery and retroperitoneum, representing metastatic lymphadenopathy from the patient's known melanoma.* (Right) *Axial CECT in a patient with severe pancreatitis shows extensive soft tissue density* ➡ *and nodularity throughout the mesentery and omentum. While almost resembling a tumor in its density and texture, these findings reflect extensive extrapancreatic necrosis related to pancreatitis.*

Diaphragmatic Insertions (Mimic)

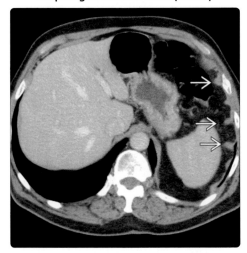

Mesenteric Hematoma (Mimic)

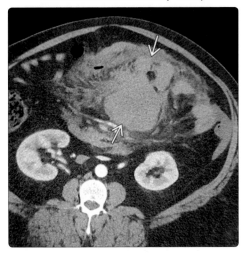

(Left) *Axial CECT shows numerous nodular densities* ➡ *that mimic peritoneal implants. These "nodules" represent finger-like slips of diaphragm as they near their abdominal wall insertions.* (Right) *Axial CECT shows a large mesenteric hematoma* ➡. *The hematoma was spontaneous and attributed to a bleeding diathesis.*

Mesothelioma

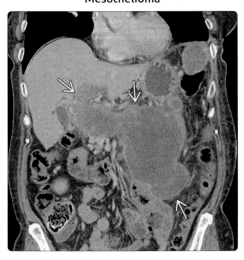

Mesothelioma

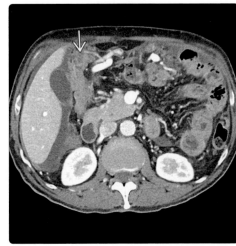

(Left) *Coronal CECT shows a hypodense mass* ➡ *in the central abdomen with extension upward into the porta hepatis, found to represent mesothelioma. Focal forms of mesothelioma have a better prognosis than diffuse forms and can be surgically resected in some instances.* (Right) *Axial CECT shows soft tissue infiltration* ➡ *in the right upper quadrant omentum with associated ascites. While this appearance most often represents carcinomatosis, this represents a rare instance of abdominal mesothelioma.*

Desmoid

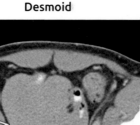

Desmoid

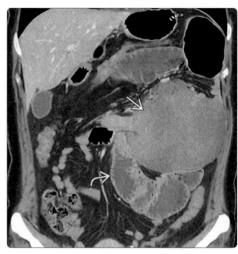

(Left) *Axial CECT shows a smooth, homogeneous soft tissue mass* ➡ *in the pelvis intimately associated with the adjacent bowel, representing a desmoid tumor.* (Right) *Coronal CECT shows a large, homogeneous soft tissue mass* ➡ *in the left abdomen causing small bowel obstruction* ➡*, representing a desmoid tumor (ostensibly related to prior surgery in this patient).*

Sclerosing Mesenteritis

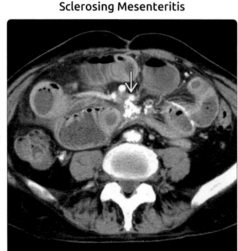

Sclerosing Mesenteritis

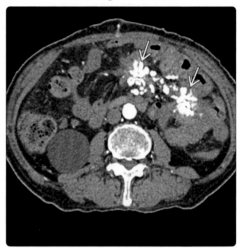

(Left) *Axial CECT shows a calcified mass* ➡ *in the central mesentery, which tethers multiple surrounding loops of bowel (resulting in a bowel obstruction). This mass was proven to represent sclerosing mesenteritis.* (Right) *Axial CECT shows a dramatic form of sclerosing mesenteritis* ➡ *in the left upper quadrant with confluent soft tissue and extensive calcification. Note the manner in which this process tethers and distorts the adjacent bowel.*

Carcinoid Tumor

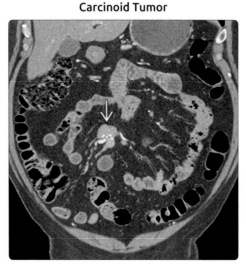

Carcinoid Tumor

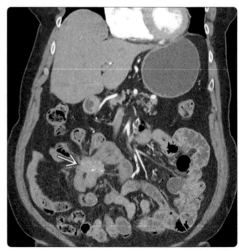

(Left) *Coronal CECT shows a soft tissue mass* ➡ *with calcification in the midmesentery found to represent a mesenteric metastasis from a carcinoid tumor. The primary tumor was found in the ileum at surgery but was not visible on CT.* (Right) *Axial CECT shows an irregularly shaped mass* ➡ *in the central mesentery with a few internal punctate calcifications and resultant tethering of the adjacent small bowel, representing a carcinoid mesenteric metastasis from a primary ileal tumor.*

Splenosis

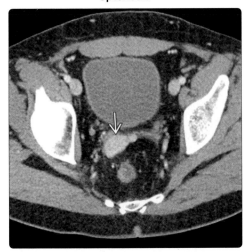

Splenosis

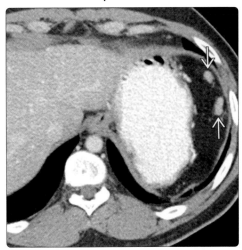

(Left) *Axial CECT shows an enhancing soft tissue nodule ➡ in the deep pelvis.* (Right) *Axial CECT in the same patient shows similar-appearing nodules ➡ in the left upper quadrant, as well as absence of the spleen, a classic constellation of findings for splenosis.*

Gastrointestinal Stromal Tumor

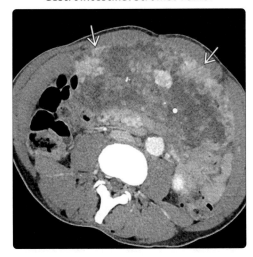

Gastrointestinal Stromal Tumor

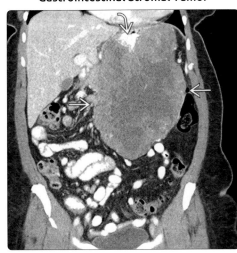

(Left) *Axial CECT shows a huge mass ➡ occupying much of the omentum and mesentery. The mass has very heterogeneous enhancement with areas of necrosis, found at surgery to represent an exophytic GIST arising from the stomach.* (Right) *Coronal CECT shows a large, heterogeneous mass ➡ ➡ arising from the stomach ➡ and projecting downward into the mesentery, representing a gastric GIST.*

Benign Mesenchymal Tumors

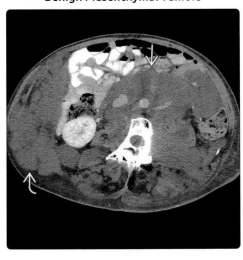

Benign Mesenchymal Tumors

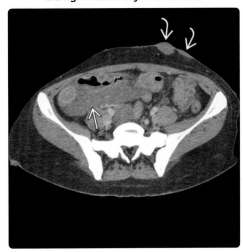

(Left) *Axial CECT in a patient with neurofibromatosis type 1 (NF1) shows extensive plexiform neurofibromas occupying a large portion of the mesentery ➡, particularly in the left abdomen, with additional lesions seen in the soft tissues ➡ and in the retroperitoneum.* (Right) *Axial CECT in a patient with NF1 shows a large, right-sided mesenteric plexiform neurofibroma ➡ surrounding vessels as well as multiple additional neurofibromas in the subcutaneous fat ➡.*

DIFFERENTIAL DIAGNOSIS

Common

- Loculated Ascites
- Abscess, Abdominal
- Pancreatic Pseudocyst
- Peritoneal Metastases
- Cystic Ovarian Neoplasm
- Lymphocele
- Visceral Organ Cysts or Cystic Neoplasms (Mimic)

Less Common

- Pseudomyxoma Peritonei
- Mesenteric Cyst
- Urachal Remnant
- Dermoid (Mature Teratoma)
- Lymphadenopathy, Cystic or Caseated
- Peritoneal Inclusion Cyst
- Endometriosis
- Hydatid Cyst
- Benign Multicystic Peritoneal Mesothelioma
- Hydrometrocolpos

ESSENTIAL INFORMATION

Key Differential Diagnosis Issues

- Correctly identifying site of origin of cystic mass is critical in generating appropriate differential diagnosis
- Any infectious, inflammatory, or neoplastic process in peritoneum may result in loculated ascites and simulate cystic mass

Helpful Clues for Common Diagnoses

- **Loculated Ascites**
  - Ascites may become loculated due to adhesions, peritonitis, or peritoneal malignancy
    - Peritonitis may be infectious (bacterial, viral, fungal, etc.) or inflammatory (e.g., bile peritonitis)
      □ Peritonitis typically associated with smooth, regular thickening and hyperenhancement of peritoneum on CT/MR (± mesenteric fat stranding)
      □ Multiple repetitive bouts of peritonitis can result in severe chronic thickening and calcification of peritoneal lining with loculated ascites, as with chronic peritoneal dialysis (abdominal cocoon)
    - Loculated ascites due to peritoneal carcinomatosis typically associated with irregular, nodular peritoneal thickening and enhancement (± discrete peritoneal soft tissue implants or omental caking)
    - Loculated ascites due to adhesions typically in patients with known history of abdominal surgeries or prior abdominal inflammatory processes
- **Abscess, Abdominal**
  - Loculated collection of fluid (usually fluid density or slightly hyperdense) with peripheral enhancement
    - Ectopic gas within fluid collection, in absence of intervention, highly suspicious for gas-forming infection or hollow-viscus perforation
    - Usually associated with fat stranding and edema in mesentery (± imaging findings of peritonitis)
- **Pancreatic Pseudocyst**

- Term used to describe fluid collections, in setting of acute edematous pancreatitis, which persist > 4 weeks
- Loculated fluid collections encapsulated by well-defined wall of granulation tissue
  - Can rarely demonstrate peripheral calcification
- Pseudocysts can occur anywhere in abdomen, including locations far from pancreas, simulating other intraperitoneal and retroperitoneal cystic masses
  - Most common in lesser sac or near pancreas
- Most (but not all) pseudocysts decrease in size or resolve over time, helping distinguish them from neoplasms
  - History of pancreatitis important for diagnosis, but some pseudocysts may require aspiration/fluid analysis to differentiate from cystic neoplasm
- **Peritoneal Metastases**
  - Tumors arising from GI tract, uterus, or ovaries are most common causes of peritoneal carcinomatosis
  - Loculated ascites is frequent with carcinomatosis and is usually associated with other signs of peritoneal malignancy, including nodular peritoneal thickening and enhancement as well as discrete tumor implants
  - Cystic primary tumors (e.g., ovarian cystadenocarcinoma) and their metastases may appear as cystic masses
- **Cystic Ovarian Neoplasm**
  - Most ovarian cystic neoplasms are of epithelial origin (with mucinous and serous subtypes most common)
  - Serous tumors more likely to be truly cystic, while mucinous neoplasms may demonstrate range of densities due to proteinaceous, hemorrhagic, or mucinous constituents
  - Internal complexity (e.g., septations, mural nodularity, papillary projections) raises concern for malignancy
- **Lymphocele**
  - Simple-appearing cyst composed of lymphatic fluid immediately adjacent to surgical clips, most commonly after lymphadenectomy or other pelvic surgery
- **Visceral Organ Cysts or Cystic Neoplasms (Mimic)**
  - Exophytic visceral organ cysts (e.g., renal cysts, etc.) or visceral organ cystic neoplasms (pancreatic cystic neoplasms, etc.) may mimic mesenteric or omental cyst

Helpful Clues for Less Common Diagnoses

- **Pseudomyxoma Peritonei**
  - Gelatinous mucinous implants throughout peritoneum due to ruptured appendiceal mucinous neoplasm
    - Term also utilized by some sources to encompass mucinous tumor implants due to other mucinous neoplasms (e.g., ovary or GI tract)
  - Low-density or cystic implants throughout peritoneum, which frequently indent liver and spleen, producing scalloped appearance
    - Implants may be associated with curvilinear calcification or other collections of loculated ascites (similar in density to individual mucinous implants)
  - Slowly progressive process frequently associated with bowel obstruction
- **Mesenteric Cyst**
  - Mesenteric cyst is generic term used to described number of benign congenital cysts (e.g., lymphangioma, enteric cyst, duplication cyst, mesothelial cyst)

- o Lymphangioma appears as thin-walled cystic lesion with either water density (~ 0 HU) or, rarely, chylous density (~ -20 HU) but no evidence of internal enhancement, soft tissue component, or nodularity
    - Often demonstrate feathery morphology with multiple loculations and septations
    - May indent and abut other structures (such as bowel or vessels) without appreciable mass effect
- o GI duplication cysts and enteric cysts appear as simple cysts along antimesenteric border of bowel
- o Mesothelial cysts are simple cysts arising in mesentery
- **Urachal Remnant**
- o Failure of urachal remnant to close during embryologic development can result in spectrum of abnormalities that can appear as cystic mass
    - Urachal cyst appears as discrete cyst at midline abdominal wall between bladder dome and umbilicus
    - Patent urachus appears as channel between bladder dome and umbilicus with tubular morphology
- o Location of cyst between dome of bladder and umbilicus is key to diagnosis with superinfection and development of urachal adenocarcinoma known complications
    - Presence of nodularity or soft tissue within remnant should raise concern for tumor
- **Dermoid Cyst (Mature Teratoma)**
- o Ovarian mass with multiple possible constituents, including fat, soft tissue, and calcification
    - May appear cystic, although measured density is typically less than simple fluid (indicating fat)
- o Multiple possible ultrasound appearances have been described, including diffusely echogenic mass with posterior shadowing (tip-of-iceberg sign), echogenic nodule within larger anechoic lesion (dermoid plug), and dot-dash pattern due to hair in lesion
- o Complications include torsion, superinfection, rupture, and malignant degeneration (very rare)
- **Lymphadenopathy, Cystic or Caseated**
- o Multiple causes of cystic, caseated, or necrotic lymph nodes include Whipple disease, mycobacterial disease, celiac sprue, and malignant lymphadenopathy
- **Peritoneal Inclusion Cyst**

- o Loculated fluid collection in pelvis resulting from peritoneal adhesions
    - Most often occurs in premenopausal women with prior gynecologic surgery or inflammatory conditions (e.g., endometriosis, pelvic inflammatory disease, etc.) that results in peritoneal scarring
- o Loculated cystic mass (usually in pelvis) conforming to geographic margins of pelvis
    - Ovary often at center of cyst due to hormonally active ovaries secreting fluid that becomes loculated
    - Internal septations within mass are frequent but no solid component or mural nodularity
- **Endometriosis**
- o Wide range of imaging appearances but often appear as complex cysts on CT, US, and MR (with typical T1 hyperintensity and T2 shading)
- **Hydatid Cyst**
- o Peritoneal hydatid cysts likely reflect sequelae of hepatic or splenic hydatid cyst rupture
- o Appearance is similar to hydatid cysts in liver/spleen with acute phase characterized by dominant cystic mass with internal daughter cysts or wavy, serpiginous internal densities (water-lily sign)
- o Chronic hydatid cysts often demonstrate extensive serpiginous internal calcification
- o Seeding of infection in entire peritoneum can give rise to entity known as peritoneal hydatidosis with multiple cystic lesions throughout abdomen
- **Benign Multicystic Peritoneal Mesothelioma**
- o Rare mesothelial neoplasm arising from peritoneum, which has no relationship with asbestos exposure
- o Unilocular or multilocular cyst(s) arising in peritoneum with predilection for pelvis and without any soft tissue component or mural nodularity
- o Benign lesion that is typically treated with surgery but with high local recurrence rates (25-50%)
- **Hydrometrocolpos**
- o Fluid distension of vaginal/uterine cavities due to distal obstruction (imperforate hymen, vaginal septum, etc.)
- o Usually diagnosed in pediatric population but very rarely encountered in young adults as well

Loculated Ascites

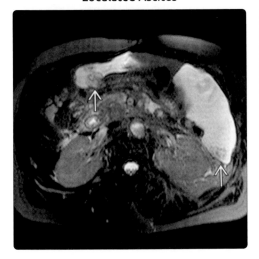

Pancreatic Pseudocyst

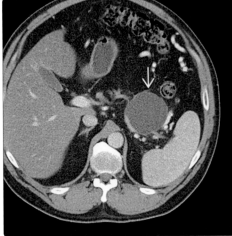

(Left) Axial T2 FS MR in a patient with metastatic appendiceal adenocarcinoma demonstrates loculated ascites in the left upper quadrant with multiple discrete peritoneal tumor implants ➡ along the margins of several loculated fluid collections. (Right) Axial CECT in a patient with a history of pancreatitis demonstrates a simple-appearing pseudocyst ➡ arising near the pancreatic tail.

Pancreatic Pseudocyst

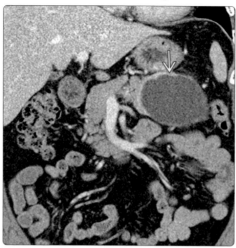

Cystic Ovarian Neoplasm

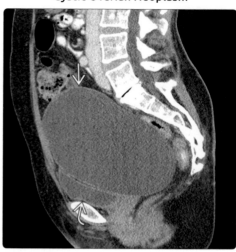

(Left) *Coronal CECT in a patient with a known history of pancreatitis demonstrates a large, simple-appearing pseudocyst* ➡ *arising in the vicinity of the pancreatic tail.* **(Right)** *Sagittal CECT demonstrates a large cystic mass* ➡ *in the pelvis representing a low-grade serous cystadenoma of the ovary. The mass arises immediately above the bladder* ➡ *and was initially confused for a distended bladder on the axial images.*

Cystic Ovarian Neoplasm

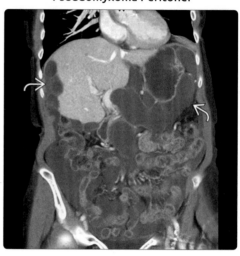

Pseudomyxoma Peritonei

(center right image)

(Left) *Axial T1 C+ FS MR demonstrates a large cystic ovarian mass* ➡ *with multiple internal septations and extensive enhancing solid component* ➡*, features strongly suggestive of malignancy. This lesion was found to represent endometrioid carcinoma at resection.* **(Right)** *Coronal volume-rendered CECT demonstrates multiple low-density gelatinous implants* ➡ *throughout the abdomen and pelvis, including multiple lesions scalloping the surface of the liver, characteristic of pseudomyxoma peritonei.*

Pseudomyxoma Peritonei

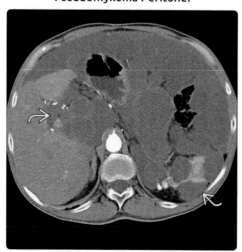

Mesenteric Cyst

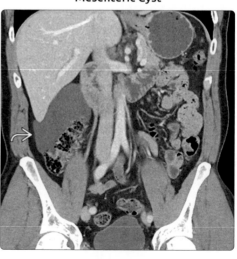

(Left) *Axial CECT demonstrates a characteristic appearance of pseudomyxoma peritonei with low-density mucinous implants* ➡ *throughout the upper abdomen, including numerous lesions invaginating into the porta hepatis and around the spleen.* **(Right)** *Coronal CECT demonstrates a large, simple-appearing, low-density cystic mass* ➡ *in the right upper abdomen, found to represent a large lymphangioma.*

Mesenteric or Omental Mass (Cystic)

Mesenteric Cyst

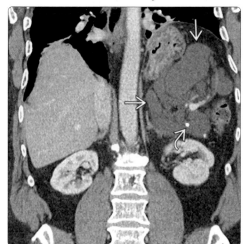

Urachal Remnant

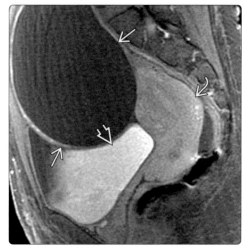

(Left) *Coronal CECT demonstrates a characteristic appearance of a lymphangioma* ➡, *which demonstrates a feathery appearance with multiple internal cystic components and some subtle calcification* ➡. (Right) *Sagittal T1 C+ FS MR shows a large urachal cyst* ➡ *that indents the dome of the bladder* ➡ *and displaces the uterus* ➡. *The bladder urine is opacified due to the IV gadolinium injection.*

Urachal Remnant

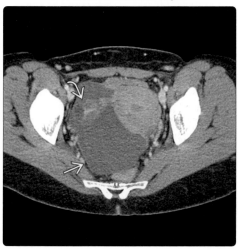

Dermoid (Mature Teratoma)

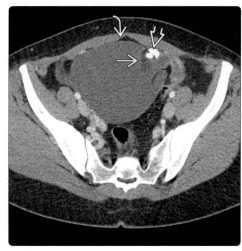

(Left) *Sagittal CECT demonstrates a large infected urachal cyst* ➡ *adjacent to the bladder* ➡, *which appears markedly thick walled with substantial surrounding inflammation.* (Right) *Axial CECT demonstrates a large dermoid* ➡ *with peripheral nodular calcification* ➡ *and small internal macroscopic fat* ➡. *The presence of macroscopic fat within an adnexal mass allows the definitive diagnosis of a dermoid.*

Peritoneal Inclusion Cyst

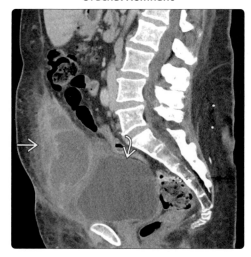

Hydatid Cyst

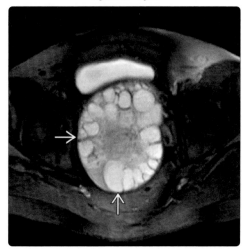

(Left) *Coronal CECT demonstrates a large fluid collection* ➡ *in the right pelvis surrounding the right ovary* ➡. *The patient had a history of Crohn disease and prior surgery, and this collection had been stable over several examinations, features compatible with a peritoneal inclusion cyst.* (Right) *Axial T2 FS MR in a patient from abroad with a known history of a hydatid cyst in the liver demonstrates a classic hydatid cyst* ➡ *in the pelvis with multiple internal daughter cysts.*

DIFFERENTIAL DIAGNOSIS

Common

- Sclerosing Mesenteritis
- Omental Infarct
- Epiploic Appendagitis
- Fat Necrosis
- Dermoid Cyst (Mature Teratoma)
- Fibrofatty Mesenteric Proliferation ("Creeping Fat") (Mimic)
- Intussusception (Mimic)

Less Common

- Liposarcoma
- Cystic Fibrosis of Pancreas (Mimic)
- Lipomatous Pseudohypertrophy of Pancreas (Mimic)
- Lipoma of Intestine
- Lipomatous Infiltration of Ileocecal Valve (Mimic)
- Pseudolipoma of Glisson Capsule
- Metastatic Malignant Teratoma
- Peritoneal Lipomatosis

ESSENTIAL INFORMATION

Key Differential Diagnosis Issues

- With rare exceptions, fat-containing lesions in peritoneal space are typically benign entities that can be specifically diagnosed based on imaging appearance
- Fat-containing masses are very common in retroperitoneum (liposarcoma, angiomyolipoma, myelolipoma), and very large retroperitoneal lesions can extend into peritoneal cavity

Helpful Clues for Common Diagnoses

- **Sclerosing Mesenteritis**
  - Idiopathic inflammatory and fibrotic disorder of mesentery (of unknown etiology) that can produce abdominal pain
    - Likely underdiagnosed cause of acute abdominal pain
  - Appearance is variable depending on stage of evolution, but usually located in jejunal mesentery (left upper quadrant)
    - Acute stage appears as subtly increased attenuation of mesenteric fat ("misty mesentery")
    - Can evolve into discrete fat-containing mass with thin pseudocapsule
      - Often contains multiple prominent subcentimeter lymph nodes with halo of surrounding spared fat (fat-halo sign)
      - Envelops vasculature without narrowing or attenuation
    - Chronic stage can develop into discrete fibrotic mass with calcification and desmoplastic reaction
      - Can be associated with bowel obstruction or venous/lymphatic obstruction
      - Can be difficult to differentiate from carcinoid tumors at this stage of evolution, although location (jejunal mesentery vs. ileal mesentery for carcinoid) can be helpful clue
- **Omental Infarct**
  - Fat necrosis of omentum due to compromised arterial blood supply, which can cause abdominal pain

- Usually idiopathic but can also be secondary to prior surgery or trauma
  - Heterogeneous, fat-containing mass in omentum with surrounding hyperdense rim (± whorled appearance of vessels leading to infarct)
    - Appears as hyperechoic mass fixed to colon with absent color flow vascularity on US
  - Most often located in right lower quadrant but can occur anywhere in omentum
  - Typically larger in appearance than epiploic appendagitis without central dot sign
  - Can be extremely large (and simulate tumor) in some cases, particularly when occurring after surgery
    - Unlike tumors, omental infarcts are associated with pain and should become smaller over time
- **Epiploic Appendagitis**
  - Acute inflammation of epiploic appendage of colon, which can cause abdominal pain
  - Small, fat-containing mass with hyperdense rim immediately adjacent to colon with mild, adjacent fat stranding
    - May demonstrate central dot sign: Thrombosed vein at center of inflamed appendage
  - Can arise anywhere in colon but usually in left lower quadrant adjacent to descending or sigmoid colon
  - Self-limited process that requires only conservative management
- **Fat Necrosis**
  - Can occur anywhere in body but typically is result of prior insult (often prior surgery or trauma)
  - Discrete, fat-containing mass with weakly enhancing capsule (but no evidence of aggressiveness or local spread) ± calcification
    - Can have variable internal attenuation (with little fat), potentially mimicking fluid collection or soft tissue mass
      - Unlike tumor, should (but not always) gradually decrease in size over time
- **Dermoid Cyst (Mature Teratoma)**
  - Most common germ cell neoplasm of ovary
  - Usually asymptomatic, but rare complications include pelvic pain, rupture, torsion, superinfection, or malignant degeneration (very rare)
  - May demonstrate various internal components on CT, including macroscopic fat, calcification, fluid attenuation, or soft tissue density
    - Presence of macroscopic fat within adnexal mass is key to diagnosis and can be easily confirmed with MR in equivocal cases
  - Multiple possible appearances on US, including tip-of-iceberg sign, dermoid plug, or dot-dash pattern
- **Fibrofatty Mesenteric Proliferation ("Creeping Fat") (Mimic)**
  - Common in longstanding Crohn disease but can be seen as sequelae of any longstanding or repetitive inflammatory process in abdomen
  - Usually found immediately adjacent to most commonly inflamed segment of bowel (typically right lower quadrant ileocolic mesentery)

- o Manifests as increased amount of mesenteric fat but does not appear as discrete mass or demonstrate defined borders
- **Intussusception (Mimic)**
  - o Mesenteric fat is drawn into intussuscipiens along with bowel (intussusceptum)
  - o When viewed in cross section, appears as crescent of fat density within intussuscipiens, which might mimic fatty mass or lipoma

Helpful Clues for Less Common Diagnoses

- **Liposarcoma**
  - o Much more common in retroperitoneum but can very rarely primarily arise in peritoneum or mesentery or extend from retroperitoneal space into peritoneum (particularly when large)
  - o Fat-containing mass with variable attenuation, depending on degree of differentiation
    - – Well-differentiated tumors more likely to show predominantly fat attenuation, whereas dedifferentiated tumors more likely to show soft tissue attenuation or other complex components
    - – Subtypes based on degree of differentiation include well-differentiated, myxoid, dedifferentiated, round cell, and pleomorphic tumors
- **Cystic Fibrosis of Pancreas (Mimic)**
  - o Complete fatty infiltration of pancreas very common in cystic fibrosis and usually seen by end of teenage years
  - o Does not appear mass-like and usually conforms to normal shape of pancreas
  - o Pancreatic insufficiency very common (~ 85%) manifestation of cystic fibrosis
  - o Other manifestations of cystic fibrosis in pancreas include simple pancreatic cysts, scattered punctate calcifications, and stigmata of chronic pancreatitis (due to repeated bouts of acute pancreatitis)
- **Lipomatous Pseudohypertrophy of Pancreas (Mimic)**
  - o Focal or diffuse, mass-like enlargement of pancreas with fatty replacement of unknown etiology (possibly related to cirrhosis or viral infection)

- o Pancreas can be severely enlarged and resemble large, fat-containing mass
- o Usually benign, incidental finding without patient symptoms
- **Lipoma of Intestine**
  - o Simple lipomas (fat-density spherical mass) may arise in stomach, small bowel, or colon (usually submucosal)
    - – Most frequent site is colon (usually right colon)
  - o Uncommon lesions that can be seen anywhere in GI tract and may very rarely cause occult GI bleeding when large and ulcerated
  - o Usually asymptomatic, incidental findings discovered at colonoscopy, surgery, or imaging
- **Lipomatous Infiltration of Ileocecal Valve (Mimic)**
  - o Fatty hypertrophy of ileocecal valve may be confused with intraluminal fatty mass
  - o Typically appears as circumferential fatty proliferation around margins of valve, rather than mass-like
  - o Incidental finding that does not require treatment
- **Pseudolipoma of Glisson Capsule**
  - o Encapsulated, fat-containing lesion located within liver capsule (possibly representing degenerated epiploic fat that is trapped by liver capsule during development)
  - o Simple, fat-containing nodule along surface of liver
- **Metastatic Malignant Teratoma**
  - o Primary malignant teratomas usually arise in anterior mediastinum or testicle in young patients
  - o Appearance of both primary tumor and metastases is variable depending on degree of differentiation, but metastases can demonstrate internal fat attenuation
- **Peritoneal Lipomatosis**
  - o Fatty proliferation can very rarely occur in peritoneum, similar to more common sites of lipomatosis in pelvis, mediastinum, and epidural space
  - o Exact etiology unknown but does have strong male predilection and is more common in obese patients
  - o Appears as diffuse, fatty proliferation without discrete capsule or mass-like margins

Sclerosing Mesenteritis

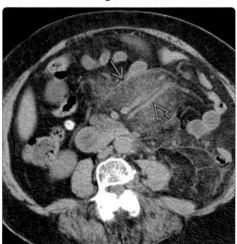

Sclerosing Mesenteritis

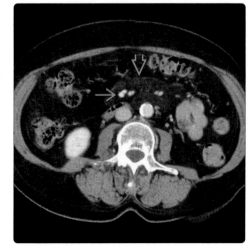

(**Left**) *Axial CECT shows heterogeneous infiltration of the mesenteric fat with a thin capsule ⇨ and mesenteric vessels ⇨ coursing through without attenuation or narrowing. This is a fairly typical appearance for sclerosing mesenteritis.* (**Right**) *Axial CECT shows infiltration of the jejunal mesentery. Note the thin capsule ⇨ around the process, as well as the fatty halo around the enlarged nodes ⇨, all of which are classic features of sclerosing mesenteritis.*

Sclerosing Mesenteritis

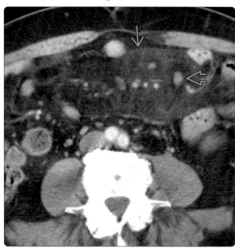

Omental Infarct

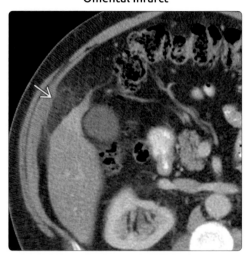

(Left) *Axial CECT shows infiltration of the small bowel mesentery with a thin surrounding pseudocapsule ⊟, as well as multiple enlarged mesenteric nodes ⊟, some of which demonstrate a subtle surrounding halo of spared fat. These findings are characteristic of sclerosing mesenteritis.* (Right) *Axial CECT shows the classic appearance of right-sided omental infarct with an oval, encapsulated, fat-containing lesion ➡ in the right abdominal omentum with surrounding fat stranding.*

Omental Infarct

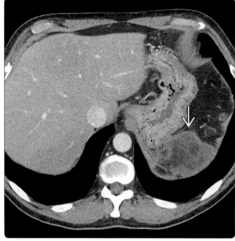

Epiploic Appendagitis

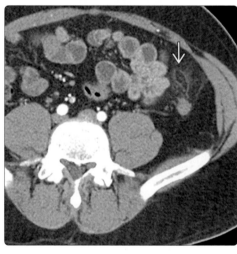

(Left) *Axial CECT in a patient status post laparoscopic distal pancreatectomy shows a large, fat-attenuation mass ➡ in the left upper quadrant with a surrounding hyperdense rim, representing a large postsurgical omental infarct/fat necrosis.* (Right) *Axial CECT shows a small, fat-containing mass ➡ abutting the left colon with subtle surrounding stranding and edema, compatible with epiploic appendagitis. This is a self-limited abnormality that does not require treatment.*

Epiploic Appendagitis

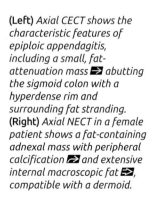

Dermoid Cyst (Mature Teratoma)

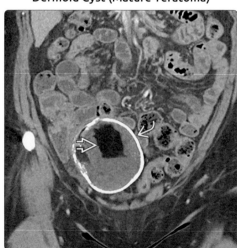

(Left) *Axial CECT shows the characteristic features of epiploic appendagitis, including a small, fat-attenuation mass ➡ abutting the sigmoid colon with a hyperdense rim and surrounding fat stranding.* (Right) *Axial NECT in a female patient shows a fat-containing adnexal mass with peripheral calcification ➡ and extensive internal macroscopic fat ⊟, compatible with a dermoid.*

Dermoid Cyst (Mature Teratoma)

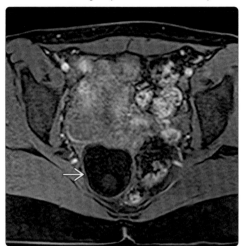

Fibrofatty Mesenteric Proliferation ("Creeping Fat") (Mimic)

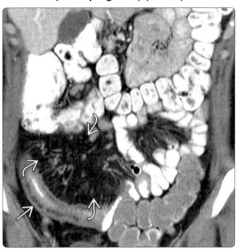

(Left) Axial T1 FS MR shows an ovarian dermoid ➡, which has signal similar to subcutaneous fat. (Right) Coronal T1 C+ MR in a patient with Crohn disease shows thickening of the terminal ileum ➡, portions of which demonstrate intramural fatty deposition related to prior inflammation. Note the extensive fibrofatty proliferation ➡ in the ileocolic mesentery, representing the sequelae of chronic Crohn-related inflammation ("creeping fat").

Liposarcoma

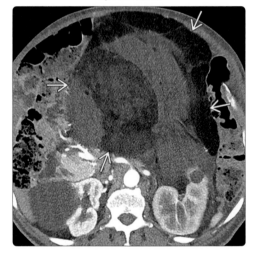

Liposarcoma

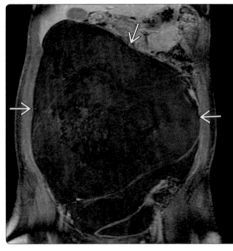

(Left) Axial CECT shows a large, encapsulated, predominantly fat-containing mass ➡ occupying much of the central abdomen with some internal complexity and soft tissue attenuation. This was found to be a well-differentiated liposarcoma at resection. (Right) Coronal T1 FS MR shows a massive, fat-containing, hyperintense mass ➡ occupying the entire abdomen. There is virtually no complexity within this mass, which was found to be a well-differentiated liposarcoma at resection.

Cystic Fibrosis of Pancreas (Mimic)

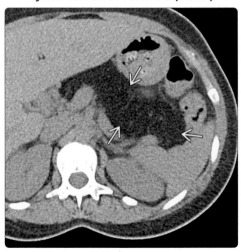

Pseudolipoma of Glisson Capsule

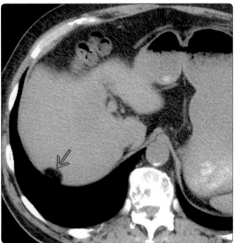

(Left) Axial NECT in a patient with cystic fibrosis shows the characteristic fatty replacement of the pancreas ➡ commonly seen in these patients by the end of their teenage years. (Right) Axial NECT shows a small, fat-attenuation lesion ➡ abutting the subcapsular surface of the liver dome, a classic appearance for a small pseudolipoma of Glisson capsule.

DIFFERENTIAL DIAGNOSIS

Common

- Lymphoma
- Metastases
- Reactive Lymphadenopathy Due to Localized Abdominal Inflammation
- Reactive Lymphadenopathy Due to Systemic Inflammation
- Postsurgical Lymphadenopathy
- Mesenteric Adenitis
- Sclerosing Mesenteritis
- Mononucleosis
- HIV/AIDS

Less Common

- Sarcoidosis
- Whipple Disease
- Celiac-Sprue Disease
- Tuberculosis and Other Infections

Rare but Important

- Castleman Disease
- Mastocytosis

ESSENTIAL INFORMATION

Key Differential Diagnosis Issues

- No consensus on size threshold for abnormal mesenteric lymph nodes, but normal nodes are typically < 5 mm in short axis
  - There is overlap in size of normal and abnormal nodes, and few mildly prominent lymph nodes may still be within normal limits
  - Multiplicity of abnormal nodes, nodal calcifications, abnormal node morphology (e.g., irregular margins, adjacent stranding), and abnormal node enhancement (e.g., hyperenhancing, necrotic, etc.) are other features that help determine if nodes are truly abnormal
    - Necrotic lymphadenopathy should raise concern for metastatic disease, tuberculosis (TB), celiac-sprue, or Whipple disease
    - Hypervascular lymphadenopathy should raise concern for Kaposi sarcoma, Castleman disease, or metastatic lymphadenopathy from hypervascular malignancies
    - Calcified lymphadenopathy may be associated with carcinoid tumor, treated/inactive disease (lymphoma or TB most common), or metastatic lymphadenopathy from mucinous malignancies
- **Generalized** mesenteric lymphadenopathy is most likely to be reactive as result of systemic infectious/inflammatory disease or lymphoma
  - Mild generalized lymphadenopathy most likely to be reactive or normal variant
  - Massive generalized mesenteric lymphadenopathy should strongly raise suspicion for lymphoma or, less commonly, metastatic disease
- **Localized** lymphadenopathy should prompt search for adjacent inflammatory process or malignancy
  - For example, RLQ lymphadenopathy should prompt concern for appendicitis, Crohn ileitis, right-sided colon cancer, carcinoid tumor, etc.

Helpful Clues for Common Diagnoses

- **Lymphoma**
  - Non-Hodgkin lymphoma much more commonly involves mesenteric nodes (~ 45% of patients) compared to Hodgkin lymphoma (~ 5-8%) and is most common malignant cause of mesenteric lymphadenopathy
  - Lymph nodes are typically substantially enlarged and may form confluent conglomerate nodal masses
    - Nodes in mesentery are of soft tissue density and often grow around bowel and vessels without causing obstruction or vascular narrowing/occlusion
    - Sandwich sign: Mesenteric nodal mass grows on both sides of vasculature, appearing similar to sandwich
  - Look for evidence of nodal (e.g., chest, abdomen, axilla, and neck) or extranodal disease elsewhere in body
  - Nodes may demonstrate calcification after treatment but virtually never calcify prior to treatment
- **Metastases**
  - Mesenteric lymphadenopathy most commonly occurs adjacent to primary GI tract malignancy
    - Common abdominal malignancies to produce adjacent mesenteric lymphadenopathy include colon cancer (most common), pancreatic cancer, carcinoid, and small bowel adenocarcinoma
    - Most of these malignancies produce lymphadenopathy of soft tissue density, although carcinoid nodal metastases tend to be hypervascular with frequent central calcification and desmoplastic reaction (spiculation and tethering of adjacent bowel/vasculature)
    - Lymph node metastases may often be 1st clue as to presence of tumor in bowel, as bowel lesion may be relatively subtle on imaging
  - Most common extraabdominal malignancies to produce generalized mesenteric lymphadenopathy are melanoma, lung cancer, and breast cancer
- **Reactive Lymphadenopathy Due to Localized Abdominal Inflammation**
  - Abdominal inflammatory disorders often result in reactive lymphadenopathy in adjacent mesentery
  - Appendicitis frequently associated with cluster of mildly enlarged nodes in RLQ mesentery
  - Crohn disease also frequently results in mild lymphadenopathy in RLQ ileocolic mesentery (usually in setting of active inflammation of ileum)
    - Look for evidence of active ileitis, including bowel wall thickening, mucosal hyperemia, fat stranding, etc.
  - Diverticulitis may result in very mild lymphadenopathy in sigmoid mesocolon
    - Significantly enlarged nodes, however, are uncommon and raise concern for malignancy
    - Colon wall thickening with regional lymphadenopathy should be considered malignancy until proven otherwise and should prompt colonoscopy
  - Infectious enteritis or colitis frequently associated with mild localized mesenteric lymphadenopathy
- **Reactive Lymphadenopathy Due to Systemic Inflammation**
  - Mesenteric nodes may be mildly enlarged in patients with underlying systemic inflammatory disorders (e.g., lupus, rheumatoid arthritis, systemic sclerosis, vasculitis)

- o Lymphadenopathy in such cases is usually very mild and found in multiple other locations
- **Postsurgical Lymphadenopathy**
  - o Mildly enlarged mesenteric lymph nodes are very common finding in immediate postoperative setting after abdominal surgery (especially involving GI tract)
  - o Lymphadenopathy usually quite minimal and should resolve in few weeks
- **Mesenteric Adenitis**
  - o Self-limited disorder usually affecting children and young adults, which may be related to underlying occult infection of terminal ileum (e.g., viral, *Yersinia*, etc.)
  - o Cluster of mildly enlarged lymph nodes in RLQ without evidence of underlying cause (e.g., appendicitis, etc.)
- **Sclerosing Mesenteritis**
  - o Probably underdiagnosed cause of persistent or recurrent abdominal pain
  - o Results in mild hazy infiltration of small bowel mesentery (misty mesentery) with prominent or mildly enlarged internal lymph nodes and halo of spared fat surrounding these lymph nodes and vessels
  - o Thin pseudocapsule surrounds infiltrated mesentery
- **Mononucleosis**
  - o Typically diagnosed in young adult with fever, malaise, and other mild constitutional symptoms
  - o Frequently associated with generalized lymphadenopathy, including mesenteric lymphadenopathy, as well as splenomegaly
- **HIV/AIDS**
  - o Direct HIV infection may result in mild mesenteric lymphadenopathy (and nodes elsewhere)
  - o Mesenteric lymphadenopathy may be manifestation of opportunistic infection (especially with CD4 < 50/mL)
    - – Both *Mycobacterium avium* (MAC) and TB can result in centrally necrotic or low-density lymph nodes (although soft tissue density nodes are also possible)
  - o Also consider malignancies in AIDS patients with low CD4 counts, including lymphoma and Kaposi sarcoma
    - – Kaposi sarcoma frequently produces hypervascular lymph nodes

Helpful Clues for Less Common Diagnoses

- **Sarcoidosis**
  - o Not infrequently involves upper abdominal organs, including hepatosplenomegaly with small, hypoenhancing nodules in liver or spleen
  - o Thoracic lymphadenopathy most common, but abdominal lymphadenopathy also possible
- **Whipple Disease**
  - o Systemic bacterial infection due to *Tropheryma whipplei*
  - o Characteristic low density (10- to 20-HU) mesenteric lymphadenopathy and small bowel wall thickening
- **Celiac-Sprue Disease**
  - o Can result in cavitating mesenteric node syndrome with low-attenuation mesenteric lymphadenopathy
  - o Nodes regress once patient placed on gluten-free diet
  - o Patients with celiac disease do have higher risk of lymphoma, and persistence of nodes, especially with soft tissue density, should raise concern for malignancy
- **Tuberculosis and Other Infections**
  - o TB lymphadenitis often associated with other manifestations of TB but can be isolated involvement
  - o Enlarged lymph nodes with frequent central necrosis
  - o Classic pattern is ileocecal wall thickening and regional lymphadenopathy, but other infections can have similar pattern (*Yersinia*, *Campylobacter*, *Salmonella*, etc.)

Helpful Clues for Rare Diagnoses

- **Castleman Disease**
  - o Benign lymphoproliferative disorder, which can be either localized or (rarely) diffuse
  - o Can result in hypervascular lymphadenopathy
- **Mastocytosis**
  - o Rare disorder that may be idiopathic or secondary to underlying hematologic malignancy that results in excessive number of mast cells
  - o Patients present with flushing, diarrhea, vomiting, abdominal pain, and skin manifestations
  - o May present with hepatosplenomegaly, small bowel wall thickening, omental infiltration, and abdominal lymphadenopathy (mesenteric or retroperitoneal)

Lymphoma

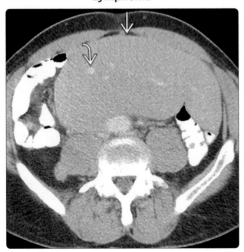

Lymphoma

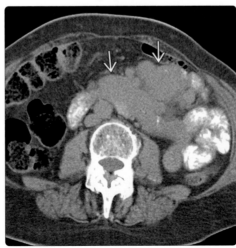

(Left) *Axial CECT shows a massive mesenteric conglomerate nodal mass ➡ that surrounds and sandwiches mesenteric vessels ⮑ without attenuation or narrowing, classic for lymphoma.* (Right) *Axial NECT shows extensive conglomerate mesenteric lymphadenopathy ➡, found to represent diffuse large B-cell lymphoma.*

Metastases

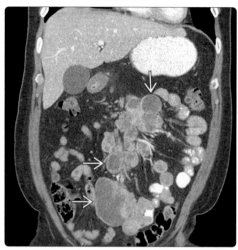

Metastases

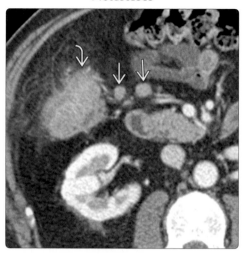

(Left) *Coronal CECT shows multiple enlarged central mesenteric lymph nodes ➡, many of which demonstrate internal necrosis, found to represent metastatic melanoma.* **(Right)** *Axial CECT shows a mass ➡ in the right colon, found to represent a primary colon adenocarcinoma with mildly enlarged lymph nodes ➡ in the adjacent ileocolic mesentery.*

Metastases

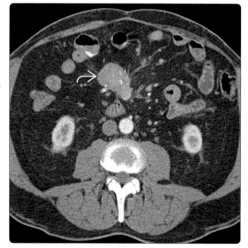

Metastases

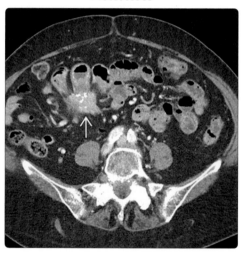

(Left) *Axial CECT shows an enhancing mesenteric mass ➡, found to be a carcinoid tumor. The primary mass in the ileum was not well visualized via imaging.* **(Right)** *Axial CECT shows a spiculated, hypervascular metastasis ➡ to the RLQ mesentery in a patient with carcinoid. Note the subtle calcification within the mass as well as the desmoplastic reaction with tethering of adjacent bowel loops.*

Reactive Lymphadenopathy Due to Localized Abdominal Inflammation

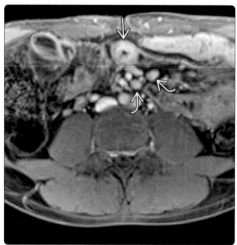

Mesenteric Adenitis

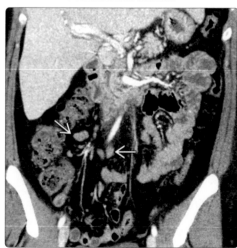

(Left) *Axial T1 C+ FS MR in a patient with Crohn disease shows thickening and hyperemia of a bowel loop ➡ due to active inflammation as well as mildly enlarged reactive lymph nodes ➡ clustered in the adjacent mesentery.* **(Right)** *Axial CECT in a young person with RLQ pain shows several nonspecific RLQ lymph nodes ➡. No appendicitis was found on CT. These findings were thought to be secondary to mesenteric adenitis.*

Sclerosing Mesenteritis

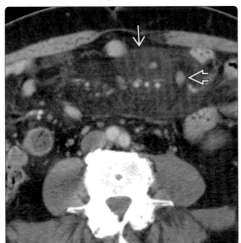

HIV/AIDS

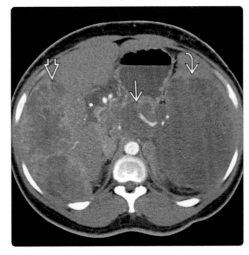

(Left) Axial CECT shows infiltration of the small bowel mesentery, set off by a pseudocapsule ➡. Multiple enlarged mesenteric nodes ➡ are present with a halo of surrounding spared fat, classic for sclerosing mesenteritis. (Right) Axial CECT in an AIDS patient shows large, heterogeneous masses in the liver ➡ and spleen ➡ as well as significant conglomerate lymphadenopathy ➡ in the upper abdomen, all of which was found to represent Kaposi sarcoma.

HIV/AIDS

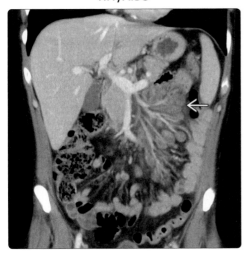

HIV/AIDS

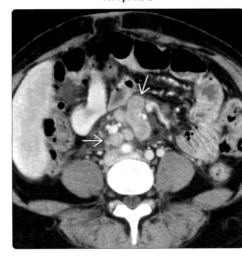

(Left) Coronal volume-rendered CECT shows innumerable mildly enlarged lymph nodes ➡ in the left abdominal mesentery, ultimately found to represent opportunistic histoplasmosis infection. (Right) Axial CECT shows mesenteric nodes ➡ with a peculiar low-density or caseated appearance, characteristic of mycobacterial infection in this AIDS patient.

Sarcoidosis

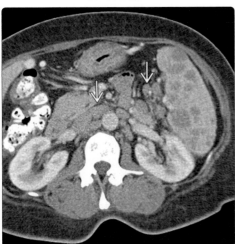

Tuberculosis and Other Infections

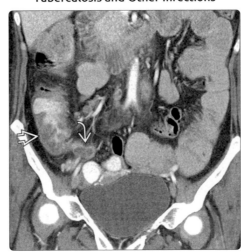

(Left) Axial CECT shows multiple small, hypodense nodules in the spleen as well as multiple enlarged upper abdominal lymph nodes ➡, all of which were found to be secondary to sarcoidosis. (Right) Coronal CECT shows a thickened, cone-shaped cecum ➡ and an immediately adjacent necrotic lymph node ➡ in the ileocolic mesentery, representing tuberculous colitis and tuberculous lymphadenitis.

DIFFERENTIAL DIAGNOSIS

Common

- Biliary Tract Calcifications
  - Gallstones
  - Porcelain Gallbladder
- Hepatic and Splenic Calcifications
  - Calcified Hepatic Masses (Primary or Metastatic)
  - Splenic and Hepatic Granulomas
  - Splenic Cysts
  - Echinococcal Cysts
  - Ischemia/Infarct
- Pancreatic Calcifications
  - Chronic Pancreatitis
  - Calcified Pancreatic Masses
- Urinary Tract and Adrenal Calcifications
  - Urolithiasis
  - Calcified Renal Masses
  - Renal Cysts
  - Renal TB
  - Adrenal Parenchymal Calcification
  - Calcified Adrenal Masses
  - Prostatic or Vas Deferens Calcification
  - Bladder Calculi
- Female Reproductive Organ Calcifications
  - Uterine Leiomyoma (Fibroid)
  - Ovarian Neoplasms
- Abdominal Wall or Soft Tissue Calcifications
  - Abdominal Injection Sites
  - Costal Cartilage Calcification (Mimic)
  - Calcified or Ossified Scar
  - Calcinosis Syndromes
- Vascular Calcifications
- Bowel Calcifications
  - Appendicolith (Fecalith)
  - Appendiceal Mucocele
- Mesenteric or Peritoneal Calcifications
  - Calcified Lymph Nodes
  - Sclerosing Peritonitis
  - Pseudomyxoma Peritonei
  - Lymphangioma
  - Sclerosing Mesenteritis

ESSENTIAL INFORMATION

Key Differential Diagnosis Issues

- Abdominal calcifications broadly divided into several types
  - **Metastatic calcification** reflects deposition of calcium salts in normal tissue (e.g., renal failure with secondary hyperparathyroidism)
    - Requires hypercalcemia and alkaline pH environment
  - **Dystrophic calcification** reflects deposition of calcium salts in tissue damaged by trauma, ischemia, infarction, infection, or tumor
  - **Ossification** reflects formation of bone in damaged tissue (e.g., ovarian teratoma or ossification within incision scar)
  - **Concretions** occur due to calcified precipitates inside vessel or hollow viscus (e.g., gallstones, renal calculi, phleboliths)

- **Conduit wall calcifications** are calcifications in wall of fluid-conducting tube (e.g., arterial calcification, aneurysm, vas deferens calcification)
  - Appear as ring-like or tram-track linear calcifications, which are often discontinuous
- **Cystic calcification** reflects wall of fluid-filled mass
- **Solid mass calcification** encompasses greatest variety of etiologies and appearances

Helpful Clues for Common Diagnoses

- **Biliary Tract Calcifications**
  - **Gallstones** vary greatly in density depending on type, ranging from soft tissue density to densely calcified
    - Only ~ 20% of stones are visible on radiographs
    - Calcium bilirubinate stones may be densely calcified and are most likely to be seen on radiographs
    - Cholesterol stones can be isoattenuating to bile and difficult to visualize on radiographs or CT
    - Gallstones can appear laminated or faceted ± internal gas (Mercedes-Benz sign)
  - **Porcelain gallbladder** represents calcification within wall of gallbladder
    - Much easier to perceive on CT but appears as thin, crescentic calcification in RUQ on radiographs
- **Hepatic and Splenic Calcifications**
  - Variety of **hepatic masses** can demonstrate calcification
    - Primary tumors: Hemangioma (central coarse calcification), adenoma (usually eccentric and secondary to prior hemorrhage), fibrolamellar hepatocellular carcinoma (coarse calcification in central scar), and conventional hepatoma
    - Metastases: Consider mucinous tumors (e.g., from colon), which produce stippled or faint calcifications
  - **Splenic and hepatic granulomas** appear as multiple punctate calcifications (easier to appreciate on CT)
    - Occur secondary to old, healed granulomatous infection (e.g., histoplasmosis, TB)
  - **Splenic cysts** may demonstrate peripheral wall calcification, which is more common with acquired (rather than congenital) cysts
  - **Echinococcal cysts** can demonstrate extensive internal whorled or serpiginous calcification in chronic phase
  - Dystrophic calcification can occur at sites of parenchymal scarring due to prior **ischemia or infarcts**
- **Pancreatic Calcifications**
  - **Chronic pancreatitis** may be associated with parenchymal/intraductal calcifications (along with dilated pancreatic duct)
  - Several types of cystic and solid **pancreatic masses** may demonstrate calcification
    - Pancreatic neuroendocrine tumor most common solid mass to calcify (usually central and coarse)
    - Mucinous cystic neoplasm (MCN), solid pseudopapillary neoplasms, serous cystadenoma, and pseudocysts are cystic masses with frequent calcification
      - MCNs often have peripheral curvilinear calcification, while serous cystadenomas may have coarse calcifications within central scar
- **Urinary Tract and Adrenal Calcifications**
  - **Urolithiasis:** All renal calculi are opaque on CT (except indinavir-induced stones)

- Only larger and calcified stones are visible on plain radiographs (urate stones are lucent)
- Stones tend to form and layer dependently within **calyceal diverticula**
  - Calcifications can be present in variety of **renal neoplasms**, including renal cell carcinoma, Wilms tumor, and multilocular cystic nephroma
  - Calcifications are common in **renal cysts** (typically thin or smooth along periphery or within septa), although Bosniak classification considers thick, irregular, or nodular calcifications as risk factors for malignancy
    - Calcifications are common with polycystic kidney disease due to cyst wall calcifications or stones
  - **Renal TB** in chronic setting can result in severe atrophy and parenchymal calcification
  - **Adrenal parenchymal calcifications** are usually coarse and typically reflect prior hemorrhage or infection (especially TB or histoplasmosis)
  - Calcifications may be present within **adrenal masses**, including myelolipoma (usually coarse calcification in mass with macroscopic fat), adrenocortical carcinoma, pheochromocytoma, and adrenal cyst
  - Dense central dystrophic **prostate calcifications** are common in aging men but can also reflect sequelae of prior prostatitis, malignancy, or benign prostatic hyperplasia (BPH)
  - **Vas deferens calcifications** appear as paired tubular "conduit" calcifications in pelvis extending midline
    - Tend to be present most often in insulin-dependent diabetic patients or in older patients
  - **Bladder stones** most often due to urinary stasis or migration of stones from upper urinary tract
- **Female Reproductive Organ Calcification**
  - Uterine calcifications usually reflect presence of **fibroids** with variety of possible appearances (e.g., whorled, flocculent, heterogeneous, popcorn)
  - **Dermoids** frequently contain calcification (representing bone or teeth), often within mural nodule
  - Calcification can also be found in **epithelial ovarian neoplasms**, especially serous malignancies
- **Abdominal Wall or Soft Tissue Calcifications**

  - **Abdominal injection sites** can develop calcification (usually as oval rim), especially common in buttocks
  - **Costal cartilage calcification (mimic)**: Irregular bilateral, symmetrical, cartilaginous calcification is more often seen in older women
  - **Calcified or ossified scar** may develop within midline surgical incision (usually with vertical orientation)
  - **Calcinosis syndromes** may produce calcifications in subcutaneous soft tissues and musculature
    - Associated with connective tissue diseases (e.g., scleroderma, CREST, lupus, dermatomyositis)
- **Vascular Calcifications**
  - Wide variety of different vascular calcifications
    - **Atherosclerotic** (tram-track morphology)
    - **Mönckeberg calcifications** in renal failure (diffuse circumferential arterial calcification)
    - Peripheral calcifications in wall of **aneurysm**
    - Linear venous calcifications due to **chronic deep venous thrombosis**
    - **Phleboliths** (small calcifications within veins, which often demonstrate lucent centers)
- **Bowel Calcifications**
  - **Fecalith** is calcification resulting from hardened fecal material and can be associated with appendicitis
  - **Appendiceal mucocele** may demonstrate curvilinear wall calcification
- **Mesenteric or Peritoneal Calcifications**
  - **Calcified lymph nodes** may result from prior TB or other granulomatous infections or, rarely, treated lymphoma
  - **Sclerosing peritonitis** is form of chronic peritonitis often resulting from prior peritoneal dialysis that manifests as extensive peritoneal thickening and calcification
  - Mucinous implants in **pseudomyxoma peritonei** may be associated with curvilinear or punctate calcifications
  - **Lymphangiomas** may demonstrate fine calcifications along their wall or within septations
  - **Sclerosing mesenteritis** in its final stages may result in LUQ calcified mass with tethering of bowel and vessels

Gallstones

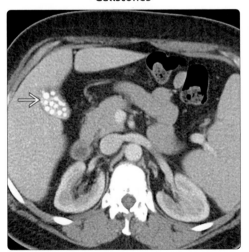

Porcelain Gallbladder

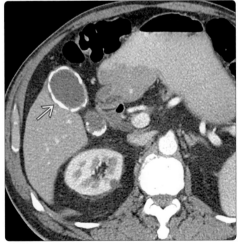

(Left) *Axial CECT shows calcified gallstones ➡ in the gallbladder. Gallstones may be of variable attenuation with calcified gallstones easiest to appreciate on CT or radiography.* **(Right)** *Axial CECT shows prominent calcification of the gallbladder wall ➡, compatible with a porcelain gallbladder. The association between porcelain gallbladder and gallbladder carcinoma is now considered somewhat debatable.*

Peritoneum and Mesentery

Calcified Hepatic Masses (Primary or Metastatic)

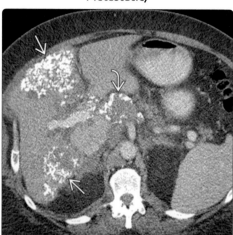

Splenic and Hepatic Granulomas

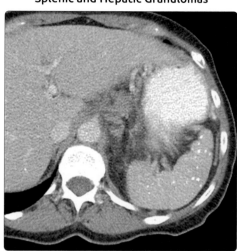

(Left) *Axial CECT shows large, heterogeneously calcified mass lesions ➡ in the liver as well as a similarly calcified lymph node mass ➡ in the gastrohepatic ligament. These findings reflect metastases from the patient's primary mucinous colon cancer.* (Right) *Axial CECT shows multiple punctate calcifications in the spleen, likely related to old, healed granulomatous disease.*

Splenic Cysts

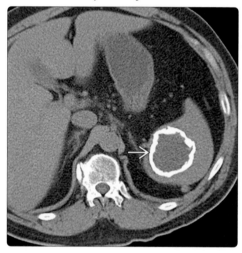

Echinococcal Cysts

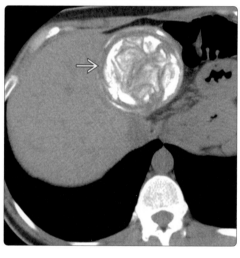

(Left) *Axial NECT shows an incidentally discovered benign splenic cyst ➡ with prominent peripheral calcification. Acquired splenic cysts are more likely to demonstrate calcification compared to congenital splenic cysts.* (Right) *Axial NECT shows a large, heavily calcified mass ➡ in the liver with a characteristically whorled or serpiginous pattern of calcification. This represents a large, chronic echinococcal cyst in a patient who had emigrated from an endemic area.*

Ischemia/Infarct

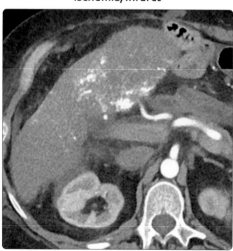

Chronic Pancreatitis

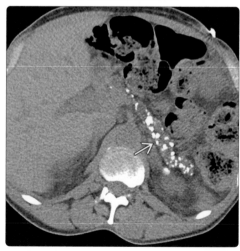

(Left) *Axial CECT in a patient status post liver transplant shows patchy areas of calcification throughout the liver parenchyma, which were found on biopsy to represent the sequelae of ischemia and rejection.* (Right) *Axial NECT shows an atrophic pancreas ➡ with extensive calcification, findings diagnostic of chronic pancreatitis.*

Calcified Pancreatic Masses

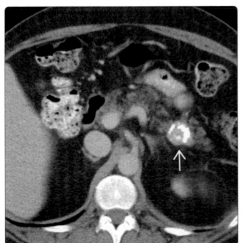

Calcified Pancreatic Masses

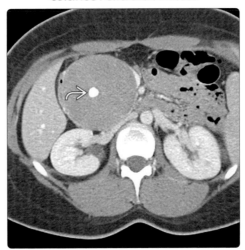

(Left) Axial CECT shows a solid, enhancing mass ➡ in the pancreatic body with internal coarse calcification, representing a pancreatic neuroendocrine tumor. (Right) Axial CECT in a young woman shows a large solid and pseudopapillary neoplasm (SPEN) with a sizable central coarse calcification ➡.

Urolithiasis

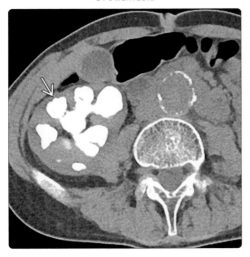

Renal Cell Carcinoma

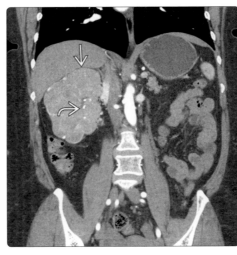

(Left) Axial NECT shows a massive staghorn renal calculus ➡ almost completely filling the right intrarenal collecting system. (Right) Coronal NECT shows a large, right-sided renal mass ➡ with subtle internal calcifications ➡, found to represent a chromophobe renal cell carcinoma at surgical resection.

Bladder Calculi

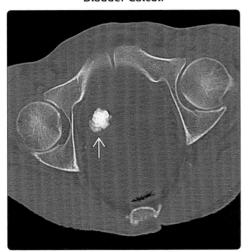

Ovarian Carcinoma

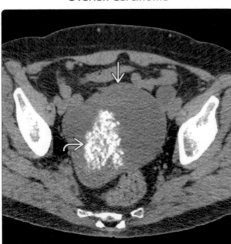

(Left) Axial NECT shows a large, high-density stone ➡ within the bladder. (Right) Axial NECT in a female patient shows a large, cystic pelvic mass ➡ with extensive calcification ➡, found to represent an ovarian cancer.

Ovarian Dermoid/Teratoma

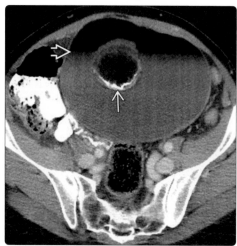

Ovarian Carcinoma

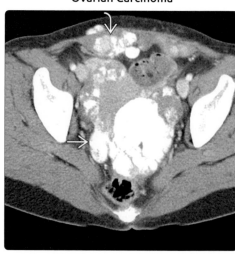

(Left) *Axial CECT shows a large pelvic mass in a young female patient with extensive internal fat, a discrete fat-fluid level* ➡ *, and internal calcification* ➡ *, compatible with a dermoid cyst.* (Right) *Axial CECT shows a large, calcified mass* ➡ *in the pelvis, representing a primary ovarian malignancy, with additional calcified tumor implants in the peritoneum and anterior pelvic wall* ➡ *.*

Abdominal Injection Sites

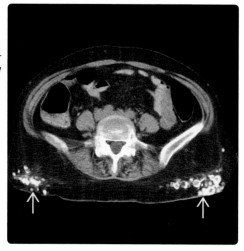

Calcified or Ossified Scar

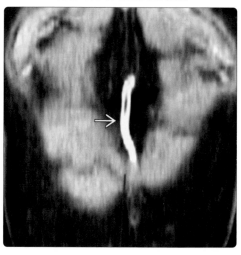

(Left) *Axial NECT shows multiple calcified injection granulomas* ➡ *in the subcutaneous fat of the buttocks.* (Right) *Coronal CECT shows a linear, ossified scar* ➡ *along a prior midline abdominal incision.*

Calcinosis Syndromes

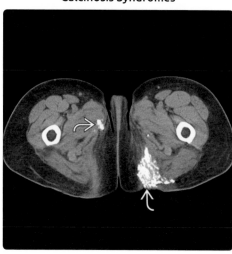

Vascular Calcifications

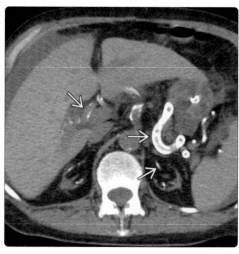

(Left) *Axial NECT shows extensive calcifications* ➡ *in the subcutaneous soft tissues and musculature of the pelvis in a patient with scleroderma.* (Right) *Axial NECT in a patient with end-stage renal disease shows shrunken, end-stage kidneys and extensive upper abdominal arterial vascular tram-track calcifications* ➡ *.*

Vascular Calcifications

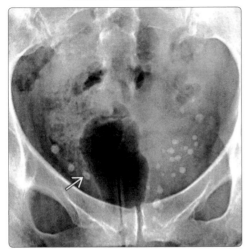

Vascular Calcifications

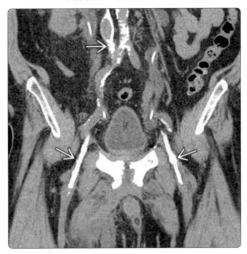

(Left) *Frontal radiograph shows multiple phleboliths in the pelvis (having their typical distribution) mainly below the iliac spines, some with central lucency ➡. (Right) Coronal NECT shows an atretic appearance of the IVC and iliac veins, with extensive linear calcification in the inferior vena cava (IVC) and external iliac veins ➡, findings compatible with the patient's known history of chronic deep venous thrombosis.*

Appendiceal Mucocele

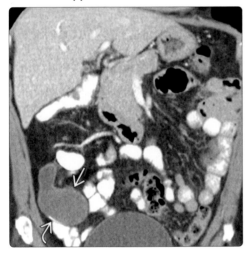

Calcified Lymph Nodes

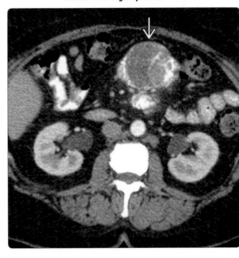

(Left) *Coronal CECT shows a large, tubular, cystic mass ➡ with subtle peripheral calcification ➡. On close inspection, this cystic mass connected with the cecum, representing a large appendiceal mucocele. (Right) Axial CECT in a patient with history of treated non-Hodgkin lymphoma shows a residual soft tissue mass ➡ with calcification in the mesentery, representing the sequelae of treatment. The mass was stable over several exams and was not metabolically active on PET.*

Sclerosing Peritonitis

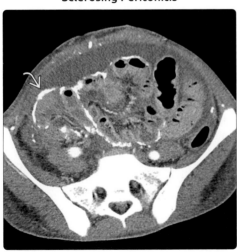

Sclerosing Mesenteritis

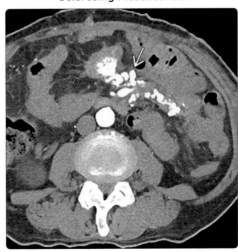

(Left) *Axial CECT shows extensive calcification ➡ of the peritoneal lining and along the surface of bowel loops (along with loculated ascites) in a patient with sclerosing peritonitis related to a prior history of peritoneal dialysis. (Right) Axial NECT shows extensive calcification ➡ in the left upper quadrant mesentery with tethering of adjacent bowel loops, representing an end-stage form of sclerosing mesenteritis.*

DIFFERENTIAL DIAGNOSIS

Common

- Normal Postoperative Pneumoperitoneum
- Barotrauma
- Iatrogenic Injuries or Complications
  o Bowel Anastomotic Leak
- Perforated Ulcer
  o Duodenal Ulcer
  o Gastric Ulcer
- Diverticulitis
- Intestinal Trauma
- Appendicitis
- Thoracic Processes (Mimics)
  o Pneumothorax
  o Subsegmental Atelectasis
  o Cystic Lung Disease
- Colonic Interposition (Mimic)
- Subphrenic Fat (Mimic)

Less Common

- Other Causes of Bowel Perforation
- Peritonitis
- Abdominal Abscess
- Pneumatosis Cystoides Intestinalis
- From Female Genital Tract
- Small Bowel Diverticula
- Foreign Body Perforation

ESSENTIAL INFORMATION

Key Differential Diagnosis Issues

- CT is significantly more sensitive than plain radiographs for detection of pneumoperitoneum and should be test of choice in cases of suspected hollow viscus perforation
- Upright or decubitus radiographs are much more sensitive than supine films for detection of free air
  o Free intraperitoneal gas is difficult to detect on supine radiographs as result of subtle radiographic findings and frequent poor image quality of portable films
- In cases with unexplained free intraperitoneal air, amount and location of gas should help guide diagnosis
  o Gas often located in proximity to site of perforation
    – Gastric/duodenal perforations typically result in free air in upper abdomen (above transverse mesocolon)
    – Jejunal, ileal, and colonic perforations result in free air below transverse mesocolon
  o Small bowel perforation usually results in only small amounts of pneumoperitoneum, while gastric and colon perforations can result in massive free air
    – Perforated ulcers and diverticulitis usually result in relatively small amounts of free air
    – Perforation of colon or misplaced feeding tubes may result in massive free air
- While pneumoperitoneum should (justifiably) raise concern for intestinal perforation, also consider benign causes of pneumoperitoneum when free air is incidental finding in asymptomatic patient

Helpful Clues for Common Diagnoses

- **Normal Postoperative Pneumoperitoneum**

---

  o Small amount of free air is normal finding after laparotomy or other invasive procedures (e.g., peritoneal dialysis, gastrostomy tube placement, etc.)
    – Seen on CT in almost 90% of patients at 3 days after surgery and 50% at 6 days
    – Typically resolves in 7-10 days but may rarely persist longer in some patients
      □ Free air may persist longer in patients with history of prior surgeries or prior bouts of peritonitis
    – Normal postoperative free air should be minimal, as **large or massive pneumoperitoneum is abnormal finding** that should raise concern for anastomotic leak or perforation
- **Barotrauma**
  o Positive pressure ventilation can lead to alveolar rupture that results in pneumothorax, pneumomediastinum, subcutaneous emphysema, pneumatosis, or pneumoperitoneum
  o Gas in pleural or mediastinal spaces may dissect into peritoneum or retroperitoneum
  o Suspect in patient on positive pressure ventilation with both pneumothorax and pneumoperitoneum
- **Iatrogenic Injuries or Complications**
  o Common causes of injury include endoscopy with bowel perforation, complicated feeding tube placement
  o Bowel anastomotic leak can be seen as complication of any intraperitoneal bowel anastomosis, often manifesting as greater than expected postoperative free air ± imaging findings of peritonitis or abscess
- **Perforated Ulcer**
  o Gastroduodenal ulcers represent most common cause of GI tract perforation
    – Gastric and duodenal ulcers have equal risk of perforation, although duodenal ulcers are 3x as common
  o Duodenal ulcer perforation typically results in ectopic gas, fluid, and fat stranding immediately adjacent to duodenal bulb
    – Gas and fluid may be both intraperitoneal and extraperitoneal (anterior pararenal space)
  o Gastric ulcer perforation often occurs into lesser sac, resulting in collection of gas, fluid, or contrast posterior to stomach with subsequent extension into peritoneal cavity through epiploic foramen (of Winslow)
- **Diverticulitis**
  o Very common cause of pneumoperitoneum in pelvis, although amount of free air usually quite minimal, as omentum walls off perforated diverticulum
    – Usually does not cause generalized peritonitis or large free air and manifests as several tiny foci of free air adjacent to inflamed colon (usually sigmoid)
  o Patients may rarely develop large pneumoperitoneum and generalized peritonitis, especially older adult patients and those using steroids
- **Intestinal Trauma**
  o Pneumoperitoneum following blunt trauma is indicative of intestinal perforation until proven otherwise with duodenum and proximal jejunum most common sites
  o Often associated with ancillary signs of bowel injury, including mesenteric hematoma and bowel wall thickening

- o Be aware that diagnostic peritoneal lavage (DPL) performed during initial clinical assessment may result in free intraperitoneal air and fluid
- **Appendicitis**
  - o Ruptured appendicitis typically produces only small amount of free air, usually in conjunction with significant free fluid (± loculated fluid collection/abscess)
  - o Appendicitis complicated by rupture in ~ 25%
- **Thoracic Processes (Mimics)**
  - o Variety of lung abnormalities may simulate pneumoperitoneum on plain radiograph due to proximity to diaphragm
    - Thin crescent of pleural air (pneumothorax) near diaphragm may simulate pneumoperitoneum
    - Plate-like, basal atelectasis may result in curvilinear density that parallels diaphragm with aerated lung below atelectasis mimicking pneumoperitoneum
    - Cystic lung disease, including bullae and other cysts near diaphragm, may simulate free air on radiographs
- **Colonic Interposition (Mimic)**
  - o a.k.a. Chilaiditi syndrome, when hepatic flexure of colon lies above liver, beneath right hemidiaphragm
  - o Not uncommonly mistaken for free air on radiographs
- **Subphrenic Fat (Mimic)**
  - o Collections of fat in subxiphoid and perihepatic regions may be quite radiolucent and may be misinterpreted as free air on radiography

Helpful Clues for Less Common Diagnoses

- **Other Causes of Bowel Perforation**
  - o Multiple other causes of bowel perforation include
    - Severe bowel distension due to severe ileus, volvulus, or obstruction
    - Bowel ischemia
    - Vasculitis (polyarteritis nodosa and Behçet disease most commonly cause small bowel perforation)
    - Severe infection or inflammatory bowel disease
    - Malignancy
      - □ Lymphoma most common malignant cause of perforation in small bowel, while adenocarcinoma most common cause in colon

- Ingested foreign bodies (e.g., bone, toothpick, etc.)
  - □ Tend to cause perforations in ileum, ileocecal region, or rectosigmoid
- Radiation therapy
- Fecal stool impaction (i.e., stercoral colitis)
- Chemotherapy or other medications (e.g., steroids)
- Penetrating trauma (e.g., knife or gunshot wounds)
  - o Small bowel perforations are much less common than colonic perforation
- **Peritonitis**
  - o Intraperitoneal gas and fluid may result from pyogenic infection with gas-forming organisms (usually enteric)
  - o Usually associated with other signs of peritonitis, including abscess or peritoneal thickening/enhancement
- **Abdominal Abscess**
  - o Gas-containing subphrenic abscess may simulate free abdominal gas on upright radiograph
- **Pneumatosis Cystoides Intestinalis**
  - o Uncommon, benign form of pneumatosis with cystic collections of gas in bowel wall
    - Most often diagnosed in patients with scleroderma and other collagen vascular disease
    - May relate to steroid use or other immunosuppressive medications
  - o Cystic intramural gas may rupture, leading to pneumoperitoneum
  - o Even though CT may appear highly concerning, patients are asymptomatic
- **From Female Genital Tract**
  - o Retrograde passage of ectopic gas into peritoneum through female genital tract may occur in variety of settings [e.g., following sexual intercourse, pelvic examination, or water sports (e.g., water skiing)]
- **Small Bowel Diverticula**
  - o Diverticula arising from duodenum or small intestine may perforate spontaneously due to small bowel diverticulitis or as result of feeding tube placement
  - o Perforation of small bowel diverticula usually results in very little free air and does not typically result in peritonitis or need for surgery

Normal Postoperative Pneumoperitoneum

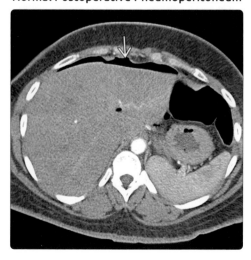

Barotrauma

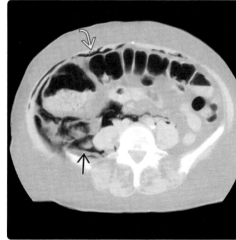

(Left) *Axial CECT acquired after abdominal surgery demonstrates a thin crescent of pneumoperitoneum ⇨ in the nondependent upper abdomen, a normal finding in the postoperative period.* **(Right)** *Axial NECT in a patient on positive-pressure ventilation and with known large bilateral pneumothoraces (not shown) demonstrates gas dissecting downward into the abdomen to involve the retroperitoneum ⇨ and intraperitoneal space ⇉, classic findings for barotrauma.*

Iatrogenic Injuries or Complications

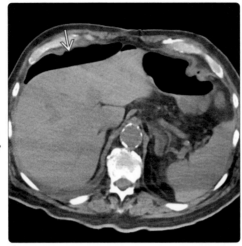

Iatrogenic Injuries or Complications

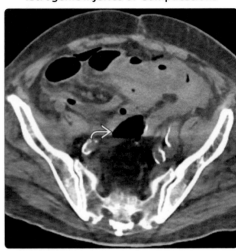

(Left) *Axial NECT after a low anterior rectal resection demonstrates greater than expected pneumoperitoneum ➡ immediately after surgery.* **(Right)** *Axial NECT in the same patient demonstrates a focal collection of ectopic gas near the rectal anastomosis ➡. While small free air is normal after surgery, large free air, as in this case, should suggest the presence of anastomotic leak. This patient required surgical revision of the rectal anastomosis.*

Iatrogenic Injuries or Complications

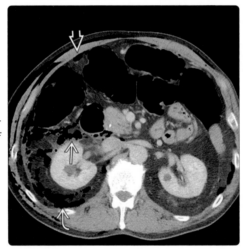

Perforated Ulcer

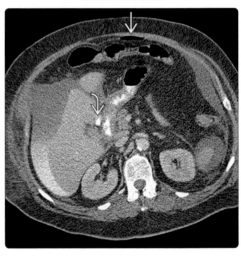

(Left) *Axial CECT after ERCP demonstrates gas tracking from the duodenum ➡ tracking into both the peritoneal ➡ and retroperitoneal ➡ spaces as well as into the subcutaneous soft tissues, representing the sequelae of duodenal perforation.* **(Right)** *Axial CECT demonstrates extravasation of enteric contrast ➡ from the duodenum along with free intraperitoneal air ➡ and large ascites (portions of which contain oral contrast material), representing a perforated duodenal ulcer.*

Perforated Ulcer

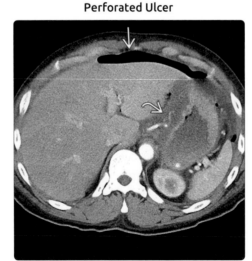

Diverticulitis

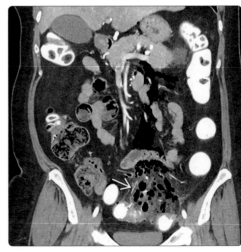

(Left) *Axial CECT demonstrates marked wall edema and thickening ➡ along the lesser curvature of the stomach as well as free intraperitoneal air ➡, representing a perforated gastric ulcer.* **(Right)** *Coronal CECT demonstrates gas and enteric contrast ➡ tracking upward from the inflamed sigmoid colon, representing perforated sigmoid diverticulitis.*

Other Causes of Bowel Perforation

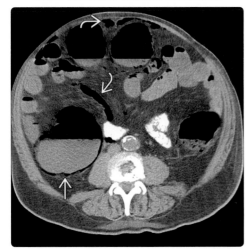

Other Causes of Bowel Perforation

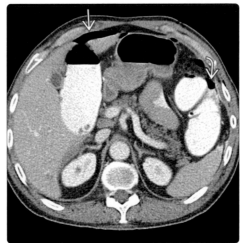

(Left) *Axial NECT demonstrates a massively dilated cecum with pneumatosis* ➡ *and multiple foci of free intraperitoneal air* ➡, *representing colonic ischemia with perforation.* (Right) *Axial CECT in a patient with multiple stab wounds demonstrates multiple foci of free air* ➡ *along with gas and ectopic enteric contrast* ➡ *immediately along the outer margin of the colon. Colonic injury was discovered at surgery.*

Pneumatosis Cystoides Intestinalis

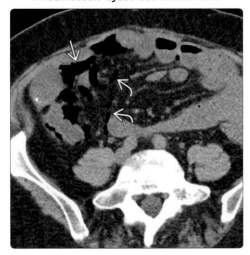

Pneumatosis Cystoides Intestinalis

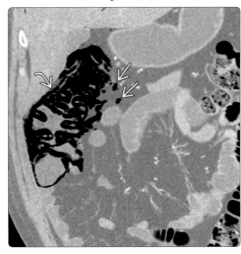

(Left) *Axial NECT in an asymptomatic patient demonstrates bubbly pneumatosis* ➡ *in the right colon with several foci of adjacent free air* ➡. *The patient was clinically doing well, and this was thought to represent benign pneumatosis.* (Right) *Coronal CECT in an asymptomatic patient on chronic steroid treatment for autoimmune disease demonstrates extensive benign pneumatosis* ➡ *throughout the right colon with resultant perforation and small adjacent free air* ➡.

Small Bowel Diverticula

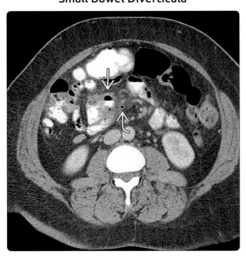

Foreign Body Perforation

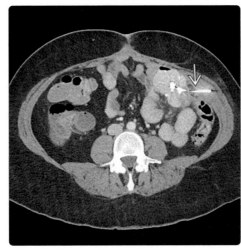

(Left) *Axial CECT in a patient with abdominal pain demonstrates an inflamed contrast-filled diverticulum* ➡ *arising from a small bowel loop as well as a tiny focus of adjacent ectopic gas* ➡, *compatible with small bowel diverticulitis.* (Right) *Axial CECT in a psychiatric patient demonstrates an intentionally ingested pin* ➡ *perforating through the small bowel into the adjacent abdominal wall. These findings required surgical intervention.*

DIFFERENTIAL DIAGNOSIS

Common

- Abdominal Trauma
- Iatrogenic Injury
- Coagulopathic Hemorrhage
- Obstetric or Gynecological Source
  - Ruptured Ovarian Cyst
  - Ruptured Ectopic Pregnancy
  - HELLP Syndrome
- Ruptured Aneurysm
- Other Nonhemorrhagic Causes of High-Attenuation Ascites

Less Common

- Neoplastic Hemorrhage
- Ruptured Spleen
- Hemorrhagic Pancreatitis

ESSENTIAL INFORMATION

Key Differential Diagnosis Issues

- Attenuation of blood products will vary depending on age of bleed
  - Acute, unclotted extravascular blood typically demonstrates attenuation of 35-45 HU
    - Blood products may demonstrate slightly lower attenuation in patients with severe anemia
    - Density of blood may also be decreased due to dilution by ascites, urine, bile, or bowel contents
  - Clotted blood is typically higher in attenuation (45-70 HU), explaining why highest density blood is usually found immediately adjacent to site of bleeding (i.e., **sentinel clot sign**)
    - Sentinel clot sign can be important clue to source of bleeding in difficult cases
    - Blood products distant from site of bleeding usually lower in attenuation
  - Active extravasation of contrast (often easiest to identify on arterial-phase imaging) may be found at sites of active bleeding with attenuation identical to blood pool
    - Identifying active extravasation critical in determining need for urgent embolization or surgery
- Clinical history is key to diagnosis, including recent trauma, recent surgery, anticoagulation, coagulopathy, and pregnancy status
  - In patients without history of trauma, look for evidence of abnormal visceral organ (organomegaly or mass) or vasculature (aneurysm, dissection) that may explain bleeding
  - Unexplained hemoperitoneum in young woman of childbearing age should always prompt correlation with β-hCG levels to exclude ruptured ectopic pregnancy
- CT is critical for diagnosis in cases of large nontraumatic hemoperitoneum, as physical exam can be misleading, and hematocrit levels may be normal in acute setting
- Abdominal hemorrhage on MR can be quite variable in signal depending on age of blood products and sequence utilized and may not follow standard signal characteristics classically described with intracranial hemorrhage

Helpful Clues for Common Diagnoses

- **Abdominal Trauma**
  - Presence of intraabdominal hemorrhage in setting of trauma should prompt careful search for solid organ or bowel injuries, particularly when acute blood seen immediately adjacent to visceral organ or bowel loop
    - Sentinel clot (heterogeneous higher density clot) may be visualized adjacent to source of bleeding
  - Most commonly injured solid organs in abdomen are spleen and liver with injuries almost always associated with adjacent hematoma
    - Hematoma in such cases usually extends downward along paracolic gutters into pelvis
  - Duodenum and proximal jejunum most common sites of bowel injury, and presence of mesenteric or interloop blood may be only clue to diagnosis
    - Hematoma in such cases more often centrally located within leaves of mesentery adjacent to bowel loops
- **Iatrogenic Injury (Complication of Surgery or Other Intervention)**
  - Diagnosis based on history of recent surgery or other intervention (biopsy, endoscopy, angiography) with blood seen in close proximity to site of intervention
  - Often associated with other postoperative findings, including pneumoperitoneum, subcutaneous gas, and free fluid
- **Coagulopathic Hemorrhage**
  - May result from anticoagulation or bleeding diathesis
  - Most common sites of spontaneous bleeding are iliopsoas compartment and rectus sheath, although hemorrhage can either originate from or track into peritoneal cavity
  - Classically associated with multiple sites of bleeding and frequent internal hematocrit levels (more common with coagulopathic hemorrhage than other causes)
- **Obstetric or Gynecologic Source**
  - Gynecologic causes are most common etiologies for nontraumatic hemoperitoneum in women of child-bearing age, particularly when hemorrhage is located in pelvis
    - Given limitations of CT in female pelvis, correlation with ultrasound and β-hCG levels may be necessary once hemorrhage is identified on CT
    - **Ruptured ovarian cyst**
      - Common cause of hemorrhage in premenopausal females with hemorrhage usually localized in pelvis immediately adjacent to adnexa
      - Hemorrhagic cyst may be directly visualized on CT as mixed-attenuation spherical mass arising from adnexa with adjacent hematoma
    - **Ruptured ectopic pregnancy**
      - Given life-threatening nature of this entity, ectopic pregnancy must be first consideration when confronted with pelvic hemorrhage in woman of child-bearing age
      - CT findings of pelvic hemorrhage in premenopausal female should prompt correlation with β-hCG levels (urine pregnancy test may be falsely negative) and ultrasound
    - **HELLP syndrome**
      - Peripartum complication of preeclampsia characterized by hemolysis, increased liver enzymes, and thrombocytopenia

□ May be associated with disseminated intravascular coagulation (DIC), hemolysis, hepatic infarction, hepatic rupture, or hemorrhage

- **Ruptured Aneurysm**
  - Bleeding aortic aneurysms usually result in retroperitoneal bleeding, although large hematoma can extend into peritoneal cavity
  - Visceral artery aneurysms usually produce intraperitoneal bleeding with splenic artery aneurysms most common (60%)
    - Disproportionately seen in female and pregnant patients with greater risk of rupture
- **Other Nonhemorrhagic Causes of High-Attenuation Ascites**
  - Bladder trauma
    - Intraperitoneal bladder rupture results in intraperitoneal fluid, which may demonstrate variable attenuation
      □ Unopacified urine is usually of water density but can appear higher in density due to combination of urine and blood or due to excretion of contrast-opacified urine into bladder
    - Most definitively diagnosed with CT cystogram after instillation of diluted contrast material into bladder
  - Vicarious excretion
    - Ascites may be minimally increased in attenuation due to prior administration of IV contrast material, especially when CT performed > 10 minutes after contrast administration
  - Gastrointestinal tract perforation
    - Ascites may be slightly hyperdense due to presence of extraluminal bowel contents
  - Peritonitis
    - Often associated with complex, loculated ascites (slightly higher in attenuation than simple fluid) and peritoneal thickening/enhancement
  - Malignant ascites
    - Often associated with other imaging features of peritoneal carcinomatosis, including peritoneal thickening/nodularity or frank tumor implants

- Ascites appears complex with slightly higher attenuation than simple fluid (10-25 HU), loculation, and internal septations

Helpful Clues for Less Common Diagnoses

- **Neoplastic Hemorrhage**
  - Any primary or metastatic tumor can bleed, although certain tumors are much more likely to present with significant bleeding
  - Most common hepatic tumors to be associated with bleeding are hepatic adenoma and hepatocellular carcinoma
    - Tumors near liver capsule most likely to present with large hemoperitoneum
    - Most other benign (i.e., hemangioma, focal nodular hyperplasia) or malignant liver lesions do not typically present with bleeding
  - Most common pancreatic tumor to present with bleeding is solid pseudopapillary neoplasm (SPEN), which is tumor most often seen in young female patients
    - Bleeding also described with neuroendocrine tumors, acinar cell carcinoma, and metastases (especially melanoma), albeit very uncommonly
  - Angiosarcoma, regardless of location (usually spleen or liver), classically associated with bleeding
  - Lung cancer, renal cell carcinoma, and melanoma most likely metastatic lesions to bleed in abdomen
- **Ruptured Spleen**
  - Enlarged spleen, most often due to infection or tumor (such as lymphoma/leukemia), is at increased risk for rupture and can result in massive hemoperitoneum
  - Mononucleosis is most common cause of spontaneous splenic rupture in Western societies and may be injured in minor trauma, such as sports activities
- **Hemorrhagic Pancreatitis**
  - Most often seen with severe necrotizing pancreatitis
    - Bleeding typically due to disruption of small vessels and capillaries by pancreatic enzymes
  - Pseudoaneurysm (most often splenic artery) must be excluded when hemorrhage seen adjacent to pancreas

Abdominal Trauma

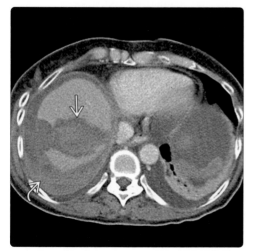

Abdominal Trauma

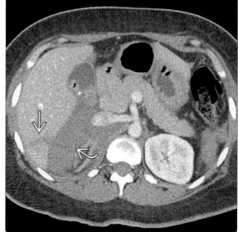

(Left) Axial CECT after trauma demonstrates a large laceration ➡ throughout the right liver with perihepatic hematoma ⬆. (Right) Axial CECT after trauma demonstrates a laceration ➡ through the right liver with immediately adjacent high-density perihepatic hematoma ⬆.

(Left) *Axial CECT in a patient with extensive splenic lacerations* ⇨ *after trauma demonstrates a classic sentinel clot sign with blood around the spleen* ⇨ *higher in density than the blood around the liver* ⇨*. The highest density blood products should be found adjacent to the site of bleeding.* (Right) *Axial CECT after trauma demonstrates extensive hemoperitoneum* ⇨ *with a large focus of active extravasation* ⇨ *in the central mesentery. Mesenteric and small bowel injury were discovered at surgery.*

Abdominal Trauma

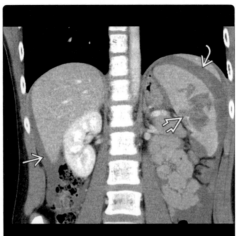

Abdominal Trauma

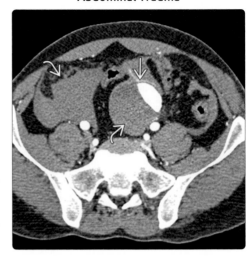

(Left) *Axial CECT after a Whipple procedure shows a hematoma* ⇨ *adjacent to the surgical bed with active extravasation* ⇨*, prompting angiographic embolization. Active bleeding from a gastroduodenal artery stump was seen at angiography.* (Right) *Axial CECT in an anticoagulated patient shows a large retroperitoneal hematoma* ⇨ *centered in the psoas muscle with extension into the right abdomen. Note the hematocrit level* ⇨ *within the hemorrhage, a common feature with coagulopathic bleeds.*

Iatrogenic Injury

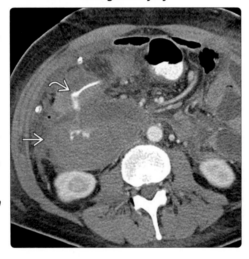

Coagulopathic Hemorrhage

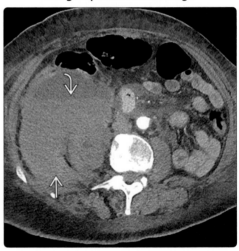

(Left) *Axial CECT shows a left adnexal cyst* ⇨ *with adjacent high-density hematoma* ⇨ *throughout the deep pelvis, compatible with bleeding secondary to a ruptured ovarian cyst.* (Right) *Axial CECT shows a large pelvic hematoma* ⇨ *with evidence of active extravasation* ⇨ *in a young female patient. In the absence of a history of trauma, these findings should prompt correlation with β-HCG levels and US to exclude a ruptured ectopic pregnancy.*

Ruptured Ovarian Cyst

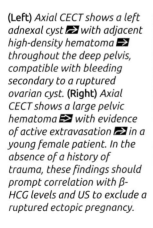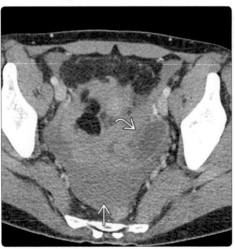

Ruptured Ectopic Pregnancy

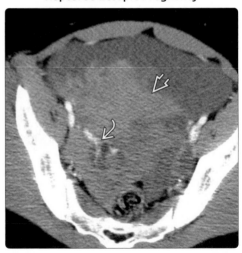

HELLP Syndrome

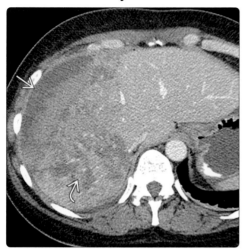

Ruptured Aneurysm

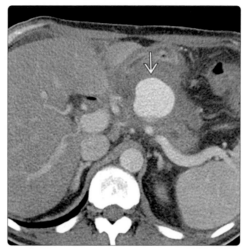

(Left) Axial CECT in a pregnant patient with HELLP syndrome demonstrates large subcapsular and perihepatic hemorrhage ➡. Note the areas of patchy hypodensity in the right hepatic lobe ➡, likely representing areas of infarction. (Right) Axial CECT demonstrates a large splenic artery aneurysm ➡ with surrounding blood as a result of rupture.

Neoplastic Hemorrhage

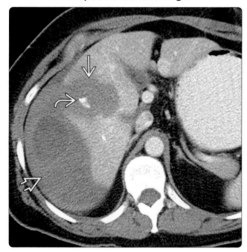

Neoplastic Hemorrhage

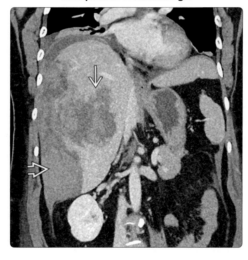

(Left) Axial CECT demonstrates a mass ➡ in the right hepatic lobe with internal active extravasation ➡ and contiguous perihepatic hematoma ➡, representing a bleeding hepatic adenoma. Adenoma and hepatocellular carcinoma are the most common liver tumors to present with bleeding. (Right) Coronal CECT demonstrates a hemorrhagic liver mass ➡ with directly contiguous perihepatic hematoma ➡. This was a young woman using oral contraceptives, and this tuned out to be a bleeding hepatic adenoma.

Neoplastic Hemorrhage

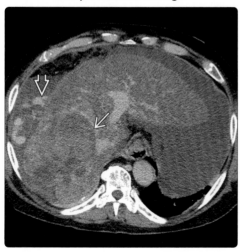

Neoplastic Hemorrhage

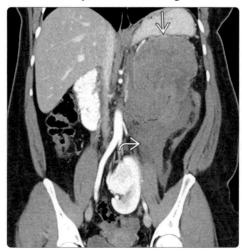

(Left) Axial CECT demonstrates large perihepatic hematoma with active extravasation ➡ secondary to rupture of a large hepatocellular carcinoma ➡ in the right hepatic lobe. (Right) Coronal CECT demonstrates a pancreatic mass ➡ with internal and surrounding hematoma ➡ tracking into the pelvis, found to be a solid pseudopapillary neoplasm (SPEN) in this young female patient.

DIFFERENTIAL DIAGNOSIS

Common

- Cirrhosis and Portal Hypertension
- Heart Failure
- Renal Failure
- Acute Pancreatitis
- Peritonitis
- Lymphoma
- Sclerosing Mesenteritis
- Acute Inflammatory Conditions of Gastrointestinal Tract
  - Diverticulitis
  - Crohn Disease
  - Ischemic Enteritis
- Postsurgical Mesenteric Infiltration
- Carcinoid Tumor

Less Common

- Mesenteric Hemorrhage
- Small Bowel Vasculitis
- Radiation Therapy
- Peritoneal Metastases and Mesothelioma
- Portomesenteric Venous Thrombosis
- Small Bowel Transplantation
- Intestinal Lymphangiectasia
- Leukemic or Lymphomatous Infiltration of Peritoneum
- Liposarcoma

ESSENTIAL INFORMATION

Key Differential Diagnosis Issues

- Misty mesentery represents increased attenuation of mesenteric fat as result of infiltration by edema (fluid), inflammation, blood, or tumor
  - Nonspecific finding with significance determined by clinical history, symptoms, and ancillary imaging findings
  - Routine follow-up for misty mesentery is **unnecessary** in absence of enlarged mesenteric lymph nodes (≥ 1 cm)
- 4 primary etiologic categories for misty mesentery depending on nature of mesenteric fat infiltration
  - **Edema**: Portal hypertension, heart failure, renal failure, hypoalbuminemia, congenital, postsurgical, radiation therapy, mesenteric vein thrombosis
  - **Inflammation**: Pancreatitis, diverticulitis, Crohn disease, sclerosing mesenteritis, peritonitis, vasculitis
  - **Hemorrhage**: Bowel or mesenteric trauma, anticoagulation, ischemic enteritis
  - **Neoplastic**: Lymphoma, leukemia, peritoneal metastases, mesothelioma

Helpful Clues for Common Diagnoses

- **Cirrhosis and Portal Hypertension**
  - Cirrhosis often results in portal hypertension and hypoproteinemia, both leading to mesenteric edema
  - Mesenteric edema becomes more conspicuous in setting of superimposed mesenteric venous thrombosis
- **Heart Failure**
  - Any form of cardiac dysfunction (e.g., CHF, constrictive pericarditis) may lead to generalized volume overload and edema (including mesenteric edema)
- **Renal Failure**

- Renal failure resulting in generalized volume overload and edema may cause mesenteric edema
- **Acute Pancreatitis**
  - Most common inflammatory cause of misty mesentery
  - Fluid and inflammation spread from inflamed pancreas both laterally (throughout anterior pararenal space) and ventrally/inferiorly (into leaves of small bowel mesentery and transverse mesocolon)
- **Peritonitis**
  - Inflammation of peritoneal lining may cause edema of adjacent mesenteric fat planes
  - Can result from either infectious (pyogenic, TB) or chemical (bile, peritoneal dialysis) peritonitis
- **Lymphoma**
  - Early Hodgkin or non-Hodgkin lymphoma can, in theory, manifest as only misty mesentery with mildly prominent mesenteric nodes
    - Nodes may rarely demonstrate fat-halo sign, leading to misdiagnosis as sclerosing mesenteritis
    - **Almost never** only manifestation of lymphoma, as there are typically legitimately enlarged nodes in mesentery or other lymph node stations
    - Studies have shown misty mesentery with normal-sized mesenteric lymph nodes (< 1 cm) carries **extremely** low risk of malignancy
  - Treated lymphoma (radiation or chemotherapy) may result in permanent infiltration of mesenteric fat planes (even though adenopathy may have resolved)
- **Sclerosing Mesenteritis**
  - Exact incidence is unknown but probably more common than conventionally thought
  - Misty mesentery with discrete borders (i.e., pseudocapsule measuring < 3 mm) and multiple prominent internal mesenteric lymph nodes
    - Classically, "halo" of spared fat with normal density surrounding both lymph nodes and vessels
    - Involved portions of mesentery may demonstrate slightly increased T2 signal on suppressed T2 MR
  - Should be diagnosis of exclusion once other causes of misty mesentery considered
- **Acute Inflammatory Conditions of Gastrointestinal Tract**
  - Any acute form of bowel inflammation will result in inflammation of adjacent mesentery with increased mesenteric attenuation
  - Increase in mesenteric attenuation tends to be localized near involved segment of bowel
  - Common inflammatory GI causes of mesenteric infiltration include diverticulitis, Crohn disease, appendicitis, and bowel ischemia
- **Postsurgical Mesenteric Infiltration**
  - Mild infiltration of mesentery is very common after abdominal surgeries (particularly surgeries of GI tract or mesentery), and this mesenteric infiltration may persist to mild degree long after surgery
- **Carcinoid Tumor**
  - May manifest as spiculated mesenteric mass [usually in right lower quadrant (RLQ)] with internal calcification
    - May result in distortion and narrowing of adjacent vasculature as well as tethering of small bowel loops (sometimes resulting in obstruction)

- May cause infiltration of RLQ mesentery due to tumor spread or lymphatic/venous obstruction
  - Tethered small bowel loops may be thickened as result of chronic venous/lymphatic obstruction
  - Primary tumor usually located in terminal ileum

Helpful Clues for Less Common Diagnoses

- **Mesenteric Hemorrhage**
  - Acute hemorrhage in mesentery results in high-density hematoma and infiltration of surrounding mesentery with blood products
  - Probably most common in setting of trauma with blood products seen as triangular collections of high-density blood between bowel loops
    - Though isolated mesenteric injury can occur, presence of mesenteric hemorrhage should prompt careful search for imaging evidence of bowel injury (i.e., bowel wall thickening, pneumoperitoneum)
  - Isolated mesenteric or intraperitoneal hemorrhage as result of coagulopathy is quite rare
    - Hemorrhage more often originates from retroperitoneum or abdominal wall musculature and tracks into peritoneal space
    - Largest amount of blood products found outside mesentery/peritoneum

- **Small Bowel Vasculitis**
  - Multiple types of vasculitis (Henoch-Schönlein, lupus, etc.) are categorized as small, medium, and large vessel
  - Can produce profound small bowel wall thickening and mucosal hyperenhancement, usually in conjunction with extensive mesenteric infiltration and hemorrhage
  - May be associated with vascular stigmata of vasculitis depending on size of vessels involved (e.g., arterial wall thickening, vascular "beading," or aneurysms)

- **Radiation Therapy**
  - Seen most in pelvic radiation for gynecologic (especially cervical cancer) or rectal malignancies
  - May cause permanent infiltration of pelvic fat planes/mesentery, often with thickening of pelvic small bowel (radiation enteritis), rectum (radiation proctitis), bladder (radiation cystitis)

- **Peritoneal Metastases and Mesothelioma**
  - Earliest signs of peritoneal malignancy may be subtle infiltration of mesentery and omentum, often with evidence of peritoneal thickening and enhancement
    - Infiltration of peritoneal fat may predate development of frank soft tissue tumor implants
  - Most common causes of peritoneal carcinomatosis are gynecologic and GI malignancies, whereas mesothelioma (very rare tumor) can appear virtually identical

- **Portomesenteric Venous Thrombosis**
  - Portal or superior mesenteric vein thrombosis can lead to mesenteric infiltration secondary to leaking of fluid from lymphatics or mesenteric hemorrhage
  - Mesenteric infiltration tends to be most conspicuous adjacent to thickened and inflamed loops of small bowel (due to venous ischemia)
  - Bowel ischemia related to venous thrombosis tends to result in particularly profound mesenteric infiltration (often with associated mesenteric hemorrhage)

- **Small Bowel Transplantation**
  - Mesenteric edema is often striking after small bowel transplant due to transection of lymphatics or rejection of transplanted bowel and its mesentery

- **Intestinal Lymphangiectasia**
  - Rare disorder that manifests as dilated lymphatics within small bowel villi, resulting in significant small bowel wall thickening, ascites, and mesenteric edema

- **Leukemic or Lymphomatous Infiltration of Peritoneum**
  - May mimic appearance of carcinomatosis with diffuse infiltration of peritoneal cavity, mass-like thickening of peritoneum, and ascites

- **Liposarcoma**
  - Primary peritoneal liposarcomas are rare, but large retroperitoneal liposarcomas can extend into peritoneum
  - Large liposarcoma could mimic appearance of sclerosing mesenteritis, as these tumors are encapsulated and demonstrate predominantly fat density with internal stranding and complexity

Cirrhosis and Portal Hypertension

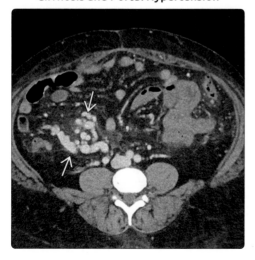

Cirrhosis and Portal Hypertension

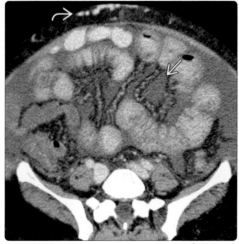

(Left) Axial CECT in a patient with cirrhosis and portal hypertension demonstrates a cluster of varices ➡ in the right aspect of the mesentery. Note the subtle, mild infiltration of the mesenteric fat throughout the abdomen, a common feature of portal hypertension. (Right) Axial CECT in a patient with cirrhosis and portal hypertension demonstrates mesenteric edema ➡, causing the mesenteric vessels and fat to stand out in contrast. Periumbilical varices ➡ and ascites are also present.

Acute Pancreatitis

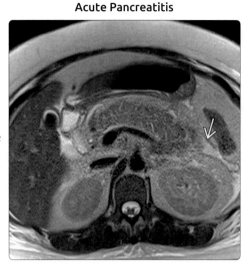

Acute Pancreatitis

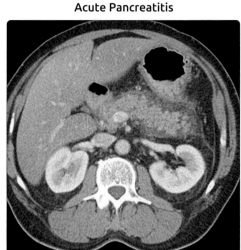

(Left) *Axial T2 MR in a patient with abdominal pain demonstrates mild pancreatic edema with peripancreatic fluid* ➡️ *tracking along the anterior pararenal space, compatible with acute pancreatitis.* (Right) *Axial CECT demonstrates an enlarged, edematous pancreas with peripancreatic free fluid and blurring of adjacent fat planes, consistent with acute pancreatitis.*

Peritonitis

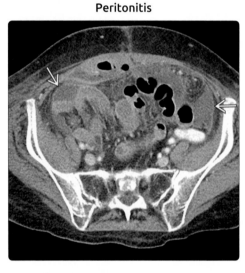

Sclerosing Mesenteritis

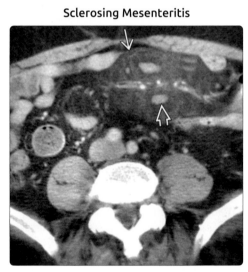

(Left) *Axial CECT in a patient with recent bowel perforation demonstrates diffuse peritonitis with mesenteric stranding and edema, diffuse peritoneal thickening and enhancement, and multiple pockets of small, loculated fluid* ➡️. (Right) *Axial CECT demonstrates infiltration of the small bowel mesentery, set off by a pseudocapsule* ➡️. *Multiple mildly enlarged mesenteric nodes are present* ➡️ *with a subtle surrounding "halo" of spared fat. These findings are classic for sclerosing mesenteritis.*

Sclerosing Mesenteritis

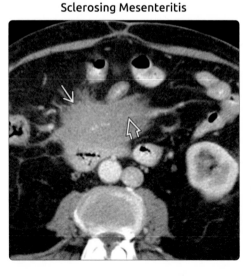

Diverticulitis

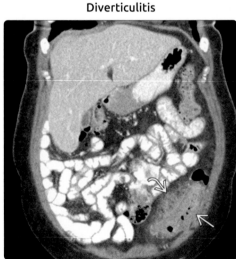

(Left) *Axial CECT shows extensive infiltration of the jejunal mesentery* ➡️ *with encasement of the mesenteric vessels* ➡️ *that results in bowel wall edema. These findings represent an advanced case of sclerosing mesenteritis.* (Right) *Coronal CECT demonstrates a markedly thickened, inflamed sigmoid colon* ➡️ *due to diverticulitis. Note the presence of stranding and infiltration* ➡️ *extending medially into the sigmoid mesocolon.*

Crohn Disease

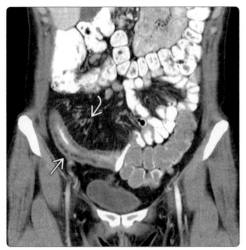

Crohn Disease

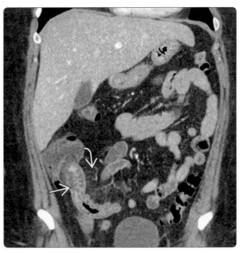

(Left) *Coronal CECT demonstrates a thickened terminal ileum ➡ with intramural fat deposition, fibrofatty proliferation in the ileocolic mesentery, and mild adjacent stranding and vasa recta engorgement ➡, representing mild Crohn ileitis superimposed on a chronic fibrostenotic stricture.* (Right) *Coronal CECT demonstrates thickening and submucosal edema of the distal ileum ➡, compatible with Crohn ileitis. There is mild infiltration ➡ of the adjacent right lower quadrant mesentery with fat stranding and inflammation.*

Ischemic Enteritis

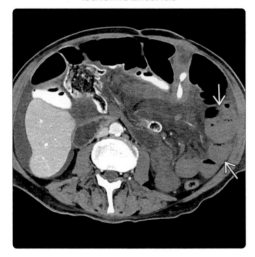

Ischemic Enteritis

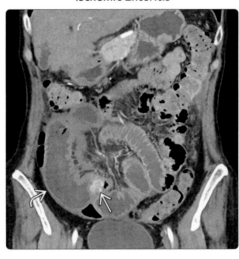

(Left) *Axial CECT demonstrates nonenhancing loops of dilated small bowel ➡ in the left upper quadrant due to bowel ischemia from an internal hernia. Notice the profound infiltration and fat stranding throughout the left upper quadrant mesentery.* (Right) *Coronal CECT demonstrates an enhancing carcinoid tumor ➡ in the small bowel, resulting in proximal bowel obstruction. The small bowel ➡ proximal to the mass is dilated, thickened, and hypoenhancing, compatible with ischemia.*

Carcinoid Tumor

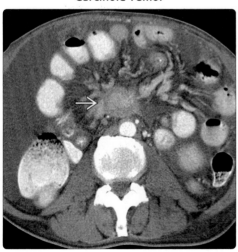

Mesenteric Hemorrhage

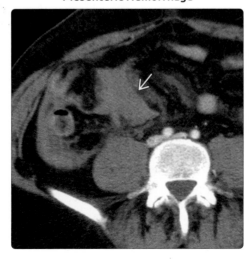

(Left) *Coronal CECT demonstrates an avidly enhancing mesenteric mass ➡, compatible with metastatic carcinoid tumor, resulting in tethering of multiple surrounding bowel loops. There is extensive surrounding infiltration of the mesentery and large ascites.* (Right) *Axial CECT demonstrates the characteristic appearance of a mesenteric injury after trauma with hematoma ➡ seen between loops of bowel in the mesentery.*

Mesenteric Hemorrhage

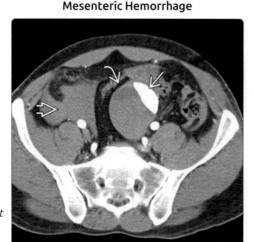

Small Bowel Vasculitis

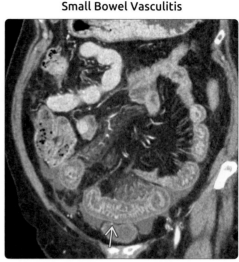

(Left) *Axial CECT in a trauma patient demonstrates mesenteric infiltration and hematoma ⮕, including a large hematoma ⮕ in the central pelvis with extensive internal active extravasation ⮕. Small bowel, colonic, and mesenteric injury were discovered at surgery.* (Right) *Coronal CECT demonstrates several markedly thickened and edematous small bowel loops ⮕ in the pelvis with adjacent mesenteric infiltration, found to represent small bowel vasculitis due to lupus.*

Radiation Therapy

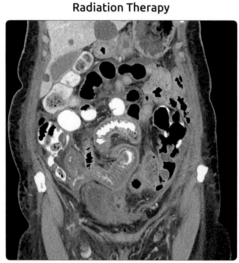

Radiation Therapy

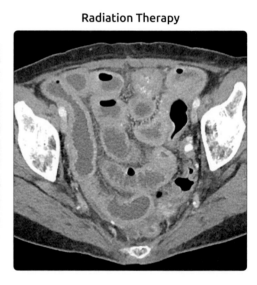

(Left) *Coronal CECT demonstrates multiple thick-walled loops of small bowel in the pelvis with submucosal edema as well as diffuse blurring of pelvic fat planes, reflecting radiation enteritis in a patient receiving treatment for cervical cancer.* (Right) *Axial CECT demonstrates multiple thick-walled, hyperenhancing loops of small bowel in the pelvis due to radiation enteritis in a patient receiving radiation therapy for a gynecologic malignancy.*

Peritoneal Metastases and Mesothelioma

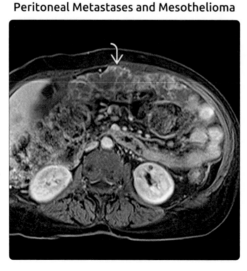

Peritoneal Metastases and Mesothelioma

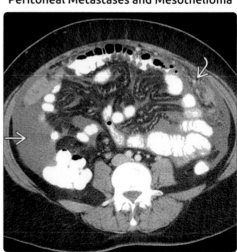

(Left) *Axial T1 C+ FS MR demonstrates extensive peritoneal carcinomatosis secondary to cholangiocarcinoma with confluent omental tumor and omental caking ⮕.* (Right) *Axial CECT demonstrates induration and thickening throughout the omentum ⮕ with associated peritoneal thickening and ascites ⮕, representing peritoneal tumor spread in a patient with primary peritoneal carcinoma.*

Peritoneal Metastases and Mesothelioma

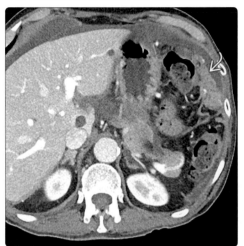

Portomesenteric Venous Thrombosis

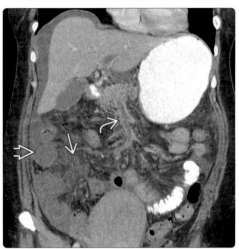

(Left) *Axial CECT shows ascites with tumor infiltration of the omentum* ➔, *caused by mesothelioma. Peritoneal carcinomatosis could have an identical appearance.* (Right) *Coronal CECT demonstrates acute thrombosis of the superior mesenteric vein* ➔ *(SMV) with resultant thickening and submucosal edema in the small bowel* ➔ *as well as extensive mesenteric stranding and ascites* ➔.

Portomesenteric Venous Thrombosis

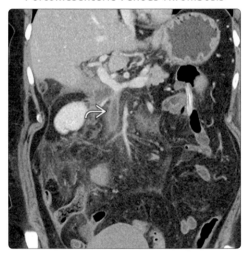

Small Bowel Transplantation

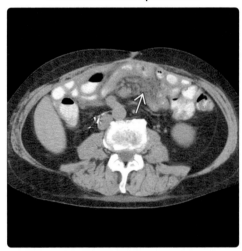

(Left) *Coronal CECT demonstrates thrombus within the SMV* ➔ *with resultant extensive infiltration of the central and right-sided mesentery.* (Right) *Axial CECT demonstrates extensive infiltration* ➔ *of the small bowel mesenteric allograft along with mural thickening of the bowel wall. Both findings are common and nonspecific in recipients of small bowel transplants and probably indicate some degree of rejection &/or lymphedema.*

Intestinal Lymphangiectasia

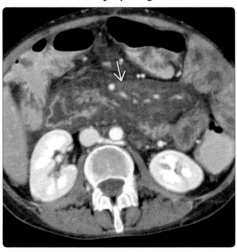

Intestinal Lymphangiectasia

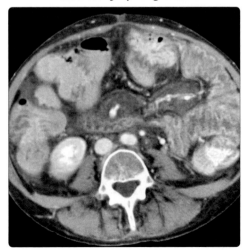

(Left) *Axial CECT shows extensive infiltration of the mesentery* ➔ *and small bowel wall thickening in a young woman with congenital lymphangiectasia of the small bowel.* (Right) *Axial CECT in the same patient once again demonstrates extensive infiltration of the mesentery with diffuse small bowel wall thickening and submucosal edema, classic imaging findings for this rare disorder.*

DIFFERENTIAL DIAGNOSIS

Common

- Hemoperitoneum
  o Traumatic Hemoperitoneum
  o Nontraumatic Causes of Hemoperitoneum
    – Gynecologic or Obstetric Sources
      □ Ruptured Ectopic Pregnancy
      □ Ruptured Ovarian Cyst
      □ Endometriosis
    – Coagulopathic Hemorrhage
      □ Retroperitoneal Hemorrhage
      □ HELLP Syndrome
  o Tumor Associated
  o Ruptured Aneurysm
  o Splenic Rupture
- Vicarious Excretion
- Bladder Trauma
- Perforation of GI Tract

Less Common

- Exudative Ascites
- Pseudomyxoma Peritonei

ESSENTIAL INFORMATION

Key Differential Diagnosis Issues

- Ascites (i.e., intraperitoneal fluid) typically shows water density (0-15 HU) and should be free flowing
  o Free-flowing ascites normally found in subphrenic spaces, Morison pouch, paracolic gutters, pouch of Douglas, and other dependent portions of abdomen
  o Most ascites is transudative (simple) with most common etiologies including liver, heart, or renal dysfunction
    – Transudative ascites almost always shows simple water density
  o Hemorrhage/hemoperitoneum shows higher attenuation on CT with unclotted blood measuring 30-45 HU and clotted blood measuring 45-70 HU
  o Simple fluid appears anechoic on US, while hemorrhage tends to demonstrate internal echoes

Helpful Clues for Common Diagnoses

- **Traumatic Hemoperitoneum**
  o Probably most common cause of hemorrhagic ascites with highest density blood products located near site of injury (sentinel clot sign)
    – Blood products further away from site of injury (lysed blood products) usually lower in attenuation
    – Look for evidence of active extravasation (with attenuation similar to blood pool), which can impact decision to undergo angiographic embolization or surgery
    – Hemorrhage may be slightly lower in attenuation than expected in patients with anemia or when hemorrhage is diluted by bile, urine, or bowel contents
  o Most common visceral traumatic injuries (in blunt trauma) causing hemoperitoneum are spleen > liver > bowel/mesentery
- **Nontraumatic Causes of Hemoperitoneum**
  o **Gynecologic or obstetric sources**
    – Hemoperitoneum in female of childbearing age (particularly when blood primarily localized in pelvis) should prompt correlation with β-HCG to exclude ruptured ectopic pregnancy
    – Other causes include ruptured ovarian hemorrhagic cyst, endometriosis or, rarely, torsion
      □ Ruptured hemorrhagic cyst, in particular, can result in large hemoperitoneum
  o **Coagulopathic hemorrhage**
    – Most often diagnosed in patients on heparin or Coumadin but also in hemophiliacs and patients with other forms of bleeding diathesis
    – Coagulopathic hemorrhage most often seen in iliopsoas compartment or rectus sheath but can occur anywhere and may extend into peritoneal cavity (but rarely limited to peritoneal cavity alone)
    – Coagulopathic hemorrhage has particular predisposition for hematocrit levels (fluid-hemorrhage level) as well as multiple sites of bleeding (out of proportion to any history of trauma)
    – HELLP syndrome: Peripartum complication of toxemia with possible manifestations including hemolysis, thrombocytopenia, hepatic infarction, hepatic rupture, and hemorrhage
  o **Tumor associated**
    – May complicate highly vascular visceral tumors with hepatic adenoma, hepatocellular carcinoma, angiosarcoma, and vascular metastases (renal cell, neuroendocrine, melanoma, choriocarcinoma) amongst tumors most often associated with bleeding
    – Hepatic tumors most likely to produce hepatic rupture with hemoperitoneum when located in subcapsular position
    – Metastases to solid organs can also rarely bleed, especially lung cancer, renal cell carcinoma, and melanoma
  o **Ruptured aneurysm**
    – Visceral artery aneurysms may rupture and produce intraperitoneal bleeding
      □ Splenic artery aneurysms are most common, particularly in female or pregnant patients
    – Aortic aneurysms produce retroperitoneal hemorrhage, which can rarely extend into peritoneum when particularly massive
  o **Splenic rupture**
    – Spleen can undergo spontaneous rupture, particularly when severely enlarged, usually due to splenic infection, infiltrative processes (such as amyloidosis or Gaucher disease), or neoplastic infiltration
    – Direct correlation between splenic size/weight and risk of rupture
    – Rupture may not be truly spontaneous, as even minor, unnoticed trauma may induce rupture when spleen is massively enlarged
- **Vicarious Excretion**
  o Increased attenuation of ascites fluid due to vicarious excretion occurs in > 50% of patients with ascites
    – Most conspicuous on scans performed > 10 minutes after intravascular administration of contrast material
    – Occurs regardless of etiology of ascites (benign or malignant)

- Smaller amounts of ascites typically exhibit greater degree of enhancement
- Mild increased attenuation of ascites seen in normal patients and does not necessarily denote renal dysfunction
- May occur more frequently and to greater extent in patients with renal impairment (and less effective renal excretion of contrast)

- **Bladder Trauma**
  - Intraperitoneal rupture of bladder or rupture of urine from ileal conduit or other postoperative bladder diversion can result in intraperitoneal ascites
    - Extravasated urine may be hyperdense when bladder instilled with contrast material (CT cystogram) or contrast excretion into bladder after IV injection

- **Perforation of GI Tract**
  - Can result in hyperdense ascites if enteric fluid contents are mixed with blood products or with oral (enteric) contrast medium

Helpful Clues for Less Common Diagnoses

- **Exudative Ascites**

- Any type of exudative ascites may exhibit slightly higher attenuation (> 15 HU) than simple fluid (but less than hemorrhage)
- Exudative ascites may be seen with variety of causes, including malignant ascites, infection, peritonitis, ischemia, pancreatitis, etc.
- Exudative ascites on US often shows complexity, including internal echoes and septations

- **Pseudomyxoma Peritonei**
  - Accumulation of gelatinous implants throughout abdomen as result of rupture of appendiceal mucinous neoplasm
  - Individual mucinous implants are slightly hyperdense to simple fluid and can result in scalloping of liver and spleen
  - Often associated with loculated ascites of similar density to mucinous implants (slightly hyperdense to simple fluid)

Traumatic Hemoperitoneum

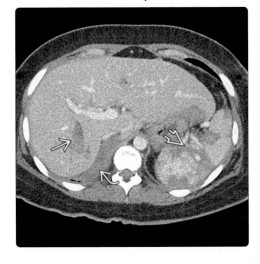

Traumatic Hemoperitoneum

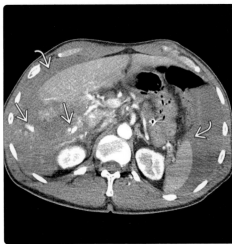

(Left) Axial CECT in a trauma patient shows hepatic ➡ and splenic ➡ lacerations with adjacent hemoperitoneum ➡. Spleen and liver injuries are the most common causes of traumatic hemoperitoneum. (Right) Axial CECT in a trauma patient shows a large laceration through the right liver with several sites of active extravasation ➡ and upper abdominal hemoperitoneum ➡. The highest density blood products are found adjacent to the liver injury (sentinel clot sign).

Traumatic Hemoperitoneum

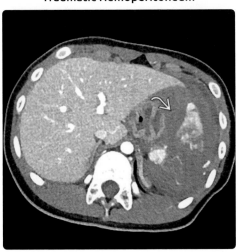

Traumatic Hemoperitoneum

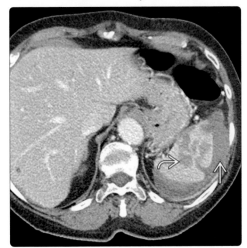

(Left) Axial CECT in a trauma patient shows a large hematoma ➡ surrounding the extensively lacerated spleen. (Right) Axial CECT shows extensive lacerations ➡ through the spleen with left upper quadrant perisplenic hematoma ➡.

(Left) *Coronal CECT in a young woman shows a hematoma in the right adnexa with additional blood tracking upward. The patient's β-HCG was negative, and US showed a ruptured hemorrhagic cyst to be the cause of the hemoperitoneum.* **(Right)** *US shows an adnexal hemorrhagic cyst with adjacent hemoperitoneum, compatible with a ruptured hemorrhagic cyst. Notably, the patient's β-HCG was negative, as a ruptured ectopic pregnancy could have a similar appearance.*

Ruptured Ovarian Cyst

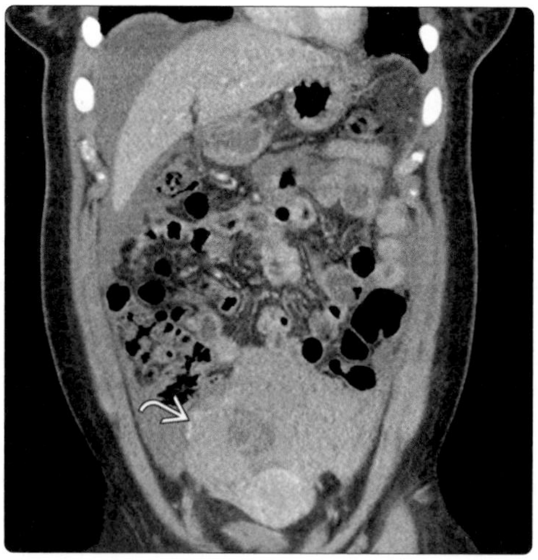

Ruptured Ovarian Cyst

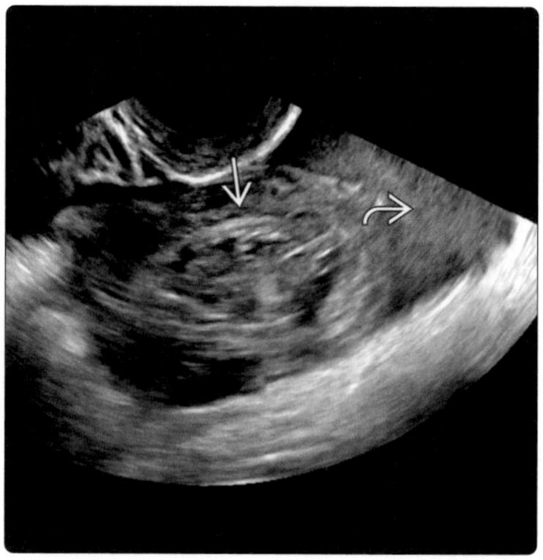

(Left) *Axial CECT shows hemoperitoneum with a sentinel clot surrounding a focus of ring-like enhancement in the pelvis. These findings were found to be secondary to a ruptured ectopic pregnancy.* **(Right)** *Axial CECT in an anticoagulated patient shows a large right-sided coagulopathic hemorrhage centered in the right psoas muscle and adjacent retroperitoneum with a large hematocrit level within the hematoma.*

Ruptured Ectopic Pregnancy

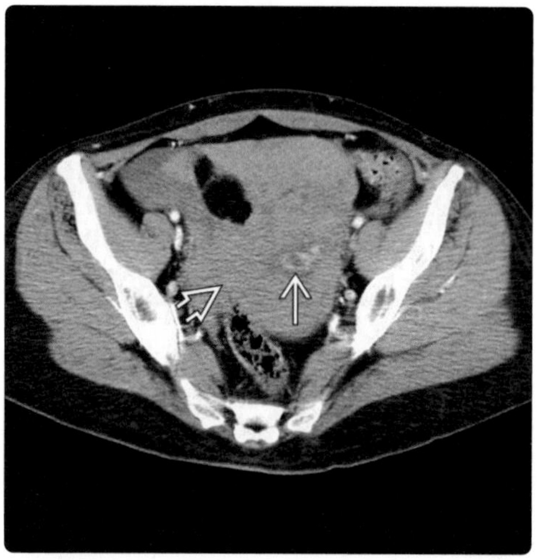

Coagulopathic Hemorrhage

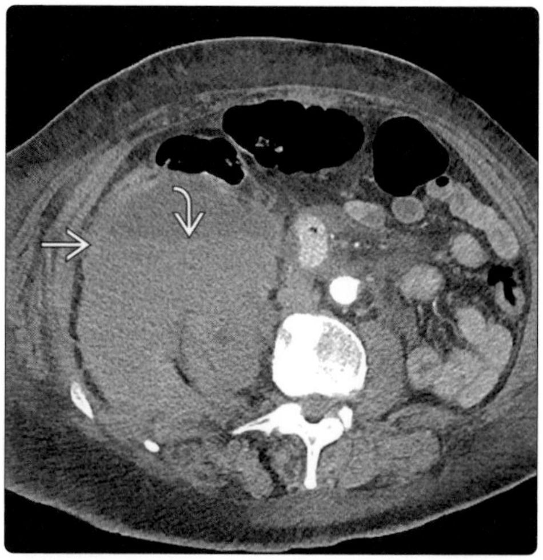

(Left) *Axial CECT in an anticoagulated patient shows right gluteal hematoma with internal hematocrit levels. Hematocrit levels are particularly common in the setting of coagulopathic bleeding.* **(Right)** *Axial CECT in a pregnant patient with HELLP syndrome shows areas of low-density infarction within the right hepatic lobe as well as a large mixed attenuation subcapsular hematoma along the margin of the right hepatic lobe.*

Coagulopathic Hemorrhage

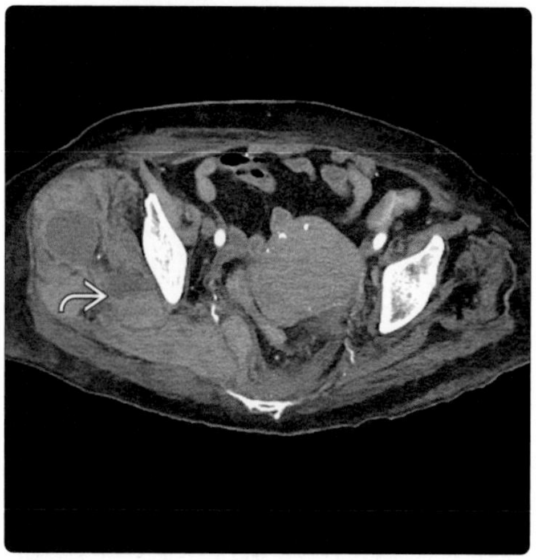

HELLP Syndrome

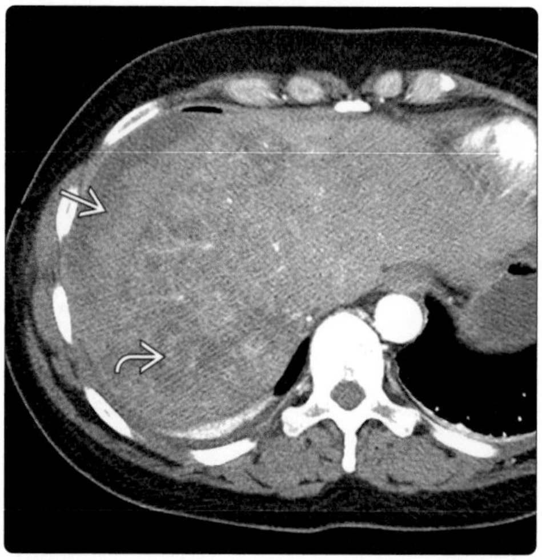

Tumor Associated

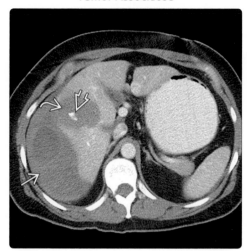

Tumor Associated

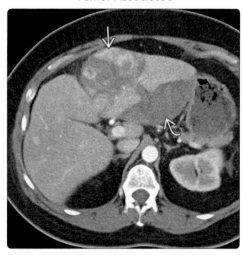

(Left) *Axial CECT shows a hemorrhagic mass* ➘ *in the right hepatic lobe with internal active extravasation* ➔. *The mass has ruptured through the liver capsule with hemorrhage tracking down the right subcapsular space* ➔. *This was found at resection to be a bleeding hepatic adenoma.* (Right) *Axial CECT shows an enhancing liver* ➔ *in the left hepatic lobe with rupture and subcapsular hematoma* ➔. *This was ultimately found to represent a bleeding hepatic adenoma at resection.*

Tumor Associated

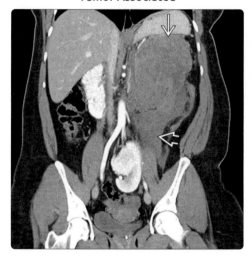

Ruptured Aneurysm

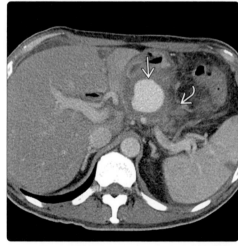

(Left) *Coronal CECT shows a large hemorrhagic mass* ➔ *in the pancreatic tail with hematoma tracking down into the left paracolic gutter and the mesentery* ➔. *These findings were found to be secondary to solid pseudopapillary neoplasm (SPEN) with rupture and hemorrhage.* (Right) *Axial CECT shows a large splenic artery aneurysm* ➔ *with ill-defined surrounding fat stranding and small hemorrhage* ➔, *representing early rupture.*

Bladder Trauma

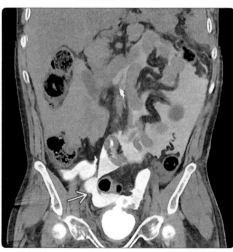

Duodenal Ulcer

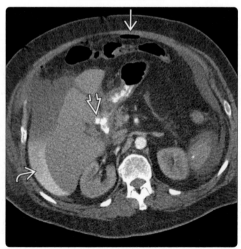

(Left) *Coronal cystogram in a trauma patient shows contrast* ➔ *surrounding bowel loops and extending up the paracolic gutters. These findings are compatible with intraperitoneal bladder rupture.* (Right) *Axial CECT shows free fluid in the upper abdomen, including hyperdense fluid* ➔ *due to extravasated enteric contrast, along with pneumoperitoneum* ➔. *These findings were secondary to a perforated ulcer with contrast directly extravasating from the duodenum* ➔.

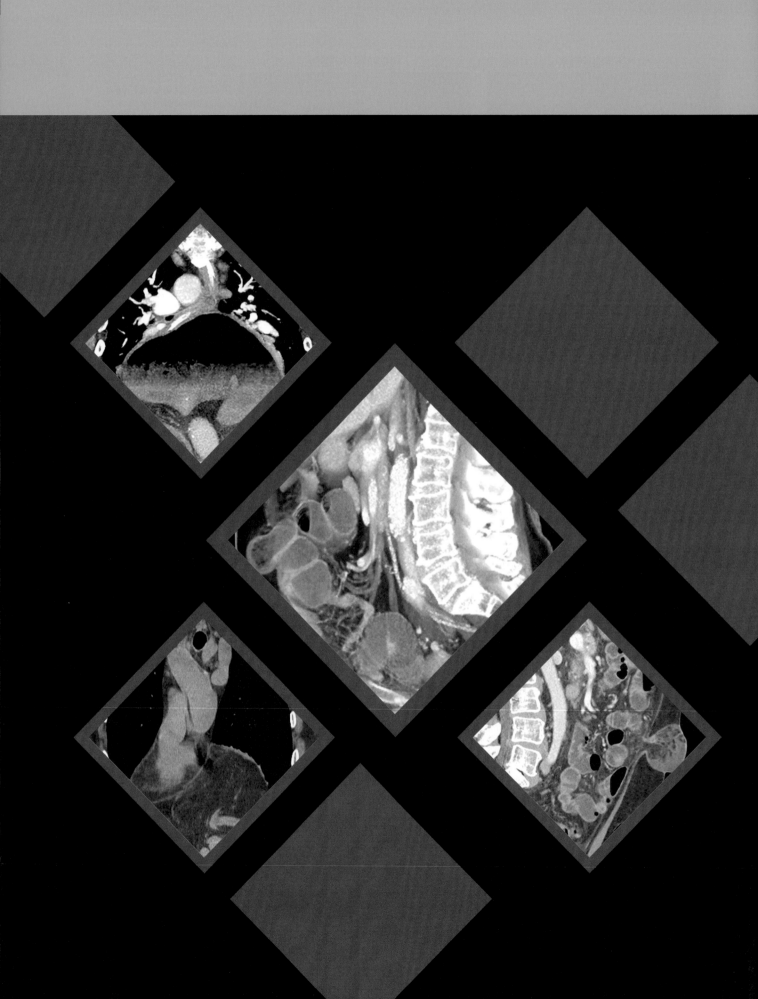

SECTION 2
Abdominal Wall

Anatomically Based Differentials

Abdominal Wall Mass	48
Mass in Iliopsoas Compartment	52
Groin Mass	54
Elevated or Deformed Hemidiaphragm	58
Defect in Abdominal Wall (Hernia)	60

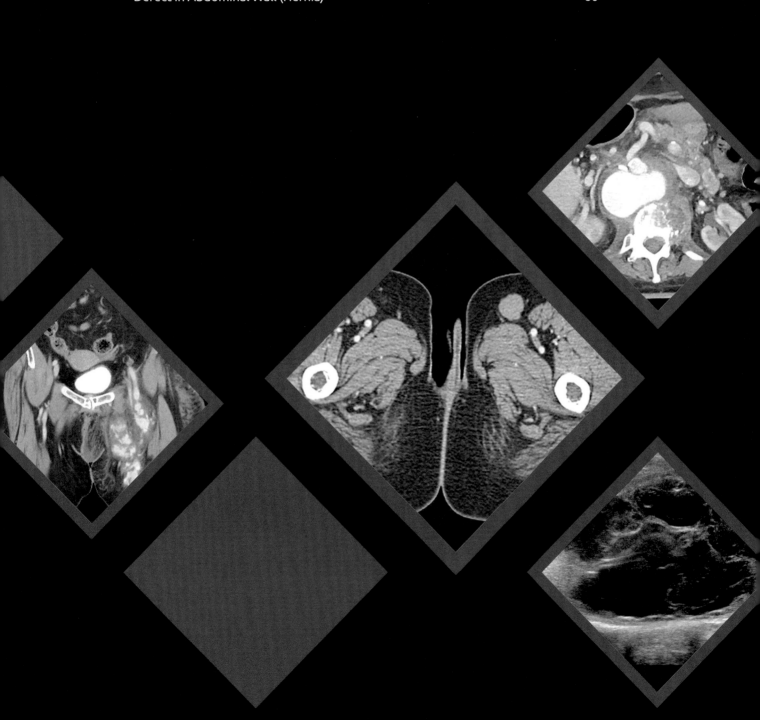

DIFFERENTIAL DIAGNOSIS

Common

- Abdominal Wall Hernias
  - Inguinal Hernia
  - Ventral Hernia
  - Umbilical Hernia
  - Spigelian Hernia
  - Femoral Hernia
  - Lumbar Hernia
- Abdominal Wall Abscess
- Sebaceous Cyst
- Lipoma
- Keloid
- Hematoma
- Paraumbilical Varices
- Injection Site
- Calcified Scar
- Muscle Asymmetry (Mimic)
- Melanoma

Less Common

- Endometriosis
- Calcinosis Syndromes
- Soft Tissue Metastases
- Lymphoma and Leukemia
- Desmoid
- Sarcoma
- Rhabdomyolysis
- Pancreatic Panniculitis
- Kaposi Sarcoma

ESSENTIAL INFORMATION

Key Differential Diagnosis Issues

- Given limitations of clinical examination, imaging plays important role in differentiating true soft tissue masses from hernias, vascular abnormalities, and normal variants
- Most soft tissue masses have nonspecific appearance and may require biopsy or excision for diagnosis

Helpful Clues for Common Diagnoses

- Abdominal Wall Hernias
  - Inguinal hernia
    - Most common external hernia, which extends into groin anterior to horizontal plane of pubic tubercle
    - Divided into direct (arises anteromedial to inferior epigastric vessels) and indirect (arises superolateral to inferior epigastric vessels) subtypes
  - Ventral hernia
    - Broad term describing acquired or congenital hernias through anterior and lateral abdominal wall
    - Midline hernias include epigastric (above umbilicus) and hypogastric (below umbilicus) hernias
    - Incisional hernias occur at prior surgical incision sites
  - Umbilical hernia
    - Hernias arising at midline in upper 1/2 of umbilical ring, which can be congenital or acquired
  - Spigelian hernia
    - Hernia through defect lateral to rectus sheath (inferior and lateral to umbilicus) often covered by external oblique muscle and aponeurosis
  - Femoral hernia
    - Groin hernia extending medial to femoral vessels with frequent compression of femoral vein
  - Lumbar hernia
    - Hernia through defect in lumbar muscle or thoracolumbar fascia
    - Can be congenital or acquired with many acquired due to incisions in flank region for renal surgery
- Abdominal Wall Abscess
  - Loculated fluid collection (± internal gas) with peripheral enhancement and surrounding edema/fat stranding
  - Presence of gas-containing abdominal wall abscess in close contiguity with bowel tethered to abdominal wall raises possibility of enterocutaneous fistula
- Sebaceous Cyst
  - Common incidental finding, appearing as small, round/oval, well-encapsulated cyst near skin surface
  - Should be low density and nonenhancing without surrounding subcutaneous edema/fat stranding
- Lipoma
  - Common incidental mass in subcutaneous tissues and between muscle planes, demonstrating uniform fat density with no internal soft tissue component
  - Differentiate from liposarcoma, which demonstrates internal complexity and soft tissue component
  - Confident diagnosis may be difficult on US, but mass should have similar echogenicity to subcutaneous fat
- Keloid
  - Benign fibrotic scar tissue or tissue overgrowth at site of soft tissue injury (i.e., surgical incision or trauma)
  - Usually asymptomatic but can be painful or pruritic
  - No clear imaging features to allow differentiation of large keloid from other soft tissue masses
- Hematoma
  - Heterogeneous, high-density blood products, which gradually evolve and become lower in density over time
  - More diffuse subcutaneous blood products may reflect subcutaneous ecchymosis
- Paraumbilical Varices
  - Common portosystemic collaterals in patients with severe cirrhosis and portal hypertension
  - Serpiginous enhancing structures that connect to recanalized paraumbilical vein near falciform ligament
  - May be visible/palpable at skin (i.e., caput medusae)
- Injection Site
  - Common incidental finding usually secondary to injection of heparin, insulin, or other medications
  - Small nodular foci with ectopic gas, blood, or fluid
  - May chronically evolve into injection granulomas, appearing as rounded or linear foci of soft tissue or calcification (most common in buttocks)
- Calcified Scar
  - Heterotopic ossification (myositis ossificans traumatica) can occur at abdominal incision sites and is most common in linea alba after midline abdominal incision
- Muscle Asymmetry (Mimic)
  - May be mistaken for mass and are common secondary to prior surgery, paralysis, myopathy, etc.

- **Melanoma**
  - 5th most common new cancer in US, but imaging typically not utilized for diagnosis of primary tumor
  - Most commonly multiple small subcutaneous nodules, although rarely presents as solitary abdominal wall mass
  - Homogeneous enhancement ± hyperintense on T1 MR

Helpful Clues for Less Common Diagnoses

- **Endometriosis**
  - Endometriosis implants may be seen within incision sites after prior C-section or hysterectomy
  - Typically appears as solid, spiculated subcutaneous mass with variable enhancement (usually hypointense on T1 and hyperintense on T2 MR)
  - May be associated with clinical history of cyclical pain (corresponding with menstruation) at incision site
- **Calcinosis Syndromes**
  - Dystrophic: Calcifications may be due to tissue injury response, such as implanted medical device, connective tissue diseases (scleroderma, dermatomyositis, CREST), severe pancreatitis, or fat necrosis
  - Metastatic: Most often in patients with calcium-phosphate imbalance (renal failure, milk-alkali syndrome)
  - Tumoral calcification: Large globular deposits of calcification near joints
- **Soft Tissue Metastases**
  - Most common malignancies to metastasize to soft tissues are melanoma and renal cell carcinoma
  - Soft tissue nodule or mass(es) in subcutaneous fat or muscle with enhancement similar to primary tumor
  - Tumor may also be implanted at site of surgery (probably more common with laparoscopic surgery) or biopsy
    - Surgical seeding can also occur with benign lesions, including uterine fibroids and ectopic splenic tissue
- **Lymphoma and Leukemia**
  - Cutaneous T-cell lymphoma (a.k.a. mycosis fungoides or Sézary syndrome)
    - Skin 2nd most common site of extranodal lymphoma (after GI tract)
    - Skin involvement may be difficult to appreciate on imaging unless unusually nodular or mass-like

  - Subcutaneous panniculitis-like T-cell lymphoma
    - Manifests as site of soft tissue induration/infiltration or as discrete nodules
  - Leukemia cutis (i.e., chloroma or granulocytic sarcoma)
  - Primary B-cell cutaneous lymphomas more likely to present as solitary isolated skin lesion
- **Desmoid**
  - Benign locally aggressive neoplasm, which can be intraabdominal or extraabdominal (e.g., abdominal wall)
  - Abdominal wall lesions most frequently arise from rectus or oblique muscles, especially at incision sites
  - Major risk factors include prior surgery, trauma, Gardner syndrome, and familial adenomatous polyposis
  - Variable appearance but typically solid, well-defined, hypoenhancing, heterogeneously high signal on T2 and low signal on T1 MR
- **Sarcoma**
  - Malignant mesenchymal soft tissue tumors, which encompass wide range of different histologic subtypes
  - May be difficult to differentiate from other soft tissue masses based on imaging alone, although most sarcomas tend to be larger and more heterogeneous with frequent necrosis (± distant metastatic disease)
- **Rhabdomyolysis**
  - Muscle necrosis in response to wide variety of causes, including crush injury, seizures, statin medications, etc.
  - Involved muscles on CT generally appear either normal or abnormally hypodense (due to edema)
  - MR more sensitive, with muscles demonstrating T2 hyperintensity and enlargement, as well as hyperenhancement (can appear ring-like or mass-like)
- **Pancreatic Panniculitis**
  - Subcutaneous fat necrosis seen with pancreatitis and pancreatic adenocarcinoma (due to ↑ serum lipase)
  - Manifest as small nodular foci of predominantly fat density on CT and hyperechoic on US
- **Kaposi Sarcoma**
  - Most common AID-related vascular neoplasm in Western world, presenting as either diffuse infiltration of skin or discrete subcutaneous nodules

Abdominal Wall Hernias

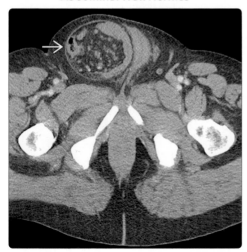

Sebaceous Cyst

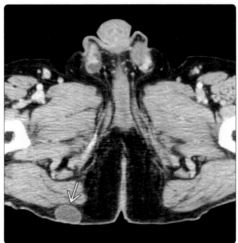

(Left) *Axial CECT shows a right inguinal hernia ➡ containing loops of nonobstructed small bowel.* **(Right)** *Axial CECT shows an encapsulated, near water density mass ➡ in the left buttock. Sebaceous cysts are a common incidental finding and, when demonstrating a classic appearance, do not require further follow-up or evaluation.*

Abdominal Wall Mass

Lipoma

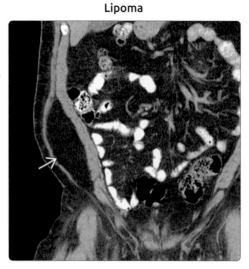

Hematoma

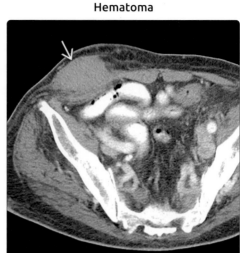

(Left) *Coronal CECT shows a large, fat-containing mass* ➡ *within the right lateral abdominal wall, compatible with a simple lipoma. Note the absence of any complexity or soft tissue component within the mass.* (Right) *Axial CECT shows an acute, high-density subcutaneous hematoma* ➡ *in a patient with recent trauma.*

Hematoma

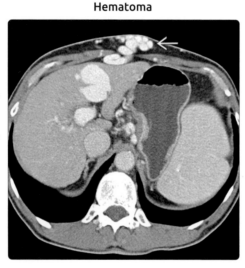

Paraumbilical Varices

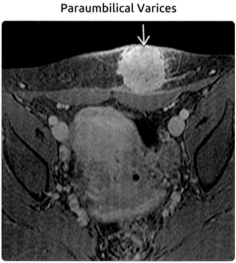

(Left) *Axial CECT in a patient with cirrhosis and portal hypertension shows subcutaneous varices* ➡ *overlying the anterior abdominal wall, representing a caput medusae.* (Right) *Axial T1 C+ MR shows an enhancing mass* ➡ *in the left anterior pelvic wall, found to represent a scar endometrioma in this patient status post prior laparoscopic pelvic surgery.*

Endometriosis

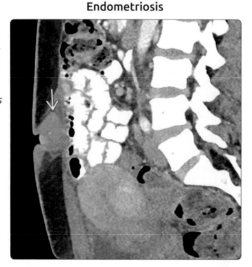

Soft Tissue Metastases

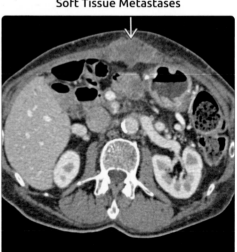

(Left) *Sagittal CECT shows a soft tissue mass* ➡ *intimately associated with the umbilicus, ultimately found at biopsy to represent endometriosis.* (Right) *Axial CECT shows a hypodense mass* ➡ *in the midline anterior abdominal wall, proven to represent a metastasis from the patient's known primary colon cancer.*

Soft Tissue Metastases

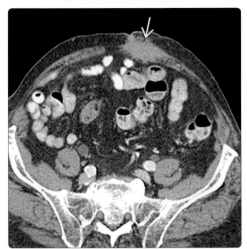

Lymphoma and Leukemia

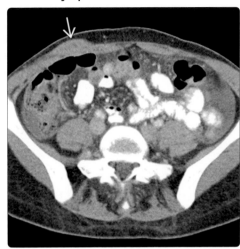

(Left) *Axial CECT shows a hypodense mass ➡ in the abdominal wall musculature, representing a metastasis from the patient's known colon cancer.* **(Right)** *Axial CECT shows a biopsy-proven chloroma ➡ in the right anterior abdominal wall in a patient with known leukemia.*

Desmoid

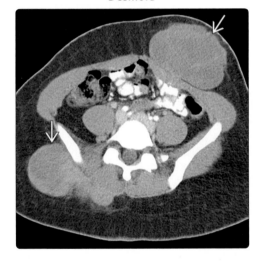

Desmoid

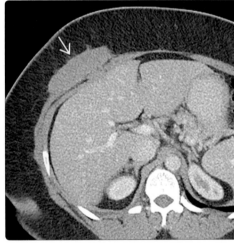

(Left) *Axial CECT shows multiple large, hypodense masses ➡ in the pelvic subcutaneous soft tissues in a patient with known familial polyposis, representing desmoid tumors.* **(Right)** *Axial CECT shows a hypodense mass ➡ in the right anterior abdominal wall, ultimately found to represent a desmoid tumor.*

Sarcoma

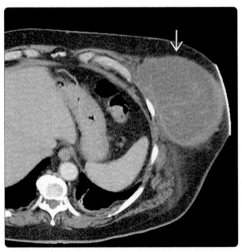

Sarcoma

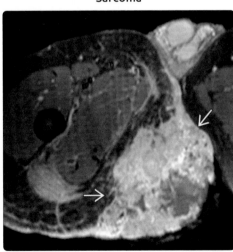

(Left) *Axial CECT shows a large, rapidly growing mass ➡ in the left anterior abdominal wall, representing a primary soft tissue sarcoma (malignant fibrous histiocytoma).* **(Right)** *Axial T1 C+ FS MR shows a highly invasive, large tumor in the buttock ➡, which enhances significantly. This lesion proved on biopsy to be a high-grade epithelioid sarcoma.*

DIFFERENTIAL DIAGNOSIS

Common
- Iliopsoas Hematoma
- Asymmetric Musculature (Mimic)
- Secondary Infection/Abscess

Less Common
- Retroperitoneal Fibrosis
- Primary Infection
- Primary Neoplasm
- Secondary Neoplasm

ESSENTIAL INFORMATION

Key Differential Diagnosis Issues
- Iliopsoas compartment masses are much more likely to result from infection or hemorrhage than from tumor
- Iliopsoas pathology often due to spread from adjacent infection (such as spine) or adjacent tumor, rather than originating within iliopsoas itself

Helpful Clues for Common Diagnoses
- **Iliopsoas Hematoma**
  - Iliopsoas is most common site for spontaneous retroperitoneal hemorrhage (usually due to bleeding diathesis or anticoagulation)
    - Presence of multiple hematocrit levels within hematoma suggests coagulopathic hemorrhage
  - Other causes include surgery, trauma, or extension of bleeding from adjacent structures (e.g., bleeding renal AML, ruptured abdominal aortic aneurysm, etc.)
  - Appearance variable depending on age of hematoma
    - Acute bleeding may simply appear as homogeneous enlargement of muscle ± hematocrit levels
    - Chronic bleeds may appear hypodense and can be difficult to differentiate from abscess
- **Asymmetric Musculature (Mimic)**
  - Iliopsoas muscles can be asymmetric in size, particularly in patients with unilateral leg amputation, paralysis, or lower extremity/spine arthritis

- **Secondary Infection/Abscess**
  - Infection and abscess formation in iliopsoas typically due to spread of infection from contiguous structures
    - Most commonly infectious spread from bone, kidney, and bowel (including appendix)
      - Paraspinal psoas abscess should prompt careful search for infectious spondylitis (TB or pyogenic)
      - Renal sources of iliopsoas infection include renal/perirenal abscess or xanthogranulomatous pyelonephritis
      - Common bowel sources of iliopsoas infection include appendicitis, diverticulitis, or Crohn disease
    - Often associated with other features of infection (fat stranding, blurring of fat planes, ectopic gas)

Helpful Clues for Less Common Diagnoses
- **Retroperitoneal Fibrosis**
  - Irregular soft tissue mass enveloping aorta, inferior vena cava, and ureters, which can involve adjacent psoas muscles
  - Variable enhancement depending on stage with hyperenhancement in early stages of disease and hypoenhancement in later stages
- **Primary Infection**
  - Iliopsoas compartment is rarely primary site of infection, except in immunocompromised patients (including HIV) and intravenous drug abusers
    - Infection usually due to *Staphylococcus aureus* and mixed gram-negative organisms
- **Primary Neoplasm**
  - Primary mesenchymal tumors (liposarcoma, fibrosarcoma, leiomyosarcoma, hemangiopericytoma, etc.) may rarely originate from iliopsoas compartment
- **Secondary Neoplasm**
  - Hematogenous metastasis (e.g., lymphoma, melanoma) to iliopsoas very rare
  - More commonly directly invaded by adjacent tumors (e.g., retroperitoneal sarcoma, lymphoma, neurogenic tumors, adjacent bone tumor, etc.)
  - Plexiform neurofibroma (in neurofibromatosis) may involve psoas compartment

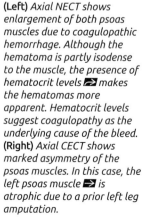

(Left) *Axial NECT shows enlargement of both psoas muscles due to coagulopathic hemorrhage. Although the hematoma is partly isodense to the muscle, the presence of hematocrit levels* ⇗ *makes the hematomas more apparent. Hematocrit levels suggest coagulopathy as the underlying cause of the bleed.* (Right) *Axial CECT shows marked asymmetry of the psoas muscles. In this case, the left psoas muscle* ⇥ *is atrophic due to a prior left leg amputation.*

Iliopsoas Hematoma

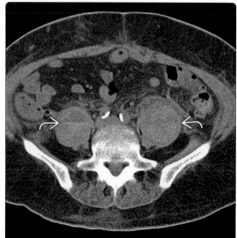

Asymmetric Musculature (Mimic)

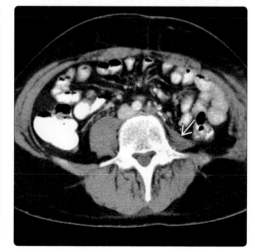

Secondary Infection/Abscess

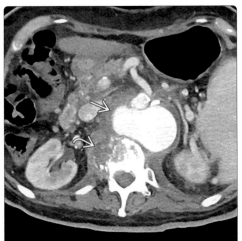

Secondary Infection/Abscess

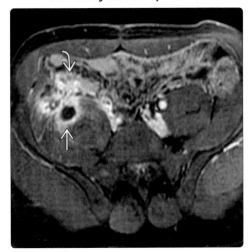

(Left) *Axial CECT shows lytic destruction of a vertebral body with an abscess ➡ extending into the right psoas muscle. Note the presence of a large mycotic aneurysm ➡ immediately anteriorly arising from the abdominal aorta.* **(Right)** *Axial T1 C+ MR shows an abscess ➡ in the iliopsoas muscle directly contiguous with phlegmonous change ➡ in the right lower quadrant due to the patient's fistulizing Crohn disease.*

Retroperitoneal Fibrosis

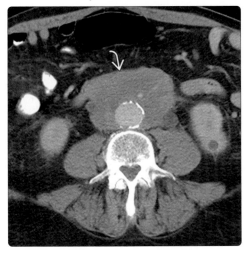

Primary Neoplasm

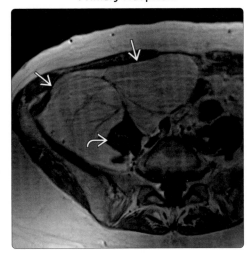

(Left) *Axial CECT shows a rind of mass-like soft tissue ➡ encasing the aorta and inferior vena cava. While more mass-like than is typical, this was found to represent retroperitoneal fibrosis.* **(Right)** *Axial T1 MR shows a large, fat-containing mass ➡ occupying much of the right hemipelvis, with the right left psoas muscle ➡ appearing stretched and distorted as a result of the retroperitoneal tumor. This was found to be a well-differentiated liposarcoma at resection.*

Secondary Neoplasm

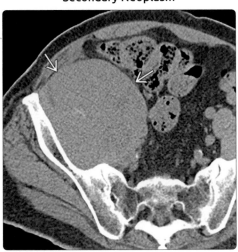

Secondary Neoplasm

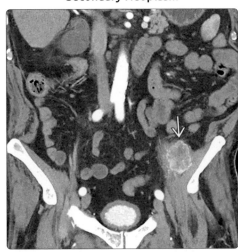

(Left) *Axial CECT shows a large, homogeneous soft tissue mass ➡ involving the right psoas and iliopsoas musculature. There were multiple enlarged lymph nodes elsewhere (not shown), and this was found to represent non-Hodgkin lymphoma.* **(Right)** *Coronal CECT shows an avidly enhancing mass ➡ with central necrosis arising in the left iliopsoas muscle, representing a metastasis related to the patient's known renal cell carcinoma.*

DIFFERENTIAL DIAGNOSIS

Common

- Inguinal Hernia
- Femoral Hernia
- Groin Hematoma
- Groin Pseudoaneurysm
- Groin Arteriovenous Fistula
- Inguinal Lymphadenopathy
- Varicocele
- Spermatic Cord Lipoma
- Mesh Hernia Repair (Mimic)

Less Common

- Cryptorchidism
- Groin Aneurysm
- Iliopsoas Bursitis
- Bone Tumor
- Inguinal Abscess

Rare but Important

- Canal of Nuck Hydrocele
- Inguinal Canal Endometriosis
- Liposarcoma
- Metastases to Inguinal Canal

ESSENTIAL INFORMATION

Key Differential Diagnosis Issues

- Although clinical exam may diagnose many common groin masses (particularly hernias), imaging often necessary for accurate diagnosis, particularly with atypical masses
  - US 1st-line modality for vascular and male reproductive (e.g., cryptorchidism, varicocele) abnormalities
  - CT and US are best options for diagnosis of groin hernias
    - US offers advantage of being able to image patients in different positions (such as standing) or during Valsalva to increase chance of visualizing hernias
  - CT or MR appropriate for suspected musculoskeletal lesions, such as bursitis or bone tumor

Helpful Clues for Common Diagnoses

- **Inguinal Hernia**
  - Divided into **direct** or **indirect** subtypes based on relationship to inferior epigastric vessels
    - Direct hernias arising anteromedial to inferior epigastric vessels
    - Indirect hernias arising superolateral to inferior epigastric vessels
  - Typically located anterior to horizontal plane of pubic tubercle with no significant mass effect on femoral vein
  - Hernia sac can contain omental fat, bowel, bladder, appendix, and other pelvic structures
  - Usually diagnosed on clinical exam, but diagnosis easily confirmed on both CT and US
- **Femoral Hernia**
  - Almost always diagnosed in older women
  - Extends medial to femoral vein and inferior to inferior epigastric vessels with mass effect on femoral vessels
  - Hernia sac located posterior and lateral to pubic tubercle
  - Highest strangulation rate among groin hernias (25-40%)
- **Groin Hematoma**

- Most often encountered after groin catheterization and should prompt search for underlying pseudoaneurysm or active extravasation, though also commonly seen in setting of inguinal or scrotal surgery and anticoagulation
  - May demonstrate active extravasation on CECT in setting of active bleeding
- **Groin Pseudoaneurysm**
  - Most often encountered after groin catheterization (3% of cases following cardiac catheterization)
  - US demonstrates cystic structure connecting to femoral artery with internal yin-yang biphasic flow
  - Often treated with compression or thrombin injection
- **Groin Arteriovenous Fistula**
  - Abnormal communication between artery and vein, which is most often iatrogenic and related to groin catheterization
  - Direct communication between femoral artery and vein may not be readily visible on US, but secondary findings can help make diagnosis (increased diastolic flow in artery, arterialized flow in vein, turbulent flow with soft tissue color bruit artifact)
- **Inguinal Lymphadenopathy**
  - Inguinal regions are common site of lymphadenopathy in many malignancies and systemic disease
  - Lymph nodes are usually mobile and easily distinguished from hernia based on clinical exam alone, although imaging can easily make distinction in difficult cases
- **Varicocele**
  - Can extend into inguinal canal (as can hydrocele) and may be thought to represent mass on clinical exam
  - US demonstrates tangle of mildly dilated vessels (≥ 3 mm) with slow flow and enlargement during Valsalva
  - May be seen on CT with tangle of dilated vessels, which communicate with dilated ipsilateral gonadal vein
  - Most often found on left side, as isolated right-sided varicocele should raise concern for obstructing mass in abdominal or pelvic cavity
- **Spermatic Cord Lipoma**
  - Can clinically mimic hernia without true hernia being present and frequently mistaken for inguinal hernia on CT/MR
  - Extremely common incidental finding at surgery (seen in 20-70% of all inguinal hernia repairs)
  - Fat-containing lesion in inguinal canal **without** any true connection to intraperitoneal fat, though differentiating spermatic cord lipoma from small inguinal hernia on any imaging modality can be extremely difficult to do with accuracy
- **Mesh Hernia Repair (Mimic)**
  - Mesh plugs used during inguinal hernia repair can appear focal and mass-like and potentially mimic lymph node or other mass
  - Ipsilateral spermatic cord often thickened as well due to surgical manipulation

Helpful Clues for Less Common Diagnoses

- **Cryptorchidism**
  - Common congenital anomaly found in up to 4% of term male babies, which can be associated with increased risk of infertility and malignancy later in life

- ○ Undescended testicle (usually are found in vicinity of groin/inguinal canal) can be palpated on physical exam in vast majority of cases
- ○ US or MR are 1st-line imaging modalities with MR offering ability to identify intraabdominal testicle
- **Groin Aneurysm**
  - ○ True atherosclerotic aneurysms of common femoral artery are rare and often associated with aneurysms elsewhere (especially aorta and popliteal arteries)
- **Iliopsoas Bursitis**
  - ○ Focal, teardrop-shaped collection of fluid immediately anterior to hip joint typically associated with hip joint pathology (such as degeneration, infection, etc.)
- **Bone Tumor**
  - ○ Any benign or malignant primary bone tumor arising from pubic rami or hip can present as groin mass with CT and MR best initial modalities for evaluation
- **Inguinal Abscess**
  - ○ Focal, rim-enhancing fluid collection with surrounding stranding and edema in patient with clinical signs and symptoms of infection

Helpful Clues for Rare Diagnoses

- **Canal of Nuck Hydrocele**
  - ○ Extremely rare condition caused by congenital incomplete obliteration of canal of Nuck (fold of parietal peritoneum that extends into inguinal canal and toward labia majora)
  - ○ Typically diagnosed in female children (and extremely rarely in female adults) as painless, fluctuant swelling in groin
  - ○ Unilocular cystic mass in groin extending along inguinal canal toward labia (without any solid or soft tissue component and usually simple in appearance)
- **Inguinal Canal Endometriosis**
  - ○ Endometriosis can rarely extend into inguinal canal (usually on right)
  - ○ Imaging appearance akin to endometriosis elsewhere with pain groin mass varying with menstrual cycle
  - ○ Incomplete closure of canal of Nuck may provide pathway for endometriosis to extend into groin

- **Liposarcoma**
  - ○ Fat-containing mass typically with solid, soft tissue components, septations, and other complexity (and with variable amounts of internal fat depending of degree of differentiation)
  - ○ Primary spermatic cord liposarcomas arise below superficial ring without extension superiorly into peritoneum
    - – Other primary sarcomas of spermatic cord (leiomyosarcoma, rhabdomyosarcoma, etc.) are also possible but far less common
  - ○ Retroperitoneal liposarcomas with secondary extension downward into inguinal canal are much less common but can clinically mimic groin hernia
- **Metastases to Inguinal Canal**
  - ○ Metastases to inguinal canal are extraordinary rare, but most common with prostate cancer, pancreatic cancer, melanoma, rhabdomyosarcoma, and pseudomyxoma peritonei

SELECTED REFERENCES

1. Piga E et al: Imaging modalities for inguinal hernia diagnosis: a systematic review. Hernia. 24(5):917-26, 2020
2. Thomas AK et al: Canal of Nuck abnormalities. J Ultrasound Med. 39(2):385-95, 2020
3. Yang DM et al: Groin abnormalities: ultrasonographic and clinical findings. Ultrasonography. 39(2):166-77, 2020

Inguinal Hernia

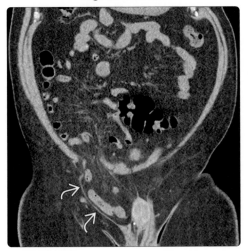

Femoral Hernia

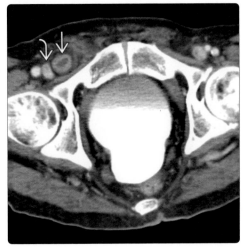

(Left) *Coronal NECT shows a large right inguinal hernia ➡ containing loops of small bowel without evidence of obstruction. In most cases, inguinal hernias can be palpated and diagnosed clinically.* **(Right)** *Axial CECT shows the characteristic position of a femoral hernia with a knuckle of bowel ➡ identified medial to the femoral vessels. Note the characteristic compression of the adjacent femoral vein ➡.*

Groin Hematoma

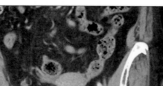

(Left) *Coronal CECT shows a large right groin hematoma with massive active extravasation of contrast ➡. This patient had recently undergone a complicated right groin catheterization with subsequent severe blood loss.*
(Right) *Longitudinal US in a patient with groin swelling after catheterization shows a large, complex hematoma ➡ with internal echoes and mixed echogenicity.*

Groin Hematoma

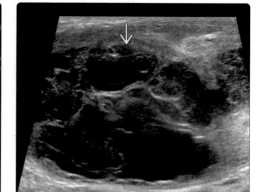

Groin Pseudoaneurysm

(Left) *Color Doppler US in a patient who had undergone recent groin catheterization shows the characteristic features of a pseudoaneurysm ➡ with a yin-yang pattern of internal color flow. Note that the pseudoaneurysm does appear to connect with the adjacent femoral artery ➡.*
(Right) *Axial CECT in a patient with a history of IV drug abuse shows a large, mycotic pseudoaneurysm ➡ of the right common femoral artery with surrounding fat stranding and edema.*

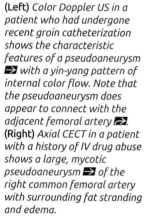

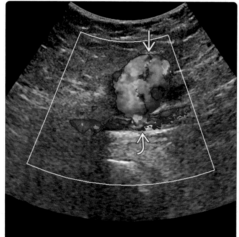

Groin Pseudoaneurysm

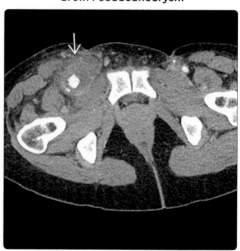

Groin Arteriovenous Fistula

(Left) *Axial CECT in a patient with swelling of the right groin after groin catheterization shows asymmetric enlargement and enhancement of the right common femoral vein ➡, while the contralateral left femoral vein ➡ is not yet opacified. This constellation of findings should rise strong concern for an AV fistula.*
(Right) *Axial CECT shows an enlarged left inguinal lymph node ➡, found to represent posttransplant lymphoproliferative disorder in this patient with a history of renal transplant.*

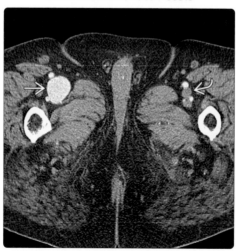

Inguinal Lymphadenopathy

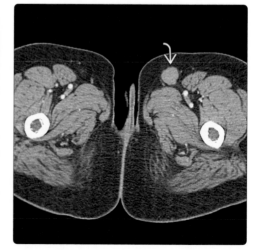

Varicocele

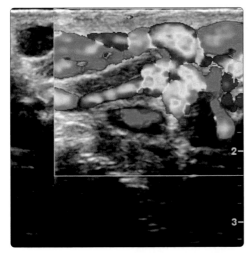

Mesh Hernia Repair (Mimic)

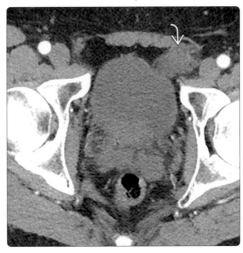

(Left) *Sagittal color Doppler US shows a classic tangle of tortuous vessels within the upper part of the scrotum. Flow and vessel dilation are accentuated by Valsalva maneuver, characteristic of a varicocele.* **(Right)** *Axial CECT shows the characteristic appearance of a mesh plug ⮕ related to prior inguinal hernia repair. This is a classic appearance, which should not be confused for pathology.*

Cryptorchidism

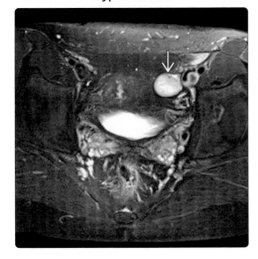

Iliopsoas Bursitis

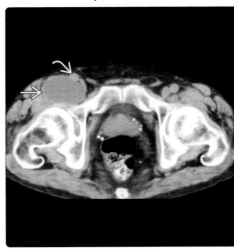

(Left) *Axial T2 FS MR in a patient with an undescended left testicle shows the T2-bright testicle ⮕ in the left pelvis. MR is the best modality for identifying an undescended testicle with an advantage over US for identifying testicles in the abdominal/pelvic cavities.* **(Right)** *Axial CECT shows the classic appearance of iliopsoas bursitis with a fluid collection ⮕ anterior to the right hip displacing the neurovascular bundle ⮕ anteriorly.*

Liposarcoma

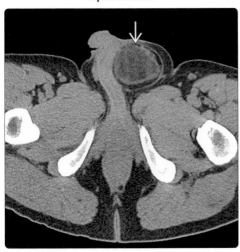

Liposarcoma

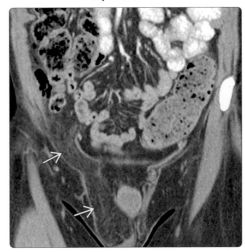

(Left) *Axial NECT shows a complex, fat-containing mass ⮕ in the left inguinal canal, found at resection to represent a primary spermatic cord liposarcoma.* **(Right)** *Coronal CECT shows a fat-containing mass ⮕ with minimal internal complexity extending from the right lower quadrant into the right inguinal canal. This represents a primary retroperitoneal liposarcoma with secondary extension into the inguinal canal.*

DIFFERENTIAL DIAGNOSIS

Common

- Paralyzed Diaphragm
- Eventration of Diaphragm
- Hiatal Hernia
- Bochdalek Hernia
- Morgagni Hernia
- Traumatic Diaphragmatic Hernia
- Subdiaphragmatic Mass
- Abdominal Abscess
- Unilateral Lung Volume Loss
- Subpulmonic Pleural Effusion (Mimic)

ESSENTIAL INFORMATION

Key Differential Diagnosis Issues

- Axial CT suboptimal for distinguishing diaphragm from spleen, liver, and muscle and identifying many diaphragmatic abnormalities
  - Multiplanar reformations critical for accurate diagnosis
- Diaphragm easier to visualize discretely on MR compared to CT and can demonstrate diaphragm in multiple planes
- Fluoroscopy and US useful for providing functional information, particularly for paralysis
  - Dynamic MR (not widely utilized) can provide functional information similar to US or fluoroscopy

Helpful Clues for Common Diagnoses

- **Paralyzed Diaphragm**
  - Normal diaphragm that fails to contract secondary to abnormalities of brain, spinal cord, neuromuscular junction, phrenic nerve, or muscle
  - US or fluoroscopy demonstrate no motion or paradoxical (upward) motion during inspiration or sniff test
- **Eventration of Diaphragm**
  - Congenital thinning/weakness of portion of diaphragm, which normally attaches to costal margin
  - Eccentric diaphragmatic contour (usually anteromedial right hemidiaphragm) ± paradoxical motion with large eventrations

- **Hiatal Hernia**
  - Herniation of abdominal contents into thoracic cavity through esophageal hiatus
  - Divided into sliding type (GE junction displaced upward through hiatus) and paraesophageal type (GE junction in normal location with stomach herniating above diaphragm)
- **Bochdalek Hernia**
  - Type of congenital diaphragmatic hernia due to defect in posterolateral diaphragm (usually on left side)
  - Hernia may contain retroperitoneal fat, bowel, kidney, stomach, spleen, or liver
- **Morgagni Hernia**
  - Type of congenital diaphragmatic hernia due to defect in retrosternal diaphragm (usually on right side)
  - Usually located in right cardiophrenic angle and most often contains just omental fat (but can contain colon, liver, small bowel, or stomach)
- **Traumatic Diaphragmatic Hernia**
  - Traumatic injury may be due to blunt or penetrating trauma
  - Multiple imaging signs of injury include dependent viscus sign, collar sign, and dangling diaphragm sign
  - Injuries both above and below diaphragm should raise concern for diaphragmatic injury
- **Subdiaphragmatic Mass**
  - Tumor, hepatomegaly, or splenomegaly can exert mass effect and raise ipsilateral diaphragm
- **Abdominal Abscess**
  - Subphrenic abscess can cause upward displacement of diaphragm due to mass effect or splinting (decreased motion of diaphragm due to pain)
- **Unilateral Lung Volume Loss**
  - Diminished unilateral lung volume (lung resection, atelectasis) will cause elevation of ipsilateral diaphragm
- **Subpulmonic Pleural Effusion (Mimic)**
  - Pleural fluid loculated in subpulmonic pleural space will displace lung upward and may simulate elevated diaphragm on radiographs (but not on cross-sectional imaging)

(Left) Coronal CECT shows marked asymmetric elevation of the left hemidiaphragm. In this case, the left diaphragm ➡ is paralyzed due to phrenic nerve involvement by the patient's mediastinal lymphoma (not shown).
(Right) Coronal CECT shows the characteristic appearance of diaphragmatic eventration with focal scalloping of the right anterior hemidiaphragm and superior protrusion of the liver at the site of eventration ➡.

Paralyzed Diaphragm

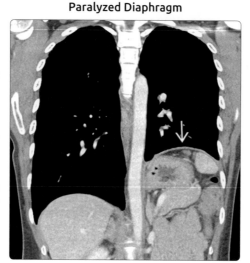

Eventration of Diaphragm

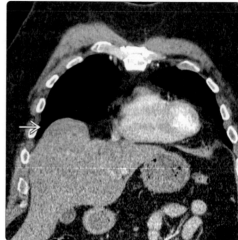

Hiatal Hernia

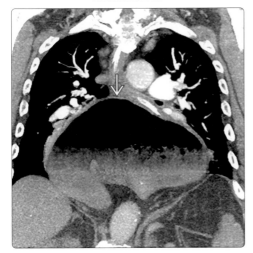

Bochdalek Hernia

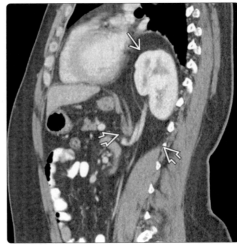

(Left) *Coronal CECT shows a large hiatal hernia with the entirety of the stomach ➡️ located within the thoracic cavity.* (Right) *Sagittal CECT shows a large Bochdalek hernia containing bowel and kidney. There is focal interruption of the hemidiaphragm ➡️ with herniation of the kidney ➡️ into the thorax.*

Morgagni Hernia

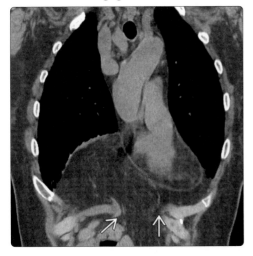

Traumatic Diaphragmatic Hernia

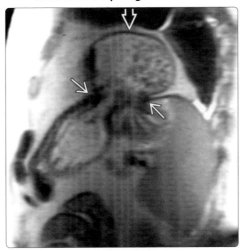

(Left) *Coronal NECT shows a characteristic Morgagni hernia with omental fat herniating into the chest through a defect ➡️ in the right anteromedial diaphragm.* (Right) *Sagittal T2 MR shows a posttraumatic defect ➡️ in the left hemidiaphragm with the stomach ➡️ herniating into the chest. Note that the diaphragm is identified as a low-signal curvilinear structure. The stomach is pinched as it traverses the defect in the diaphragm.*

Traumatic Diaphragmatic Hernia

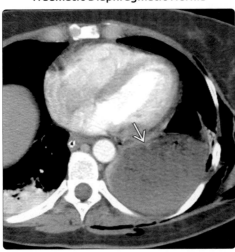

Subpulmonic Pleural Effusion (Mimic)

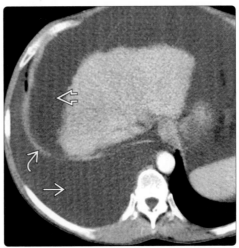

(Left) *Axial CECT shows the fallen viscus sign associated with traumatic diaphragmatic injury. Note that the stomach ➡️ lies in the chest and has fallen medially and posteriorly to lie against the lung and the posteromedial chest wall.* (Right) *Axial CECT shows a pleural effusion ➡️ below the lung and lateral to the diaphragm ➡️. Ascites ➡️ lies medial to the diaphragm and adjacent to the cirrhotic liver.*

DIFFERENTIAL DIAGNOSIS

Common

- Inguinal Hernia
- Femoral Hernia
- Ventral Hernia
  - Epigastric Hernia
  - Hypogastric Hernia
  - Incisional Hernia
- Spigelian Hernia
- Lumbar Hernia
- Umbilical Hernia
- Subcutaneous Abdominal Wall Mass (Mimic)
  - Subcutaneous Hematoma (Mimic)
  - Subcutaneous Abscess (Mimic)
  - Inguinal Lymphadenopathy (Mimic)
  - Soft Tissue Neoplasm (Mimic)
  - Cryptorchidism (Mimic)
- Enterocutaneous Fistula (Mimic)

Less Common

- Obturator Hernia
- Traumatic Abdominal Wall Hernia
- Sciatic Hernia
- Perineal Hernia
- Spermatic Cord Lipoma or Liposarcoma (Mimic)

ESSENTIAL INFORMATION

Key Differential Diagnosis Issues

- CT is most accurate imaging modality for diagnosis of hernias and associated complications
- US can be helpful for determining reducibility of hernias, as well as diagnosis of hernias, which are transiently reducible
  - Offers advantage of scanning patient in upright position or with Valsalva maneuver to elicit hernia
  - Efficacy of US for hernias is debatable in literature, and CT should certainly be 1st-line modality in patients with acute presentation or concerns for hernia-related complications
    - US should be reserved for nonurgent presentation in outpatient setting
- Evaluate any hernia for presence of complications, including bowel involvement, obstruction, and ischemia
  - Different types of hernias are associated with very different risks of complications
- Descriptive terms used to describe abdominal wall hernias
  - **Interparietal** (i.e., interstitial) hernia: Hernia sac is located in fascial planes between abdominal wall muscles without entering subcutaneous soft tissues
  - **Richter** hernia: Entirety of bowel circumference does not herniate (just antimesenteric border of bowel)

Helpful Clues for Common Diagnoses

- **Inguinal Hernia**
  - Most common type of external hernia (~ 80%) with indirect hernias typically congenital (due to weakness of processus vaginalis), and direct hernias usually acquired due to abdominal wall weakness
    - Hernia seen in groin region anterior to horizontal plane of pubic tubercle

- Do not result in compression of femoral vessels (unlike femoral hernia)
  - **Direct** hernias: Hernia sac arises anteromedial to inferior epigastric vessels
  - **Indirect** hernia: Hernia sac arises superomedial to inferior epigastric vessels
    - 5x more common than direct hernias
    - Complications more common with indirect hernias
- **Femoral Hernia**
  - Most commonly seen in older female patients (especially > 80 years) but much less common than inguinal hernias
  - Hernia extends into femoral canal medial to femoral vein and inferior to inferior epigastric vessels with frequent compression of femoral vein
  - Hernia sac located posterior and lateral to pubic tubercle
  - Very high risk of complications (incarceration, strangulation) and mortality compared to inguinal hernias
- **Ventral Hernia**
  - General term encompassing hernias extending through anterior and lateral abdominal wall
    - Can be acquired or congenital
  - **Epigastric** hernias occur at midline through linea alba above umbilicus, while **hypogastric** hernias occur at midline below umbilicus
  - **Incisional** hernias occur through any prior surgical incision site
    - Most often occur within a few months (usually first 4 months) of surgery but can occur at later time points as well
    - **Parastomal hernias** (considered type of incisional hernia) are quite common adjacent to ileostomy or colostomy
      - Parastomal hernias tend to slowly develop and enlarge over time and are very common with end-colostomies (48%) and end-ileostomies (28%) but much less common with loop ileostomies (6%)
  - Even if asymptomatic, most ventral hernias get larger over time with increasing risk of complications, making surgical treatment advisable
- **Spigelian Hernia**
  - Hernia extending through defect in aponeurosis of internal oblique and transverse abdominal muscles
  - Arise along lateral margin of rectus abdominis muscles, at level of arcuate line, inferior and lateral to umbilicus
  - Usually congenital in children and acquired in adults (prior surgery, obesity, pregnancies, etc. are risk factors)
  - High risk of strangulation and incarceration
- **Lumbar Hernia**
  - Hernia extends through defect in lumbar muscle or thoracolumbar fascia (usually below 12th rib and above iliac crest)
    - Can herniate through superior (Grynfeltt-Lesshaft) or inferior (petit) lumbar triangles
  - Most (80%) are acquired, usually due to surgical incisions (especially renal surgery)
  - Complications uncommon due to typically large neck, which makes incarceration/strangulation uncommon
- **Umbilical Hernia**
  - Hernia at midline extends through umbilical ring (usually upper 1/2 of umbilicus)

- Can be congenital (diagnosed in infancy) or acquired (usually in middle age)
  - Congenital type 8x more common in Black patients but most resolve spontaneously by 4-6 years of age
  - Acquired hernias associated with obesity, multiparity, and ascites
- Very common and usually small/asymptomatic, but larger or symptomatic hernias may require repair
- **Subcutaneous Abdominal Wall Mass (Mimic)**
  - Any subcutaneous or intramuscular mass may be superficially mistaken for hernia on clinical examination, although distinction should be obvious on imaging
  - Consider inguinal lymphadenopathy, abdominal wall tumors, cryptorchidism (especially in children), abscess, hydrocele, varicocele, or hematoma as entities that may be mistaken for hernia on physical examination
- **Enterocutaneous Fistula (Mimic)**
  - Gas- or contrast-filled tract from intraabdominal bowel loop into anterior abdominal wall may be confused for hernia
    - Bowel loops often tethered to anterior abdominal wall at site of fistula
  - Careful examination illustrates lack of true abdominal wall defect

Helpful Clues for Less Common Diagnoses

- **Obturator Hernia**
  - Rare type of hernia extending through obturator foramen into superolateral obturator canal
    - Usually involves loop of ileum but can involve any pelvic viscera
  - Typically seen in older female patients (especially older or multiparous females) secondary to either pelvic floor defect or pelvic floor laxity
  - High risk of complications (incarceration, strangulation) and mortality
- **Traumatic Abdominal Wall Hernia**
  - Hernia in anterior abdominal wall developing at site of focal trauma
  - Majority occur in lower abdomen with iliac crest region very common due to seat belt injuries

- Most commonly seen in young children < 10 years due to bicycle injury (e.g., handlebar hernia) but can also be seen in adults after high-energy trauma (e.g., motor vehicle collisions)
- **Sciatic Hernia**
  - Very uncommon hernia involving herniation of bowel loop through greater sciatic foramen laterally into subgluteal region
  - Occurs most often in female patients, likely as result of piriformis muscle atrophy
  - Can result in symptoms of sciatica as result of compression of sciatic nerve
- **Perineal Hernia**
  - Uncommon hernia with hernia sac extending anteriorly through urogenital diaphragm (most common) or posteriorly between levator ani and coccygeus muscles
  - Usually diagnosed in older women (> 50 years of age) with history of prior surgery in deep pelvis/perineum, prior pregnancies, obesity, or ascites
- **Spermatic Cord Lipoma or Liposarcoma (Mimic)**
  - Uncommon fat-containing mass arising in spermatic cord, which can extend into scrotum inferiorly or inguinal canal/retroperitoneum superiorly
  - When extending into inguinal canal, can mimic inguinal hernia, but lesion typically appears expansile and mass-like
  - Liposarcomas will often demonstrate internal complexity (or even soft tissue component) depending on degree of dedifferentiation
    - Well-differentiated liposarcomas may appear largely fat attenuation and are more apt to be confused for inguinal hernia containing omental fat
    - Usually appear hyperechoic on US (particularly when well differentiated) with similar echogenicity to subcutaneous fat

Inguinal Hernia

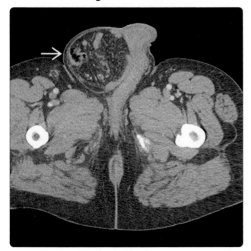

Inguinal Hernia

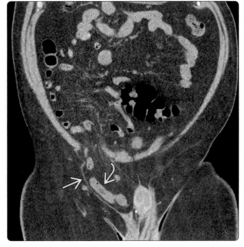

(Left) Axial CECT shows a large right inguinal hernia ➔ containing multiple loops of small bowel without evidence of obstruction. Inguinal hernias account for the vast majority of external hernias. (Right) Coronal NECT shows a classic right inguinal hernia ➔ containing loops of small bowel ➔ without evidence of obstruction.

Defect in Abdominal Wall (Hernia)

Femoral Hernia

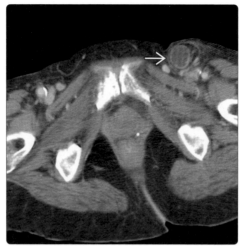

Ventral Hernia

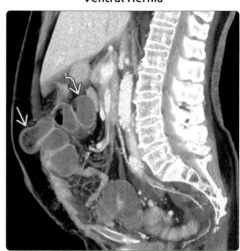

(Left) *Axial CECT shows a herniated bowel loop ➡ in the left groin. Note the close relationship of the hernia to the femoral vessels at the level of the symphysis pubis, characteristic of a femoral hernia.* **(Right)** *Sagittal volume-rendered CECT shows a ventral hernia containing loops of small bowel ➡. The small bowel proximal to the hernia sac is dilated ➡, compatible with small bowel obstruction.*

Ventral Hernia

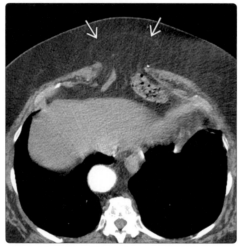

Spigelian Hernia

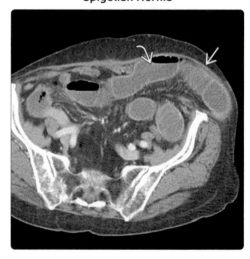

(Left) *Axial CECT in a patient with a history of prior thoracic surgery shows a fat-containing ventral hernia ➡ arising in the upper abdomen. Ventral hernias occurring above the umbilicus, as in this case, are termed epigastric hernias.* **(Right)** *Axial CECT shows a left abdominal spigelian hernia ➡ with multiple dilated loops of small bowel ➡, compatible with small bowel obstruction.*

Lumbar Hernia

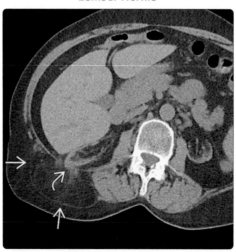

Lumbar Hernia

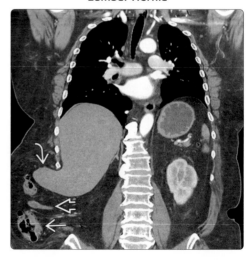

(Left) *Axial NECT shows a large lumbar hernia ➡ in the right flank containing a portion of the right kidney ➡.* **(Right)** *Coronal CECT shows a large lumbar hernia containing colon ➡, small bowel ➡, as well as a portion of the right hepatic lobe ➡. Lumbar hernias are often secondary to prior surgical incisions and are particularly common after renal surgeries.*

Umbilical Hernia

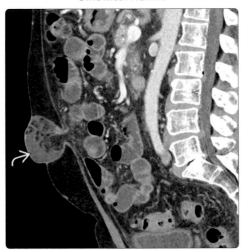

Enterocutaneous Fistula (Mimic)

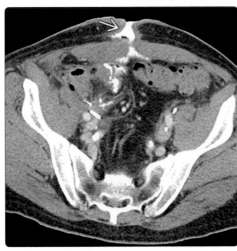

(Left) *Sagittal CECT shows an umbilical hernia containing ascites ⇗ in a patient with cirrhosis and portal hypertension.* (Right) *Axial CECT shows an enterocutaneous fistula with enteric contrast directly extending from the small bowel into the anterior abdominal wall ⇒.*

Obturator Hernia

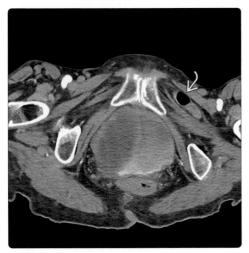

Traumatic Abdominal Wall Hernia

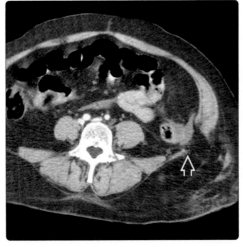

(Left) *Axial CECT shows a loop of small bowel ⇗ lying between the obturator externus and pectineus muscles, compatible with an obturator hernia.* (Right) *Axial CECT in a trauma patient shows disruption of the musculofascial plane ⇒ near the insertion into the iliac crest and thoracolumbar fascia. Note the presence of adjacent subcutaneous hematoma. The spleen was also lacerated (not shown). These findings are compatible with a traumatic hernia.*

Spermatic Cord Lipoma or Liposarcoma (Mimic)

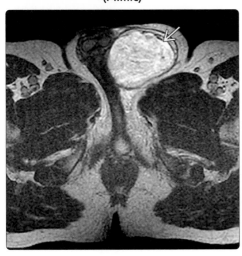

Spermatic Cord Lipoma or Liposarcoma (Mimic)

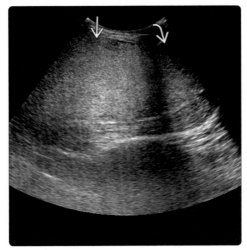

(Left) *Axial T1 MR shows a large mass with fat signal ⇒ extending through the inguinal canal into the left scrotum. This was found to be a spermatic cord liposarcoma at resection.* (Right) *Sagittal US in the same patient shows that the mass ⇒ is very echogenic as a result of its fatty component, a fairly common appearance for these lesions, and extends down to just above the testicle ⇗.*

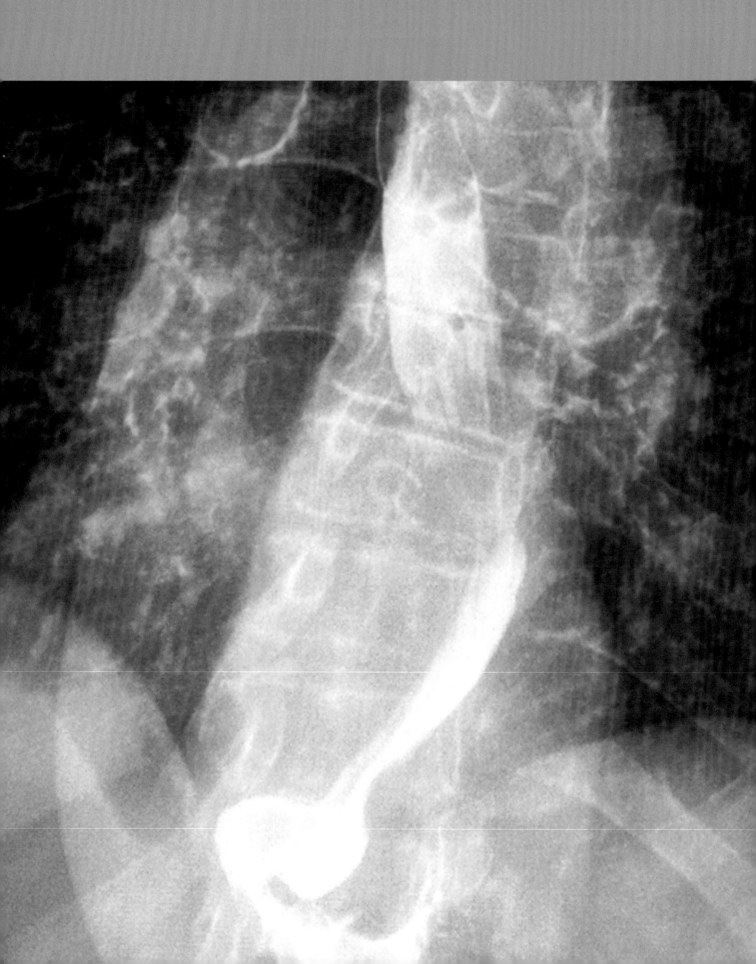

SECTION 3
Esophagus

Generic Imaging Patterns

Intraluminal Mass, Esophagus   66
Extrinsic Mass, Esophagus   68
Lesion at Pharyngoesophageal Junction   72
Esophageal Ulceration   74
Mucosal Nodularity, Esophagus   76
Esophageal Strictures   78
Dilated Esophagus   80
Esophageal Outpouchings (Diverticula)   82
Esophageal Dysmotility   84

Clinically Based Differentials

Odynophagia   86

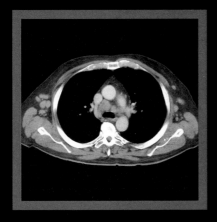
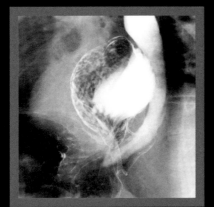

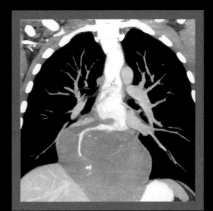
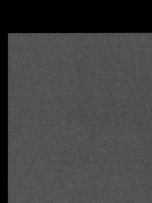

DIFFERENTIAL DIAGNOSIS

Common

- Esophageal Carcinoma
- Esophageal Foreign Body
- Intramural Benign Esophageal Tumors

Less Common

- Thrombosed Esophageal Varix ± Hemorrhage
- Inflammatory Polyp, Esophagus
- *Candida* Esophagitis
- Viral Esophagitis
- Abscess
- Papilloma, Esophagus

Rare but Important

- Fibrovascular Polyp
- Esophageal Metastases and Lymphoma
- Esophageal Adenoma
- Esophageal Gastrointestinal Stromal Tumor

ESSENTIAL INFORMATION

Key Differential Diagnosis Issues

- Intraluminal masses usually have irregular surface and acute angles with wall

Helpful Clues for Common Diagnoses

- **Esophageal Carcinoma**
  - Most common tumor of esophagus
  - Luminal narrowing with nodular, ulcerated mucosa
- **Esophageal Foreign Body**
  - Check for history of sudden onset of dysphagia
  - Usually lodges just above point of physiologic or pathologic narrowing
    - e.g., Schatzki ring, web, or carcinoma
  - Repeat barium esophagram or endoscopy after removal or passage of foreign body
- **Intramural Benign Esophageal Tumors**
  - Leiomyoma > lipoma > gastrointestinal stromal tumor > neuroma, neurofibroma, and others

- Peristalsis may draw mass into esophageal lumen, simulating intraluminal mass
- Overlying mucosa may ulcerate

Helpful Clues for Less Common Diagnoses

- **Thrombosed Esophageal Varix ± Hemorrhage**
  - May be indistinguishable from carcinoma (varicoid carcinoma)
  - Look for confirmatory evidence of cirrhosis and portal hypertension (uphill varices seen distally) vs. proximally located downhill varices from superior vena cava obstruction
- **Inflammatory Polyp, Esophagus**
  - Polypoid protuberance just above esophagogastric junction
  - Appears as single, prominent fold or rounded mass
  - Associated with hiatal hernia, reflux
- ***Candida* or Viral Esophagitis**
  - May result in intraluminal sloughed cells, organisms, and debris that appear as mass
  - Usually occurs in immune-suppressed patient
    - Opportunistic infections
- **Papilloma, Esophagus**
  - Benign; small (0.5-1.5 cm)

Helpful Clues for Rare Diagnoses

- **Fibrovascular Polyp**
  - Rare benign mass arises from cervical esophagus but grows into giant, sausage-like polypoid mass that may fill much of esophageal lumen
  - CT may show elements of fat and soft tissue within mass; 7-20 cm
  - Patients may have history of regurgitating sausage-like mass
- **Esophageal Metastases and Lymphoma**
  - Gastric, breast, or lung cancer may extend into wall or lumen of esophagus
  - Other metastases and lymphoma are rare
- **Esophageal Gastrointestinal Stromal Tumor**
  - Usual appearance is that of intramural mass

Esophageal Carcinoma

Esophageal Carcinoma

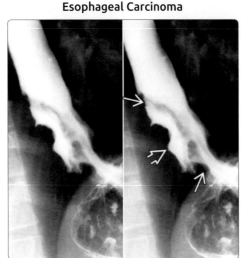
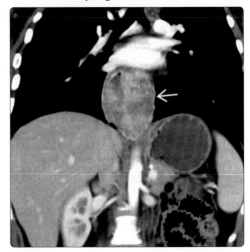

(Left) Esophagram shows a mass in the distal esophagus with the tumor causing a filling defect ➡ and the ulceration causing a collection of barium ➡ within the mass. (Right) Coronal CECT in a 21-year-old woman shows an expansile, heterogeneous distal esophageal mass ➡. Resection was performed, and pathology showed malignant glomus tumor.

Esophageal Foreign Body

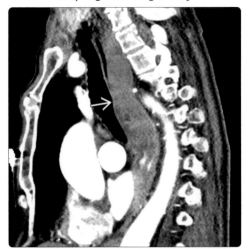

Esophageal Foreign Body

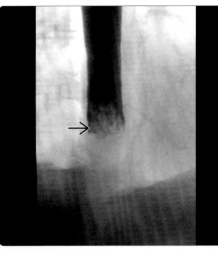

(Left) *Sagittal CECT in an 80-year-old man with hematemesis shows a large endoluminal mass ➡, a blood clot seen on endoscopy. The source of bleeding was an ulcer.* (Right) *Esophagram shows a filling defect ➡ within the distal esophagus and complete obstruction to distal flow of barium. Endoscopic finding was a bolus of meat stuck above a Schatzki ring.*

Inflammatory Polyp, Esophagus

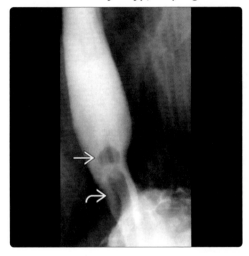

Candida Esophagitis

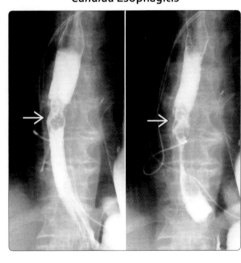

(Left) *Esophagram shows a polypoid lesion in the distal esophagus ➡ that is contiguous with a nodular, thickened fold ➡ traversing the esophagogastric junction.* (Right) *Esophagram shows an irregular filling defect ➡ closely simulating an esophageal cancer. At endoscopy, this was a mass of inflammatory debris in a patient with Candida esophagitis.*

Fibrovascular Polyp

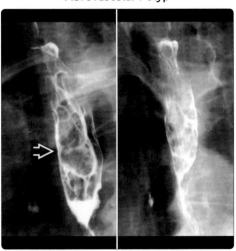

Esophageal Metastases and Lymphoma

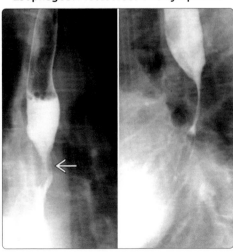

(Left) *Esophagram shows a huge mass ➡ that originates in the cervical esophagus and fills most of the lumen.* (Right) *Esophagram shows abrupt narrowing of the midesophagus. The tapered margins and intact mucosal folds ➡ correctly suggest an extrinsic process, lung cancer, rather than primary tumor.*

DIFFERENTIAL DIAGNOSIS

Common

- Left Main Bronchus and Aortic Arch
- Aortic Aneurysm
- Left Atrial Enlargement
- Hiatal Hernia
- Mediastinal Lymph Nodes
- Aberrant Right Subclavian Artery
- Cervical or Thoracic Osteophytes
- Enlarged Thyroid
- Esophageal Varices
- Lung Cancer

Less Common

- Intramural (Mesenchymal) Esophageal Tumors
- Esophageal Carcinoma (Mimic)
- Gastric Carcinoma (Mimic)
- Gastrointestinal Duplication Cyst
- Bronchogenic Cyst
- Metastases and Lymphoma, Esophagus

ESSENTIAL INFORMATION

Key Differential Diagnosis Issues

- Extrinsic lesions: Smooth, intact mucosa and obtuse angles at indentation
- Entire lumen may be displaced or compressed
- Extrinsic masses are usually easily recognized on CT
  - Multiplanar reformations are especially helpful

Helpful Clues for Common Diagnoses

- **Left Main Bronchus and Aortic Arch**
  - Normal indentations along left lateral margin
  - Most apparent in left posterior oblique position
- **Aortic Aneurysm**
  - Usually indents distal esophagus obliquely, just above diaphragm
- **Left Atrial Enlargement**
  - Especially if enlarged

- Displaces distal 1/3 of esophagus posteriorly
- **Hiatal Hernia**
  - Paraesophageal hernias displace or compress esophagus
- **Mediastinal Lymph Nodes**
  - Enlarged by benign or malignant disease
  - Usually most apparent in midesophagus
- **Aberrant Right Subclavian Artery**
  - Either aberrant right or left subclavian artery may compress posterior wall of esophagus
  - Easily recognized on CECT
- **Enlarged Thyroid**
  - Goiter may extend into mediastinum
    - Look for cervicothoracic mass with increased attenuation on CT
- **Esophageal Varices**
  - Large or thrombosed varices often simulate mediastinal mass

Helpful Clues for Less Common Diagnoses

- **Intramural (Mesenchymal) Esophageal Tumors**
  - Leiomyoma, gastrointestinal stromal tumor, lipoma, etc.
  - Often difficult on barium esophagram to distinguish extrinsic from intramural mass
    - Classic finding for intramural mass would be smooth mucosal surface; right angle interface with lumen
  - Usually easier with CT
- **Esophageal Carcinoma (Mimic)**
  - Submucosal extension and mediastinal spread may mimic extrinsic lesion
- **Gastric Carcinoma (Mimic)**
  - Spread into submucosal esophagus and thoracic nodes
- **Bronchogenic Cyst**
  - Spherical subcarinal mass; nonenhancing contents; most commonly located in middle mediastinum
  - May appear hyperdense or T1 hyperintense
- **Metastases and Lymphoma, Esophagus**
  - Both are much less common than metastases to mediastinal nodes
  - Direct invasion of esophagus from lung cancer is not rare

---

(Left) Esophagram shows a normal esophagus with indentations along the left anterolateral wall by the aortic knob ➡ and left main bronchus ⬈. (Right) Esophagram in an older man shows extrinsic indentation ➡ along the posterior wall of the distal esophagus by a dilated, ectatic aorta. Note sternal wires ➚ from a prior coronary artery graft procedure.

Left Main Bronchus and Aortic Arch

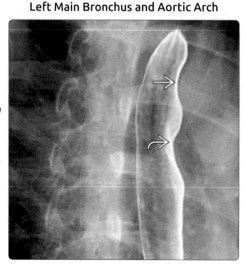

Aortic Aneurysm

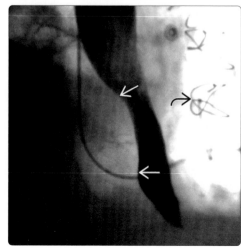

Left Atrial Enlargement

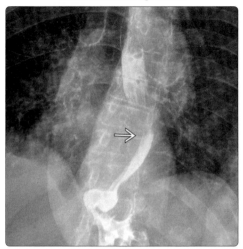

Left Atrial Enlargement

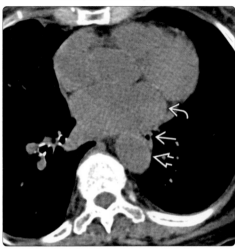

(Left) *Esophagram in an 82-year-old woman shows displacement of the distal esophagus* ➡️. (Right) *Axial CECT in the same patient shows a displaced esophagus* ➡️ *due to mass effect from an enlarged left atrium* ➡️ *and a tortuous aorta* ➡️.

Mediastinal Lymph Nodes

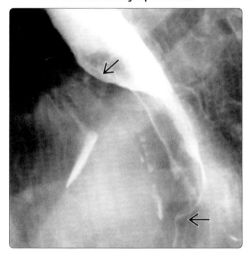

Mediastinal Lymph Nodes

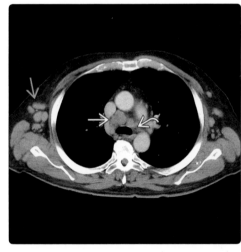

(Left) *Esophagram shows a broad indentation* ➡️ *of the anterior wall of the midesophagus by enlarged mediastinal nodes; this is metastases from primary lung cancer.* (Right) *Axial CECT shows displacement and compression of the esophagus* ➡️ *by mediastinal lymphadenopathy* ➡️. *Other nodal groups were enlarged* ➡️ *in the chest and abdomen, typical of leukemia or lymphoma. Chronic lymphocytic leukemia was confirmed.*

Aberrant Right Subclavian Artery

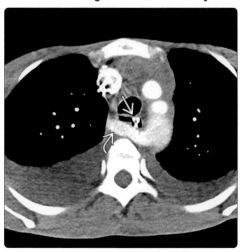

Aberrant Right Subclavian Artery

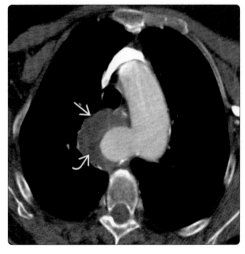

(Left) *Axial CECT shows an aberrant right subclavian artery* ➡️ *arising from the aortic arch and crossing between the spine and the esophagus, within which an enteric feeding tube* ➡️ *is seen. Unrelated mediastinal adenopathy and pleural effusions are also present.* (Right) *Axial CECT in a patient with dysphagia and a mediastinal mass shows aneurysmal dilation of an aberrant right subclavian artery* ➡️ *that compressed and displaced the esophagus. The aneurysm lumen contains thrombus* ➡️.

Cervical or Thoracic Osteophytes

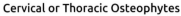
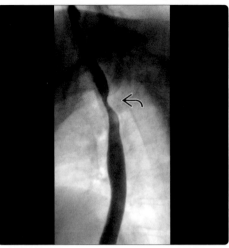

Cervical or Thoracic Osteophytes

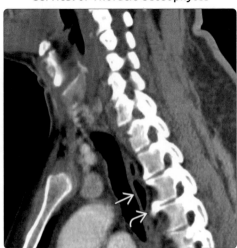

(Left) *Esophagram in a 49-year-old man shows the barium-filled esophagus with a smooth indentation along its posterior wall ⟾. A primary intramural esophageal tumor was suspected. CT showed no mass, but there was prominent osteophytes at this level.* (Right) *Sagittal CECT in the same patient shows prominent osteophytes at the T3-T4 level ⟾ accounting for the indentation and narrowing of the esophagus ⟾. Extrinsic indentation by osteophytes more commonly occurs at the lower cervical level.*

Enlarged Thyroid

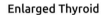
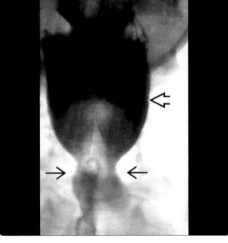

Esophageal Varices

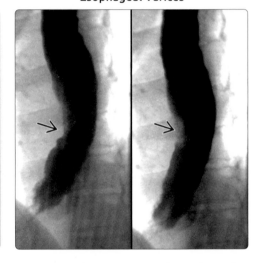

(Left) *Esophagram shows persistent dilation of the pharynx ⟾ even after passage of the barium bolus. The proximal esophagus is narrowed ⟾. CT showed an enlarged thyroid gland.* (Right) *Esophagram shows fixed serpiginous intramural filling defects ⟾ in the esophagus due to sclerosed varices.*

Intramural (Mesenchymal) Esophageal Tumors

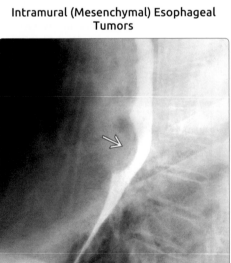
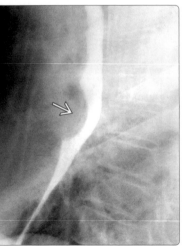

Intramural (Mesenchymal) Esophageal Tumors

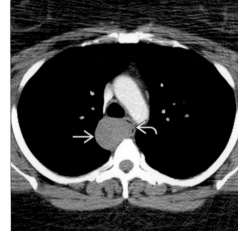

(Left) *Esophagram shows a mass causing eccentric narrowing of the distal lumen. The mass forms obtuse angles with the wall, and the esophageal folds and mucosa are intact ⟾. An esophageal leiomyoma was removed thoracoscopically.* (Right) *Axial CECT shows a soft tissue density mass ⟾ displacing but not obstructing the esophageal lumen ⟾. Benign esophageal leiomyoma was confirmed at resection.*

Intramural (Mesenchymal) Esophageal Tumors

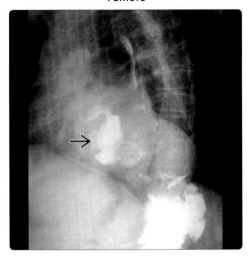

Intramural (Mesenchymal) Esophageal Tumors

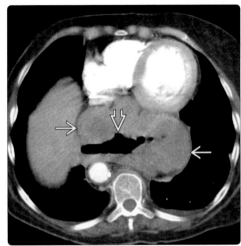

(Left) Esophagram in a young man with dysphagia shows an irregular collection of barium ➡ within the ulcerated cavity of a mass. This was an esophageal gastrointestinal stromal tumor. (Right) Axial CECT in the same patient shows a huge esophageal mass ➡ with a large central ulceration ➡ that contains gas due to communication with the esophageal lumen. This was a gastrointestinal stromal tumor of the esophagus.

Bronchogenic Cyst

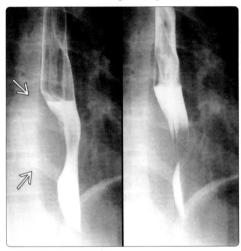

Bronchogenic Cyst

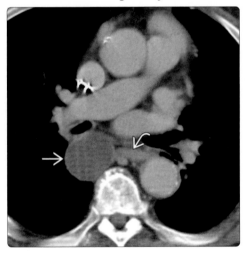

(Left) Esophagram shows eccentric narrowing of the distal esophageal lumen by a mass ➡ that forms obtuse angles as it meets the barium-filled lumen. The overlying esophageal mucosa and folds are intact. This was a bronchogenic cyst. (Right) Axial CECT shows a water density mediastinal mass ➡ arising just below the tracheal carina and indenting the esophagus ➡.

Bronchogenic Cyst

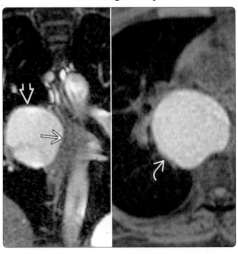

Metastases and Lymphoma, Esophagus

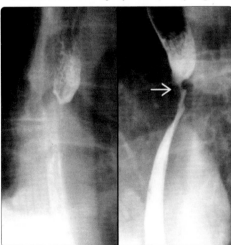

(Left) MR in a 49-year-old woman shows extrinsic mass effect on the esophagus ➡ by a T2-hyperintense bronchogenic cyst ➡. The cyst is also T1 hyperintense ➡ due to hemorrhagic fluid. (Right) Esophagram shows abrupt but smooth tapering ➡ of the esophagus at the carinal level with intact mucosal folds, indicating extrinsic involvement and direct invasion from lung cancer.

DIFFERENTIAL DIAGNOSIS

Common

- Achalasia, Cricopharyngeal
- Cervical Osteophytes
- Muscular Disorders
  - Myasthenia Gravis

Less Common

- Esophageal Webs
- Esophageal Carcinoma
- Esophagitis, Drug Induced
- Neck Mass
- Neck Hematoma
- Postradiation Therapy for Neck Malignancy
- Cervical Lymphadenopathy

ESSENTIAL INFORMATION

Key Differential Diagnosis Issues

- Determine which side(s) of lumen are indented
  - Cricopharyngeal muscle indents posterior wall
  - Webs usually arise from anterolateral walls
  - Thyroid masses usually encircle anterior and lateral walls

Helpful Clues for Common Diagnoses

- **Achalasia, Cricopharyngeal**
  - Smooth indentation of posterior wall at C5-C6 vertebral level
  - May be intermittent or persistent finding
  - Prominent or persistent contraction may result in dilated pharynx with retained barium
  - Usually associated with various forms of esophageal dysmotility
- **Cervical Osteophytes**
  - May or may not be ossified
  - Indent posterior wall of esophagus, often at several levels
  - Usually asymptomatic but may be large enough to cause dysphagia

- Postoperative changes (**cervical laminectomy**, **fusion**) may have similar effects on esophagus
  - Patients with metallic plate at site of fusion often have symptomatic dysphagia
  - Even in absence of marked mass effect upon esophageal lumen

Helpful Clues for Less Common Diagnoses

- **Esophageal Webs**
  - Thin, shelf-like indentation of lumen
  - May be congenital or acquired
    - e.g., as result of scarring from epidermolysis bullosa
  - May be associated with glossitis and iron-deficiency anemia (Plummer-Vinson syndrome)
  - Arise from anterolateral wall, unlike more common causes of posterior wall indentation
- **Esophageal Carcinoma**
  - Irregular mucosal surface
    - Early lesion: Plaque-like lesions; flat, sessile polyps
  - Eccentric or concentric narrowing of lumen
- **Esophagitis, Drug Induced**
  - Oral medications may have impaired passage through pharyngoesophageal junction
  - May result in esophageal spasm, ulceration, stricture
  - Ask about medications (especially tetracycline and cardiac drugs)
  - Patients usually have abrupt onset of odynophagia (painful swallowing)
- **Neck Mass**
  - Any paraesophageal mass may indent esophagus
  - Near pharyngoesophageal junction, most common are thyroid and parathyroid masses
  - Others to consider include aneurysms, retropharyngeal abscess
  - US, CT, and MR can narrow or establish diagnosis

Achalasia, Cricopharyngeal

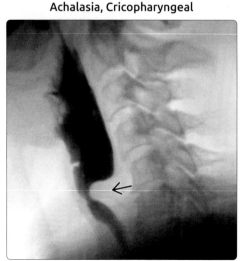

Achalasia, Cricopharyngeal

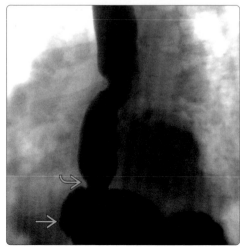

(Left) Rapid-sequence esophagram of the pharynx during swallowing in this woman with gastroesophogeal reflux disease (GERD) and dysphagia shows prominence and spasm of the cricopharyngeal muscle ➡ at the level of the C5-C6 vertebral disc space. (Right) Esophagram of the lower esophagus in the same patient shows a type 1 hiatal hernia ➡, a patulous gastroesophageal junction ➡, and free reflux. In this case, cricopharyngeal achalasia is probably related to reflux esophagitis.

Cervical Osteophytes

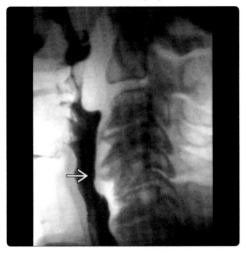

Esophageal Webs

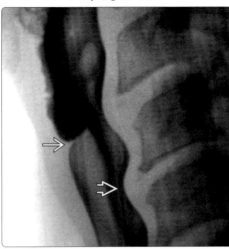

(Left) *Esophagram shows indentation of the posterior wall of the pharyngoesophageal junction by cervical osteophytes* ➡. (Right) *Esophagram shows a thin, shelf-like indentation* ➡ *of the anterolateral wall of the pharyngoesophageal junction. The pharynx is mildly dilated above this web. Posterior osteophytes* ➡ *(unossified) are also noted.*

Esophageal Carcinoma

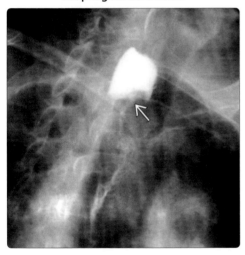

Esophagitis, Drug Induced

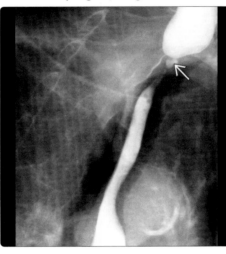

(Left) *Esophagram shows an apple core, abrupt, high-grade obstructing lesion* ➡ *at the thoracic inlet.* (Right) *Esophagram shows a tight stricture and ulceration* ➡ *at the pharyngoesophageal junction caused by oral medication. Pills more commonly stick at points of physiologic narrowing, such as the aortic knob.*

Neck Mass

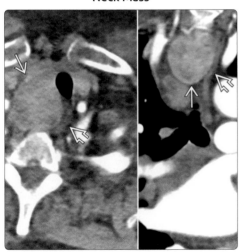

Neck Mass

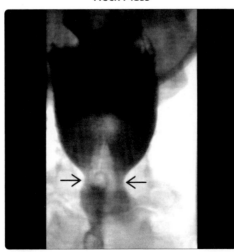

(Left) *Axial (left) and coronal (right) CECT in an 86-year-old woman with dysphagia shows a large, benign thyroid nodule* ➡ *with smooth mass effect and displacement of the esophagus* ➡. (Right) *Esophagram in a patient with thyromegaly due to autoimmune thyroiditis shows distention of the pharynx and compression of the proximal esophagus* ➡.

DIFFERENTIAL DIAGNOSIS

Common

- Reflux Esophagitis
- *Candida* Esophagitis
- Drug-Induced Esophagitis
- Viral Esophagitis

Less Common

- Caustic Esophagitis
- Radiation Esophagitis
- Nasogastric Intubation
- Crohn Disease
- Esophageal Cancer

Rare but Important

- Behçet Disease
- Epidermolysis Bullosa Dystrophica and Pemphigoid

ESSENTIAL INFORMATION

Key Differential Diagnosis Issues

- History is often key (e.g., AIDS, caustic ingestion, other known diseases)

Helpful Clues for Common Diagnoses

- **Reflux Esophagitis**
  - Most common etiology
  - Shallow, punctate, or linear ulcers
  - Check for gastroesophageal reflux
  - Hiatal hernia is common
  - Peptic stricture is common in those with ulceration
- *Candida* **Esophagitis**
  - Ulcers with cobblestone, shaggy, or snakeskin appearance with confluent plaques
  - Odynophagia in immunocompromised patients
  - Often have oral thrush (*Candida*)
  - Discrete plaques with longitudinal orientation
- **Drug-Induced Esophagitis**
  - Ulceration

- Solitary or localized cluster of tiny ulcers distributed circumferentially on normal background mucosa
- Giant, flat ulcers
  - Usually near aortic arch or left main bronchus
  - Odynophagia in patients taking oral medications (tetracycline, KCl, heart medications)
  - Abrupt onset of symptoms
- **Viral Esophagitis**
  - Herpes, CMV, HIV
  - Superficial, often large, usually flat ulcerations on normal mucosa
  - Odynophagia in immunocompromised patient

Helpful Clues for Less Common Diagnoses

- **Caustic Esophagitis**
  - Immediate ulceration and spasm
  - Often leads to long stricture of esophagus
  - Acute severe phase (1-4 days): Narrowed lumen with irregular contour/ulcerations
  - Ulcer granulation phase (5-28 days): More defined ulcers; spasm
  - Cicatrization and scarring (3-4 weeks): Strictures, sacculations, pseudodiverticula
- **Nasogastric Intubation**
  - Long-term nasogastric tube leads to reflux and direct trauma to esophagus
  - May cause shallow or long ulcers ± stricture
- **Crohn Disease**
  - Usually in patients with advanced disease
  - Aphthous ulcers (as in stomach and bowel)

Helpful Clues for Rare Diagnoses

- **Behçet Disease**
  - Ulceration of oral, esophageal, and genital mucosa
  - Associated vasculitis
- **Epidermolysis Bullosa Dystrophica and Pemphigoid**
  - Esophageal strictures, most in upper 1/3 of esophagus; may be multiple, webs
  - Long history of disease
    - Diagnosis is already known

(Left) *Esophagram shows a stricture and large ulcer* ➡ *at the gastroesophageal junction with shortened esophagus and hiatal hernia.* (Right) *Esophagram shows a shaggy or tree bark surface of the esophagus due to diffuse ulceration and raised plaques, typical of severe Candida esophagitis.*

Reflux Esophagitis

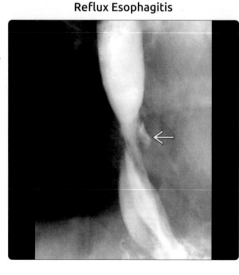

Candida **Esophagitis**

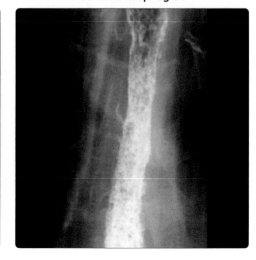

Drug-Induced Esophagitis

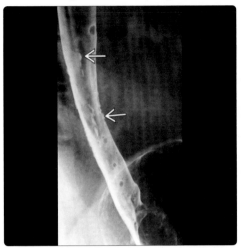

Viral Esophagitis

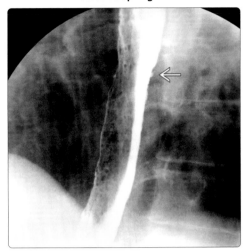

(Left) *Esophagram shows multiple shallow ulcerations ➡ due to tetracycline-induced esophagitis.* (Right) *Esophagram shows multiple small, superficial ulcers ➡ due to herpes esophagitis.*

Caustic Esophagitis

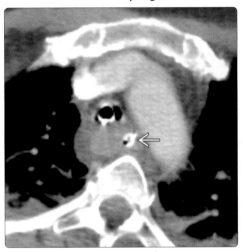

Radiation Esophagitis

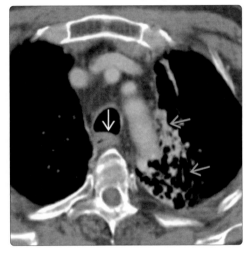

(Left) *Axial CECT in a patient with recent ingestion of lye as a suicide attempt shows massive thickening of the esophageal wall with its lumen marked by nasogastric tube ➡. An endotracheal tube is also noted with widespread pulmonary infiltrates.* (Right) *Axial CECT in a patient who had external beam radiation therapy for left upper lobe lung cancer shows damage to the lungs ➡ along the radiation port. The esophageal wall is thick and the lumen is narrowed ➡, also due to radiation-induced injury.*

Radiation Esophagitis

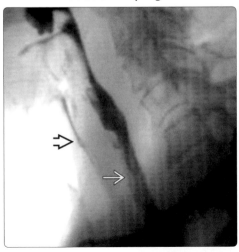

Epidermolysis Bullosa Dystrophica and Pemphigoid

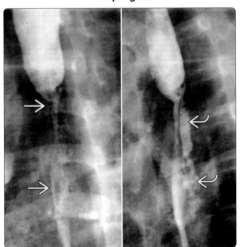

(Left) *Esophagram in a patient with lung cancer and radiation-induced esophagitis shows a luminal narrowing ➡ and mucosal ulceration of the proximal esophagus along with aspiration of barium ➡ into the trachea.* (Right) *Esophagram shows an ulcerated stricture of the midesophagus ➡ due to epidermolysis. Following balloon dilation of the stricture, the esophagus was perforated with extraluminal contrast extravasation noted ➡.*

DIFFERENTIAL DIAGNOSIS

Common

- Reflux Esophagitis
- *Candida* Esophagitis
- Viral Esophagitis
- Glycogenic Acanthosis
- Artifact: Undissolved Gas Granules, Bubbles (Mimics)

Less Common

- Barrett Esophagus
- Esophageal Carcinoma

Rare but Important

- Papillomatosis, Esophageal
- Acanthosis Nigricans
- Cowden Disease
- Leukoplakia

ESSENTIAL INFORMATION

Key Differential Diagnosis Issues

- Consider clinical setting
  - Symptoms, age of patient, AIDS, etc.

Helpful Clues for Common Diagnoses

- **Reflux Esophagitis**
  - Poorly defined nodules; granular mucosa
  - Usually affects distal 1/3 of esophagus
  - Gastroesophageal (GE) reflux, hiatal hernia
- *Candida* **Esophagitis**
  - Discrete plaques with longitudinal orientation and ulcers; cobblestone, shaggy, or snakeskin appearance with confluent plaques
  - May be localized or diffuse
  - Odynophagia in immunocompromised patient
    - May look like tree bark
- **Glycogenic Acanthosis**
  - Numerous small nodules or plaques
  - Less well-defined than candidiasis
  - Asymptomatic lesions of no clinical importance

- **Artifact: Undissolved Gas Granules, Bubbles (Mimics)**
  - Transient finding, usually with 1st swallows during air-contrast esophagram

Helpful Clues for Less Common Diagnoses

- **Barrett Esophagus**
  - Fine surface nodularity is characteristic but difficult to distinguish from other causes
  - Associated GE reflux and hiatal hernia
  - Long segment: > 3 cm above GE junction
    - Due to more severe reflux disease
    - Hiatal hernia in almost all patients
    - Associated esophageal ulceration, stricture
    - Greater cancer risk in long- vs. short-segment type
  - Short segment: Columnar epithelium ≤ 3 cm above GE junction
    - Due to less severe reflux disease
    - More common than long segment
- **Esophageal Carcinoma**
  - Superficial spreading carcinoma can appear as poorly defined, coalescent nodules or plaques
  - Localized more often than diffuse
  - Often asymptomatic

Helpful Clues for Rare Diagnoses

- **Papillomatosis, Esophageal**
  - More commonly affects larynx
  - Related to HPV infection
- **Cowden Disease**
  - Tiny nodules = hamartomatous polyps
  - Hereditary with associated tumors of skin, gastrointestinal tract, and thyroid
- **Leukoplakia**
  - Common in mouth, rare in esophagus
  - Hyperkeratosis, dysplasia on biopsy

Reflux Esophagitis

Reflux Esophagitis

(Left) Spot film from an esophagram shows a stricture at the esophagogastric junction ➡, a small hiatal hernia ➡, and nodular mucosal surface ➡ of the esophagus, all due to gastroesophageal reflux disease (GERD). (Right) Spot film from an esophagram shows a peptic stricture ➡ of the esophagus along with a small hiatal hernia ➡. Nodularity of the esophageal mucosa is less evident with full distention of the lumen.

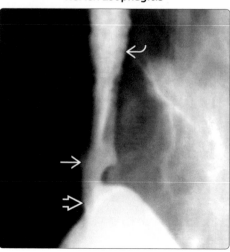
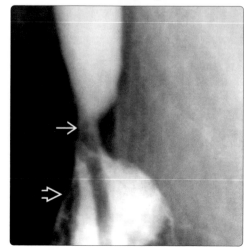

Candida Esophagitis

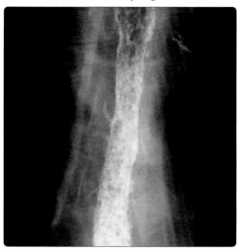

Candida Esophagitis

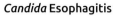
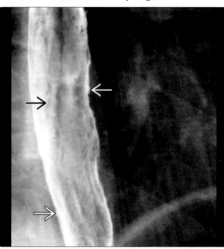
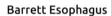

(Left) *Esophagram shows a shaggy tree bark appearance of the esophagus due to ulcerations and plaques from Candida esophagitis.* (Right) *Spot film from an esophagram shows multiple superficial ulcerations ➡ and raised plaques ➡ in a patient with AIDS. This is viral esophagitis but is indistinguishable from C. esophagitis by imaging alone.*

Artifact: Undissolved Gas Granules, Bubbles (Mimics)

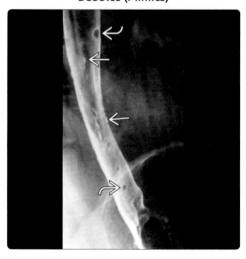

Barrett Esophagus

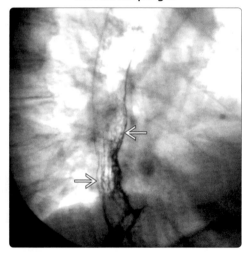

(Left) *Spot film from an esophagram shows multiple radiolucent filling defects ➡ that represent gas bubbles that are adherent to the esophageal surface. Also present are multiple ulcerations ➡ due to tetracycline-induced esophagitis.* (Right) *Spot film from an esophagram shows nodular distal esophageal mucosa ➡ due to Barrett esophagus. A hiatal hernia and reflux were also demonstrated.*

Esophageal Carcinoma

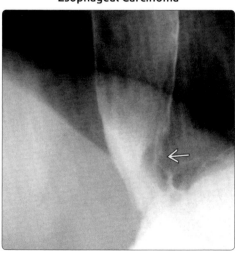

Papillomatosis, Esophageal

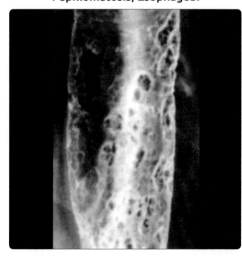

(Left) *Spot film from an esophagram shows nodular thickened folds ➡ in the distal esophagus and fundus of stomach. These nodules are much larger than those seen in most infectious conditions.* (Right) *Esophagram shows clusters of small, irregular nodules that represent biopsy-proven squamous papillomas.*

DIFFERENTIAL DIAGNOSIS

Common

- Reflux Esophagitis
- Barrett Esophagus
- Esophageal Carcinoma
- Scleroderma, Esophagus
- Spasm
- Extrinsic Compression (Mimic)

Less Common

- Esophageal Metastases and Lymphoma
- Radiation Esophagitis
- Caustic Esophagitis
- Drug-Induced Esophagitis
- *Candida* Esophagitis
- Nasogastric Intubation
- Sclerotherapy of Esophageal Varices

Rare but Important

- Crohn Disease
- Graft-vs.-Host Disease
- Glutaraldehyde-Induced Injury
- Epidermolysis and Pemphigoid
- Esophagitis, Eosinophilic

ESSENTIAL INFORMATION

Key Differential Diagnosis Issues

- History is key (e.g., radiation therapy, caustic or drug ingestion, bone marrow transplant)

Helpful Clues for Common Diagnoses

- **Reflux Esophagitis**
  - Peptic stricture of distal 1/3
  - Hiatal hernia, reflux, short esophagus
  - Often with ulceration
  - Short, smooth, tapered, symmetric or asymmetric
- **Barrett Esophagus**
  - Distal or midesophagus
  - Often with ulceration

- Short or moderate length, symmetric or asymmetric
- **Esophageal Carcinoma**
  - Middle 1/3 (50%), lower 1/3 (30%), and upper 1/3 (20%)
  - Abrupt narrowing, apple core
  - Irregular nodular surface; ulceration
  - Moderate length; asymmetric
  - Absent peristalsis through length of tumor
- **Scleroderma, Esophagus**
  - Distal 1/3
  - Short or moderate length; symmetric taper
  - Diminished or absent peristalsis
    - Mild to moderate dilatation of esophagus
  - Correlate with pulmonary and skin findings

Helpful Clues for Less Common Diagnoses

- **Esophageal Metastases and Lymphoma**
  - Lung or gastric cancer may invade esophagus
  - Hematogenous metastases and lymphoma are rare
  - Nodal metastases in mediastinum may compress esophagus
- **Radiation Esophagitis**
  - Long stricture of midesophagus
  - Check for history of radiation therapy (lymphoma, lung, or breast cancer)
- **Caustic Esophagitis**
  - Long, high-grade stricture
- **Nasogastric Intubation**
  - Mimics caustic ingestion stricture

Helpful Clues for Rare Diagnoses

- **Glutaraldehyde-Induced Injury**
  - Agent used to sterilize endoscopes is very caustic, and thorough instrument cleansing is advised to minimize risk of injury

SELECTED REFERENCES

1. Chung JH et al: Imaging features of systemic sclerosis-associated interstitial lung disease. J Vis Exp. (160), 2020
2. Elsherif SB et al: Role of precision imaging in esophageal cancer. J Thorac Dis. 12(9):5159-76, 2020

Barrett Esophagus

Spasm

(Left) *Esophagram shows a stricture and ulceration* ➜ *of the distal 1/3 of the esophagus.* (Right) *Moderate to severe esophageal spasm in the midesophagus* ➜ *is associated with episodes of retching and mild gastroesophageal reflux.*

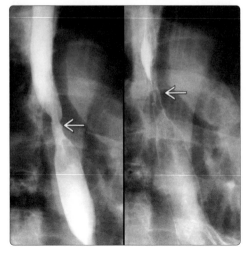
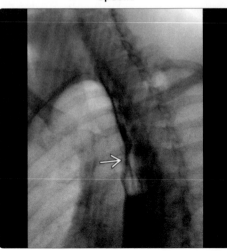

Esophageal Carcinoma

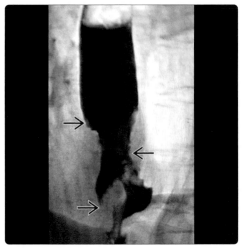

Scleroderma, Esophagus

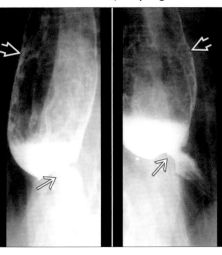

(Left) *Esophagram shows an apple core narrowing* ➡ *of the distal esophagus with nodular, destroyed mucosal surface.* (Right) *Esophagram shows a tight stricture of the distal esophagus* ➡ *with a markedly dilated, atonic esophagus* ➡. *The appearance mimics achalasia, but the stricture is more abrupt and irregular.*

Esophageal Metastases and Lymphoma

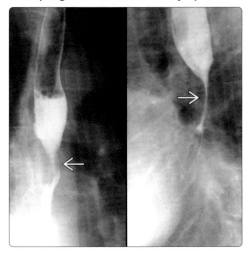

Radiation Esophagitis

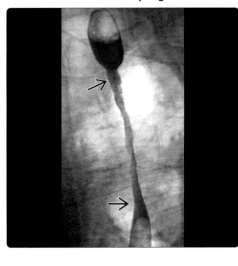

(Left) *Esophagram shows a tight but smoothly tapered stricture* ➡ *of the midesophagus due to direct invasion by lung cancer.* (Right) *Esophagram shows a long stricture* ➡ *of the midesophagus 8 months after radiation therapy for right lung cancer and mediastinal lymph node metastases.*

Caustic Esophagitis

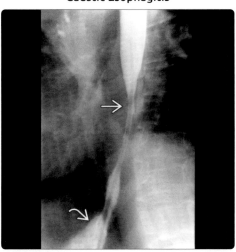

Drug-Induced Esophagitis

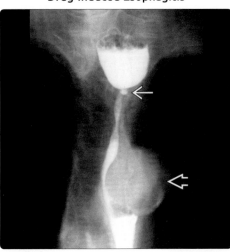

(Left) *Esophagram shows a long, smooth stricture* ➡ *of the distal 1/2 of the esophagus with a shortened esophagus causing hiatal hernia* ➡. (Right) *Esophagram shows a high-grade stricture and ulceration* ➡ *of the proximal esophagus, just above the aortic knob* ➡, *in this older woman with odynophagia.*

Esophagus

DIFFERENTIAL DIAGNOSIS

Common

- Achalasia, Esophagus
- Scleroderma, Esophagus
- Postvagotomy State
- Fundoplication Complications
- Reflux Esophagitis
- Esophageal Carcinoma
- Hiatal Hernia (Mimic)
- Postesophagectomy (Mimic)

Less Common

- Gastric Carcinoma
- Metastases and Lymphoma, Esophageal
- Chagas Disease

ESSENTIAL INFORMATION

Key Differential Diagnosis Issues

- Check for history of prior surgery
  - Esophagectomy (Ivor-Lewis and variations)
  - Fundoplication
  - Vagotomy

Helpful Clues for Common Diagnoses

- **Achalasia, Esophagus**
  - Primary motility disorder; aperistaltic
  - Grossly dilated esophagus; often elongated
  - Ends in smooth taper; "bird beak"
  - Onset in younger patients (20-40 years), progresses with age
- **Scleroderma, Esophagus**
  - Collagen vascular disorder of skin, smooth muscle
    - Most common sites: Esophagus > duodenum > anorectal > small bowel > colon
  - Diminished or absent peristalsis
  - Stricture and esophageal dilation are late findings
  - More common in women
- **Postvagotomy State**

- Vagotomy often performed for acid peptic disease
- Reflux (peptic) stricture may contribute to dilation
  - But lumen is rarely significantly dilated
- **Fundoplication Complications**
  - Fundoplication wrap may be excessively tight, impairing esophageal emptying
  - Especially common in older adults, who also have presbyesophagus (nonspecific esophageal dysmotility)
- **Reflux Esophagitis**
  - Esophagitis may cause diminished peristalsis
  - Peptic stricture contributes to dilation
- **Esophageal Carcinoma**
  - Narrowed lumen may cause dilation of esophagus upstream
- **Hiatal Hernia (Mimic)**
  - Intrathoracic part of stomach may be mistaken for dilated esophagus
    - More likely to be mistaken on axial CT imaging
    - Coronal reformation can help to clarify
- **Postesophagectomy (Mimic)**
  - Ivor-Lewis or similar operations
  - Mobilization of stomach to create gastric tube/conduit that will replace resected esophagus
  - May be mistaken for dilated esophagus on esophagram, CT, etc.

Helpful Clues for Less Common Diagnoses

- **Gastric Carcinoma**
  - Cancer arising in gastric cardia or fundus may invade distal esophagus submucosa
  - Involvement of intramural nerves may result in diminished peristalsis
  - Tumor may also narrow lumen of distal esophagus
- **Chagas Disease**
  - Parasitic disease common in South America and Mexico

(Left) *Upright spot film from an esophagram shows a markedly dilated esophagus with very delayed emptying, indicated by the persistent air-fluid contrast levels ➡. The esophagus narrows at the esophagogastric junction to a tapered bird beak appearance ➚. **(Right)** Upright spot film from an esophagram shows marked dilation and atony of the esophagus with stasis of barium and a tight stricture ➡ at the gastroesophageal junction. The appearance mimics achalasia, but clinical features are usually very different.*

Achalasia, Esophagus

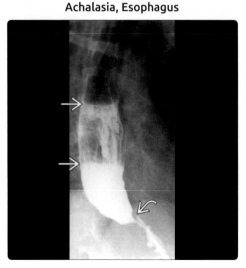

Scleroderma, Esophagus

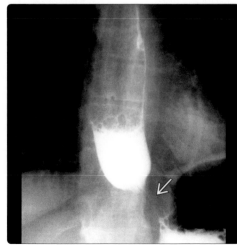

Postvagotomy State

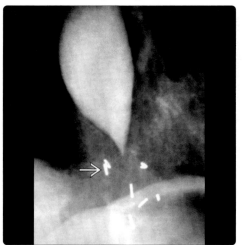

Fundoplication Complications

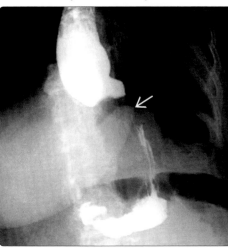

(Left) *Spot film from an esophagram shows a dilated esophagus with a smooth-tapered stricture just above the esophagogastric junction. Note the clips from vagotomy* ⊞. (Right) *Upright spot film from a esophagram in an older adult woman shows a dilated esophagus with stasis of food and barium. The esophageal lumen is tightly compressed at the site of the fundoplication* ⊞.

Esophageal Carcinoma

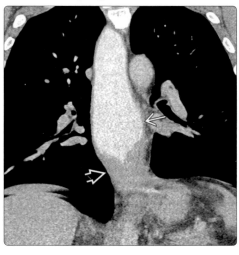

Hiatal Hernia (Mimic)

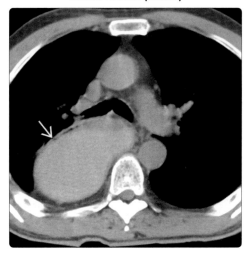

(Left) *Coronal portal venous phase CECT shows a dilated esophagus with an abrupt cutoff* ⊞ *and shouldering due to a circumferential mass* ⊞ *in the distal esophagus. Pathology showed poorly differentiated adenocarcinoma.* (Right) *Axial NECT shows a dilated tubular structure* ⊞ *in the thorax containing oral contrast. On axial CT, it would be difficult to recognize this as a hiatal hernia and not a dilated esophagus.*

Postesophagectomy (Mimic)

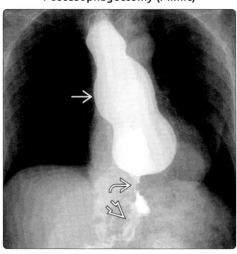

Gastric Carcinoma

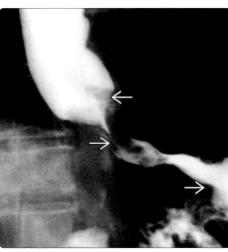

(Left) *Esophagram shows massive dilation of the gastric conduit* ⊞, *pulled into the chest to replace a resected portion of the esophagus. The conduit is not redundant, but it is mechanically obstructed by narrowing as it traverses diaphragmatic hiatus* ⊞. *The subdiaphragmatic stomach* ⊞ *is collapsed and normal.* (Right) *Esophagram shows a dilated esophagus with abrupt narrowing at the gastroesophageal junction. A mass causes constriction of the gastric cardia and fundus* ⊞ *and extends into submucosa of the esophagus.*

DIFFERENTIAL DIAGNOSIS

Common
- Zenker Diverticulum
- Traction Diverticulum
- Pulsion Diverticulum
- Hiatal Hernia (Mimic)
- Postesophagectomy (Mimic)
- Fundoplication Complications (Mimic)

Less Common
- Killian-Jamieson Diverticulum
- Intramural Pseudodiverticulosis
- Boerhaave Syndrome (Mimic)

ESSENTIAL INFORMATION

Key Differential Diagnosis Issues
- Most diverticula are pulsion and are associated with abnormalities of esophageal peristalsis

Helpful Clues for Common Diagnoses
- **Zenker Diverticulum**
  - Outpouching from posterior wall of pharyngoesophageal junction; just above cricopharyngeus muscle
  - Usually starts at C5-C6 vertebral level
    - May extend caudally into upper mediastinum
  - Increased prevalence with aging and dysmotility conditions
  - Regurgitation or emptying of barium into hypopharynx
- **Traction Diverticulum**
  - Usually midesophagus near carina
  - Acquired due to adherence to subcarinal or perihilar granulomatous lymph nodes
  - Tented or triangular in shape with pointed tip, wide mouth on esophagogram
    - Diverticulum tends to empty when esophagus is collapsed (because it contains all layers) vs. pulsion diverticula that remains filled after most of barium is emptied due to lack of muscle

- **Pulsion Diverticulum**
  - Saccular, often large, outpouching
  - Distal (epiphrenic) is most common
    - Usually smooth, rounded contour and wide neck from side of distal esophagus; right side > left
  - Strongly associated with esophageal motility disturbances (e.g., presbyesophagus, diffuse esophageal spasm)
  - Easily mistaken for hiatal hernia and vice versa
- **Postesophagectomy (Mimic)**
  - Ivor-Lewis and other procedures for distal esophagectomy and gastric pull through
  - Gastric conduit pulled into chest and anastomosed to stump of esophagus
    - Anastomosis is usually above carina
  - Outpouching at anastomosis or dilation of gastric conduit may mimic diverticulum or dilated esophagus
    - Look for rugae to distinguish stomach from esophagus
- **Fundoplication Complications (Mimic)**
  - Barium may fill portions of fundal wrap, resembling diverticulum
    - Rugae within collection identify it as stomach

Helpful Clues for Less Common Diagnoses
- **Killian-Jamieson Diverticulum**
  - Originate from anterolateral wall of cervical esophagus; opening below cricopharyngeus muscle
  - Higher, more anterior and usually smaller than Zenker diverticulum
- **Intramural Pseudodiverticulosis**
  - Barium trapped in dilated excretory ducts of deep mucous glands
  - Multiple, tiny (1- to 4-mm depth), flask-like outpouchings
- **Boerhaave Syndrome (Mimic)**
  - May result in paraesophageal collection of gas, fluid, or contrast medium

(Left) *Esophagram shows a moderate-sized diverticulum ➡ originating at the pharyngoesophageal junction that extends into the upper mediastinum. Posterior indentation of the cricopharyngeus muscle is also seen ➡. (Right) Esophagram shows an outpouching ➡ from the midesophagus (carinal level). Note the calcified perihilar lymph nodes ➡.*

Zenker Diverticulum

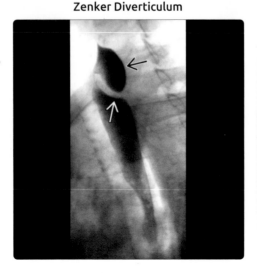

Traction Diverticulum

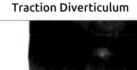
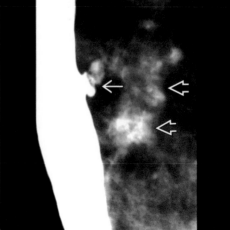

Pulsion Diverticulum

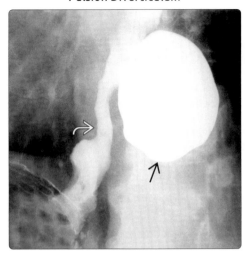

Pulsion Diverticulum

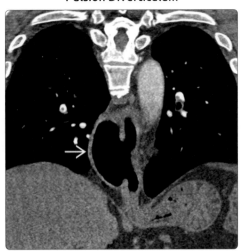

(Left) *Esophagram shows an unusually large pulsion diverticulum ⮕ projecting from the middistal esophagus. Primary esophageal peristalsis was markedly diminished, and deep tertiary contractions were noted ⮕.* (Right) *Coronal CECT shows a large pulsion diverticulum ⮕ projecting laterally from the distal esophagus.*

Fundoplication Complications (Mimic)

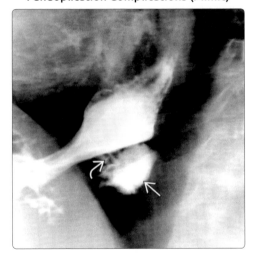

Killian-Jamieson Diverticulum

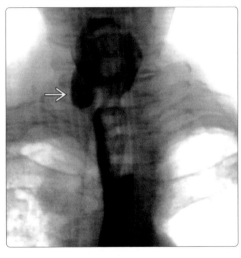

(Left) *Esophagram shows a collection of barium ⮕ within the fundoplication wrap, which has slipped into the thorax. Note the rugal folds ⮕, identifying it as stomach rather than a leak.* (Right) *Esophagram shows an outpouching ⮕ from the anterolateral wall of the cervical esophagus, a Killian-Jamison diverticulum.*

Intramural Pseudodiverticulosis

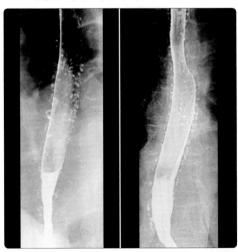

Boerhaave Syndrome (Mimic)

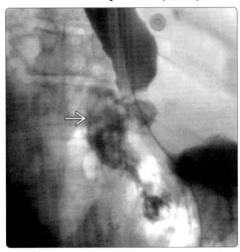

(Left) *Esophagram shows innumerable tiny, flask-shaped outpouchings of barium within the wall of the esophagus.* (Right) *Esophagram shows an irregular collection of contrast and gas ⮕ in the lower mediastinum, which has leaked out of the perforated distal esophagus.*

DIFFERENTIAL DIAGNOSIS

Common

- Presbyesophagus
- Diffuse Esophageal Spasm
- Achalasia, Esophagus
- Scleroderma, Esophagus
- Reflux Esophagitis
- Surgical Complications
  - Fundoplication Complications
  - Postvagotomy State

Less Common

- Neuromuscular Disorders
- Esophageal Carcinoma
- Gastric Carcinoma

ESSENTIAL INFORMATION

Key Differential Diagnosis Issues

- Manometry and barium esophagram are complementary

Helpful Clues for Common Diagnoses

- **Presbyesophagus**
  - Nonspecific esophageal motility disorder
  - Increased prevalence with aging
  - Decreased primary peristalsis; frequent tertiary (nonpropulsive) contractions
- **Diffuse Esophageal Spasm**
  - Intermittent disruption of primary peristalsis with focally obliterative secondary or tertiary contractions
  - May impart corkscrew appearance to esophagram
  - May cause chest pain simulating angina
- **Achalasia, Esophagus**
  - Absent primary peristalsis
  - May have tertiary contractions early in disease
  - Dilated esophagus ending in tapered bird beak deformity
- **Scleroderma, Esophagus**
  - Multisystem collagen vascular disease

- Early disease: Nonperistaltic esophagus with patulous gastroesophageal (GE) junction
- Late disease: Dilated esophagus with peptic stricture at GE junction; simulates achalasia
- **Reflux Esophagitis**
  - Esophagus is often foreshortened (spasm of longitudinal muscles)
    - Esophageal lumen is usually not very dilated
  - Distal peptic stricture; possible ulcerations and nodular mucosa
  - Esophagitis itself impairs normal peristalsis
- **Surgical Complications**
  - Fundoplication or vagotomy may result in narrowed distal esophagus and poor esophageal emptying

Helpful Clues for Less Common Diagnoses

- **Neuromuscular Disorders**
  - Diseases, such as multiple sclerosis, ALS, and myasthenia gravis, may impair esophageal motility
- **Esophageal Carcinoma**
  - Combination of luminal narrowing and submucosal nerve plexus destruction
- **Gastric Carcinoma**
  - Carcinoma of gastric fundus may invade esophageal submucosa
    - Look for nodular, fixed folds in fundus on UGI or CT
    - Endoscopy is mandatory to evaluate for this possibility

Presbyesophagus

Diffuse Esophageal Spasm

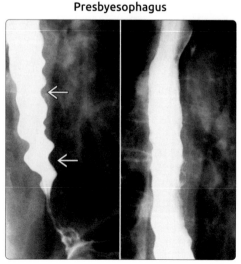 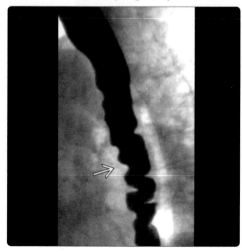

(Left) Spot films from an esophagram in this older man with dysphagia and food sticking show inconstant tertiary contractions ➡. Primary peristalsis was absent. These are typical features of nonspecific esophageal dysmotility (presbyesophagus). (Right) Spot film from an esophagram shows persistent deep contractions of the esophagus in an older adult patient with dysphagia and chest pain. This has been described as a corkscrew esophagus ➡.

Achalasia, Esophagus

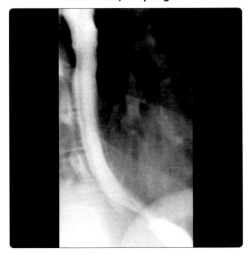

Scleroderma, Esophagus

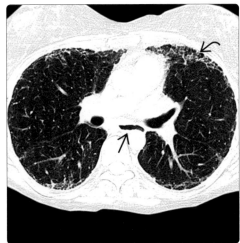

(Left) *Esophagram in a 28-year-old woman who had been treated with Heller myotomy shows a normal-caliber esophagus that emptied readily in the upright position. Upright positioning is inadequate to evaluate esophageal dysmotility.* **(Right)** *Axial CT in a 49-year-old woman with scleroderma is shown. Dilated esophagus ➡ with typical subpleural interstitial fibrosis is ➡ present.*

Scleroderma, Esophagus

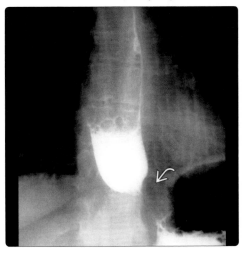

Reflux Esophagitis

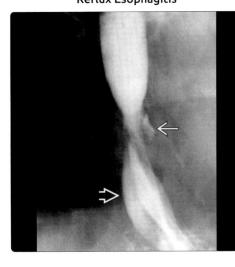

(Left) *A single film from a barium esophagram shows a dilated, atonic esophagus with a tight stricture at the gastroesophageal (GE) junction ➡. The esophagus was slow to empty, even in this upright position. This patient also had typical skin and intestinal features of scleroderma.* **(Right)** *Spot film from an esophagram shows a deep ulcer ➡ at the GE junction and a shortened esophagus with hiatal hernia ➡. Primary peristalsis was minimal.*

Fundoplication Complications

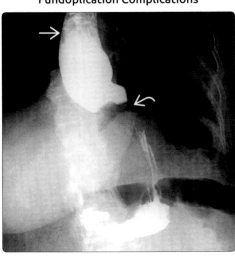

Postvagotomy State

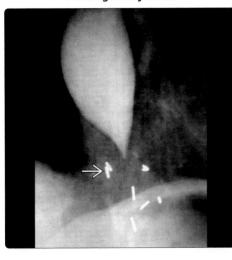

(Left) *A subsequent esophagram in this older woman who had fundoplication for GE reflux disease (GERD) shows a markedly dilated esophagus with retention of food ➡ and a very tight lumen at the site of the fundoplication ➡. Esophageal peristalsis was minimal.* **(Right)** *Spot film from an esophagram shows a dilated esophagus with a smooth, distal, tapered obstruction. Esophageal peristalsis was minimal. Note the clips ➡ from vagotomy.*

Esophagus

DIFFERENTIAL DIAGNOSIS

Common

- Pharyngitis
- Reflux Esophagitis
- *Candida* Esophagitis
- Viral Esophagitis
- Drug-Induced Esophagitis
- Esophageal Foreign Body

Less Common

- Caustic Esophagitis
- Radiation Esophagitis

ESSENTIAL INFORMATION

Key Differential Diagnosis Issues

- Odynophagia: Pain on swallowing
  - Almost always indicates mucosal irritation or ulceration
- Clinical setting and history are key elements in differential diagnosis

Helpful Clues for Common Diagnoses

- **Pharyngitis**
  - Inflammation of pharyngeal mucosa associated with several common viral and bacterial infections
  - This is clinical, not radiographic, diagnosis
- **Reflux Esophagitis**
  - Distal ulcers/erosions, hiatal hernia, reflux
- ***Candida* Esophagitis**
  - Common cause of odynophagia in immunocompromised patients (can occur in immunocompetent as well)
  - Usually associated with oral thrush
  - Shaggy esophageal surface; raised plaques and shallow ulcers
- **Viral Esophagitis**
  - Usually causes shallow ulcers on otherwise normal esophageal mucosal surface
  - Occurs in immunocompromised patients
- **Drug-Induced Esophagitis**
  - Causes sudden onset of severe odynophagia

- More common in older adult patients
- Often caused by antibiotics and cardiac medications
  - Ulceration, spasm, stricture at sites of normal luminal narrowing (aortic arch, left main bronchus, retrocardiac region)
- **Esophageal Foreign Body**
  - Fish or chicken bones often scratch pharynx (e.g., pyriform sinuses) or esophagus when swallowed
  - May be sufficiently radiopaque to visualize in radiography
  - May need to have patient swallow cotton swab soaked in barium to identify luminal projection of foreign body

Helpful Clues for Less Common Diagnoses

- **Caustic Esophagitis**
  - Odynophagia is severe and immediate following ingestion of strong acid or alkaline material
  - May prevent immediate evaluation by barium esophagram
  - CT is good alternative to demonstrate esophageal wall thickening, any evidence of perforation, aspiration pneumonitis

Reflux Esophagitis

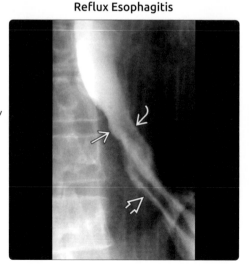

Candida Esophagitis

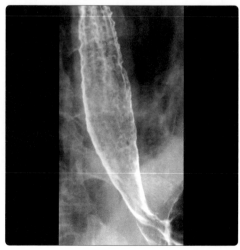

(Left) *Spot film from an esophagram shows a small hiatal hernia ⇨ and a shortened esophagus with a distal esophageal stricture ⇨ and a broad-based ulcer ⇨.* (Right) *Spot film from an esophagram shows a markedly irregular mucosal surface due to raised plaques and superficial ulcerations.*

Viral Esophagitis

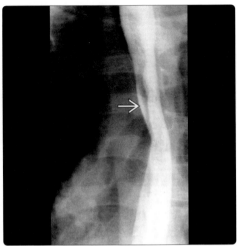

Viral Esophagitis

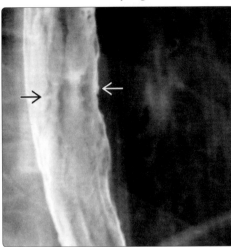

(Left) *Spot film from an esophagram shows a large, shallow ulcer* ⮕ *in an otherwise normal esophagus in a patient with AIDS, HIV-induced ulceration.* (Right) *Spot film from an esophagram shows both superficial ulcerations* ⮕ *and raised plaques* ⮕, *proven to be due to viral (herpes) esophagitis but indistinguishable from Candida esophagitis by imaging.*

Drug-Induced Esophagitis

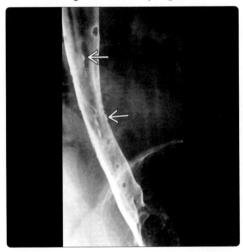

Esophageal Foreign Body

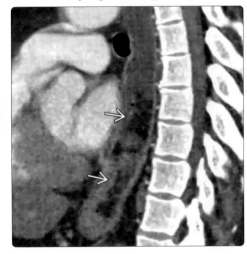

(Left) *Spot film from an esophagram shows multiple ulcerations* ⮕ *due to tetracycline in a middle-aged woman with severe odynophagia.* (Right) *Sagittal CECT in a patient with chest pain after a steak dinner is shown. Note dilated esophagus containing areas of low attenuation* ⮕, *consistent with fat in the steak meat.*

Caustic Esophagitis

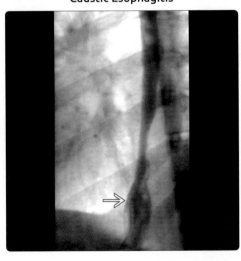

Radiation Esophagitis

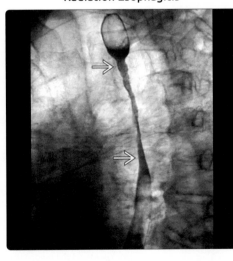

(Left) *Spot film from an esophagram shows a long stricture and shortening of the distal 2/3 of the esophagus, the result of lye ingestion several days earlier. The stomach* ⮕ *is pulled up into the chest as a result of spasm of the longitudinal esophageal muscles.* (Right) *Spot film from an esophagram shows a long stricture* ⮕ *of the midesophagus due to radiation injury following treatment for lung cancer with mediastinal lymphadenopathy.*

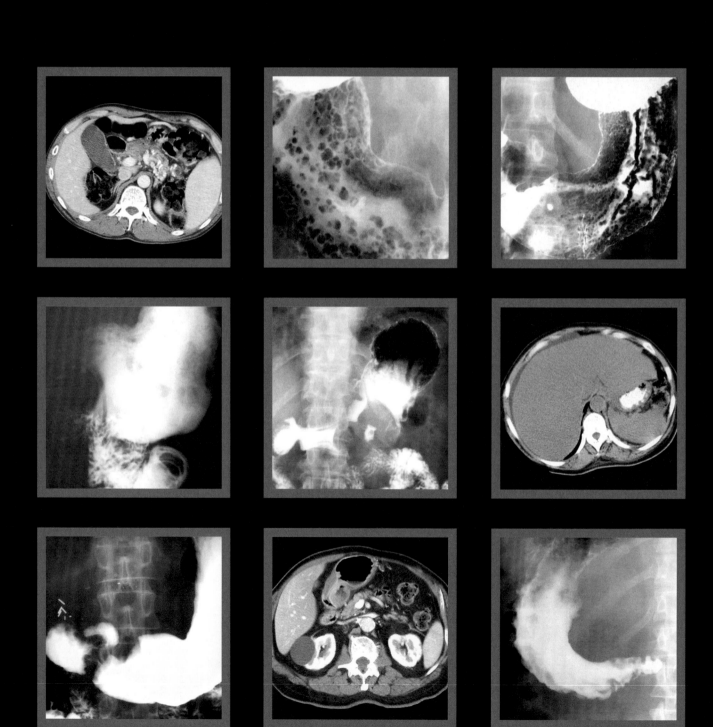

SECTION 4
Stomach

Generic Imaging Patterns

Gastric Mass Lesions   90
Intramural Mass, Stomach   96
Target or Bull's-Eye Lesions, Stomach   98
Gastric Ulceration (Without Mass)   100
Intrathoracic Stomach   102
Thickened Gastric Folds   104
Gastric Dilation or Outlet Obstruction   110
Linitis Plastica, Limited Distensibility   114

Clinically Based Differentials

Epigastric Pain   118
Left Upper Quadrant Mass   124

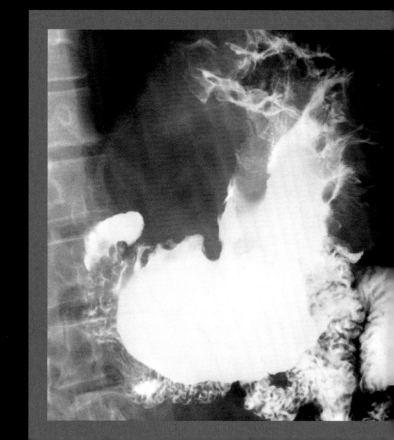

DIFFERENTIAL DIAGNOSIS

Common

- Gastric Carcinoma
- Hyperplastic Polyps
- Artifacts
  - Air (Gas) Bubbles
  - Apposed Walls of Stomach
- Adenomatous Polyp
- Bezoar (Mimic)
- Perigastric Mass (Mimic)
  - Splenomegaly and Hypersplenism
  - Renal Cell Carcinoma
  - Exophytic Hepatic Mass
  - Splenosis
- Gastric Varices

Less Common

- Gastrointestinal Stromal Tumor, Gastric
- Intramural Gastric Tumors
- Gastric Metastases and Lymphoma
- Gardner Syndrome
- Hamartomatous Polyposis Syndromes
- Other Mesenchymal Tumors
- Ectopic Pancreatic Tissue
- Hematoma, Gastric
- Duplication Cyst, Stomach
- Neuroendocrine Tumor

ESSENTIAL INFORMATION

Key Differential Diagnosis Issues

- Primary gastric mucosal lesion
  - Irregular surface; acute angles with inner wall of stomach
- Intramural mass lesion
  - Smooth mucosal surface; sharp obtuse angle with inner wall
- Extrinsic mass lesion
  - Smooth mucosal surface; shallow obtuse angles with gastric wall

Helpful Clues for Common Diagnoses

- **Gastric Carcinoma**
  - Variable morphologic features
  - Nodular folds, polypoid mass, ulceration are common in advanced disease
  - Lack of peristalsis and limited distensibility of affected part of stomach are key features on fluoroscopy [upper GI (UGI) series]
  - CT usually shows extension outside stomach (lymphatic, direct invasion, liver metastasis)
- **Hyperplastic Polyps**
  - Round, small (< 1 cm), sessile polyps; most common polyps
  - Usually multiple in fundus and body
  - Not premalignant
- **Artifacts**
  - **Air (gas) bubbles**
    - Swallowed air or dissolving gas granules may simulate small polypoid lesions on UGI series
  - **Apposed walls of stomach**
    - On air contrast UGI series, anterior and posterior walls of stomach may temporarily "stick together"
    - May mimic mass lesion in barium pool or mass coated with barium
- **Adenomatous Polyp**
  - Usually solitary, lobulated, or on stalk; > 1 cm
  - Usually in antrum
  - Considered premalignant
- **Bezoar (Mimic)**
  - History of prior surgery (e.g., partial gastrectomy), psychiatric disease
  - Adolescent girls may chew on ends of their hair; resulting in trichobezoar
  - Large, movable mass that fills stomach
  - Mottled appearance is result of air bubbles retained in interstices of mass
- **Perigastric Mass (Mimic)**
  - Mass arising from any adjacent structure may simulate gastric mass
  - On UGI series, extrinsic masses are especially likely to simulate intramural masses of stomach
  - On CT or MR, look for fat plane separating stomach from extrinsic mass
    - Multiplanar imaging is often useful
    - Look for claw sign indicating origin from extragastric organ
- **Gastric Varices**
  - In patient with portal hypertension or splenic vein occlusion
  - Easy to recognize on CECT; may mimic tumor on NECT or UGI series

Helpful Clues for Less Common Diagnoses

- **Gastrointestinal Stromal Tumor, Gastric**
  - Most common cause of large, exophytic mass arising from gastric wall
  - Mucosa stretched over mass, may ulcerate
  - CT: Large, exophytic mass with central necrosis; may contain gas, oral contrast medium
  - May be benign or malignant
- **Intramural Gastric Tumors**
  - Any component of gastric wall may give rise to benign or malignant tumor
    - Schwannoma, hemangioma, neuroendocrine, etc.
  - Gastric lipoma is most common lesion, recognized by fat content
  - May arise in gastric antrum; may prolapse through pylorus, causing intermittent obstruction
- **Gastric Metastases and Lymphoma**
  - Metastases may be nodular (e.g., melanoma, Kaposi sarcoma) or infiltrative/linitis plastica (e.g., breast)
  - Lymphoma: Usually massive, confluent thickening of gastric wall, regional or widespread adenopathy
    - Wall thickening from lymphoma usually exceeds that caused by carcinoma
    - Gastric outlet from lymphoma is uncommon to rare
- **Gardner Syndrome**
  - Familial adenomatous polyposis of colon + osteomas, desmoid tumors, adrenal, thyroid, and liver carcinomas, etc.
  - May also have adenomatous polyps in stomach

- Less common than colonic and small bowel polyps
- **Hamartomatous Polyposis Syndromes**
  - Peutz-Jeghers syndrome, Cronkite-Canada, Cowden, etc.
  - Hamartomatous polyps more common in small bowel and colon
    - Usually multiple, small, broad-based masses
    - Usually not carpeting bowel (unlike familial polyposis)
  - Polyps are not premalignant, but patients are at increased risk for carcinomas of GI tract (as well as of pancreas, breast, reproductive tract)
- **Ectopic Pancreatic Tissue**
  - Typical appearance is small mass along greater curvature of antrum
  - May have central umbilication (opening of primitive pancreatic duct)
- **Hematoma, Gastric**
  - From blunt or penetrating trauma
  - Prior placement of percutaneous gastrostomy tube should be considered
  - Hyperdense on CT
- **Duplication Cyst, Stomach**
  - May or may not communicate with stomach
  - May have water density or more proteinaceous contents (hyperdense on CT and hyperintense on T1 MR)
  - No enhancement of contents after contrast administration

Alternative Differential Approaches

- Causes of multiple gastric masses
  - Hyperplastic polyps
  - Gastric metastases and lymphoma
  - Gardner syndrome
  - Hamartomatous polyposis syndromes

SELECTED REFERENCES

1. Foley KG et al: Opportunities in cancer imaging: a review of oesophageal, gastric and colorectal malignancies. Clin Radiol. 76(10):748-62, 2021
2. Ahmed M: Gastrointestinal neuroendocrine tumors in 2020. World J Gastrointest Oncol. 12(8):791-807, 2020
3. Anderson AC et al: Multimodality imaging of gastric pathologic conditions: a primer for radiologists. Radiographics. 40(3):707-8, 2020
4. Ren Y et al: Multiple metabolic parameters and visual assessment of 18F-FDG uptake heterogeneity of PET/CT in advanced gastric cancer and primary gastric lymphoma. Abdom Radiol (NY). 45(11):3569-80, 2020

Gastric Carcinoma

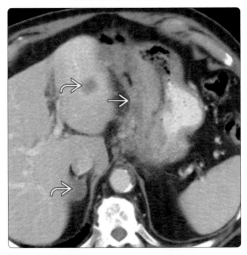

Gastric Carcinoma

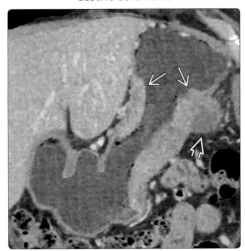

(Left) *Axial CECT in a 72-year-old man shows an eccentric, soft tissue density mass* ➡ *growing along the lesser curve of the stomach. Note the hepatic and adrenal metastases* ⊇. **(Right)** *Coronal CECT in a patient with gastric adenocarcinoma shows an annular gastric lesion* ➡, *which extends beyond the gastric lumen* ⊋.

Gastric Carcinoma

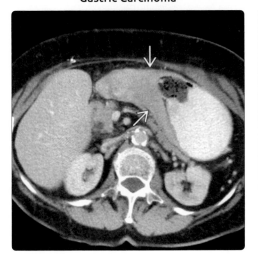

Air (Gas) Bubbles

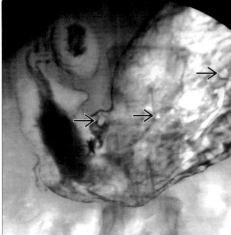

(Left) *Axial CECT shows soft tissue density infiltration of the wall of the distal stomach* ➡ *with gastric outlet obstruction suggested by the presence of retained food within the stomach. These are typical findings indicating the scirrhous, fibrotic character of many gastric carcinomas.* **(Right)** *Upper GI series shows what seem to be multiple barium-lined polyps* ⊇, *but these were mobile and transient, representing air bubbles. Upper endoscopy results were normal.*

Hyperplastic Polyps

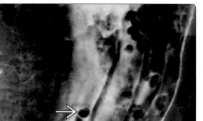

Hyperplastic Polyps

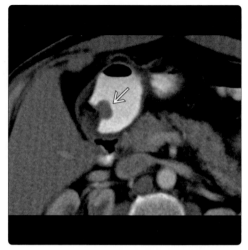

(Left) *Upper GI series shows multiple sharply defined polyps ➡ of similar small size, typical of hyperplastic polyps.* **(Right)** *Axial CECT shows a smooth, well-defined, hyperplastic polyp is present in the gastric antrum ➡. The lesion is well defined by oral contrast. The location and singularity is unusual for a hyperplastic polyp.*

Adenomatous Polyp

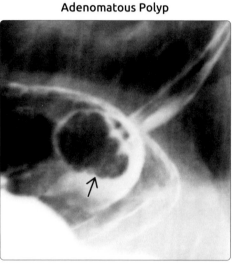

Adenomatous Polyp

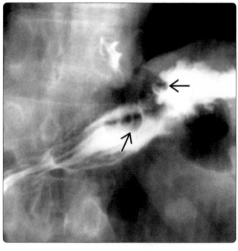

(Left) *Upper GI series shows a well-defined, sessile polyp ➡ just caudal to the esophagogastric junction, proven to be an adenomatous polyp on endoscopy and resection.* **(Right)** *Upper GI series shows several sessile and pedunculated gastric polyps ➡ in an older woman, which proved to be adenomatous polyps with villous architecture.*

Adenomatous Polyp

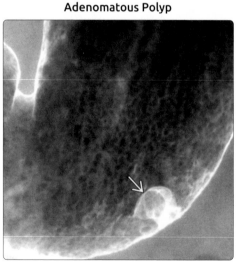

Adenomatous Polyp

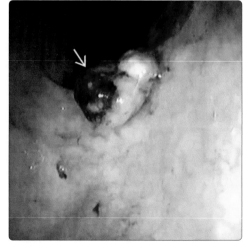

(Left) *Upper GI series in a 65-year-old woman shows a well-defined, sessile polyp ➡ with acute angles at its interface with the gastric wall.* **(Right)** *Endoscopy in the same patient shows an ulcerated mass ➡ that was proven to be a benign adenoma. A band was placed around the base of the polyp, and it was resected at endoscopy.*

Bezoar (Mimic)

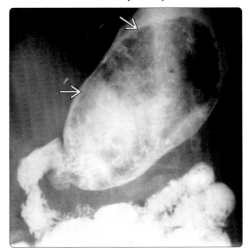

Perigastric Mass (Mimic)

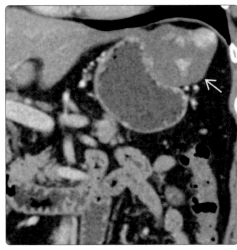

(Left) *Upper GI series shows a large, mobile filling defect or mass* ➡ *within the stomach. This patient had a prior vagotomy and distal antrectomy (Billroth 1 procedure) for peptic ulcer disease.* (Right) *Coronal CECT shows indentation of the stomach from an exophytic hepatic hemangioma* ➡ *mimicking a gastric mass. Note obtuse angles and intact gastric mucosa.*

Splenosis

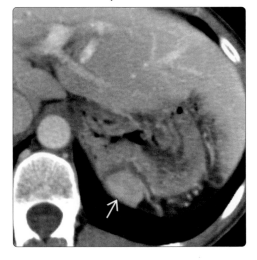

Gastric Varices

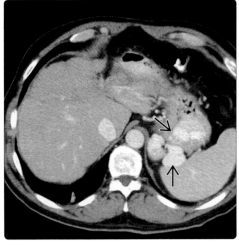

(Left) *Axial CECT shows an intramural mass* ➡ *(splenosis) in a patient who had splenectomy for traumatic splenic rupture some years previously.* (Right) *Axial CECT shows large varices* ➡ *that distort the fundus of the stomach in a patient with cirrhosis and portal hypertension. On an unenhanced CT or an upper GI series, these could mimic a neoplastic mass.*

Gastrointestinal Stromal Tumor, Gastric

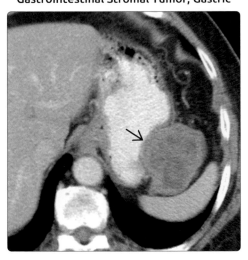

Gastrointestinal Stromal Tumor, Gastric

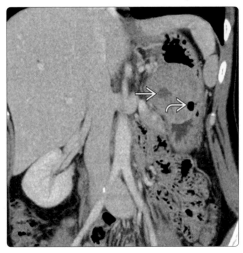

(Left) *Axial CECT shows a classic intramural mass* ➡ *with obtuse angles and intact gastric mucosa. Central necrosis in the mass is a clue to its etiology (gastric GI stromal tumor).* (Right) *Coronal CECT in a young woman shows a large, intramural gastric mass with central necrosis* ➡ *and air* ➡.

Intramural Gastric Tumors

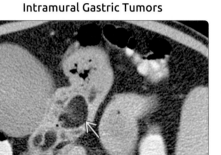

Gastric Metastases and Lymphoma

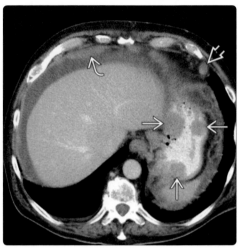

(Left) *Axial NECT shows one* ➡ *of several fat-density masses (lipomas) within the stomach but actually arising from the gastric wall. Intramural masses of the stomach and GI tract are frequently drawn into the gut lumen by peristalsis.* **(Right)** *Axial CECT in a patient with melanoma shows several intramural gastric masses* ➡, *along with metastases to nodes* ➡ *and the peritoneal surface* ➡.

Gastric Metastases and Lymphoma

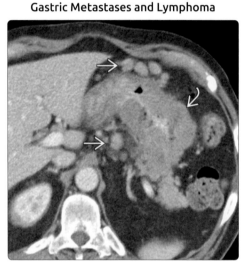

Gastric Metastases and Lymphoma

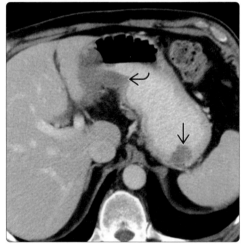

(Left) *Axial CECT shows circumferential, marked, soft tissue density thickening of the gastric wall* ➡ *and extensive perigastric lymphadenopathy* ➡, *typical features of gastric lymphoma.* **(Right)** *Axial CECT shows 2 soft tissue density masses in the stomach representing gastric lymphoma. One is a sessile polyp* ➡, *and the other is a bulky, circumferential antral mass* ➡.

Gastric Metastases and Lymphoma

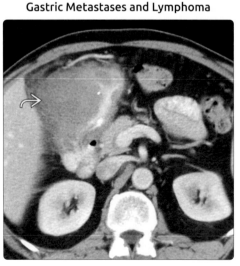

Gardner Syndrome

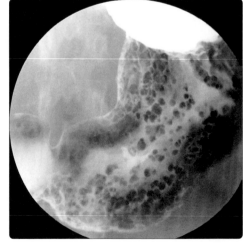

(Left) *Axial CECT shows a bulky, circumferential antral mass* ➡ *that is due to gastric lymphoma. There was no gastric outlet obstruction due to the soft nature of lymphomatous masses.* **(Right)** *Upper GI series shows innumerable small polyps that are larger and more irregular than usually seen with hyperplastic polyps. These are adenomatous (premalignant) polyps in a patient with familial polyposis (Gardner syndrome).*

Hamartomatous Polyposis Syndromes

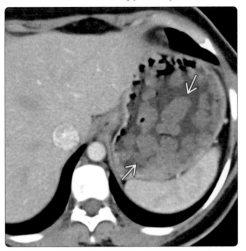

Hamartomatous Polyposis Syndromes

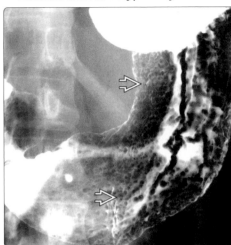

(Left) *Axial CECT in a patient with familial polyposis shows innumerable small polyps throughout the stomach ➔. These are larger, more numerous, and more irregular in shape than most hyperplastic polyps.* **(Right)** *Upper GI series shows innumerable small gastric polyps ➔ of similar size. In the general population, these would probably be hyperplastic polyps, but this patient has Peutz-Jeghers syndrome, and these are hamartomatous polyps.*

Hamartomatous Polyposis Syndromes

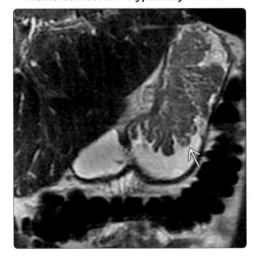

Other Mesenchymal Tumors

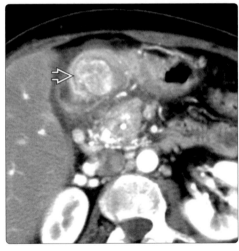

(Left) *Coronal T2 HASTE MR shows a large, sessile, hamartomatous polyp in the stomach ➔ associated with Peutz-Jeghers syndrome.* **(Right)** *Axial CECT shows a highly vascular mass ➔ in the posterior wall of the stomach as an incidental finding in a patient who had CT evaluation for chronic pancreatitis. This was surgically proven neurilemmoma.*

Duplication Cyst, Stomach

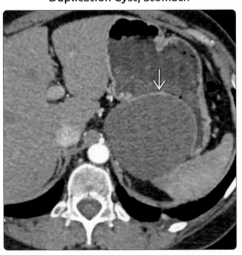

Neuroendocrine Tumor

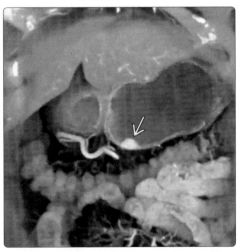

(Left) *Axial CT shows a round, cystic structure of fluid attenuation with a thin wall ➔ within the stomach, consistent with a duplication cyst.* **(Right)** *Hypervascular mass arising in the greater curvature of the stomach ➔ was a small carcinoid tumor.*

DIFFERENTIAL DIAGNOSIS

Common

- Gastric Varices
- Pancreatic Pseudocyst
- Gastric GI Stromal Tumor
- Metastases and Lymphoma, Gastric

Less Common

- Intramural Gastric Tumors
  - Lipoma
  - Neuroendocrine Tumor
  - Glomus Tumor
  - Leiomyoma
  - Schwannoma
  - Hemangioma
- Gastric Intramural Hematoma
- Heterotopic (Ectopic) Pancreatic Tissue
- Accessory Spleen or Splenosis
- Gastric Duplication Cyst

ESSENTIAL INFORMATION

Key Differential Diagnosis Issues

- It is often difficult to distinguish intramural from extrinsic masses
  - Even mucosal lesions (e.g., gastric carcinoma) may have overlapping features

Helpful Clues for Common Diagnoses

- **Gastric Varices**
  - CECT: Tortuous, tubular enhancing vessels in portal hypertension or splenic vein occlusion
- **Pancreatic Pseudocyst**
  - Indents posterior wall of stomach
  - Gastric mucosal folds overlying pseudocyst are often thickened due to inflammation
- **Gastric GI Stromal Tumor**
  - Well-circumscribed, subepithelial mass with large exophytic component
  - Often hypervascular with central necrosis

- May have mucosal ulceration
- **Metastases and Lymphoma, Gastric**
  - May be nodular and multiple (melanoma, Kaposi sarcoma) or diffuse (breast cancer)
    - May spread to stomach by direct extension (e.g., from pancreas), hematogenous (melanoma and breast), or via peritoneal seeding of gastric serosal surface (ovarian, uterine, GI primaries)
  - Lymphoma: Usually large, homogeneous tumor that does not obstruct stomach

Helpful Clues for Less Common Diagnoses

- **Intramural Gastric Tumors**
  - Lipoma; characteristic fat density
  - Other mesenchymal tumors (neuroma, fibroma, hemangioma, etc.)
    - Any component of gastric wall may give rise to benign or malignant tumor
    - Except for lipoma, have overlapping and nonspecific imaging features
    - Neuroendocrine tumor, glomus tumors, and hemangiomas are often hypervascular
    - Leiomyoma: Homogeneous, hypoenhancing small masses in gastric cardia; may calcify
- **Gastric Intramural Hematoma**
  - Following endoscopy, biopsy, percutaneous endoscopic gastrostomy (PEG) tube placement, or blunt trauma
- **Heterotopic (Ectopic) Pancreatic Tissue**
  - Small mural nodule along greater curvature of antrum with central umbilication (central barium-filled pit)
- **Accessory Spleen or Splenosis**
  - May indent or implant on gastric wall
  - Splenosis, following traumatic rupture of spleen, may implant anywhere on peritoneal surface
  - Multiphasic CECT or MR show same enhancement as spleen
  - Focal uptake on Tc heat-damaged RBC radionuclide scan is diagnostic
- **Gastric Duplication Cyst**
  - Rare; may or may not communicate with gastric lumen

Gastric Varices

Pancreatic Pseudocyst

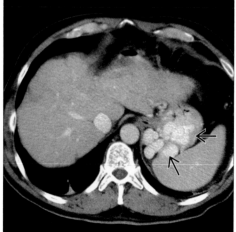 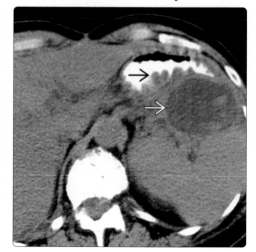

(Left) Axial CECT shows massive varices ➡ that deform the fundus of the stomach. On NECT or upper GI series, these would appear as a soft tissue density intramural mass. (Right) Axial NECT shows a pseudocyst ➡ that indents the posterior gastric wall. Note the thickened gastric folds ➡, suggesting intramural involvement by the pseudocyst.

Metastases and Lymphoma, Gastric

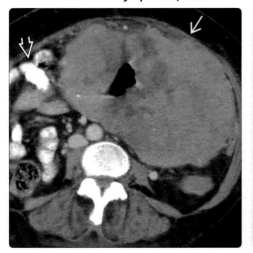

Metastases and Lymphoma, Gastric

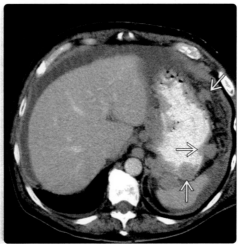

(Left) Axial CECT shows a large, circumferential soft tissue mass ⮕ that envelopes the gastric antrum but does not cause gastric outlet obstruction with passage of contrast into the small bowel ⮕. These are typical findings for gastric lymphoma. (Right) Axial CECT shows peritoneal and gastric wall metastases as discrete nodules ⮕ in this patient with metastatic melanoma. Omental metastases and malignant ascites were also evident.

Intramural Gastric Tumors

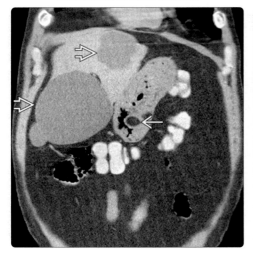

Glomus Tumor

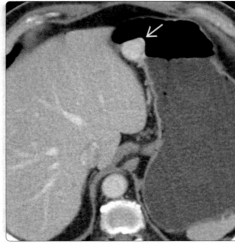

(Left) Coronal NECT shows a fat-density mass ⮕, a lipoma, within the gastric wall. There are 2 large benign cysts ⮕ in the liver as unrelated lesions. (Right) Axial CECT shows a hypervascular intramural mass ⮕ arising in the wall of the gastric antrum. Pathology showed glomus tumor.

Leiomyoma

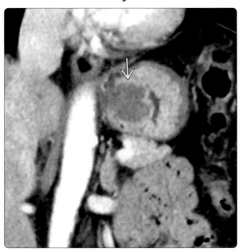

Heterotopic (Ectopic) Pancreatic Tissue

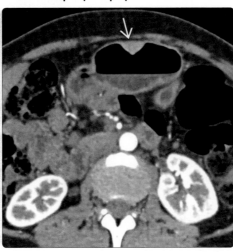

(Left) Coronal CECT shows a hypoenhancing mass within the stomach wall ⮕ in the region of the gastric cardia. (Right) Axial CECT shows the intramural mass in the gastric antrum with endoluminal growth ⮕ was heterotopic pancreatic tissue. The mass does not have any anatomic or vascular connection with the main pancreas.

DIFFERENTIAL DIAGNOSIS

Common

- Gastric Metastases
- Gastric Lymphoma
- Kaposi Sarcoma

Less Common

- Gastric GI Stromal Tumor
- Gastric Carcinoma
- Ectopic Pancreatic Tissue
- Carcinoid, Stomach
- Mesenchymal Tumors
  - Schwannoma

ESSENTIAL INFORMATION

Key Differential Diagnosis Issues

- Target or bull's-eye lesions are raised nodules or masses with central ulceration
  - Etiology is submucosal mass with ulceration of overlying mucosa
  - Highly suggestive of malignant gastric lesion (or ectopic pancreas)
    - Multiple lesions are almost always malignant
  - Target lesions are different from aphthous lesions (shallow erosions with small edematous mound; seen in gastritis)

Helpful Clues for Common Diagnoses

- **Gastric Metastases**
  - Most common cause of bull's-eye pattern of metastases is malignant melanoma
- **Gastric Lymphoma**
  - GI tract lymphoma can also cause bull's-eye lesions
    - Stomach is most common site
- **Kaposi Sarcoma**
  - Usually in homosexual men with AIDS
  - Stomach is most common site of GI tract involvement

Helpful Clues for Less Common Diagnoses

- **Gastric GI Stromal Tumor**
  - Stomach is most common site of GI stromal tumor
  - Usual appearance: Large exophytic mass arising from gastric wall
  - Erosion of overlying mucosa can result in bull's-eye appearance
    - Gas, fluid, and oral contrast medium may enter central necrotic area of GI stromal tumor
- **Gastric Carcinoma**
  - Rarely appears as single target lesion
  - Central ulceration is common, but surrounding tissue is more irregular and nodular than with other etiologies
- **Ectopic Pancreatic Tissue**
  - Usually single umbilicated lesion in gastric antrum
  - Does not result in multiple bull's-eye lesions
- **Carcinoid, Stomach**
  - From chromograffin cells in gastric mucosa
  - Does not produce carcinoid syndrome
  - Increased frequency in Zollinger-Ellison syndrome and atrophic gastritis
- **Mesenchymal Tumors**
  - **Schwannoma**
    - Rare, mostly benign
    - May be associated with neurofibromatosis
    - Slow-growing and mostly asymptomatic
      □ May present with bleeding and abdominal pain
    - CT: Mostly exophytic with homogeneous enhancement
    - Central ulcer can be seen in 25-50% of cases, secondary to mucosal ischemia

Gastric Metastases

Gastric Lymphoma

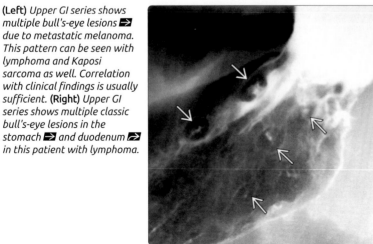
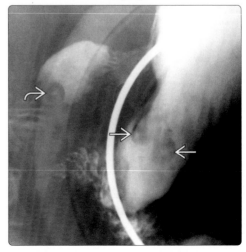

(Left) Upper GI series shows multiple bull's-eye lesions ➡ due to metastatic melanoma. This pattern can be seen with lymphoma and Kaposi sarcoma as well. Correlation with clinical findings is usually sufficient. (Right) Upper GI series shows multiple classic bull's-eye lesions in the stomach ➡ and duodenum ➡ in this patient with lymphoma.

Gastric Lymphoma

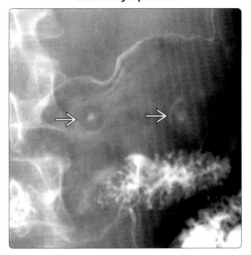

Gastric GI Stromal Tumor

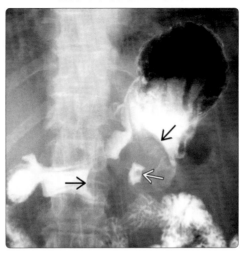

(Left) *Upper GI series shows classic bull's-eye lesions ➡ in the stomach on this air-contrast study with small masses and central umbilication.* (Right) *Upper GI series shows a large intramural mass ➡ with a central ulceration ➡, a typical appearance for a gastric GI stromal tumor (GIST). This lesion would be considered by many to be too large to constitute a bull's-eye lesion.*

Gastric Carcinoma

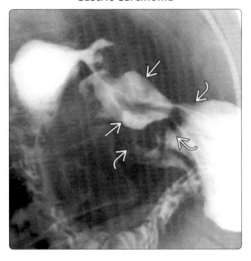

Ectopic Pancreatic Tissue

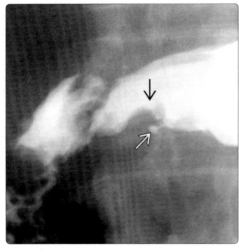

(Left) *Upper GI series shows a large ulcer ➡ (persistent collection of barium) within a larger mass ➡. This is not what is usually referred to as a bull's-eye lesion, but it is very suggestive of gastric carcinoma.* (Right) *Upper GI series in a 36-year-old man shows a pathognomonic appearance of an ectopic pancreas with a small mural mass ➡ in the antrum with an umbilication ➡, representing the orifice of a primitive pancreatic duct.*

Ectopic Pancreatic Tissue

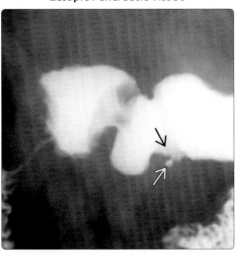

Mesenchymal Tumors

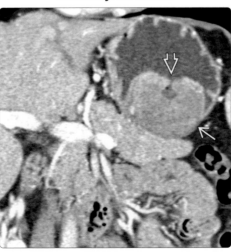

(Left) *Upper GI series in a 60-year-old woman shows a typical small intramural mass ➡ along the greater curve of the antrum with a central umbilication ➡, representing filling of a rudimentary pancreatic duct.* (Right) *Coronal CECT shows a homogeneously enhancing mass within the gastric lumen ➡. The lesion appears as a target lesion on barium studies and endoscopy due to the central ulceration ➡. Pathology showed a schwannoma.*

DIFFERENTIAL DIAGNOSIS

Common

- NSAID-Induced Gastritis
- Gastritis (Other Causes)
- Gastric Ulcer

Less Common

- Gastric Carcinoma
- Zollinger-Ellison Syndrome
- Crohn Disease
- Caustic Gastroduodenal Injury

ESSENTIAL INFORMATION

Key Differential Diagnosis Issues

- Gastritis is, by far, most common cause of gastric erosions or ulcerations

Helpful Clues for Common Diagnoses

- **NSAID-Induced Gastritis**
  - NSAIDs, including aspirin
  - Gastric erosion may be varioliform, linear, or serpiginous
  - Erosions may be clustered along dependent surface of stomach, distal body, or antrum
  - Distal 1/2 of greater curvature
- **Gastritis (Other Causes)**
  - Other medications, alcohol, uremia, idiopathic
  - Appearance similar to NSAID-induced gastritis, regardless of etiology
  - CT shows thick gastric wall, submucosal edema, shallow erosions
- **Gastric Ulcer**
  - Deeper erosion, into submucosa or even through wall of stomach
  - Often associated with *Helicobacter pylori* infection
  - Ulcers are usually found along lesser curvature or posterior wall of antrum or body
  - Ulcer projects beyond expected contour of stomach (on upper GI series and CT imaging)

- May cause perforation, often through posterior gastric wall into lesser sac
  - Look for enteric contrast medium, gas, blood within lesser sac
  - Usually much more evident on CT than on upper GI series

Helpful Clues for Less Common Diagnoses

- **Gastric Carcinoma**
  - Often causes ulceration; usually mass with irregular nodular folds around ulcer crater
  - Uneven shape; irregular or asymmetric edges; interruption and clubbing of radiating folds on en face view
  - Usually on greater curvature
  - Nodular, clubbed, fused, or amputated folds
  - Carman meniscus sign: Ulcer crater and radiolucent elevated border on profile view
  - Does not project beyond contour of stomach
  - Superficial or early cancer may have no visible mass
    - This form is rarely ulcerated
  - CT: Soft tissue density, nodular thickening of gastric wall
    - Infiltration of omentum, nodal, peritoneal, or liver metastases are often seen
- **Zollinger-Ellison Syndrome**
  - Gastrin-producing islet cell (neuroendocrine) tumor of pancreas
  - Intractable; multiple ulcers in stomach, duodenum, even proximal jejunum
  - CT: Hypervascular pancreatic mass (arterial phase), thick gastric folds, metastases
- **Crohn Disease**
  - May induce aphthoid erosions in stomach
  - Chronic involvement: Ram's horn contraction of distal body and antrum

NSAID-Induced Gastritis

Gastritis (Other Causes)

(Left) Spot film from an upper GI series shows thickened antral folds with linear erosions ➡ along the peaks of the folds, diagnostic of some form of gastritis. (Right) Spot film from an upper GI series shows superficial rounded and linear erosions ➡ (superficial ulcerations). On endoscopy, these were interpreted as erosive gastritis, cause not specified.

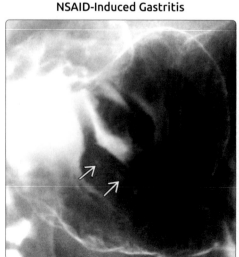

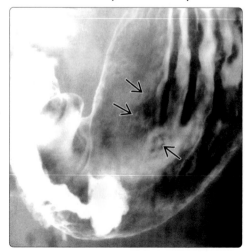

Gastric Ulcer

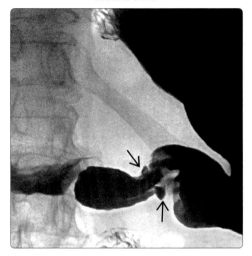

Gastric Ulcer

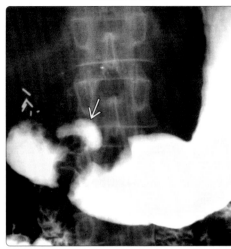

(Left) *Spot film from an upper GI series shows contraction of the antrum and thickened folds that extend to the edges of 2 discrete ulcers* ➡. (Right) *Spot film from an upper GI series shows a fixed collection of barium* ➡ *extending beyond the confines of the gastric wall. This was a perforated prepyloric ulcer. Note spasm and distortion of the antrum.*

Gastric Ulcer

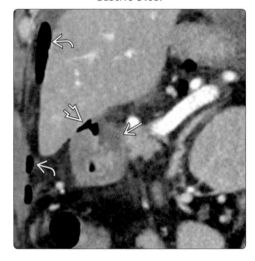

Gastric Carcinoma

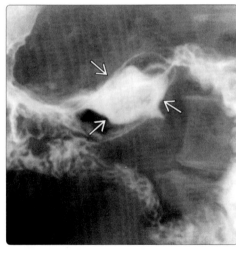

(Left) *Sagittal CECT of a gastric ulcer shows submucosal edema* ➡, *the site of perforation* ➡, *and free intraperitoneal air* ➡. (Right) *Prone oblique spot film from an upper GI series shows a large antral ulcer* ➡ *(fixed collection of barium). The surrounding mass is less evident, although fluoroscopy showed a stiff, nonperistaltic distal body and antrum that was found to be a large carcinoma at surgery.*

Zollinger-Ellison Syndrome

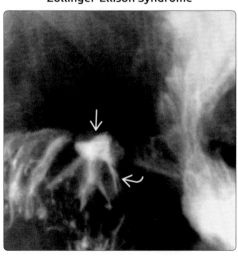

Crohn Disease

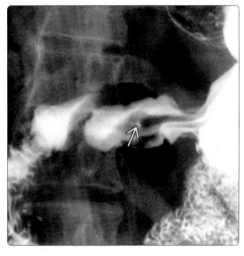

(Left) *Spot film from an upper GI series shows an ulcer* ➡ *at the site of a gastroenteric anastomosis following partial gastrectomy and vagotomy for ulcers. Note the folds* ➡ *radiating to edge of ulcer. Recurrent ulcers were a common feature of Zollinger-Ellison syndrome prior to improved diagnosis and therapy.* (Right) *Upper GI series shows an aphthous erosion* ➡ *of a thickened antral fold in a young man with proven Crohn gastritis who also had small bowel involvement.*

DIFFERENTIAL DIAGNOSIS

Common

- Hiatal Hernia
- Postesophagectomy
- Achalasia, Esophagus (Mimic)

Less Common

- Postoperative Fluid Collection (Mimic)
- Pulsion Diverticulum, Esophagus (Mimic)

ESSENTIAL INFORMATION

Key Differential Diagnosis Issues

- Dilated esophagus from any etiology may be mistaken for intrathoracic stomach (or vice versa)
  - Look for evidence of surgery (suture lines; portions of stomach missing from abdomen)
- Postoperative conditions can mimic or cause intrathoracic stomach
  - Ivor-Lewis or other type of esophagectomy with gastric pull-through
  - Gastric conduit (intrathoracic stomach) mimics dilated esophagus
- Epiphrenic esophageal diverticulum can mimic stomach on upper GI series, CT, or MR

Helpful Clues for Common Diagnoses

- **Hiatal Hernia**
  - Paraesophageal hernias may result in much or all of stomach lying in thorax
  - Type I: "Sliding"; gastroesophageal (GE) junction and cardia above diaphragm
  - Type II: Herniation of fundus through hiatus; GE junction below diaphragm (rare)
  - Type III: Most common type of paraesophageal hernia; GE junction and fundus ± body of stomach in chest
  - Type IV: Intrathoracic stomach; GE junction and most of stomach in chest
  - **CT useful in distinguishing between gastric volvulus and hiatal hernia**

- Types III and IV paraesophageal hernias have increased risk for gastric volvulus
  - Organoaxial volvulus: Rotation of stomach around its longitudinal axis
  - Mesenteroaxial volvulus: Rotation of stomach about its mesenteric (short) axis
  - Gastric volvulus with obstruction demands immediate decompression
- **Postesophagectomy**
  - Common surgical procedure for esophageal carcinoma
  - Much of stomach is pulled into thorax to replace resected portion of esophagus
    - Esophagogastric anastomosis is created in thorax, above level of tracheal carina (sometimes lower neck)
    - Distention and slow emptying of conduit are relatively common complications of procedure
  - Esophagogastric anastomosis is usually near thoracic inlet or carina
- **Achalasia, Esophagus (Mimic)**
  - May result in marked dilation of esophagus
  - Bird beak deformity: Dilated esophagus with smooth, symmetric, tapered narrowing at esophagogastric region
  - Distended lumen with air-fluid levels may simulate intrathoracic stomach, especially on axial CT
  - Length of narrowed segment < 3.5 cm; widest diameter upstream is > 4 cm

Helpful Clues for Less Common Diagnoses

- **Postoperative Fluid Collection (Mimic)**
  - Following esophagectomy, fundoplication, or repair of large hiatal hernia
  - May result in large collection of fluid ± gas that may simulate intrathoracic stomach
- **Pulsion Diverticulum, Esophagus (Mimic)**
  - Epiphrenic diverticula may be large
  - Retention of food, fluid, and gas simulates stomach
  - Associated with older adults; esophageal dysmotility syndromes

Hiatal Hernia

Hiatal Hernia

(Left) Coronal CECT shows massive dilation of the herniated stomach ➡, representing a large type III or even IV paraesophageal hernia with gastric volvulus. (Right) Axial CECT in this older woman with chest pain and retching shows a large type IV paraesophageal hernia ➡ (intrathoracic stomach). Note the compressed, atelectatic lung ➡.

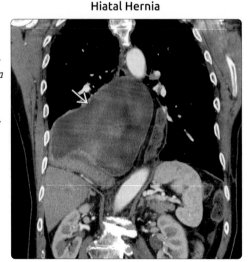

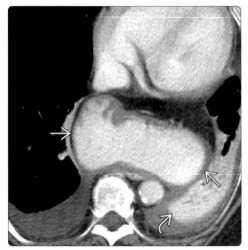

Postesophagectomy

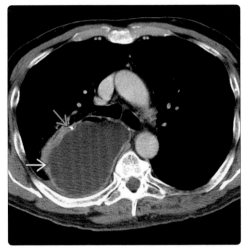

Postesophagectomy

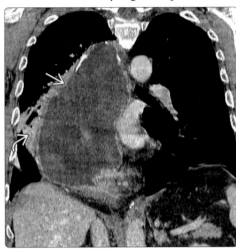

(Left) *Axial CECT in this 66-year-old man status post Ivor-Lewis esophagectomy shows a dilated gastric conduit ➡. Note the staple line ⇨ along the margin of the conduit.* **(Right)** *Coronal CECT in the same patient shows massive dilation of the gastric conduit (intrathoracic stomach) ➡ along with aspiration pneumonitis in the right lower lobe ➡.*

Achalasia, Esophagus (Mimic)

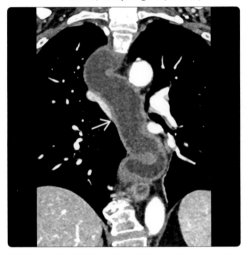

Postoperative Fluid Collection (Mimic)

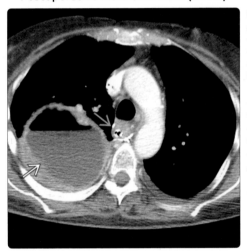

(Left) *Coronal CECT shows a grossly dilated, tortuous esophagus with a sigmoid appearance ➡ in this example of longstanding achalasia.* **(Right)** *Axial CECT in a patient who has had an Ivor-Lewis esophagectomy, a loculated collection of gas and fluid ➡ represents a large empyema due to an anastomotic leak but could be easily mistaken for a dilated gastric conduit. The nondilated conduit ⇨ is in its expected position.*

Pulsion Diverticulum, Esophagus (Mimic)

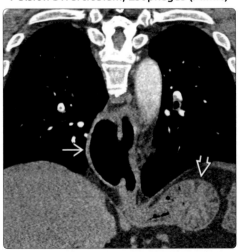

Pulsion Diverticulum, Esophagus (Mimic)

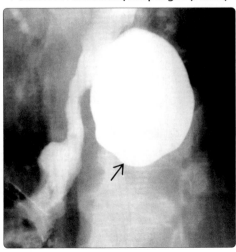

(Left) *Coronal CECT shows a large epiphrenic diverticulum ➡ in the distal esophagus. Note the presence of a normal stomach ➡.* **(Right)** *Esophagram shows a large epiphrenic pulsion diverticulum ⇨ and signs of esophageal dysmotility in this older man with dysphagia.*

DIFFERENTIAL DIAGNOSIS

Common

- Gastritis
- Gastric Ulcer
- Portal Hypertension, Varices
- Gastric Carcinoma
- Pancreatitis, Acute
  o Pancreatic Pseudocyst
- Portal Hypertensive Gastropathy

Less Common

- Gastric Metastases and Lymphoma
- Ménétrier Disease
- Zollinger-Ellison Syndrome
- Caustic Gastroduodenal Injury
- Crohn Disease
- Polyposis Syndromes Involving Stomach
- Candidiasis

Rare but Important

- Tuberculosis
- Radiation Gastritis
- Amyloidosis
- Eosinophilic Gastritis
- Chemotherapy-Induced Gastritis
- Sarcoidosis

ESSENTIAL INFORMATION

Key Differential Diagnosis Issues

- CT helps to narrow differential diagnosis by showing disease beyond stomach
  o e.g., metastatic tumor, signs of pancreatitis
- CT can show nature of submucosal thickening that is usual source of thick folds
  o Edema: Near-water attenuation = inflammatory or infectious
  o Soft tissue density = more likely to be neoplastic
    - Carcinoma, lymphoma, or metastases
- Correlation with history is important
  o e.g., history of pancreatitis, Crohn disease, extragastric malignancy

Helpful Clues for Common Diagnoses

- **Gastritis**
  o Symptomatic with abdominal pain
  o Causes: NSAIDs, alcohol, *Helicobacter pylori*
  o Antrum affected most commonly
  o Look for erosions, especially along rugal folds; limited distensibility
  o Erosive gastritis: Multiple punctate or slit-like collections of barium
  o NSAID induced: Linear or serpiginous erosions clustered in body on or near greater curvature
- **Gastric Ulcer**
  o Folds of uniform thickness radiate from edge of ulcer crater
  o Look for extraluminal gas or enteric contrast medium
- **Portal Hypertension, Varices**
  o Varices mostly in fundus

- Portal hypertensive gastropathy can affect entire stomach
  o Associated with portal hypertension (cirrhosis, splenomegaly, ascites)
  o Also caused by splenic vein occlusion (pancreatic carcinoma, chronic pancreatitis)
  o CECT: Usually distinguishes varices from other etiologies of thickened folds, shows underlying cause
    - Varices enhance like vessels on portal venous-phase CECT
    - Thick folds enhance like wall of stomach
- **Gastric Carcinoma**
  o Irregular, nodular, thickened folds
  o Submucosa of soft tissue density
  o Limited distensibility and peristalsis
    - These findings are more evident on upper GI series (fluoroscopy) than on CT
  o CT usually shows extragastric spread of tumor
    - Enlarged nodes, liver metastases, omental seeding
- **Pancreatitis, Acute**
  o Fold thickening of posterior wall of stomach, adjacent to pancreas
  o CT signs of pancreatitis: Enlarged gland, peripancreatic infiltration, fluid collections
  o **Pancreatic pseudocyst**
    - Back wall of stomach is often draped over pseudocyst
    - Gastric folds in contact with pseudocyst are thickened

Helpful Clues for Less Common Diagnoses

- **Gastric Metastases and Lymphoma**
  o Lymphoma
    - Massive nodular thickening of folds but usually normal distensibility
    - No outlet obstruction
  o Metastases may cause nodular intramural masses, ± ulceration, ± limited distensibility
    - Breast cancer especially likely to result in thick folds, limited distensibility
- **Ménétrier Disease**
  o Massive fold thickening in fundus and body
    - Antrum is usually spared
  o Hypersecretion of protein; hyposecretion of acid
    - May result in dilution and poor coating of barium on upper GI series
- **Zollinger-Ellison Syndrome**
  o Hypersecretion of acid and thick folds, multiple and recurrent ulcers at unusual locations
  o Gastrin-secreting neuroendocrine (islet cell) tumor of pancreas
    - CECT often shows hypervascular pancreatic tumor
  o May be part of multiple endocrine neoplasia syndrome
- **Caustic Gastroduodenal Injury**
  o Ingestion of strong alkali or acid
  o Acute findings = massive wall edema ± ulceration of mucosa
    - Difficult and potentially dangerous to perform upper GI series; CT shows pertinent findings in esophagus and stomach, including wall injury and possible perforation
  o End result is often perforation or linitis plastica appearance of stomach

- **Crohn Disease**
  - May cause gastritis with erosions and thickened folds
  - Multiple aphthous ulcers
  - Advanced disease → large ulcers, thickened folds, nodular or cobblestone mucosa
    - Longstanding involvement may cause ram's horn appearance
      - Nondistensible distal body and antrum with tapered curve toward pylorus
- **Polyposis Syndromes Involving Stomach**
  - Familial adenomatous polyposis (FAP) syndrome
    - > 50% of patients have gastric adenomatous or fundic gland polyps
  - Polyposis may mimic thickened folds
  - More nodular appearance
  - Presence of polyps elsewhere in GI tract

Helpful Clues for Rare Diagnoses

- **Tuberculosis**
  - Classic appearance is thickened folds and limited distensibility of stomach and duodenum
  - Relatively common in some populations (e.g., Native Americans)
- **Radiation Gastritis**
  - Nonspecific fold thickening and limited distensibility
  - History of upper abdominal radiation therapy is essential to diagnosis
- **Amyloidosis**
  - Look for evidence of systemic amyloid
  - Usually involves antrum
- **Eosinophilic Gastritis**
  - Mostly affects antrum
  - Check for peripheral blood eosinophilia
  - History of allergic diseases
- **Chemotherapy-Induced Gastritis**
  - Usually due to inadvertent perfusion of stomach during hepatic arterial infusion of floxuridine
- **Sarcoidosis**
  - Usually affects antrum
  - Check for pulmonary and hepatic involvement

Gastritis

Gastritis

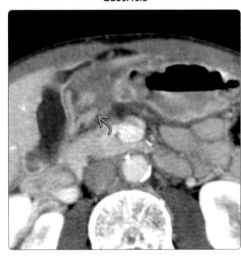

(Left) *Axial CECT in a 54-year-old man with acute gastritis shows a thickened and hyperemic gastric wall* ➡️. (Right) *Axial CECT in the same patient shows the base of the duodenal bulb* ➡️ *is indented, and edematous gastric folds are herniating into the bulb.*

Gastritis

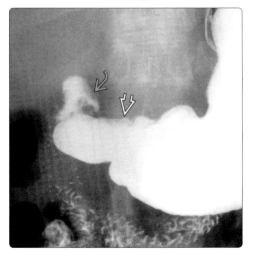

Gastritis

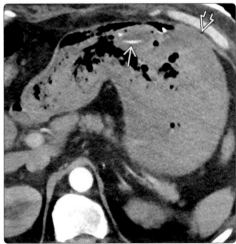

(Left) *Spot film from an upper GI series in the same patient shows a nondistensible antrum with thickened, nodular folds* ➡️, *and herniation of gastric folds into the duodenal bulb* ➡️. (Right) *Axial CECT in a patient with active gastric bleeding shows gastric extravasation of contrast* ➡️ *from a branch of the left gastric artery. Apparent wall thickening* ➡️ *is hemorrhage in the gastric lumen.*

Gastric Ulcer

Portal Hypertension, Varices

(Left) *Axial NECT in a 64-year-old man shows free intraperitoneal gas* ➜ *and extravasation of gastric contrast medium* ➜, *indicating a perforated gastric ulcer.* **(Right)** *Axial CECT shows active bleeding* ➜ *(extravasation of IV contrast) into the stomach due to portal hypertensive gastropathy from cirrhosis. Note the thick folds* ➜.

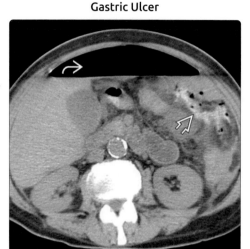

Gastric Carcinoma

Gastric Carcinoma

(Left) *Axial CECT in an older adult woman with early satiety shows gastric wall thickening* ➜ *of soft tissue density through the distal body and antrum. Note signs of gastric outlet obstruction.* **(Right)** *Spot film from an upper GI series in an older adult woman with early satiety and weight loss shows markedly thickened, nodular folds* ➜ *in the gastric body and antrum with lack of distensibility. No peristalsis was seen at fluoroscopy through the affected area.*

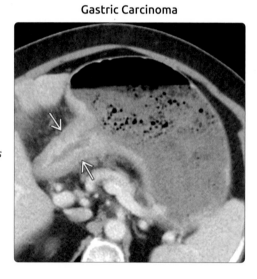
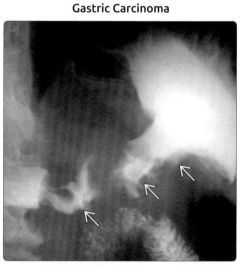

Gastric Carcinoma

Gastric Carcinoma

(Left) *Axial CECT in an older Asian man shows a circumferential soft tissue density mass* ➜ *that narrows the lumen of the gastric antrum with an abrupt transition from the distended, thin-walled proximal stomach. An irregular collection of gas and particulate material* ➜ *is noted within the antral mass.* **(Right)** *Axial CECT in the same patient shows a circumferential mass in the gastric antrum* ➜ *that appears as wall thickening due to poorly differentiated gastric adenocarcinoma with signet-ring cell features.*

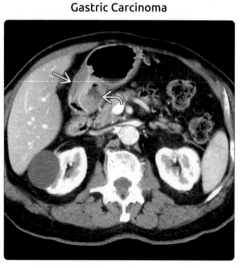
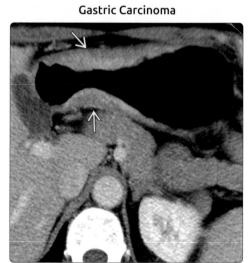

Pancreatitis, Acute

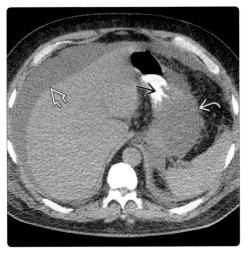

Pancreatic Pseudocyst

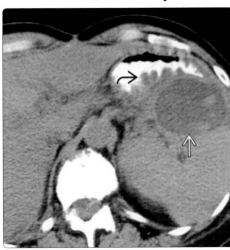

(Left) *Axial NECT in an older man with acute pancreatitis shows ascites* ➡️, *a lesser sac fluid collection* ➡️, *and thickened gastric folds along the greater curvature* ➡️. **(Right)** *Axial NECT in a 65-year-old woman shows a pancreatic pseudocyst* ➡️ *that displaces the posterior wall of the stomach and results in thickened gastric folds* ➡️.

Gastric Metastases and Lymphoma

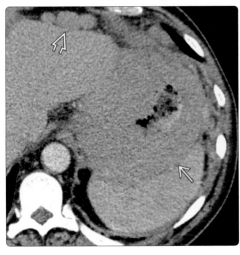

Gastric Metastases and Lymphoma

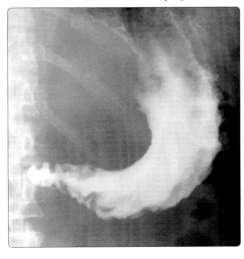

(Left) *Axial CECT shows a patient with diffuse gastric wall thickening* ➡️ *and cardiophrenic lymphadenopathy* ➡️ *secondary to MALT lymphoma.* **(Right)** *Spot film from an upper GI series in an older woman with fever and weight loss due to gastric lymphoma demonstrates marked thickening and blunting of the gastric folds but nearly normal distensibility and no obstruction.*

Gastric Metastases and Lymphoma

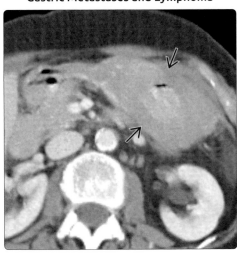

Gastric Metastases and Lymphoma

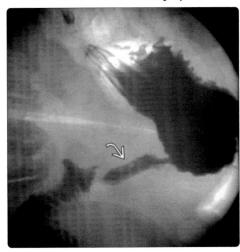

(Left) *Axial CECT in an older woman with gastric lymphoma shows a soft tissue density mass* ➡️ *that diffusely infiltrates the gastric wall. There was no sign of outlet obstruction.* **(Right)** *Spot film from an upper GI series in an older woman with metastatic breast cancer and early satiety shows a scirrhous lesion of the gastric antrum* ➡️ *that delays gastric emptying.*

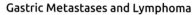

(Left) *Axial CECT in a patient with breast cancer shows gastric distention and retention of food. The antrum is nondistensible and infiltrated with a soft tissue density mass* ➡ *due to metastasis, though the imaging findings are indistinguishable from primary gastric carcinoma.* (Right) *Upper GI series shows massive fold thickening* ➡ *limited to the gastric fundus and body with sparing of the antrum. There are indirect signs of excess fluid secretion with poor coating of the gastric mucosa by the barium.*

Gastric Metastases and Lymphoma

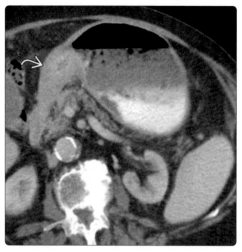

Ménétrier Disease

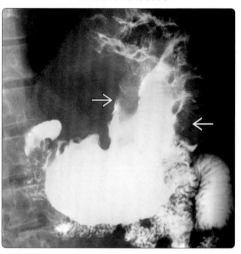

(Left) *Axial CECT in a 71-year-old woman shows massive fold thickening* ➡ *that was limited to the gastric fundus and body, mimicking the appearance of cerebral folds. Note the absence of a tumor mass.* (Right) *Axial CECT in a man with intractable ulcer symptoms shows hyperemia and fold thickening of the stomach* ➡. *A small gastrinoma in the pancreas (not shown) was responsible for Zollinger-Ellison syndrome.*

Ménétrier Disease

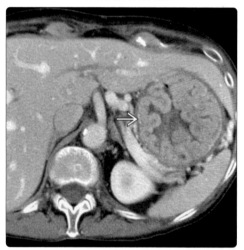

Zollinger-Ellison Syndrome

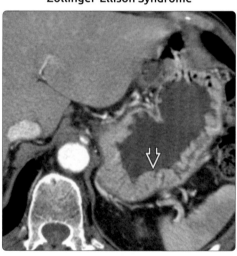

(Left) *Arterial-phase CECT shows thickened gastric folds* ➡ *secondary to gastrin-producing neuroendocrine tumor (gastrinoma) in the pancreatic body* ➡. (Right) *Axial CECT in a young woman who drank lye in a suicide attempt shows marked fold thickening, submucosal edema, and luminal narrowing of the stomach* ➡. *Similar findings were present in the esophagus, along with aspiration pneumonitis.*

Zollinger-Ellison Syndrome

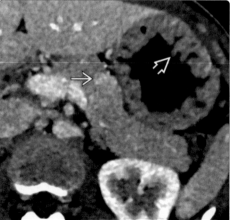

Caustic Gastroduodenal Injury

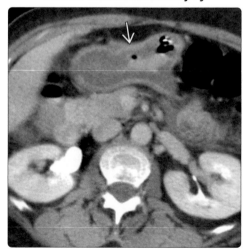

Crohn Disease

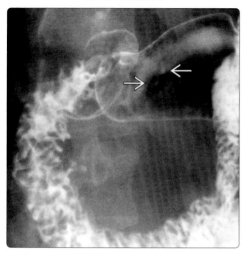

Crohn Disease

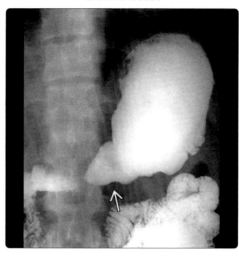

(Left) *Upper GI series in a young woman with Crohn gastritis shows incomplete distensibility of the antrum, thickened folds, and several shallow ulcerations (aphthous erosions)* ➡. *Endoscopic biopsy and correlation with clinical findings indicated that these were due to Crohn disease.* (Right) *Upper GI series in a 24-year-old man with chronic Crohn disease of the stomach and bowel shows decreased distensibility of the stomach with a ram's horn shape of the contracted body and antrum* ➡. *Also note thickened folds.*

Polyposis Syndromes Involving Stomach

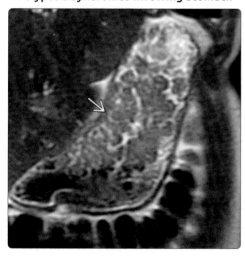

Polyposis Syndromes Involving Stomach

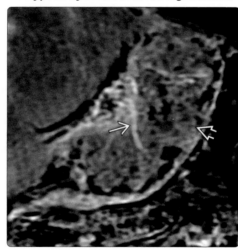

(Left) *Coronal T2 FS MR shows a large, hamartomatous polyp* ➡ *that appears as hypertrophic gastric folds.* (Right) *Coronal postcontrast MR in the same patient demonstrates vascularity* ➡ *of the hamartomatous polyp* ➡.

Candidiasis

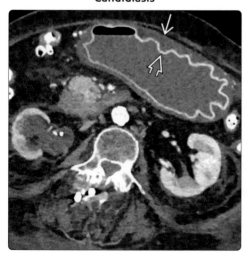

Amyloidosis

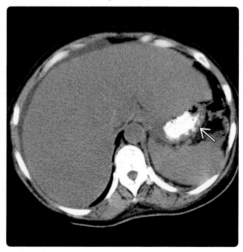

(Left) *Axial CECT in an immunocompromised patient shows gastric wall thickening* ➡ *and mucosal hyperenhancement* ➡ *from gastritis secondary to candidiasis.* (Right) *Axial NECT shows hepatosplenomegaly and thickened gastric folds due to amyloidosis* ➡. *Liver biopsy and endoscopy were used to confirm the histologic diagnoses.*

DIFFERENTIAL DIAGNOSIS

Common

- Gastric or Duodenal Ulcer
  - Gastritis
  - Peritonitis (Ruptured Peptic Ulcer)
- Gastric Carcinoma
- Gastroparesis
- Postoperative State, Stomach
  - Gastric Bezoar
  - Fundoplication Complications
  - Post Whipple Procedure
  - Post Vagotomy
- Gastric Volvulus
- Gastric Ileus
- Small Bowel Obstruction (Proximal)
- Aerophagia
- Carbonated Beverages
- Posttraumatic

Less Common

- Pancreatitis, Acute
- Pancreatitis, Chronic
- Metastases, Gastric
- Duodenal Mass or Stricture
  - Duodenal Carcinoma
  - Annular Pancreas
  - Metastases, Duodenal
- Gastric Polyps
- Muscular Disorder (Muscular Dystrophy, Cerebral Palsy)

Rare but Important

- Infiltrating Lesions
  - Crohn Disease (Gastric)
  - Chagas Disease
  - Sarcoidosis, Gastric
  - Tuberculosis, Gastroduodenal
  - Syphilis, Stomach
  - Amyloidosis
  - Electrolyte Imbalance
  - Scleroderma

ESSENTIAL INFORMATION

Key Differential Diagnosis Issues

- Look for mass or stricture in stomach or proximal bowel
- Recent onset of gastric outlet obstruction without long preceding history of "ulcer pain" should suggest malignant etiology

Helpful Clues for Common Diagnoses

- **Gastric or Duodenal Ulcer**
  - Peptic ulcers account for 2/3 of cases of gastric outlet obstruction
  - Prepyloric or duodenal ulcer may cause spasm, edema, and scarring that obstruct gastric outlet
    - Gastritis (many etiologies) is uncommon cause of outlet obstruction
    - Distinguished from ulcer by shallow mucosal erosions
  - Outlet obstruction is late finding

- Should be preceded by long history of pain attributable to peptic ulcer disease
- **Gastric Carcinoma**
  - 2nd most common cause of gastric outlet obstruction
    - Accounts for almost 1/3 of cases of gastric outlet obstruction
  - Involvement of antrum may obstruct outlet
  - Gastric carcinoma is often scirrhous
    - "Hard," inflexible mass that limits distensibility and peristalsis
    - Lack of peristalsis is most evident at fluoroscopic upper GI series
- **Gastroparesis**
  - Common sequela of diabetes, narcotic analgesics
  - Flaccid stomach without peristalsis
  - Radionuclide gastric-emptying study is best diagnostic tool
- **Postoperative State, Stomach**
  - **Gastric bezoar**
    - Increased prevalence following vagotomy and partial gastric resection
    - Look for large, heterogeneous mass that fills stomach but is freely movable
      - Mass conforms to shape of stomach
      - May be difficult to distinguish from food from recent meal
  - **Fundoplication complications**
    - Limits ability to belch
    - May result in distention of stomach with swallowed air
      - "Gas bloat" syndrome
  - **Post Whipple procedure**
    - Delayed gastric emptying and distention: One of most common postoperative complications after Whipple
    - On fluoroscopy, mild delay of gastric emptying: > 15-20 min of contrast emptying from stomach; severe delay: > 1-h delay in emptying of contrast to jejunum
- **Gastric Volvulus**
  - Intrathoracic stomach (paraesophageal hernia, type IV)
  - May twist on itself
    - Organoaxial or mesenteroaxial volvulus
  - More important to determine if gastric outlet is obstructed
    - Obstruction may constitute surgical emergency or require endoscopic decompression
- **Gastric Ileus**
  - Usually accompanied by dilation of small and large bowel
  - Common sequela of
    - Trauma
    - Postoperative state (usually abdominal surgery)
    - Electrolyte disorder
    - Narcotic analgesic use

Helpful Clues for Less Common Diagnoses

- **Pancreatitis, Acute**
  - Gastric dilatation from several possible etiologies
    - Duodenal inflammation
    - Pain (ileus)
    - Narcotics
- **Pancreatitis, Chronic**
  - May result in stricture of 2nd portion of duodenum

- o Chronic pancreatic pseudocysts can also contribute to functional gastric outlet obstruction
- **Metastases, Gastric**
  - o Metastases to stomach may cause scirrhous reaction
  - o Breast cancer is most common etiology
  - o Lymphoma of stomach (or duodenum) rarely causes outlet obstruction
- **Duodenal Mass or Stricture**
  - o Any process that narrows lumen of duodenum may result in "gastric outlet obstruction" and distention
  - o Examples
    - – Duodenal carcinoma: Scirrhous circumferential or intraluminal mass
    - – Annular pancreas: Characteristic appearance of pancreatic tissue encircling 2nd portion of duodenum
    - – Metastases: Carcinomatous metastases or direct invasion from adjacent tumor (e.g., pancreatic carcinoma)
- **Gastric Polyps**
  - o Antral polyp may prolapse through and obstruct pylorus
  - o Leads to intermittent outlet obstruction

Helpful Clues for Rare Diagnoses
- **Infiltrating Lesions**
  - o May cause narrowing of gastric antrum and subsequent outlet obstruction
  - o Multiple possible etiologies
    - – Crohn disease
    - – Sarcoidosis
    - – Tuberculosis
    - – Syphilis
    - – Amyloidosis

Gastric or Duodenal Ulcer

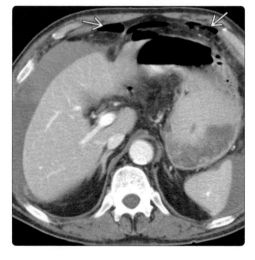

Gastric or Duodenal Ulcer

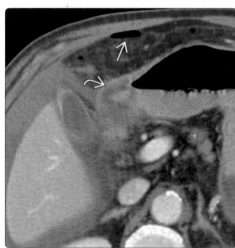

(Left) *Axial CECT in an older man shows ascites and free intraperitoneal gas ➡. The stomach is distended.* (Right) *Axial CECT in an older man shows free intraperitoneal gas ➡, prepyloric antral wall thickening ➡, and luminal narrowing accounting for gastric outlet obstruction. At surgery, a perforated prepyloric ulcer was found and "patched."*

Gastric Carcinoma

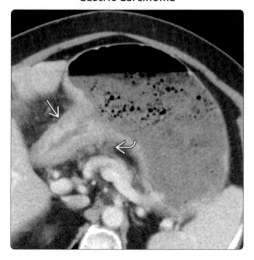

Gastroparesis

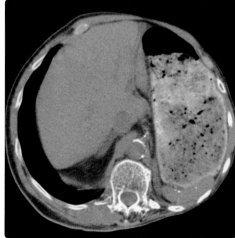

(Left) *Axial CECT shows circumferential thickening of the gastric antrum ➡ of soft tissue attenuation. Note the distended stomach with food debris and perigastric nodes ➡.* (Right) *Axial NECT in a man with gastroparesis due to diabetes shows massive distention of the stomach and retained food debris with no obstructing mass or ulcer.*

Fundoplication Complications

(Left) *Supine radiograph in a young man who had recent fundoplication demonstrates marked distention of the stomach and moderate distention of bowel.* **(Right)** *Upper GI series in a young man who had recent fundoplication was obtained following placement of an NG tube* ➡ *and shows less gastric distention but a persistent ileus* ➡. *The combination of an ileus and the prevention of reflux of gas into the esophagus due to the fundoplication can result in marked distention of the stomach.*

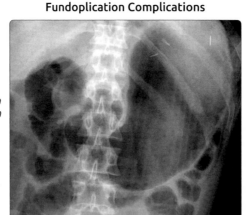

Fundoplication Complications

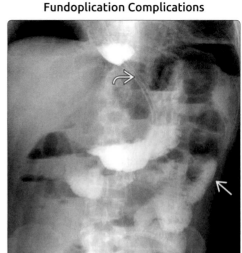

Post Whipple Procedure

(Left) *Severe gastric distention* ➡ *post pancreaticoduodenectomy (Whipple) is seen. Delayed gastric emptying is not uncommon after this type of surgery.* **(Right)** *Upper GI series shows a small stomach, the result of a prior antrectomy (Billroth 1 procedure) with vagotomy clips seen* ➡. *The stomach is distended with a bezoar of undigested vegetable matter.*

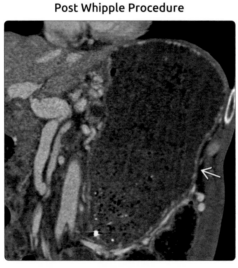

Gastric Bezoar

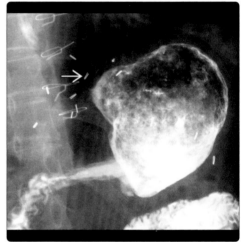

Gastric Volvulus

(Left) *Axial CECT in a older woman with chest pain and vomiting shows the distended stomach* ➡ *within a hernia sac in the right thorax, and it is rotated on its long axis.* **(Right)** *Upper GI series in an older woman with chest pain confirms the organoaxial volvulus of the stomach* ➡. *The stomach is distended and rotated along its long axis.*

Gastric Volvulus

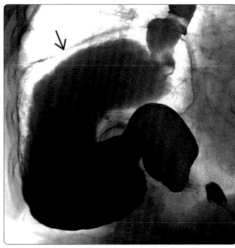

Pancreatitis, Chronic

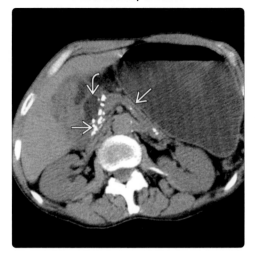

Pancreatitis, Chronic

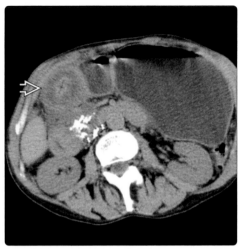

(Left) *Axial NECT in a 59-year-old man with alcoholic chronic pancreatitis shows distention of the stomach and evidence of chronic pancreatitis (parenchymal atrophy and calcifications)* ➡. *The wall of the 2nd portion of duodenum is thickened, and the lumen is compressed, in part, by a pseudocyst* �);. **(Right)** *Axial NECT in the same patient shows gastric distention and calcifications in the head of the pancreas from chronic pancreatitis. Note the mural thickening of the antrum and duodenum* ➡ *from acute exacerbation of pancreatitis.*

Duodenal Mass or Stricture

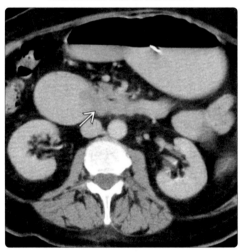

Metastases, Gastric

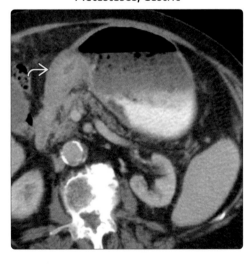

(Left) *Axial CECT shows dilation of the stomach and duodenum with abrupt narrowing of the 3rd portion of the duodenum* ➡. *There is an intramural mass that constricts the lumen of the duodenum. At surgery, metastatic breast cancer was confirmed.* **(Right)** *Axial CECT shows gastric distention and food debris from outlet obstruction. The antral wall is thickened and the lumen narrowed* ➡ *due to metastatic breast cancer.*

Annular Pancreas

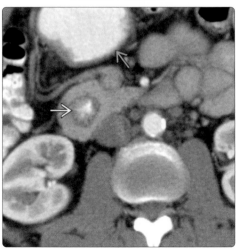

Gastric Polyps

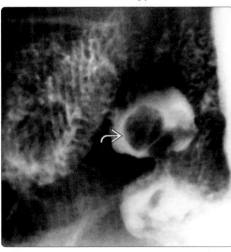

(Left) *Axial CECT shows the 2nd portion of duodenum* ➡ *completely encircled and compressed by pancreatic tissue. Note the distended stomach* ➡. **(Right)** *Upper GI series shows a polyp* ➡ *within the duodenal bulb that has its base in the prepyloric antrum. It periodically herniated through the pylorus, causing partial gastric outlet obstruction.*

DIFFERENTIAL DIAGNOSIS

Common
- Gastric Carcinoma
- Metastases and Lymphoma, Gastric

Less Common
- Gastritis
- Intramural Gastric Hematoma
- Caustic Gastroduodenal Injury
- Peritoneal Metastases
- Opportunistic Infection, Gastric
- Perigastric Adhesions

Rare but Important
- Crohn Disease, Gastric
- Following Gastric Freezing
- Syphilis, Stomach
- Radiation-Induced Gastritis
- Infiltrative Granulomatous Diseases
  - Tuberculosis
  - Sarcoidosis
  - Amyloidosis

ESSENTIAL INFORMATION

Key Differential Diagnosis Issues
- Linitis plastica is descriptive term, not pathologic diagnosis
  - Refers to rigid, nondistensible "leather bottle" stomach
  - **Usually due to 1 of 3 etiologies**
    - **Gastric carcinoma**
    - **Metastases** to stomach
      - Especially breast cancer
    - **Caustic gastric injury**
  - Many more etiologies for mild to moderate nondistensibility of stomach
    - Malignant neoplasm
      - Primary carcinoma or lymphoma, or metastatic to stomach or peritoneal surfaces
    - Gastritis
      - Many infectious and inflammatory types
    - Iatrogenic
      - Radiation therapy or gastric freezing for control of variceal bleeding
    - Diffuse infiltrative, granulomatous diseases
      - TB, sarcoid, syphilis, amyloidosis

Helpful Clues for Common Diagnoses
- **Gastric Carcinoma**
  - Most common cause worldwide
  - May invade and diffusely infiltrate submucosal layer
    - Often produces scirrhous, fibrotic response
  - May have minimal mucosal or intraluminal component
    - Can be missed on endoscopy and biopsy
  - Gastric wall is usually only moderately thickened (1-2 cm)
  - Peristalsis and distensibility are markedly diminished
    - Often most striking finding
    - Best recognized on fluoroscopic upper GI series
    - Gastric outlet obstruction may also occur
      - Look for distention of proximal portions of stomach

      - Retention of food from prior meals
  - Patients complain of early satiety and weight loss rather than pain
- **Metastases and Lymphoma, Gastric**
  - Some metastases cause scirrhous infiltration of gastric wall and fibrotic reaction
  - May cause linitis plastica appearance that is indistinguishable from gastric carcinoma
  - **Breast cancer** is most common primary source for this pattern
    - In North America, breast metastases may be more common cause of linitis plastica than gastric carcinoma
    - Markedly thickened gastric wall with enhancement, folds preserved
  - **Lymphoma** often diffusely infiltrates gastric wall but usually only causes mild limitation of gastric distention
    - Rarely causes linitis plastica or gastric outlet obstruction
    - Gastric wall is typically more diffusely thickened, and to greater degree, > 3 cm with lymphoma

Helpful Clues for Less Common Diagnoses
- **Gastritis**
  - Many etiologies
    - Limited ability to suggest specific etiology based on imaging findings
    - May have superficial erosions or ulceration of mucosa
    - Gastric folds are thickened, especially in antrum with incomplete distensibility
      - Folds may prolapse through pylorus into duodenal bulb
    - Erosive gastritis, complete or varioliform erosions (most common type): Gastric antrum; multiple punctate or slit-like collections of barium
    - NSAID-related gastropathy: Subtle flattening and deformity of greater curvature of antrum
    - Antral gastritis: Thickened folds, spasm, or decreased distensibility; prolapse of antral mucosa through pylorus
    - *Helicobacter pylori* gastritis: Antrum, body, or, occasionally, fundus; diffuse or localized
    - Granulomatous gastritis, Crohn disease: Antrum and body; multiple aphthous ulcers
    - Granulomatous gastritis, tuberculosis: Lesser curvature of antrum or pylorus, antral narrowing → obstruction
    - Eosinophilic gastritis: Antrum and body; mucosal nodularity, thickened folds, antral narrowing and rigidity
    - CT shows low-density edematous submucosa
      - Distinguished from soft tissue density seen with malignant infiltration of gastric wall
      - Mucosal hyperenhancement also suggests gastritis
- **Caustic Gastroduodenal Injury**
  - Often accompanied by similar injury to esophagus
  - Accidental or intentional ingestion of strong alkali (lye), acid, or formaldehyde
  - Acute findings
    - Gastric atony and delayed emptying
    - Striking wall thickening and edema

- Subacute or chronic findings
  - Perforation of stomach
  - Marked loss of gastric, size, distensibility, and peristalsis
    - □ Classic linitis plastica appearance
- **Peritoneal Metastases**
  - Serosal surface of stomach may be coated with peritoneal metastases, limiting distensibility
  - Peritoneal and omental metstases and malignant ascites can compress stomach
  - Usual sources: Ovarian, endometrial, GI tract cancers, pseudomyxoma peritonei
  - CT is much better than radiography or upper GI series in detecting and characterizing these findings

Helpful Clues for Rare Diagnoses

- **Crohn Disease, Gastric**
  - Uncommonly affects stomach; usually in patients with small bowel &/or colon involvement as well
  - Acute
    - Gastric fold thickening and erosions

- Similar appearance as other causes of gastritis
  - Chronic
    - Limited distensibility of stomach
    - Conical contraction of antrum with ram's horn configuration
- **Following Gastric Freezing**
  - Gastric infusion of iced saline may be used to control GI bleeding
  - If used excessively, can freeze stomach and lead to scarring
- **Infiltrative Granulomatous Diseases**
  - All are rare and probably indistinguishable by imaging alone
    - Syphilis
    - Sarcoidosis
    - TB
    - Amyloidosis
  - All tend to cause fold thickening and limited distention without gastric erosions or ulceration

Gastric Carcinoma

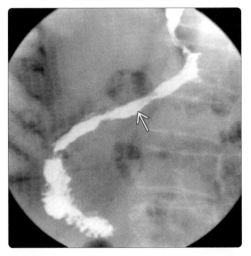

Gastric Carcinoma

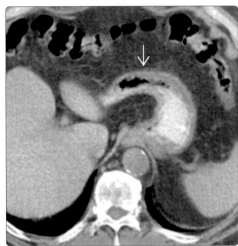

(Left) *Spot film from an upper GI series in an 82-year-old man shows a remarkably contracted and nondistensible stomach ➡ due to diffusely infiltrative gastric carcinoma; this is a classic linitis plastica appearance.* (Right) *Axial NECT in the same patient shows the contracted stomach ➡ due to diffusely infiltrative gastric carcinoma. As depicted by CT, there was no spread beyond the stomach at gastric resection.*

Gastric Carcinoma

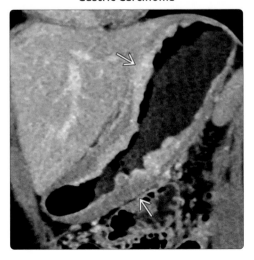

Gastric Carcinoma

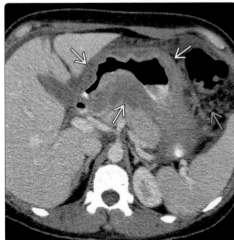

(Left) *Coronal CECT shows fixed distention of the stomach due to an infiltrative nodular gastric adenocarcinoma involving the greater part of the stomach ➡.* (Right) *Axial CECT in a 40-year-old woman shows circumferential soft tissue density thickening of the gastric wall ➡, causing fixed narrowing of the gastric lumen. Peritoneal metastases ➡ are also evident.*

Gastric Carcinoma

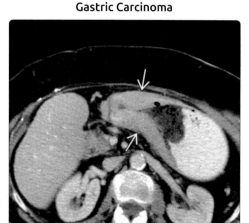

Gastric Carcinoma

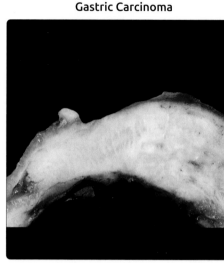

(Left) Axial CECT in an 81-year-old woman shows diffuse tumor infiltration ➡ and lack of distensibility of the gastric antrum and distal body. Retained food debris and distention of the proximal stomach indicate gastric outlet obstruction. (Right) Surgical photo in the same patient shows the gross appearance of the resected stomach with extensive pale-colored tumor infiltration and fibrosis throughout the gastric wall that accounts for the scirrhous nature of this tumor.

Metastases and Lymphoma, Gastric

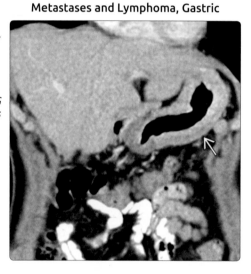

Metastases and Lymphoma, Gastric

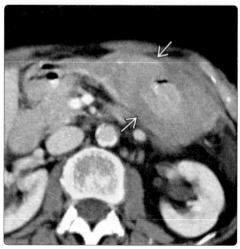

(Left) Coronal CECT in a 49-year-old woman shows diffuse thickening of the gastric wall ➡ and fixed narrowing of the gastric lumen due to metastatic breast cancer to the stomach. (Right) Axial FDG PET in the same patient shows FDG avidity in the stomach wall ➡ due to metastatic breast cancer.

Metastases and Lymphoma, Gastric

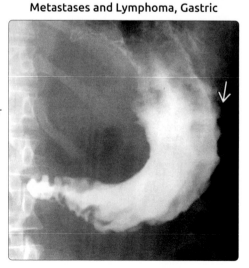

Metastases and Lymphoma, Gastric

(Left) Spot film from an upper GI series in a 75-year-old man with gastric lymphoma shows diffusely thickened and nodular folds ➡, and mildly reduced distention of the stomach but no gastric outlet obstruction. (Right) Axial CECT in the same patient shows diffuse, marked soft tissue density thickening of the gastric wall ➡ due to lymphoma. There was no clinical or radiographic evidence of gastric outlet obstruction.

Gastritis

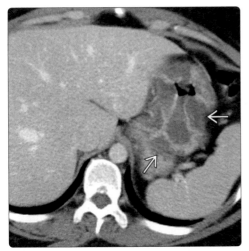

Caustic Gastroduodenal Injury

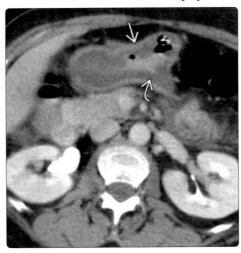

(Left) *Axial CECT shows striking gastric intramural edema* ➡, *causing wall thickening and luminal narrowing of the entire stomach in a 30-year-old man with NSAID-induced gastritis that resolved with antacids and cessation of analgesic use.* **(Right)** *Axial CECT shows wall thickening and nondistensibility of the body and antrum* ➡ *with an edematous submucosal layer* ➡ *in a 67-year-old woman who ingested lye a few days prior to this CT scan.*

Caustic Gastroduodenal Injury

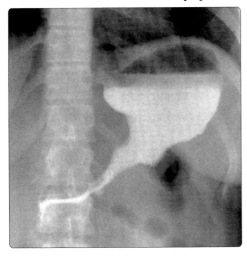

Peritoneal Metastases

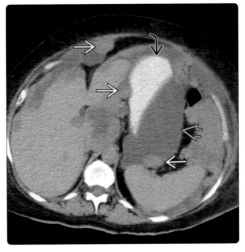

(Left) *Upright film from an upper GI series hows a shrunken, nondistensible stomach with evidence of gastric outlet obstruction in a 24-year-old man 2 weeks after ingestion of lye (strong alkali) in a suicide attempt.* **(Right)** *Axial CECT in a woman with metastatic endometrial carcinoma shows compression of the stomach* ➡ *by nodular peritoneal metastases* ➡ *and malignant ascites, involving the lesser sac* ➡ *and general peritoneal cavity.*

Peritoneal Metastases

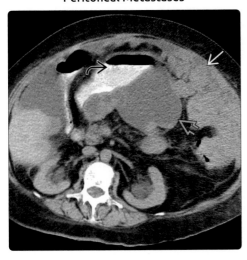

Crohn Disease, Gastric

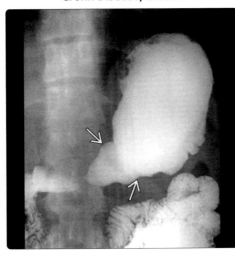

(Left) *Axial CECT in a woman with endometrial cancer shows a large omental cake of tumor* ➡ *and malignant lesser sac ascites* ➡ *that compress the stomach* ➡. **(Right)** *Frontal upper GI series shows a conical antrum* ➡ *and reduced distensibility of the stomach due to chronic Crohn gastritis.*

DIFFERENTIAL DIAGNOSIS

Common

- Functional Dyspepsia
- Acute Esophageal Inflammation
  - Reflux Esophagitis
  - Drug-Induced Esophagitis
- Acute Gastroduodenal Inflammation
  - Duodenal Ulcer
  - Gastric Ulcer
  - Gastritis
- Acute Biliary Inflammation
  - Acute Cholecystitis
  - Choledocholithiasis
  - Ascending Cholangitis
  - Sphincter of Oddi Dysfunction
- Pancreatic Inflammation
  - Acute Pancreatitis
  - Chronic Pancreatitis
  - Autoimmune (IgG4) Pancreatitis
- Bowel Inflammation or Obstruction
  - Acute Appendicitis
  - Small Bowel Obstruction
  - Crohn Disease
- Hepatic Inflammation or Tumor
  - Viral and Alcoholic Hepatitis
  - Steatosis/Steatohepatitis
  - Hepatic Abscess (Pyogenic, Amebic, Hydatid)
  - Hepatic Cysts and Polycystic Liver
  - Hepatic Metastases
  - Hepatocellular Carcinoma
- Abdominal Hernia (External and Internal)
  - Hiatal Hernia
  - Ventral Hernia
  - Transmesenteric Internal Hernia
  - Paraduodenal Hernia
- Coronary Artery Disease

Less Common

- Esophageal Foreign Body
- Esophageal Carcinoma
- Gastric Carcinoma
- Gastric Metastases
- Gastrointestinal Stromal Tumor, Stomach
- Pancreatic Ductal Carcinoma
- Pancreatic Serous (Microcystic) Adenoma
- Solid and Pseudopapillary Neoplasm, Pancreas
- Hepatic Adenoma

ESSENTIAL INFORMATION

Key Differential Diagnosis Issues

- Choice of initial imaging study should be on basis of clinical judgment
  - Barium upper gastrointestinal (UGI) series: Best for GERD, peptic ulcer disease
  - US: Good choice when acute biliary abnormality is considered likely
  - CT: Best for most other considerations

- Some etiologies are clinically apparent (trauma, postoperative, HELLP syndrome, etc.)
  - Not included on this list of differential diagnoses

Helpful Clues for Common Diagnoses

- **Functional Dyspepsia**
  - Pain or discomfort in absence of demonstrable structural or physiologic abnormalities
  - Probably due to abnormal motility, sensation, perception
- **Acute Esophageal Inflammation**
  - **Reflux esophagitis**
    - Irregular ulcerated mucosa of distal esophagus on barium esophagram
    - Often associated with hiatal hernia
  - **Drug-induced esophagitis**
    - Acute onset of odynophagia due to erosive effect of pill within esophagus
- **Acute Gastroduodenal Inflammation**
  - **Duodenal or gastric ulcer**
    - Wall thickening, extraluminal gas, or contrast medium
    - Complications: Perforation, hemorrhage, gastric outlet obstruction
  - **Gastritis**
    - Heterogeneous group of disorders causing inflammation of gastric mucosa
    - UGI: Antral fold thickening, erosions, limited distensibility
    - CECT: Mucosal enhancement, submucosal edema
- **Acute Biliary Inflammation**
  - **Acute cholecystitis**
    - 95% caused by stone obstructing cystic duct
    - US: Gallstone(s), distended gallbladder with thick wall; positive Murphy sign
    - CT: Same, + pericholecystic inflammation ± signs of perforation
  - **Choledocholithiasis**
    - 95% of bile duct stones are due to passage from gallbladder into common bile duct (CBD)
      - Imaging: Discrete, low-signal filling defect within bile duct on MRCP
      - MRCP superior to US or CT for visualizing stones
  - **Ascending cholangitis**
    - Due to gallstones or biliary-enteric communication
    - Irregular contour, branching pattern, dilation of bile ducts
    - Pneumobilia, hyperenhancement of biliary mucosa
  - **Sphincter of Oddi dysfunction**
    - Due to papillary stenosis or sphincter of Oddi dyskinesia
    - Opioids may cause spasm of sphincter of Oddi
    - Diagnosis by ERCP, Tc-HIDA, or MR cholangiography
- **Pancreatic Inflammation**
  - **Acute pancreatitis**
    - Enlarged pancreas, peripancreatic fluid or infiltrated fat planes, and thickened fascia
    - Heterogeneous enhancement on CECT, nonenhancing necrotic areas
  - **Chronic pancreatitis**
    - Atrophy of gland, dilated main duct, intraductal calculi
  - **Autoimmune (IgG4) pancreatitis**

- Part of spectrum of IgG4-related sclerosing diseases (including sclerosing cholangitis)
- **Bowel Inflammation or Obstruction**
  - ○ **Acute appendicitis**
    - Early inflammation may cause nausea, epigastric pain, followed by right lower quadrant pain and tenderness
    - Thick-walled appendix with inflamed periappendiceal fat, ± ileal mesenteric lymphadenopathy
  - ○ **Small bowel obstruction**
    - Many causes (adhesions, hernias, cancer, etc.)
    - Infectious or inflammatory enteritis
  - ○ **Crohn disease**
    - Segmental involvement, skip areas
    - Favors distal small bowel
    - Mucosal and mesenteric hyperemia, submucosal edema, lymphadenopathy
- **Hepatic Inflammation or Tumor**
  - ○ **Viral and alcoholic hepatitis**
    - Starry-sky appearance: Increased echogenicity of portal venous walls
    - Hepatomegaly, gallbladder wall thickening, periportal lucency
  - ○ **Steatosis/steatohepatitis**
    - Are common causes for epigastric/right upper quadrant discomfort and abnormal liver function tests
  - ○ **Hepatic abscess (pyogenic, amebic, hydatid)**
    - Each has characteristic appearance on imaging and unique demographic features
    - Pyogenic
      - □ Cluster of grapes, multiseptate
    - Amebic
      - □ Usually solitary, thick capsule
    - Hydatid
      - □ Spherical outer cyst with daughter cysts inside
      - □ Cyst wall or contents (hydatid sand) may be calcified or echogenic
  - ○ **Hepatic metastases**
    - Any large mass may be symptomatic (epigastric or right upper quadrant pain)

- Especially those that break through hepatic capsule or cause hemorrhage
- **Abdominal Hernia (External and Internal)**
  - ○ Have characteristic clinical and imaging features
- **Coronary Artery Disease**
  - ○ Inferior wall ischemia/infarction may present by epigastric pain in absence of chest pain

Helpful Clues for Less Common Diagnoses

- **Esophageal Foreign Body**
  - ○ Abrupt onset of chest and epigastric pain, inability to swallow food
  - ○ Food bolus stuck above Schatzki ring or other type of stricture
- **Esophageal Carcinoma**
  - ○ May cause symptomatic esophageal stricture
- **Gastric Carcinoma**
  - ○ May be symptomatic due to ulcerated surface or gastric outlet obstruction
  - ○ Soft tissue density thickening of wall, narrowing of lumen
    - ± nodal, peritoneal, hepatic metastases
- **Gastric Metastases**
  - ○ Carcinomatous metastases (e.g., from breast, lung) may cause linitis plastica or gastric outlet obstruction similar to primary gastric cancer
- **Gastrointestinal Stromal Tumor, Stomach**
  - ○ Usually exophytic submucosal mass with central necrosis
  - ○ May contain gas and oral contrast medium if eroded into lumen
- **Pancreatic Ductal Carcinoma**
  - ○ 75% of all pancreatic tumors; usually in pancreatic head
  - ○ Irregular, heterogeneous, poorly enhancing mass with abrupt obstruction of pancreatic duct ± CBD (double duct sign)
  - ○ Extensive local invasion and regional metastases

Reflux Esophagitis

Gastric Ulcer

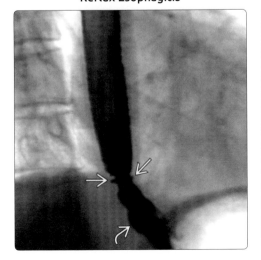
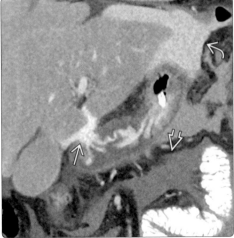

(Left) *Esophagram shows a type 1 hiatal hernia ➜ with a stricture at the esophagogastric junction. Two outpouchings ➜ indicate ulcerations of the mucosa.* (Right) *Coronal CECT in a 65-year-old man with severe abdominal pain shows the antral gastric wall defect ➜ with extraluminal positive oral contrast ➜ and free fluid ➜. Endoscopy revealed a perforated ulcer.*

Gastritis

Gastritis

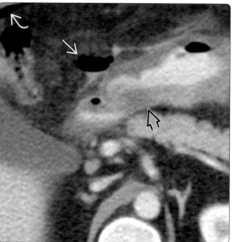

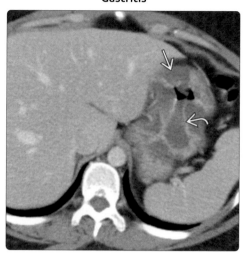

(Left) *Axial CECT shows free intraperitoneal gas* . *The gastric wall is thickened, probably due to gastritis. Just ventral to the duodenal bulb and antrum are small collections of extraluminal gas and oral contrast medium, confirming the source of perforation.* (Right) *Axial CECT in a young athlete taking large doses of NSAIDs shows marked gastric wall thickening due to submucosal edema and mucosal hyperemia.*

Acute Cholecystitis

Acute Pancreatitis

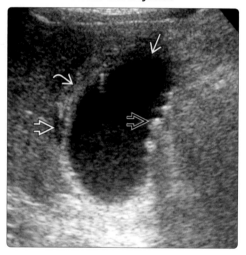

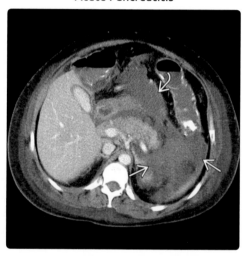

(Left) *US shows a distended gallbladder with diffuse wall thickening, multiple gallstones, and pericholecystic fluid. Sonographic Murphy sign was positive.* (Right) *Axial CECT shows extensive peripancreatic inflammation and exudation of fluid throughout the mesentery and anterior pararenal space, essentially diagnostic of acute pancreatitis.*

Chronic Pancreatitis

Autoimmune (IgG4) Pancreatitis

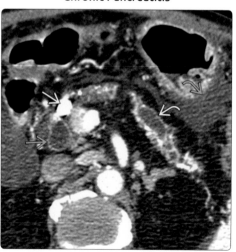

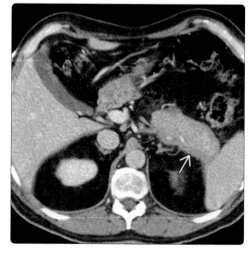

(Left) *Axial CECT shows marked dilation of the pancreatic duct with parenchymal atrophy and calcifications. The common bile duct is also dilated. Peripancreatic fluid suggests acute on chronic pancreatitis.* (Right) *Axial CECT in a man with weight loss and epigastric pain shows diffuse infiltration and enlargement of the pancreas with loss of its normal fatty lobulation. There is a halo or capsule of edematous tissue around the pancreas, typical for autoimmune pancreatitis.*

Small Bowel Obstruction

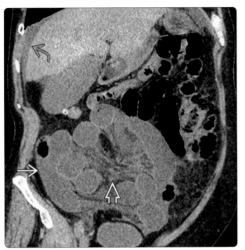

Crohn Disease

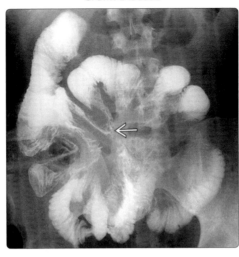

(Left) *Coronal CECT shows small bowel (SB) segments ➡ that are dilated out of proportion to others, typical of a closed-loop obstruction. The mesenteric vessels are twisted and dilated ➡ with extensive infiltration of the mesentery and ascites ➡, indicative of bowel ischemia.* (Right) *Marked angulation of SB segments with partial obstruction ➡ is shown. The bowel loops seem to be drawn toward a central point in the mesentery. This patient has chronic Crohn disease with extensive mesenteric and bowel scarring.*

Viral and Alcoholic Hepatitis

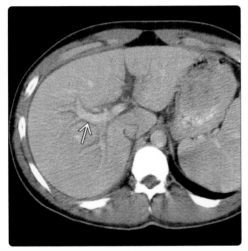

Viral and Alcoholic Hepatitis

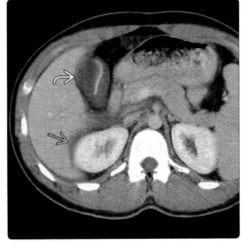

(Left) *Axial CECT in a young man with epigastric and right upper quadrant pain due to viral and alcoholic hepatitis shows periportal edema as a collar of low density surrounding the vessels ➡.* (Right) *Axial CECT in the same patient shows striking thickening of the gallbladder wall with the lumen almost completely collapsed ➡. A small amount of ascites is noted ➡. Any cause of acute hepatic engorgement, including steatohepatitis, may cause pain and abnormal liver function.*

Hepatic Abscess (Pyogenic, Amebic, Hydatid)

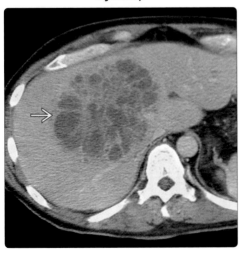

Hepatic Metastases

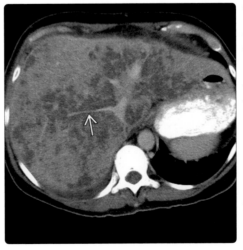

(Left) *Axial CECT in a man with fever and upper abdominal pain shows a multiloculated mass ➡ typical of a pyogenic abscess. The abscess was caused by subacute diverticulitis with portal venous septic thrombophlebitis.* (Right) *Axial CECT in a woman with a history of breast cancer, now with epigastric pain, shows hepatomegaly and innumerable, poorly defined, coalescent, perivascular, and perihepatic, low-attenuation metastases. The right hepatic vein ➡ is compressed.*

Hepatocellular Carcinoma

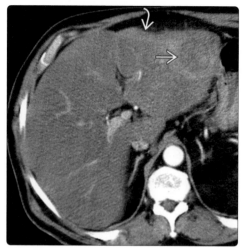

Hiatal Hernia

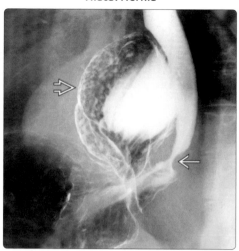

(Left) *Axial CECT in a man with acute epigastric pain shows a heterogeneous, enhancing, encapsulated left lobe hepatic mass ➡. High-attenuation fluid ➡ surrounding the mass and extending through the hepatic capsule represents spontaneous rupture with bleeding.* (Right) *Spot film from an upper GI series demonstrates a type 3 paraesophageal hiatal hernia, in which the gastroesophageal junction ➡ and fundus ➡ lie within the thorax.*

Hiatal Hernia

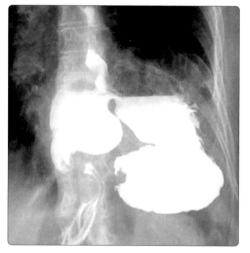

Ventral Hernia

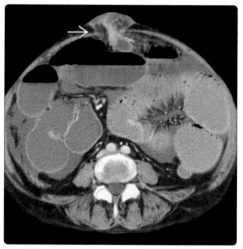

(Left) *Spot film from an upper GI series shows an "upside down" stomach, located entirely within the thorax, an organoaxial volvulus.* (Right) *Axial CECT shows a ventral hernia ➡ that contains a strangulated segment of bowel, resulting in SB obstruction.*

Transmesenteric Internal Hernia

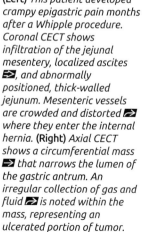
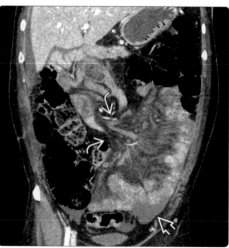

Gastric Carcinoma

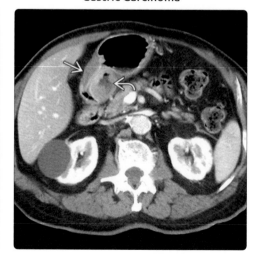

(Left) *This patient developed crampy epigastric pain months after a Whipple procedure. Coronal CECT shows infiltration of the jejunal mesentery, localized ascites ➡, and abnormally positioned, thick-walled jejunum. Mesenteric vessels are crowded and distorted ➡ where they enter the internal hernia.* (Right) *Axial CECT shows a circumferential mass ➡ that narrows the lumen of the gastric antrum. An irregular collection of gas and fluid ➡ is noted within the mass, representing an ulcerated portion of tumor.*

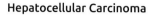

Gastric Metastases

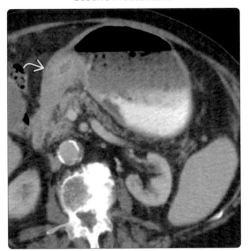

Gastrointestinal Stromal Tumor, Stomach

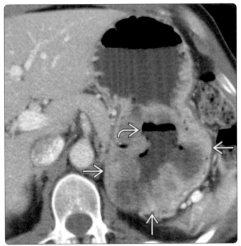

(Left) *Axial CECT shows soft tissue density and circumferential thickening of the gastric antrum* ➔, *resulting in gastric outlet obstruction. The appearance is indistinguishable from primary gastric carcinoma, but this obstruction was due to metastatic breast cancer.* (Right) *Axial CECT shows a large, exophytic mass* ➔ *arising from the posterior wall of the stomach. The center of the tumor is necrotic with an air-fluid level* ➔, *indicating communication with the gastric lumen.*

Pancreatic Ductal Carcinoma

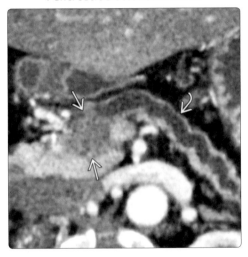

Pancreatic Serous (Microcystic) Adenoma

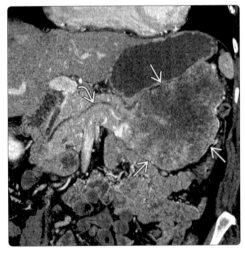

(Left) *Curved planar reformatted CT in an older man with weight loss and epigastric and back pain shows marked pancreatic parenchymal atrophy and dilation of the pancreatic duct* ➔ *ending abruptly at a hypodense mass* ➔ *in the pancreatic head.* (Right) *Coronal CECT in an older woman with epigastric pain shows a large, encapsulated, low-density mass* ➔ *arising from the pancreatic body and consisting of innumerable tiny cysts. The pancreatic duct* ➔ *is normal, and no "invasive" features are evident.*

Solid and Pseudopapillary Neoplasm, Pancreas

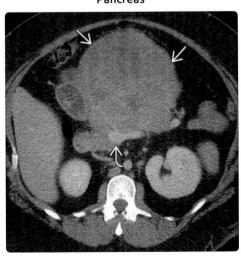

Hepatic Adenoma

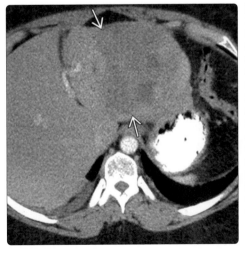

(Left) *Axial CECT in a young woman with epigastric pain and a palpable mass shows an abdominal mass* ➔ *that lies ventral to the splenic-portal venous confluence* ➔. *The mass is well encapsulated and mostly solid but has large foci of central low density, likely representing necrosis.* (Right) *Axial CECT in a young woman with acute onset of epigastric pain shows a large, heterogeneous hepatic mass* ➔. *NECT (not shown) demonstrated foci of hemorrhage within the mass.*

DIFFERENTIAL DIAGNOSIS

Common

- Splenomegaly and Splenic Masses
- Hepatomegaly and Hepatic Masses
- Gastric Masses and Distention
  - Gastroparesis
  - Gastric Carcinoma
  - Metastases and Lymphoma, Gastric
  - Gastrointestinal Stromal Tumor
  - Gastric Bezoar
- Pancreatic Masses
  - Pancreatic Pseudocyst
  - Mucinous Cystic Neoplasm
  - Serous Cystadenoma
  - Solid and Papillary Neoplasm, Pancreas
  - Pancreatic Neuroendocrine Tumor (PanNET)
- Adrenal Masses
  - Adrenal Carcinoma
  - Adrenal Metastases and Lymphoma
  - Adrenal Cyst
  - Pheochromocytoma
- Abdominal Abscess
- Peritoneal Metastases
- Ascites (Loculated)
- Renal Masses
  - Renal Cyst
  - Renal Cell Carcinoma
  - Renal Angiomyolipoma

Less Common

- Gastric Diverticulum
- Retroperitoneal Sarcoma
- Pseudomyxoma Peritonei
- Abdominal Wall Masses
  - Abdominal Wall Hernia (Mimic)
  - Abdominal Wall Hematoma (Mimic)
- Gastric Volvulus

ESSENTIAL INFORMATION

Key Differential Diagnosis Issues

- Determine whether mass arises from abdominal wall (e.g., hematoma or hernia) or within abdomen
- Distention, enlargement, or mass of any upper abdominal viscus may be perceived as left upper quadrant (LUQ) mass
- For large mass, determination of organ of origin may be difficult
  - Look for claw sign
    - Mass arising from solid organ will replace and distort part of its contour

Helpful Clues for Common Diagnoses

- **Splenomegaly and Splenic Masses**
  - Any cause of splenomegaly may result in palpable or radiographically evident LUQ mass
  - Consider accessory spleen and splenosis, which may cause enlarging mass(es) after splenectomy
    - These should have same attenuation and enhancement pattern as normal spleen

- Heterogeneous enhancement on arterial phase, homogeneous on venous phase on CECT
    - Tc-99m-labeled heat-damaged RBC scan is definitive imaging study
  - Also consider splenic masses, metastases, and lymphoma
- **Hepatomegaly and Hepatic Masses**
  - Enlarged left lobe of liver is often perceived or palpated as epigastric or LUQ mass
  - On axial CT images, may appear to be separated from remainder of liver, as heart indents cephalic surface of liver
  - Any mass in left lobe of liver or exophytic may be palpable LUQ mass
    - Common: Metastases, hepatocellular carcinoma, focal nodular hyperplasia, hemangioma
- **Gastric Masses and Distention**
  - Any gastric tumor [carcinoma, lymphoma, gastrointestinal stromal tumor (GIST), metastases] may result in LUQ mass
    - Exophytic masses (e.g., GIST) may not have obvious gastric origin
    - View multiplanar reformations
  - Also consider gastric distention (gastroparesis, volvulus, gastric outlet obstruction) and gastric bezoar
- **Pancreatic Masses**
  - Usually displace splenic vein posteriorly and may obstruct it (ductal cancer and chronic pancreatitis)
  - Pseudocyst is most common symptomatic large cystic mass
    - Check for history of pain, elevated pancreatic enzymes
    - Will typically change size over short-term follow-up (days to weeks), unlike cystic tumors
  - Consider serous (microcystic) cystadenoma in older adult
  - Mucinous cystic neoplasm in middle-aged women
  - Solid and papillary neoplasm in young women
  - Pancreatic ductal cancer usually does not cause palpable mass
    - Hypovascular lesion causing pancreatic ± biliary ductal obstruction is more common
  - Pancreatic metastases and lymphoma are not rare
  - Nonsyndromic PanNETs may come to clinical attention as incidental finding on imaging for unrelated reason
    - Typically large (> 10 cm) at presentation
- **Adrenal Masses**
  - Usually displace splenic vein ventrally
  - Cyst, adenoma, carcinoma, myelolipoma, metastases, pheochromocytoma
  - Most have characteristic appearance but must consider clinical and laboratory findings
    - Cyst: Water density, no enhancement
    - Adenoma: < 10 HU attenuation on NECT; absolute percentage washout > 60% on adrenal protocol CT, loses signal on opposed-phase GRE images
    - Adrenal cortical carcinoma: Heterogeneous appearance, > 5 cm
    - Pheochromocytoma: Heterogeneous, brightly enhancing; may be bright on T2WI MR
- **Abdominal Abscess**

- Left subphrenic space is common location for seroma, fat necrosis (especially after laparoscopic distal pancreatectomy) or pus after trauma or surgery (e.g., splenectomy)
- **Ascites (Loculated)**
  - Loculated collection of fluid may simulate LUQ mass
  - Malignant ascites, especially pseudomyxoma peritonei, may appear heterogeneous and exert mass effect
    - May cause scalloped surface of liver and spleen; displace other organs
- **Renal Masses**
  - Look for claw sign of expansile renal mass
    - Focal loss of renal parenchyma with other parenchyma draped around mass
    - Includes cysts, renal cell carcinoma, oncocytoma, angiomyolipoma, metastases (plus renal abscess)
    - Cyst: Water density, no enhancement, sonolucent, acoustic enhancement deep to cyst
    - Renal cell carcinoma: Heterogeneous enhancing lesion
    - Angiomyolipoma: Foci of fat, prominent blood vessels

- Infiltrating renal masses
  - Transitional cell carcinoma, lymphoma, renal infections (pyelonephritis and xanthogranulomatous pyelonephritis)
  - Renal vein thrombosis may simulate infiltrative mass

Helpful Clues for Less Common Diagnoses

- **Retroperitoneal Sarcoma**
  - Most common is liposarcoma
    - Usually has foci of variable attenuation, including some of near-fat density
  - Distinguishing liposarcoma from renal angiomyolipoma or adrenal myelolipoma
    - Liposarcoma is less vascular and displaces retroperitoneal organs but does not arise from them (e.g., no claw sign in kidney)
- **Abdominal Wall Masses**
  - External hernias and hematomas may be mistaken for LUQ mass
  - Most hernias have characteristic features allowing easy diagnosis

Splenomegaly and Splenic Masses

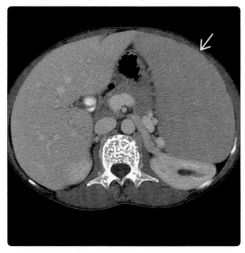

Splenomegaly and Splenic Masses

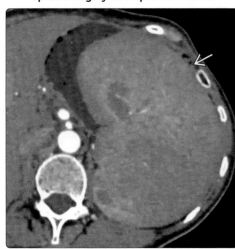

(Left) Axial CECT in a young man with thalassemia shows compression of the stomach by a massively enlarged spleen ➡ and liver. (Right) Axial CECT shows an enlarged spleen with heterogeneous appearance ➡ secondary to lymphomatous infiltration from chronic lymphocytic leukemia.

Hepatomegaly and Hepatic Masses

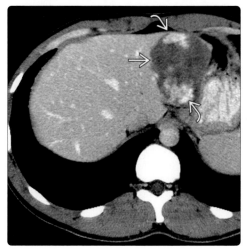

Gastroparesis

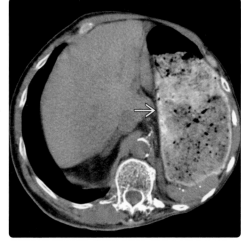

(Left) Axial CECT in a patient with a palpable left upper quadrant (LUQ) mass in the portal venous phase shows centripetal, discontinuous enhancement of the mass ➡ with the enhanced portions of the mass ➡ remaining isodense with blood pool, consistent with hemangioma. (Right) Axial CECT in a 62-year-old man with diabetes shows a massively enlarged stomach ➡ filled with particulate debris, fluid, and gas, typical signs of gastroparesis.

Gastrointestinal Stromal Tumor

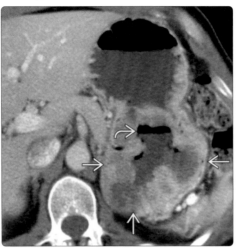

Pancreatic Pseudocyst

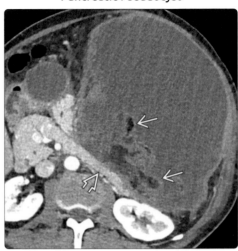

(Left) *Axial CECT shows a large, exophytic mass ➡ arising from the posterior gastric wall. The gastric origin is suggested by the presence of an air-fluid level ➡ within the necrotic center of the mass, indicating communication with the gastric lumen.* (Right) *Axial CECT in a patient with acute pancreatitis shows a large left abdominal fluid collection with areas of fat necrosis ➡ and a normal-appearing pancreas ➡, consistent with necrotizing pancreatitis with extrapancreatic necrosis alone.*

Mucinous Cystic Neoplasm

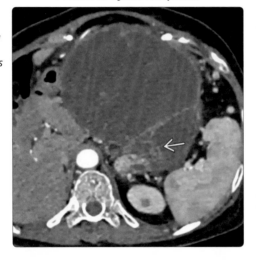

Serous Cystadenoma

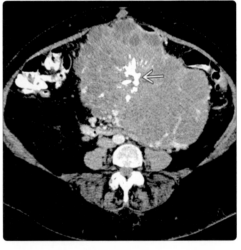

(Left) *Axial CECT shows a large LUQ cystic mass with multiple septations ➡ arising from the body and tail of the pancreas, typical for mucinous cystic neoplasm.* (Right) *Axial CECT in a 72-year-old woman demonstrates a large, predominantly cystic mass in the abdomen with a calcified central scar ➡, pathognomonic for serous cystadenoma.*

Solid and Papillary Neoplasm, Pancreas

Pancreatic Neuroendocrine Tumor (PanNET)

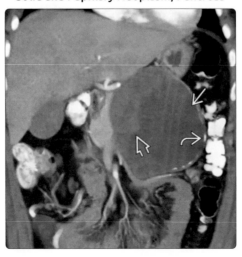

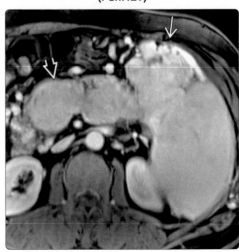

(Left) *Coronal CECT in a 30-year-old woman shows a solid and papillary neoplasm. Note the cystic ➡ and solid ➡ components as well as capsular calcifications ➡.* (Right) *Axial T1 C+ MR in a 55-year-old man with an aggressive pancreatic neuroendocrine tumor in the LUQ ➡ with enhancing tumor thrombus in the splenic and portal veins ➡ is shown.*

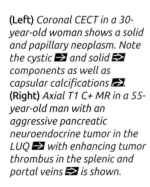

Adrenal Carcinoma

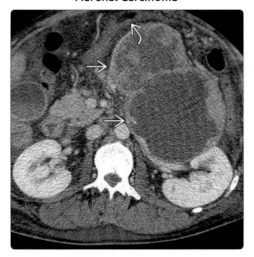

Abdominal Abscess

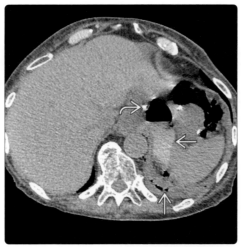

(Left) Axial CECT in a woman with Cushing syndrome shows a large, hypervascular mass ➡️ with extensive necrosis that displaces the stomach ➡️ and kidney without seeming to arise from either. Splenic vein and pancreas were displaced ventrally, helping to distinguish from pancreatic mass. (Right) Axial CECT in a woman who was febrile s/p gastric bypass surgery shows a complex LUQ mass. Near pouch-enteric anastomosis ➡️ is a large collection of gas, fluid, and enteric contrast medium ➡️ filling much subphrenic space.

Peritoneal Metastases

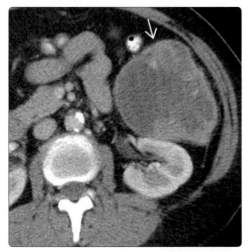

Peritoneal Metastases

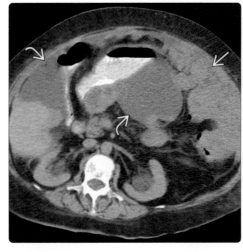

(Left) Axial CECT in a 55-year-old woman with metastatic sarcoma seen as a large LUQ mass ➡️ is shown. (Right) Axial CECT shows a classic omental cake ➡️ and malignant, loculated ascites ➡️ due to metastatic endometrial carcinoma.

Pseudomyxoma Peritonei

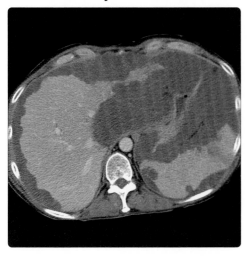

Abdominal Wall Hematoma (Mimic)

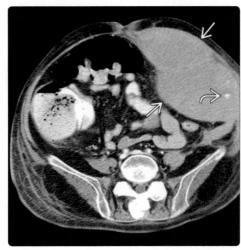

(Left) Axial CECT shows a classic scalloped surface of the liver and spleen and complex ascites filling the abdomen, and presenting as a doughy LUQ mass (metastatic appendiceal mucinous carcinoma). (Right) Axial CT shows a massive rectus sheath hematoma ➡️ with foci of active extravasation ➡️, representing spontaneous hemorrhage due to anticoagulation medication.

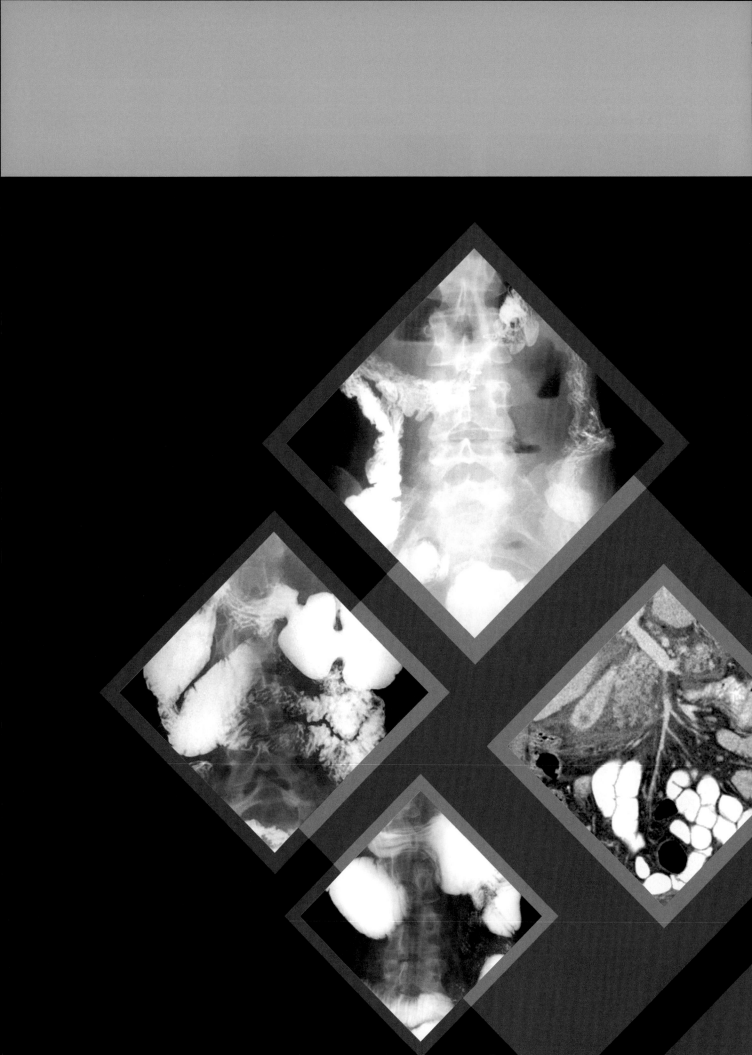

SECTION 5
Duodenum

Generic Imaging Patterns

Duodenal Mass   130

Dilated Duodenum   136

Thickened Duodenal Folds   138

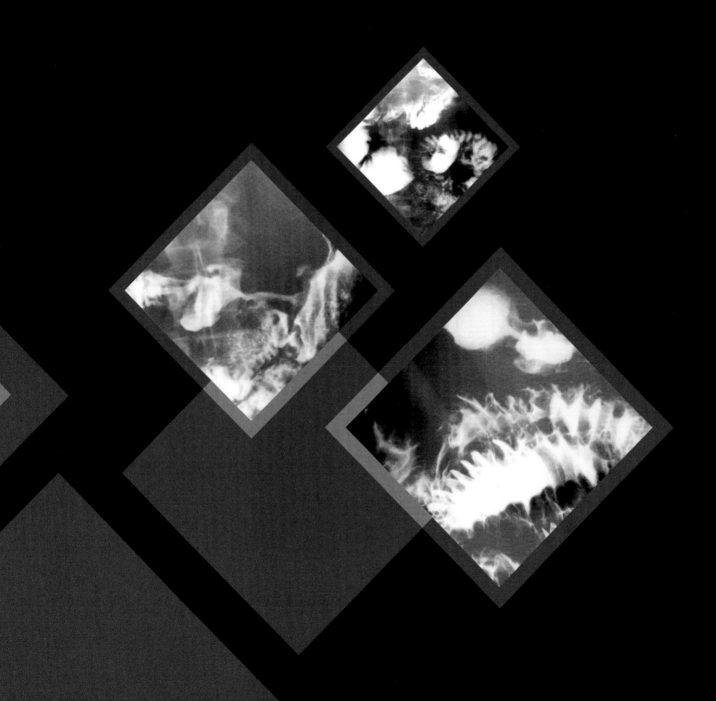

DIFFERENTIAL DIAGNOSIS

Less Common

- Intraluminal Duodenal Lesions
  - Duodenal Polyps
  - Duodenal Carcinoma
  - Prominent Duodenal Ampulla Mimicking Mass
  - Brunner Gland Hyperplasia ± Groove Pancreatitis
  - Carcinoid Tumor
- Intramural Duodenal Lesions
  - Mesenchymal Tumors
  - Metastases and Lymphoma
  - Duodenal Hematoma
  - Duplication Cyst
  - Choledochocele
- Extrinsic Pancreatic Masses
  - Pancreatic Pseudocyst
  - Pancreatic Ductal Adenocarcinoma
  - Annular Pancreas
  - Ampullary Tumor
  - Pancreatic Serous Adenoma
  - Pancreatic Intraductal Papillary Mucinous Neoplasm
  - Pancreatic Neuroendocrine Tumor
- Extrinsic Gallbladder Lesion
  - Acute Cholecystitis
  - Gallbladder Carcinoma
  - Hydrops or Empyema of Gallbladder
- Extrinsic Renal Mass
  - Renal Cell Carcinoma
  - Renal Cyst
  - Renal Angiomyolipoma
- Extrinsic Colon Mass
  - Colon Carcinoma
  - Infectious Colitis
- Extrinsic Hepatic Mass
  - Hepatomegaly
  - Hepatic Metastases
  - Hepatocellular Carcinoma

ESSENTIAL INFORMATION

Key Differential Diagnosis Issues

- Barium upper GI (UGI) series may suggest diagnosis or indicate finding
  - Barium UGI and endoscopy are best for mucosal/intrinsic duodenal lesions
- CT, MR, or US (including endoscopic US) are essential to characterize nature of intramural or extrinsic lesions
  - Use multiplanar reconstructions to delineate organ of origin

Helpful Clues for Less Common Diagnoses

- Intraluminal Duodenal Lesions
  - e.g., Brunner gland, hamartomatous and adenomatous polyps
    - Best evaluated by UGI or endoscopy
  - Duodenal polyps
    - Duodenal polyps are much less common than gastric
    - Adenomatous polyps (most common)
      □ Single, lobulated, or cauliflower-like surface

- Hyperplastic polyps
  □ Multiple small, sessile polyps uniform in size
- Hamartomas: Cluster of broad-based polyps
  □ Can occur as part of Peutz-Jeghers syndrome (PJS)
  - Duodenal carcinoma
    - Best diagnostic clue: Irregular intraluminal mass or apple core lesion at or distal to ampulla of Vater
    - Usually causes luminal obstruction
  - Prominent duodenal ampulla mimicking mass
    - Incidentally noted on CT or MR/MRCP performed for evaluation of biliary and pancreatic ductal evaluation
    - Normal ampulla ≤ 10 mm; in absence of biliary &/or pancreatic ductal dilation, heterogeneous enhancement or irregularity; normal finding
  - Brunner gland hyperplasia ± groove pancreatitis
    - Duodenal wall thickening with solitary or multiple nodules in proximal duodenum
    - Can be seen in association with groove pancreatitis
      □ Chronic pancreatitis-associated changes maybe present in adjacent pancreatic head
      □ Mass or soft tissue thickening in pancreaticoduodenal groove and cystic duodenal wall thickening is highly suggestive of groove pancreatitis
      □ May lead to partial obstruction of minor papilla
      □ Mimics pancreatic ductal carcinoma clinically and on imaging
- Intramural Duodenal Lesions
  - Mesenchymal tumors
    - Arising from any component of wall (fat, muscle, nerve, etc.)
    - GI stromal tumors (GIST) commonly arise in duodenum
      □ Hyperenhancing solid component; necrotic center
      □ May erode into lumen of duodenum (gas and enteric contents within GIST)
  - Metastases and lymphoma
    - Soft tissue density mass thickening wall, ± luminal obstruction
    - Metastatic carcinomas usually cause obstruction
    - Lymphomas usually do not cause obstruction
      □ May actually have aneurysmal dilation of bowel lumen
  - Duodenal hematoma
    - Following trauma or anticoagulant therapy
    - High attenuation (> 60 HU) thickens wall, narrows lumen
  - Duplication cyst
    - Quite rare in adults
    - Often water attenuation
    - May compress &/or communicate with lumen
  - Choledochocele
    - Choledochocele (type III): Fusiform dilation of distal common bile duct within duodenal wall may appear as mass
      □ MRCP may help delineate it accurately
- Extrinsic Pancreatic Masses
  - Pancreatic pseudocyst
    - In patient with history of pancreatitis and pain, consider pseudocyst

- ○ **Ampullary tumor**
  - – Small mass usually causing obstruction of common bile and pancreatic ducts (double duct sign)
- ○ **Pancreatic serous cystadenoma**
  - – Encapsulated mass in older adult with innumerable, tiny, cystic components
  - – Sponge or honeycomb appearance
  - – No invasive features
  - – May grow over time
- ○ **Pancreatic intraductal papillary mucinous neoplasm**
  - – Dilation of main ± side branch pancreatic ducts
  - – Usually causes bulging of ampulla of Vater (fishmouth ampulla)
- ○ **Pancreatic neuroendocrine tumor**
  - – Usually small and hypervascular; rarely cause mass effect on duodenum
  - – Gastrinomas may lie within duodenal wall
- • **Extrinsic Gallbladder Lesion**
- ○ **Acute cholecystitis**
  - – Distended gallbladder often compresses lateral wall of 2nd portion of duodenum

- ○ **Gallbladder carcinoma**
  - – Tumor may displace or encase 2nd portion of duodenum
  - – Invasion of liver, obstruction of bile ducts often evident on US, CT, or MR
- • **Extrinsic Renal Mass**
  - ○ Any benign or malignant mass may displace 2nd portion of duodenum
- • **Extrinsic Colon Mass**
  - ○ Infectious or neoplastic mass may displace 2nd portion of duodenum
  - ○ Diagnosis is usually evident by combination of CT and clinical findings
- • **Extrinsic Hepatic Mass**
  - ○ Hepatomegaly or hepatic mass (especially exophytic)
  - ○ May displace 2nd portion of duodenum

Duodenal Polyps

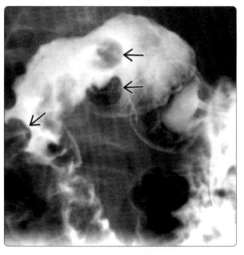

Duodenal Polyps

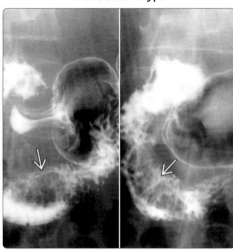

(Left) *Upper GI series shows multiple polypoid filling defects ⇨ in the duodenal bulb and the 2nd portion of the duodenum. Endoscopy and biopsy revealed Brunner gland hyperplasia and hamartomatous change in this patient with hyperacidity.* (Right) *Upper GI series shows a long, polypoid filling defect ⇨ within the lumen of the 2nd and 3rd portions of the duodenum. Surgical resection confirmed benign adenomatous polyp.*

Duodenal Polyps

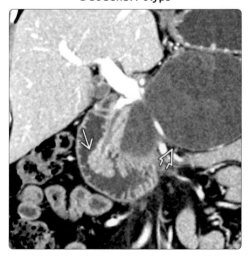

Duodenal Carcinoma

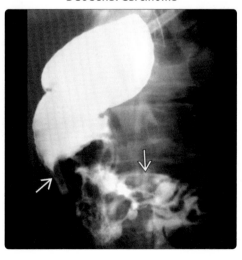

(Left) *Coronal CECT in a middle-aged woman shows acute pancreatitis with pseudocyst formation ⇨ secondary to an obstructing ampullary mass ⇨. The mass was surgically removed, and pathology showed tubulovillous adenoma with high-grade dysplasia.* (Right) *Upper GI series in a patient with familial adenomatous polyposis syndrome shows an apple core appearance of a mass ⇨ in the 2nd and 3rd portions of the duodenum with irregular, destroyed mucosal pattern.*

Duodenal Carcinoma

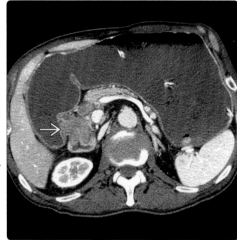

Mesenchymal Tumors

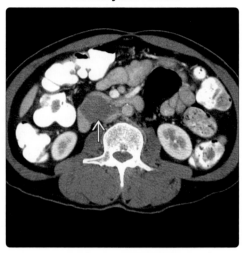

(Left) *Axial CECT shows massive dilation of the stomach, indicating gastric outlet obstruction. A mass ➡ in the proximal duodenum is causing the obstruction. The tumor invades the head of the pancreas, but the bile duct and pancreatic duct were not obstructed.* (Right) *Axial CECT shows a homogeneous, soft tissue density mass ➡ within the wall of the duodenum, proven leiomyoma. The wall of the duodenum seems wrapped around the mass, but the duodenal lumen is not obstructed.*

Mesenchymal Tumors

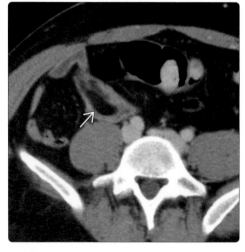

Mesenchymal Tumors

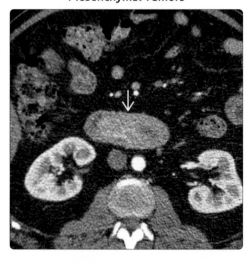

(Left) *Axial CECT shows a fat density mass ➡ within the lumen of the duodenum, even though this lipoma arose from the duodenal wall.* (Right) *Axial CECT shows a cylindrical, enhancing mass ➡ within the lumen of the 3rd portion of the duodenum without signs of bowel obstruction. This was a paraganglioma, arising from the duodenal wall.*

Mesenchymal Tumors

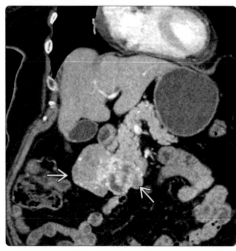

Mesenchymal Tumors

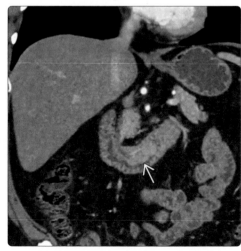

(Left) *Coronal CECT shows a lobulated, heterogeneous mass ➡ arising from the 2nd portion of the duodenum. Portions of the mass are hypervascular, while others appear necrotic, which are all typical features of a duodenal GI stromal tumor.* (Right) *Coronal CECT shows a gangliocytic paraganglioma as a mass in the 3rd portion of the duodenum ➡.*

Metastases and Lymphoma

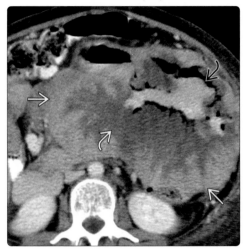

Metastases and Lymphoma

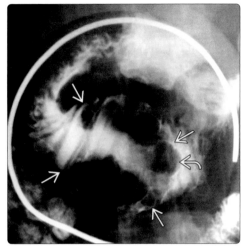

(Left) *Axial CECT shows classic aneurysmal dilation of the 4th portion of the duodenum* ➡ *with a huge, soft tissue density mass* ➡ *(lymphoma) with central necrosis* ➡, *communicating with the duodenal lumen. Note the absence of bowel obstruction or gastric distention.* (Right) *Upper GI series shows aneurysmal dilation* ➡ *of the 3rd portion of the duodenum with a large intraluminal component* ➡ *due to malignant melanoma. Lymphoma can appear identical.*

Metastases and Lymphoma

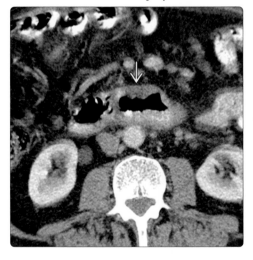

Metastases and Lymphoma

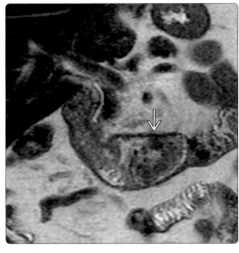

(Left) *Coronal CECT shows diffuse, large B-cell lymphoma of the 3rd portion of the duodenum with wall thickening and a dilated lumen without obstruction* ➡. (Right) *Axial T2 MR in the same patient shows a focally dilated 3rd portion of the duodenum* ➡ *with wall thickening, the characteristic appearance of lymphoma.*

Metastases and Lymphoma

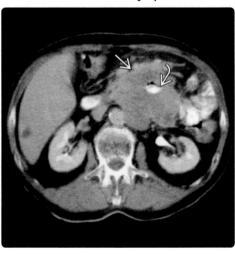

Metastases and Lymphoma

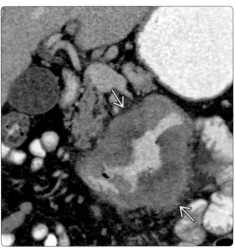

(Left) *Axial CECT shows a large soft tissue mass* ➡ *encasing, but not obstructing, the duodenum* ➡ *in this patient with posttransplant lymphoproliferative disease.* (Right) *Coronal CECT shows a large, annular mass involving the 3rd and 4th portions of the duodenum* ➡. *The aneurysmal dilation appearance is usually associated with lymphoma; however, this lesion turned out to be metastatic melanoma.*

Prominent Duodenal Ampulla Mimicking Mass

(Left) Curved planar reformatted CT shows a protruding, mildly hypodense ampulla measuring 8 mm ➡. The common bile duct is mildly dilated ➡. The patient is status post cholecystectomy. (Right) Coronal T2 MR in a 22-year-old man shows a fluid-filled duplication cyst within the duodenal lumen ➡. Surgical resection was performed due to obstructive symptoms.

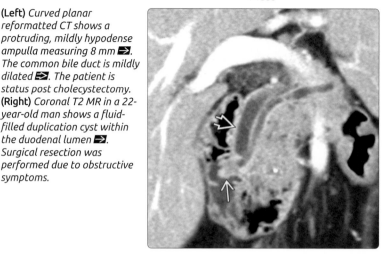

Duplication Cyst

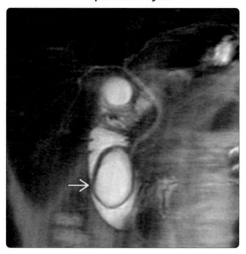

Duplication Cyst

(Left) Axial CECT in a 9-month-old infant shows 2 thick-walled cystic masses ➡, proven to be represent duplication cysts. (Right) Multiplanar reformation CECT in a 58-year-old woman shows dilation of the common duct ➡, ending in a choledochocele ➡ that causes a water density filling defect within the duodenal lumen.

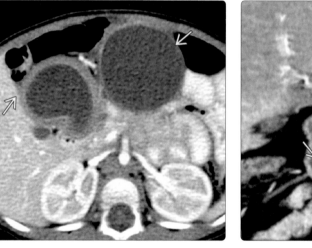

Choledochocele

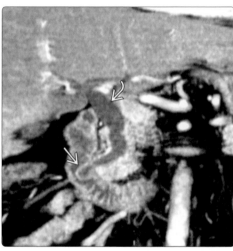

Ampullary Tumor

(Left) Coronal CECT in this older woman with painless jaundice shows an ampullary mass ➡ causing obstruction of both the pancreatic ➡ and common bile ➡ ducts, classic findings of ampullary carcinoma. (Right) Coronal CECT in a 46-year-old woman with early satiety and weight loss shows a hypodense mass ➡ arising from the uncinate process that encased the superior mesenteric vein and the 3rd portion of the duodenum, characteristic of pancreatic ductal carcinoma.

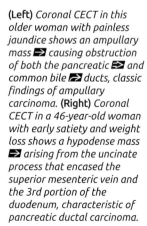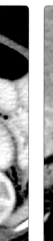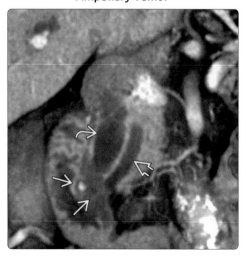

Pancreatic Ductal Adenocarcinoma

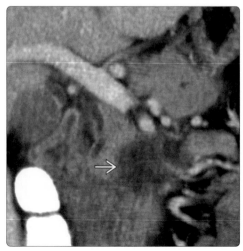

Brunner Gland Hyperplasia ± Groove Pancreatitis

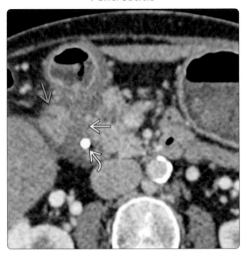

Pancreatic Intraductal Papillary Mucinous Neoplasm

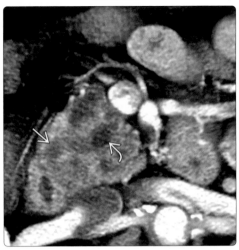

(Left) *Axial CECT shows a low-density "mass"* ➡ *between the pancreatic head and the 2nd portion of the duodenum* ➡. *Biliary obstruction was treated with a stent* ➡. *Surgery confirmed groove pancreatitis, though pancreatic carcinoma may have a similar appearance.* (Right) *Axial CECT in a patient with jaundice shows dilation of the main and side branches of the pancreatic duct* ➡, *typical of intraductal papillary mucinous neoplasm. There is a hypodense, solid mass* ➡ *that obstructed CBD, found to be pancreatic ductal carcinoma.*

Pancreatic Serous Adenoma

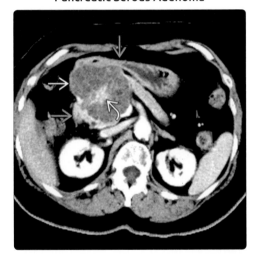

Annular Pancreas

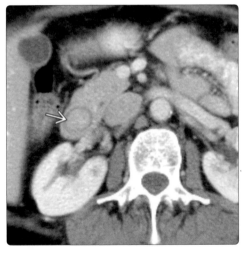

(Left) *Axial CECT in an older, asymptomatic woman shows a mass* ➡ *in the pancreatic head that displaces the stomach and duodenum* ➡. *The mass is composed of small cysts separated by thin, fibrous septa with a "scar"* ➡ *in the center of the mass.* (Right) *Axial CECT in a young man with early satiety shows that the 2nd portion of the duodenum* ➡ *is completely encircled by pancreatic tissue with narrowing of its lumen.*

Pancreatic Pseudocyst

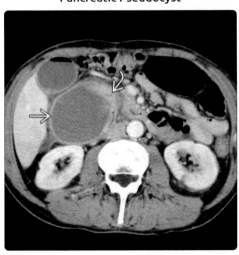

Duodenal Hematoma

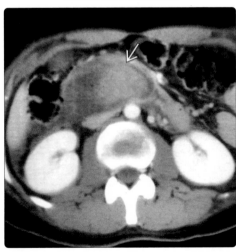

(Left) *Axial CECT in a man with recurrent pancreatitis shows a cystic mass* ➡ *that lies lateral to, and distorts the lumen of, the 2nd portion of the duodenum* ➡, *characteristic of intramural pseudocyst.* (Right) *Axial CECT in an adolescent boy with blunt trauma shows a heterogeneously high-attenuation mass* ➡ *within the wall of the duodenum, representing intramural hematoma. This resolved within 1 week with nonoperative management.*

DIFFERENTIAL DIAGNOSIS

Common

- Ileus
- Small Bowel Obstruction
- Pancreatitis, Acute
- Superior Mesenteric Artery Syndrome
- Postvagotomy
- Scleroderma, Intestinal
- Celiac-Sprue Disease

Less Common

- *Strongyloides*
- Zollinger-Ellison Syndrome

ESSENTIAL INFORMATION

Key Differential Diagnosis Issues

- Fluoroscopy and CT/MR have complementary roles in evaluation of duodenal dilation
  - Fluoroscopy is better at assessing dynamic changes, peristalsis, effect of positioning
  - Also better at identifying mucosal or constricting lesions
- CT better at showing extrinsic compression and disease beyond duodenum

Helpful Clues for Common Diagnoses

- **Ileus**
  - Duodenum dilated along with small bowel (SB) and colon
  - No transition from dilated to nondilated bowel (in general)
    - It is not uncommon for descending colon to be less dilated than remaining colon or SB in cases of ileus
  - Common etiologies
    - Postoperative, metabolic imbalance, medication
- **Small Bowel Obstruction**
  - Dilation of SB "downstream" from duodenum, "upstream" from obstructing lesion
- **Pancreatitis, Acute**
  - Often causes focal ileus of adjacent bowel with dilated lumen
  - May narrow lumen of 2nd and 3rd portions of duodenum
- **Superior Mesenteric Artery Syndrome**
  - 3rd duodenum becomes compressed as it passes between aorta and superior mesenteric artery (SMA)
  - Common in thin, bedridden patients, especially with recent weight loss
  - Look for linear crossing defect on 3rd duodenum (barium upper GI study)
    - Narrow angle between aorta and SMA on CT, MR angiography
      - Aorto-SMA angle < 22-25°, aortomesenteric distance < 8-10 mm in sagittal plane
- **Postvagotomy**
  - Stomach and duodenum become dilated, atonic
  - Result of loss of parasympathetic innervation
- **Scleroderma, Intestinal**
  - Dilated, decreased peristalsis; "megaduodenum"
  - Look for characteristic changes in esophagus, SB, skin
    - Hidebound appearance of SB folds
      - Thin and closely spaced
    - Esophagus: Dilated, atonic, ± distal stricture
- **Celiac-Sprue Disease**
  - Look for dilated SB with decreased folds in jejunum (reversed fold pattern) and signs of malabsorption
  - May also have transient intussusceptions, "conformation" of SB flaccid, dilated segments
  - Correlate with clinical evidence of gluten intolerance

Helpful Clues for Less Common Diagnoses

- *Strongyloides*
  - Causes thickened or effaced folds in duodenum and SB
  - May cause lead pipe appearance of same segments
- **Zollinger-Ellison Syndrome**
  - Thickened folds, increased secretions, ulcerations in stomach and duodenum
  - Gastrin-producing islet cell tumor

(Left) Coronal CECT shows dilated proximal small bowel segments, including duodenum and jejunum ➡, while distal small bowel ➡ is collapsed; obstruction due to adhesions ➡ is also seen. (Right) Axial CECT shows dilation of the stomach and 2nd portion of duodenum ➡. Peripancreatic inflammation is evident, and there is a collection of gas and fluid, an infected collection ➡. Common duct stent ➡ is also seen.

Small Bowel Obstruction

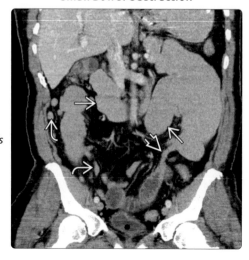

Pancreatitis, Acute

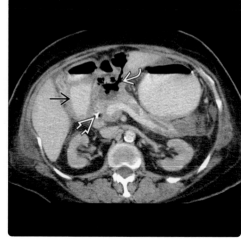

Superior Mesenteric Artery Syndrome

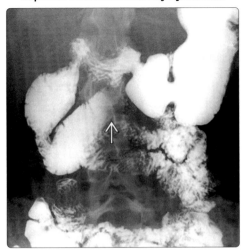

Superior Mesenteric Artery Syndrome

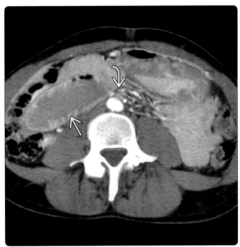

(Left) *Frontal small bowel follow-through shows marked dilation of the 2nd and 3rd portions of duodenum with abrupt narrowing as it crosses the spine with a vertical straight line demarcation ➡. **(Right)** Axial CECT shows marked dilation of the duodenum ➡, which is compressed with luminal narrowing as it passes between the aorta and the root of the mesenteric vessels ➡.*

Scleroderma, Intestinal

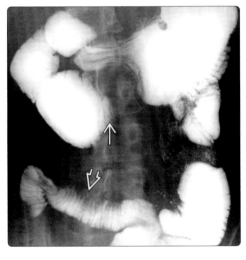

Scleroderma, Intestinal

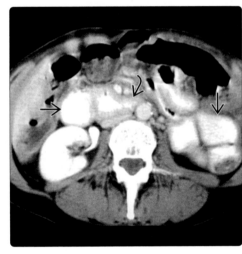

(Left) *Small bowel follow-through shows marked dilation of the duodenum up to where it crosses the spine ➡. The appearance is similar to superior mesenteric artery syndrome, but the abnormal, closely spaced fold pattern of the small bowel ➡ helps to confirm the diagnosis of scleroderma. **(Right)** Axial CECT shows a dilated lumen ➡ of the duodenum and small bowel with fold thickening of the duodenal wall ➡, proven to be scleroderma.*

Celiac-Sprue Disease

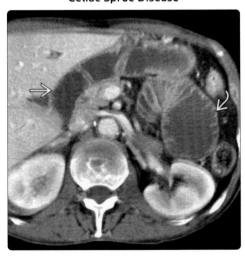

Zollinger-Ellison Syndrome

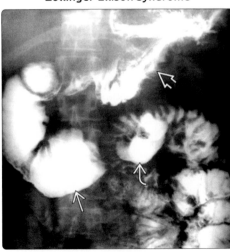

(Left) *Axial CECT shows fluid distention of dilated duodenum ➡ and jejunum, and some atrophy of the jejunal folds ➡. **(Right)** Spot film from an upper GI series shows a dilated duodenum ➡ and thick gastric folds ➡ with dilution of the barium, due to excess fluid (acid). A large jejunal ulcer ➡ is seen. A pancreatic neuroendocrine tumor (gastrinoma) was subsequently found.*

DIFFERENTIAL DIAGNOSIS

Common

- Duodenitis
- Duodenal Ulcer
- Brunner Gland Hyperplasia
- Acute Pancreatitis
- Duodenal Hematoma and Laceration
- Chronic Renal Failure

Less Common

- Zollinger-Ellison Syndrome
- Opportunistic Intestinal Infections
- Caustic Gastroduodenal Injury
- Crohn Disease
- Celiac-Sprue Disease
- Metastases and Lymphoma, Duodenal
- Duodenal Varices

ESSENTIAL INFORMATION

Key Differential Diagnosis Issues

- Barium UGI and CT: Complementary studies
  - Fluoroscopic studies are often better for intrinsic duodenal disease
  - CT excels at showing paraduodenal etiologies (e.g., pancreatitis)
- Imaging findings are uncommonly pathognomonic (e.g., duodenal varices); need clinical correlation

Helpful Clues for Common Diagnoses

- **Duodenitis**
  - Inflammation without frank ulceration
  - Same etiologies as gastritis, often coexisting gastritis and duodenitis
  - Occasionally see aphthous erosions on barium UGI
  - CECT: Mural thickening of duodenum ± adjacent inflammation
  - Delayed gastric emptying or outlet obstruction
- **Duodenal Ulcer**

- Discrete ulcer crater with marked spasm of wall and distortion of lumen
- ± extraluminal gas, fluid, enteric contrast medium
- **Brunner Gland Hyperplasia**
  - Thick, nodular folds in duodenal bulb
  - Usually associated with duodenitis and sometimes with groove pancreatitis (cystic changes in medial wall)
- **Acute Pancreatitis**
  - Thick folds, widening of C loop
  - Signs of pancreatitis are usually evident on CT
- **Duodenal Hematoma and Laceration**
  - Thick spiculated folds
  - Etiologies: Focal, epigastric trauma or anticoagulation
- **Chronic Renal Failure**
  - Thick, nodular folds

Helpful Clues for Less Common Diagnoses

- **Zollinger-Ellison Syndrome**
  - Gastrin-producing islet cell tumor often evident on CECT
  - Thick folds and ulcers of stomach and duodenum
- **Opportunistic Intestinal Infections**
  - Giardiasis, strongyloides, cryptosporidiosis
  - More common in immunosuppressed patients
  - Thickened and nodular or effaced folds + spasm, excess fluid, diarrhea
- **Caustic Gastroduodenal Injury**
  - Esophagus and stomach are usually more affected
- **Crohn Disease**
  - Thickened folds, ulceration, spasm
  - Usually with known disease in small bowel
- **Celiac-Sprue Disease**
  - Usually with small bowel disease
  - Reversed fold pattern: Effaced jejunal folds; prominent ileal folds
- **Duodenal Varices**
  - Portal hypertension &/or portal vein occlusion
  - Duodenal (and gastroesophageal) varices are evident on CECT

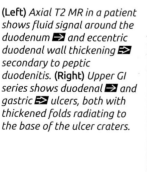

(Left) Axial T2 MR in a patient shows fluid signal around the duodenum ➡ and eccentric duodenal wall thickening ⇉ secondary to peptic duodenitis. (Right) Upper GI series shows duodenal ➡ and gastric ⇉ ulcers, both with thickened folds radiating to the base of the ulcer craters.

Duodenitis

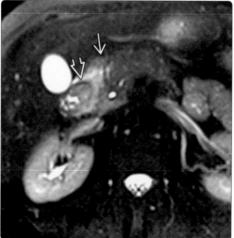

Duodenal Ulcer

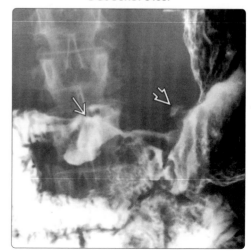

Brunner Gland Hyperplasia

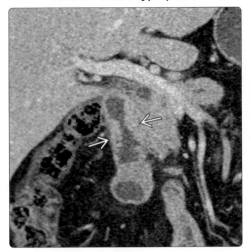

Acute Pancreatitis

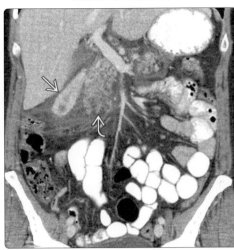

(Left) *Coronal CT shows circumferential duodenal wall thickening* ➡ *mimicking an annular duodenal carcinoma. Histopathology post pancreaticoduodenectomy revealed groove pancreatitis with inflammatory changes in the duodenal wall, including Brunner gland hyperplasia.* (Right) *Coronal CECT shows infiltrative changes around the pancreatic head* ➡ *with mural thickening and luminal narrowing of the 2nd portion of duodenum* ➡*, which shares the anterior pararenal space with the pancreas.*

Duodenal Hematoma and Laceration

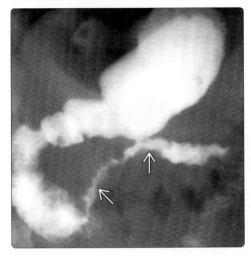

Zollinger-Ellison Syndrome

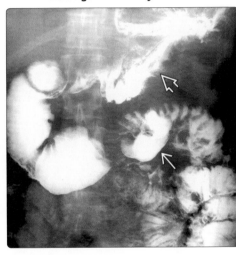

(Left) *Upper GI series shows thickened folds and narrowed lumen* ➡ *of the distal duodenum, due to spontaneous coagulopathic hemorrhage into the duodenal wall in this 70-year-old woman on Coumadin therapy.* (Right) *Upper GI series shows a large distal duodenal or jejunal ulcer* ➡*, a dilated, partially obstructed 2nd portion of the duodenum, and thickened folds with excess fluid (acid) in the stomach* ➡*.*

Metastases and Lymphoma, Duodenal

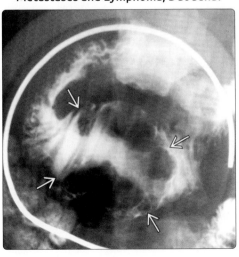

Duodenal Varices

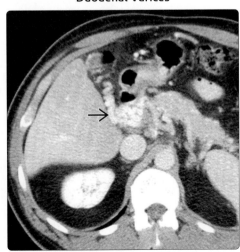

(Left) *Upper GI series shows aneurysmal dilation of the lumen and thickening of the folds of the 3rd portion of duodenum, due to an intramural mass* ➡ *(metastatic melanoma).* (Right) *Axial CECT shows a collection of varices* ➡ *around the 2nd duodenum and pancreatic head in this man with cirrhosis and portal vein thrombosis with cavernous transformation of the portal vein.*

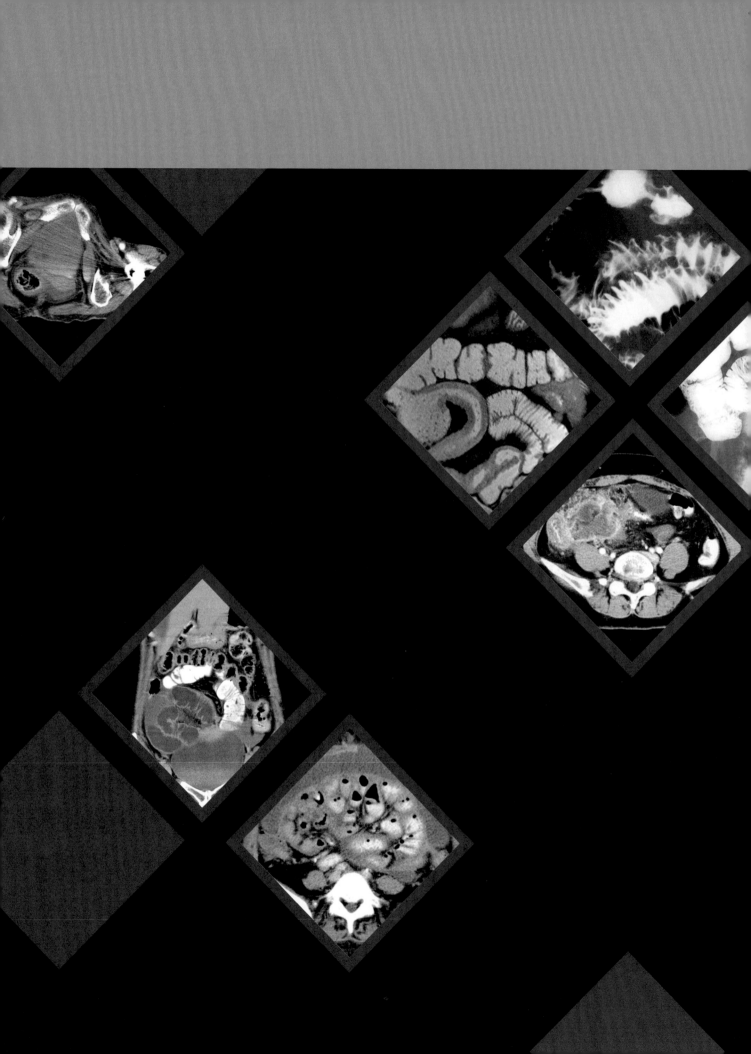

SECTION 6
Small Intestine

Generic Imaging Patterns

Multiple Masses or Filling Defects, Small Bowel   142
Cluster of Dilated Small Bowel   144
Aneurysmal Dilation of Small Bowel Lumen   146
Stenosis, Terminal Ileum   148
Segmental or Diffuse Small Bowel Wall Thickening   150
Pneumatosis of Small Intestine or Colon   156

Clinically Based Differentials

Occult GI Bleeding   160
Small Bowel Obstruction   164

DIFFERENTIAL DIAGNOSIS

Common

- Food, Pills
- Lymphoid Follicles, Small Bowel
- Intestinal Parasitic Disease

Less Common

- Intestinal Metastases and Lymphoma
- Intramural Benign Intestinal Tumors
- Hamartomatous Polyposis Syndromes
- Gardner Syndrome
- Familial Polyposis

ESSENTIAL INFORMATION

Key Differential Diagnosis Issues

- Most filling defects are food or pills

Helpful Clues for Common Diagnoses

- **Food, Pills**
  - Pills usually have recognizable round or oval shape
  - Corn and other vegetables are common sources of filling defects
  - Especially common in older adult, edentulous patients
  - Food materials with high amount of sugar (candies) may appear hyperdense on CT
- **Lymphoid Follicles, Small Bowel**
  - Prevalent in distal small bowel (SB), especially in children
  - Uniform size (2-4 mm), ill-defined borders due to submucosal location
- **Intestinal Parasitic Disease**
  - Common in some developing countries
  - Linear filling defects, thickened proximal SB folds, ileocecal ulcerations
  - Ascariasis: Curvilinear filling defects up to 35 cm on SB follow-through (SBFT)
    - Double-contrast sign representing *Ascaris* worm with barium ingestion
  - Giardiasis and cryptosporidiosis: Thickened duodenal and jejunal folds on SBFT

Helpful Clues for Less Common Diagnoses

- **Intestinal Metastases and Lymphoma**
  - Rarely as numerous as in polyposis syndromes
  - Both can lead to multiple polyps, may ulcerate → bull's-eye (target) lesions
  - Lymphoma: Thickened bowel wall and folds; adenopathy seen
  - Melanoma most common etiology of SB metastases
- **Intramural Benign Intestinal Tumors**
  - Any mesenchymal component of SB wall
  - GI bleeding, intestinal obstruction, intussusception
  - Lipoma is most commonly recognized due to fat density on CT
    - Most common cause of SB intussusception (symptomatic)
  - Multiple neurofibromas in neurofibromatosis in type 1 (NF1)
  - Leiomyoma: Calcifications and necrosis are common in this rare tumor
- **Hamartomatous Polyposis Syndromes**
  - Peutz-Jeghers syndrome: Jejunum and ileum > duodenum > colon > stomach
    - Mucocutaneous pigment lesions, lips and skin
  - Cowden disease: Polyps from esophagus to colon; colonic polyps > SB
  - Cronkhite-Canada syndrome: All GI tract except esophagus; most in distal stomach
- **Gardner Syndrome**
  - Adenomatous polyps in colon, SB, stomach
  - Extracolonic neoplasms (osteomas, ampullary tumors, desmoids; adrenal, thyroid, liver carcinomas)
- **Familial Polyposis**
  - Adenomas in colon > stomach > duodenum > SB

SELECTED REFERENCES

1. Wu M et al: Peutz-Jeghers syndrome. StatPearls, 2021
2. Wu ZY et al: Cronkhite-Canada syndrome: from clinical features to treatment. Gastroenterol Rep (Oxf). 8(5):333-42, 2020

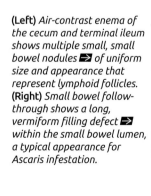

(Left) Air-contrast enema of the cecum and terminal ileum shows multiple small, small bowel nodules ➡ of uniform size and appearance that represent lymphoid follicles. (Right) Small bowel follow-through shows a long, vermiform filling defect ➡ within the small bowel lumen, a typical appearance for Ascaris infestation.

Lymphoid Follicles, Small Bowel

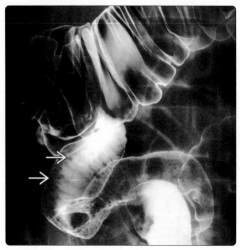

Intestinal Parasitic Disease

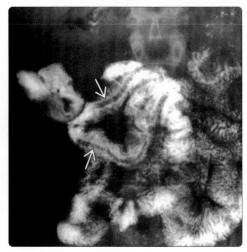

Intestinal Metastases and Lymphoma

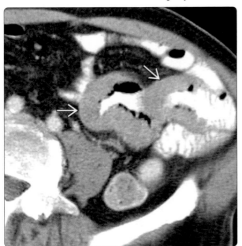

Intestinal Metastases and Lymphoma

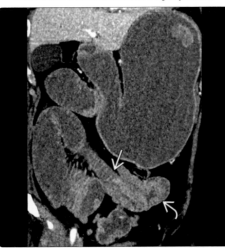

(Left) *Axial CECT shows 2 of many small bowel metastases ➔ from melanoma with intramural masses and mucosal ulceration.* (Right) *Coronal CECT in a patient with small bowel obstruction due to intussusception secondary to metastatic melanoma shows intussusceptum ➔ and intussuscipiens ➔. A discrete lesion is not visible, and metastatic melanoma was found at surgery.*

Intramural Benign Intestinal Tumors

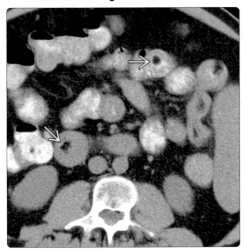

Intramural Benign Intestinal Tumors

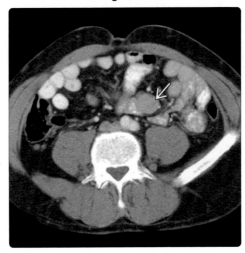

(Left) *Axial NECT shows 2 of several fat density lesions ➔ within the small bowel, diagnostic of lipomas. These appear to be intraluminal, though they arise in the bowel wall, subsequently being drawn into the lumen by peristalsis.* (Right) *Axial CECT shows one of several soft tissue density nodules ➔ within the SB wall, representing neurofibromas, in a patient with neurofibromatosis.*

Hamartomatous Polyposis Syndromes

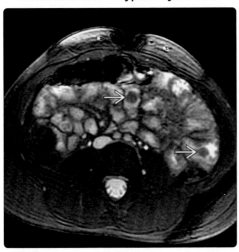

Gardner Syndrome

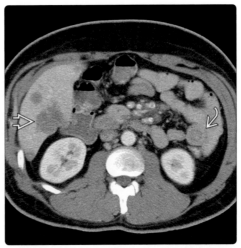

(Left) *MR enterography in this 12-year-old boy with Peutz-Jeghers syndrome shows 2 ➔ of many small bowel hamartomatous polyps.* (Right) *Axial CECT in a patient with Gardner syndrome shows a small bowel intussusception ➔ but not the adenomatous polyp that was the likely cause. Liver metastases ➔ are present from a colon carcinoma (not shown).*

DIFFERENTIAL DIAGNOSIS

Common

- Simple Small Bowel Obstruction
- Focal ileus
- Closed Loop Small Bowel Obstruction
- External Hernia

Less Common

- Peritoneal Metastases
- Sclerosing Peritonitis
- Transmesenteric Postoperative Hernia
- Paraduodenal Hernia
- Transplantation, Small Intestine
- Other Types of Internal Hernia
- Afferent Loop Syndrome

ESSENTIAL INFORMATION

Key Differential Diagnosis Issues

- Check for internal or external hernia
  - Ask about predisposing conditions, e.g., prior Roux-en-Y gastric bypass or liver transplantation
- Check for peritoneal infection or tumor

Helpful Clues for Common Diagnoses

- **Simple Small Bowel Obstruction**
  - Gas and fluid-distended small bowel (SB) loops (> 3 cm) proximal to collapsed loops
  - Transition zone but no mass, hernia, or other visible cause = adhesive SB obstruction
  - Dilated SB leading into hernia, collapsed SB coming out of hernia = hernia as etiology of SB
- **Closed Loop Small Bowel Obstruction**
  - Markedly distended segment of fluid-filled SB
  - Bowel proximal and distal to closed loop usually not dilated
  - Stretched mesenteric vessels converging toward site of obstruction
  - Distended SB loops appear as balloons on strings
- **External Hernia**

- Gas- and fluid-filled bowel loops, omental fat, and vessels in ventral, inguinal, or other external hernia sac

Helpful Clues for Less Common Diagnoses

- **Peritoneal Metastases**
  - Serosal metastases encase and obstruct SB
  - Look for soft tissue density thickening of SB walls &/or mesenteric leaves
- **Sclerosing Peritonitis**
  - Results from chronic peritoneal dialysis (uncommonly)
    - Even more rarely as result of infected ascites (bacterial, TB, or fungal peritonitis)
  - Fibrotic and often calcified serosal encasement of SB (cocoon)
- **Transmesenteric Postoperative Hernia**
  - Protrusion of SB loops through congenital or acquired defect of mesentery
  - Cluster of dilated SB loops with distorted mesenteric vessels; hernia usually not encapsulated
- **Paraduodenal Hernia**
  - Protrusion of bowel loops through congenital paraduodenal fossae
  - Left paraduodenal hernia (75%): Lateral to 4th part of duodenum, between pancreas and stomach
  - Right paraduodenal hernia (25%): Via jejunal mesentericoparietal fossa of Waldeyer
  - Cluster of dilated bowel loops in abnormal location with crowded, distorted mesenteric vessels
- **Transplantation, Small Intestine**
  - Usually accompanied by considerable mesenteric infiltration and scarring
- **Afferent Loop Syndrome**
  - Plain films and barium fluoroscopic exams often miss this complication, as afferent loop is fluid-distended and oral contrast medium does not enter it
  - CT shows dilation of afferent loop and any complications (e.g., dilated bile ducts, recurrent tumor, ischemia, perforation)

Simple Small Bowel Obstruction

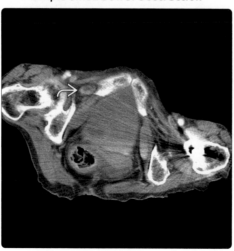

Closed Loop Small Bowel Obstruction

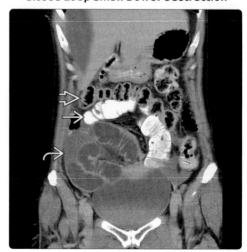

(Left) *Axial CECT in an older adult woman with dilated proximal and mid small bowel (SB), at the point of transition, shows there is a segment of SB ➡ that has herniated through the obturator canal with the strangulated segment lying between the pectineus and obturator muscles. This is a classic obturator hernia.* **(Right)** *Coronal CECT shows a radial distribution of the closed loops ➡, which are dilated out of proportion to proximal SB ➡ or colon ➡.*

Peritoneal Metastases

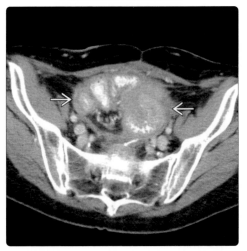

Sclerosing Peritonitis

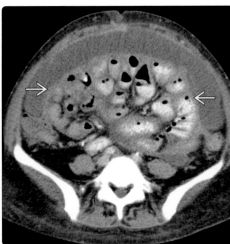

(Left) *Axial CECT shows a tight cluster of SB* ➥ *that produced a functional SB obstruction due to peritoneal (serosal) metastases from ovarian carcinoma that encased the bowel.* (Right) *Axial CECT shows a cluster of SB that produced chronic symptoms of SB obstruction in a patient with renal failure on chronic ambulatory peritoneal dialysis, who developed sclerosing peritonitis. Note peritoneal thickening* ➥*, encasing SB.*

Transmesenteric Postoperative Hernia

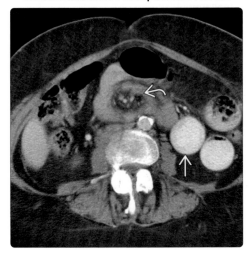

Paraduodenal Hernia

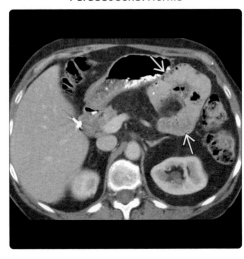

(Left) *Axial CECT in a patient s/p Roux-en-Y gastric bypass shows the Roux limb and proximal SB* ➥ *are dilated while the distal SB and colon are collapsed. Note twisting of the SB mesenteric root* ➥*. The jejunal anastomotic staple line was displaced, and mesenteric vessels were distorted.* (Right) *Axial CECT shows a sac-of-bowel appearance* ➥ *of proximal bowel segments to the left of the ligament of Treitz, displacing the stomach forward. Their mesenteric vessels are displaced toward the center of the hernia.*

Transplantation, Small Intestine

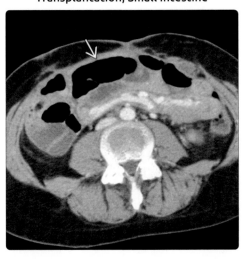

Afferent Loop Syndrome

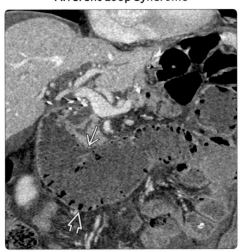

(Left) *Axial CECT shows mild dilation of the SB allograft* ➥*, along with infiltration of its mesentery, both common and nonspecific findings.* (Right) *Coronal CECT in a patient s/p total gastrectomy with Roux-en-Y reconstruction for gastric cancer shows a dilated afferent loop* ➥*, concerning for afferent loop syndrome, with extensive pneumatosis* ➥ *in the wall of the dilated afferent loop, consistent with ischemia, a complication of afferent loop syndrome.*

DIFFERENTIAL DIAGNOSIS

Common

- Lymphoma, Small Bowel
- Metastases, Small Bowel
- Bowel-Bowel Anastomosis

Less Common

- Gastrointestinal Stromal Tumor
- Small Bowel Obstruction
- Diverticula, Small Bowel
- Primary Adenocarcinoma

Rare but Important

- Duplication Cyst, Gastrointestinal Tract

ESSENTIAL INFORMATION

Key Differential Diagnosis Issues

- Luminal dilation plus intramural mass = infiltrative malignancy, such as lymphoma, metastases, or gastrointestinal tumor
- CT enterography is best protocol with multiplanar reformation

Helpful Clues for Common Diagnoses

- **Lymphoma, Small Bowel**
  - Classic etiology of aneurysmal dilation
  - Destroys myenteric plexus &/or wall of small bowel (SB)
    - Necrotic tumor may form cavity in communication with bowel lumen
    - Destruction of nerves in bowel wall allows dilation of lumen
  - Danger of free perforation into peritoneal cavity if tumor is treated with chemo- or radiation therapy
- **Metastases, Small Bowel**
  - Malignant melanoma is especially likely to cause aneurysmal dilation, similar to lymphoma
  - Usually see other metastases to bowel, mesentery, etc.
  - Bull's-eye or target lesions; intussusception
  - May arise many years after primary tumor removal

- **Bowel-Bowel Anastomosis**
  - Common after prior SB resection, creation of Roux loop, or to bypass stricture
  - Look for staple line at anastomosis

Helpful Clues for Less Common Diagnoses

- **Gastrointestinal Stromal Tumor**
  - Most common mesenchymal neoplasm in SB
  - Duodenum and jejunum 2nd most common site (after stomach)
  - Large, exophyte mass arising from bowel wall
  - Ulceration of mucosa and central necrosis of tumor are common
  - May result in intratumoral gas and contrast media, resembling aneurysmal dilation
  - Aggressive tumors: Tumor size > 10 cm, irregular or invasive border, necrosis, internal air or enteric contrast
- **Small Bowel Obstruction**
  - Chronically dilated SB may attain large diameter (> 6 cm)
  - Preservation of normal SB folds distinguishes this from aneurysmal dilation related to neoplastic infiltration
- **Diverticula, Small Bowel**
  - Outpouchings from duodenum are very common
  - These are uncommon, but not rare, throughout remainder of SB
  - Perforation of SB diverticula can result in "SB diverticulitis" with abscess cavity
- **Primary Adenocarcinoma**
  - Annular or eccentric mass causing intussusception or obstruction
  - ↑ risk with celiac and Crohn disease, polyposis syndromes
  - Annular or eccentric mass causing intussusception or obstruction

Helpful Clues for Rare Diagnoses

- **Duplication Cyst, Gastrointestinal Tract**
  - Can arise from SB or any portion of gastrointestinal tract
  - May communicate with SB lumen, rarely simulating dilated lumen or aneurysmal dilation

(Left) Spot film from a small bowel (SB) follow-through shows a large mass ➡ that encases but does not obstruct a segment of jejunum. Note aneurysmal dilation ➡ (tumor necrosis that fills with barium). (Right) Axial NECT shows a large mass ➡ that encases but does not obstruct the jejunum with central necrosis of the mass that fills with gas ➡ from the SB lumen.

Lymphoma, Small Bowel

Lymphoma, Small Bowel

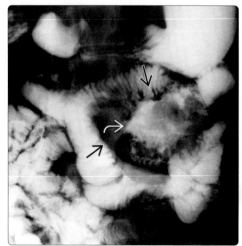

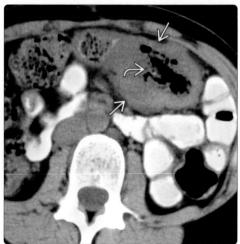

Metastases, Small Bowel

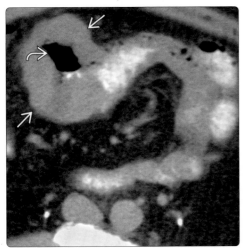

Gastrointestinal Stromal Tumor

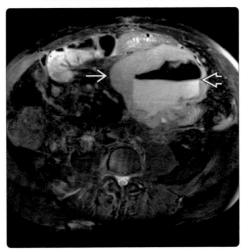

(Left) *Axial NECT in a patient with melanoma metastatic to the SB shows a soft tissue mass* ➡ *that encases but does not obstruct the SB with a central necrotic cavity* ➡ *that fills with gas and enteric contrast.* **(Right)** *Axial T2 FS MR shows a high-grade gastrointestinal stromal tumor (GIST) with aneurysmal dilation of the bowel* ➡ *and an air-fluid level* ➡.

Bowel-Bowel Anastomosis

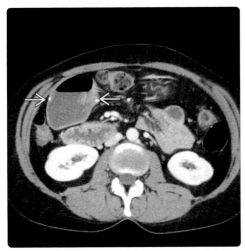

Diverticula, Small Bowel

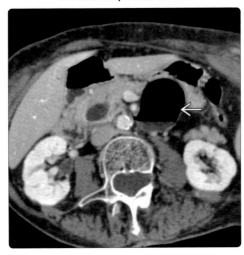

(Left) *Axial CECT shows focal dilation of the SB without evidence of obstruction. The metallic staple line* ➡ *helps to identify this as the site of a side-to-side SB anastomosis.* **(Right)** *Axial CECT shows one of several duodenal and jejunal diverticula* ➡ *with a thin wall and an air-fluid level present.*

Duplication Cyst, Gastrointestinal Tract

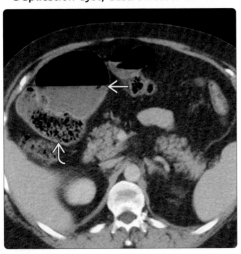

Primary Adenocarcinoma

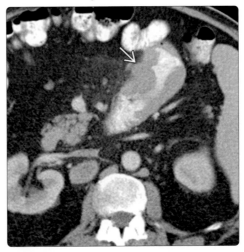

(Left) *Axial CECT shows a cystic structure that communicates with the SB lumen (air-fluid level)* ➡ *and causes partial SB obstruction (note SB feces sign)* ➡. *This was a duplication cyst of the ileum.* **(Right)** *Axial CECT in a 63-year-old man with abdominal pain shows an annular endoluminal mass in a dilated jejunum* ➡. *The mass was resected, and pathology showed an adenocarcinoma.*

DIFFERENTIAL DIAGNOSIS

Common

- Crohn Disease
- Infectious Enteritis
- Acute Appendicitis

Less Common

- Ulcerative Colitis (Backwash Ileitis)
- Abdominal Abscess
- Cecal Carcinoma
- Carcinoid Tumor
- Tuberculosis
- Metastases and Lymphoma, Intestinal
- Radiation Enteritis
- Small Bowel Carcinoma

ESSENTIAL INFORMATION

Key Differential Diagnosis Issues

- Stenosis (stricture) of terminal ileum is much less common than simple wall thickening but may be difficult to distinguish between these on single imaging study

Helpful Clues for Common Diagnoses

- **Crohn Disease**
  - Terminal ileum usually initial site of involvement
  - Small bowel follow-through (SBFT): Longitudinal and transverse ulcerations, aphthous lesions in small bowel (SB) and colon
  - CT/MR: Wall thickening, luminal narrowing, mesenteric lymphadenopathy, and fibrofatty proliferation
    - Mucosal and mesenteric hyperemia = acute inflammation
- **Infectious Enteritis**
  - *Yersinia* (gram-negative bacterium) produces radiographic findings similar to Crohn disease
    - Usually resolves quickly without stricture
  - Other bacterial and viral organisms can cause enteritis, often with cluster of mildly enlarged mesenteric nodes
- **Acute Appendicitis**

- SB and colon adjacent to inflamed appendix often have reactive wall thickening and luminal narrowing
    - Usually not true stricture
    - May result in functional SB obstruction
  - Key is to identify abnormal appendix on CT, US, or MR
- **Ulcerative Colitis (Backwash Ileitis)**
  - Lesions are usually continuous and almost always involve rectum
  - Fistulas, abscesses, and strictures are much less common

Helpful Clues for Less Common Diagnoses

- **Abdominal Abscess**
  - Pus from any abdominal or pelvic source (appendicitis, diverticulitis, adnexal abscess)
    - May bathe distal ileum, causing wall thickening and spasm
  - Fold thickening and luminal narrowing simulates primary SB inflammation
- **Cecal Carcinoma**
  - May extend into distal SB wall, serosa
  - CT may show peritoneal and liver metastases
- **Carcinoid Tumor**
  - Common in appendix, distal SB
  - CT shows mesenteric mass (± calcification) usually more evident than primary tumor
    - Primary tumor and metastases are usually hypervascular
  - Marked desmoplastic infiltration of SB mesentery
- **Tuberculosis**
  - May involve cecum and terminal ileum
  - Look for signs of peritonitis and caseated nodes on CT
- **Radiation Enteritis**
  - Usually pelvic SB loops, not terminal ileum
- **Small Bowel Carcinoma**
  - Short segment stricture with overhanging edges (apple core)
  - Typically results in SB obstruction
  - Regional nodal and liver metastases

Crohn Disease

Crohn Disease

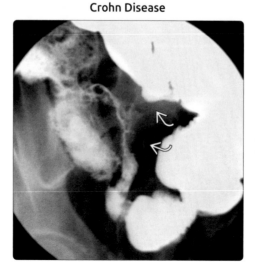
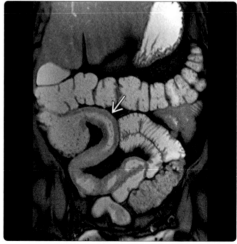

(Left) *Small bowel follow-through shows luminal narrowing and mucosal ulceration of the distal ileum and ascending colon. Also noted are mass effect and fistulas ➵ in the mesenteric fat.* **(Right)** *Coronal T2 FS MR in a 48-year-old man with Crohn disease shows wall thickening of the terminal ileum ➔, along with luminal narrowing.*

Infectious Enteritis

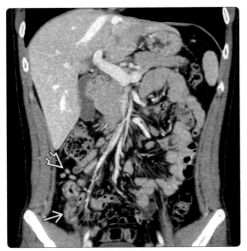

Acute Appendicitis

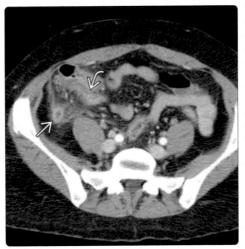

(Left) *Coronal CECT in a young woman with acute right lower quadrant pain and fever shows luminal narrowing, mucosal hyperenhancement, and submucosal edema in the terminal ileum ➡ and cecum, along with mesenteric lymphadenopathy ➡. The appendix was normal. All signs and symptoms resolved without treatment.* **(Right)** *Axial CECT shows a dilated lumen and thickened wall of the appendix ➡ with inflammatory infiltration of the mesenteric fat and secondary inflammation of the terminal ileum ➡.*

Ulcerative Colitis (Backwash Ileitis)

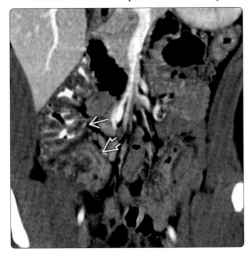

Abdominal Abscess

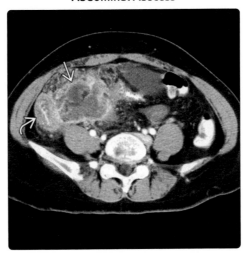

(Left) *Coronal venous-phase CECT shows wall thickening of the cecum ➡ extending to the terminal ileum, which shows narrowed lumen ➡ referred to as backwash ileitis.* **(Right)** *Axial CECT shows a RLQ abscess ➡ with mural thickening and luminal narrowing of the cecum ➡ and terminal ileum. A perforated appendix was found at surgery.*

Cecal Carcinoma

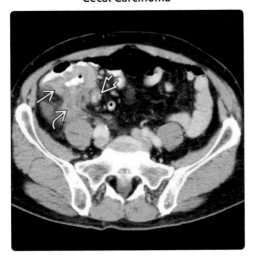

Tuberculosis

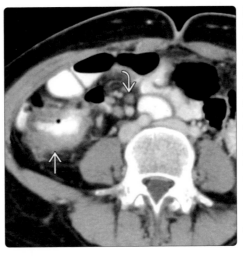

(Left) *Axial CECT shows a soft tissue density mass that causes circumferential thickening of the cecal wall ➡ and obstruction of the base of the appendix ➡. There is infiltration of adjacent fat planes and the wall of the terminal ileum ➡.* **(Right)** *Axial CECT shows mural thickening and luminal narrowing of the cecum ➡ and terminal ileum with mesenteric adenopathy ➡. This is proven ileocecal tuberculosis in a young woman who is an immigrant from Southeast Asia.*

DIFFERENTIAL DIAGNOSIS

Common

- Crohn Disease
- Shock Bowel (Systemic Hypotension)
- Portal Hypertension
- Ischemic Enteritis
- Infectious Enteritis
- Mesenteric Adenitis/Enteritis
- Chemotherapy-Induced Enteritis
- Celiac-Sprue Disease

Less Common

- Opportunistic Intestinal Infections
- Graft-vs.-Host Disease
- Vasculitis, Small Intestine
- Angioedema, Intestinal
- Carcinoid Tumor
- Intramural Hemorrhage
- Hypoalbuminemia (e.g., Hepatic Cirrhosis, Nephrotic Syndrome)
- Radiation Enteritis
- Metastases and Lymphoma, Intestinal
- Endometriosis

Rare but Important

- Lymphangiectasia, Intestinal
- Whipple Disease
- Mastocytosis

ESSENTIAL INFORMATION

Key Differential Diagnosis Issues

- Characterize wall thickening by
  - **Length and degree of involvement**
    - Focal (< 10-cm) length of involvement
      - Neoplasm, endometriosis, Crohn disease
    - Segmental (< 40-cm) length
      - Most common; least specific
    - Diffuse (> 40-cm) length of involvement
      - Systemic processes (shock, portal hypertension, vasculitis)
  - **Attenuation of submucosal layer**
    - Air: Pneumatosis (exclude ischemia)
    - Fat: Normal variant, inactive Crohn; cytoreductive chemotherapy
    - Edema/water: Infection, inflammation, or ischemia
    - Blood (> 60 HU): Intramural hemorrhage
  - **Pattern of enhancement** (homo- or heterogeneous)
    - Heterogeneous suggests neoplastic
  - **Associated findings**
    - Vessel engorgement or thrombosis
    - Lymphadenopathy, edema, ascites
    - Extraintestinal sites of tumor
    - History or signs of shock, portal hypertension, or immunosuppression
  - **Degree of mucosal enhancement**
    - Normal [similar to remainder of small bowel (SB)]
    - Increased and often thickened
      - Infection (e.g., opportunistic)
      - Inflammation (e.g., Crohn disease, vasculitis, angioedema)
    - Decreased = ischemia
- **Optimal CT technique**
  - Distend SB lumen by water or neutral contrast agent
  - Rapid IV contrast medium administration (4-5 mL/sec)
  - Multiplanar viewing (especially coronal)

Helpful Clues for Common Diagnoses

- **Crohn Disease**
  - Segmental distribution with skip lesions
  - Submucosal attenuation: Edema in acute; fat density in chronic
  - Mucosal hyperenhancement: Marked in sites of active inflammation
  - Associated findings: Mesenteric hyperemia, fibrofatty proliferation, lymphadenopathy
- **Shock Bowel (Systemic Hypotension)**
  - Diffuse distribution with marked wall thickening
  - Submucosal attenuation: Water density
  - Mucosal hyperenhancement: Intense
  - Associated findings: Mesenteric edema, flattened inferior vena cava
- **Portal Hypertension**
  - Diffuse distribution
  - Associated findings: Cirrhosis, ascites, splenomegaly
- **Ischemic Enteritis**
  - Segmental with marked wall thickening in venous obstruction
  - Attenuation: Air (infarction) to edema to blood density
  - Enhancement: Intense mucosal in venous thrombosis; absent in arterial thrombosis
  - Associated findings: Thrombosis of mesenteric vessels, ascites, and ileus
    - Minimal wall thickening in arterial occlusion
- **Infectious Enteritis**
  - In previously healthy individuals, usually self-limited
    - Variety of pathogens (bacteria, protozoa, viruses, etc.)
  - Distribution: Long segmental
    - *Giardia*: Duodenum and jejunum
    - *Yersinia, Campylobacter*: Distal ileum and cecum
  - Mucosal hyperenhancement and submucosal edema
  - Associated: Mesenteric adenopathy and diarrhea (liquid bowel contents)
- **Mesenteric Adenitis/Enteritis**
  - Form of infectious enteritis
  - Occurs in children and young adults presenting with acute right lower quadrant pain
  - Cluster of enlarged ileac mesenteric nodes may be only finding
  - Terminal ileum and cecum may appear inflamed
- **Chemotherapy-Induced Enteritis**
  - Diffuse or predominantly distal ileum
  - CT: Submucosal edema and hyperemia of mucosa and serosa (target sign)
- **Celiac-Sprue Disease**
  - Most common disease causing malabsorption pattern
    - Dilated, fluid-distended SB, appearing flaccid
    - SB segments indent and conform to each other

- – Decreased fold height in jejunum; increased in ileum (reversed fold pattern)
- – Short-segment intussusceptions

Helpful Clues for Less Common Diagnoses
- **Opportunistic Intestinal Infections**
  - o Segmental with moderate thickening
  - o Associated findings
    - – History of AIDS or transplantation
    - – Lymphadenopathy (low density in mycobacterial disease)
- **Graft-vs.-Host Disease**
  - o Usually diffuse
  - o Attenuation: Water to soft tissue
  - o Associated findings: Skin and liver involvement
  - o By imaging alone, it is difficult or impossible to distinguish graft-vs.-host disease (GVHD) from opportunistic SB infection
- **Vasculitis, Small Intestine**
  - o Segmental or diffuse with moderate to marked thickening
  - o Attenuation: Air to water to soft tissue to blood
    - – Pneumatosis may be due to ischemia or from medications (steroids)
  - o Associated findings: Skin and subcutaneous purpura (Henoch-Schönlein), visceral ischemic lesions (lupus, polyarteritis)
- **Angioedema, Intestinal**
  - o Congenital or associated with medications (e.g., ACE inhibitors), hepatitis, etc.
  - o Involves long segment of jejunum &/or ileum
  - o Imaging findings are entirely reversible, seen only during acute phase
  - o Associated findings: Ascites (almost always)
- **Carcinoid Tumor**
  - o Segmental, usually distal ileum
  - o Mural mass and mesenteric metastases are hyperenhancing (distinctive feature)
  - o Associated findings: Liver metastases
    - – Mesenteric mass with calcification

- – Desmoplastic effect on adjacent SB loops
- **Intramural Hemorrhage**
  - o Segmental with marked thickening
  - o Attenuation: Blood density (> 60 HU)
  - o Associated findings: Signs of trauma or coagulopathic bleeding
- **Radiation Enteritis**
  - o Segmental in pelvis
  - o Associated findings: Evidence of surgery &/or brachytherapy beads in pelvis
- **Metastases and Lymphoma, Intestinal**
  - o Segmental or diffuse (lymphoma)
  - o Multifocal discrete (metastases, e.g., melanoma)
    - – Marked thickening at sites of tumor
  - o Associated findings: Other metastatic foci (e.g., liver, spleen); lymphadenopathy, splenomegaly (lymphoma)
- **Endometriosis**
  - o Focal to segmental with skip areas
  - o Attenuation: Soft tissue or blood density
  - o Associated findings: Pelvic mass; characteristic features of blood on MR

Helpful Clues for Rare Diagnoses
- **Lymphangiectasia, Intestinal**
  - o Diffuse distribution
  - o Submucosal and mesenteric edema (marked)
  - o Ascites and lower extremity edema
  - o Diarrhea (fluid distention of SB and colon)
- **Whipple Disease**
  - o Thickened proximal SB folds and low-density mesenteric lymphadenopathy
    - – Most often affects distal duodenum and jejunum, but ileum can be involved in severe cases
- **Mastocytosis**
  - o Systemic proliferation of mast cells
  - o Thickened folds throughout SB with fluid-distended lumen
  - o Associated: Mixed sclerotic and lytic lesions, skin lesions, hematologic disorders

Crohn Disease

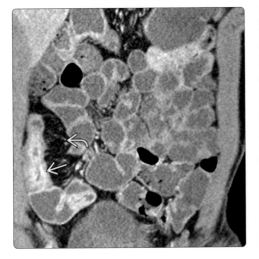

Shock Bowel (Systemic Hypotension)

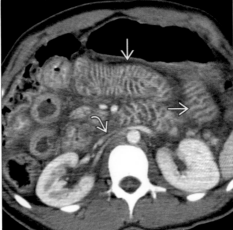

(Left) Coronal CECT shows a thick-walled terminal ileum ➡ with hyperenhancing mucosa and a narrowed lumen. Within the ileal mesentery, there are engorged blood vessels and a proliferation of fibrofatty tissue ➡. (Right) Note the intense enhancement of the small bowel (SB) mucosa ➡ and kidneys along with marked edema/infiltration of the mesentery. Also note the "collapsed cava" ➡ and renal veins due to hypovolemia.

Portal Hypertension

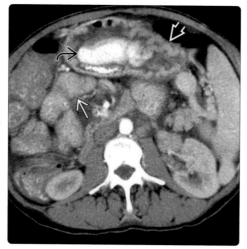

Ischemic Enteritis

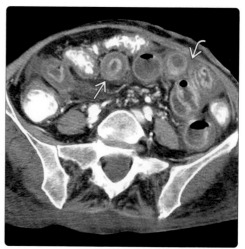

(Left) Axial CECT shows diffuse SB wall edema ⇨ due to cirrhosis and portal hypertension. Associated findings include gastric varices ⇨ causing active bleeding into the gastric lumen ➔. (Right) Axial CECT shows marked mural thickening ⇨ of a long segment of SB due to ischemia following a hypotensive episode. Interloop ascites is also noted ⇨.

Ischemic Enteritis

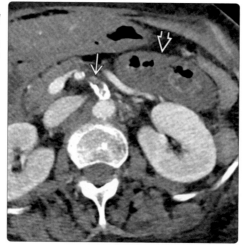

Infectious Enteritis

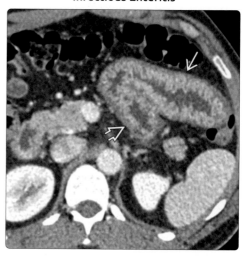

(Left) Axial CECT shows wall thickening of a jejunal loop ⇨ secondary to ischemia from a partially occlusive thrombus in the superior mesenteric artery ⇨. (Right) Axial CECT in an HIV patient with nausea, vomiting, and diarrhea who had a positive stool antigen test for Giardia shows jejunal fold thickening ⇨ and submucosal edema ⇨, consistent with giardiasis.

Mesenteric Adenitis/Enteritis

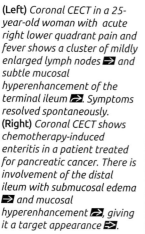

Chemotherapy-Induced Enteritis

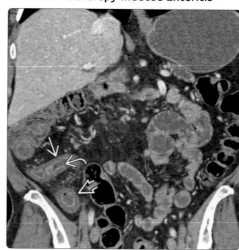

(Left) Coronal CECT in a 25-year-old woman with acute right lower quadrant pain and fever shows a cluster of mildly enlarged lymph nodes ⇨ and subtle mucosal hyperenhancement of the terminal ileum ⇨. Symptoms resolved spontaneously. (Right) Coronal CECT shows chemotherapy-induced enteritis in a patient treated for pancreatic cancer. There is involvement of the distal ileum with submucosal edema ⇨ and mucosal hyperenhancement ⇨, giving it a target appearance ⇨.

Celiac-Sprue Disease

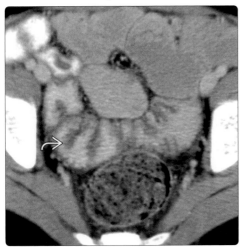

Celiac-Sprue Disease

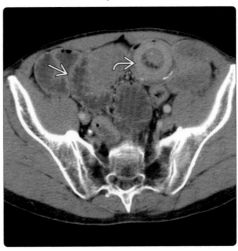

(Left) *Axial CECT in a young man shows fluid distention of the SB. The fold pattern of the jejunum is abnormally effaced, resembling the expected pattern of the ileum. Conversely, the ileal fold pattern is abnormally prominent �'. Endoscopic biopsy and response to a gluten-free diet confirmed the diagnosis of celiac disease. (Right) Axial CECT in a 69-year-old man shows fluid distention of the SB and prominent ileal folds ➡. A short-segment intussusception ➡ is noted.*

Opportunistic Intestinal Infections

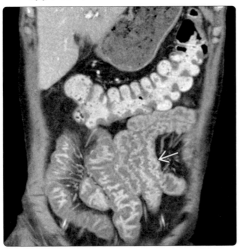

Graft-vs.-Host Disease

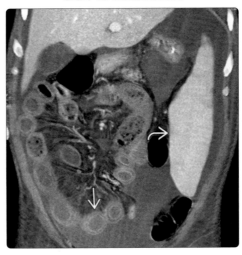

(Left) *Coronal CT in a woman with acute severe diarrhea following lung transplantation for cystic fibrosis shows diffuse SB mucosal hyperenhancement and submucosal edema ➡ (proven CMV enteritis). (Right) Coronal CECT in a man with bone marrow transplantation for myelofibrosis who developed a rash and abdominal pain with diarrhea shows diffuse SB submucosal edema ➡ along with ascites and splenomegaly ➡. It is difficult to distinguish graft-vs.-host disease from opportunistic infection by CT alone.*

Vasculitis, Small Intestine

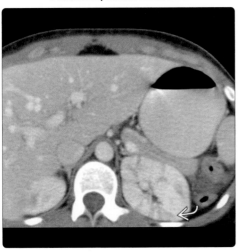

Vasculitis, Small Intestine

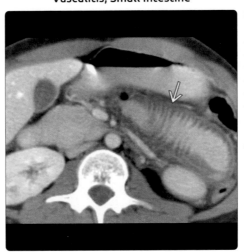

(Left) *Axial CECT in a young woman with abdominal pain shows wedge-shaped and striated zones of decreased attenuation ➡ within the kidneys and ascites. (Right) Axial CECT in the same patient shows long segmental wall thickening of the jejunum ➡. The combination of the patient's young age and renal and SB involvement suggested vasculitis, and polyarteritis was confirmed.*

Angioedema, Intestinal

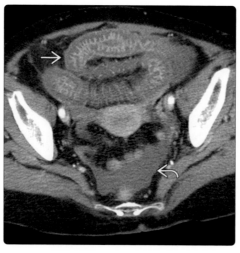

Angioedema, Intestinal

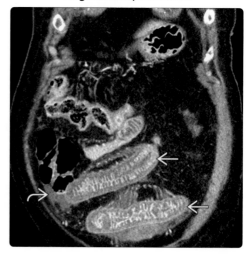

(Left) *Axial CECT in an older woman with repeated bouts of laryngeal edema and severe abdominal pain shows long segmental SB wall edema ➡ and ascites ➡. (Right) Coronal CECT in the same patient shows long segmental SB submucosal edema ➡ and ascites ➡. This was attributed to the use of ACE inhibitor medication, and symptoms and signs resolved with withdrawal of this medication.*

Carcinoid Tumor

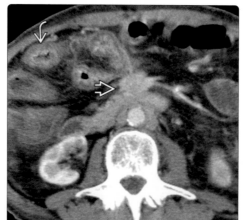

Carcinoid Tumor

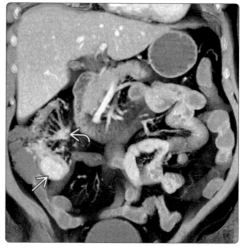

(Left) *Axial CECT in a 64-year-old man shows a hypervascular mesenteric mass ➡ due to nodal metastases. Note the SB wall edema ➡ and tethering due to the desmoplastic effect of the tumor on mesenteric veins and lymphatics. (Right) Coronal CECT in a 54-year-old man shows a hypervascular mass ➡ in the distal ileum with associated mesenteric metastasis ➡ having a characteristic desmoplastic effect on adjacent bowel.*

Intramural Hemorrhage

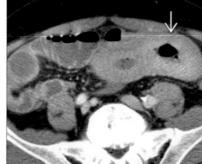

Radiation Enteritis

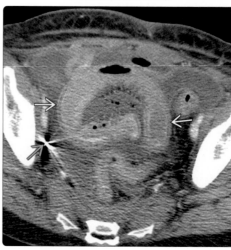

(Left) *Axial CT shows segmental mural thickening of the jejunum ➡, representing intramural hematoma due to coagulopathic hemorrhage in a patient who was on warfarin therapy. The submucosal attenuation was 60 HU. (Right) Axial CECT in a woman with cervical carcinoma shows wall edema of pelvic SB segments ➡, along with ascites. Surgical clips ➡ are from lymph node dissection at the time of hysterectomy. The SB lumen is also dilated. At surgery, an ischemic stricture and radiation enteritis were confirmed.*

Metastases and Lymphoma, Intestinal

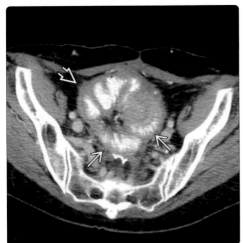

Metastases and Lymphoma, Intestinal

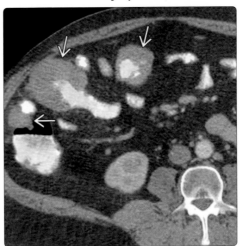

(Left) *Axial CECT in a woman with metastatic ovarian cancer shows loculated, malignant ascites ➡ and a cluster of SB loops with thickened folds due to serosal metastases ➡.* (Right) *Axial CECT shows marked soft tissue density wall thickening in several segments of SB ➡. In spite of the large masses, there is no luminal obstruction, typical findings of SB lymphoma.*

Lymphangiectasia, Intestinal

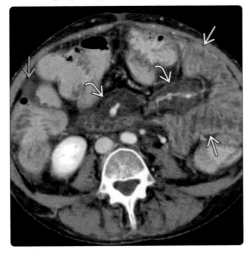

Lymphangiectasia, Intestinal

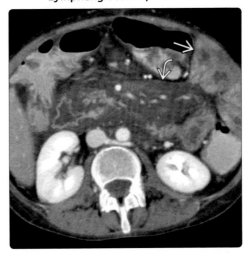

(Left) *Axial CECT in a 36-year-old woman with chronic diarrhea shows ascites ➡ and submucosal edema throughout much of the small intestine ➡. More striking is the edema in the root and leaves of mesentery ➡.* (Right) *Axial CECT in a young woman with chronic diarrhea shows diffuse SB wall edema ➡ and striking infiltration of the SB mesentery ➡.*

Mastocytosis

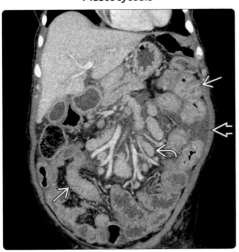

Mastocytosis

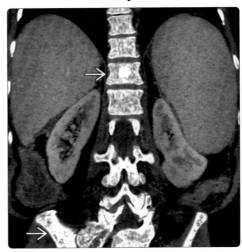

(Left) *Coronal CECT in a 64-year-old woman shows widespread abdominal lymphadenopathy ➡, ascites ➡, and diffuse SB submucosal edema ➡.* (Right) *Coronal CECT in the same patient shows hepatosplenomegaly and multifocal sclerosis of the axial skeleton ➡, all due to systemic mastocytosis.*

DIFFERENTIAL DIAGNOSIS

Common

- Ischemic Enteritis and Colitis
- Medication-Induced Pneumatosis
- Postoperative State, Bowel
- Post Endoscopy
- Pseudopneumatosis (Mimic)
- Pulmonary Disease
  - Barotrauma, Abdominal Manifestations
    - Asthma
    - Chronic Obstructive Pulmonary Disease
    - Cystic Fibrosis
    - Ventilator
- Small Bowel Obstruction
- Necrotizing Enterocolitis

Less Common

- Pneumatosis Cystoides Intestinalis
- Intestinal Trauma
- Small Bowel Transplantation
- Inflammatory Bowel Disease
- Toxic Megacolon
- Graft-vs.-Host Disease
- Caustic Gastroduodenal Injury
- Gas in Wall of Ileal Conduit
- Scleroderma
- Autoimmune Disease
  - Lupus
  - Polyarteritis Nodosa
  - Celiac Sprue
  - Polymyositis
  - Dermatomyositis

ESSENTIAL INFORMATION

Key Differential Diagnosis Issues

- Pneumatosis is radiographic finding, not disease process
  - To determine its significance, must correlate with
    - Patient history
    - Clinical signs and symptoms
      - Nonischemic causes: Patients are often asymptomatic
      - Bowel ischemia: Nausea, abdominal pain, distention, melena, fever, vomiting, cough (depending on etiology)
      - If pneumatosis is due to ischemia, patient will be very ill
      - Check for laboratory abnormalities (acidosis, leukocytosis, elevated serum amylase)

Helpful Clues for Common Diagnoses

- **Ischemic Enteritis and Colitis**
  - Best imaging tool: Dual-phase CECT with multiplanar reformations without enteric contrast medium
  - Findings vary by acuity, etiology, and severity
  - Spherical or linear collections of gas in submucosa of affected bowel
    - Thrombus may not always be visible
  - Often associated with portal venous gas
    - Portal venous gas collects in liver periphery

- Small bowel (SB) ischemia is usually due to occlusion of superior mesenteric artery or superior mesenteric vein
  - Acute arterial thromboembolic: Emboli to superior mesenteric artery from cardiac sources most commonly; affects right colon ± small bowel
  - Mesenteric venous thrombosis: Marked submucosal edema of affected colon (right > left) ± small bowel
  - Colonic ischemia more often due to hypoperfusion; not thrombotic
    - Rectum is rarely affected by ischemic colitis
  - Dilated bowel lumen (ileus), thickened wall, abnormal enhancement
  - Ascites; may be of blood density (> 35 HU)
- **Medication-Induced Pneumatosis**
  - Corticosteroids, chemotherapy, antirejection medications
  - Any organ or bone marrow transplant recipient
  - Medications may cause tiny perforations of mucosa by inducing atrophy of submucosal lymphoid follicles
  - ↑ mucosal permeability, ↓ immune system → bacterial gas enters bowel wall
- **Postoperative State, Bowel**
  - Bowel-to-bowel anastomosis
  - Gastrostomy, jejunostomy tubes
  - Either may cause gas to leak from bowel lumen into wall
  - Patients are usually asymptomatic unless there is leak of other bowel contents or associated SB obstruction
- **Post Endoscopy**
  - Upper or lower endoscopy
  - Also after barium or hydrogen peroxide enema
  - Mucosal disruption and ↑ luminal pressure → bowel distention → air dissection into wall
- **Pseudopneumatosis (Mimic)**
  - Gas may be trapped against inner wall of bowel, simulating pneumatosis
  - Very common in cecum, ascending colon
    - Usually not seen above air-feces level within colon
  - SB feces sign (in SB obstruction or cystic fibrosis)
    - Gas may be trapped within lumen, up against inner wall of SB
- **Pulmonary Disease**
  - Investigate history of
    - Asthma
    - Chronic obstructive pulmonary disease
    - Pulmonary fibrosis
    - Cystic fibrosis
    - Ventilator
  - Partial bronchial obstruction and coughing leads to alveolar rupture
  - Gas dissects down into peribronchial and perivascular tissue planes of mediastinum, hiatus of esophagus and aorta allows access to retroperitoneum and mesentery, into bowel wall
  - Further progression to subserosa and submucosa of bowel wall
- **Small Bowel Obstruction**
  - Gas may enter wall of SB, especially if there has been prior SB surgery or intrinsic SB disease (e.g., Crohn disease)
  - Check for signs of closed loop obstruction

- – Disproportionate dilation of cluster of SB loops, engorged vessels, ascites, infiltrated mesentery
- – Pneumatosis with these signs = bowel infarction
- o Correlate with clinical and laboratory evidence of bowel ischemia
- • **Necrotizing Enterocolitis**
  - o Common cause of pneumatosis in neonates

Helpful Clues for Less Common Diagnoses

- • **Pneumatosis Cystoides Intestinalis**
  - o Idiopathic, asymptomatic, usually colonic
  - o Usually appears as large gas cysts in wall of colon
    - – Bubble-like
    - – May be mistaken for polyps if gas density is not appreciated
- • **Intestinal Trauma**
  - o Serosa of bowel may be avulsed (degloving injury)
  - o Leads to devascularization and ischemia of bowel
  - o Rarely, may be transient finding not indicative of bowel injury
- • **Small Bowel Transplantation**
  - o Patients frequently develop benign pneumatosis
  - o Many potential causes
    - – Medications
    - – Bowel-to-bowel anastomoses
    - – Rejection
    - – Infarction
  - o Often requires endoscopic evaluation to distinguish from ischemia
- • **Inflammatory Bowel Disease**
  - o Crohn disease, ulcerative colitis, others
  - o Any disease that causes ulceration of bowel mucosa can cause pneumatosis
  - o Patients are often on steroid medications that may also cause pneumatosis
- • **Graft-vs.-Host Disease**
  - o Bone marrow transplant recipients
  - o Clinical triad: Damage to gut, skin, liver
  - o Pneumatosis does not necessarily indicate ischemia

- – Patients are receiving medications (steroids, immunosuppression) associated with benign pneumatosis
- • **Caustic Gastroduodenal Injury**
  - o Usually limited to esophagus and stomach
  - o Duodenum may also be injured
  - o Mucosal or transmural necrosis may cause pneumatosis &/or perforation of bowel
- • **Gas in Wall of Ileal Conduit**
  - o Following cystectomy
  - o Ureters may be anastomosed to ileal conduit
  - o Nonischemic gas may collect transiently within bowel wall
  - o Check for gas-forming infection of urine (may release gas into lumen, or, rarely, into wall of conduit)
- • **Scleroderma**
  - o Plus other forms of mixed connective tissue disease
  - o Intramural gas may result from bowel disease itself, associated medications (e.g., corticosteroids), or ischemia
    - – Must correlate with clinical and laboratory evidence of disease exacerbation or ischemia
  - o Pathognomonic: Hidebound sign of small bowel (or stack of coins sign)
    - – Dilated jejunal lumen with crowded, thin, circular folds
  - o ± transient, nonobstructive intussusceptions
  - o Marked dilatation of SB (particularly 2nd and 3rd parts of duodenum and jejunum)
  - o Delayed barium transit time

SELECTED REFERENCES

1. im J et al: Pneumatosis intestinalis, StatPearls 2021
2. Blom T et al: Treatment-related toxicities during anti-GD2 immunotherapy in high-risk neuroblastoma patients. Front Oncol. 10:601076, 2020
3. Lassandro G et al: Intestinal pneumatosis: differential diagnosis. Abdom Radiol (NY). 47(5):1529-40, 2020
4. Spencer K et al: Extensive small bowel pneumatosis and ischemia during dinutuximab therapy for high-risk neuroblastoma. Pediatr Blood Cancer. 67(4):e28147, 2020

Ischemic Enteritis and Colitis

Ischemic Enteritis and Colitis

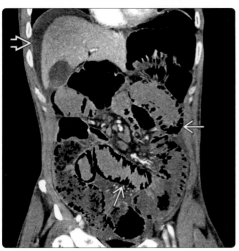

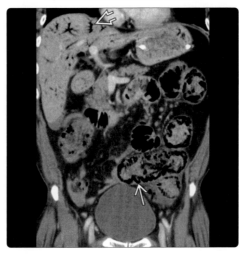

(Left) Coronal CECT shows extensive pneumatosis ➡ throughout the small bowel. Also note dilation of the bowel lumen and ascites ➡, findings that help to confirm that pneumatosis is likely due to bowel ischemia. (Right) Coronal CECT shows small bowel pneumatosis ➡ with extensive portal venous air ➡ in this patient with small bowel ischemia.

(Left) *Supine radiograph in this patient who had a bone marrow transplant shows extensive colonic pneumatosis ➡ but no small bowel dilation. The patient remained essentially asymptomatic, and the pneumatosis was attributed to his immunosuppressive medications.* **(Right)** *Axial CECT in the same patient shows extensive colonic pneumatosis ➡ but neither ascites nor ileus. The patient remained well, and the pneumatosis slowly resolved without other intervention.*

Medication-Induced Pneumatosis

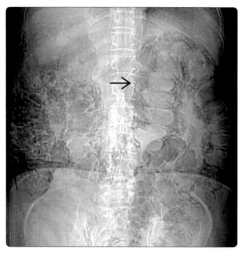

Medication-Induced Pneumatosis

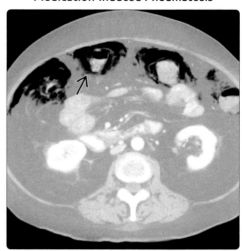

(Left) *Axial CECT shows pneumatosis ➡ near the site of prior bowel resection ➡ but also within bowel that is some distance removed from the operative site ➡. The patient had signs of sepsis, and ischemia was confirmed at surgery.* **(Right)** *Axial CECT shows gas trapped against the wall of the ascending colon ➡, simulating pneumatosis. Note that this finding is not present in the nondependent colon, where the fluid stool is not in contact with the bowel wall.*

Postoperative State, Bowel

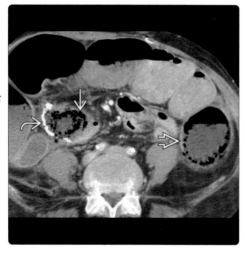

Pseudopneumatosis (Mimic)

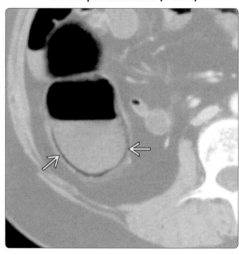

(Left) *Axial CECT shows extensive gas dissecting throughout the abdomen ➡, some of which may be in bowel wall, due to barotrauma in this patient on positive pressure ventilation.* **(Right)** *Coronal NECT in a young woman with an adhesive small bowel obstruction shows marked luminal dilation and pneumatosis ➡ within proximal small bowel segments. At surgery, the dilated bowel returned to normal appearance following release of adhesions and was not resected.*

Barotrauma, Abdominal Manifestations

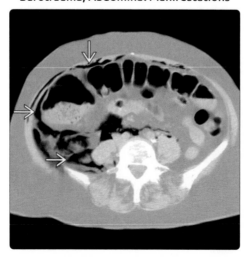

Small Bowel Obstruction

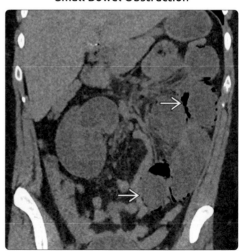

Pneumatosis Cystoides Intestinalis

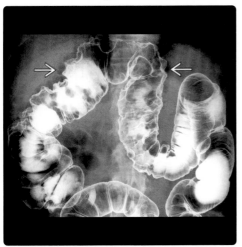

Small Bowel Transplantation

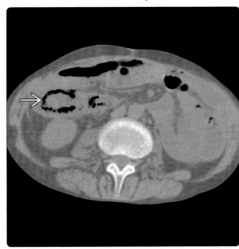

(Left) *Air-contrast enema shows gas cysts ➡ within the wall of otherwise normal colon in an asymptomatic man with idiopathic primary colonic pneumatosis.* (Right) *Small bowel allograft is dilated with a thickened wall and pneumatosis ➡, raising concern for infarction. On endoscopy (through the ileostomy), the small bowel mucosa appeared normal.*

Inflammatory Bowel Disease

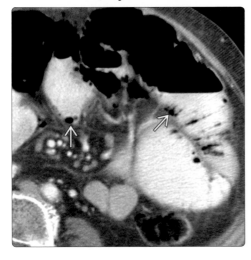

Toxic Megacolon

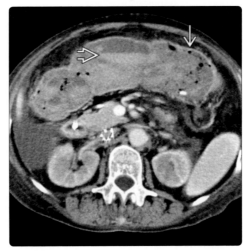

(Left) *In this patient with prior bowel resection for Crohn disease, gas is seen in the wall of dilated loops of the small intestine ➡ in the upper abdomen. Pneumatosis here could be due to ischemia, medication, Crohn disease, or bowel obstruction. At surgery, the bowel was determined to be ischemic but not infarcted.* (Right) *Axial CECT shows a grossly dilated transverse colon with loss of haustration. There is gas within the wall of the colon ➡, hemorrhagic debris within the lumen ➡, and ascites. All findings confirmed at colectomy.*

Graft-vs.-Host Disease

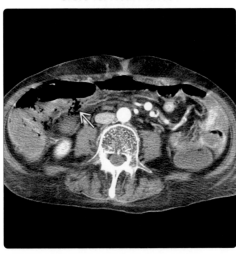

Scleroderma

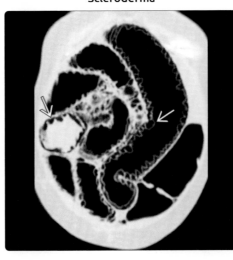

(Left) *Axial CECT in a 64-year-old man who had a bone marrow transplant for leukemia shows pneumatosis ➡ within segments of the small bowel and colon. This patient had both graft-vs.-host disease and CMV infection of the small bowel. It is often difficult or impossible to distinguish these 2 entities on imaging.* (Right) *Coronal CT in a patient with scleroderma shows cystic pneumatosis through multiple loops of small bowel ➡ associated with the disease.*

Small Intestine

DIFFERENTIAL DIAGNOSIS

Common

- Vascular Ectasia, Intestinal
- Crohn Disease

Less Common

- Carcinoid Tumor
- Gastrointestinal Stromal Tumor
- Metastases and Lymphoma, Intestinal
- Small Bowel Carcinoma
- Aortoenteric Fistula
- Ischemic Enteritis
- Vasculitis, Small Intestine
- Mesenteric Varices
- Intramural Benign Tumor, Intestinal
- Radiation Enteritis

ESSENTIAL INFORMATION

Key Differential Diagnosis Issues

- **Occult GI bleeding** = loss of blood with no source identified by endoscopy
  - Small intestine is most common site
  - CT and capsule endoscopy are complementary for diagnosis
- **Overt GI bleeding** = hematemesis, melena, or hematochezia
  - Bleeding site is usually detectable by endoscopy
  - Common sources: Gastric and duodenal ulcers, esophageal varices, tumors of esophagus, stomach, or colon
- Optimal CT technique = CT enterography
  - Distend bowel with water (preferred) or VoLumen
  - Rapid (4-6 mL/s) bolus of IV contrast
  - Multiplanar reformations and multiphasic imaging
    - Arterial phase (~ 20- to 30-s delay) is mandatory
    - Venous phase (60 s) is useful to see pooling of intraluminal opacified blood

Helpful Clues for Common Diagnoses

- **Vascular Ectasia, Intestinal**
  - Angioectasia: Most commonly occurs in colon, 15% in small bowel
  - Coronal MIP helpful for diagnosis
- **Crohn Disease**
  - Usually abdominal symptoms (pain, diarrhea) unlike most other causes of obscure GI bleeding

Helpful Clues for Less Common Diagnoses

- **Carcinoid Tumor**
  - Hypervascular mass in ileum with mesenteric metastasis and desmoplasia
- **Gastrointestinal Stromal Tumor**
  - Bulky mass, exophytic [small bowel (SB) < duodenum < stomach]
  - Central ulceration in communication with lumen
- **Metastases and Lymphoma, Intestinal**
  - Bull's-eye (target) or circumferential mass
  - May cause aneurysmal dilation of lumen (melanoma and lymphoma)
  - Uncommonly cause luminal obstruction
- **Small Bowel Carcinoma**
  - Constricting lesion, usually causes obstruction
- **Aortoenteric Fistula**
  - Complication of graft repair of aortic aneurysm
  - CTA: Focal wall thickening of 3rd portion of duodenum
  - Appears adherent to proximal portion of aortic graft
  - ± extraluminal gas bubbles, active bleeding into lumen
- **Ischemic Enteritis**
  - Superior mesenteric artery or vein; closed-loop SB obstruction
  - Abnormal enhancement and thickening of SB wall
  - Infiltrated mesentery, ascites, especially with venous thrombosis
- **Vasculitis, Small Intestine**
  - Segmental involvement, thick SB folds
- **Mesenteric Varices**
  - In portal hypertension
  - Usually at site of prior bowel surgery

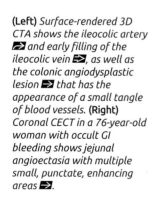

(Left) Surface-rendered 3D CTA shows the ileocolic artery ➡ and early filling of the ileocolic vein ➡, as well as the colonic angiodysplastic lesion ➡ that has the appearance of a small tangle of blood vessels. (Right) Coronal CECT in a 76-year-old woman with occult GI bleeding shows jejunal angioectasia with multiple small, punctate, enhancing areas ➡.

Vascular Ectasia, Intestinal

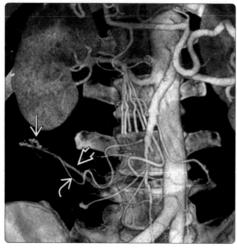

Vascular Ectasia, Intestinal

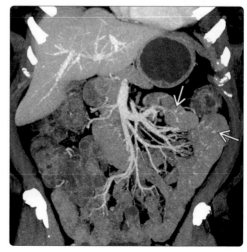

Vascular Ectasia, Intestinal

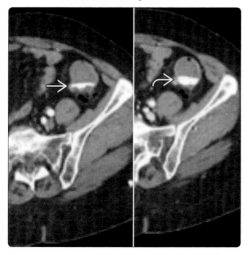

Crohn Disease

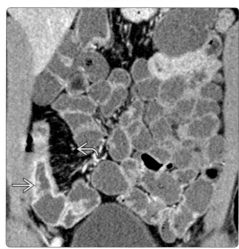

(Left) *Dual-phase CT helps make the diagnosis of active extravasation. Note the contrast extravasation in the colon on the arterial phase* ➡ *with contrast pooling on the venous phase* ➡, *confirming the diagnosis of active bleeding.* (Right) *Coronal CECT enterography shows mucosal hyperenhancement* ➡ *and wall thickening of the terminal ileum with engorged feeding vessels* ➡ *and fibrofatty proliferation of the adjacent mesenteric fat, diagnostic of acute or chronic Crohn disease.*

Carcinoid Tumor

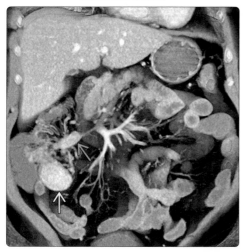

Gastrointestinal Stromal Tumor

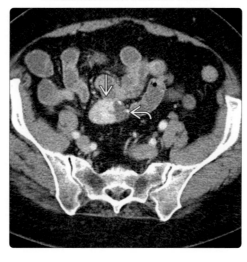

(Left) *Coronal 3D-reformatted CECT shows a distal ileal mass* ➡, *a hypervascular mesenteric metastasis* ➡, *and desmoplastic response within the mesentery.* (Right) *Axial CECT enterography shows a brightly enhancing mass* ➡ *arising from the ileum. Within the lumen of the affected segment of bowel, there are high-density foci of extravasated contrast material* ➡, *indicating active bleeding from the mass.*

Gastrointestinal Stromal Tumor

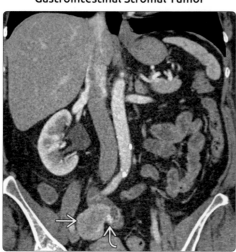

Metastases and Lymphoma, Intestinal

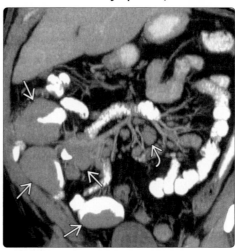

(Left) *Coronal CECT shows a partially exophytic, hypervascular mass* ➡ *arising from the small bowel wall with active bleeding into the bowel lumen* ➡. (Right) *Coronal CECT shows multifocal small bowel wall masses* ➡ *without bowel obstruction. Also noted is extensive mesenteric lymphadenopathy* ➡, *classic features of intestinal non-Hodgkin lymphoma, though metastatic melanoma could have a similar appearance.*

Metastases and Lymphoma, Intestinal

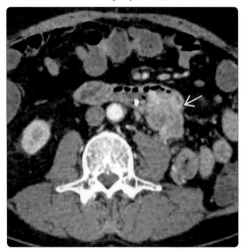

Small Bowel Carcinoma

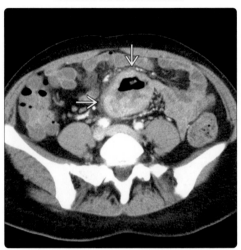

(Left) *Axial CECT in a patient s/p left nephrectomy for renal cell carcinoma with occult GI bleeding shows a hypervascular mass* ➡ *in the jejunum, consistent with metastatic disease.* **(Right)** *Axial CECT shows a complex mass* ➡ *arising from the bowel wall and invading the surrounding mesentery. An unusual feature of this primary small bowel carcinoma is the lack of luminal obstruction.*

Aortoenteric Fistula

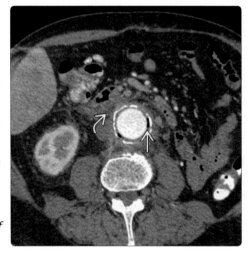

Aortoenteric Fistula

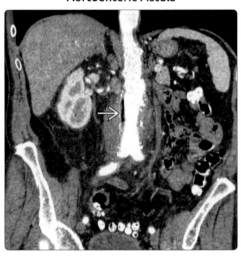

(Left) *Axial CECT in a patient presenting with fever and occult GI bleeding s/p surgical repair of an abdominal aortic aneurysm (AAA) shows the native, calcified aortic wall wrapped around the synthetic graft. Between the graft and the aortic wall are collections of gas* ➡*, indicating infection &/or fistula to gut. There is a rind of soft tissue density surrounding the aorta and the 3rd portion of the duodenum* ➡*.* **(Right)** *Coronal CECT shows soft tissue and gas* ➡ *surrounding an aortic graft months after surgical repair of an AAA.*

Small Bowel Carcinoma

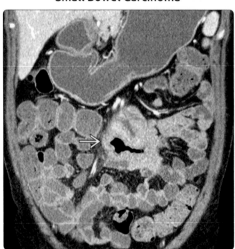

Ischemic Enteritis

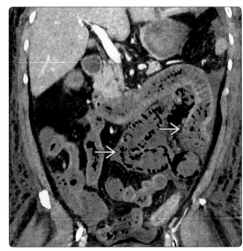

(Left) *Coronal CECT shows a mass* ➡ *arising from the bowel wall and invading adjacent tissues. Hypovascularity of the mass is a typical feature of a primary adenocarcinoma, but the absence of bowel obstruction is less common.* **(Right)** *Coronal CECT in a man with acute abdominal pain, acidosis, and hematochezia shows dilated small bowel segments with pneumatosis* ➡ *and ascites, suggesting bowel infarction.*

Ischemic Enteritis

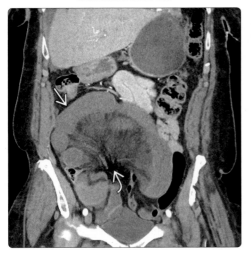

Intramural Benign Tumor, Intestinal

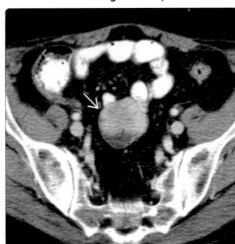

(Left) *Patient with crampy abdominal pain and hematochezia shows segmental dilation of fluid-distended small bowel and pinching of mesenteric vessels and bowel* ➡*, lacking mucosal enhancement of the dilated small bowel segments* ➡ *and infiltration of the mesentery, all findings indicating closed-loop small bowel obstruction with bowel ischemia.* **(Right)** *Axial CECT shows a heterogeneous mass* ➡ *in the wall of distal small bowel. The mass, a leiomyoma, caused chronic GI bleeding but not obstruction.*

Vasculitis, Small Intestine

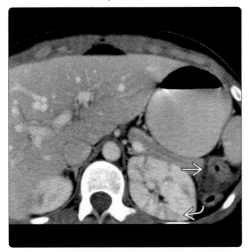

Vasculitis, Small Intestine

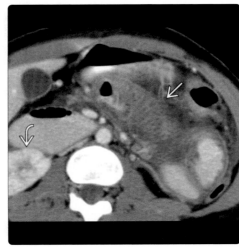

(Left) *Axial CECT in a young woman with severe abdominal pain shows wedge-shaped and striated zones of decreased attenuation* ➡ *within the kidneys. Small bowel wall thickening and ascites are also noted* ➡. **(Right)** *Axial CECT in the same patient shows a striated nephrogram* ➡, *ascites, and marked thickening of the wall of the jejunum* ➡. *The finding of "inflammatory" or hemorrhagic injury to the bowel wall and kidneys in a young patient is strongly suggestive of vasculitis (polyarteritis nodosa in this case).*

Mesenteric Varices

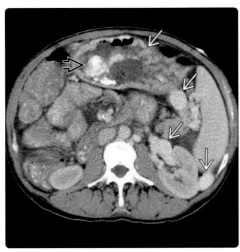

Radiation Enteritis

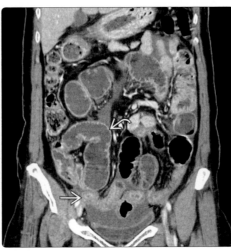

(Left) *Axial CECT in a patient with cirrhosis and portal vein thrombosis shows ascites and extensive varices* ➡. *Also noted is a hyperdense collection* ➡ *within the stomach representing active bleeding from gastric varices.* **(Right)** *Coronal CECT in a woman with radiation enteritis following treatment for endometrial carcinoma shows ascites and dilation of the mid small bowel* ➡. *The small bowel segments within the pelvis have a narrowed lumen and a thickened wall, characterized by submucosal edema* ➡.

Small Intestine

DIFFERENTIAL DIAGNOSIS

Common

- Adhesions
- External Hernias
  - Femoral Hernia
  - Inguinal Hernia
  - Obturator Hernia
  - Ventral Hernia
- Peritoneal Metastases
- Crohn Disease
- Malrotation, Bands
- Cystic Fibrosis

Less Common

- Intestinal Metastases and Lymphoma
- Carcinoid Tumor
- Small Bowel Carcinoma
- Iatrogenic; Small Bowel Intubation
  - Iatrogenic Injury: Feeding Tubes
- Internal Hernias
  - Transmesenteric Internal Hernia
  - Paraduodenal Hernia
- Intussusception
- Intestinal Trauma
- Gallstone Ileus
- Vasculitis
- Radiation Enteritis
- Ischemic Enteritis
- Afferent Loop Syndrome

Rare but Important

- Intestinal Parasitic Disease
- Meckel Diverticulum

ESSENTIAL INFORMATION

Key Differential Diagnosis Issues

- **3 most common causes**
  - **Adhesions, hernias, and cancer**
  - Metastasis to bowel serosa (peritoneal carcinomatosis) is more common cause of small bowel obstruction (SBO) than primary bowel neoplasm
- Obstruction vs. ileus
  - Obstruction: Abrupt transition from dilated to nondilated bowel
    - Air-fluid levels at varying heights
    - Obstructing process is usually evident on CT (except for adhesions)
  - Ileus: No or gradual transition from dilated to nondilated bowel
    - Descending colon often collapsed in ileus; do not mistake for obstruction if there is no pathologic process in proximal descending colon
    - **Ileus plus ascites is especially likely to mimic bowel obstruction**
      - Retroperitoneal colonic segments (ascending, descending colon, and rectum) will be collapsed
      - Bowel segments on mesentery (SB transverse and sigmoid colon) are dilated disproportionately

- **Important to distinguish simple from closed loop obstruction**
- Signs of closed loop SBO
  - Segmental dilation of fluid-distended SB out of proportion to more proximal or distal SB
  - **Whirl sign** due to tightly twisted mesenteric vessels
  - **Balloons on strings**: Dilated SB tethered by stretched mesenteric vessels
  - **Beak sign**: Fusiform tapering at point of torsion/obstruction
  - Mesenteric infiltration, diminished mucosal enhancement, and ascites suggest ischemia and indicate urgent need for surgery

Helpful Clues for Common Diagnoses

- **Adhesions**
  - Most common cause of SBO in adults
    - Usually result of prior abdominal surgery
  - Adhesions themselves are not identified on CT
    - No obstructing mass or other cause identified
  - Sharp transition, acute angulation of bowel
- **External Hernias**
  - Any defect in abdominal or pelvic muscles or fascial boundary (inguinal, ventral, spigelian, obturator, etc.)
    - Most can be identified and distinguished by CT criteria
  - Many patients have hernias that are not etiology of bowel obstruction
    - Key to diagnosing hernia as etiology of SB obstruction
      - Dilated bowel enters hernia; collapsed bowel leaves hernia
- **Peritoneal Metastases**
  - Peritoneal-serosal metastases are most common malignant cause of SBO
  - Primary sites in GI and GYN tracts are most common
    - Almost any malignancy may metastasize to peritoneum and serosa
- **Crohn Disease**
  - Favors terminal ileum, may have skip lesions
  - Mesenteric fatty proliferation and cluster of small nodes
- **Malrotation, Bands**
  - Usually diagnosed in childhood
  - Midgut volvulus may occur in adults
    - SB loops are often twisted with whirl sign in volvulus
    - Volvulus may also occur in transmesenteric internal hernia and adhesive closed loop obstruction
- **Cystic Fibrosis**
  - Children or adults may develop SBO due to thick secretions in SB
  - **Distal intestinal obstruction syndrome**
    - Stool distended distal SB
    - Almost unique to cystic fibrosis
    - Optimally managed by aggressive laxatives and enemas, avoiding surgery

Helpful Clues for Less Common Diagnoses

- **Intestinal Metastases and Lymphoma**
  - Metastasis to bowel itself; intra- or retroperitoneal segments
  - From any primary, especially melanoma, lung or breast cancer

- Lymphoma is less likely to cause SBO than carcinoma (primary or metastatic)
- **Carcinoid Tumor**
  - SBO due to tumor itself or mesenteric metastases and desmoplasia; Ileum is most common site
- **Small Bowel Carcinoma**
  - Apple core lesion: Short, circumferential soft tissue density thickening of wall, narrowing of lumen
- **Iatrogenic; Small Bowel Intubation**
  - If balloon-tipped catheter is used for enteral feeding, it may lead to intussusception &/or obstruction
- **Internal Hernias**
  - **Transmesenteric internal hernia**
    - Protrusion of small bowel through congenital or acquired defect in mesentery
    - Usually follows surgery in which Roux limb has been created; e.g., liver transplantation, Roux-en-Y gastric bypass
    - Cluster of dilated SB loops with distorted mesenteric vessels
      - □ Dilated bowel lies adjacent to abdominal wall, displacing colon medially
  - **Paraduodenal hernia**
    - Protrusion of SB loops through congenital or acquired defect in mesentery
      - □ Left side more common (75%) than right (25%)
      - □ Look for spherical or ovoid cluster of dilated SB between pancreatic body and posterior gastric wall
      - □ Mesenteric vessels are crowded and distorted
- **Intussusception**
  - Short, transient, nonobstructing intussusception is of no clinical concern, usually idiopathic
  - Longer, obstructing intussusception in adult is usually associated with lead mass
- **Intestinal Trauma**
  - Blunt injury of bowel &/or hematoma in bowel wall may cause luminal narrowing and obstruction
  - Check for evidence of anticoagulation
  - Children more prone to duodenal and SB intramural hematomas than adults

- **Gallstone Ileus**
  - Triad of intraluminal stone, SB obstruction, biliary gas
  - Almost always in older adult women
- **Vasculitis**
  - Henoch-Schönlein purpura and others
  - Cause bowel wall hemorrhage &/or edema, luminal narrowing or dilation (upstream)
  - Angioedema can produce identical findings
    - Check for C1 esterase deficiency, use of ACE inhibitors
- **Radiation Enteritis**
  - Irregular fold thickening and luminal narrowing, usually in pelvic SB loops
  - Ask about history of prior radiation for pelvic malignancy
- **Ischemic Enteritis**
  - Causes: Superior mesenteric artery or superior mesenteric vein thrombosis; closed loop SBO
  - Acute: Fold thickening, submucosal edema, hemorrhage, pneumatosis
  - Chronic: Stricture with tapered margins
- **Afferent Loop Syndrome**
  - Afferent loop (AL) becomes obstructed by adhesions, recurrent tumor, internal hernia, etc.
  - Plain films and barium fluoroscopic exams often miss this complication, as AL is fluid-distended and oral contrast medium does not enter AL
  - CT shows dilation of AL and any complications (e.g., dilated bile ducts, recurrent tumor, ischemia, perforation)

Helpful Clues for Rare Diagnoses

- **Intestinal Parasitic Disease**
  - Ascariasis is common cause of SB obstruction in some developing countries
  - Mass of tangled worms may obstruct SB lumen
- **Meckel Diverticulum**
  - Inverted Meckel diverticulum may cause distal SB intussusception and obstruction
  - Inflammation due to perforated Meckel diverticulum may cause SBO

Adhesions

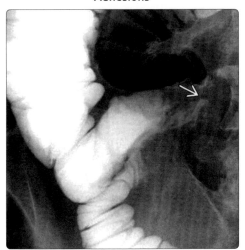

Adhesions

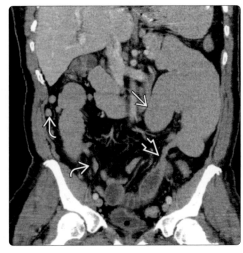

(Left) Spot film from a contrast enema shows angulation and distortion of small bowel (SB) folds directed toward the point of obstruction ➡. There is an abrupt change in caliber of the SB. Retrograde injection of barium showed prior colectomy. (Right) Coronal CECT shows dilated proximal SB loops ➡ with collapsed distal SB ➡ and colon. At the point of transition ➡ there is no mass, hernia, etc.

Small Intestine

(Left) *Axial CECT in an older woman shows fluid-distended SB segments* ➡️ *in the pelvis. The distended bowel could be followed into a femoral hernia, while collapsed SB* ➡️ *returns from this site.* **(Right)** *Axial CECT in the same patient with SB obstruction (SBO) due to femoral hernia shows the close relationship of the hernia* ➡️ *to the femoral vessels at the level of the symphysis pubis as well as compression of the femoral vein* ➡️*.*

Femoral Hernia

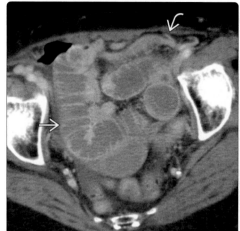

Femoral Hernia

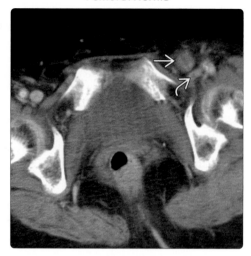

(Left) *Axial CECT shows a right inguinal hernia* ➡️ *containing SB with mild dilation of bowel upstream from the hernia. Note that the hernia contents extend anterior to the femoral vessels.* **(Right)** *Axial CECT in an older woman shows dilated proximal* ➡️ *and collapsed distal* ➡️ *SB loops with an obturator hernia as the point of obstruction (not shown).*

Inguinal Hernia

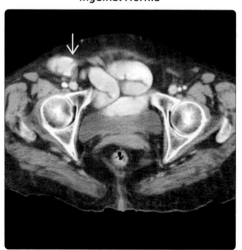

Obturator Hernia

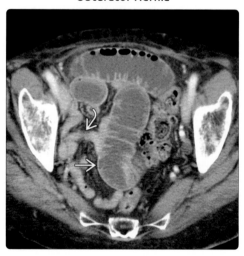

(Left) *Axial CECT in an older woman shows a segment of distal SB* ➡️ *herniated between the obturator externus* ➡️ *and pectineus* ➡️ *muscles, resulting in an SBO.* **(Right)** *Axial CECT shows a ventral hernia* ➡️ *with markedly dilated bowel leading into the hernia and collapsed bowel* ➡️ *leaving it. Also note ascites* ➡️*. A segment of ischemic bowel was resected as the hernia was repaired.*

Obturator Hernia

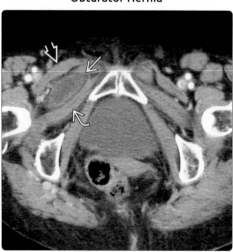

Ventral Hernia

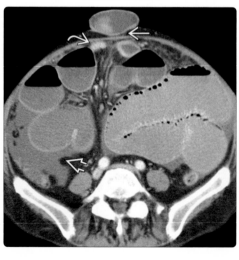

Peritoneal Metastases

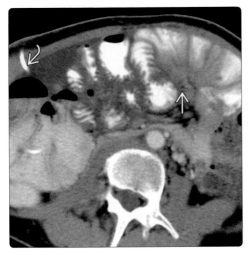

Crohn Disease

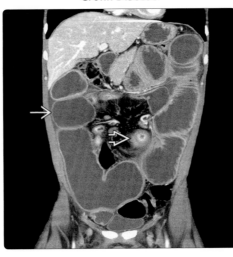

(Left) *Axial CECT in a woman with functional SBO due to ovarian carcinoma metastatic to the peritoneum shows abnormal clustering and angulation of small bowel segments* ➡ *with wall thickening. A peritoneal drainage catheter* ➡ *was inserted to drain ascites.* (Right) *Coronal CECT shows marked dilation of SB* ➡ *proximal to SB loops that have active and chronic Crohn disease, marked by mucosal enhancement, wall thickening, and luminal narrowing* ➡.

Cystic Fibrosis

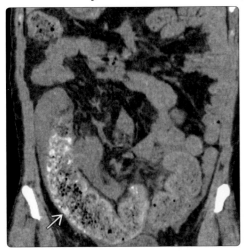

Intestinal Metastases and Lymphoma

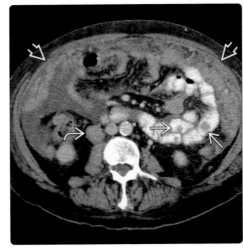

(Left) *Coronal CECT shows a relatively collapsed proximal SB and colon. The distal ileum is dilated and distended with feces-like inspissated material* ➡. *These are classic features of distal intestinal obstruction syndrome, which is almost unique to patients with cystic fibrosis.* (Right) *Axial CECT shows classic widespread metastases from melanoma, including to the SB* ➡, *lymph nodes* ➡, *and omentum with both nodular and diffuse metastases seen* ➡.

Intestinal Metastases and Lymphoma

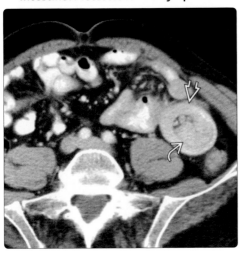

Small Bowel Carcinoma

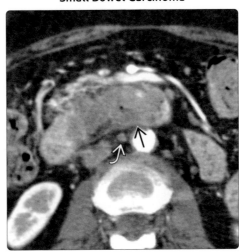

(Left) *Axial CECT shows a SB intussusception* ➡ *causing a partial SBO. The lead mass was a metastatic melanoma* ➡ *deposit in the bowel wall.* (Right) *Axial CECT shows a mass in the 3rd portion of the duodenum* ➡, *causing partial obstruction. Also evident is regional lymphadenopathy* ➡.

(Left) *Axial CECT shows the balloon of an enteric feeding tube* ➡ *inflated inappropriately within the SB, causing SBO.* (Right) *Axial CECT in a patient who had a Roux-en-Y gastric bypass procedure shows displacement of the jejunal anastomotic suture line* ➡ *from its expected left midabdominal location. The Roux limb and proximal SB are dilated* ➡, *displaced, and twisted around their mesentery* ➡ *at the site of the mesenteric hernia.*

Iatrogenic; Small Bowel Intubation

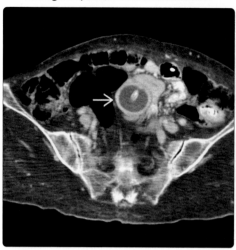

Transmesenteric Internal Hernia

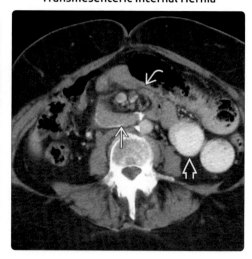

(Left) *Coronal CECT shows a cluster of SB segments that are not dilated but appear to be confined within a sac* ➡. *Note the crowding and displacement of the mesenteric vessels* ➡ *in the center of this cluster.* (Right) *Axial CECT shows a distal SB intussusception* ➡ *due to an inverted or intraluminal Meckel diverticulum.*

Paraduodenal Hernia

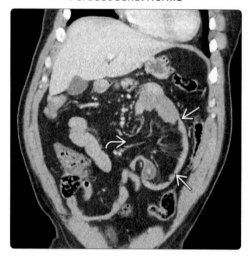

Meckel Diverticulum

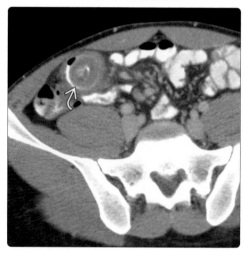

(Left) *Axial CECT shows a long-segment intussusception* ➡ *involving the terminal ileum with functional SBO. Note the bowel-within-bowel appearance and the presence of mesenteric fat within the lumen of the intussuscipiens. The lead mass was an inverted or intraluminal Meckel diverticulum.* (Right) *Coronal CECT in a 63-year-old man post total gastrectomy with Roux-en-Y reconstruction for gastric cancer shows a dilated afferent loop* ➡, *consistent with afferent loop syndrome.*

Intussusception

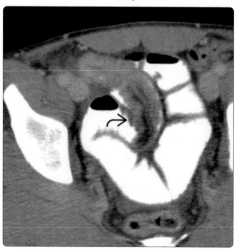

Afferent Loop Syndrome

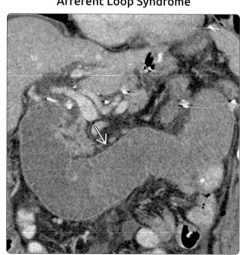

Gallstone Ileus

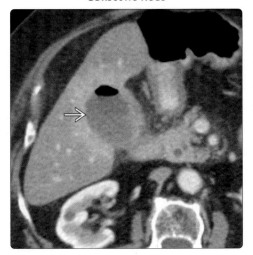

Gallstone Ileus

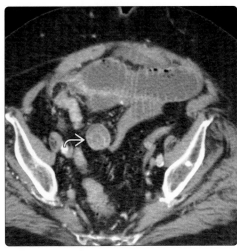

(Left) Axial CECT shows gas within a thick-walled gallbladder ➡ and enhancement of the adjacent liver due to inflammation. SBO was also present in this older woman. (Right) Axial CECT shows a large, laminated gallstone ➡ at the point of SBO in the distal small bowel. Gas was present in the gallbladder of this older woman.

Vasculitis

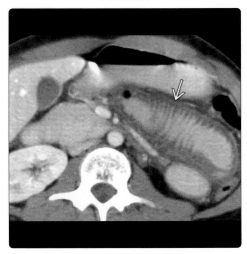

Radiation Enteritis

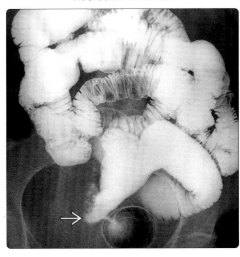

(Left) Axial CECT shows luminal dilation and wall thickening ➡ of the jejunum due to polyarteritis nodosa. (Right) Spot film from a SB follow-through shows an abrupt angulation and stricture ➡ of the distal SB, simulating an adhesive SBO. At surgery, a radiation-induced stricture was found, due to prior therapy for uterine carcinoma.

Radiation Enteritis

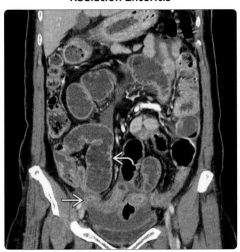

Ischemic Enteritis

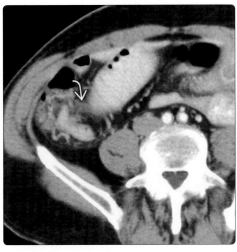

(Left) Coronal CECT in a woman with radiation enteritis following treatment for endometrial carcinoma shows dilation of the proximal and mid SB ➡. In contrast, the SB segments within the pelvis have a narrowed lumen and a thickened wall ➡, characterized by submucosal edema. (Right) Axial CECT shows a distal SB stricture ➡ with SBO due to acute and chronic bowel ischemia, proven at surgery.

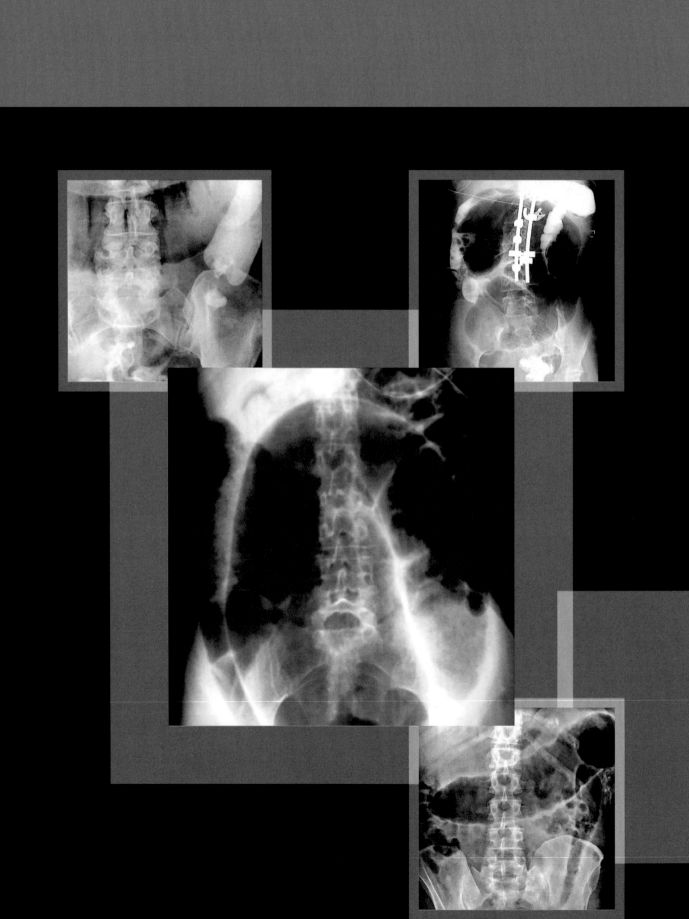

SECTION 7
Colon

Generic Imaging Patterns

Solitary Colonic Filling Defect   172
Multiple Colonic Filling Defects   174
Mass or Inflammation of Ileocecal Area   176
Colonic Ileus or Dilation   182
Toxic Megacolon   186
Rectal or Colonic Fistula   188
Segmental Colonic Narrowing   194
Colonic Thumbprinting   198
Colonic Wall Thickening   200
Smooth Ahaustral Colon   206

Clinically Based Differentials

Acute Right Lower Quadrant Pain   208
Acute Left Abdominal Pain   214

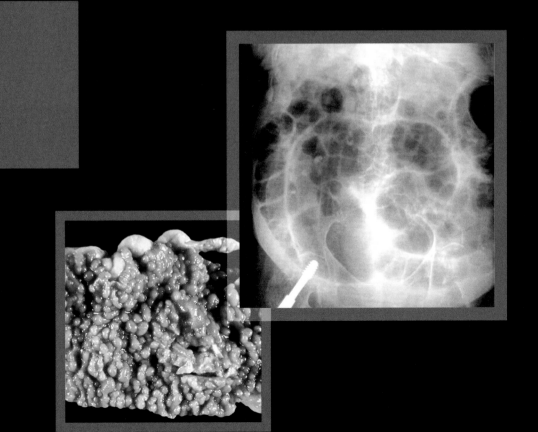

DIFFERENTIAL DIAGNOSIS

Common

- Colonic Polyps
- Colon or Rectal Carcinoma
- Villous Adenoma
- Feces

Less Common

- Inverted Appendical Stump
- Endometrioma
- Metastases and Lymphoma, Colonic
- Tuberculoma
- Ameboma
- Intramural Hematoma
- Solitary Rectal Ulcer Syndrome
- Foreign Body
- Varix, Hemorrhoidal
- Diverticulitis
- Mesenchymal Tumor

ESSENTIAL INFORMATION

Key Differential Diagnosis Issues

- Determine if intraluminal or mucosal lesion
  - Or if intramural or extrinsic mass

Helpful Clues for Common Diagnoses

- **Colonic Polyps**
  - Adenomatous > hyperplastic > hamartomatous
  - Adenomas are more likely to present as solitary filling defect than are other types
  - Hyperplastic polyps: Most commonly appear as smooth round sessile nodules measuring < 5 mm in rectosigmoid colon
  - Hamartomatous polyps: Variable in size but will not present as carpet lesion
- **Colon or Rectal Carcinoma**
  - Sessile or pedunculated polyp or apple core lesion
  - Rectal cancer: Semiannular (saddle- or C-shaped) lesion
- **Villous Adenoma**
  - Larger, sessile polyps with barium trapped in frond-like projections, resulting in granular pattern
    - Without causing obstruction
  - ↑ lobulation, reticulation, or granulation in polyp usually associated with greater villous component
  - Most commonly occur in rectum

Helpful Clues for Less Common Diagnoses

- **Inverted Appendiceal Stump**
  - May appear as discrete polyp in cecal tip
  - Often indistinguishable from other polyps by imaging alone
- **Endometrioma**
  - Implants may cause intramural mass in sigmoid or any part of colon
  - May appear as apple core lesion, closely simulating colon cancer
    - Consider this in any female of reproductive age
    - CT shows eccentric, extraluminal component better than barium enema
- **Metastases and Lymphoma, Colonic**
  - Usually drop mets or direct invasion
  - Usually eccentric mural mass, anterior wall of rectum
- **Tuberculoma and Ameboma**
  - Either can cause apple core lesion indistinguishable from colon carcinoma
- **Intramural Hematoma**
  - From blunt or penetrating trauma
- **Foreign Body**
  - May cause intramural hematoma, perforation
  - History is key
- **Varix, Hemorrhoidal**
  - May simulate rectal carcinoma, especially if thrombosed
- **Diverticulitis**
  - May cause mass effect and spasm simulating colorectal cancer
- **Mesenchymal Tumor**
  - Lipoma, neuroma, fibroma, hemangioma, gastrointestinal stromal tumor (GIST)
    - Rectal GIST is being recognized more frequently

(Left) *A spot film from an air-contrast barium enema shows a small, fixed filling defect ➡ in the barium pool, a typical appearance of a polyp.* **(Right)** *A pedunculated polyp (on a stalk) ➡ is seen on this endoluminal 3D image from a CT colonography study.*

Colonic Polyps

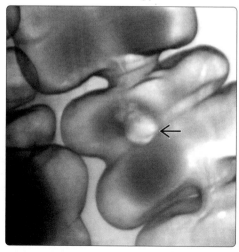

Colonic Polyps

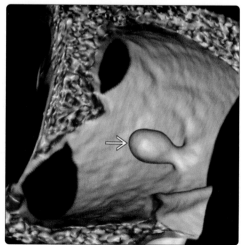

Solitary Colonic Filling Defect

Colonic Polyps

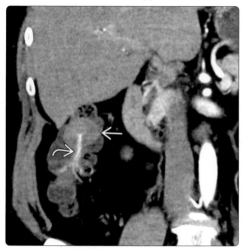

Colon or Rectal Carcinoma

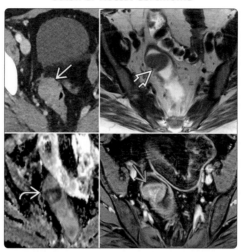

(Left) *A pedunculated polyp ➡ in the colon in a patient with juvenile polyposis is shown. Note the stalk of the feeding vessel ➡.* (Right) *Fullness ➡ seen on CT in the rectum is better seen on T2 due to the presence of rectal gel as a polypoid lesion ➡. The mass shows diffusion restriction ➡ and enhancement ➡. Pathology showed invasive adenocarcinoma in a tubular adenoma.*

Colon or Rectal Carcinoma

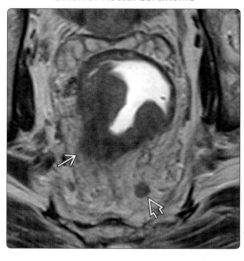

Inverted Appendical Stump

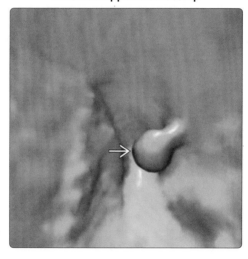

(Left) *Axial high-resolution T2 MR shows a saddle-shaped mass in the rectum with 10-mm extension into the mesorectal fat ➡, consistent with a T3c lesion. A suspicious lymph node in the mesorectum with a round shape measures 6 mm ➡.* (Right) *This 3D surface-rendered image from a CT colonography shows a small, polypoid lesion ➡ in the cecal tip. Other than by its typical location, this inverted appendiceal stump is indistinguishable from other benign polyps.*

Tuberculoma

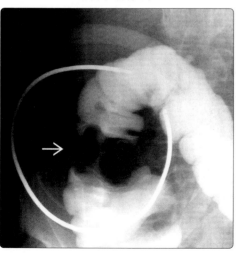

Mesenchymal Tumor

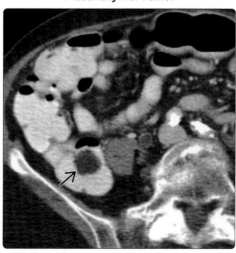

(Left) *A spot film from a barium enema shows a classic apple core constricting lesion ➡ in the ascending colon that is indistinguishable from that often seen with a primary colon carcinoma. At surgical resection, the lesion proved to be due to tuberculous infection of the colon.* (Right) *Axial CECT shows a spherical fat density mass ➡ within the cecum, a typical lipoma.*

DIFFERENTIAL DIAGNOSIS

Common

- Feces
- Air Bubbles
- Colonic Polyps
- Colon Carcinoma
- Ulcerative Colitis

Less Common

- Familial Polyposis
- Gardner Syndrome
- Metastases and Lymphoma, Colonic
- Pseudomembranous Colitis, Diverticulitis
- Lymphoid Follicles (Mimic)
- Hemorrhoids
- Diverticulosis (Mimic)
- Mesenchymal Tumor, Colon
- Pneumatosis (Mimic)
- Endometriosis
- Colonic Varices
- Urticaria, Colon
- Colonic Parasites

ESSENTIAL INFORMATION

Key Differential Diagnosis Issues

- Check if defects are movable (gas or feces)

Helpful Clues for Common Diagnoses

- **Feces**
  - Usually more irregular in shape and size
  - Usually well coated by barium
  - Usually contains air bubbles
- **Air Bubbles**
  - On barium enema (BE)
    - Usually not problem on CT colonography
  - Key is change in shape, size, location with positioning
- **Colonic Polyps**
  - Smooth-surfaced intraluminal small mass on CT colonoscopy or BE
  - 3 types defined by C-RADS nomenclature: Sessile: Broad-based with width > height; pedunculated: Polyp with separate stalk; Flat: Polyp with vertical height < 3 mm
    - Polyps > 1 cm are often neoplastic (benign or malignant) adenomas and resected
    - Management of 6- to 9-mm polyps debatable and can be managed with either CT surveillance or polypectomy
    - Small polyps of uniform size in younger patients are often hyperplastic: (< 5 mm), often multiple
      - Can be safely disregarded
  - Location: Cecum (4%), ascending colon (6%), hepatic flexure (4%), transverse (2%), splenic flexure (8%), descending (20%), sigmoid (41%), rectum (23%)
- **Colon Carcinoma**
  - Rarely multifocal but commonly found with other polyps
- **Ulcerative Colitis**
  - Along with granulomatous colitis (Crohn), may result in inflammatory polyps
  - May grow into filiform, pedunculated appearance
  - Associated with increased risk of colon cancer

Helpful Clues for Less Common Diagnoses

- **Familial Polyposis and Gardner Syndrome**
  - Often innumerable adenomatous polyps, may carpet colon
  - Other syndromes may result in multiple adenomatous hamartomatous or hyperplastic polyps
- **Pseudomembranous Colitis**, Diverticulitis
  - Any infectious or inflammatory colitis may result in thickened folds that might be mistaken for polypoid lesions
- **Lymphoid Follicles (Mimic)**
  - Small (2-4 mm), submucosal, numerous; more in right colon
- **Diverticulosis (Mimic)**
  - On air-contrast enema, barium-lined diverticulum may simulate barium-coated polyp

---

*(Left) Contrast enema shows innumerable filling defects of varying size in the ascending colon, which is the typical appearance of stool in an unprepped colon. **(Right)** Contrast enema shows a pedunculated polyp ⊅ on a long stalk ⧊. Also note diverticula ⊅, some filled with air and some with air, that might be mistaken for polyps.*

Feces

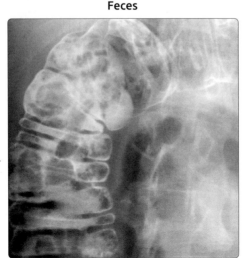

Colonic Polyps

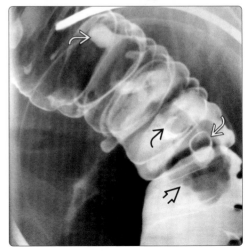

Colonic Polyps

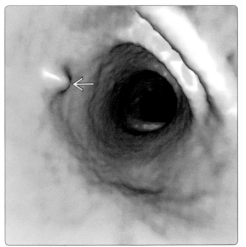

Colonic Polyps

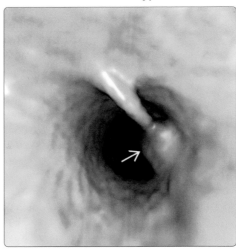

(Left) CT colonography in a 74-year-old man shows a small, probably hyperplastic polyp ➡ of no clinical concern. (Right) CT colonography in the same patient shows a pedunculated polyp ➡ that was removed at colonoscopy and proved to be benign.

Colon Carcinoma

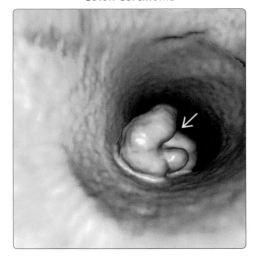

Ulcerative Colitis

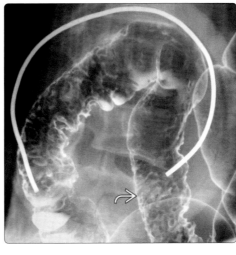

(Left) CT colonography in an older patient with multiple small, hyperplastic polyps shows a large, sessile, polypoid mass ➡. This was removed at left hemicolectomy and proved to be primary colon carcinoma. (Right) Contrast enema in a patient with chronic but quiescent ulcerative colitis shows multiple filiform polyps ➡ within the colon.

Familial Polyposis

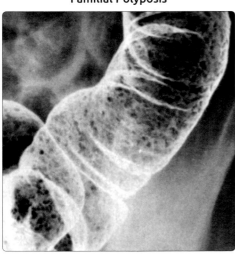

Pneumatosis (Mimic)

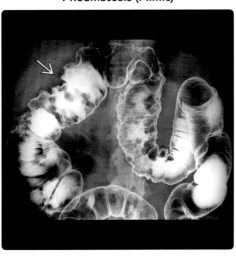

(Left) Contrast enema shows thousands of small polyps carpeting the surface of the colon. (Right) Contrast enema shows what appear to be numerous polyps throughout the colon. These are due to intramural blebs of gas ➡ from idiopathic pneumatosis in this asymptomatic patient.

DIFFERENTIAL DIAGNOSIS

Common

- Crohn Disease
- Appendicitis
- Prominent Ileocecal Valve
  - Lipomatous Infiltration of Ileocecal Valve
  - Lipoma of Ileocecal Valve
- Colon Carcinoma
- Mesenteric Adenitis
- Infectious Ileocolitis

Less Common

- Carcinoid Tumor
- Cecal Diverticulitis
- Metastases and Lymphoma, Intestinal
- Appendiceal Carcinoma
- Intussusception
- Mucocele of Appendix
- Typhlitis (Neutropenic Colitis)
- Tuberculosis, Colon
- Cecal Volvulus
- Endometriosis
- Ischemic Colitis
- Amebiasis

ESSENTIAL INFORMATION

Key Differential Diagnosis Issues

- CT: Optimal for evaluation of intra- and extramural disease in right lower quadrant (RLQ)
  - Try to characterize distribution of disease, nature of wall thickening, and associated findings
  - Fat density mural thickening
    - Normal variant or quiescent inflammatory bowel disease
  - Water density
    - Acute inflammation or ischemia
  - Soft tissue density: Least specific
    - Infection
    - Ischemia
    - Inflammation
    - Tumor
- Barium studies: Optimal for mucosal detail
  - e.g., early inflammatory changes of Crohn disease

Helpful Clues for Common Diagnoses

- **Crohn Disease**
  - Most common inflammatory process of terminal ileum and cecum
  - Homogeneous attenuation of thickened bowel wall on CECT
    - > 15 mm suspicious for neoplasm
  - Mural stratification lost: Indistinct mucosa, submucosa, muscularis propria
  - Mesenteric fibrofatty proliferation
  - Enlarged mesenteric lymph nodes
  - Mucosal and mesenteric hyperemia
    - Comb or caterpillar sign of engorged mesenteric vessels = active inflammation
- **Appendicitis**

- Medial wall of cecum and terminal ileum may be thickened by inflammation starting in appendix
- Appendiceal wall is thickened and lumen usually distended
- Often have cluster of mildly enlarged nodes, especially with subacute inflammation
- May have associated abscess following perforation of appendix
- **Prominent Ileocecal Valve**
  - Often normal variant
  - Submucosal fat is usually evident on CT within lips of valve
  - Lipoma is benign neoplasm common in this area
    - Spherical mass of fat
    - Usually seen as eccentric mass near ileocecal valve
- **Colon Carcinoma**
  - Cecum accounts for 10% of colon adenocarcinomas
  - Usually bulky mass without obstruction, outgrowing blood supply → necrosis
    - Surface irregularity identifies mucosal origin
  - May occlude base of appendix
    - May simulate appendicitis clinically and on imaging (dilated lumen of appendix)
  - Adjacent lymphadenopathy is common
    - Also look for peritoneal and hepatic metastases
- **Mesenteric Adenitis**
  - Common in children and adolescents
  - Idiopathic, self-limited inflammation, cluster of enlarged nodes in RLQ
  - Ileal ± cecal wall thickening, sometimes with regional ileus
  - Often much more evident on coronal reformatted CT
- **Infectious Ileocolitis**
  - Causes acute diarrhea
  - Common causative agents
    - *Yersinia*
    - *Campylobacter*
    - *Salmonella*
  - Mural thickening of cecum and terminal ileum
  - Mucosal hyperenhancement and submucosal edema
  - RLQ adenopathy
  - Imaging findings indistinguishable from mesenteric adenitis (may be same disease)

Helpful Clues for Less Common Diagnoses

- **Carcinoid Tumor**
  - Thickening of distal ileal wall and mesenteric mass
    - Mesenteric mass often has focus of calcification
    - Desmoplastic response in mesentery
      - □ Small bowel loops and mesenteric vessels may have stellate configuration and distorted course
    - Primary mass and metastases are hypervascular
- **Cecal Diverticulitis**
  - Can usually identify other diverticula and normal appendix
  - Cecal wall thickened with adjacent inflammatory changes
  - No mucosal hyperemia or submucosal edema
    - Distinguishes this from colitis
- **Metastases and Lymphoma, Intestinal**

Mass or Inflammation of Ileocecal Area

- o Lymphoma may cause dramatic bowel wall thickening
  - – Often circumferential, multifocal
  - – Rarely obstructs bowel lumen or vessels (unlike carcinoma)
  - o May have significant adenopathy or involvement of other organs
- **Intussusception**
  - o Due to tumor or inflammation of ileum or ileocecal valve
  - o May identify mass within lumen
  - o Intraluminal crescent of intussuscepted ileal mesenteric fat
  - o Ileocecal intussusceptions in adults are usually obstructive and due to lead mass (neoplastic, benign or malignant)
- **Mucocele of Appendix**
  - o Round or oval, thin-walled, cystic mass near tip of cecum
  - o May have curvilinear calcifications in wall
  - o Low-grade appendiceal mucinous neoplasm (LAMN): Progressive contrast enhancement of mural nodules
  - o Mucinous adenocarcinoma: Large, irregular mass with thickened nodular wall

- **Typhlitis (Neutropenic Colitis)**
  - o Presents as fever, RLQ tenderness in immunosuppressed patient
  - o Massive mural thickening of cecal ± ascending colon wall
  - o Cecal distention, circumferential wall thickening
  - o Mucosal hyperenhancement and submucosal edema (marked)
  - o Infiltration of pericolonic fat
  - o Less common: Pneumatosis, extraluminal gas and fluid (perforation)
  - o ± dilated adjacent bowel loops (paralytic ileus)
- **Tuberculosis, Colon**
  - o Gastrointestinal infection generally follows pulmonary infection
    - – Obtain chest x-ray in suspected cases
  - o Symptoms more chronic than in other causes of infectious colitis
  - o Involvement varies from mild thickening to apple-core lesion
  - o Mesenteric adenopathy common

Crohn Disease

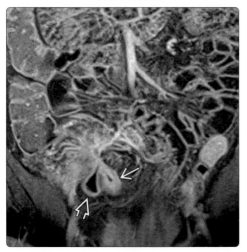

Crohn Disease

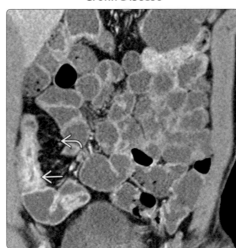

(Left) *Coronal T1 C+ FS MR shows acute inflammation of the terminal ileum with wall thickening and mucosal hyperenhancement ➡. Sacculation of the terminal ileum at the antimesenteric border ➡ is a feature of Crohn disease.* **(Right)** *Coronal CECT shows mucosal hyperenhancement, wall thickening, and luminal narrowing of terminal ileum ➡. Note mesenteric fatty proliferation and hyperemia ➡.*

Crohn Disease

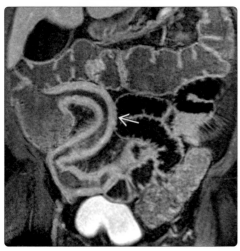

Crohn Disease

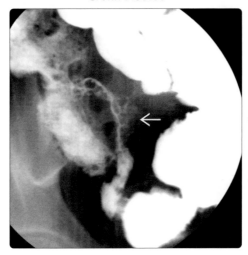

(Left) *Coronal T1 C+ MR in a 48-year-old man with Crohn disease shows mucosal hyperenhancement of a thickened terminal ileum ➡, consistent with acute inflammation.* **(Right)** *SBFT shows classic findings in a 19-year-old man with luminal narrowing and wall thickening of the terminal ileum and cecum, cobblestone mucosal ulcerations, and sinus tracks ➡ into the thickened mesenteric fat.*

Appendicitis

Appendicitis

(Left) *Coronal CECT in a 34-year-old woman with acute right lower quadrant (RLQ) pain shows generalized infiltration of the fat planes around the cecal tip and terminal ileum. An appendicolith* ➡ *is noted within the base of a thickened appendix.* (Right) *Coronal CECT in the same patient shows the dilated appendix* ➡ *along with regional adenopathy* ➡.

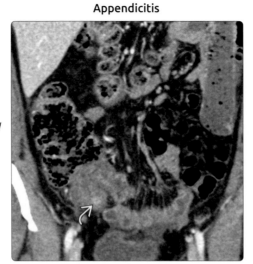

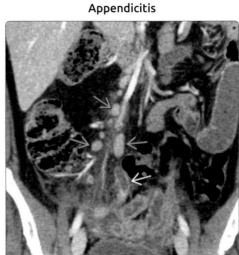

Appendicitis

Appendicitis

(Left) *Axial CECT shows a dilated lumen and thickened wall of the retrocecal appendix* ➡ *with infiltration of its mesenteric fat.* (Right) *Axial CECT shows an abscess* ➡ *medial to a thick-walled cecum* ➡, *both the result of appendiceal perforation.*

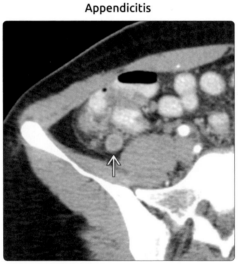

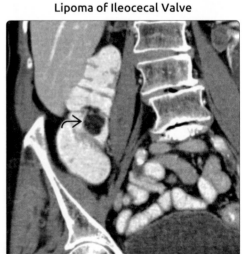

Lipomatous Infiltration of Ileocecal Valve

Lipoma of Ileocecal Valve

(Left) *Axial CECT shows lipomatous infiltration of both lips of the ileocecal valve* ➡ *as the terminal ileum* ➡ *enters the colon.* (Right) *Coronal CECT shows a spherical, fat density mass* ➡ *in the ascending colon in this patient with lipoma.*

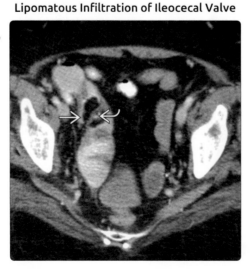

Colon Carcinoma

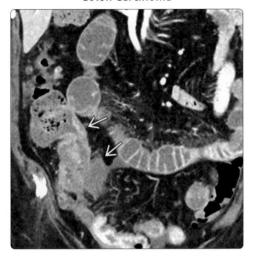

Colon Carcinoma

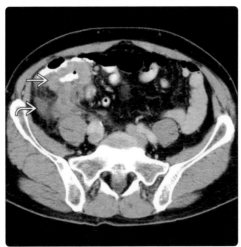

(Left) *Coronal CECT in a 73-year-old woman with Crohn disease and invasive adenocarcinoma shows mucinous features involving the terminal ileum and cecum* ➡. *Colorectal cancer risk is increased in inflammatory bowel disease.* (Right) *Axial CECT shows circumferential thickening of the wall of the cecum* ➡. *A dilated appendix was seen along with local lymphadenopathy* ➡ *and omental metastases. This patient presented with signs and symptoms of appendicitis.*

Mesenteric Adenitis

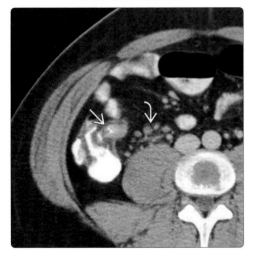

Mesenteric Adenitis

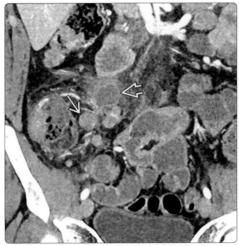

(Left) *Axial CECT shows mild thickening of the wall of the terminal ileum* ➡ *and a cluster of slightly enlarged nodes* ➡. *The appendix was normal.* (Right) *In this patient with Salmonella infection, note mesenteric adenopathy* ➡ *and a small abscess in the ileocecal region* ➡.

Carcinoid Tumor

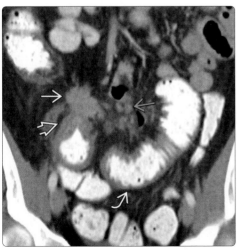

Metastases and Lymphoma, Intestinal

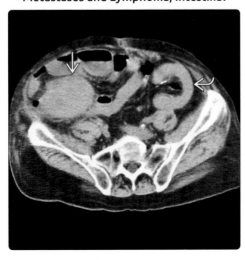

(Left) *Coronal CECT in a 47-year-old woman with small bowel carcinoid shows a spiculated mass in the mesentery* ➡, *in the ileocecal area, which has ileal wall thickening* ➡ *and upstream dilation* ➡ *due to partial obstruction. An adjacent cluster of lymph nodes* ➡ *was also positive for tumor upon resection.* (Right) *Axial NECT shows a soft tissue mass* ➡ *in the ileocecal region in this renal transplant* ➡ *recipient with lymphoma (posttransplant lymphoproliferative disorder) of the appendix.*

(Left) *Axial CECT shows a normal appendix ➡ and a cecal diverticulum ➡ with pericolonic inflammatory changes ➡.* **(Right)** *Axial CECT shows a normal appendix ➡ and extensive pericecal inflammatory infiltrates ➡. Unlike colitis, most of the inflammation is outside the colonic lumen.*

Cecal Diverticulitis

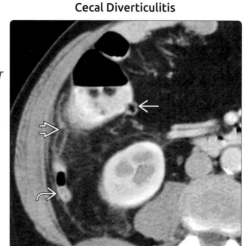

Cecal Diverticulitis

(Left) *Axial CECT shows an ileocolic intussusception ➡ and the lead mass, an appendiceal mucocele ➡ in the transverse colon.* **(Right)** *Axial CECT shows an ileocolic intussusception ➡ with the lead mass in the transverse colon, a mucocele ➡.*

Intussusception

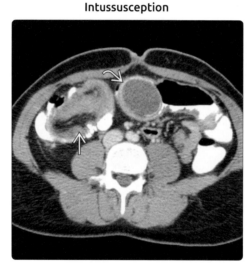

Intussusception

(Left) *Coronal CECT shows a water density mass in the appendix with curvilinear calcifications ➡, consistent with mucocele.* **(Right)** *Gross pathology shows a bivalved, mucin-filled mucocele ➡, which was the lead mass causing intussusception.*

Mucocele of Appendix

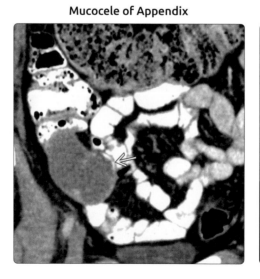

Mucocele of Appendix

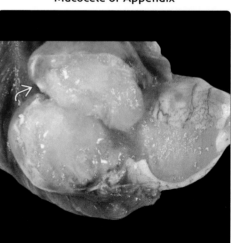

Typhlitis (Neutropenic Colitis)

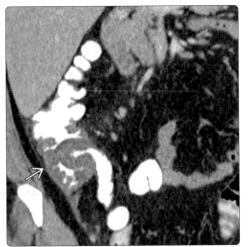

Typhlitis (Neutropenic Colitis)

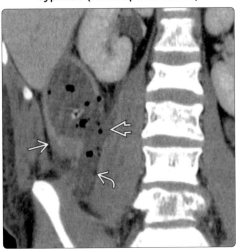

(Left) *Coronal CECT in a 36-year-old man with acute myeloid leukemia and severe neutropenia shows circumferential wall thickening localized to the cecum* ➡, *consistent with typhlitis.* (Right) *Coronal CECT in a patient with neutropenic colitis (typhlitis) and severe neutropenia due to high-dose chemotherapy shows wall thickening of the cecum* ➡ *with discontinuity of the wall* ➡ *and extraluminal bowel content along the right psoas* ➡, *consistent with perforation.*

Typhlitis (Neutropenic Colitis)

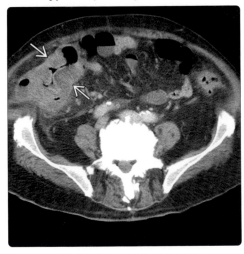

Ischemic Colitis

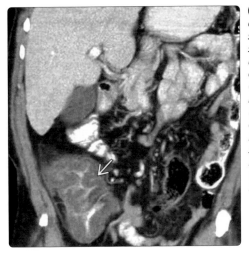

(Left) *Axial CECT in an older adult man with leukemia shows mesenteric and massive submucosal edema* ➡ *limited to the wall of the ascending colon and cecum.* (Right) *Coronal CECT shows marked mural thickening ("thumbprinting")* ➡ *of the cecum and ascending colon. Note the compressed lumen, submucosal edema, and intense mucosal enhancement. These findings indicate ischemia or inflammation.*

Tuberculosis, Colon

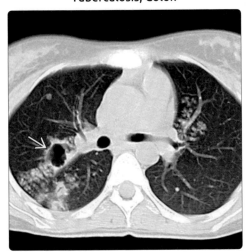

Tuberculosis, Colon

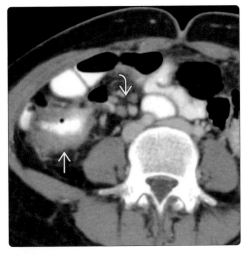

(Left) *Axial CECT shows active cavitary pulmonary tuberculosis* ➡ *in a young woman with ileocecal tuberculosis.* (Right) *Axial CECT in the same patient shows a thick-walled cecum and terminal ileum* ➡ *with mesenteric lymphadenopathy* ➡ *in this young female immigrant from India with tuberculosis (enteric and pulmonary).*

DIFFERENTIAL DIAGNOSIS

Common

- Ileus
  - Ogilvie Syndrome
- Colorectal Carcinoma
- Sigmoid Volvulus
- Cecal Volvulus
- Diverticulitis
- Fecal Impaction, Stercoral Colitis

Less Common

- Ischemic Colitis
- Toxic Megacolon
- Endocrine Disorders
- Neuromuscular Disorders

ESSENTIAL INFORMATION

Key Differential Diagnosis Issues

- Do not assume colonic dilation is ileus without considering rectal or distal colonic obstruction
- Use prone or decubitus film to visualize gas through rectum

Helpful Clues for Common Diagnoses

- **Ileus**
  - Most common cause of colonic distention
  - Usually accompanied by small bowel dilation
  - Many potential causes, including postoperative state, electrolyte or endocrine imbalance, and medications
  - **Ogilvie syndrome**
    - Colonic pseudoobstruction without mechanical cause
    - Disproportionate dilation of cecum and ascending colon
      - □ Cecal diameter > 12 cm (on plain supine radiographs) is considered at risk for perforation
- **Colorectal Carcinoma**
  - Most common cause of colonic obstruction in adults
  - Soft tissue density mass; short-segment obstruction
    - Obstruction more common in distal colon
- **Sigmoid Volvulus**

- Very elongated, dilated sigmoid, folded back on itself
  - Coffee bean, football shape
- Entire colon is dilated but less than sigmoid
- **Cecal Volvulus**
  - Ascending colon twists on mesentery; becomes obstructed, dilated, displaced toward left upper quadrant
  - Distal colon is not dilated
- **Diverticulitis**
  - Inflammation narrows lumen
  - Long segment involvement with pericolonic infiltration
- **Fecal Impaction, Stercoral Colitis**
  - Common in older patients
  - Look for stercoral colitis
    - Large, impacted mass of stool in rectosigmoid colon
    - Can lead to mucosal ulceration and wall perforation
    - Gas or discontinuity in colorectal wall, perirectal infiltration

Helpful Clues for Less Common Diagnoses

- **Ischemic Colitis**
  - May result in stricture (chronically) or spasm (acutely)
    - Colon dilated up to ischemic segment
  - Most common form is hypoperfusion affecting left side of colon ("watershed areas")
- **Toxic Megacolon**
  - Best diagnostic clue: Dilated colon with air-fluid levels and abnormal mucosal and transverse fold patterns
    - Transverse colonic folds may be thickened (edema or hemorrhage) or lost (sloughed mucosa and submucosa)
  - Requires urgent discussion with referring physician
    - Patients with toxic megacolon are extremely ill and often require urgent colectomy
- **Endocrine Disorders**
  - Hypothyroidism, diabetes, other endocrine and metabolic disorders
  - May cause ileus or colonic inertia
- **Neuromuscular Disorders**
  - Spinal cord injury, multiple sclerosis, Parkinson, etc.

Ileus

Ogilvie Syndrome

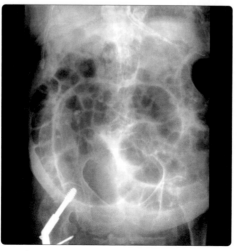
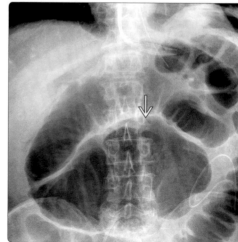

(Left) *Supine radiograph shows diffuse dilation of large and small bowel without transition in an older woman recently postoperative for hip fracture stabilization.* (Right) *Supine radiograph taken 1 day after surgery shows a medially displaced, dilated cecum and ascending colon* ➡ *with generalized distention of the colon. The cecum measures 15 cm in diameter and is folded upon itself without apparent volvulus.*

Colorectal Carcinoma

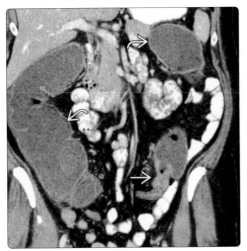

Colorectal Carcinoma

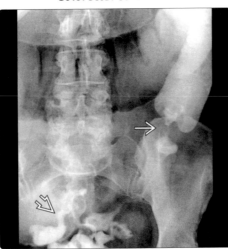

(Left) *Coronal CECT in a man with abdominal distention and hematochezia shows a classic apple core lesion* ➡ *causing obstruction of the descending colon and distention of the more proximal colon* ➡.
(Right) *Contrast enema in a man with abdominal distention and hematochezia shows a classic apple core lesion* ➡ *of the descending colon, causing high-grade obstruction. The sigmoid colon* ➡ *and small bowel are collapsed.*

Sigmoid Volvulus

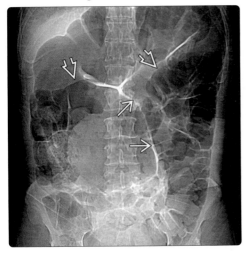

Sigmoid Volvulus

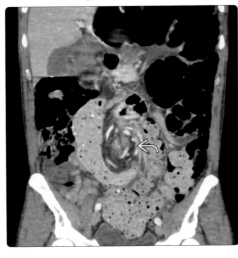

(Left) *Supine radiograph in a 59-year-old man shows marked dilation of the colon, especially the sigmoid colon. The sigmoid is folded back upon itself, and the apposed walls of the sigmoid colon* ➡ *form the "seam" of the football shape. The sigmoid extends into the upper abdomen above the transverse colon* ➡, *another useful sign in identifying colonic segments.* (Right) *Coronal CECT in the same patient shows twisting and engorgement of the sigmoid mesocolon and its vessels* ➡.

Sigmoid Volvulus

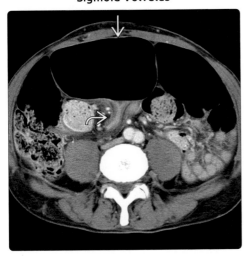

Sigmoid Volvulus

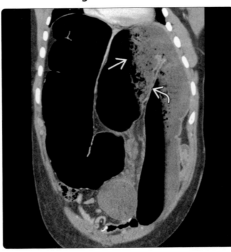

(Left) *Axial CECT shows massively dilated and redundant sigmoid* ➡, *along with twisting and displacement of the inferior mesenteric vessels supplying this segment of bowel* ➡.
(Right) *Coronal reformatted CECT shows a dilated and obstructed sigmoid colon with fecalization* ➡. *Note the apposed walls* ➡.

Colonic Ileus or Dilation

Cecal Volvulus

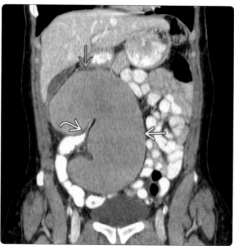

Cecal Volvulus

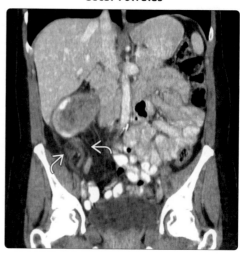

(Left) *Coronal CECT in a female patient shows a markedly distended cecum*  *and contrast-filled terminal ileum entering the ileocecal valve* ➔. *The base of the cecum* ➯ *is directed upward.* **(Right)** *Coronal CECT in the same patient shows that the ileocolic mesentery is twisted (whorled) within the right lower quadrant* ➔, *confirming cecal volvulus.*

Diverticulitis

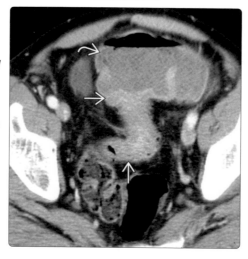

Fecal Impaction, Stercoral Colitis

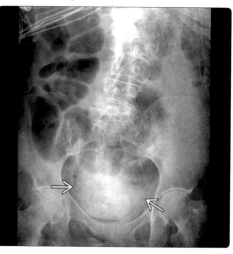

(Left) *Axial CECT shows marked dilation of the colon* ➔ *with abrupt transition to a short segment of luminal narrowing and wall thickening in the sigmoid colon* ➔. *Neither diverticula nor pericolonic inflammatory changes are evident, but diverticulitis was confirmed as the cause of the obstructing mass.* **(Right)** *Supine radiograph in an older woman with chronic constipation and acute, severe abdominal pain shows colonic distention and fecal impaction in the rectum* ➔.

Fecal Impaction, Stercoral Colitis

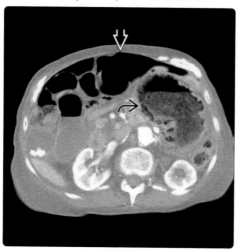

Fecal Impaction, Stercoral Colitis

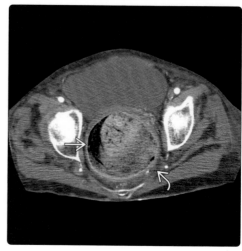

(Left) *Axial CECT in an older patient shows free intraperitoneal gas* ➔ *and massive distention of the left colon with gas and impacted feces* ➯. **(Right)** *Axial CECT in the same patient shows distention of the rectum with impacted feces* ➔. *Infiltration of the perirectal fat* ➔ *suggests stercoral ulceration, confirmed at surgery.*

Ischemic Colitis

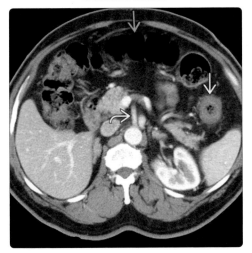

Ischemic Colitis

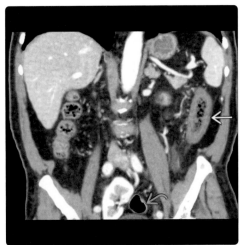

(Left) *Axial CECT in an older man who developed acute abdominal pain and distention after hip replacement surgery shows distended colon ➡ that narrowed abruptly at splenic flexure. Descending colon ➡ is thick walled with submucosal edema. Mesenteric vessels ➡ are patent.* (Right) *Coronal CECT in the same patient shows wall thickening and luminal narrowing of the descending colon ➡ with sparing of the rectum ➡, typical features of ischemic colitis.*

Toxic Megacolon

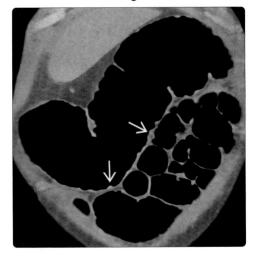

Toxic Megacolon

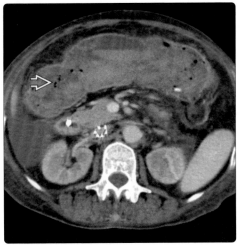

(Left) *Coronal CECT in a 63-year-old hospitalized man with Clostridium difficile colitis who presented with worsening abdominal pain shows a dilated transverse colon measuring up to 8 cm with multiple pseudopolyps ➡.* (Right) *Axial CECT in a woman with acute abdominal pain and bloody diarrhea due to Clostridium difficile colitis shows massive dilation of the colon with loss of haustration and intraluminal, high-density material representing hemorrhage and sloughed mucosa ➡.*

Toxic Megacolon

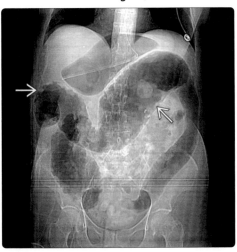

Toxic Megacolon

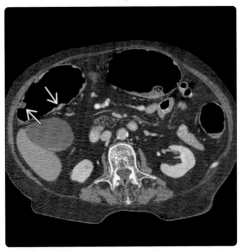

(Left) *Supine radiograph in a woman with chronic Crohn colitis shows marked dilation of the transverse colon with a featureless, ahaustral appearance. There is some irregularity of the luminal surface ➡, suggesting mucosal sloughing or pseudopolyps.* (Right) *Axial CECT in a woman with Crohn colitis unresponsive to medical therapy shows the colonic dilation and ahaustral appearance with marked thinning of the wall, suggesting risk of perforation. Note the tags of inflamed mucosa or pseudopolyps ➡.*

DIFFERENTIAL DIAGNOSIS

Common

- Ulcerative Colitis
- Crohn Colitis
- Infectious Colitis
- Colonic Ileus (Mimic)

Less Common

- Ischemic Colitis

ESSENTIAL INFORMATION

Key Differential Diagnosis Issues

- Any etiology of severe colitis may result in toxic megacolon
  - Infectious colitis is likely more common cause than ulcerative colitis
- Diagnosis of toxic megacolon is based on imaging & clinical features
- **Best diagnostic clue: Dilated colon with air-fluid levels & abnormal mucosal & transverse fold patterns**
  - > 6 cm on CT, often > 8 cm (as measured on supine radiograph)
- **CT is best imaging tool (contrast enema is contraindicated)**
  - Loss of normal colonic folds & mucosal pattern is characteristic
    - Mucosal islands or pseudopolyps cause irregular surface contour
  - Colonic wall may be thickened or abnormally thin
  - May show hemorrhage within colonic lumen; no formed stool
  - Presence of ascites &/or pneumoperitoneum are critical prognostic signs
  - Urgent colectomy is usually mandatory
- Clinical findings
  - Patients appear toxic, very ill
  - Patients with ulcerative colitis usually have known diagnosis

- Patients with infectious or ischemic colitis may develop toxic megacolon without preceding history of bowel disease

Helpful Clues for Common Diagnoses

- **Ulcerative or Crohn Colitis**
  - Colonic wall is usually not markedly thickened; may be paper thin
  - Crohn (granulomatous) colitis usually occurs with longstanding Crohn involvement of small bowel as well
- **Infectious Colitis**
  - *Clostridium difficile* (pseudomembranous) or others
    - Colonic wall is usually markedly thickened with submucosal edema
    - Mucosal hyperenhancement may evolve to lack of enhancement & mucosal sloughing
  - *Escherichia coli, Campylobacter*, typhoid, & amebic colitis are among other reported causes of infectious colitis with toxic megacolon
- **Colonic Ileus (Mimic)**
  - Colonic ileus may occur ± small bowel involvement
  - Causes include: Postoperative, electrolyte disturbances, medications
  - Normal fold & mucosal pattern are preserved
    - Distinguishes ileus from toxic megacolon
  - Acute & severe dilation (> 12 cm on radiography; 10 cm on CT) increases risk of ischemic & perforation
    - Colonic obstruction is not necessary

Helpful Clues for Less Common Diagnoses

- **Ischemic Colitis**
  - Uncommon to rare etiology of toxic megacolon
  - Most common form of ischemic colitis is hypoperfusion
    - Typically results in colonic wall thickening in splenic flexure or sigmoid distribution
      - Watershed zones of overlapping SMA-IMA arterial supply
  - Thromboembolic arterial occlusion more often in SMA distribution
    - More likely to result in colonic infarction but uncommonly preceded by toxic megacolon

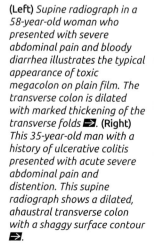

(Left) *Supine radiograph in a 58-year-old woman who presented with severe abdominal pain and bloody diarrhea illustrates the typical appearance of toxic megacolon on plain film. The transverse colon is dilated with marked thickening of the transverse folds* ➡. **(Right)** *This 35-year-old man with a history of ulcerative colitis presented with acute severe abdominal pain and distention. This supine radiograph shows a dilated, ahaustral transverse colon with a shaggy surface contour* ➡.

Ulcerative Colitis

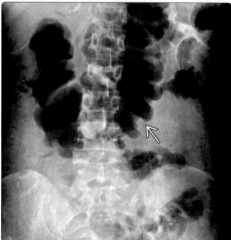

Ulcerative Colitis

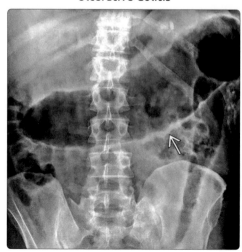

Ulcerative Colitis

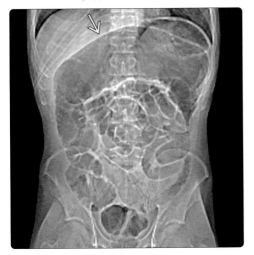

Ulcerative Colitis

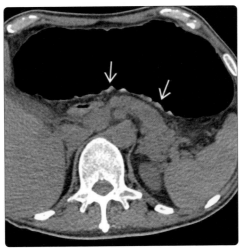

(Left) *Coronal CT in a 43-year-old man with ulcerative colitis and abdominal pain shows that the large bowel is severely dilated* ➡. **(Right)** *Axial CT in the same patient shows a dilated large bowel (up to 9 cm) with multiple pseudopolyps* ➡. *Patient underwent total colectomy due to worsening symptoms.*

Crohn Colitis

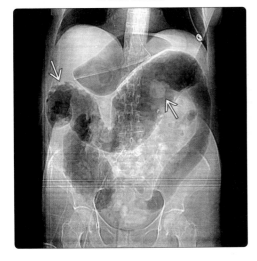

Crohn Colitis

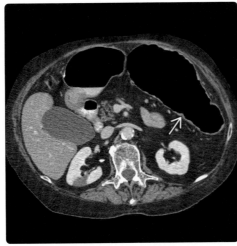

(Left) *In this woman with chronic Crohn (granulomatous) colitis, a supine film shows marked dilation of the transverse colon with a featureless ahaustral appearance. There is some irregularity of the luminal surface* ➡, *suggesting mucosal sloughing or pseudopolyps.* **(Right)** *In this woman with Crohn colitis, axial CECT shows the colonic dilation and ahaustral appearance with marked thinning of the wall, which suggests risk of perforation. Note the tags of inflamed mucosa or pseudopolyps* ➡.

Infectious Colitis

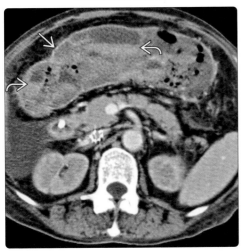

Infectious Colitis

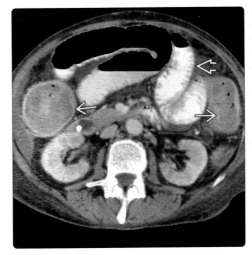

(Left) *In this patient with Clostridium difficile colitis, axial CECT shows a dilated transverse colon* ➡ *with pneumatosis, intraluminal bleeding* ➡, *and sloughed mucosa. The colonic wall is thin; ascites is present.* **(Right)** *In this patient with C. difficile colitis, axial CECT shows a generalized ileus* ➡. *The colon* ➡ *is massively distended with blood and debris, and its wall is relatively thin. Soon after this scan, the colon perforated, and a total colectomy was required.*

DIFFERENTIAL DIAGNOSIS

Common

- Diverticulitis
- Crohn Disease
- Postoperative State, Bowel
- Pelvic Malignancy
  - Colon Carcinoma
  - Rectal Cancer
  - Cervical and Uterine Carcinoma
  - Endometrial Carcinoma
  - Ovarian Cancer
  - Bladder Carcinoma
  - Prostate Carcinoma
- Bladder Instrumentation (Mimic)

Less Common

- Cystitis (Mimic)
  - Emphysematous Cystitis
- Abdominal or Pelvic Abscess
- Infectious Colitis
- Trauma, Colorectal or Vaginal
- Foreign Body

ESSENTIAL INFORMATION

Key Differential Diagnosis Issues

- Gas in urinary bladder may be due to
  - Colovesical or enterovesical fistula
  - Gas-forming infection within bladder or its wall (emphysematous cystitis)
  - Instrumentation that introduces gas into bladder (e.g., catheterization)
  - Check for extensive coliform bacterial infection of urine, pneumaturia
- Surgical resection of any pelvic mass predisposes to fistulas
  - Especially if followed or preceded by radiation therapy
  - Even resection of benign process (e.g., uterine fibroids, endometrioma)
  - Fistulas may develop years later, often due to diverticulitis
- All low rectal anastomoses are prone to leak
  - Resulting perianastomotic abscess can fistulize into any pelvic space, organ, or skin
  - Perianastomotic collection of gas and fluid is presumptive evidence of anastomotic leak
  - Rectal administration of contrast material at fluoroscopy or CT should be considered to document or exclude fistula
    - Generally much more successful than oral administration of contrast
    - Alternatives
      - Contrast-enhanced MR
      - Contrast injection into cutaneous fistula opening
      - Contrast injection into bladder (cystogram) with fluoroscopic or CT evaluation
- Abdominal or pelvic abscesses of any etiology may erode into gut, bladder, vagina, or skin

Helpful Clues for Common Diagnoses

- **Diverticulitis**

- Most common etiology for colonic fistulas in industrialized nations
- Infection can spread to any pelvic structure
  - Examples
    - Fistula to skin
    - Bladder
    - Vagina
    - Hip joint
- Diverticulitis may cause infection of pelvic scar (e.g., from hysterectomy) leading to colovaginal fistula

- **Crohn Disease**
  - Most common cause of enteric (small bowel) fistulas
    - Can also cause colonic fistulas in setting of Crohn (granulomatous) colitis
  - St Jame's University Hospital (SJUH) grading for perianal fistulas on MR
    - Grade 1: Simple intersphincteric fistula
    - Grade 2: Intersphincteric fistula with a secondary tract or abscess
    - Grade 3: Simple transsphincteric fistulae
    - Grade 4: Complicated transsphincteric process with secondary tract or abscess
    - Grade 5: Complicated abscess with supra or translevator component

- **Postoperative State, Bowel**
  - Any pelvic surgery or resection (e.g., rectal, hysterectomy, cesarean section)
    - Examples
      - Rectal
      - Hysterectomy
      - Cesarean section
    - Low anterior resection or sigmoid resection for rectosigmoid carcinoma
      - Low colorectal anastomosis within 5 cm from anal verge
    - Creation of ileal pouch with ileoanal anastomosis following colectomy
    - May occur post radiation
  - Infection of scar by diverticulitis may cause fistula
  - Leak at rectal or colonic anastomosis may lead to abscess and then fistula
    - This is quite common in patients who have anastomotic leaks from low rectal anastomoses

- **Colon Carcinoma**
  - Usually from sigmoid or rectum
  - Fistula may be spontaneous or follow surgery, radiation, or chemotherapy
  - Especially likely in older, diabetic, and debilitated patients

- **Rectal carcinoma**
  - Risk factors: Tumors > 5 cm, locally advanced tumors requiring neoadjuvant therapy, stage IV rectal cancer
  - My develop fistula with vagina, presacral area etc.

- **Cervical and Uterine Carcinoma**
  - Advanced stage may invade bladder, rectum, or colon
  - Fistula usually follows surgery or therapy
  - Tumor may "bridge" or connect 2 pelvic viscera
    - Subsequent necrosis of tumor may open the connection

- Benign scar results from resection of cervical/uterine carcinoma
  - Scar may become infected (e.g., from diverticulitis)
  - May result in colovaginal fistula
- **Bladder Carcinoma**
  - Fistula from local invasion by tumor itself or following therapy
  - Same mechanisms as for gynecologic tumors
    - Tumor or benign scar tissue may form bridge to bowel or other organs
- **Bladder Instrumentation (Mimic)**
  - Foley catheter, cystoscopy, etc.

Helpful Clues for Less Common Diagnoses
- **Cystitis**
  - Can cause or mimic fistula
  - Gas-forming infection in urine or bladder may be mistaken for colovesical fistula
- **Abdominal or Pelvic Abscess**
  - Abdominal or pelvic abscess may erode into bladder, vagina, colon, &/or skin

- Postoperative abscesses are most common cause
- Reported as etiologies
  - Tuboovarian
  - Appendiceal
  - Other pelvic abscesses
- **Trauma, Colorectal or Vaginal**
  - May create communication between pelvic viscera directly
  - Or may lead to infection with subsequent fistula
    - Examples
      - Foreign body insertion into rectum or vagina
      - Complex pelvic fractures
      - Stab wounds to pelvis
- **Foreign Body**
  - In bladder, vagina, or rectum, can lead to fistula
    - Chronic inflammation and infection cause adherence between viscera and tissue breakdown

Diverticulitis

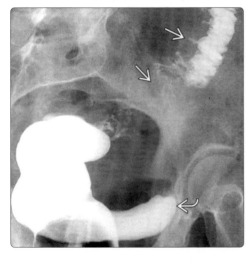

Diverticulitis

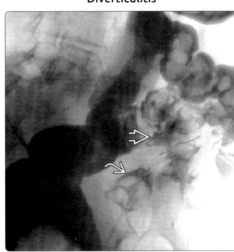

(Left) Spot film from a contrast enema in a middle-aged woman with recurrent urinary tract infections shows extensive sigmoid diverticulitis ➡ with filling of the urinary bladder ➡ via a fistulous track. (Right) Spot film from a contrast enema in the same patient shows contrast extravasation ➡ from the sigmoid colon and a fistula to the bladder, represented by contrast opacification of urine surrounding the Foley catheter balloon ➡.

Diverticulitis

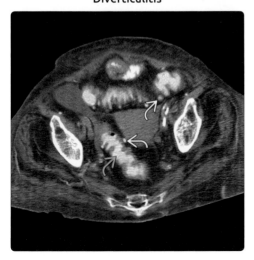

Diverticulitis

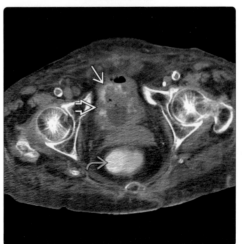

(Left) Axial NECT in an older adult woman with urosepsis shows extensive sigmoid diverticular disease ➡. Contrast medium had been instilled into the rectosigmoid colon ➡. (Right) Axial NECT in the same patient shows the contrast-opacified rectum ➡. Within the bladder ➡ is some of the rectal contrast medium ➡, along with gas, debris, and the Foley balloon. Diverticulitis was the source of the colovesical fistula.

Colon

(Left) *Axial CECT in a a 50-year-old woman who developed a foul vaginal discharge years after a hysterectomy for benign uterine fibroids shows contrast material injected by tube into the rectum ⮧ that opacifies the vagina ⮧, indicating a fistula.* **(Right)** *Sagittal CECT in a woman with a colovaginal fistula due to diverticulitis shows contrast administered into the rectum ⮧, filling the vagina ⮧ via a fistulous tract ➡.*

Diverticulitis

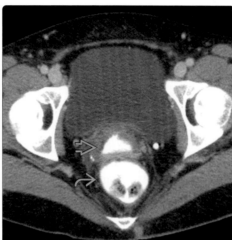

Diverticulitis

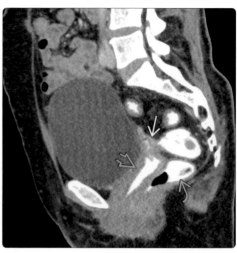

(Left) *Axial CECT performed after rectal administration of contrast medium in an older adult woman with foul vaginal discharge shows gas, fluid, and contrast medium within the rectum ⮧ and uterine lumen ⮧, indicating a colouterine fistula.* **(Right)** *Coronal CECT in the same patient shows extensive sigmoid diverticulitis ➡ and an adjacent collection of gas and fluid that is within the lumen of the uterus ⮧. Surgery confirmed a colouterine fistula caused by diverticulitis.*

Diverticulitis

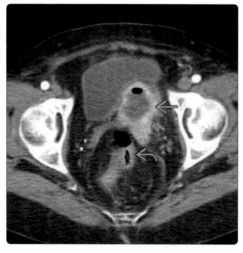

Diverticulitis

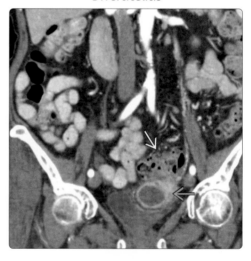

(Left) *Axial NECT in a 47-year-old woman who had recurrent urinary tract infections following sigmoid resection for diverticulitis shows gas within the left ureter ➡ and renal collecting system.* **(Right)** *Axial NECT in the same patient shows gas in the distal ureter ➡, which appears adherent to the site of the stapled anastomosis ➡ of the sigmoid colon. Diverticulitis with coloureteral fistula was confirmed.*

Diverticulitis

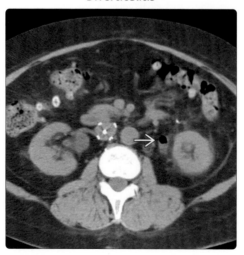

Diverticulitis

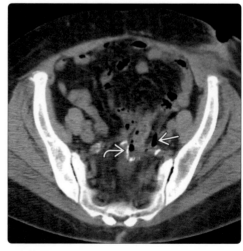

Diverticulitis

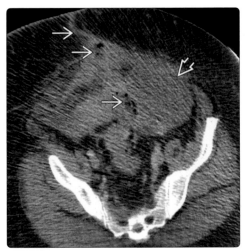

Diverticulitis

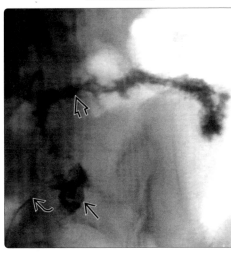

(Left) *Axial NECT in an obese young woman who has a tender, warm lesion in her abdominal wall with a foul-smelling discharge shows a walled-off abscess ⊟ adjacent to the sigmoid colon. There is a tract of gas and fluid ⊟ leading to the anterior abdominal wall defect.* (Right) *In the same patient, injection of a catheter ⊟ inserted into the abdominal wall defect opacifies an abscess cavity ⊟ and the sigmoid colon lumen ⊟, confirming a colocutaneous fistula from diverticulitis.*

Crohn Disease

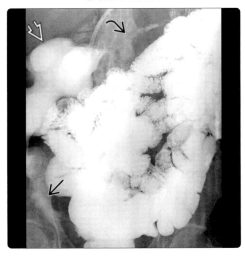

Crohn Disease

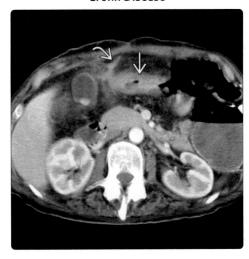

(Left) *This 64-year-old man with Crohn disease developed a feculent fistula to the skin of his anterior abdominal wall. A barium small bowel follow-through shows strictures ⊟ of the transverse colon and terminal ileum ⊟ with a dilated segment of colon ⊟ in between.* (Right) *In the same patient with Crohn disease and feculent discharge from his abdominal wall, axial CECT shows a stricture and inflammation of the transverse colon ⊟ but also shows the fistula ⊟ to the anterior abdominal wall.*

Crohn Disease

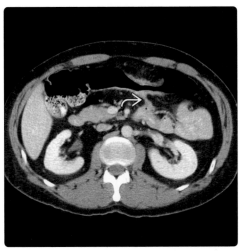

Crohn Disease

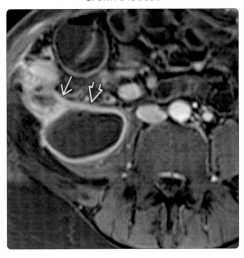

(Left) *Axial CECT in a patient with chronic Crohn disease shows a fistula ⊟ connecting inflamed small bowel to the colon. This "short circuit" between the midsmall bowel and the transverse colon resulted in massive loss of fluid and electrolytes.* (Right) *Axial T1 C+ FS MR in a 41-year-old man with Crohn disease shows a psoas abscess ⊟, which is communicating with the adjacent ascending colon ⊟.*

Crohn Disease

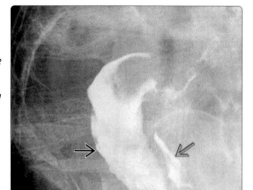

Crohn Disease

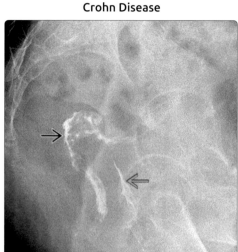

(Left) *Lateral spot film from a contrast enema in a 54-year-old woman with Crohn colitis shows opacification of the rectosigmoid colon* ➡ *and the vagina* ➡ *through a fistulous tract* ➡ *starting low in the rectum. The image is obscured by contrast spilling onto sheets.* (Right) *Repeat film in the same patient after removal of the stained sheets clearly shows contrast medium in the rectum* ➡ *and vagina* ➡.

Crohn Disease

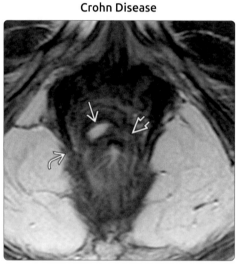

Crohn Disease

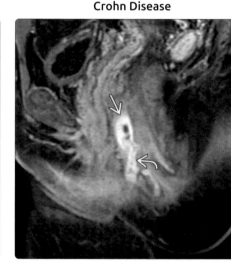

(Left) *Axial T2 HASTE MR shows a grade 2 fistula-in-ano in a patient with history of Crohn disease. Note a small fluid collection* ➡ *between the internal* ➡ *and external sphincters* ➡. (Right) *Sagittal T1 C+ FS MR in the same patient shows the rim enhancing fluid collection* ➡ *along with an inferior fistulous tract that demonstrates enhancement* ➡, *indicative of active inflammation.*

Postoperative State, Bowel

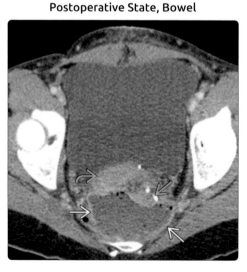

Postoperative State, Bowel

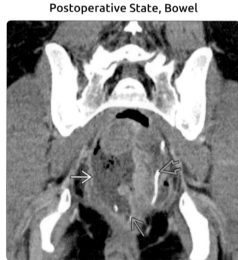

(Left) *This young woman had a colectomy with ileoanal anastomosis for ulcerative colitis. CT shows an encapsulated collection of gas and fluid (abscess)* ➡ *at the anal anastomotic staple line* ➡, *presumptive evidence of an anastomotic leak. The vagina* ➡ *abuts the abscess.* (Right) *Coronal CECT in the same patient shows the abscess* ➡ *and anal* ➡ *and pouch anastomotic* ➡ *staple lines. She subsequently developed a colovaginal fistula.*

Colon Carcinoma

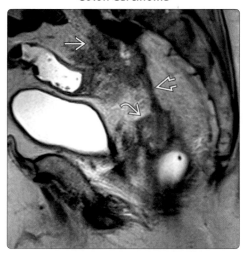

Rectal Cancer

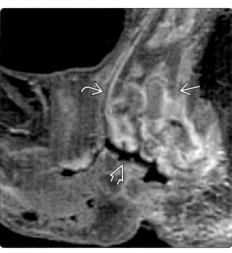

(Left) *Sagittal T2 HASTE MR in a 70-year-old man with invasive squamous cell cancer of the sigmoid colon* ➡ *shows a malignant fistula* ➡ *communicating with perirectal metastases* ➡. **(Right)** *Patient with a large rectal cancer* ➡ *treated with chemoradiation has an MR obtained for foul-smelling discharge from the vagina* ➡ *due to the development of a rectovaginal fistula* ➡.

Cervical and Uterine Carcinoma

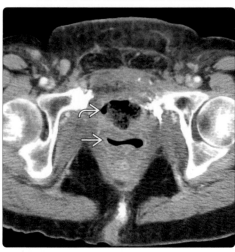

Cystitis (Mimic)

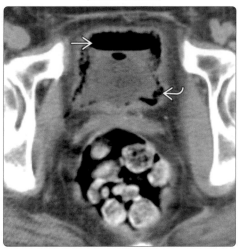

(Left) *Axial CECT shows gas in the vagina* ➡ *and bladder* ➡ *due to rectovaginal and rectovesical fistulas due to cervical carcinoma, status post resection and radiation therapy.* **(Right)** *Axial NECT shows gas within the lumen* ➡ *and wall of the bladder* ➡ *due to emphysematous cystitis. This might be mistaken for a fistula to the colon.*

Trauma, Colorectal or Vaginal

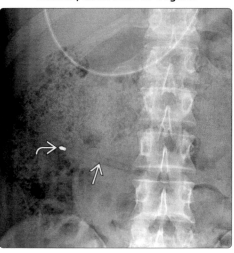

Trauma, Colorectal or Vaginal

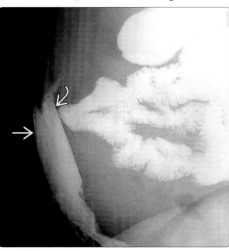

(Left) *This young man developed a cutaneous fistula after stabbing himself in the abdomen with a Bic pen, which he pushed into the abdomen. Radiograph shows the faint outline of the plastic pen* ➡ *and its metal tip* ➡. **(Right)** *Lateral view from a small bowel follow-through in a man with a self-inflicted stab wound shows a segment of small bowel that is tethered to the anterior abdominal wall* ➡ *with extravasation of barium into a bag* ➡ *that overlies anterior abdominal wall wound, confirming the enterocutaneous fistula.*

DIFFERENTIAL DIAGNOSIS

Common

- Colon Carcinoma
- Diverticulitis or Diverticulosis
- Ischemic Colitis
- Colonic Metastases and Lymphoma
- Colonic Spasm
- Peristalsis
- Infectious Colitis
- Ulcerative Colitis
- Crohn (Granulomatous) Colitis

Less Common

- Pancreatitis
- Extrinsic or Intramural Masses
  - Endometriosis
  - Uterine Fibroid
  - Pericolic Abscess
  - Gastrointestinal Stromal Tumor (GIST)
- Postoperative Stricture
- Cathartic Abuse
- Typhlitis (Neutropenic Colitis)
- Rectal Mucosal Prolapse
- Tuberculosis, Colon
- Amebic Colitis
- Radiation Colitis
- Intramural Hematoma, Colon

ESSENTIAL INFORMATION

Key Differential Diagnosis Issues

- Important to describe length, site, and nature of narrowed segment
  - Abrupt narrowing with shoulders or apple core appearance = carcinoma until proven otherwise
    - May rarely result from infectious or ischemic etiology
  - Longer strictures with smooth, tapered margins are usually benign
- Colon may be narrowed by extrinsic inflammatory process, such as pancreatitis, cholecystitis, abscess, endometriosis
  - Also by extrinsic mass (e.g., uterine fibroid) or even distended urinary bladder
- Barium enema shows strictures and mucosal lesions better than CT
  - CT shows extracolonic processes better

Helpful Clues for Common Diagnoses

- **Colon Carcinoma**
  - Most common cause of colonic stricture and obstruction in adults
  - Short segment of narrowing (< 10 cm)
    - Usually little pericolonic infiltration
  - Regional lymphadenopathy suggests carcinoma (or infection)
- **Diverticulitis or Diverticulosis**
  - Usually causes longer segment (> 10 cm) narrowing, more pericolonic inflammation, no lymphadenopathy
  - Luminal narrowing is often due to circular muscle hypertrophy

- Best seen on contrast enema as irregular indentation of lumen (cog wheel)
- Does not imply active inflammation or spasm
- Is not relieved by administration of glucagon

- **Ischemic Colitis**
  - May be acute, subacute, or chronic
  - Might follow hypoperfusion episode or arterial or venous occlusion
    - Imaging findings vary according to etiology and acuity of ischemia
    - Arterial thrombosis/embolism usually causes small bowel ischemic injury limited to distribution of superior mesenteric artery with limited bowel wall/mesenteric edema
    - Hypoperfusion is most common etiology for colonic ischemia
      - Usual manifestation is wall thickening and luminal narrowing of watershed segments of colon
      - Splenic flexure > sigmoid colon
- **Colonic Metastases and Lymphoma**
  - Can be hematogenous or lymphatic spread or direct invasion
    - e.g., from duodenum, stomach, kidneys, gallbladder, uterus, prostate
  - Most common is direct invasion from primary pelvic malignancy
    - e.g., cervical, endometrial, prostatic
  - Drop metastases = intraperitoneal spread of tumor
    - Common site is to pouch of Douglas (rectovesical or rectouterine recess)
      - Mass indents anterior wall of rectum and can be palpated on physical exam
- **Colonic Spasm**
  - May exactly simulate carcinoma on imaging
  - Give IV glucagon to relieve spasm; repeat imaging
- **Peristalsis**
  - May appear as area of narrowing on single image
  - Usually absent on 2nd phase of multiphasic study (dual-phase CT or MR)
- **Infectious Colitis**
  - Tuberculosis and amebic colitis can cause apple core lesion exactly like carcinoma
  - Lymphogranuloma venereum
    - Caused by *Chlamydia trachomatis*
    - Rectosigmoid involvement due to anal intercourse
    - Luminal narrowing, mucosal ulceration, perirectal abscess, rectal fistula, perirectal fat stranding on CT
  - Other infectious colitides
    - *Clostridium difficile* and *Campylobacter colitis* usually involve entire colon but may be segmental
- **Ulcerative or Granulomatous Colitis**
  - May result in diffuse or segmental stricture of colon
    - Short, focal stricture should raise concern for colon carcinoma as complication of chronic colitis

Helpful Clues for Less Common Diagnoses

- **Pancreatitis**
  - Inflammation often spreads laterally within anterior pararenal space to contact proximal descending colon

- Colon cutoff sign = proximal descending colon is narrowed due to spasm and inflammation caused by pancreatitis
  - Transverse colon is gas distended
- **Endometriosis**
  - Endometrial tissue may implant on any part of intraperitoneal bowel
    - Involves rectosigmoid area in 75-95% of cases
  - Typical findings: Extrinsic mass effect on anterior wall of rectosigmoid junction
    - Less common: Polypoid mass, annular constricting lesion
      - Indistinguishable for primary colonic carcinoma
- **Gastrointestinal Stromal Tumor (GIST)**
  - Hypo- or hypervascular, well-circumscribed, mass on arterial-phase CECT images; central ulceration and necrosis are common
  - Cavitation in lesion may collect air trapped in necrotic ulcer in nondependent portion, which is called Torricelli-Bernoulli crescentic necrosis sign
  - Sometimes hemorrhagic
  - Often exophytic
    - May not be visible on endoscopy if completely exophytic
  - Tumors with large intraluminal component may mimic primary gastric carcinoma
- **Postoperative Stricture**
  - Usually web-like, short strictured segment with smooth edges
  - Anastomosis often marked by surgical staple line
- **Cathartic Abuse**
  - Due to chronic use of stimulant laxatives
  - Results in neuromuscular damage of colon
  - Ahaustral colon (simulates chronic ulcerative colitis)
    - Irregular and transient segmental narrowing, primarily in ascending and transverse colon
- **Typhlitis (Neutropenic Colitis)**
  - Luminal narrowing and wall thickening of cecum and ascending colon
  - Due to polymicrobial infiltration of colonic wall

- Encountered only in severely neutropenic patients
  - Leukemia, bone marrow transplant recipient
- **Rectal Mucosal Prolapse**
  - Solitary rectal ulcer syndrome
    - Traumatic or ischemic ulceration of rectal mucosa associated with disordered evacuation
  - Usually in women with pelvic floor laxity
    - MR defecography: Complete visualization of pelvic organs and supporting structures of all 3 compartments
  - Repeated episodes of rectal prolapse injure anterolateral walls of rectum, leading to edema and ulceration
    - Proximal rectum ± sigmoid telescopes into distal rectum, rarely through anus
    - Contributes to sensation of incomplete evacuation
    - 3 types: Intrarectal, intraanal, extraanal (rectal prolapse)
    - ± anterior rectocele (very common cause of incomplete evacuation in women)
  - May also cause spasm, mural thickening (colitis cystica profunda), stricture
  - Diagnosed on barium enema, MR defecography, or sigmoidoscopy
- **Radiation Colitis**
  - Usually follows radiation therapy for pelvic primary malignancy (e.g., cervical or prostate carcinoma)
  - Leads to long stricture of rectosigmoid colon with tapered margins

Colon Carcinoma

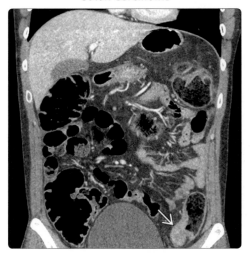

Diverticulitis or Diverticulosis

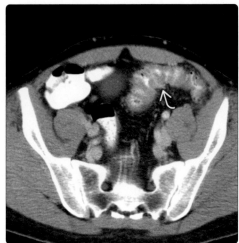

(Left) Coronal CECT shows a colonic obstructing lesion ➡️ as a classic apple core carcinoma with a short segment and soft tissue density thickening of the colonic wall. (Right) Axial CECT shows luminal narrowing and wall thickening of the sigmoid colon ➡️ due to circular muscle hypertrophy.

Ischemic Colitis

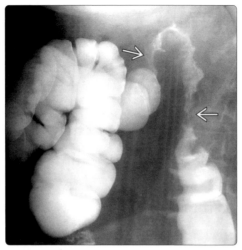

Colonic Spasm

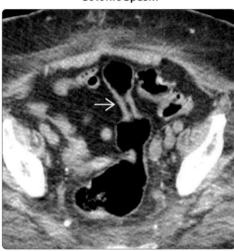

(Left) *Spot film from a contrast enema shows luminal narrowing and fold thickening of the splenic flexure region of colon ➡. This is a characteristic location and appearance for hypoperfusion etiology ischemic colitis.* (Right) *Axial CECT shows an apparent stricture ➡ of the sigmoid colon. This was normal at colonoscopy and probably represented simple spasm. Note normal wall thickness and no infiltration of adjacent fat.*

Infectious Colitis

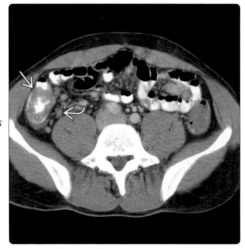

Infectious Colitis

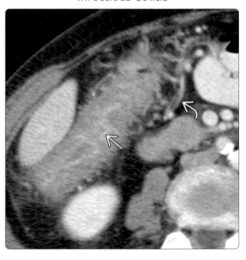

(Left) *Axial CECT shows luminal narrowing and wall thickening of the ascending colon ➡ due to Yersinia colitis. Also note some mesocolic lymphadenopathy ➡.* (Right) *Axial CECT in an older adult patient with bloody diarrhea shows pancolitis. The colonic lumen is narrowed ➡ with submucosal edema and mucosal and mesenteric hyperemia ➡. Campylobacter was the responsible organism.*

Ulcerative Colitis

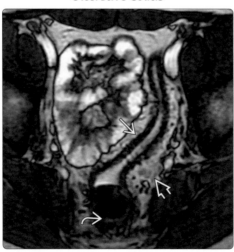

Ulcerative Colitis

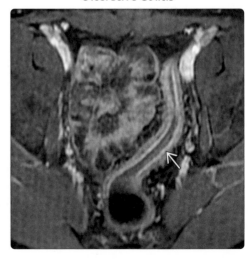

(Left) *Axial T2 MR in a 26-year-old man with an acute flair of ulcerative colitis shows moderate wall thickening causing luminal narrowing ➡. Mild edema in the wall ➡ is indicative of acute inflammation. Loss of haustration of the sigmoid colon and surrounding fibrofatty proliferation ➡ is suggestive of longstanding disease.* (Right) *Axial T1 C+ FS MR shows mucosal hyperenhancement ➡, consistent with acute inflammation in the setting of chronic disease.*

Ulcerative Colitis

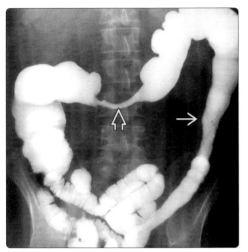

Pancreatitis

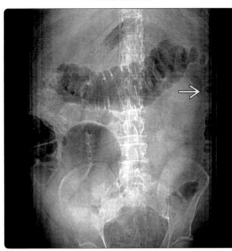

(Left) *Frontal film from a contrast enema shows a shortened ahaustral left colon* ➡ *due to chronic ulcerative colitis. The short, focal stricture in the transverse colon is a carcinoma* ➡. *Note the abrupt proximal margin.* (Right) *Supine radiograph shows dilation of the transverse colon with abrupt narrowing of the anatomic splenic flexure* ➡ *due to pancreatitis that had spread to the colon. This is a classic plain film finding of pancreatitis called the colon cutoff sign.*

Uterine Fibroid

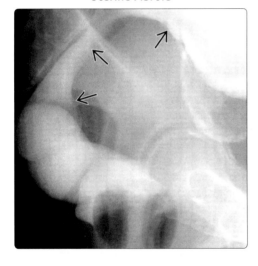

Cathartic Abuse

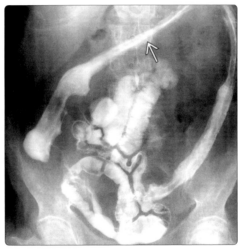

(Left) *Spot film from a contrast enema shows narrowing of the rectosigmoid colon* ➡ *due to an extrinsic mass. This proved to be a large uterine fibroid (leiomyoma).* (Right) *Supine film from a contrast enema shows focal and long strictures of the colon due to chronic laxative abuse* ➡.

Tuberculosis, Colon

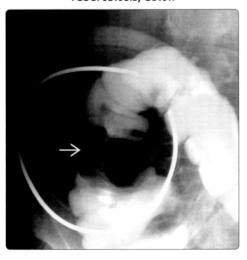

Radiation Colitis

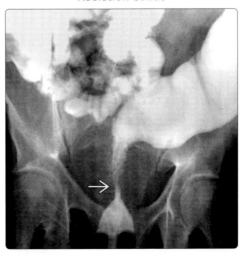

(Left) *Contrast enema shows a classic apple core lesion of the ascending colon, indistinguishable from carcinoma. It was proven at surgery to be due to tuberculous infection of the colon* ➡. (Right) *Spot film from a contrast enema shows a high-grade stricture* ➡ *of the rectum that resulted from radiation therapy for a sacral metastatic focus.*

DIFFERENTIAL DIAGNOSIS

Common

- Infectious Colitis
  - Pseudomembranous Colitis
- Ischemic Colitis
- Portal Hypertensive Colopathy
- Ulcerative Colitis

Less Common

- Typhlitis (Neutropenic Colitis)
- Chemical Proctocolitis
- Diverticulitis
- Intramural Hematoma, Colon
- Metastases & Lymphoma, Colonic
- Pneumatosis

ESSENTIAL INFORMATION

Key Differential Diagnosis Issues

- Thumbprinting describes rounded thickening of transverse colonic folds; usually due to edema
- Basically same differential diagnosis as for submucosal edema, as seen on CT
  - However, generally requires more extensive thickening to cause thumbprinting
- Neoplasm (primary or metastatic) rarely causes thumbprinting

Helpful Clues for Common Diagnoses

- **Infectious Colitis**
  - Infectious (including *Clostridium difficile*) colitis is most common cause of marked submucosal edema (thumbprinting)
  - *Campylobacter*, *Escherichia coli*, staphylococcal, amebic, *Strongyloides*, etc. in general population
  - Cytomegalovirus & others in immune suppressed
  - **Pseudomembranous colitis**
    - Caused by *C. difficile* infection of colon
    - Has become most common cause of thumbprinting

- Endemic in hospitalized patients, usually those on antibiotic therapy
- **Ischemic Colitis**
  - Often due to hypoperfusion (favors splenic flexure & sigmoid)
  - May be due to venous thrombosis
    - Arterial embolism or thrombosis rarely causes thumbprinting
- **Portal Hypertensive Colopathy**
  - Cirrhosis ± portal vein thrombosis
  - Often leads to marked colonic edema
  - Usually favors right side of colon
- **Ulcerative Colitis**
  - Or Crohn (granulomatous) colitis
  - Look for ulceration of mucosa
  - Usually causes less submucosal edema than infectious colitis

Helpful Clues for Less Common Diagnoses

- **Typhlitis (Neutropenic Colitis)**
  - Neutropenic colitis in severely neutropenic patients
  - Usually limited to cecum & ascending colon
- **Chemical Proctocolitis**
  - From glutaraldehyde, used to clean colonoscopes
- **Diverticulitis**
  - Wall thickening may be due to infection, pericolonic abscess, &/or circular muscle hypertrophy (**myochosis coli**)
  - Not truly thumbprinting nor submucosal edema
- **Intramural Hematoma, Colon**
  - Following trauma or anticoagulation
- **Metastases & Lymphoma, Colonic**
  - Rare cause of thumbprinting
  - Lymphoma more likely than metastases to cause multifocal sites of wall thickening
    - Will be soft tissue (not water) density on CT
- **Pneumatosis**
  - Usually benign, idiopathic, entity limited to rectosigmoid colon
  - Presence of gas cysts in wall of colon is diagnostic

Infectious Colitis

Infectious Colitis

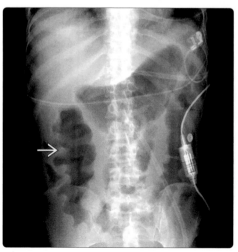
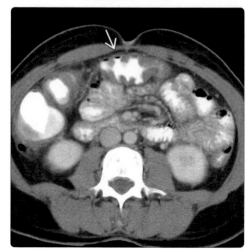

(Left) *Supine radiograph shows classic thumbprinting of the ascending colon ➡ due to cytomegalovirus colitis in a young man with AIDS.* (Right) *In this previously healthy young woman, CT shows massive, pancolonic, submucosal edema, imparting a thumbprinting appearance to the transverse colon ➡. Campylobacter was the responsible organism.*

Pseudomembranous Colitis

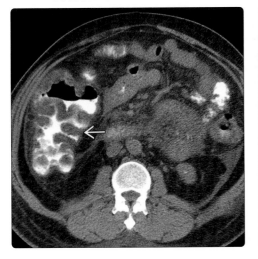

Ischemic Colitis

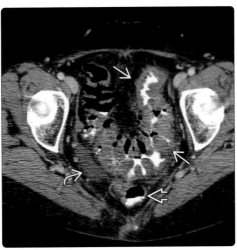

(Left) In this renal transplant recipient with acute C. diff colitis, CT shows massive thickening of the wall of the entire colon (pancolitis) with some segments having a thumbprinted appearance ➡. In spite of prompt diagnosis & treatment, toxic megacolon developed & resulted in total colectomy. (Right) This older adult patient had acute onset of hematochezia & abdominal pain after a hypotensive episode. CT shows ascites ➡ & thumbprinting of the sigmoid colon ➡ but sparing of the rectum ➡, typical features of hypoperfusion ischemic colitis.

Portal Hypertensive Colopathy

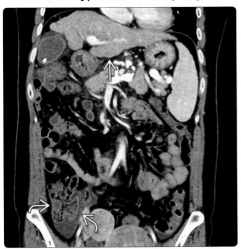

Ulcerative Colitis

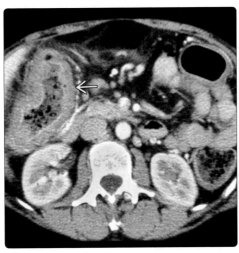

(Left) Coronal CECT in a 55-year-old asymptomatic woman with hepatic cirrhosis ➡ is shown. Colonic wall thumbprinting due to submucosal edema ➡ is secondary to portal colopathy. (Right) Axial CECT shows marked thickening of the colonic wall, especially the ascending colon, with intense mucosal hyperenhancement ➡. This degree of wall thickening is unusual for ulcerative colitis.

Typhlitis (Neutropenic Colitis)

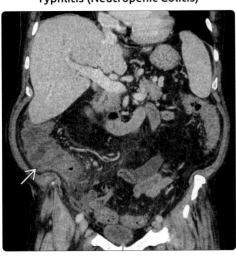

Pneumatosis

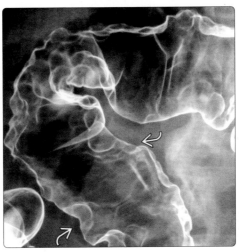

(Left) In this older man with acute leukemia, coronal CT shows massive submucosal edema ➡ limited to the wall of the ascending colon & cecum. These are typical features of typhlitis or neutropenic colitis. (Right) Spot film from an air-contrast barium enema shows thumbprinted pattern. The presence of gas blebs ➡ in the colonic wall indicates benign colonic pneumatosis in this asymptomatic patient.

DIFFERENTIAL DIAGNOSIS

Common

- Diverticulitis
- Infectious Colitis
  - Pseudomembranous Colitis
- Ischemic Colitis
- Ulcerative and Crohn Colitis
- Colon Carcinoma
- Portal Hypertensive Colopathy
- Endometriosis

Less Common

- Obesity (Mimic)
- Typhlitis (Neutropenic Colitis)
- Chemical Proctocolitis
- Colonic Metastases and Lymphoma
- Intramural Hemorrhage
- Pneumatosis of Colon
- Hemolytic Uremic Syndrome
- Angioedema, Intestinal

ESSENTIAL INFORMATION

Key Differential Diagnosis Issues

- **Characterize length and site of involvement**
  - Focal (< 10 cm): Neoplasm, endometriosis, rarely amebic or TB
  - Segmental (10-15 cm): Diverticulitis most common
  - Right colon and small intestine: Crohn disease, embolic or thrombotic, ischemic, portal colopathy, infectious
  - Watershed areas (splenic flexure &/or sigmoid): Hypoperfusion, ischemia
  - Pancolonic with sparing of small intestine: Infectious or ulcerative colitis (not ischemic)
  - Pancolonic sparing rectum: Infectious (not ischemic or ulcerative)
- **Characterize attenuation of submucosal layer**
  - Air density: Pneumatosis (various causes, including ischemia)
  - Fat density: Chronic ulcerative or granulomatous colitis, obesity
  - Near-water density: Inflammation or ischemia (not neoplastic)
  - Soft tissue density: Diverticulitis, inflammation, ischemia, tumor
  - High attenuation (> 60 HU): Hemorrhage

Helpful Clues for Common Diagnoses

- **Diverticulitis**
  - Wall is thickened over 10-15 cm in length by edema and smooth muscle hypertrophy (myochosis coli)
    - Usually no distinct submucosal layer of low density
  - Diverticula, pericolonic infiltration ± gas and fluid
- **Infectious Colitis**
  - Long segmental or pancolitis
    - Mucosal hyperemia and marked submucosal edema
  - Difficult to distinguish among etiologies from imaging alone
  - **Pseudomembranous colitis**
    - Most impressive wall thickening among colitides

- □ Submucosal edema with compressed lumen and intense mucosal enhancement may result in accordion sign or thumbprinting
- □ Accordion sign: Alternating bands of enhancing mucosa and submucosal edema with compressed lumen
- – Segmental or pancolitis
- – Caused by *Clostridium difficile* toxin, endemic in health care facilities
  - □ No longer confined to hospitalized patients who have received broad-spectrum antibiotics

- **Ischemic Colitis**
  - Most common in watershed regions when caused by hypoperfusion
    - Splenic flexure > sigmoid colon
  - Embolic or thrombotic arterial occlusion more commonly affects small intestine and right side of colon
    - Arterial occlusive ischemia usually does not cause much wall thickening
  - Rectum is rarely affected by ischemic colitis
- **Ulcerative and Crohn Colitis**
  - Acute: Wall edema, pericolonic infiltration, mesenteric hyperemia (comb or caterpillar sign)
    - Submucosal edema usually less marked than with infectious colitis
  - Chronic: Submucosal layer is fat density
  - Ulcerative colitis favors rectum and distal colon
  - Granulomatous (Crohn) colitis favors distal ileum with skip areas in small bowel and colon; perianal involvement (fistulas)
- **Colon Carcinoma**
  - Wall thickening is soft tissue attenuation
  - Usually short segment involvement (< 10 cm)
    - Apple core lesion
    - Right-sided colon cancers often bulkier; less likely to obstruct
  - Often with regional adenopathy (strong predictor of cancer with lymphatic spread)
  - Look for hepatic and peritoneal metastases
- **Portal Hypertensive Colopathy**
  - Edema of colonic wall ± small bowel
    - Portal hypertensive colopathy, not inflammatory
  - Look for signs of cirrhosis, ascites
  - May occur with heart and renal failure
- **Endometriosis**
  - Implants on colonic wall closely mimic primary colon cancer
    - Short segment, soft tissue density
    - Narrowing, possibly obstructing, colonic lumen
    - May be multifocal, especially in sigmoid colon
  - Correlate with periodic symptoms in young women
  - ± hyperintense on T1 MR

Helpful Clues for Less Common Diagnoses

- **Obesity (Mimic)**
  - Fatty infiltration of submucosal layer may be asymptomatic finding of no significance
  - Ask about history of prior colitis
- **Typhlitis (Neutropenic Colitis)**
  - Neutropenic colitis
  - Leukemia and bone marrow transplant patients

- Limited to cecum and ascending colon
- Wall thickening is marked; wall may perforate
  - Extraluminal gas &/or fluid is ominous sign; usually requires surgery
- **Chemical Proctocolitis**
  - Glutaraldehyde used to sterilize endoscopes
  - If not thoroughly washed from surface of scope, can damage colonic mucosa
- **Colonic Metastases and Lymphoma**
  - Wall thickening is soft tissue density
  - Quite rare; less common than small bowel involvement
- **Intramural Hemorrhage**
  - Uncommon in colon
  - Etiologies: Trauma (including endoscopy), anticoagulation
  - Attenuation is greater than soft tissue (may be apparent only on NECT)
- **Pneumatosis of Colon**
  - Spherical or linear air density
  - From infarction, idiopathic pneumatosis cystoides, or other causes of "benign" pneumatosis

- Steroid and immunosuppressive/chemotherapy medications are common etiology
- **Hemolytic Uremic Syndrome**
  - Primarily disease of infants and small children
  - Caused by toxin of *Escherichia coli* (or other organisms)
  - Diarrhea, hemolytic anemia, thrombocytopenia, acute renal failure
- **Angioedema, Intestinal**
  - Inherited deficiency of inhibitor of C1 esterase (part of complement cascade)
  - Similar pathology can be induced by reactions to medications (e.g., ACE inhibitors) and in some patients with viral hepatitis
  - Small bowel involvement more common than colonic

SELECTED REFERENCES

1. Gu L et al: Computed tomography angiography of gastrocolic vein trunk by morphological filtering technique in right colon cancer. Ther Clin Risk Manag. 17:1-7, 2021
2. Antonelli M et al: Clostridioides difficile (formerly Clostridium difficile) infection in the critically ill: an expert statement. Intensive Care Med. 46(2):215-24, 2020

Diverticulitis

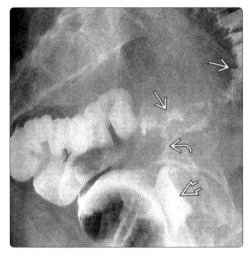

Diverticulitis

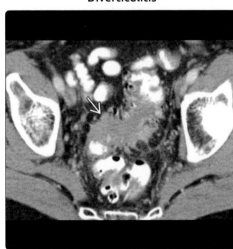

(Left) *In this 63-year-old woman who had a temporary colostomy for diverticulitis, a contrast enema was performed 6 months later in anticipation of reanastomosing her colon. This shows extensive diverticulosis of the sigmoid colon* ➡ *and a fistulous track* ➡ *to the vagina* ➡. **(Right)** *Myochosis coli* ➡ *is shown in a patient with diverticulosis. There is circular muscle hypertrophy that is commonly present along with diverticulosis.*

Infectious Colitis

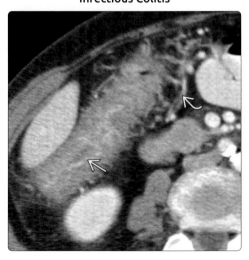

Infectious Colitis

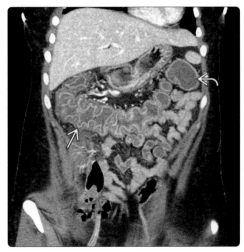

(Left) *Axial CECT shows marked thickening of the colonic wall with intense mucosal enhancement* ➡ *and mesenteric hyperemia* ➡. *The entire colon was involved but not the small bowel in this case of Campylobacter colitis.* **(Right)** *Coronal CECT in an 18-year-old woman with acute bloody diarrhea shows panproctocolitis with marked submucosal edema* ➡. *Fluid within the left side of the colon* ➡ *indicates a diarrheal state. This was Escherichia coli colitis due to ingestion of a contaminated hamburger.*

Pseudomembranous Colitis

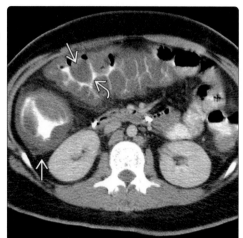

Ischemic Colitis

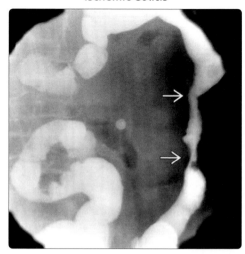

(Left) *Axial CECT in a 15-year-old boy hospitalized with pancreatitis shows Clostridium difficile pancolitis with an accordion sign caused by submucosal edema ➡ compressing and separating the enhanced mucosal folds ➡. **(Right)** Contrast enema in a woman with recent cardiac arrest shows a stricture ➡ of the proximal descending colon, the classic watershed distribution of the hypoperfusion ischemic colitis.*

Ischemic Colitis

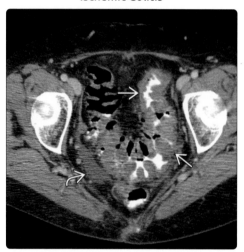

Ischemic Colitis

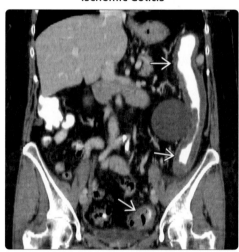

(Left) *This 69-year-old woman with cardiac disease developed acute pain and hematochezia following a hypotensive episode. Axial CECT shows submucosal edema that was limited to the descending and sigmoid colon ➡ and ascites ➡. **(Right)** Coronal CECT in the same patient shows wall thickening of the descending and sigmoid colon ➡, classic for the hypoperfusion etiology of ischemic colitis.*

Ulcerative and Crohn Colitis

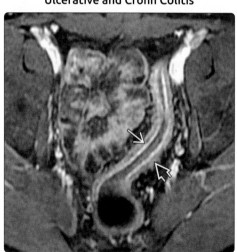

Ulcerative and Crohn Colitis

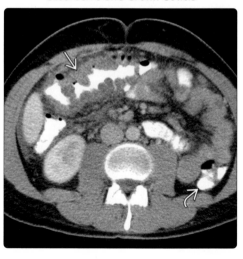

(Left) *Axial T1 C+ FS MR in a 26-year-old man with an acute ulcerative colitis shows moderate wall thickening ➡ and mucosal hyperenhancement ➡, consistent with acute inflammation in the setting of chronic disease. **(Right)** Axial CECT in a young man with recurrent pain and diarrhea shows massive thickening of the wall of the right side of the colon ➡ with relative sparing of the descending colon ➡ and rectum (not shown). Endoscopic biopsy revealed granulomatous (Crohn) colitis.*

Colon Carcinoma

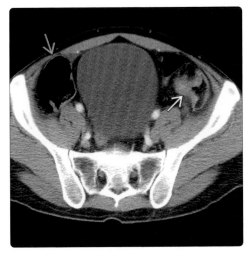

Colon Carcinoma

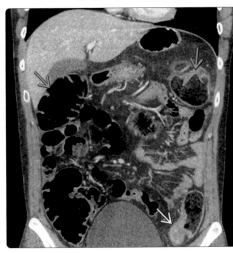

(Left) *Axial CECT in a 31-year-old man with symptoms of colonic obstruction shows a grossly dilated colon ⮕ with stool and gas, ending abruptly at an apple core lesion ⮕ at the junction of the descending and sigmoid colon.* (Right) *Coronal CECT in a 31-year-old man with constipation and hematochezia shows a grossly dilated colon ⮕ ending abruptly at an apple core lesion ⮕ at the junction of the descending and sigmoid colon, a typical appearance for primary colon carcinoma.*

Colon Carcinoma

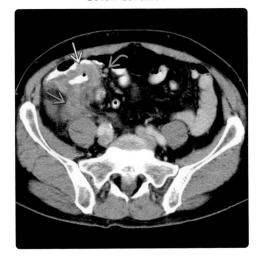

Colon Carcinoma

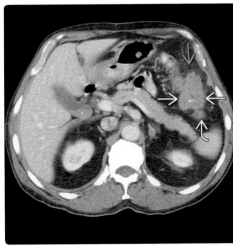

(Left) *Axial CECT in a patient with acute right lower quadrant pain shows a circumferential, bulky, cecal mass ⮕ that had obstructed the base of the appendix. Transmural invasion ⮕, lymphadenopathy ⮕, and peritoneal metastases (not shown) were evident.* (Right) *Axial CECT in a man with weight loss shows a focal, circumferential, colonic soft tissue density mass ⮕. Transmural infiltration is evident ⮕ along with omental or mesenteric tumor ⮕.*

Portal Hypertensive Colopathy

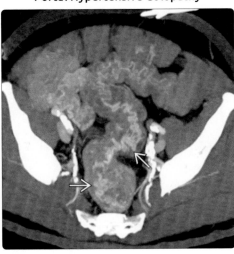

Portal Hypertensive Colopathy

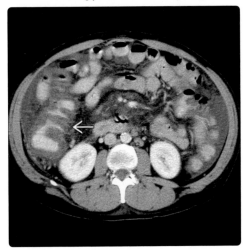

(Left) *Axial CECT in a patient with portal hypertension due to hepatic cirrhosis, presenting with rectal bleeding, shows multiple rectal varices ⮕ serving as the cause.* (Right) *Axial CECT in a 60-year-old man with cirrhosis shows colonic wall thickening ⮕ due to portal hypertensive colopathy.*

Endometriosis

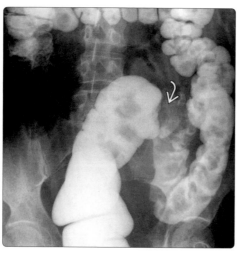

Endometriosis

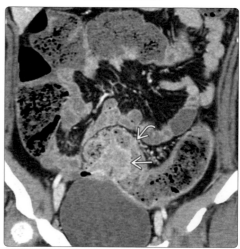

(Left) *Contrast enema in a young woman with symptoms of colonic obstruction shows partial obstruction to retrograde filling and a tight, short stricture* ➡️*. The more proximal colon is distended with stool and gas. Colon carcinoma was the primary concern, but endometriosis was confirmed.* (Right) *Coronal CECT in a young woman with symptoms of colonic obstruction shows a colonic stricture* ➡️ *with an eccentric, soft tissue density mass* ➡️ *representing endometriosis.*

Endometriosis

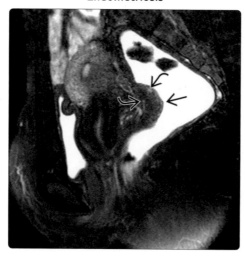

Obesity (Mimic)

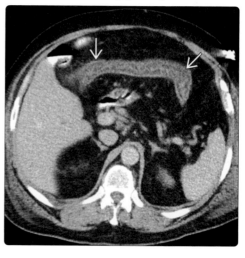

(Left) *Sagittal T2 FS MR in a 31-year-old woman with cyclical pelvic pain shows a solid, deep, infiltrating, hypointense endometriotic implant* ➡️ *with small, hyperintense, cystic foci* ➡️*, representing dilated ectopic endometrial glands.* (Right) *Axial CECT shows apparent thickening of the wall of the transverse colon* ➡️ *with submucosal fat-density proliferation. There was no history of colitis in this patient; this is a normal variant in obese and some older adult patients.*

Typhlitis (Neutropenic Colitis)

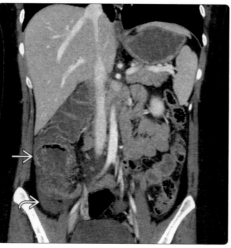

Typhlitis (Neutropenic Colitis)

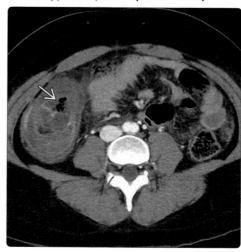

(Left) *Coronal CECT in a woman with neutropenia, fever, and right lower quadrant pain due to chemotherapy shows mucosal enhancement and marked submucosal edema* ➡️ *limited to the cecum and ascending colon. Ascites* ➡️ *raised concern for perforation, confirmed at surgery.* (Right) *Axial CECT in a woman with chemotherapy-induced neutropenic colitis shows marked submucosal edema and pneumatosis* ➡️ *in the ascending colon.*

Typhlitis (Neutropenic Colitis)

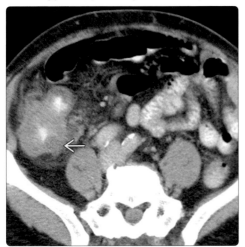

Typhlitis (Neutropenic Colitis)

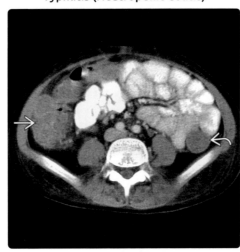

(Left) *Axial CECT shows submucosal edema and luminal narrowing ➡ limited to the ascending colon and cecum.* **(Right)** *Axial CECT in an 11-year-old boy with acute leukemia shows marked submucosal edema in the wall of the cecum ➡. The descending colon ➡ is filled with fluid but otherwise normal.*

Colonic Metastases and Lymphoma

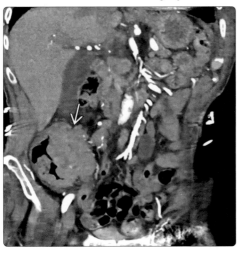

Colonic Metastases and Lymphoma

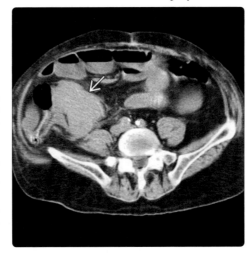

(Left) *Coronal CECT in a patient 15 years post cardiac transplant shows a cecal mass ➡ causing luminal narrowing secondary to posttransplant lymphoproliferative disorder (PTLD).* **(Right)** *Axial NECT shows a soft tissue density mass ➡ in the cecum and appendix, representing lymphoma (PTLD) in a renal transplant recipient.*

Pneumatosis of Colon

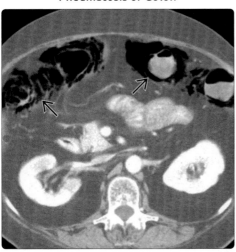

Pneumatosis of Colon

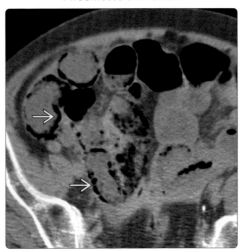

(Left) *Axial CECT shows extensive gas density in the colonic submucosa ➡, representing benign pneumatosis in a young woman with leukemia, presumably due to steroid and antirejection medications.* **(Right)** *Axial CECT shows extensive pneumatosis ➡ in the small bowel and colon due to acute embolic infarction. The ileus helps to confirm the ischemic etiology, but correlation with clinical signs of bowel ischemia is essential.*

DIFFERENTIAL DIAGNOSIS

Common

- Ulcerative Colitis
- Cathartic Abuse
- Crohn Disease (Granulomatous Colitis)
- Senescent Change, Colon
- Toxic Megacolon

Less Common

- Ischemic Colitis
- Radiation Colitis
- Amyloidosis
- Schistosomiasis

ESSENTIAL INFORMATION

Key Differential Diagnosis Issues

- Haustra should always be present in proximal colon but can be absent normally in distal colon
  - Haustra are sacculations of colonic lumen separated by colonic (semilunar) folds

Helpful Clues for Common Diagnoses

- **Ulcerative Colitis**
  - Areas affected; rectum only (30%), rectum and distal colon colon (40%), pancolitis (30%)
    - Terminal ileum affected in minority of patients
  - Usually in chronic, burned-out phase
  - Colon may appear smooth and tubular with loss of usual transverse folds and haustra
  - Colon may be foreshortened and straightened
    - Picture frame or lead pipe appearance
  - Look for evidence of active inflammation on current or prior studies (barium enema, CT, endoscopy)
  - MR: Subacute and chronic phases: Fibrosis → wall thickening; perirectal fat deposition → widening of presacral space
- **Cathartic Abuse**
  - Can also occur with chronic enema abuse
    - Results in neuromuscular damage

- Look for bizarre contractions and spasm of right colon; no ulcerations
- Colon length is usually normal, not shortened
- Other features: Colonic dilatation and spasm, pseudostrictures, patulous ileocecal valve

- **Crohn Disease (Granulomatous Colitis)**
  - Chronic phase of granulomatous colitis can resemble burned-out ulcerative colitis
- **Senescent Change, Colon**
  - Older persons often have loss of colonic folds, especially in descending colon
  - Unlike with chronic colitis, colon is not foreshortened
  - Asymptomatic and uncertain etiology
    - Some are probably due to chronic laxative and enema use
- **Toxic Megacolon**
  - Colon (especially transverse) loses normal transverse folds
  - Lumen is dilated
  - Surface irregularity = ulceration, sloughed mucosa, inflammatory pseudopolyps
  - Wall may be thin or thickened; more apparent on CT
  - Medical/surgical emergency; may perforate

Helpful Clues for Less Common Diagnoses

- **Ischemic Colitis**
  - Usually in healing or healed phase
  - Segmental loss of folds and haustra
  - Often affects splenic flexure and sigmoid colon
- **Radiation Colitis**
  - Usually takes weeks or months to develop
  - Sigmoid colon most affected following radiation therapy for pelvic malignancies

Ulcerative Colitis

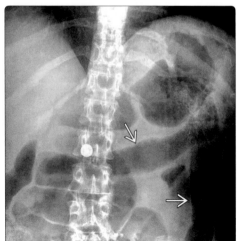

Ulcerative Colitis

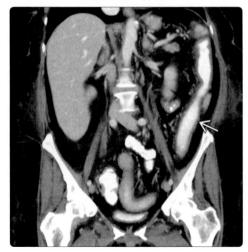

(Left) Supine radiograph shows a shortened transverse and descending colon ➡ in a patient with chronic ulcerative colitis but no current evidence of severe exacerbation. (Right) Coronal CECT in a 66-year-old woman with longstanding ulcerative colitis shows a featureless descending colon with wall thickening ➡.

Ulcerative Colitis

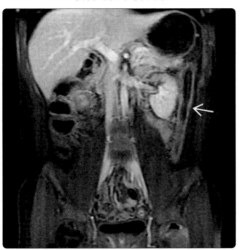

Cathartic Abuse

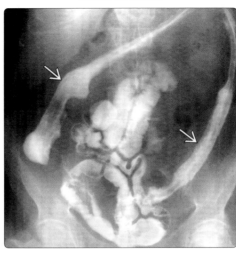

(Left) *Coronal T1 C+ FS MR in a 26-year-old man with ulcerative colitis shows a featureless descending colon ➡. (Right) Contrast enema in an older woman with chronic laxative use shows an ahaustral colon ➡ but no significant shortening. Intermittent segmental contractions were observed at fluoroscopy.*

Senescent Change, Colon

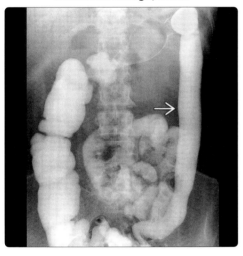

Toxic Megacolon

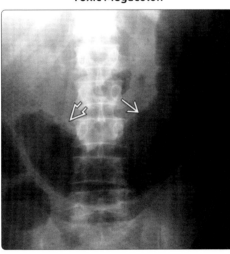

(Left) *Contrast enema shows an ahaustral distal transverse and descending colon ➡ in an older patient with no history or clinical symptoms of colitis. (Right) Supine radiograph shows a dilated ahaustral transverse colon ➡ with a suggestion of mucosal irregularity ➡. Only correlation with clinical input (severe abdominal pain and guarding) distinguishes this as toxic megacolon rather than ileus.*

Toxic Megacolon

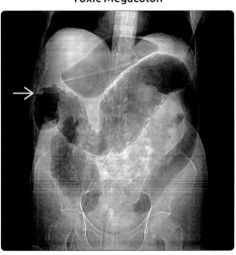

Radiation Colitis

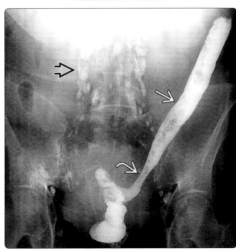

(Left) *Supine radiograph shows a shortened, ahaustral colon due to chronic granulomatous colitis (Crohn disease). Note the pseudopolyps ➡ and gross dilation of the transverse colon, which along with severe acute symptoms indicates toxic megacolon. (Right) Contrast enema shows a shortened, ahaustral left side of colon ➡ with a short stricture ➡. Note lymphangiographic opacification of retroperitoneal nodes ➡.*

DIFFERENTIAL DIAGNOSIS

Common

- Appendicitis
- Urolithiasis (Renal Calculi)
- Pelvic Inflammatory Disease
- Pyelonephritis
- Crohn Disease
- Infectious Colitis
- Mesenteric Enteritis/Adenitis

Less Common

- Diverticulitis
- Omental Infarct
- Epiploic Appendagitis
- Cholecystitis
- Gynecologic and Obstetric Causes
  o Ruptured Corpus Luteum
  o Uterine Fibroids
  o Hemorrhagic Ovarian Cyst
  o Ovarian Torsion
  o Endometriosis
  o Ruptured Ectopic Pregnancy
- Ischemic Enteritis
- Ischemic Colitis
- Colon Carcinoma
- Appendiceal Carcinoma
- Pancreatitis, Acute
- Foreign Body Perforation
- Abdominal Wall Trauma

Rare but Important

- Intussusception
- Meckel Diverticulitis
- Typhlitis (Neutropenic Colitis)
- Mucocele of Appendix

ESSENTIAL INFORMATION

Key Differential Diagnosis Issues

- Young men: Appendicitis, mesenteric enteritis/adenitis, epiploic appendagitis, omental infarction, acute pancreatitis, Crohn disease
- Young women: Also consider obstetric and gynecologic etiologies, cholecystitis, pyelonephritis
- Older adults: Cancer and bowel ischemia become more common considerations

Helpful Clues for Common Diagnoses

- **Appendicitis**
  o Dilated, thick-walled, blind-ending tube arising from cecal tip
  o Appendicolith in 1/3 to 1/2 of patients
  o Periappendiceal inflammation
- **Urolithiasis (Renal Calculi)**
  o Stones in renal pelvis or ureter
  o Dilated collecting system/ureter
  o Renal swelling → forniceal rupture → perirenal fat stranding
- **Pelvic Inflammatory Disease**
  o 2nd most common etiology in young women

o Loss of fat planes in pelvis
o Inflamed, pus-distended fallopian tubes
o Possible tuboovarian abscess
- **Pyelonephritis**
  o More common in girls, young women
  o Wedge-shaped or striated nephrogram; urothelial enhancement
- **Crohn Disease**
  o Thick wall, narrow lumen of distal ileum
  o Fibrofatty proliferation of mesentery
  o Cluster of right lower quadrant (RLQ) mesenteric nodes
  o Mesenteric hyperemia; engorged vessels; comb sign
- **Infectious Colitis**
  o Multiple possible pathogens, especially in immunocompromised patients
  o *Clostridium difficile* (pseudomembranous) colitis is endemic in health care facilities
  o Many other potential causes (*Campylobacter, Escherichia coli*, amebic, etc.)
  o Focal, segmental, or pancolitis with wall edema, pericolonic inflammation
  o Mucosal hyperenhancement, submucosal edema
- **Mesenteric Enteritis/Adenitis**
  o Distal small bowel (SB) may be inflamed in infectious ileitis (*Yersinia*, viral, *Campylobacter*)
    – Affected SB wall thickening
    – Mucosal hyperenhancement with submucosal edema
  o Cluster of mildly enlarged (~ 5 mm) nodes in RLQ
    – Without inflammation of appendix
  o Common in children and adolescents

Helpful Clues for Less Common Diagnoses

- **Diverticulitis**
  o May arise from cecum, ascending colon, or redundant sigmoid colon
  o Can usually identify diverticula and adjacent inflammation
    – Inflammation is **pericolonic**
    – No mucosal hyperemia or submucosal edema (unlike colitis)
- **Omental Infarct**
  o > 95% of primary type occur near ascending colon
  o 3- to 8-cm, rounded mass of heterogeneous fat density with enhancing "capsule" and adjacent inflammation
    – May see whorled vessels within lesion
    – Little or no inflammation of colon or small bowel
- **Epiploic Appendagitis**
  o Small (2-4 cm) oval of fat density with capsule and inflammation near colon
    – Central dot = occluded venule
  o More common in sigmoid and descending colon
- **Cholecystitis**
  o Inflamed, distended gallbladder may project into RLQ
    – Perforated cholecystitis may extend inflammation to adjacent organs, including ascending colon
- **Gynecologic and Obstetric Causes**
  o **Uterine fibroids**
    – May infarct, twist or bleed, leading to acute pain
  o **Hemorrhagic ovarian cyst or ovarian torsion**

- High-attenuation (CT) or echogenic (US) material within spherical adnexal mass in young women
- Ovarian torsion: Enlarged, edematous ovary ± absence of Doppler flow on US
○ **Endometriosis**
  - Often multifocal, affecting pelvic bowel segments
  - Soft tissue density mass, often with inflammatory and obstructive signs
  - Chronic or episodic pain with menses in young woman
  - May be T1 hyperintense on MR
○ **Ruptured ectopic pregnancy**
  - Life threatening
  - Always consider in woman of reproductive age
  - Check β-hCG pregnancy test
  - 1st imaging evaluation of pregnant patient should be by US
  - Hyperdense blood in pelvis on CT
- **Ischemic Enteritis**
  ○ Embolic or thrombotic occlusion of ileocolic artery
  ○ Thrombosis of ileocolic or superior mesenteric vein
    - Venous thrombosis is usually in patient with prothrombotic condition
- **Ischemic Colitis**
  ○ Right colon involved with superior mesenteric artery (SMA) thromboembolic disease
    - More common hypoperfusion ischemic colitis affects left colon preferentially
  ○ Mucosal hypoenhancement ± pneumatosis
- **Colon or Appendiceal Carcinoma**
  ○ Cecal carcinoma may obstruct appendix, mimic appendicitis
    - May also perforate with extraluminal gas and fluid
  ○ Look for mass in cecal or appendiceal lumen
    - Omental or mesenteric nodular mass indicates malignancy
- **Pancreatitis, Acute**
  ○ Inflammation may spread to ascending colon, simulating colitis
  ○ Characteristic inflammation of peripancreatic tissue and lab findings are key

- **Foreign Body Perforation**
  ○ Ingested foreign body (e.g., toothpick or animal bone)
  ○ Terminal ileum is most common site of obstruction or perforation of ingested foreign body
  ○ Look for radiopaque, thin structure (bone), though others are lucent
  ○ Perforation results in inflammatory infiltration of bowel and mesentery
    - ± extraluminal gas and fluid
- **Abdominal Wall Trauma**
  ○ Hematoma or rectus muscle strain may mimic intraabdominal source of RLQ pain

Helpful Clues for Rare Diagnoses

- **Intussusception**
  ○ Ileocecal is most common site
  ○ Long segment, obstructing intussusception in adult usually has lead mass
  ○ Target-shaped, bowel-within-bowel appearance
- **Meckel Diverticulitis**
  ○ Blind-ending pouch containing particulate debris, often enteroliths
  ○ Located ~ 100 cm from ileocecal valve, pointed toward midline
- **Typhlitis (Neutropenic Colitis)**
  ○ Neutropenic colitis in severely immunocompromised patients
  ○ Massive wall thickening, submucosal edema of cecum and ascending colon
- **Mucocele of Appendix**
  ○ Oval, cystic lesion arising from tip of cecum
    - May have eggshell calcification
  ○ May torse or cause intussusception

Appendicitis

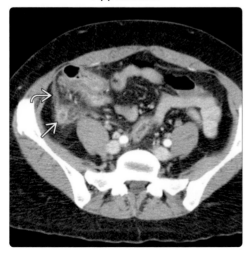

Appendicitis

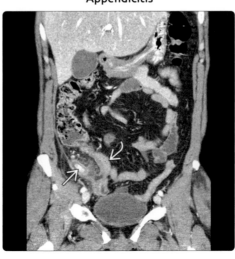

(Left) Axial CECT shows a dilated, thick-walled appendix ➔ with inflammation of the surrounding fat planes ➔. (Right) Coronal CECT shows an appendicolith ➔ within the dilated, inflamed appendix. Note surrounding inflammatory changes, including extrinsic inflammation of terminal ileum ➔.

Urolithiasis (Renal Calculi)

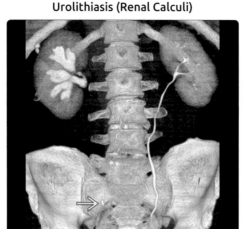

Pyelonephritis

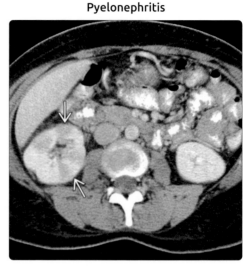

(Left) *Coronal CECT shows dilation of the right renal collecting system and delayed opacification of the right ureter due to an obstructing ureteral calculus ➡. Both were evident on NECT as well.*
(Right) *Axial CECT shows wedge-shaped and striated zones ➡ of decreased enhancement of the right kidney along with infiltration of the perirenal space.*

Pelvic Inflammatory Disease

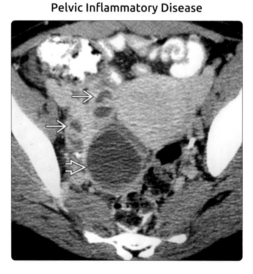

Crohn Disease

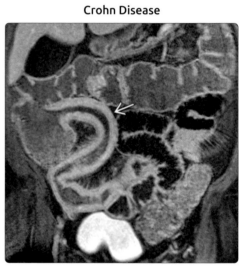

(Left) *Axial CECT shows a convoluted, dilated right pyosalpinx ➡ and a tuboovarian abscess ➡.*
(Right) *Coronal T1 C+ MR in a 48-year-old man with Crohn disease shows mucosal hyperenhancement of a thickened terminal ileum ➡, consistent with acute inflammation.*

Crohn Disease

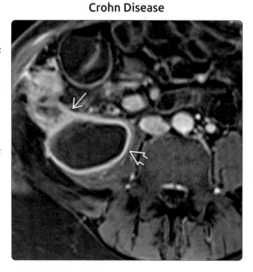

Mesenteric Enteritis/Adenitis

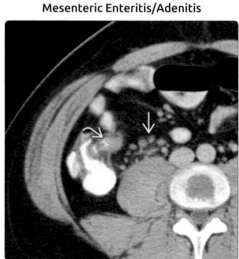

(Left) *Axial T1 C+ FS MR in a 41-year-old man with Crohn disease shows a psoas abscess ➡ communicating with the adjacent ascending colon ➡.*
(Right) *Axial CECT shows mild thickening of the wall of the terminal ileum ➡ and a cluster of minimally enlarged mesenteric nodes ➡, which resolved spontaneously in this 24-year-old woman.*

Diverticulitis

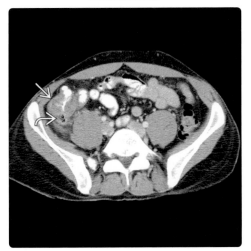

Diverticulitis

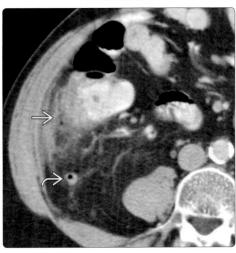

(Left) *Axial CECT shows wall thickening of the cecum* ➡ *and diverticula* ➥ *with adjacent inflammation.* (Right) *Axial CECT shows cecal wall thickening and infiltration of adjacent fat* ➡. *Note normal appendix* ➥. *Cecal diverticula were seen on adjacent sections.*

Omental Infarct

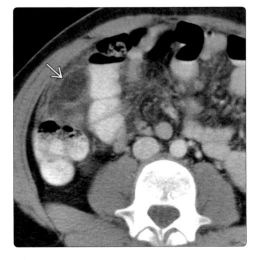

Epiploic Appendagitis

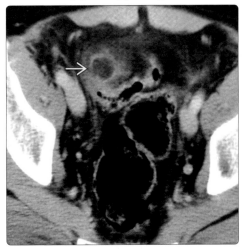

(Left) *Axial CECT shows a large, oval, fat density lesion* ➡ *adjacent to the ascending colon with inflammation of the surrounding fat.* (Right) *Axial CECT shows a small, oval, fat density lesion* ➡ *adjacent to the colon in the right lower quadrant (RLQ) with inflammation of adjacent fat.*

Cholecystitis

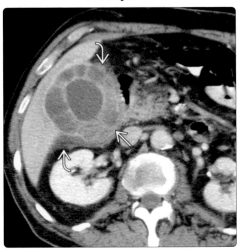

Ruptured Corpus Luteum

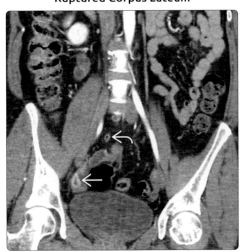

(Left) *In this patient with acute cholecystitis and perforation, axial CECT shows a thick-walled gallbladder* ➡ *with adjacent inflammation and septate fluid collections* ➥. (Right) *In this young woman with acute RLQ pain, CT shows a spherical lesion with a brightly enhancing wall* ➡ *and a small amount of adjacent, higher than water density fluid. The appendix* ➡ *is normal.*

Uterine Fibroids

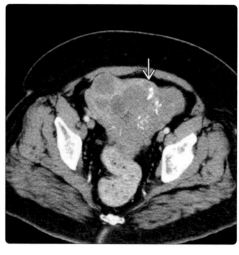

Hemorrhagic Ovarian Cyst

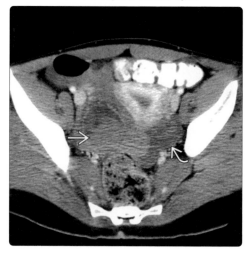

(Left) *Axial CECT shows multiple subserosal fibroids (leiomyomas) with cystic and calcified degeneration ➡ in a 51-year-old woman presenting with acute RLQ pain.* (Right) *Axial CECT shows clot within a right adnexal cyst ➡ and adjacent sentinel clot with hemoperitoneum ➡.*

Endometriosis

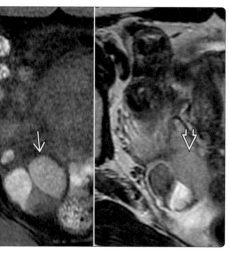

Ischemic Enteritis

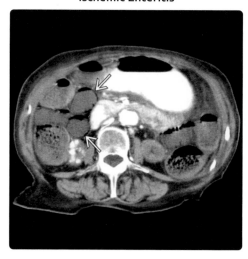

(Left) *Axial MR in a 27-year-old woman with RLQ pain shows an endometrioma with areas of increased T1 signal ➡, some of which show T2 shading ➡.* (Right) *Axial CECT shows diffuse ileus and gas within the wall of the distal small bowel ➡. Infarcted bowel was found at surgery.*

Ischemic Colitis

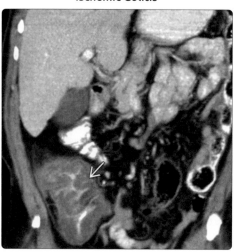

Colon Carcinoma

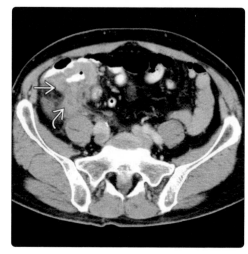

(Left) *Coronal CECT shows marked cecal mural thickening with submucosal edema ➡ and luminal narrowing. This would be difficult to distinguish from infectious colitis by CT alone.* (Right) *Axial CECT shows circumferential thickening of the wall of the cecum ➡ with a distended appendix ➡. Omental metastases were noted on adjacent sections.*

Appendiceal Carcinoma

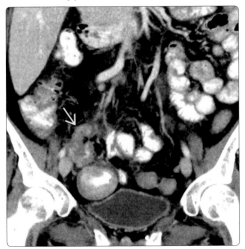

Intussusception

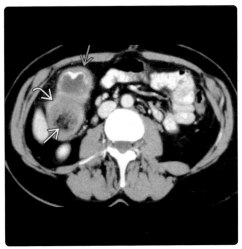

(Left) Coronal CECT in a 56-year-old woman with RLQ pain shows soft tissue thickening in the appendix ➡ with adjacent fat stranding due to invasive, poorly differentiated adenocarcinoma, which metastasized to the adjacent bowel loops and the peritoneum. (Right) Axial CECT shows an ileocolic intussusception ➡ due to an appendiceal mucocele ➡. Note the small bowel mesenteric fat ➡ within the lumen of the ascending colon.

Meckel Diverticulitis

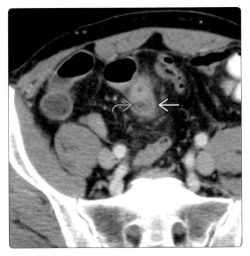

Typhlitis (Neutropenic Colitis)

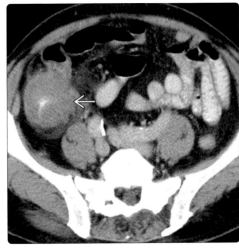

(Left) In this patient with a perforated Meckel diverticulum, axial CECT shows a blind-ending pouch ➡ arising from the distal small bowel containing a laminated stone ➡ with inflammation of the surrounding fat. (Right) Axial CECT shows marked mural thickening of the ascending colon ➡ in an older man receiving chemotherapy for acute myelogenous leukemia.

Mucocele of Appendix

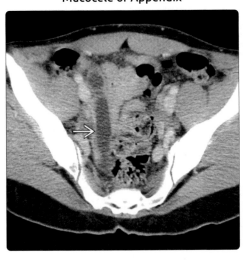

Mucocele of Appendix

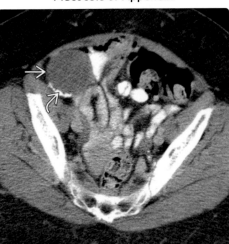

(Left) Axial CECT shows a very distended, elongated appendix ➡ in a 46-year-old woman with only vague RLQ pain, identified as mucocele of appendix at surgical pathology. (Right) Axial CECT shows a pericecal mass ➡ with eggshell, though incomplete, calcification ➡.

DIFFERENTIAL DIAGNOSIS

Common

- Diverticulitis
- Colon Carcinoma
- Epiploic Appendagitis
- Acute Colitis
  - Infectious Colitis
  - Ischemic Colitis
  - Ulcerative or Crohn Colitis
  - Fecal Impaction/Stercoral Colitis
- Gynecologic Causes
  - Adnexal Torsion
  - Endometriosis
  - Salpingitis
  - Tuboovarian Abscess
  - Uterine Fibroids
- Urolithiasis
- Sigmoid Volvulus

Less Common

- Sclerosing Mesenteritis (Panniculitis)
- Abdominal Abscess
- Peritonitis
- Renal Pathology
  - Acute Pyelonephritis
  - Renal Infarction
  - Renal Hemorrhage
- Coagulopathic ("Retroperitoneal") Hemorrhage
- External Hernias
  - Ventral Hernia
  - Spigelian Hernia
  - Inguinal Hernia
- Omental Infarct
- Appendicitis (Rare)

Rare but Important

- Bladder Fistulas

ESSENTIAL INFORMATION

Key Differential Diagnosis Issues

- Most etiologies are of bowel origin, but consider genitourinary
- Do not forget to check mesentery, omentum, and abdominal wall
- CECT is imaging modality of choice
  - In women, pregnancy and gynecologic etiologies are taken into account and investigation is supplemented with pelvic US

Helpful Clues for Common Diagnoses

- **Diverticulitis**
  - Most common cause in middle-aged and older adults
    - Can affect patients as young as 25 years old
  - Usually long (10-15 cm) segment of wall thickening, luminal narrowing, pericolonic infiltration
  - Extraluminal collections of gas or fluid help confirm diagnosis
    - Look for complications (abscesses, fistulas, obstruction)

- **Colon Carcinoma**
  - Usually short segment without much pericolonic infiltration
  - Regional lymphadenopathy has strong association with carcinoma, rarely seen in diverticulitis
  - Acute symptoms may be due to colonic obstruction ± colitis proximal to obstructing mass
- **Epiploic Appendagitis**
  - Small, oval, fatty lesion (2-4 cm) with infiltration of omental fat
  - Lies immediately adjacent to colonic surface
  - Important to distinguish from diverticulitis and colitis
    - Epiploic appendagitis resolves without specific treatment
- **Acute Colitis**
  - **Infectious colitis**
    - Usually diffuse, pancolonic with impressive submucosal edema (accordion sign)
    - Hyperenhancing mucosa and engorged mesenteric vessels
    - May be segmental, including distal colon
    - Very common, especially in hospitalized patients, and those in nursing homes
  - **Ischemic colitis**
    - Hypoperfusion is most common etiology
    - Wall thickening and luminal narrowing
    - Splenic flexure, descending and sigmoid colon are affected
    - Rectum is spared (unlike ulcerative and infectious colitis)
    - Ask about prior hypotensive episode or cardiac disease
  - **Ulcerative or Crohn colitis**
    - Favors rectum and distal colon
    - Colonic wall is usually not very thickened with ulcerative colitis
    - Look for loss of haustral pattern, infiltration of pericolonic fat
    - Ask about history of prior episodes
  - **Fecal impaction/stercoral colitis**
    - Impacted stool can lead to stercoral ulceration with erosion through colonic wall
    - Look for wall perforation, perirectal infiltration, free air
- **Gynecologic Causes**
  - Many, including adnexal infection and masses, torsed ovary, endometriosis, etc.
  - US preferred and 1st-line modality for evaluation
  - Look for evidence of mass &/or inflammation centered on adnexa rather than bowel
  - Enlarged edematous ovary ± absence of Doppler flow→ torsion
  - **Uterine fibroids**
    - May torse, undergo degeneration or infarction, lead to acute pain
    - Heterogeneous soft tissue masses within enlarged uterus, ± focal calcifications within masses
- **Urolithiasis**
  - Distal left ureteral stone may cause left lower quadrant (LLQ) pain
  - Diagnosis usually evident on CT

- – Ureteral calculus, hydronephrosis, perinephric stranding
- **Sigmoid Volvulus**
  - o Very elongated and dilated sigmoid colon, folded back on itself (coffee bean or football sign)
  - o Colon proximal to sigmoid will be dilated but not as much as sigmoid
  - o CT will show twisting of vessels in base of sigmoid mesocolon

Helpful Clues for Less Common Diagnoses

- **Sclerosing Mesenteritis (Panniculitis)**
  - o Being diagnosed much more commonly as cause of recurrent abdominal pain, usually poorly localized
  - o "Misty mesentery" with cluster of jejunal mesenteric nodes, with surrounding thin capsule, ± calcifications
  - o Often with history of prior similar episodes
  - o May respond to steroid therapy or resolve on its own
- **Abdominal Abscess**
  - o Usually in postoperative patient or following appendicitis, diverticulitis
  - o Loculated, rim-enhancing collection of fluid ± gas
- **Peritonitis**
  - o Often result of infected ascites or bowel perforation
    - – Perforated appendicitis, diverticulitis are most common
- **Renal Pathology**
  - o **Acute pyelonephritis**
    - – Swollen kidney with striated or wedge-shaped foci of heterogeneous enhancement
    - – Infiltrated perirenal fat; thickened, enhancing urothelium
  - o **Renal infarction**
    - – Wedge-shaped or global parenchymal nonenhancement
    - – Cortical rim sign in subacute infarct (enhanced renal capsule)
  - o **Renal hemorrhage**
    - – Spontaneous hemorrhage of renal cell carcinoma or other large neoplasm (e.g., angiomyolipoma)

- – Hemorrhage may also be post renal biopsy
- – Assess for underlying mass and active extravasation
- **Coagulopathic ("Retroperitoneal") Hemorrhage**
  - o Most common sites: Iliopsoas and rectus muscle compartments
    - – Often extends into adjacent retroperitoneal spaces
  - o Look for hematocrit sign, multiple sites of bleeding, active extravasation
- **External Hernias**
  - o **Ventral hernia**
    - – At site of prior laparotomy or laparoscopic incision or port
    - – Herniation of omental fat or bowel may cause focal LLQ pain
  - o **Spigelian hernia**
    - – Through defect in aponeuroses of internal oblique and transverse abdominal muscles
    - – Just lateral to rectus sheath and caudal to umbilicus
    - – External oblique muscle and aponeurosis cover herniated fat ± bowel
  - o **Inguinal hernia**
    - – Herniation and obstruction of descending colon is especially likely to be perceived as LLQ pain
- **Omental Infarct**
  - o Primary omental infarction occurs near **ascending colon**
  - o Secondary form may occur anywhere near site of surgery, infection, radiation, etc.
  - o Heterogeneous fatty mass, larger than epiploic appendagitis
    - – Usually farther removed from surface of colon than for epiploic appendagitis
  - o Usually resolves without specific treatment
  - o As complication of laparoscopic distal pancreatectomy
    - – Occurs in left upper quadrant
    - – May mimic mass
- **Appendicitis (Rare)**
  - o Appendix may be very long or may arise from malrotated colon; leads to left-sided symptoms

---

Diverticulitis

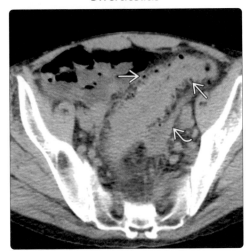

Diverticulitis

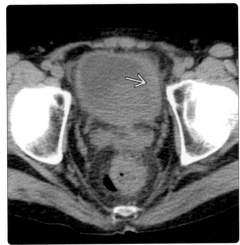

(Left) In this 40-year-old man with left lower quadrant (LLQ) pain, axial CECT shows extensive wall thickening and diverticulosis of the sigmoid colon ➔ and surrounding inflammation, including thickening at the root of the sigmoid mesocolon ➔, indicating diverticulitis. (Right) In this 40-year-old man with diverticulitis, inflammatory thickening of the adjacent wall of the bladder ➔ raises concern for development of a colovesical fistula.

Colon Carcinoma

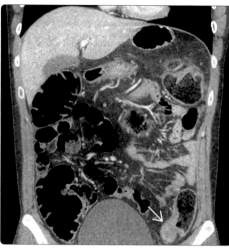

Epiploic Appendagitis

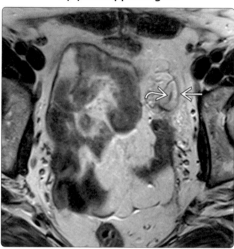

(Left) *Coronal CECT shows a grossly dilated colon ending abruptly at an apple core lesion ➡ at the junction of the descending and sigmoid colon.* (Right) *Axial T2 MR in a 61-year-old woman with LLQ pain shows a 2-cm ovoid fatty lesion adjacent to the sigmoid colon with a hypointense rim ➡ and a central hypointense area ➡ representing the central dot sign, suggestive of engorged or thrombosed vascular pedicle within the inflamed epiploic appendage.*

Infectious Colitis

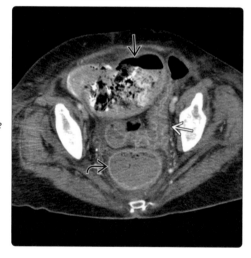

Infectious Colitis

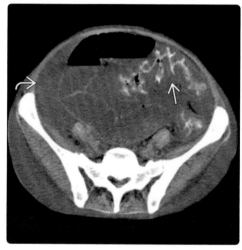

(Left) *Axial CECT shows marked distention of the proximal colon ➡. The remaining colon and rectum ➡ were fluid distended with hyperenhancing mucosa and submucosal edema ➡. The patient developed toxic megacolon, and colectomy confirmed Clostridium difficile colitis.* (Right) *In this young man with AIDS, axial CECT shows marked mural thickening and mucosal hyperenhancement of the sigmoid colon ➡ along with ascites ➡ and small bowel dilation. CMV colitis was confirmed and proved fatal.*

Ischemic Colitis

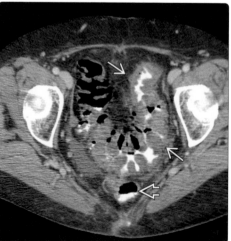

Ulcerative or Crohn Colitis

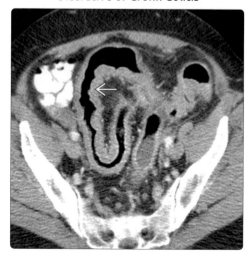

(Left) *Axial CECT in an older adult woman with cardiac disease (who developed acute pain and hematochezia) shows marked mural thickening of the sigmoid and descending colon ➡ with sparing of the rectum ➡, typical features of ischemic colitis.* (Right) *Axial CECT shows mural thickening of the sigmoid colon ➡ and loss of normal haustration. This was an acute flare of chronic ulcerative colitis.*

Fecal Impaction/Stercoral Colitis

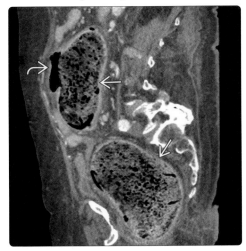

Adnexal Torsion

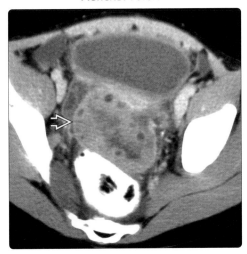

(Left) *Sagittal CECT in an older woman with chronic constipation who developed acute abdominal pain shows massive distention of the rectosigmoid colon with impacted feces ➡. Stercoral ulceration ➡ resulted in perforation of the colon and death.* (Right) *Axial CECT shows an enlarged ovary ➡ identified by the presence of normal follicles. The ovary is swollen and poorly enhancing due to torsion and ischemia.*

Endometriosis

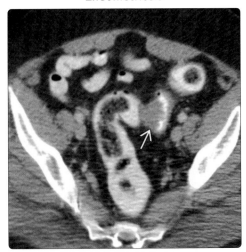

Tuboovarian Abscess

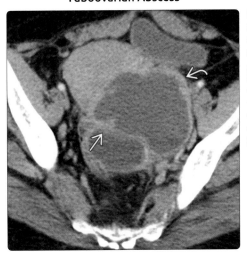

(Left) *Axial CECT shows focal eccentric narrowing and mass effect in the sigmoid colon ➡ simulating colon cancer, later proven to be endometriosis.* (Right) *Axial venous-phase CECT in a 43-year-old woman with LLQ pain and fever shows a left-sided tuboovarian abscess with a thick septation ➡ and a capsule ➡.*

Sigmoid Volvulus

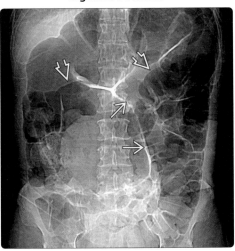

Sigmoid Volvulus

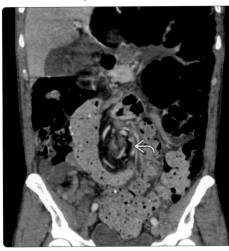

(Left) *In this 59-year-old man, a supine radiograph of the abdomen shows marked dilation of the sigmoid colon, which is folded back upon itself. The apposed walls of the redundant sigmoid colon ➡ form the "seam" of the football (or coffee bean) shape. The sigmoid extends into the upper abdomen above the transverse colon ➡.* (Right) *Coronal CECT in the same patient shows dramatic twisting and displacement of the base of the sigmoid colon and its mesentery ➡.*

Sclerosing Mesenteritis (Panniculitis)

Abdominal Abscess

(Left) *Axial venous-phase CECT shows a calcified soft tissue mass* ➡️ *with desmoplastic reaction in the root of the mesentery, consistent with sclerosing mesenteritis.* **(Right)** *Axial CECT shows a walled-off collection of fluid and gas* ➡️*, a typical abscess. Extensive sigmoid diverticulosis is seen* ➡️*, plus pericolic infiltration* ➡️*, typical signs of diverticulitis.*

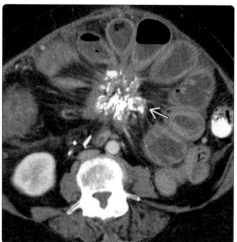

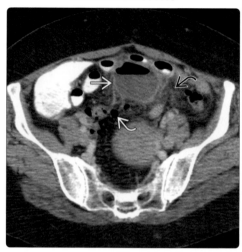

Peritonitis

Renal Infarction

(Left) *In this patient with cirrhosis and abdominal pain, axial CECT shows enhancement and thickening of the parietal and visceral peritoneum* ➡️ *and intraperitoneal gas* ➡️*. Drains* ➡️ *were placed to drain the infected ascites.* **(Right)** *Coronal arterial-phase T1 C+ FS MR in this man with sudden onset of LLQ and flank pain shows no perfusion of the cortex and medulla of most of the upper pole of the left kidney* ➡️*, which is due to spontaneous renal artery dissection.*

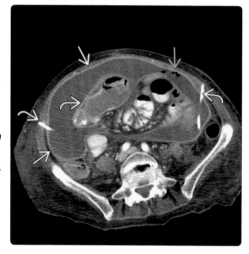

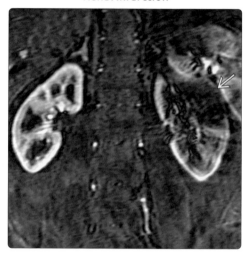

Renal Hemorrhage

Coagulopathic ("Retroperitoneal") Hemorrhage

(Left) *Axial T1 C+ FS MR shows subcapsular hemorrhage* ➡️ *post renal biopsy. Active extravasation of contrast* ➡️ *is seen on the arterial phase. Contrast pooling* ➡️ *on the delayed phase is also present.* **(Right)** *Axial CECT shows a massive rectus sheath hematoma with foci of active bleeding* ➡️ *and some extension into the retroperitoneal spaces* ➡️*.*

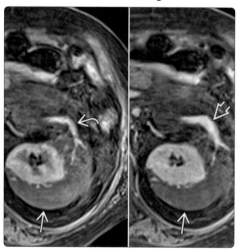

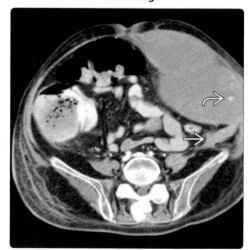

Ventral Hernia

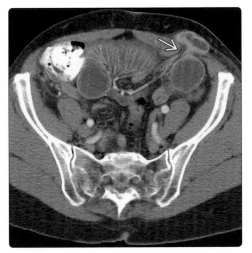

Spigelian Hernia

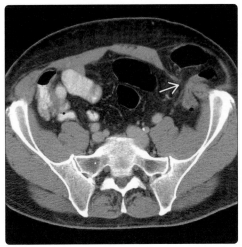

(Left) *This patient developed acute LLQ pain 2 weeks after an uneventful laparoscopic appendectomy. Axial CECT shows herniation of a segment of small bowel through one of the laparoscopy ports ➡, resulting in small bowel obstruction.* (Right) *Axial CECT shows herniation of the descending colon through a defect ➡ in the aponeurosis of the transverse abdominal and internal oblique muscles, lateral to the rectus sheath.*

Inguinal Hernia

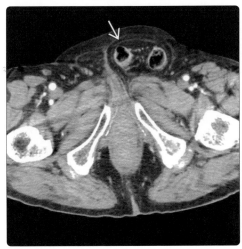

Inguinal Hernia

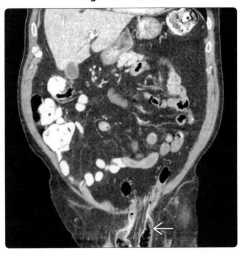

(Left) *Axial CECT shows the colon and fat within a large left inguinal hernia ➡ that extends into the scrotum.* (Right) *Coronal CECT shows the colon ➡ and fat within a large left inguinal hernia extending into the scrotum.*

Omental Infarct

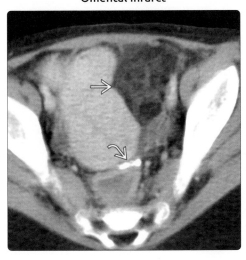

Omental Infarct

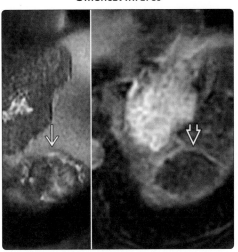

(Left) *Axial CECT shows a mottled fat density mass ➡ in the LLQ in an adolescent who had a recent colectomy; note the anastomotic staple line ➡. This omental infarct caused local pain, tenderness, and mass effect.* (Right) *In this patient with distal pancreatectomy and splenectomy for pancreatic tail ductal adenocarcinoma, MR of the left upper quadrant region shows an omental infarct as an area of heterogeneity ➡ on T2 with absence of enhancement ➡ on T1 C+ imaging.*

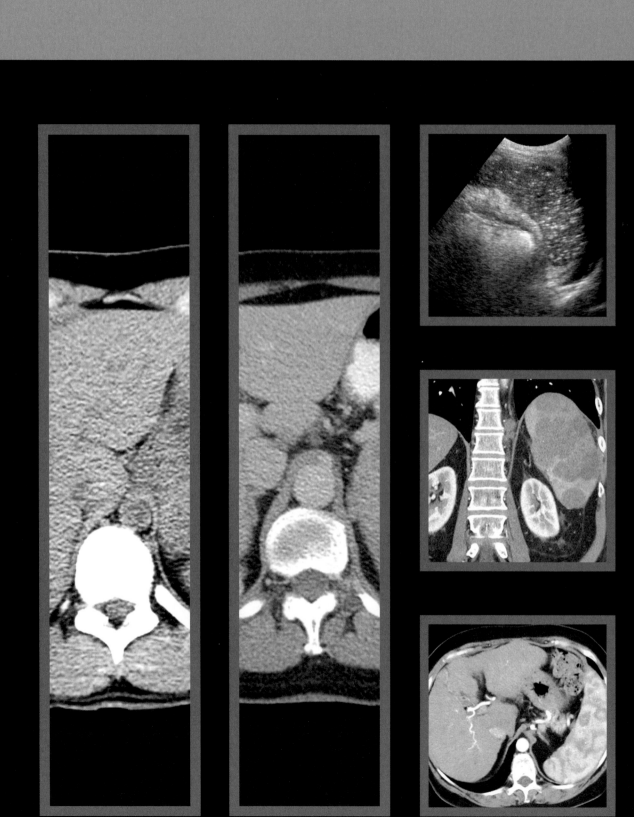

SECTION 8
Spleen

Generic Imaging Patterns

Splenomegaly   222
Multiple Splenic Calcifications   226
Solid Splenic Mass or Masses   228
Cystic Splenic Mass   230

Modality-Specific Imaging Findings

<u>Computed Tomography</u>
    Diffuse Increased Attenuation, Spleen   232

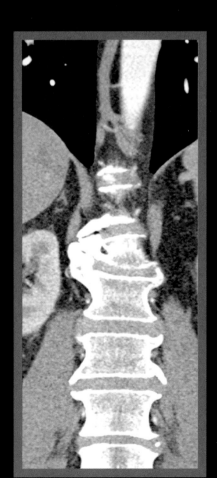

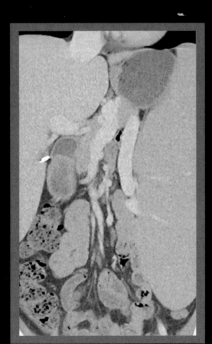

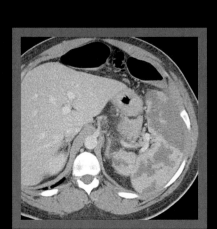

DIFFERENTIAL DIAGNOSIS

Common

- Cirrhosis With Portal Hypertension
- Congestive Heart Failure
- Hematologic Disorders
  - Hemoglobinopathies
  - Leukemia
  - Myeloproliferative Disorders
  - Myelofibrosis
- Mononucleosis
- AIDS
- Splenic Lymphoma
- Sarcoidosis
- Splenic Trauma
- Systemic Infection and Abscesses
  - IV Drug Abuse

Less Common

- Primary Splenic Tumors and Metastases
- Splenic Vein Occlusion
- Splenic Infarction
- Malaria
- Collagen Vascular Diseases
- Storage Diseases
  - Amyloidosis
  - Glycogen Storage Disease

ESSENTIAL INFORMATION

Key Differential Diagnosis Issues

- Splenomegaly can usually be attributed to 1 of 5 general etiologies
  - **Congestion**
    - Right heart failure
    - Cirrhosis with portal hypertension
    - Portal or splenic vein thrombosis
  - **Hematologic disorders**
    - Polycythemia vera
    - Leukemia
    - Myelofibrosis
    - Hemoglobinopathies
    - Acute infarction
  - **Inflammatory/infectious**
    - Mononucleosis
    - Hepatitis
    - AIDS
    - IV drug abuse
    - Sarcoidosis
    - Collagen vascular disease
    - Malaria
  - **Space-occupying masses**
    - Cyst
    - Lymphoma and metastases
    - Benign tumors
  - **Infiltrative diseases**
    - Gaucher disease
    - Diabetes
    - Amyloidosis
    - Glycogen storage disease
    - Hemosiderosis
- Normal spleen size is heavily influenced by age, sex, and body size, although length of 12 cm has traditionally been used as numerical cut-off
- Splenic index (length x width x height in cm) can also be used as means for diagnosing splenomegaly (> 480 suggests splenomegaly)

Helpful Clues for Common Diagnoses

- **Cirrhosis With Portal Hypertension**
  - One of most common causes of splenomegaly in daily practice
  - Cirrhotic liver morphology (e.g., capsular nodularity, widened fissures, caudate hypertrophy) with stigmata of portal hypertension (e.g., varices, ascites, mesenteric edema, etc.)
  - Punctate foci of low T1 and T2 signal may be present in spleen due to siderotic nodules (Gamna-Gandy bodies)
- **Congestive Heart Failure**
  - Very common cause of splenomegaly in daily practice, usually on basis of right heart failure
  - Associated with imaging features of right-sided cardiac dysfunction [e.g., cardiomegaly, dilated inferior vena cava (IVC), hepatic veins, reflux of contrast into IVC on arterial phase, etc.]
- **Hematologic Disorders**
  - Wide variety of hematologic disorders can result in splenomegaly, including hemoglobinopathies (e.g., sickle cell disease, thalassemia, spherocytosis), myelofibrosis, polycythemia vera, or leukemia
  - Sickle cell disease is most common and can result in enlarged spleen in acute setting, which gradually shrinks and calcifies due to autoinfarction
  - Look for other imaging findings of hematologic disorders, such as abnormal bones, extramedullary hematopoiesis, etc.
  - Asymptomatic splenomegaly may be only sign of chronic myelogenous leukemia (CML)
  - Myelofibrosis and CML, in particular, are known for producing massive splenomegaly
- **Mononucleosis**
  - Acute infection with Ebstein-Barr virus very common cause of splenomegaly in young adolescents
  - May be associated with lymphadenopathy, including in upper abdomen, as well as mild symptomatology (sore throat, fever)
  - Can rarely result in splenic rupture (either spontaneous or after minimal trauma)
- **AIDS**
  - Spleen commonly enlarged due to chronic viremia or opportunistic infection
  - Close attention must be paid to concurrent lymphadenopathy, as splenomegaly may also result from lymphoma (common in AIDS patients)
  - Splenomegaly alone cannot predict whether HIV patient has AIDS
- **Splenic Lymphoma**
  - Lymphoma (non-Hodgkin or Hodgkin) is common cause of splenomegaly and may or may not be associated with discrete lesions
    - Most common pattern is splenomegaly with diffuse infiltration and no focal mass

- Splenomegaly can be associated with innumerable tiny miliary lesions or discrete, hypodense masses
- Spleen may harbor lymphoma (or leukemia) without splenomegaly, and splenomegaly in lymphoma patient does not necessarily always suggest lymphomatous involvement

- **Sarcoidosis**
  - Splenic involvement generally manifests as mild splenomegaly, sometimes with innumerable small, hypodense nodules (on CT, US, or MR)
  - Other ancillary imaging features include hepatomegaly, similar small hypodense hepatic lesions, upper abdominal lymphadenopathy (especially periportal nodes), and thoracic involvement (mediastinal and hilar lymphadenopathy, lung involvement)
  - Think of this diagnosis in completely asymptomatic patient with mildly enlarged spleen and multiple small splenic/liver nodules

- **Splenic Trauma**
  - Not diagnostic dilemma on CT, but splenic trauma with perisplenic hematoma may be misinterpreted as splenomegaly on radiograph or US

- **Systemic Infection and Abscesses**
  - Spleen is often enlarged in patients with persistent bacteremia or viremia (e.g., IV drug users, patients with hepatitis, sepsis)
  - IV drug users commonly have mild splenomegaly, probably on basis of chronic, low-level sepsis from injections

Helpful Clues for Less Common Diagnoses

- **Primary Splenic Tumors and Metastases**
  - Primary splenic tumors encompass broad range of benign (hemangioma, lymphangioma, hamartoma, etc.) and malignant (e.g., angiosarcoma) lesions, which are often not easily distinguishable based on imaging
  - Splenic metastases relatively uncommon, especially in absence of metastatic disease elsewhere
  - Space-occupying masses in spleen (primary tumors or metastases) very uncommonly produce splenomegaly, instead usually replacing splenic parenchyma

- **Splenic Vein Occlusion**
  - Splenomegaly probably on basis of splenic congestion secondary to impaired outflow via splenic vein
  - Spleen often shows heterogeneous enhancement and may develop frank splenic infarct
  - Most common causes are chronic pancreatitis and pancreatic adenocarcinoma in tail

- **Splenic Infarction**
  - Acute infarction can result in splenic enlargement, although conversely, splenomegaly from any etiology does predispose to splenic infarction
  - Chronic focal or global splenic infarction leads to volume loss and scarring in spleen

- **Malaria**
  - Splenomegaly can be impressive in malarial infection
  - Repetitive bouts of malaria can result in massive splenomegaly due to abnormal immune response (hyperreactive malarial splenomegaly)
  - Very common cause of splenomegaly worldwide but uncommon in Western world

- **Collagen Vascular Diseases**
  - Variety of collagen vascular diseases (e.g., rheumatoid arthritis, scleroderma, dermatomyositis, polyarteritis) can result in splenomegaly
  - Felty syndrome: Rheumatoid arthritis, splenomegaly, and granulocytopenia

- **Storage Diseases**
  - **Amyloidosis**
    - Metabolic disease associated with deposition of abnormal proteins in 1 or more organs
    - May be primary or associated with other diseases (multiple myeloma, lymphoma, osteomyelitis, rheumatoid arthritis)
    - Often causes hepatosplenomegaly
  - **Glycogen Storage Disease**
    - Many related metabolic diseases, all caused by enzymatic defect that alters metabolism of glycogen, resulting in its storage in various tissues

Cirrhosis With Portal Hypertension

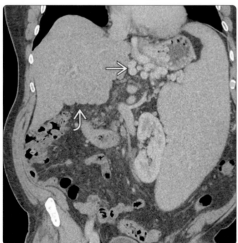

Cirrhosis With Portal Hypertension

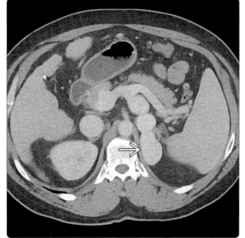

(Left) Coronal CECT shows a mildly cirrhotic liver with nodularity ➡ along its undersurface. Note the enlarged spleen as well as perigastric varices ➡, features of portal hypertension. (Right) Axial CECT shows a cirrhotic liver with capsular nodularity and widened fissures as well as mild splenomegaly and upper abdominal varices ➡ due to portal hypertension, one of the most common causes of splenomegaly in daily practice.

Cirrhosis With Portal Hypertension

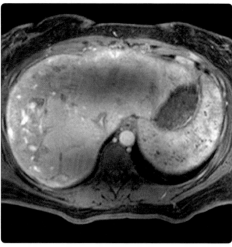

Hematologic Disorders

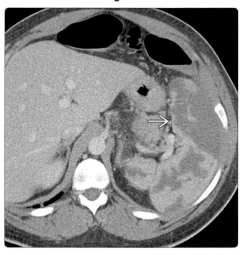
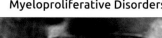

(Left) *Axial T2 FS MR shows an unusual-appearing liver with differential signal between the periphery and center secondary to chronic Budd-Chiari syndrome. The spleen is mildly enlarged with small, hypointense foci representing Gamna-Gandy bodies due to portal hypertension.* (Right) *Axial CECT in a young patient with sickle cell disease shows a mildly enlarged spleen ➡ with multiple splenic infarcts. Over time, sickle cell patients can demonstrate a small, calcified, autoinfarcted spleen.*

Hemoglobinopathies

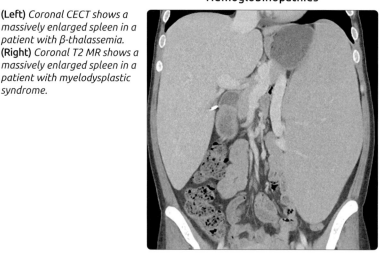

Myeloproliferative Disorders

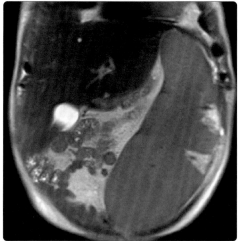

(Left) *Coronal CECT shows a massively enlarged spleen in a patient with β-thalassemia.* (Right) *Coronal T2 MR shows a massively enlarged spleen in a patient with myelodysplastic syndrome.*

Mononucleosis

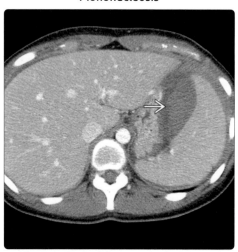

Splenic Lymphoma

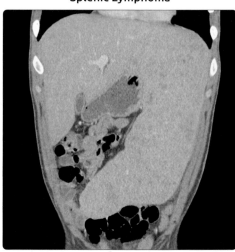

(Left) *Axial CECT shows an enlarged spleen with no apparent parenchymal lesion but with surrounding high-density hematoma ➡. These findings reflect spontaneous splenic rupture due to mononucleosis infection.* (Right) *Coronal CECT in a patient with non-Hodgkin lymphoma shows a massively enlarged spleen with innumerable tiny, hypodense, nodular foci representing lymphomatous involvement in this case.*

Splenic Lymphoma

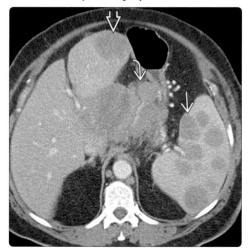

Splenic Lymphoma

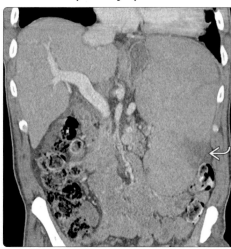

(Left) *Axial CECT shows splenomegaly with multiple hypodense, discrete splenic masses* ➡ *as well as extensive abdominal lymphadenopathy* ➡ *and a similar-appearing lesion in the liver* ➡. *These findings were found to be secondary to Hodgkin lymphoma.* (Right) *Coronal CECT shows an enlarged, heterogeneous spleen with areas of ill-defined infarction* ➡, *but without any clearly definable lesions, in this patient with non-Hodgkin lymphoma.*

Sarcoidosis

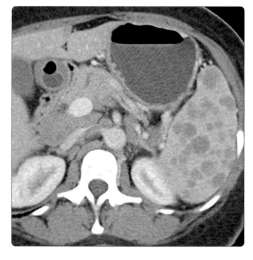

Splenic Vein Occlusion

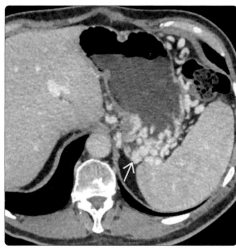

(Left) *Axial CECT shows mild splenomegaly with multiple low-density lesions in the spleen. The patient was asymptomatic, and this was found to be a manifestation of sarcoidosis.* (Right) *Axial CECT shows mild splenomegaly with extensive, isolated perigastric and intragastric varices* ➡. *These findings were found to be secondary to splenic vein occlusion due to a pancreatic tail ductal adenocarcinoma (not shown).*

Splenic Infarction

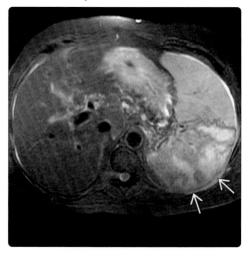

Splenic Infarction

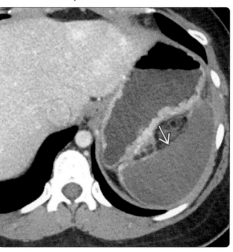

(Left) *Axial T2 FS MR shows splenomegaly with a large, hyperintense splenic infarct* ➡. (Right) *Axial CECT shows a diffusely low-density spleen* ➡ *secondary to global infarction.*

Multiple Splenic Calcifications

DIFFERENTIAL DIAGNOSIS

Common

- Healed Granulomatous Infection
- Sarcoidosis
- Vascular Abnormalities (Mimic)
- *Pneumocystis carinii*
- Splenic Infarction
- Splenic Cyst

Less Common

- Echinococcal (Hydatid) Cyst
- Healed Splenic Abscess
- Splenic Hematoma
- Primary Splenic Neoplasms
- Systemic Lupus Erythematosus

ESSENTIAL INFORMATION

Key Differential Diagnosis Issues

- Punctate splenic calcifications usually attributable to healed granulomatous disease (histoplasmosis, TB, etc.)

Helpful Clues for Common Diagnoses

- **Healed Granulomatous Infection**
  - Most common cause of punctate splenic calcifications is healed granulomatous infection (histoplasmosis, TB, brucellosis, toxoplasmosis, candidiasis, fungal infections)
  - **Histoplasmosis** is probably most common cause (in USA) for multiple (> 6) small, rounded calcifications
    - Calcifications with histoplasmosis tend to be larger and more numerous compared to other granulomatous infections
    - Similar calcifications in liver, lung, and thoracic lymph nodes may be present
  - **Tuberculosis** usually does not produce as many calcified granulomas as with histoplasmosis
    - May be associated with calcifications of liver, adrenal glands, and mesenteric nodes
  - **Brucellosis** may produce very large, focal calcifications (> 1 cm) or rim-calcified lesions with lucent center

- **Sarcoidosis**
  - Small, discrete hypodense nodules may be seen in spleen (&/or liver) in earlier stages of disease, which evolve chronically into punctate calcifications
- **Vascular Abnormalities (Mimic)**
  - Atherosclerosis may cause parallel (tram-track) splenic artery calcification, which simulate splenic calcifications
  - Splenic artery aneurysm may produce rounded eggshell calcifications near splenic hilum
- *Pneumocystis carinii*
  - *P. carinii* pneumonia infection can result in multiple tiny calcifications throughout spleen &/or liver
- **Splenic Infarction**
  - Splenic infarcts can result in splenic parenchymal scarring with peripheral subcapsular calcification or triangular calcification with apex pointed toward center of spleen
  - Sickle cell disease results in autoinfarcted spleen, which is small and diffusely calcified after multiple infarctions
- **Splenic Cyst**
  - Can demonstrate thin, peripheral eggshell calcification or thick, irregular peripheral calcification, both of which are more common with acquired cysts

Helpful Clues for Less Common Diagnoses

- **Echinococcal (Hydatid) Cyst**
  - Hydatid cysts are less frequent in spleen compared to liver or peritoneal cavity but may demonstrate either peripheral calcification or wavy, serpiginous internal calcification in chronic setting
- **Healed Splenic Abscess**
  - Any form of splenic infection may heal with calcified scar
- **Splenic Hematoma**
  - Old, resolved sites of intrasplenic hematoma may result in parenchymal calcification
- **Primary Splenic Neoplasms**
  - Lymphangiomas and hemangiomas may demonstrate calcification and may be multiple
- **Systemic Lupus Erythematosus**
  - May rarely be associated with multiple discrete splenic calcifications (which can be quite extensive)

Healed Granulomatous Infection

Healed Granulomatous Infection

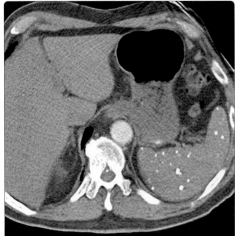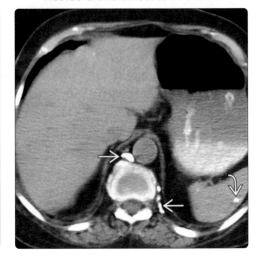

(Left) Axial CECT shows multiple punctate calcifications in the spleen, almost certainly on the basis of a healed granulomatous infection. The most common cause of such calcifications in the USA is histoplasmosis. (Right) Axial NECT shows several punctate calcified splenic granulomas ➔ in an older woman who also had calcified abdominal nodes ➔ and renal and adrenal lesions (not shown) from TB.

Sarcoidosis

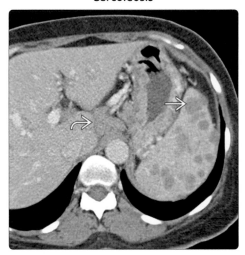

Vascular Abnormalities (Mimic)

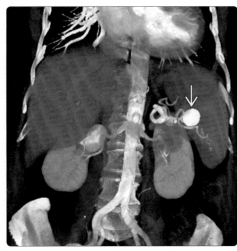

(Left) Axial CECT in a patient with sarcoidosis shows multiple small, hypodense nodules ➡ in the spleen, as well as enlarged upper abdominal lymph nodes ➡. Multiple splenic calcifications may be seen in the more chronic setting of sarcoidosis. (Right) Coronal volume-rendered CECT shows a splenic artery aneurysm ➡ projecting over the spleen in the left upper quadrant. While the diagnosis is obvious on CT, this could conceivably be mistaken for a splenic calcification on plain radiographs.

Pneumocystis carinii

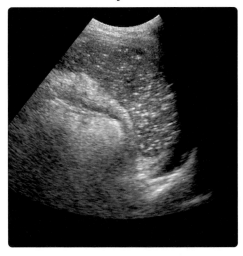

Splenic Infarction

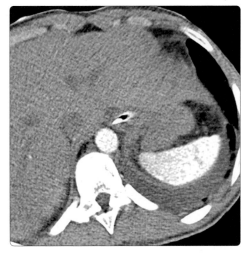

(Left) Transverse US of the spleen shows innumerable punctate calcifications of the spleen in an HIV/AIDS patient with Pneumocystis infection. (Right) Axial NECT in a patient with sickle cell disease shows a small, atrophic spleen with diffuse calcification as a result of multiple prior episodes of splenic infarction.

Splenic Cyst

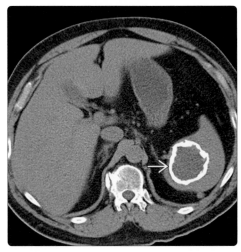

Echinococcal (Hydatid) Cyst

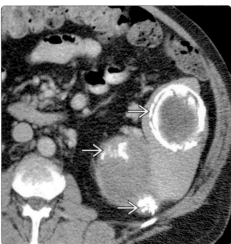

(Left) Axial NECT shows a splenic cyst ➡ with thick, peripheral calcification. Calcification is more common in acquired splenic cysts (compared to congenital splenic cysts). (Right) Axial CECT shows multiple low-density lesions ➡ in the spleen, some of which have calcified walls, representing hydatid cysts in an older man who had similar lesions in his liver and peritoneal cavity.

Solid Splenic Mass or Masses

DIFFERENTIAL DIAGNOSIS

Common
- Splenic Metastases and Lymphoma
- Splenic Trauma (Mimic)
- Splenic Infarction (Mimic)
- Perfusion Artifact (Mimic)

Less Common
- Sarcoidosis
- Splenic Infection and Abscess
- Primary Splenic Tumors
- Splenic Peliosis

ESSENTIAL INFORMATION

Key Differential Diagnosis Issues
- Most solid splenic masses are benign, incidental findings that require no further evaluation or follow-up
- Most splenic masses demonstrate nonspecific imaging features, so suspicious lesions (based on imaging or clinical features) may require biopsy or splenectomy for diagnosis

Helpful Clues for Common Diagnoses
- **Splenic Metastases and Lymphoma**
  - Splenic metastases are almost always present in setting of widespread metastatic disease; isolated splenic metastases are exceedingly uncommon
    - Most common primary tumors are breast, lung, ovary, stomach, and melanoma
  - Lymphoma most common splenic malignancy: Usually secondary (with disease elsewhere) rather than primary
    - Imaging patterns include dominant solitary mass, multiple discrete lesions, innumerable tiny nodules, or splenomegaly without discrete lesions
    - Lesions usually solid, hypoenhancing, and homogeneous without necrosis or calcification
- **Splenic Trauma (Mimic)**
  - Intrasplenic hematoma could mimic hyperdense mass
  - Clinical history, presence of splenic laceration, and perisplenic hematoma should suggest correct diagnosis

- **Splenic Infarction (Mimic)**
  - Splenic infarct typically appears as wedge-shaped area of hypoperfusion extending to capsule but rarely appears rounded or mass-like mimicking hypodense mass
- **Perfusion Artifact (Mimic)**
  - Heterogeneous splenic enhancement (moiré pattern) on arterial-phase images can mimic mass but should disappear on venous-/delayed-phase images

Helpful Clues for Less Common Diagnoses
- **Sarcoidosis**
  - Hepatosplenomegaly with multiple small, hypoenhancing nodules in liver and spleen
  - Often associated with upper abdominal and thoracic lymphadenopathy ± sarcoid-related lung findings
- **Splenic Infection and Abscess**
  - Fungal microabscesses (usually in immunocompromised or HIV/AIDS patients) appear as multiple small, hypodense nodules (usually just a few mm)
- **Primary Splenic Tumors**
  - Most primary splenic tumors are incidental findings, and specific diagnosis may not be possible based on imaging
  - Most common benign splenic masses include hemangioma, lymphangioma, and hamartoma
    - Hemangioma demonstrates prominent peripheral vascularity with delayed enhancement, lymphangioma appears primarily cystic, and hamartoma is nonspecific solid, isoattenuating mass
  - Most common primary malignancies of spleen are lymphoma and angiosarcoma
    - Angiosarcoma is extremely rare, aggressive malignancy with propensity for bleeding
      - ☐ Lesions may superficially resemble hemangiomas with frequent necrotic degeneration ± calcification
- **Splenic Peliosis**
  - Very rare entity (more often reported in liver) characterized by multiple blood-filled spaces in spleen
    - Usually associated with anabolic steroids, hematologic disorders, and chronic diseases (e.g., TB, AIDS)
  - Usually appears as multiple small, hypoattenuating lesions on CT/MR ± internal hematocrit levels

Splenic Metastases and Lymphoma

Splenic Metastases and Lymphoma

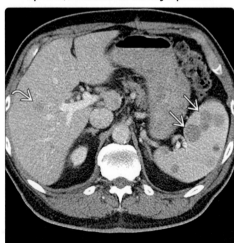

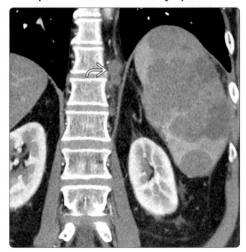

(Left) Axial CECT in a patient with melanoma shows numerous metastases ➡ in the spleen, as well as some more subtle metastases in the liver ➡. (Right) Coronal CECT shows multiple homogeneous, hypodense, solid masses throughout the spleen, found to represent lymphoma. Note the presence of some associated retrocrural lymphadenopathy ➡.

Splenic Trauma (Mimic)

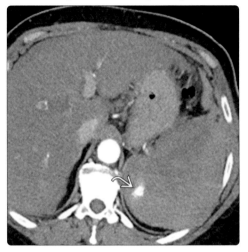

Splenic Infarction (Mimic)

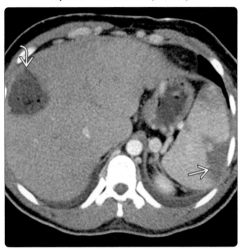

(Left) *Axial CECT in a trauma patient shows a large, hyperdense splenic hematoma replacing nearly the entire spleen with a focus of active extravasation* ➽. **(Right)** *Axial CECT in a patient after Whipple procedure shows wedge-shaped infarcts* ➾ *in the spleen, as well as an infarct in the liver* ➘, *thought to be on the basis of septic emboli.*

Perfusion Artifact (Mimic)

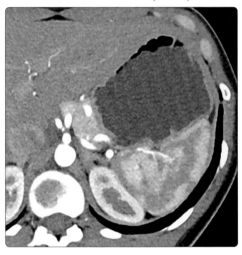

Sarcoidosis

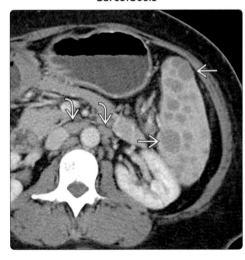

(Left) *Axial CECT shows heterogeneous enhancement of the spleen, a common normal variant on arterial-phase CECT, especially in patients such as this who have cirrhosis and portal hypertension. The spleen appeared normal on portal venous-phase CECT.* **(Right)** *Axial CECT in an asymptomatic patient being imaged for unrelated reasons shows multiple small, solid, hypodense nodules* ➾ *in the spleen, as well as upper abdominal lymphadenopathy* ➘, *found to represent sarcoidosis.*

Splenic Infection and Abscess

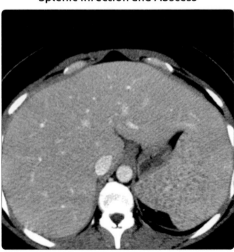

Primary Splenic Tumors

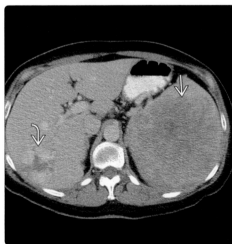

(Left) *Axial CECT shows innumerable small, hypodense foci in the spleen and, more subtly, in the liver. Both the liver and spleen are enlarged. These findings were found to represent mycobacterial infection.* **(Right)** *Axial CECT shows a large, heterogeneous splenic mass* ➾, *found to represent a primary splenic angiosarcoma. Note the presence of an enhancing metastasis* ➾ *in the liver, the most common location for metastatic disease in this aggressive malignancy.*

DIFFERENTIAL DIAGNOSIS

Common

- Splenic Cyst
- Splenic Trauma
- Splenic Infarction

Less Common

- Splenic Metastases and Lymphoma
- Splenic Infection and Abscess
- Splenic Tumors
- Pancreatic Pseudocyst

ESSENTIAL INFORMATION

Key Differential Diagnosis Issues

- While most cystic lesions of spleen are benign, metastases and lymphoma can appear low density/cystic

Helpful Clues for Common Diagnoses

- **Splenic Cyst**
  - Can be congenital (i.e., true epidermoid cyst) or acquired (e.g., trauma, infection, infarction, hematoma, etc.)
  - Usually incidental finding but can rarely be symptomatic due to size and mass effect
  - Can be entirely simple in appearance or demonstrate internal septations, necrotic debris, or peripheral calcification (either thin/eggshell or thick/irregular)
    - Should not have solid or enhancing components
  - Congenital and acquired cysts may be indistinguishable, but calcification is more common in acquired cysts
- **Splenic Trauma**
  - Acute intrasplenic hematoma is typically hyperdense on CT and may be associated with splenic laceration
  - Chronic hematoma may appear low density/cystic, while associated laceration may no longer be apparent
- **Splenic Infarction**
  - Typical appearance is wedge-shaped area of hypoperfusion at periphery of spleen but can rarely appear rounded or mass-like (and mimic cyst)

- Can evolve over time into cystic lesion, usually with immediately adjacent parenchymal scarring

Helpful Clues for Less Common Diagnoses

- **Splenic Metastases and Lymphoma**
  - Splenic metastases are rare and almost always associated with metastatic disease elsewhere
    - Isolated metastases to spleen extremely uncommon
    - Some malignancies may produce low-density or cystic metastases, including melanoma, breast cancer, ovarian cancer, and endometrial cancer
  - Splenic lymphoma usually secondary (with additional disease elsewhere) rather than primary
    - Can appear as solitary dominant mass, multiple discrete lesions, innumerable tiny nodules, or splenomegaly without discrete lesions
    - Lesions typically homogeneously hypovascular on CT and can be confused for cysts
- **Splenic Infection and Abscess**
  - Pyogenic abscesses may occur due to bacteremia, septic emboli, or infection of hematoma/infarct
    - Cystic mass with thick wall ± air-fluid levels or gas
    - Less often multiloculated compared to liver abscesses
  - Echinococcal cysts are very rare in USA but appear as complex cystic masses with internal daughter cysts or internal serpiginous linear densities (water-lily sign)
  - Fungal microabscesses usually in immunocompromised patients and appear as multiple small (few mm in size), hypodense lesions
- **Splenic Tumors**
  - Primary splenic tumors are uncommon with lymphangiomas and hemangiomas most common
    - Appearance of these lesions extremely variable, and specific diagnosis often not possible based on imaging
  - Lymphangiomas are thin-walled, simple-appearing cysts, although other lesions (including hemangiomas) can demonstrate cystic or necrotic components
- **Pancreatic Pseudocyst**
  - Pseudocysts can arise in pancreatic tail and spread into splenic hilum via splenorenal ligament
    - Over time, pseudocyst may invaginate into spleen

(Left) Coronal CECT shows a large, simple-appearing splenic cyst ➡. In many cases, it is not possible to differentiate congenital and acquired splenic cysts on imaging. (Right) Coronal CECT shows a splenic cyst ➡ with thick, peripheral calcification. Splenic calcifications are more common in acquired splenic cysts but may be seen in congenital cysts as well.

Splenic Cyst

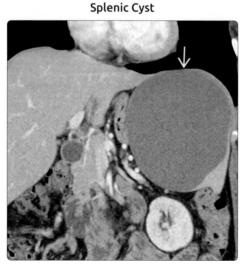

Splenic Cyst

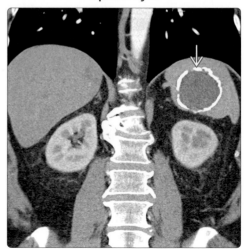

Cystic Splenic Mass

Splenic Infarction

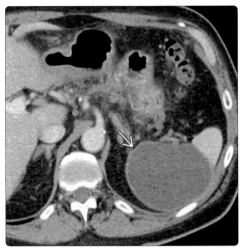

Splenic Metastases and Lymphoma

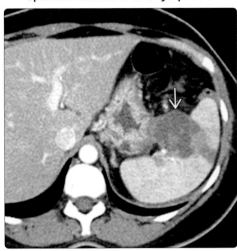

(Left) *Axial CECT shows a well-defined cyst* ➡ *in the spleen resulting from a splenic infarct a few weeks earlier.* **(Right)** *Axial CECT shows a low-density mass* ➡ *involving the spleen and splenic hilum, representing a metastasis in this patient with metastatic ovarian cancer. Ovarian cancer is one of several malignancies (such as breast cancer, endometrial cancer, and melanoma) with metastases that can appear low density or even cystic.*

Splenic Metastases and Lymphoma

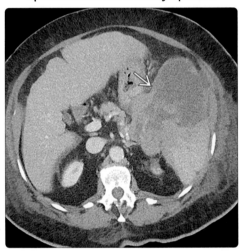

Splenic Infection and Abscess

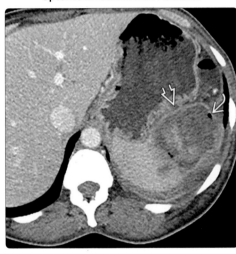

(Left) *Axial CECT shows a large, infiltrative mass* ➡ *in the spleen, portions of which appear to relatively low in density and even cystic, ultimately found to represent non-Hodgkin lymphoma.* **(Right)** *Axial CECT in a patient with HIV and sepsis shows a thick-walled fluid collection* ➡ *containing internal ectopic gas* ➡, *representing a splenic abscess.*

Splenic Tumors

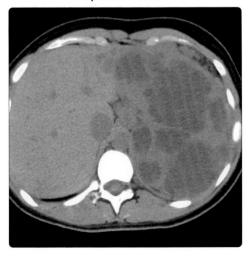

Pancreatic Pseudocyst

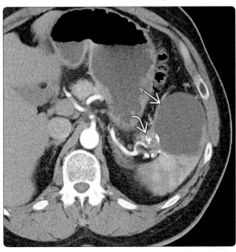

(Left) *Axial CECT shows innumerable cystic masses within an enlarged spleen, found to represent lymphangiomas at resection. The low attenuation and complexity of these lesions are typical for lymphangioma, though they cannot be considered diagnostic.* **(Right)** *Axial CECT in a patient shows a pseudocyst* ➡ *in the pancreatic tail directly invaginating into the spleen. Note the calcifications* ➡ *in the pancreatic tail, revealing the patient's history of chronic pancreatitis.*

DIFFERENTIAL DIAGNOSIS

Common

- Secondary Hemochromatosis
- Splenic Infarction
  - Sickle Cell Anemia

Less Common

- Opportunistic Infection
- Thorotrast
- Systemic Lupus Erythematosus
- Amiodarone Therapy

ESSENTIAL INFORMATION

Key Differential Diagnosis Issues

- Spleen is often used as reference standard on CT and MR by which to recognize liver pathology
  - Splenic attenuation not typically altered by metabolic processes other than calcification and iron deposition
- MDCT
  - Normal attenuation of spleen on NECT is roughly 10 HU lower than liver and usually between 40-60 HU on NECT
- MR
  - Normal spleen typically demonstrates signal lower than liver and slightly greater than muscle on T1
  - Normal spleen typically demonstrates higher signal than liver on T2

Helpful Clues for Common Diagnoses

- Secondary Hemochromatosis
  - Primary hemochromatosis is inherited autosomal recessive disorder resulting in ↑ dietary iron absorption
    - Involved organs include heart, liver, and pancreas
    - Primary hemochromatosis **does not** result in abnormal spleen MR signal intensity or CT density
  - Secondary hemochromatosis (i.e., hemosiderosis) results from frequent blood transfusions, hemoglobinopathies, portacaval shunt, etc.

- Results in deposition of iron in reticuloendothelial system, including spleen, liver, and bone marrow without associated end-organ damage
- CT shows increased attenuation of liver and spleen, although CT is much less sensitive for mild degrees of iron deposition compared to MR
- MR shows decreased signal in liver (± spleen) relative to muscle on T1 and T2 as well as signal loss on in-phase GRE (compared to out of phase) MR
  - Superparamagnetic effects of iron lead to shortening of T1, T2, and T2*, resulting in signal loss directly proportional to degree of iron deposition
- Splenic Infarction
  - Hemoglobinopathies and other causes of splenic infarction can result in segmental or subcapsular infarction, which may calcify
  - Sickle cell anemia results in repeated episodes of splenic infarctions, which by adulthood can result in small, diffusely calcified spleen (autosplenectomy)

Helpful Clues for Less Common Diagnoses

- Opportunistic Infection
  - Healed phase of many splenic infections results in multifocal calcifications (histoplasmosis, mycobacterial diseases, CMV, herpes, other granulomatous infections)
  - Diffuse calcification can result from *Pneumocystis carinii*, but now rare since advent of antiretroviral therapy
  - Look for similar involvement of liver, lymph nodes, and adrenal glands
- Thorotrast
  - Intravascular angiographic contrast agent last used in 1950s because of its strongly carcinogenic properties
  - Taken up by spleen (and to lesser extent liver) resulting in diffuse hyperdensity of affected organs, as well as parenchymal atrophy and scarring
- Systemic Lupus Erythematosus
  - Can result in unique pattern of diffuse splenic calcification (without atrophy)
- Amiodarone Therapy
  - Diffusely increased splenic and hepatic attenuation can be present even in absence of clinical signs of toxicity

(Left) Axial NECT shows subtly increased attenuation of both the liver and spleen in this patient who had received multiple transfusions due to multiple myeloma. (Right) Axial T2 MR shows diffuse low signal throughout the liver and spleen, both of which demonstrate lower signal than the paraspinal musculature. These findings reflect hemosiderosis on the basis of multiple transfusions.

Secondary Hemochromatosis

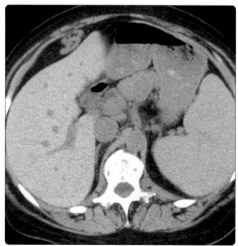

Secondary Hemochromatosis

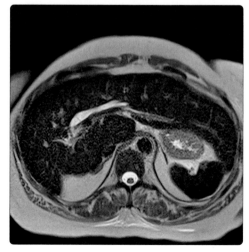

Secondary Hemochromatosis

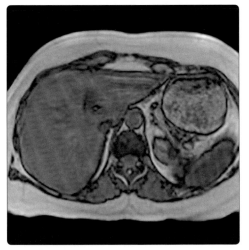

Secondary Hemochromatosis

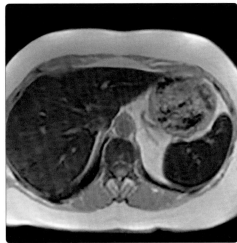

(Left) *Axial opposed-phase GRE MR shows fairly normal signal in both the liver and spleen.* (Right) *Axial in-phase GRE MR in the same patient shows diffuse loss of signal in both the liver and spleen, another finding consistent with iron deposition in these organs. Note that the pattern of signal loss on these dual-echo images is the opposite of fatty deposition. Unlike steatosis, which results in signal loss on opposed-phase images, iron results in signal loss on in-phase images.*

Sickle Cell Anemia

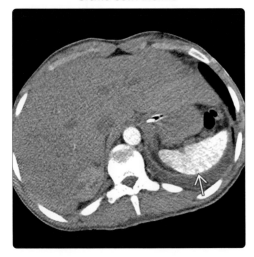

Opportunistic Infection

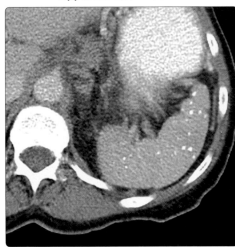

(Left) *Axial NECT in a patient with sickle cell disease shows an atrophic spleen ➡ with diffuse calcification, compatible with splenic autoinfarction. This is a relatively common finding in sickle cell patients by adulthood.* (Right) *Axial CECT in an asymptomatic patient shows numerous small splenic calcifications. Incidental splenic calcifications are a common finding and most often reflect the sequelae of healed granulomatous infection.*

Opportunistic Infection

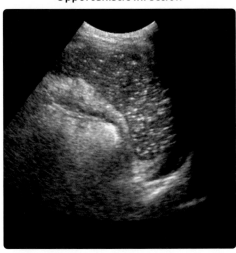

Opportunistic Infection

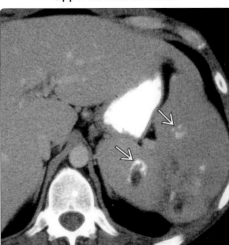

(Left) *Transverse US in an HIV/AIDS patient shows extensive echogenic calcifications throughout the spleen, compatible with the patient's history of Pneumocystis carinii pneumonia infection.* (Right) *Axial CECT in an HIV patient with Pneumocystis pneumonia shows multiple calcifications ➡ within the spleen, some of which surround low-density abscesses.*

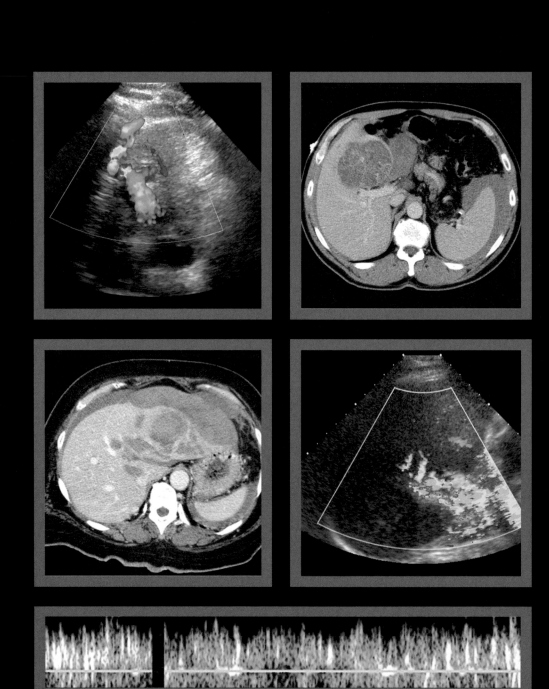

SECTION 9
Liver

Generic Imaging Patterns

Liver Mass With Central or Eccentric Scar   236
Focal Liver Lesion With Hemorrhage   240
Liver "Mass" With Capsular Retraction   244
Fat-Containing Liver Mass   246
Cystic Hepatic Mass   248
Focal Hypervascular Liver Lesion   252
Liver Mass With Mosaic Enhancement   258
Mosaic or Patchy Hepatogram   262
Hepatic Calcifications   266
Liver Lesion Containing Gas   270
Portal Venous Gas   274
Widened Hepatic Fissures   276
Dysmorphic Liver With Abnormal Bile Ducts   278
Focal Hyperperfusion Abnormality (THAD or THID)   282
Periportal Lucency or Edema   288

Modality-Specific Imaging Findings

Magnetic Resonance Imaging

Multiple Hypointense Liver Lesions (T2WI)   294
Hyperintense Liver Lesions (T1WI)   298
Liver Lesion With Capsule or Halo on MR   304

Computed Tomography

Multiple Hypodense Liver Lesions   308
Focal Hyperdense Hepatic Mass on Nonenhanced CT   314
Widespread Low Attenuation Within Liver   318

Ultrasound

Focal Hepatic Echogenic Lesion ± Acoustic Shadowing   322
Hyperechoic Liver, Diffuse   328
Hepatomegaly   330
Diffusely Abnormal Liver Echogenicity   334
Anechoic Liver Lesion   336
Hypoechoic Liver Mass   340
Echogenic Liver Mass   344
Target Lesions in Liver   348
Multiple Hypo-, Hyper- or Anechoic Liver Lesions   350
Hepatic Mass With Central Scar   354
Periportal Lesion   356
Irregular Hepatic Surface   360
Portal Vein Abnormality   362

DIFFERENTIAL DIAGNOSIS

Common

- Focal Nodular Hyperplasia
- Hepatic Cavernous Hemangioma

Less Common

- Hepatocellular Carcinoma
- Hepatic Adenoma
- Hepatic Metastases
- Fibrolamellar (Hepatocellular) Carcinoma
- Cholangiocarcinoma (Intrahepatic, Peripheral)
- Epithelioid Hemangioendothelioma

Rare but Important

- Nodular Regenerative Hyperplasia

ESSENTIAL INFORMATION

Key Differential Diagnosis Issues

- Characterize size of scar, pattern of mass enhancement, associated findings
  - Fibrolamellar carcinoma is almost always solitary; cholangiocarcinoma and focal nodular hyperplasia (FNH) are usually solitary; others are commonly multiple

Helpful Clues for Common Diagnoses

- **Focal Nodular Hyperplasia**
  - Larger FNH lesions (> 3 cm) usually have small central scar ± thin radiating septa
  - Homogeneous enhancement of **mass** on arterial phase, isodense (isointense) to liver on all other phases
  - Central **scar** bright on T2WI; shows delayed persistent enhancement on CT and by intravascular contrast agents on MR
    - Scar will not enhance on delayed gadoxetate (Eovist/Primovist)-enhanced scans and has prolonged enhancement on hepatobiliary phase
- **Hepatic Cavernous Hemangioma**

- Large hemangiomas (> 5 cm) commonly have fibrotic nonenhancing scar that may calcify; nonscarred portions have typical nodular enhancement

Helpful Clues for Less Common Diagnoses

- **Hepatocellular Carcinoma**
  - Large tumors, especially in noncirrhotic liver, may resemble fibrolamellar carcinoma
    - Heterogeneous hypervascular mass with washout
    - Central necrosis or scar (scar is rarely calcified in hepatocellular carcinoma)
  - Vascular invasion and metastases are common
- **Hepatic Adenoma**
  - Low-density foci due to fat (signal drop out on chemical shift MR), necrosis, old hemorrhage; not scar
  - Distinction from FNH best made by Eovist-enhanced MR
- **Hepatic Metastases**
  - Target appearance; necrosis, not scar
  - Calcification can be seen with mucinous carcinoma metastases (e.g., colon, ovarian)
- **Fibrolamellar (Hepatocellular) Carcinoma**
  - Large, heterogeneous mass on all phases of imaging
    - Scar is large and often (> 60%) calcified
  - Aggressive signs noted at presentation in > 60%
    - Local invasion (vessels, bile ducts); metastases
- **Cholangiocarcinoma (Intrahepatic, Peripheral)**
  - Focal necrosis or fibrosis may resemble scar
  - Often has extensive fibrous stroma
    - With typical delayed persistent enhancement
  - Overlying capsular retraction, hepatic volume loss, biliary and portal venous obstruction
- **Epithelioid Hemangioendothelioma**
  - Multiple, coalescent, peripheral nodules
  - Target or lollipop appearance on CECT or MR; capsular retraction over lesions
- **Nodular Regenerative Hyperplasia**
  - Multiacinar form of nodular regenerative hyperplasia (large regenerative nodules) may have central scar
  - Usually multiple, < 4 cm in diameter
  - Usually in patients with Budd-Chiari syndrome

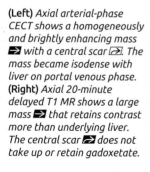

(Left) *Axial arterial-phase CECT shows a homogeneously and brightly enhancing mass* ➡ *with a central scar* ➦. *The mass became isodense with liver on portal venous phase.* **(Right)** *Axial 20-minute delayed T1 MR shows a large mass* ➡ *that retains contrast more than underlying liver. The central scar* ➦ *does not take up or retain gadoxetate.*

Focal Nodular Hyperplasia

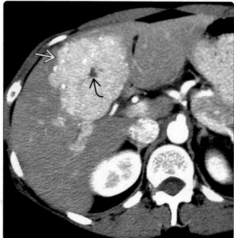

Focal Nodular Hyperplasia

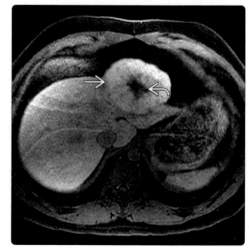

Hepatic Cavernous Hemangioma

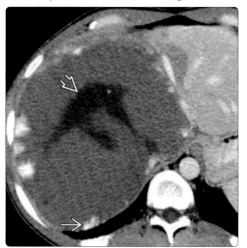

Hepatic Cavernous Hemangioma

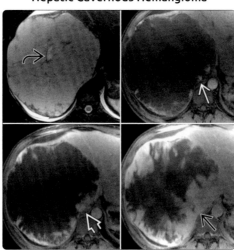

(Left) *Axial CECT shows a large mass with peripheral nodular enhancement ➡ isodense to vessels. A central scar ➡, with a small focus of calcification, did not fill in on delayed imaging. These are typical features of giant hemangiomas.* **(Right)** *Axial T2 MR shows a large, hyperintense mass with a central scar ➡ that is very bright, typical of a large hemangioma with progressive nodular enhancement on arterial ➡, venous ➡, and delayed ➡ phases.*

Hepatocellular Carcinoma

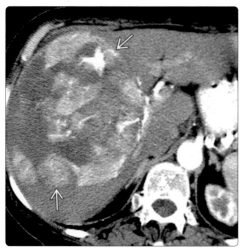

Hepatocellular Carcinoma

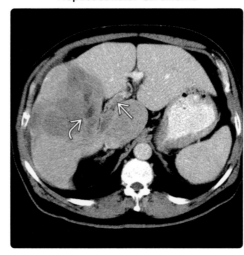

(Left) *Axial arterial-phase CECT in an older woman shows a large, heterogeneous, hypervascular mass ➡ with foci of necrosis, giving it a mottled or mosaic appearance. The age of the patient and absence of calcification favored conventional hepatocellular carcinoma (HCC), as opposed to fibrolamellar HCC, confirmed on biopsy.* **(Right)** *Axial CECT shows a large mass with an eccentric scar ➡ or necrotic area. Tumor invasion of portal vein ➡ helps to identify this as HCC.*

Hepatic Adenoma

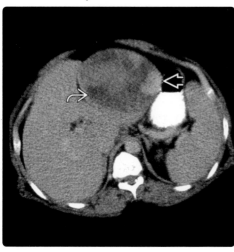

Hepatic Adenoma

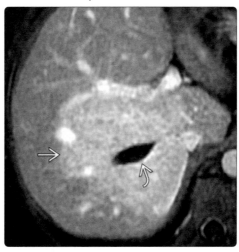

(Left) *Axial NECT shows a heterogeneous mass in the left lobe. At resection, the focus of high attenuation ➡ was hemorrhage, and the lower density foci ➡ were necrosis and fibrosis.* **(Right)** *Axial venous-phase T1 C+ MR shows a large, enhancing mass ➡ with a central nonenhancing scar ➡.*

Hepatic Metastases

Hepatic Metastases

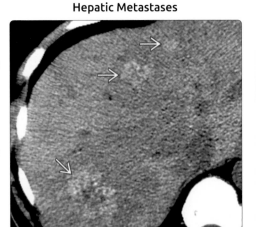

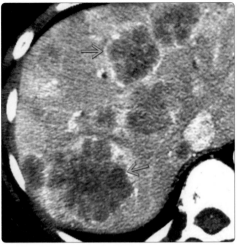

(Left) *Axial NECT in this older patient with colon cancer shows shows multiple lesions with faint central calcification* ➡. **(Right)** *Axial portal venous-phase CECT in this older patient with colon cancer shows multiple metastases* ➡ *with central, low-density necrosis or fibrosis. The faint calcification is more difficult to recognize on contrast-enhanced imaging.*

Fibrolamellar (Hepatocellular) Carcinoma

Fibrolamellar (Hepatocellular) Carcinoma

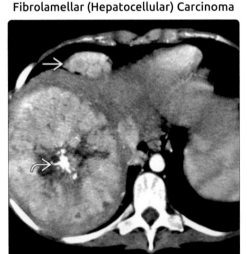

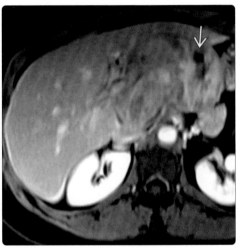

(Left) *Axial CECT in a 22-year-old man shows a heterogeneous, hypervascular mass with a large, calcified central scar* ➡. *Note the similar enhancement of tumor in a cardiophrenic node* ➡. **(Right)** *Axial T1 C+ FS MR in a young woman with a large, heterogeneously enhancing left hepatic lobe fibrolamellar HCC shows a central necrotic scar* ➡.

Cholangiocarcinoma (Intrahepatic, Peripheral)

Cholangiocarcinoma (Intrahepatic, Peripheral)

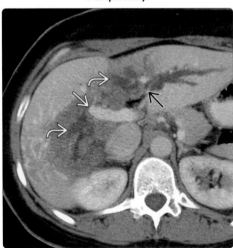

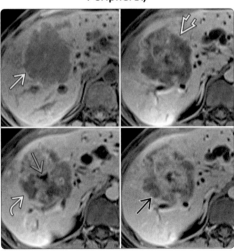

(Left) *Axial CECT shows a large hepatic mass with foci of scar or necrosis* ➡. *Capsular retraction and occlusion of the portal vein* ➡ *and bile duct* ➡ *help confirm cholangiocarcinoma.* **(Right)** *Axial T1 C+ FS MR shows a large, hypointense mass* ➡ *with progressive enhancement on arterial* ➡, *portal venous* ➡, *and delayed* ➡ *phases due to fibrotic changes and a nonenhancing central scar* ➡.

Epithelioid Hemangioendothelioma

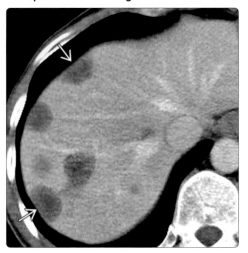

Epithelioid Hemangioendothelioma

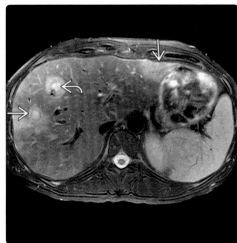

(Left) *Axial CECT in a young woman shows multiple peripheral hypovascular lesions with a target appearance. The subcapsular lesions are associated with retraction of the overlying liver capsule* ➡️. (Right) *Axial T2 FS MR in a young woman shows multiple peripheral and confluent masses* ➡️, *many with hyperintense central necrosis or scar* ➡️. *These are typical features of hepatic epithelial hemangioendothelioma.*

Nodular Regenerative Hyperplasia

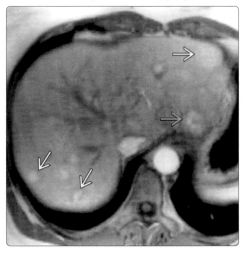

Nodular Regenerative Hyperplasia

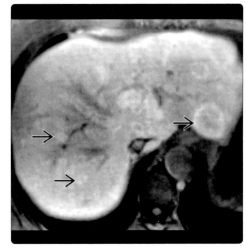

(Left) *Axial arterial-phase T1 C+ MR in a hypercoagulable patient shows multiple hypervascular foci* ➡️. *Some of the lesions seem to have a hypointense rim, while others have a hypointense central scar* ➡️. (Right) *Axial T1 C+ MR in a hypercoagulable patient 2 hours after IV administration of gadobenate dimeglumine shows persistent uptake and retention of the agent within the nodules* ➡️, *indicating functional hepatocytes and deficient biliary ducts within the lesions.*

Nodular Regenerative Hyperplasia

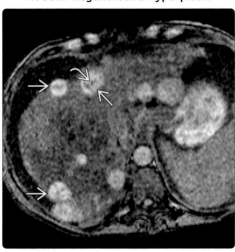

Nodular Regenerative Hyperplasia

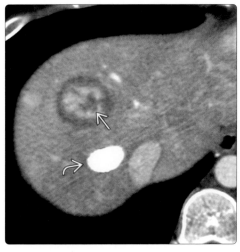

(Left) *Axial T1 C+ MR in a patient with Budd-Chiari syndrome shows multiple hypervascular nodules* ➡️, *some of which have a central scar* ➡️. *These multiple large, regenerative nodules (nodular regenerative hyperplasia) confirmed transplantation.* (Right) *Axial CECT in a patient with Budd-Chiari syndrome and nodular regenerative hyperplasia shows a central scar* ➡️ *and doughnut-like enhancement. Transjugular intrahepatic portosystemic shunt (TIPS) is also seen* ➡️.

DIFFERENTIAL DIAGNOSIS

Common

- Hepatic Trauma
- Hepatic Adenoma
- Hepatocellular Carcinoma
- Hepatic Cyst
- Autosomal Dominant Polycystic Disease, Liver

Less Common

- Coagulopathic Hemorrhage, Liver
- Hepatic Metastases
- HELLP Syndrome
- Amyloidosis

ESSENTIAL INFORMATION

Key Differential Diagnosis Issues

- Hemorrhage may be detected as heterogeneous high attenuation (> 60 HU on NECT), or high-intensity foci on T1WI and T2WI
- Bleeding may include subcapsular and intraperitoneal extension

Helpful Clues for Common Diagnoses

- **Hepatic Trauma**
  - Blunt or penetrating (including biopsies, TIPS, etc.)
  - Hepatic lacerations usually have linear or stellate configuration
  - Location: Right lobe (75%), left lobe (25%)
  - Best imaging tool: Dual-phase CT in hemodynamically stable patients
- **Hepatic Adenoma**
  - Foci of hemorrhage within tumor is common feature on MR, less common on CT
  - Spontaneous bleeding within or around hepatic mass in young female without cirrhosis is almost diagnostic of adenoma
  - Other signs of adenoma
    - Lipid or fat content
    - Multiplicity

- Encapsulation
- **Hepatocellular Carcinoma**
  - Spontaneous hemorrhage within tumor is uncommon
  - Spontaneous rupture through capsule is relatively common for large hepatocellular carcinoma (HCC)
  - Other signs of HCC
    - Occurrence within cirrhotic liver
    - Hypervascularity with washout
    - Encapsulation
- **Hepatic Cyst**
  - Isolated or part of autosomal dominant polycystic disease
  - Clotted blood in cyst may be mistaken for tumor but will not show enhancement

Helpful Clues for Less Common Diagnoses

- **Coagulopathic Hemorrhage, Liver**
  - Spontaneous intrahepatic or perihepatic hemorrhage is rare manifestation of coagulopathy or anticoagulant therapy
  - Spherical hematoma within liver may simulate tumor
  - Others signs of coagulopathic hemorrhage
    - Hematocrit sign (fluid level) within hematoma
    - Multiple sites of bleeding
    - Favored sites: Iliopsoas and rectus muscles
- **Hepatic Metastases**
  - Hemorrhage is uncommon, usually associated with hypervascular metastases
  - May occur following chemotherapy or transhepatic ablation of metastatic lesions
  - Most commonly: Lung cancer, renal cell carcinoma, pancreatic neuroendocrine tumor, and melanoma
- **HELLP Syndrome**
  - Hemolysis, elevated liver enzymes, low platelets
  - Severe variation of toxemia of pregnancy
  - Intrahepatic or subcapsular fluid collection (hematoma)
    - Occasionally active extravasation
  - Wedge-shaped areas of infarction
- **Amyloidosis**
  - Hepatocellular rupture extremely rare

(Left) *Axial CECT in a trauma victim shows a broad hepatic laceration* ➡ *with foci of active bleeding* ➡ *and hemoperitoneum* ➡. *Note adjacent rib fractures* ➡.
(Right) *Axial NECT in a patient with a falling hematocrit following liver biopsy shows high-density blood in a linear tract deep within the liver* ➡, *representing the biopsy site and depth. Also note the extension as a subcapsular hematoma, the lentiform collection lateral to the liver* ➡.

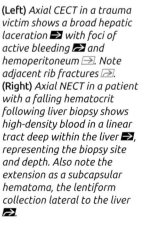
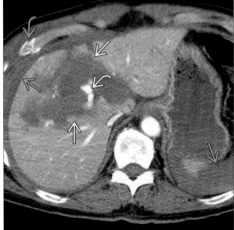

Hepatic Trauma

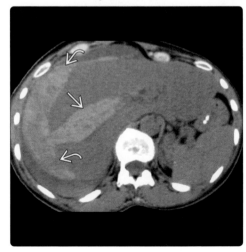

Hepatic Trauma

Hepatic Adenoma

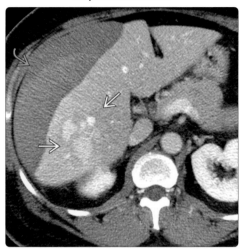

Hepatic Adenoma

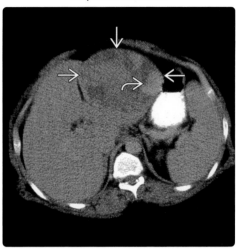

(Left) *Axial CECT in a young woman shows a hypervascular mass* ➡️ *in the right lobe with a large, spontaneous subcapsular hematoma* ⟋. (Right) *Axial NECT in a young woman with acute pain shows a mass* ➡️ *in the lateral segment with high-attenuation material* ⟋ *centrally due to an acute hematoma.*

Hepatic Adenoma

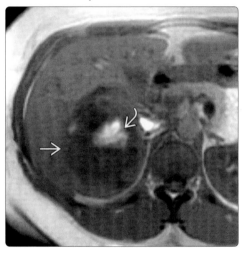

Hepatocellular Carcinoma

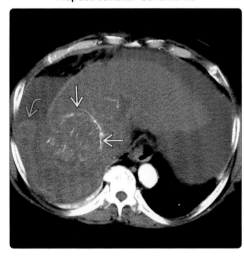

(Left) *Axial T1 MR in a young woman shows a hepatic mass* ➡️ *containing several hyperintense foci* ⟋ *that represent hemorrhage. The foci were hyperintense on T2 as well, distinguishing hemorrhage from fat as the etiology.* (Right) *Arterial-phase CECT in a man with cirrhosis and sudden right upper quadrant (RUQ) pain shows tumor vessels within a poorly defined, hypervascular mass* ➡️. *Ascites and a sentinel clot* ⟋ *overlying the hepatic mass are seen. Spontaneous rupture of hepatocellular carcinoma was the etiology.*

Hepatocellular Carcinoma

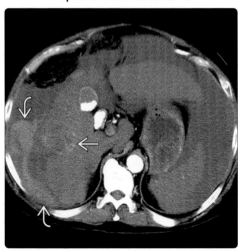

Hepatocellular Carcinoma

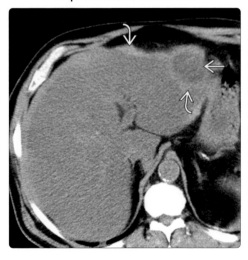

(Left) *Arterial-phase CECT in the same patient shows part of the hypervascular mass* ➡️, *as well as the ascites and sentinel clot* ⟋ *overlying the site of the capsular rupture. A catheter angiogram confirmed bleeding hepatocellular carcinoma. It was treated with coil embolization.* (Right) *Axial NECT in a 60-year-old man with alcoholic liver disease and sudden RUQ pain shows a hyperdense sentinel clot* ➡️ *within and around the liver as well as a spherical hepatic mass* ➡️.

Hepatocellular Carcinoma

Hepatic Cyst

(Left) *Coronal CECT in a woman with cirrhosis and sudden RUQ pain shows a heterogeneous, encapsulated mass* ➡ *that was hyperdense on arterial phase. There is generalized ascites but also a sentinel clot* ➡ *over the mass, indicating the source of bleeding.* (Right) *Axial CECT shows a large mass with a thin wall, characteristic of a simple cyst. Within the cyst is a heterogeneous focus of higher attenuation* ➡, *suggestive of acute hemorrhage. Other sections showed hemorrhagic ascites.*

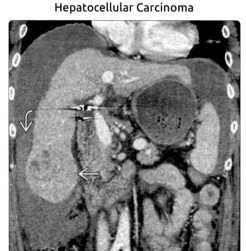

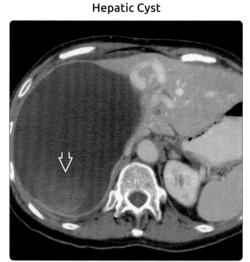

Hepatic Cyst

Hepatic Cyst

(Left) *Grayscale ultrasound shows a hepatic cyst* ➡ *containing a heterogeneous organizing hematoma with fibrin strands* ➡. (Right) *Axial FS T2 MR shows a large, complex cystic mass with dependent settling of material* ➡ *that is hypointense on T2, indicating subacute hemorrhage.*

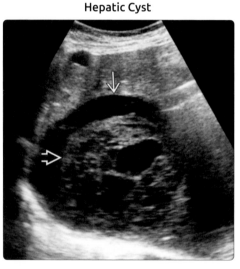

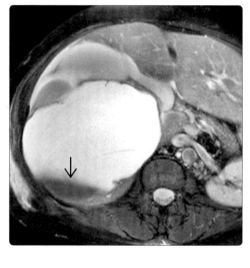

Autosomal Dominant Polycystic Disease, Liver

Coagulopathic Hemorrhage, Liver

(Left) *Axial T1 GRE opposed-phase MR shows many cysts within an enlarged liver. Many of the cysts are of water intensity* ➡ *(dark on this T1), while others* ➡ *are bright, due to hemorrhage.* (Right) *Axial CECT shows signs of coagulopathic hemorrhage, including the hematocrit sign* ➡, *active bleeding* ➡, *and multiple sites of bleeding, including hepatic* ➡ *and renal* ➡.

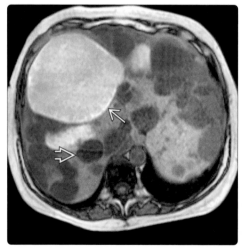

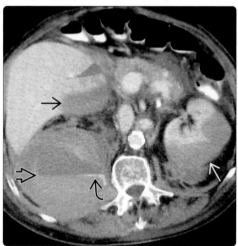

Coagulopathic Hemorrhage, Liver

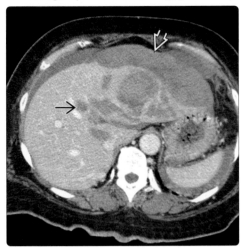

Hepatic Metastases

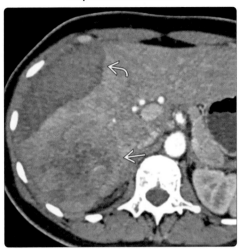

(Left) *Axial CECT in a patient who was taking anticoagulant medication shows hepatic defects that resemble fracture planes* ➡, *but there was no history of trauma. A subcapsular hematoma* ➡ *and hemoperitoneum are also shown. All findings resolved with withdrawal of the medication. No underlying hepatic mass or other pathology was found.* (Right) *Axial CECT shows a large metastatic lesion in the liver* ➡ *from a pancreatic neuroendocrine tumor with a subcapsular hematoma* ➡ *from spontaneous bleeding.*

Hepatic Metastases

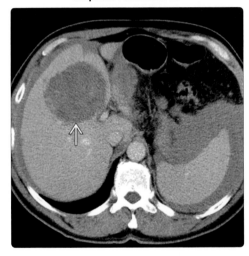

Hepatic Metastases

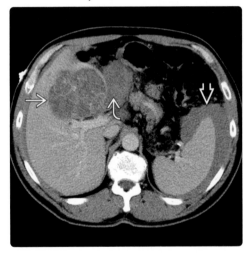

(Left) *Axial CECT in a 55-year-old man with melanoma shows metastasis to the liver* ➡ *that is peculiarly heterogeneous and high density, perhaps indicating bleeding within the metastasis.* (Right) *Axial CECT in a patient with metastatic melanoma and acute RUQ pain shows a hepatic mass* ➡. *Immediately adjacent to this metastasis is a heterogeneous sentinel clot* ➡, *strongly suggesting bleeding from the metastases. Also noted is an extensive hemoperitoneum* ➡ *with an attenuation of 35 HU.*

HELLP Syndrome

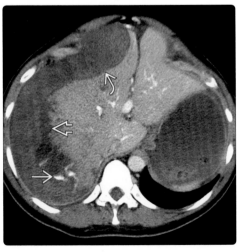

HELLP Syndrome

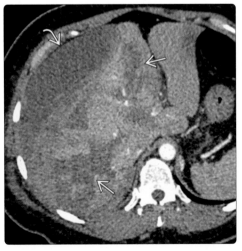

(Left) *Axial CECT in a young woman with toxemia and sudden RUQ pain shows a massive subcapsular and perihepatic hematoma* ➡, *along with active bleeding* ➡ *and heterogeneous enhancement of the hepatic parenchyma* ➡. (Right) *Axial CECT in a postpartum woman with RUQ pain shows a large, subcapsular hematoma* ➡ *and hepatic infarcts* ➡.

DIFFERENTIAL DIAGNOSIS

Common

- Focal Confluent Fibrosis
- Cholangiocarcinoma (Peripheral, Intrahepatic)
- Metastases and Lymphoma, Hepatic
- Hepatocellular Carcinoma
- Peritoneal Metastases (Mimic)

Less Common

- Epithelioid Hemangioendothelioma
- Hepatic Cavernous Hemangioma
- Primary Sclerosing Cholangitis
- Inflammatory Pseudotumor, Liver

ESSENTIAL INFORMATION

Key Differential Diagnosis Issues

- Capsular retraction: Focal hepatic volume loss, usually associated with fibrotic scarring
  - Any hepatic tumor that has undergone necrosis or fibrosis is likely to demonstrate this finding
  - Any process that obstructs intrahepatic bile ducts or portal veins may cause this
    - e.g., cholangiocarcinoma; any form of chronic cholangitis
  - Benign and malignant processes may have similar imaging features

Helpful Clues for Common Diagnoses

- Focal Confluent Fibrosis
  - Common finding in advanced cirrhosis
  - Characteristic location (in segments 8 and 4) and shape (wedge-shaped with capsular retraction and volume loss)
  - Hyperintense on T2WI and shows delayed, persistent enhancement like all fibrotic lesions and does not wash out (↓ in enhancement)
- Cholangiocarcinoma (Peripheral, Intrahepatic)
  - Marked volume loss of liver distal to tumor
  - Often obstructs bile ducts and vessels
  - Delayed, persistent enhancement

- Look for satellite tumors and peritoneal metastases
- Metastases and Lymphoma, Hepatic
  - Untreated mets rarely cause hepatic volume loss or capsular retraction
  - Effective treatment of peripheral hepatic metastases or lymphoma results in volume loss and capsular retraction
  - Breast mets: May result in liver scarring and volume loss (pseudocirrhosis)
- Hepatocellular Carcinoma
  - Hepatocellular carcinoma following treatment (ablation, transarterial chemoembolization) often results in capsular retraction
- Peritoneal Metastases (Mimic)
  - Metastases to peritoneum or hepatic capsule
    - May indent liver surface and simulate capsular retraction
    - Pseudomyxoma peritonei: "Scalloping" of liver and spleen by low-attenuation masses

Helpful Clues for Less Common Diagnoses

- Epithelioid Hemangioendothelioma
  - Rare tumor but classically causes multiple, peripheral, confluent hepatic masses with overlying capsular retraction
  - Target or lollipop appearance on CECT or MR
- Hepatic Cavernous Hemangioma
  - Common tumor that rarely causes capsular retraction
  - Capsular retraction may result from fibrosis (hyalinization) of hemangioma
    - Especially within cirrhotic liver
- Primary Sclerosing Cholangitis
  - Peripheral hepatic fibrosis and volume loss with rounded contours of liver
  - Focal areas of hepatic injury may be mistaken for or mask cholangiocarcinoma
- Inflammatory Pseudotumor, Liver
  - May be indistinguishable from peripheral or hilar cholangiocarcinoma
  - Peripheral lesions result in capsular retraction; show delayed enhancement

Focal Confluent Fibrosis

Cholangiocarcinoma (Peripheral, Intrahepatic)

(Left) Pre- (A) and postcontrast T1 C+ MR images show an area of decreased T1 signal ⇨ and progressive enhancement ⇨ through the arterial (B), venous (C), and delayed (D) phases, indicative of a fibrotic process that is consistent with confluent fibrosis. Capsular retraction ⇨ is seen. (Right) Axial T1 C+ FS MR images show a left lobe liver lesion hypointense on T1 precontrast ⇨ with peripheral enhancement on arterial-phase ⇨ and progressive enhancement on venous ⇨ and delayed phases ⇨. Note capsular retraction ⇨.

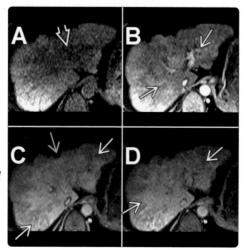

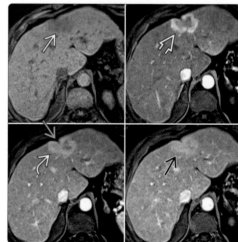

Metastases and Lymphoma, Hepatic

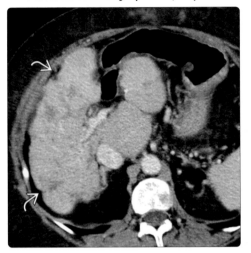

Hepatocellular Carcinoma

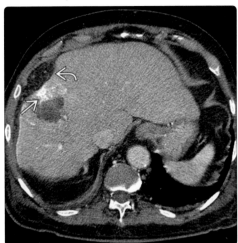

(Left) *Axial CECT shows a pseudocirrhotic-appearing liver in a woman whose hepatic metastases from breast cancer have responded to treatment, with fibrosis and volume loss and with capsular retraction* ➡. **(Right)** *Axial CECT in this patient who had hepatocellular carcinoma (treated with chemoembolization) shows a necrotic mass with retained Lipiodol* ➡. *Retraction of the liver capsule* ➡ *indicates volume loss of the tumor and adjacent liver.*

Peritoneal Metastases (Mimic)

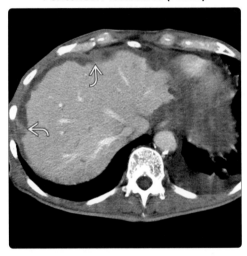

Epithelioid Hemangioendothelioma

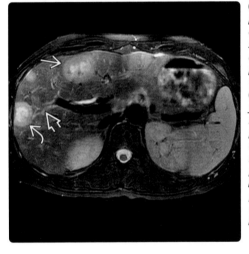

(Left) *Axial CECT in this patient with appendiceal carcinoma shows a scalloped surface of the liver* ➡ *due to extrinsic compression by peritoneal metastases (pseudomyxoma peritonei).* **(Right)** *Axial FS T2 MR in a 38-year-old woman shows several masses with the typical peripheral location and target appearance* ➡. *Capsular retraction over one of the peripheral lesions is present* ➡. *The lollipop sign is also present with the tumor mass and adjacent occluded vein* ➡.

Primary Sclerosing Cholangitis

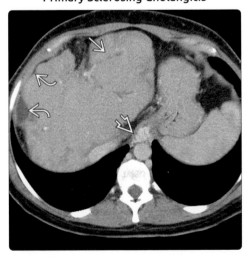

Inflammatory Pseudotumor, Liver

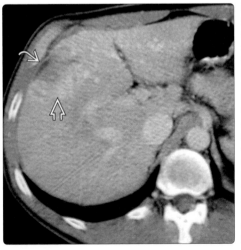

(Left) *Axial CECT shows a small liver with concave margins* ➡ *due to cirrhosis resulting from chronic primary sclerosing cholangitis. Note irregularly dilated intrahepatic bile ducts* ➡ *and esophageal varices* ➡. **(Right)** *Axial delayed-phase CECT shows a hepatic mass with delayed, persistent enhancement* ➡ *and retraction of the overlying capsule* ➡. *While the CT findings suggest a peripheral (intrahepatic) cholangiocarcinoma, the resected lesion proved to be an inflammatory pseudotumor.*

DIFFERENTIAL DIAGNOSIS

Common

- Patchy Steatosis (Fatty Liver) (Mimic)
- Pericaval Fat Deposition

Less Common

- Hepatocellular Carcinoma
- Hepatic Adenoma
- Hepatic Metastases
- Hepatic Angiomyolipoma
- Alcohol-Ablated Liver Tumors (Mimic)
- Fat Within Hepatic Surgical Defect (Mimic)

Rare but Important

- Teratoma or Liposarcoma
- Focal Nodular Hyperplasia
- Xanthomatous Lesions in Langerhans Cell Histiocytosis

ESSENTIAL INFORMATION

Key Differential Diagnosis Issues

- Compare attenuation (CT), intensity (MR), echogenicity (US) of lesion to internal standards
  - e.g., sites of fat and fluid
    - Many lesions simulate fat on 1 modality or sequence but not others

Helpful Clues for Common Diagnoses

- **Patchy Steatosis (Fatty Liver) (Mimic)**
  - Focal steatosis is usually closer to water attenuation, not fat, on CT
    - Vessels traverse lesion undisturbed
    - Along fissures and ligaments within liver
    - Geographic shape: Often lobar, segmental, or wedge-shaped
    - Predisposing factors: Alcoholism, diabetes mellitus, obesity, malnutrition, protein malabsorption, and acquired porphyria cutanea tarda
    - Can be seen post partial or complete pancreatectomy or islet transplantation

- Multifocal hepatic steatosis as variant of fatty liver
  - May have peripheral areas of steatosis with isodense/isointense central areas
  - May have surrounding increased T2 signal and hyperenhancement due to active inflammation
- **Pericaval Fat Deposition**
  - Normal variant
  - May simulate fatty mass in liver or inferior vena cava

Helpful Clues for Less Common Diagnoses

- **Hepatocellular Carcinoma**
  - Usually small foci of fat
- **Hepatic Adenoma**
  - MR shows evidence of fat (lipid) in 35-75% of adenomas; CT < 20%
- **Hepatic Metastases**
  - From liposarcoma, malignant teratoma
- **Hepatic Angiomyolipoma**
  - In 6% of patients with tuberous sclerosis
  - Look for fat-containing angiomyolipomas and cysts in kidneys
- **Alcohol-Ablated Liver Tumors (Mimic)**
  - Alcohol has fat attenuation on CT
- **Fat Within Hepatic Surgical Defect (Mimic)**
  - Omental fat may herniate or be placed into site of resection, ablation

Helpful Clues for Rare Diagnoses

- **Teratoma or Liposarcoma**
  - Primary teratoma of liver extremely rare
  - Retroperitoneal teratoma (or liposarcoma) may indent or invade liver
  - Look for fat, fluid, calcification, soft tissue
- **Focal Nodular Hyperplasia**
  - Fat within focal nodular hyperplasia is vary rare
  - May accompany diffuse steatosis
- **Xanthomatous Lesions in Langerhans Cell Histiocytosis**
  - Langerhans cell histiocytosis is malabsorption disorder of variable severity
  - Hepatic lesions usually periportal location

(Left) A case of mass-like patchy steatohepatitis is shown. Note fat attenuation on NECT ➡ with corresponding signal loss on out-of-phase T1 MR ➡. Bright T2 signal in the area ➡ is due to inflammation. Traversing vessels can be seen on postcontrast T1 MR ➡ due to the "soft" nature of this pseudomass. (Right) Axial CECT shows fat density ➡ surrounding the inferior vena cava, a normal variant. Also present are cirrhosis, regenerative nodules, and varices.

Patchy Steatosis (Fatty Liver) (Mimic)

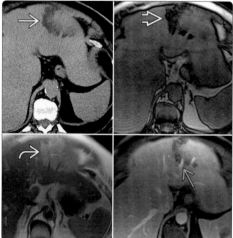

Pericaval Fat Deposition

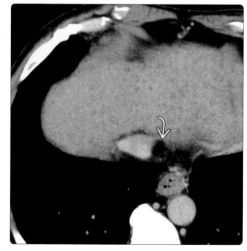

Fat-Containing Liver Mass

Hepatocellular Carcinoma

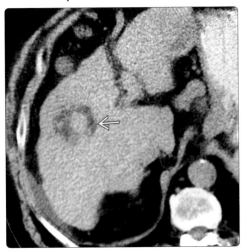

Hepatocellular Carcinoma

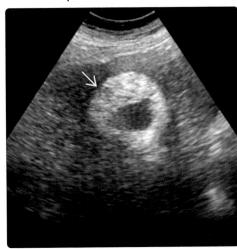

(Left) *Axial NECT shows a cirrhotic liver with a focal mass* ➡ *that has some foci of very low attenuation, indicating fatty metamorphosis. Other portions of the mass showed bright enhancement, washout, and encapsulation, typical features of a hepatocellular carcinoma.* (Right) *Sagittal US shows a very echogenic mass* ➡ *with decreased through transmission, representing hepatocellular carcinoma with fatty metamorphosis.*

Hepatic Adenoma

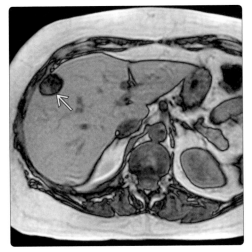

Hepatic Metastases

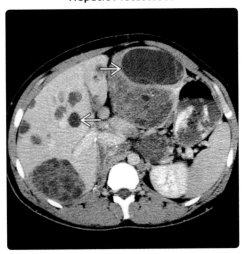

(Left) *Axial T1 MR shows a focal mass* ➡ *that was almost isointense to liver on the in-phase T1 MR with marked signal loss on this opposed-phase image, indicating lipid content. The lesion was hypervascular and encapsulated, typical features of adenoma in a young woman without cirrhosis.* (Right) *Axial CECT shows multiple metastases from testicular malignant teratoma, some with fat attenuation* ➡.

Hepatic Angiomyolipoma

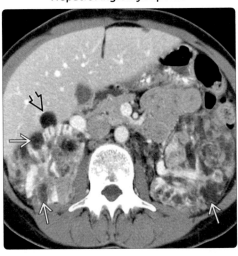

Teratoma or Liposarcoma

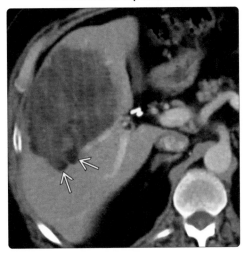

(Left) *Axial CECT shows 1* ➡ *of several fatty hepatic masses in addition to innumerable angiomyolipomas in the kidneys* ➡ *in this patient with tuberous sclerosis.* (Right) *Axial CECT in a patient with primary liposarcoma of the liver is shown. Note a large mass with areas of fat attenuation* ➡.

DIFFERENTIAL DIAGNOSIS

Common

- Hepatic Cyst
- Autosomal Dominant Polycystic Disease, Liver
- Hepatic Pyogenic Abscess
- Biliary Hamartomas
- Metastases, Hepatic
- Hepatic Amebic Abscess
- Biloma/Seroma
- Steatosis (Fatty Liver) (Mimic)

Less Common

- Hepatic Candidiasis
- Hepatic Hydatid Cyst
- Biliary Cystadenoma/Carcinoma
- Biliary Intraductal Papillary Mucinous Neoplasm
- Hepatocellular Carcinoma
- Caroli Disease
- Undifferentiated Hepatic Sarcoma
- Intrahepatic Pseudocyst
- Hepatic Inflammatory Pseudotumor
- Ciliated Hepatic Foregut Cyst

ESSENTIAL INFORMATION

Key Differential Diagnosis Issues

- Any mural nodularity or debris level within cyst should raise concern for tumor, abscess, or hematoma
- Essential to compare current study with prior studies to observe for interval change
  - Simple cysts change size only slowly
  - Abscesses change quickly
  - Treated tumors may simulate cysts [especially gastrointestinal stromal tumor (GIST)]

Helpful Clues for Common Diagnoses

- **Hepatic Cyst**
  - Water attenuation, no visible wall
    - No enhancement of cyst contents
    - MR: Very bright on T2, dark on T1 imaging; no enhancement or mural nodularity
    - US: Sonolucent with acoustic enhancement; no visible wall or nodularity
    - Hemorrhage within simple cyst can be difficult to distinguish from cystic neoplasm
  - 1 or 2 thin septa may be seen
  - Often multiple, of varying sizes
- **Autosomal Dominant Polycystic Disease, Liver**
  - Many cysts of varying sizes
  - Intracyst bleeding results in high-attenuation fluid and calcified cyst walls
  - 2 forms of polycystic liver disease (PLD): Isolated PLD and PLD in association with polycystic kidney disease (PKD)
  - Cannot diagnose autosomal dominant polycystic liver disease just by presence of numerous hepatic cysts
    - Requires cysts in other organs, family history, or genetic testing
- **Hepatic Pyogenic Abscess**
  - Multiloculated, multiseptate cluster of complex cysts
  - Wall and septa may show contrast enhancement
  - Double target sign: Pus surrounded by pyogenic membrane surrounded by edema
- **Biliary Hamartomas**
  - Mimic cysts on CT and MR
  - Multiple small (1-1.5 cm), low-attenuation lesions ± echogenic nodules in walls
  - Lack of larger cystic lesions and cysts in other organs distinguishes this from autosomal dominant polycystic disease
  - Should be considered as likely diagnosis in setting of innumerable small, slightly complex "cysts" in healthy patient
- **Metastases, Hepatic**
  - Most common etiologies
    - Ovarian primary, sarcomas, GIST, etc. after treatment
      - GIST metastasis treated with Gleevec may mimic simple cyst (check history and prior studies)
    - Squamous cell metastases and mucinous adenocarcinoma mets may appear cystic
  - Most have mural nodularity on CT, US, and MR
- **Hepatic Amebic Abscess**
  - Solitary, peripheral, round or ovoid mass
  - Imaging appearance, clinical presentation, and serology are diagnostic
- **Biloma/Seroma**
  - Following trauma, partial liver resection, radiofrequency ablation
  - In setting of liver transplantation, may result from hepatic artery thrombosis with biliary necrosis
    - Biloma in hepatic allograft is ominous finding
- **Steatosis (Fatty Liver) (Mimic)**
  - Focal deposits may be near-water density on NECT (but echogenic, not cystic, on US)
  - MR also definitive, showing selective signal dropout from focal steatotic areas on opposed-phase GRE imaging

Helpful Clues for Less Common Diagnoses

- **Hepatic Candidiasis**
  - Innumerable microabscesses (< 1 cm) with target or wheel appearance
  - Occur in immune-compromised patients
  - Fungal and mycobacterial opportunistic organisms may cause similar appearance
- **Hepatic Hydatid Cyst**
  - Solitary or multiple
  - Discrete peripheral wall ± calcification
  - Mother cyst contains hydatid matrix/sand, daughter cysts
    - Daughter cysts may be smaller spheres within larger cyst or appear as thick septations
- **Biliary Cystadenoma/Carcinoma**
  - Asymptomatic until large
  - Solitary, multiseptate mass with discrete enhancing wall and septa
    - Rarely have no visible septa
  - Complete resection of all parts of tumor essential to prevent recurrence
  - Typically in middle-aged women
- **Biliary Intraductal Papillary Mucinous Neoplasm**
  - Intraductal papillary mucinous neoplasm

- – Analogous to pancreatic intraductal papillary mucinous neoplasm
  - o Tumor within bile duct may rarely produce mucin that distends ducts and may simulate cystic mass
  - o May see nodular, enhancing component (worrisome for cholangiocarcinoma)
- **Hepatocellular Carcinoma**
  - o Spontaneous necrosis (or following treatment) may simulate cystic mass
  - o Usually have solid component with arterial hyperenhancement and delayed washout
- **Caroli Disease**
  - o Cystic dilation of intrahepatic bile ducts
  - o Communication with bile ducts is key feature, distinguishing it from other cystic masses
    - – Recommend MRCP or ERCP
  - o Central dot sign: Dilated ducts surrounding portal vein radicle
- **Undifferentiated Hepatic Sarcoma**
  - o Rare tumor with very aggressive clinical course

- o Typical appearance is large (usually > 10 cm), solitary, encapsulated mass
- o Peripheral hypervascular solid component
- o Often has large complex, cystic spaces with focal hemorrhage
- o Paradoxical appearance: Predominantly solid appearance on US and cystic-like appearance on CT/MR due to high water content of prominent myxoid stroma
- **Intrahepatic Pseudocyst**
  - o May dissect into liver along portal triads
  - o Check for imaging and clinical evidence of pancreatitis
- **Hepatic Inflammatory Pseudotumor**
  - o a.k.a. inflammatory myofibroblastic tumor
  - o Relatively rare with variable appearance
    - – Usually resemble cholangiocarcinoma with delayed, persistent enhancement
    - – Rarely has multiseptate, cystic appearance
- **Ciliated Hepatic Foregut Cyst**
  - o Rare congenital anomaly
  - o Typically small (< 3 cm), cystic mass in segment IV of liver
  - o May appear complex or solid on US

Hepatic Cyst

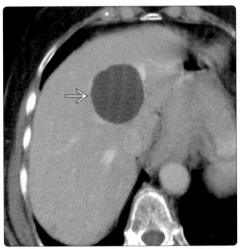

Autosomal Dominant Polycystic Disease, Liver

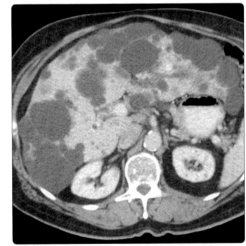

(Left) Axial CECT in a 79-year-old woman shows a spherical liver mass ➔ with water density, homogeneous contents. No internal debris or wall irregularities are present. (Right) Axial CECT shows innumerable hepatic cysts of water attenuation and varying size, causing hepatomegaly. Only a few small renal cysts are present, and renal function is normal.

Hepatic Pyogenic Abscess

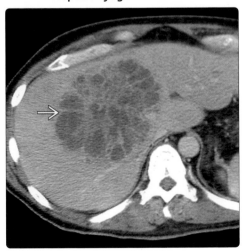

Biliary Hamartomas

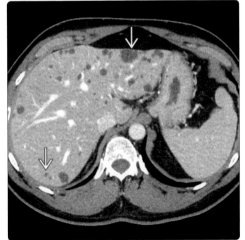

(Left) Axial CECT shows a liver mass with innumerable septa and slightly higher than water density contents ➔. Needle aspiration yielded a small quantity of pus, and a catheter was inserted for drainage. The etiology was subacute diverticulitis. (Right) Axial CECT in a 53-year-old man shows innumerable small, cystic lesions ➔ throughout the liver, ranging in size from 2-15 mm. The lesions are often not perfectly spherical, and many have visible nodular enhancement within their walls.

Biliary Hamartomas

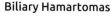

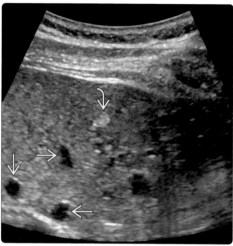

Biliary Hamartomas

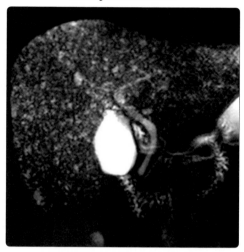

(Left) *US shows only the lesions > 10 mm as cystic structures* ➡, *while the smaller lesions are hyperechoic* ➡ *to background liver. All are typical features of biliary hamartomas.* (Right) *Coronal MRCP shows innumerable small, T2-hyperintense lesions that do not communicate with the biliary tree.*

Metastases, Hepatic

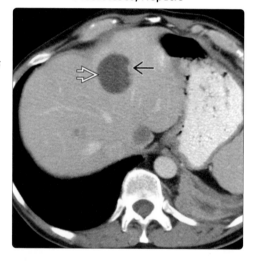

Hepatic Amebic Abscess

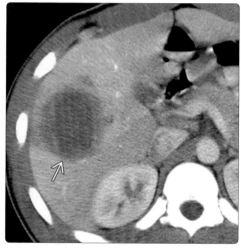

(Left) *Axial CECT shows several hypodense hepatic masses, including 1 cystic lesion* ➡. *The subtle mural nodule* ➡ *is the clue that this is a neoplasm (metastatic thyroid cancer).* (Right) *Axial CECT shows a shaggy, encapsulated, solitary cystic mass* ➡ *with nonenhancing contents, representing a typical amebic abscess. The imaging appearance, clinical presentation, and serology usually suffice for diagnosis.*

Biloma/Seroma

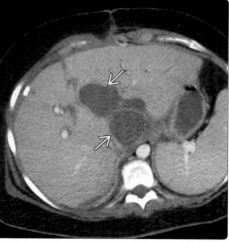

Hepatic Candidiasis

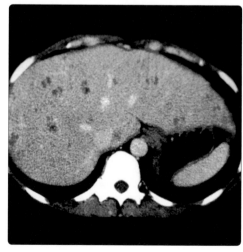

(Left) *Axial CECT 3 weeks after a blunt traumatic liver laceration shows a lobulated, cystic lesion* ➡ *that represents a combination of walled-off bile and blood, also known, respectively, as biloma and seroma. Clinical history and comparison with prior CT scans provide confident diagnosis.* (Right) *Axial CECT in a febrile, immune-suppressed patient shows innumerable small, hypodense lesions in the liver with irregular walls. Other opportunistic hepatic infections may have a similar appearance.*

Hepatic Hydatid Cyst

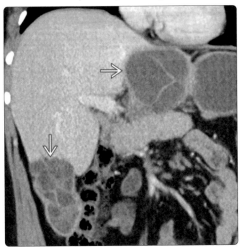

Biliary Cystadenoma/Carcinoma

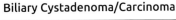
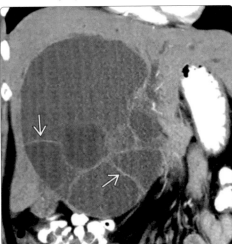

(Left) *Coronal CECT in immigrant from Middle East shows 2 large, multiseptate, cystic masses* ➡. *Within outer pericyst are multiple daughter cysts or scolices. Imaging appearance, coupled with serology, is usually sufficient for diagnosis.* (Right) *Coronal CECT in a middle-aged woman shows complex, cystic mass, lobulated margins, enhancing wall and septa* ➡. *These findings with no other known tumor could be considered sufficiently diagnostic of biliary cystadenoma to warrant resection without further evaluation.*

Biliary Intraductal Papillary Mucinous Neoplasm

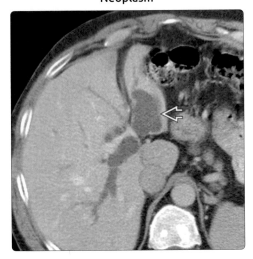

Caroli Disease

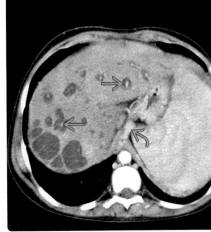

(Left) *Axial CECT of biliary IPMN with cholangiocarcinoma shows dilated intrahepatic bile ducts and a cystic mass* ➡. *ERCP showed opacification of the cyst with contrast and the presence of surface nodularity within the bile ducts.* (Right) *Axial CECT in a woman with portal hypertension due to congenital hepatic fibrosis and Caroli disease shows splenomegaly, varices* ➡, *and multiple hepatic cysts. These represent dilated intrahepatic bile ducts, draped around the central dot of accompanying portal veins* ➡.

Undifferentiated Hepatic Sarcoma

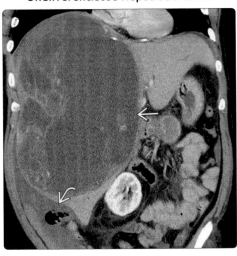

Ciliated Hepatic Foregut Cyst

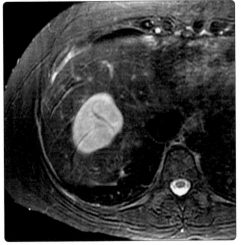

(Left) *Coronal CECT in a man with RUQ pain shows a huge, multiseptate, cystic mass* ➡ *with enhancing peripheral components. Intraperitoneal blood* ➡ *was due to capsular rupture of this undifferentiated primary hepatic sarcoma.* (Right) *Axial T2 MR in a 29-year-old woman with a solid-appearing mass on US shows a complex, cystic-appearing mass in segment 4 that had no enhancement on other sequences. Resection proved ciliated hepatic foregut cyst.*

DIFFERENTIAL DIAGNOSIS

Common

- Hepatic Cavernous Hemangioma
- Focal Nodular Hyperplasia
- Arterioportal Shunt
- Transient Hepatic Attenuation Difference
- Hepatocellular Carcinoma
- Hepatic Metastases
- Hepatic Adenoma

Less Common

- Hereditary Hemorrhagic Telangiectasia
- Nodular Regenerative Hyperplasia
- Fibrolamellar Hepatocellular Carcinoma
- Cholangiocarcinoma (Peripheral)
- Hepatic Angiomyolipoma
- Angiosarcoma, Liver
- Superior Vena Cava Obstruction, Abdominal Manifestations
- Peliosis Hepatis

ESSENTIAL INFORMATION

Key Differential Diagnosis Issues

- Critical to characterize morphology and hemodynamics of hepatic lesions to derive specific diagnosis; examples
  - Cavernous hemangioma, arterioportal shunt, arteriovenous malformation (AVM): Isodense to blood vessels on all phases of imaging
  - Focal nodular hyperplasia (FNH): Nearly isodense (isointense) to liver on nonenhanced, portal venous and delayed phases; homogeneously hyperdense on arterial phase
  - Hepatocellular carcinoma (HCC): Hypodense to liver on NECT, portal venous and delayed-phase imaging; heterogeneously hyperdense on arterial phase
  - Cholangiocarcinoma: Hypodense on NECT, hypo-, iso-, or hyperdense on arterial phase, hyperdense on delayed-phase imaging

Helpful Clues for Common Diagnoses

- **Hepatic Cavernous Hemangioma**
  - Small ("capillary") or flash-filling hemangiomas may enhance quickly and homogeneously
    - May have peripheral transient hepatic attenuation differences (THAD) or transient hepatic intensity differences (THID) changes on arterial phase
  - Enhanced portions of all hemangiomas remain nearly isodense to blood vessels on all phases of imaging (CT and MR)
  - Nodular, discontinuous peripheral enhancement with progressive centripetal fill in for larger hemangiomas
- **Focal Nodular Hyperplasia**
  - Common (~ 2-5%) among young women
  - Homogeneous bright enhancement on arterial phase of enhancement
  - Central scar seen in 2/3 of FNH > 3 cm
  - Nearly isodense (and isointense) to normal liver or nonenhanced, portal venous, delayed images
- **Arterioportal Shunt**
  - Common cause of small, usually peripheral, hypervascular foci within cirrhotic liver

- Usually ≤ 1.5 cm [e.g., cirrhotic arterioportal (AP) shunts]
  - Isodense (and isointense) to liver on nonenhanced portal venous and delayed imaging
  - May result from percutaneous biopsy, percutaneous catheter placement, or other trauma
  - Wedge-shaped area of hyperattenuation with straight margins seen during arterial phase of CECT or MR
  - Becomes isodense to hepatic parenchyma during portal venous phase of CECT or gadolinium-enhanced MR
  - No abnormality on corresponding precontrast T1 and T2 images
  - Look for early filling of portal vein branch
- **Transient Hepatic Attenuation Difference**
  - Peripheral wedge-shaped hypervascular lesion seen only on arterial-phase imaging (CT or MR)
  - Usually due to obstruction of portal vein branch with compensatory increased arterial flow to involved liver
  - Can usually ignore small subcapsular lesion
    - Larger or segmental transient hepatic attenuation difference lesion usually due to mass causing occlusion or compression of portal vein branch (e.g., metastases, HCC, large benign mass, abscess)
- **Hepatocellular Carcinoma**
  - Usually heterogeneously hyperdense on arterial phase with washout to hypoattenuating on portal venous and delayed imaging
  - Look for signs of cirrhosis and invasion of veins and bile ducts
- **Hepatic Metastases**
  - Usually from endocrine primary, melanoma, or renal cell carcinoma
  - Multiplicity, heterogeneity, ring enhancement favor malignancy
- **Hepatic Adenoma**
  - In young women on oral contraceptives or individuals on anabolic steroids
  - Usually heterogeneously hypervascular
  - Often with foci of fat, necrosis, hemorrhage (more evident on MR than on CT)

Helpful Clues for Less Common Diagnoses

- **Hereditary Hemorrhagic Telangiectasia**
  - Part of multiorgan fibrovascular dysplasia (Osler-Weber-Rendu)
    - Telangiectasias and AVMs in liver and other organs (lungs, GI tract, brain, etc.)
    - Patients present with nosebleeds, GI bleeding, hemoptysis
    - Liver: Large hepatic arteries and draining veins with "vascular masses"
    - Heterogeneous enhancement of liver during arterial phase
    - **FNH in patients with hereditary hemorrhagic telangiectasia is 100x more prevalent than general population**
- **Nodular Regenerative Hyperplasia**
  - In Budd-Chiari, congenital heart disease (after Fontan procedure)
  - "Large regenerative nodules" (multiacinar form of nodular regenerative hyperplasia) are common

- o Usually multiple, 1-3 cm; resemble FNH on imaging and pathology
- o Patients with Budd-Chiari also have hepatic and perihepatic venous collaterals that may appear as hypervascular lesions
- **Fibrolamellar Hepatocellular Carcinoma**
  - o Large, heterogeneous tumor with calcification within large scar
  - o 2/3 have metastases at time of diagnosis (nodal, lung)
  - o Usually diagnosed in young adults or children
- **Cholangiocarcinoma (Peripheral)**
  - o Occasionally hypervascular
  - o Look for delayed, persistent enhancement and capsular retraction (not seen in HCC)
- **Hepatic Angiomyolipoma**
  - o Nonfatty portions of mass are hypervascular
  - o Only 50% of hepatic angiomyolipomas (AMLs) have macroscopic fat evident on CT
    - – These are difficult to distinguish from other tumors
  - o May be associated with renal AMLs, ± tuberous sclerosis complex (10%)

- **Angiosarcoma, Liver**
  - o Associated with industrial toxins
  - o Bizarre enhancement patterns; may resemble hemangioma
  - o Multiple lesions in liver and spleen
- **Superior Vena Cava Obstruction, Abdominal Manifestations**
  - o Collateral veins running along diaphragm may pass through liver to inferior vena cava
  - o Broad area of hypervascularity in left lobe on arterial phase; no mass effect
  - o 2 routes: Superior vena cava → superficial epigastric vein → umbilical vein → left portal vein and superior vena cava → internal mammary vein → inferior phrenic vein → portal vein
- **Peliosis Hepatis**
  - o Clinical setting (e.g., AIDS, chronic illness, medications), also *Bartonella* infection
  - o Arterial phase: Early globular, vessel-like enhancement; portal phase: Centrifugal or centripetal enhancement without mass effect on hepatic vessels

Hepatic Cavernous Hemangioma

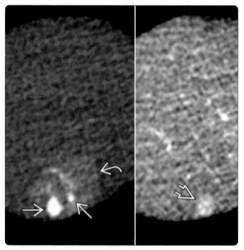

Focal Nodular Hyperplasia

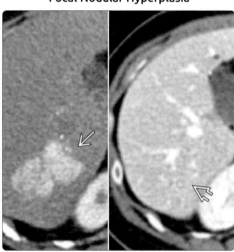

(Left) Axial arterial-phase CECT shows 2 incidentally noted hyperenhancing lesions in the hepatic dome ➡ with adjacent transient hepatic attenuation differences (THAD) ➡, consistent with flash-filling hemangiomas. There is contrast retention on the venous phase ➡. (Right) Axial CECT in a young woman with a right lobe mass shows cloud-like hyperenhancement ➡ on the arterial phase. The mass blends in imperceptibly on the portal venous phase ➡, consistent with focal nodular hyperplasia (FNH). A clear central scar is not visible.

Focal Nodular Hyperplasia

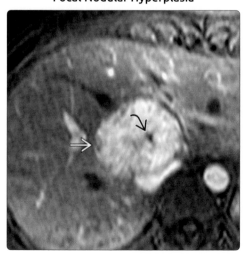

Focal Nodular Hyperplasia

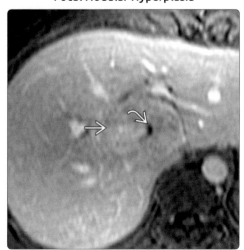

(Left) Axial arterial-phase T1 C+ FS MR shows homogeneous bright enhancement of a hepatic mass ➡ in this young woman. Note the central scar ➡. (Right) Axial portal venous-phase T1 C+ FS MR shows the FNH ➡ is nearly isointense with normal liver. The central small scar ➡ is still well seen and not yet showing delayed enhancement.

Arterioportal Shunt

(Left) *Axial arterial-phase CECT in a cirrhotic patient shows hyperdensity ➡ within the left lobe, which became isodense on portal venous phase. Early filling of the left portal vein ➡ is due to an arterioportal fistula from a biopsy.* **(Right)** *Multiple wedge-shaped, hyperenhancing foci are present mostly in the periphery of the liver ➡ in a patient with hepatitis C cirrhosis on the arterial-phase T1 MR. There are no corresponding areas of abnormality ➡ on the venous phase.*

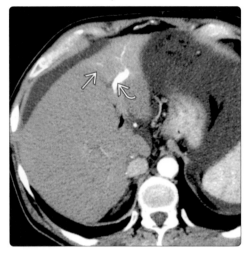

Arterioportal Shunt

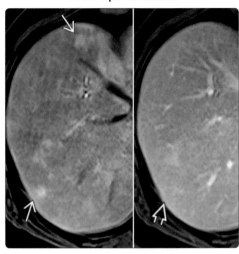

Transient Hepatic Attenuation Difference

(Left) *Arterial-phase CECT in a man with hepatic metastases from pancreatic cancer shows peripheral, wedge-shaped zones of hepatic hyperperfusion ➡ that became isodense to liver on the portal venous phase; this is THAD.* **(Right)** *Axial portal venous-phase CECT in the same patient shows the multiple hypodense, spherical metastases ➡ that caused the THADs seen on arterial-phase CECT. THAD lesions often result from occlusion of portal vein branches by tumor.*

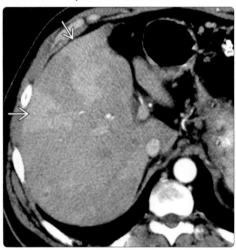

Transient Hepatic Attenuation Difference

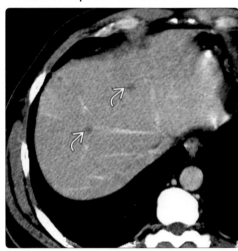

Hepatocellular Carcinoma

(Left) *Axial arterial-phase CECT in a man with cirrhosis shows a heterogeneously hypervascular mass ➡ that "washed out" to become hypodense on portal venous phase, characteristic findings of hepatocellular carcinoma (HCC).* **(Right)** *In a patient with hepatitis C virus cirrhosis, a hyperintense mass ➡ on T2 MR that restricts diffusion ➡ shows arterial hyperenhancement ➡ and washout on the venous phase ➡ with capsular enhancement, consistent with HCC.*

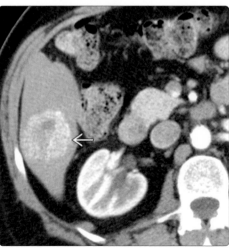

Hepatocellular Carcinoma

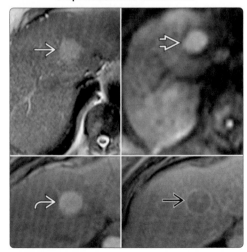

Hepatic Metastases

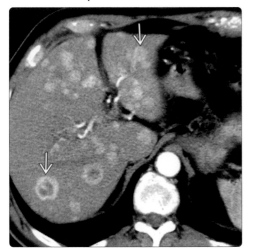

Hepatic Metastases

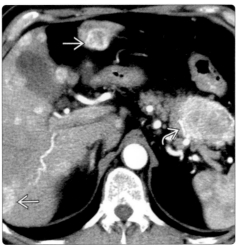

(Left) *Axial arterial-phase CECT in a man with a pancreatic endocrine tumor shows innumerable hypervascular metastases ➡, some of which are ring enhancing.* (Right) *Axial arterial-phase CECT shows hypervascular hepatic metastases ➡. The primary neuroendocrine tumor of the pancreas (malignant glucagonoma) is also evident as a hypervascular mass ➡.*

Hepatic Adenoma

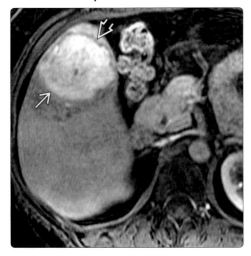

Hepatic Adenoma

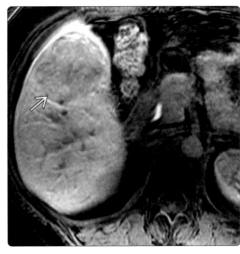

(Left) *Axial T1 C+ FS MR in a young woman in the arterial phase following bolus injection of gadoxetate (Eovist) shows a hypervascular mass ➡ that has a capsule ➡.* (Right) *Axial delayed-phase image of the Eovist-enhanced MR study in the same patient shows the mass ➡ as heterogeneously hypointense to the normal liver. The final diagnosis was hepatic adenoma of the inflammatory subtype.*

Hereditary Hemorrhagic Telangiectasia

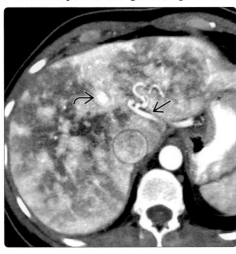

Hereditary Hemorrhagic Telangiectasia

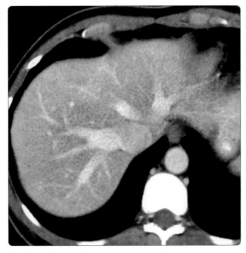

(Left) *Axial arterial-phase CECT in a middle-aged man with a family history of hereditary hemorrhagic telangiectasia (HHT) shows heterogeneous enhancement of the hepatic parenchyma, enlarged, tortuous hepatic arteries ➡, and early opacification of enlarged hepatic veins ➡ and the inferior vena cava (IVC).* (Right) *Axial portal venous-phase CECT in the same patient shows homogeneous enhancement of the liver with dilated hepatic veins and IVC.*

(Left) *Axial arterial-phase CECT in a patient with Budd-Chiari syndrome shows many small hypervascular masses ➡ (large regenerative nodules). Note the occluded IVC ➡, ascites, and a dysmorphic liver.* **(Right)** *Axial portal venous-phase CECT in the same patient shows persistent hypervascularity of the large regenerative nodules ➡ (nodular regenerative hyperplasia). Note the occluded IVC ➡ and collateral veins ➡.*

Nodular Regenerative Hyperplasia

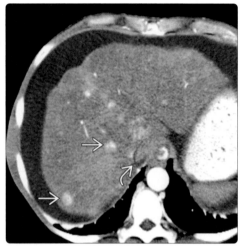

Nodular Regenerative Hyperplasia

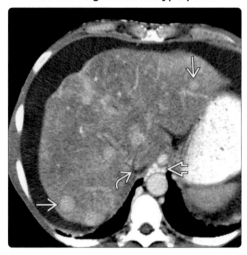

(Left) *Axial arterial-phase CECT in a 22-year-old man shows a mass ➡ that is lobulated and encapsulated with a large, calcified central scar ➡. The mass is heterogeneously hypervascular ➡.* **(Right)** *In the same patient, the hepatic mass ➡ remains heterogeneous on portal venous-phase imaging. The liver does not appear to be cirrhotic. Porta hepatis lymphadenopathy was noted on other images.*

Fibrolamellar Hepatocellular Carcinoma

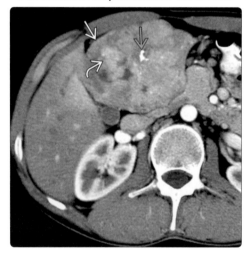

Fibrolamellar Hepatocellular Carcinoma

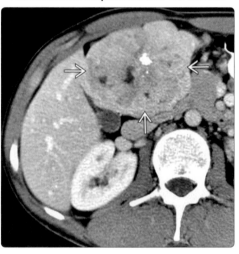

(Left) *Axial arterial-phase CECT in a 67-year-old woman shows a large mass with foci of hypervascularity ➡. Enlarged nodes ➡ in the porta hepatis enhance in a similar manner.* **(Right)** *Axial delayed-phase CECT in the same patient shows heterogeneous, persistent foci of enhancement ➡ that are hyperdense to liver and blood vessels, unlike what would be expected of a cavernous hemangioma. Cholangiocarcinoma was confirmed on biopsy and resection.*

Cholangiocarcinoma (Peripheral)

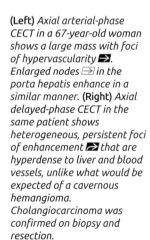
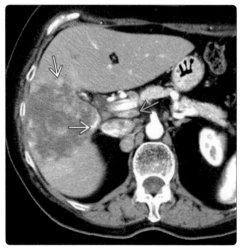

Cholangiocarcinoma (Peripheral)

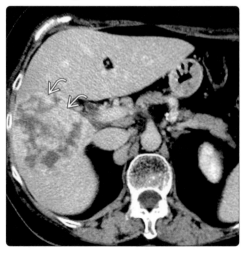

Hepatic Angiomyolipoma

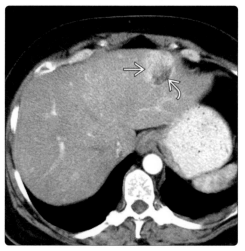

Angiosarcoma, Liver

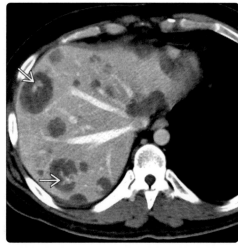

(Left) *Axial arterial-phase CECT shows a hypervascular mass ➦ that also has foci of fat attenuation ➦. Similar angiomyolipomas were present in the kidneys. While these were unsuspected findings, this patient may have a forme fruste of tuberous sclerosis complex.* **(Right)** *Axial CECT shows multiple tumor masses throughout the liver with peculiar eccentric enhancement and hypervascular foci ➦. Similar lesions were present in the spleen and grew rapidly with a fatal outcome within several months.*

Superior Vena Cava Obstruction, Abdominal Manifestations

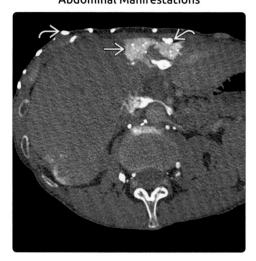

Superior Vena Cava Obstruction, Abdominal Manifestations

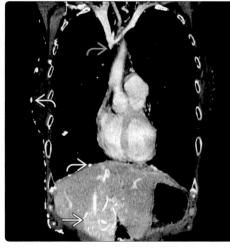

(Left) *In this 60-year-old woman with superior vena cava (SVC) occlusion, axial arterial-phase CECT shows bright enhancement of portions of the left hepatic lobe ➦ along with collateral veins ➦ in the chest wall and capsular surface of the liver. The liver was homogeneous on venous-phase CECT.* **(Right)** *Coronal arterial-phase CECT in the same patient shows the occluded SVC ➦, collateral veins ➦, and the resulting early enhancement of the medial segment of liver ➦.*

Peliosis Hepatis

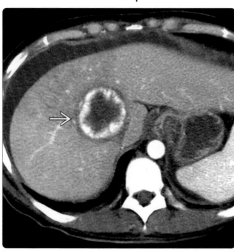

Peliosis Hepatis

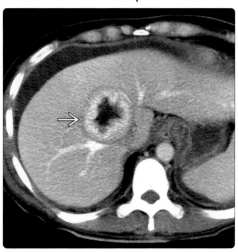

(Left) *Axial CECT shows continuous ring enhancement ➦ on this arterial-phase image. Also note ascites.* **(Right)** *Axial CECT shows progressive fill-in ➦ of the peliosis lesion in a pattern that is similar to that of cavernous hemangioma, although hemangiomas usually have nodular enhancement.*

DIFFERENTIAL DIAGNOSIS

Common

- Hepatocellular Carcinoma
- Metastatic Disease

Less Common

- Hepatic Adenoma
- Fibrolamellar Hepatocellular Carcinoma
- Cholangiocarcinoma
- Combined Hepatocellular Carcinoma-Cholangiocarcinoma

Rare but Important

- Undifferentiated Hepatic Sarcoma
- Solitary Fibrous Tumor
- Hepatic Angiosarcoma
- Primary or Metastatic Liposarcoma

ESSENTIAL INFORMATION

Key Differential Diagnosis Issues

- Presenting as large, heterogeneous mass with multiple smaller nodules or compartments with variable degree of enhancement
  - May have nodule-within-nodule appearance
  - These nodules or compartments are randomly located within larger lesion
- Often incidental
- Usually malignant
- Patient's age and sex may help with narrowing down diagnosis
- Think of unusual appearance of usual diagnosis first rather than rare diagnosis
- Contrast-enhanced multiphase MR may help to assess overall enhancement pattern of mass
- Microscopic fat on chemical shift imaging may help narrow down diagnosis
- Biopsy may be necessary for lesions with overlapping features

Helpful Clues for Common Diagnoses

- **Hepatocellular Carcinoma**
  - Hepatocellular carcinoma (HCC) arising in cirrhotic liver
    - Heterogeneous arterial enhancement with venous washout in large lesions
    - Capsular enhancement on venous and delayed images
  - HCC arising in noncirrhotic liver
    - Bimodal age distribution, peaks in 2nd and 7th decades of life
      □ Fibrolamellar HCC in younger patients
    - Often as large, solitary mass or dominant mass with satellite lesions
    - Size range: 2-23 cm (average: ~ 12 cm)
    - Right lobe more common
    - Well-differentiated → encapsulated with distinct margins, poorly differentiated and aggressive tumors → nonencapsulated, poorly circumscribed
    - ± central/peripheral calcification in fibrolamellar HCC
    - Necrosis, hemorrhage
    - Microscopic &/or macroscopic fat
    - Possible focal intrahepatic biliary dilatation due to mass effect

- More aggressive and direct invasion of adjacent structures or metastasis more common in noncirrhotic patients than in cirrhotic patients

- **Metastatic Disease**
  - Usually multiple; solitary less common
  - Primary malignancy history usually known
  - Large lesions likely from colorectal cancer
    - Assess colon well on imaging or recommend colonoscopy if no known history of primary malignancy
    - May be heterogeneous due to necrosis &/or calcifications from mucinous primary

Helpful Clues for Less Common Diagnoses

- **Hepatic Adenoma**
  - Size range: 6-30 cm
  - Encapsulation seen in ~ 20%
  - Hemorrhage within tumor best seen on NECT as hyperdense foci
  - Calcification: Focal, present in ~ 5%
  - Intratumoral fat
    - Signal dropout on chemical-shift imaging
  - Hypervascularity
    - Most intense and persistent in inflammatory subtype of hepatic adenoma (HA)
  - Heterogeneous signal intensity on MR
    - ↑ signal intensity (due to fat and recent hemorrhage) more evident on MR than CT
    - ↓ signal intensity (necrosis, calcification, old hemorrhage)
    - Rim (fibrous pseudocapsule): Hypointense on T2 imaging

- **Fibrolamellar Hepatocellular Carcinoma**
  - Heterogeneously enhancing, large, lobulated mass with hypointense central scar and radial septa
  - Age range: 5-69 years (mean: 23 years)
  - More common in left lobe
  - Intrahepatic (80%), pedunculated (20%)
  - Central scar and septa (~ 75%): Markedly hypodense
    - Central scar: Avascular
    - Calcification and necrosis are common (> 50%)
  - Nodal metastases (> 50%)
  - Lung metastases common
  - Size range: 5-20 cm (mean: 13 cm)
  - Satellite nodules are often present
  - Slow-growing tumor that usually arises in normal (noncirrhotic) liver
  - Usually, α-fetoprotein levels are normal

- **Cholangiocarcinoma**
  - Peripheral (intrahepatic) variety
  - Usually, diffuse hypoenhancement, peripheral rim enhancement, or diffuse hyperenhancement
    - Can be heterogeneous enhancement
  - Usually large (> 5 cm) at diagnosis with lobulated margins
  - Punctate, stippled, chunky calcifications (18%)
  - Bile ducts will be dilated upstream from tumor
  - Satellite nodules
  - Progressive, gradual, and concentric filling (centripetal) on delayed-phase images

- o Substantial delayed enhancement (i.e., greater than that of liver parenchyma) is common (74%)
- o Infiltrative hepatic mass with capsular retraction and delayed persistent enhancement (contrast-enhanced CT and MR)
- o T2 MR: Hyperintense periphery (cellular tumor) + large central hypointensity (fibrosis), hyperintense foci in center may represent necrosis, mucin
- o DWI MR: Target sign with peripheral hyperintensity due to restriction
- o Metastases to regional lymph nodes, peritoneum

Helpful Clues for Rare Diagnoses

- **Undifferentiated Hepatic Sarcoma**
  - o Majority of patients are children (ages 6-10)
  - o Large (usually > 10 cm), encapsulated, spherical mass
  - o May have peripheral rim of viable, hypervascular tumor
  - o Often has large, complex cystic spaces with focal hemorrhage
  - o Central necrosis, hemorrhage, cystic degeneration
    - – These areas are heterogeneously bright on both T1 and T2 MR
  - o May show signs of vascular invasion
  - o Large subcapsular tumors may rupture and bleed
  - o Lung and osseous metastases are most common
  - o Paradoxical appearance: Predominantly solid appearance on US and cystic-like appearance on CT/MR due to high water content of prominent myxoid stroma
- **Solitary Fibrous Tumor**
  - o Predominantly in women
  - o Usually large at presentation
  - o Well defined, heterogeneously enhancing
  - o ± necrosis
  - o Capsule
  - o Early arterial enhancement in hypervascular component
  - o Enhancement persists into venous and delayed phases in fibrous component
  - o Cystic changes
  - o Calcifications

- o Diffusion restriction on ADC map usually not as marked as tumor
- **Hepatic Angiosarcoma**
  - o Heterogeneous, hypervascular, multifocal malignancy
  - o Multifocal hypervascular masses in liver ± spleen, other organs
  - o Usually have serpiginous areas of hypervascularity
  - o May have peripheral and delayed enhancement simulating hemangiomas
  - o Single or multiple hepatic masses with variable necrosis
  - o T1 MR: Low signal; hyperintense areas due to hemorrhage (if present)
  - o T2 MR: Bright, usually less than hemangioma; hypointense areas due to hemorrhage (if present)
  - o Aggressive features: Blurry boundaries, bleeding, heterogeneity on all sequences (including DWI and hepatobiliary-phase contrast), rapid growth
  - o Diagnosis is rarely established by imaging alone
  - o Rupture in 15-27%

SELECTED REFERENCES

1. Mantripragada S et al: Cholangiocarcinoma - part 2, tumoral and nontumoral mimics and imaging features helpful in differentiation. Curr Probl Diagn Radiol. 51(3):362-74, 2022
2. Desai A et al: Hepatocellular carcinoma in non-cirrhotic liver: a comprehensive review. World J Hepatol. 11(1):1-18, 2019
3. Keraliya AR et al: Solitary fibrous tumors: 2016 imaging update. Radiol Clin North Am. 54(3):565-79, 2016
4. Gaddikeri S et al: Hepatocellular carcinoma in the noncirrhotic liver. AJR Am J Roentgenol. 203(1):W34-47, 2014

Hepatocellular Carcinoma

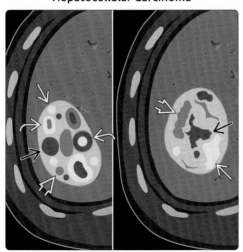

Hepatocellular Carcinoma

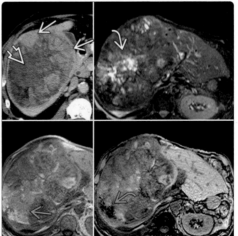

(Left) Graphic shows large liver lesions containing multiple nodules and areas of hyper- ➡, hypo- ➡, mixed ➡, and nonenhancement ➡. (Right) Composite image in a 65-year-old man with no history of cirrhosis shows a large mass containing areas of mosaic enhancement ➡ with areas of necrosis on both CT ➡ and T2 MR ➡, hemorrhage on T1 in-phase MR ➡, and signal dropout on T1 out-of-phase MR ➡, a typical appearance of hepatocellular carcinoma in older patients without cirrhosis.

Liver Mass With Mosaic Enhancement

Hepatocellular Carcinoma

(Left) *Composite image in a 70-year-old man with no history of cirrhosis shows a large, heterogeneous mass with areas of mixed signal intensity on T2 MR ➡, signal dropout on out-of-phase MR ⮫, areas of increased signal intensity on T1 MR ➡, and areas of mosaic enhancement on T1 C+ MR ➡. **(Right)** Axial CECT shows a large liver lesion with heterogeneous, mosaic enhancement and nodular areas of iso- ➡ and hypoenhancement ➡ from primary mucinous colon cancer. Another lesion is also noted ➡.*

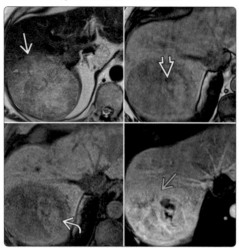

Metastatic Disease

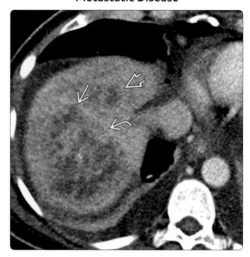

Metastatic Disease

(Left) *Axial CECT shows a large, heterogeneous mass in the right lobe of the liver with mosaic enhancement and nodular increased ➡ and decreased ➡ enhancement. Pathology showed metastatic disease from uterine leiomyosarcoma. **(Right)** Composite image in a 35-year-old woman shows a mass with restricted diffusion on DWI MR ➡, mosaic enhancement on venous phase ➡, slight hypointensity on in-phase ➡, and signal dropout on out-of-phase MR of the lesion ➡ and the liver ➡, findings seen in HNF1A-mutated adenoma.*

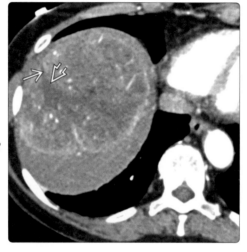

Hepatic Adenoma

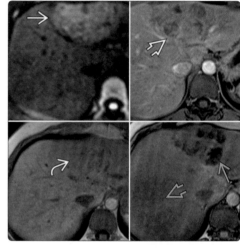

Fibrolamellar Hepatocellular Carcinoma

(Left) *Composite image in a 37-year-old woman shows a large, left hepatic lobe mass that is heterogeneously hyperintense on T2 MR ➡, has hemorrhagic products on T1 MR ➡, and shows mosaic enhancement on arterial- ➡ and venous- ➡ phase T1 C+ MR. **(Right)** Coronal CECT shows a large, heterogeneous mass in the right lobe of the liver with mosaic enhancement and nodular areas of increased ➡ and decreased ➡ enhancement.*

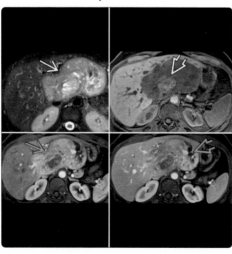

Fibrolamellar Hepatocellular Carcinoma

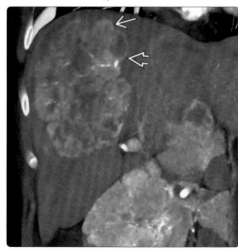

Liver Mass With Mosaic Enhancement

Fibrolamellar Hepatocellular Carcinoma

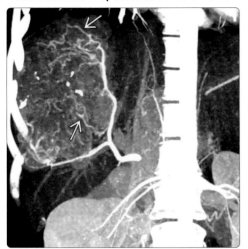

Cholangiocarcinoma

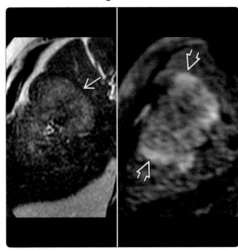

(Left) Coronal CECT MIP shows increased vascularity due to neovascularization ➡. (Right) Axial T2 MR in a 69-year-old man with an incidentally noted mass on chest CT shows a mildly hyperintense mass in the right lobe ➡ with peripheral diffusion restriction ➡.

Cholangiocarcinoma

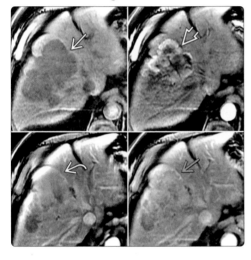

Undifferentiated Hepatic Sarcoma

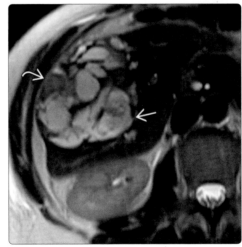

(Left) Axial pre- and postcontrast T1 MR in the same patient shows a hypointense mass ➡ with mosaic arterial enhancement ➡ that progressively fills in on portal venous- ➡ and delayed-phase ➡ imaging. Findings are consistent with cholangiocarcinoma, confirmed on biopsy. (Right) Axial T2 MR in a 47-year-old woman shows a large hepatic mass in the right lobe. The mass is heterogeneous with hyper- ➡ and hypointense ➡ areas.

Undifferentiated Hepatic Sarcoma

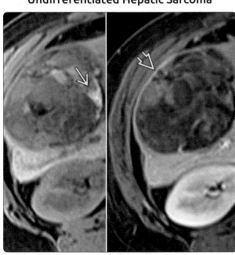

Solitary Fibrous Tumor

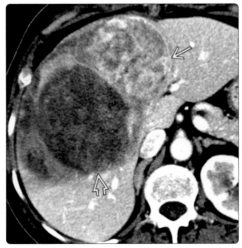

(Left) Axial pre- and postcontrast T1 MR in the same patient shows a hypointense mass with areas of hemorrhage ➡ and mosaic enhancement ➡. (Right) Axial CECT shows a large central liver mass with mosaic enhancement and areas of hyper- ➡ and hypoenhancement ➡.

DIFFERENTIAL DIAGNOSIS

Common

- Passive Hepatic Congestion
- Steatosis (Fatty Liver)
- Cirrhosis
- Hepatitis

Less Common

- Budd-Chiari Syndrome
- Hereditary Hemorrhagic Telangiectasia
- Congenital Hepatic Fibrosis
- Primary Biliary Cholangitis
- Hepatic Sarcoidosis
- Congenital Heart Disease
- Hepatic Lymphoma
- Hepatic Metastases
- Systemic Hypervolemia

ESSENTIAL INFORMATION

Key Differential Diagnosis Issues

- Mosaic liver: Enhances heterogeneously without discrete masses

Helpful Clues for Common Diagnoses

- **Passive Hepatic Congestion**
  - Most common cause; congestive heart failure, tricuspid insufficiency, constrictive pericarditis
  - Hepatic veins and inferior vena cava are engorged
- **Steatosis (Fatty Liver)**
  - May cause diffuse or multifocal hypodensity within liver
  - Favors areas around hepatic veins, fissures, and ligaments
  - Hepatic vessels pass through low-density foci without being displaced or compressed
  - Selective signal dropout on opposed-phase GRE is diagnostic of steatosis
- **Cirrhosis**
  - Fibrosis, regenerating nodules, steatosis all contribute to heterogeneity of liver

- Hepatic veins normal; portal flow may be hepatofugal (reversed)
  - Widened fissures, surface nodularity
- **Hepatitis**
  - Acute viral, alcoholic, or toxic injury
  - Enlarged liver with periportal lymphedema
    - Gallbladder wall edema is also common
  - Hepatic and portal veins: Normal caliber and flow

Helpful Clues for Less Common Diagnoses

- **Budd-Chiari Syndrome**
  - Obstruction of hepatic veins &/or inferior vena cava
  - Small veins (rather than dilated as in passive hepatic congestion)
  - Intrahepatic and perihepatic venous collaterals
- **Hereditary Hemorrhagic Telangiectasia**
  - Osler-Weber-Rendu
  - Numerous arteriovenous malformations and telangiectasias connect arteries and veins
  - Large hepatic arteries and veins
- **Congenital Hepatic Fibrosis**
  - Dysmorphic liver, big arteries, portal hypertension
  - May coexist with Caroli disease, choledochal cysts, renal fibrocystic disease
- **Primary Biliary Cholangitis**
  - Periportal halo (seen in 1/4 patients) → significant fibrosis: Hypointense on T1, hyperintense on T2 MR
  - Heterogeneous T2 signal and postcontrast enhancement
- **Hepatic Sarcoidosis**
  - May simulate or cause cirrhosis
  - Hypodense granulomas and lymphadenopathy
- **Hepatic Lymphoma and Metastases**
  - Homogeneous enlargement of liver ± subtle focal masses
  - Especially common with lymphoma, metastatic breast, and melanoma
- **Systemic Hypervolemia**
  - Excessive IV hydration: Periportal lymphedema and, less often, heterogeneous hepatogram

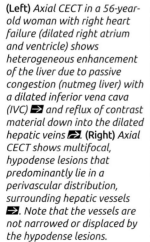

(Left) *Axial CECT in a 56-year-old woman with right heart failure (dilated right atrium and ventricle) shows heterogeneous enhancement of the liver due to passive congestion (nutmeg liver) with a dilated inferior vena cava (IVC)* ➡ *and reflux of contrast material down into the dilated hepatic veins* ➡. **(Right)** *Axial CECT shows multifocal, hypodense lesions that predominantly lie in a perivascular distribution, surrounding hepatic vessels* ➡. *Note that the vessels are not narrowed or displaced by the hypodense lesions.*

Passive Hepatic Congestion

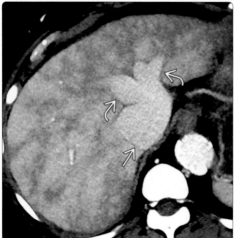

Steatosis (Fatty Liver)

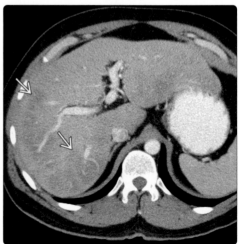

Steatosis (Fatty Liver)

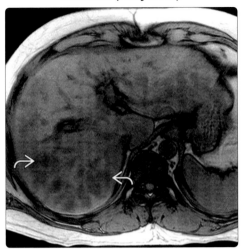

Steatosis (Fatty Liver)

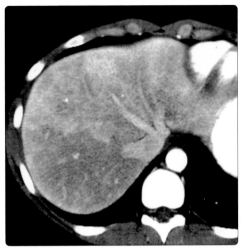

(Left) *Axial opposed-phase GRE MR in a patient with multifocal steatosis clearly shows signal dropout from each of the perivascular foci of steatosis ➘. In-phase GRE MR showed no apparent lesions.* (Right) *Axial CECT shows a patchy appearance of liver, but blood vessels traverse the hypodense areas without deviation or compression, characteristic features of steatosis.*

Cirrhosis

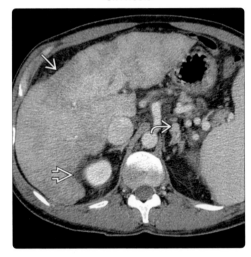

Hepatitis

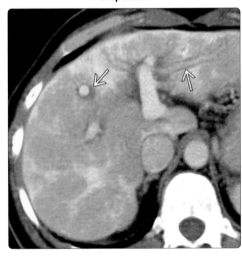

(Left) *Axial CECT in a 47-year-old man with alcoholic cirrhosis shows a heterogeneous liver with ascites ➘, varices ➘, and capsular retraction ➘ overlying a focus of focal confluent fibrosis.* (Right) *Axial CECT shows heterogeneous enhancement of the liver and periportal lymphedema ➘. Biopsy showed severe acute and chronic viral hepatitis.*

Budd-Chiari Syndrome

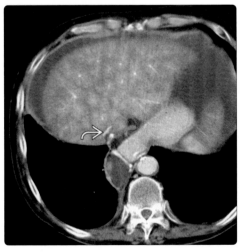

Budd-Chiari Syndrome

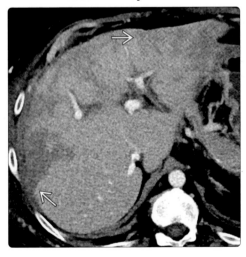

(Left) *Axial CECT in an older adult man who is hypercoagulable due to lung cancer shows massive ascites, heterogeneous mosaic enhancement of the liver parenchyma, and marked narrowing of the IVC ➘. No patent hepatic veins are identified.* (Right) *Axial CECT in a 32-year-old man with Budd-Chiari syndrome shows heterogeneous enhancement of the liver ➘, which can be seen in the chronic phase of the disease.*

Budd-Chiari Syndrome

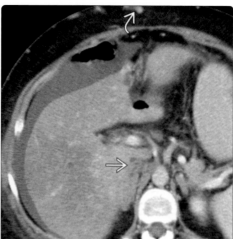

Budd-Chiari Syndrome

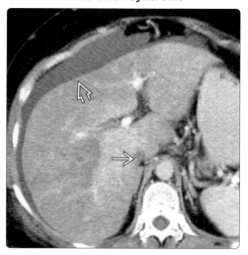

(Left) *Axial CECT in a 45-year-old woman with factor V Leiden deficiency shows a heterogeneous liver with the central right lobe and caudate enhancing normally and the peripheral right and left lobes enhancing poorly. Ascites and collateral veins ➡ are noted. The IVC is thrombosed ➡.* (Right) *Axial CECT in a 45-year-old woman with subacute Budd-Chiari syndrome shows an occluded IVC ➡ and ascites ➡. The liver is dysmorphic with normal density but has a hypertrophied caudate lobe. Peripheral liver has lower density.*

Hereditary Hemorrhagic Telangiectasia

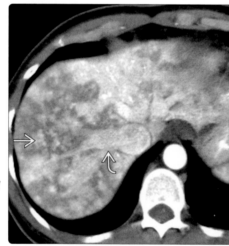

Hereditary Hemorrhagic Telangiectasia

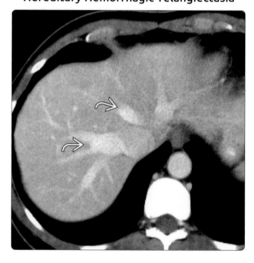

(Left) *Axial arterial-phase CECT in a middle-aged man with hereditary hemorrhagic telangiectasia shows heterogeneous enhancement of the hepatic parenchyma due to telangiectasias and arteriovenous malformations ➡, causing early filling of enlarged hepatic veins ➡.* (Right) *Axial portal venous-phase CECT in the same patient shows a more homogeneous parenchymal enhancement, dilated IVC, and hepatic veins ➡.*

Primary Biliary Cholangitis

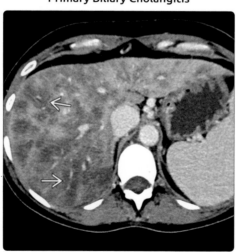

Primary Biliary Cholangitis

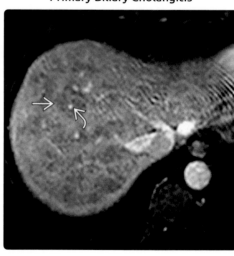

(Left) *Axial CECT shows a periportal halo sign ➡ around the portal veins due to fibrosis centered around the portal triads, which are surrounded by regenerating nodules.* (Right) *Axial portal venous-phase T1 C+ MR shows a periportal halo sign ➡ around the portal veins ➡.*

Congenital Hepatic Fibrosis

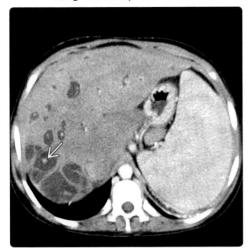

Congenital Hepatic Fibrosis

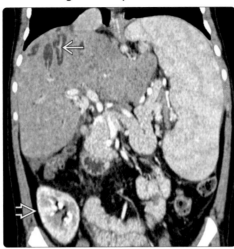

(Left) *Axial CECT in a 40-year-old woman with congenital hepatic fibrosis and Caroli disease, accounting for her portal hypertension, shows a dysmorphic liver and the central dot sign ➡, representing portal vein surrounded by dilated intrahepatic ducts.* (Right) *Coronal CECT in the same patient shows dilated, deformed intrahepatic bile ducts ➡, characteristic of Caroli disease. Note renal allograft ➡, necessitated by congenital renal fibrocystic disease.*

Hepatic Sarcoidosis

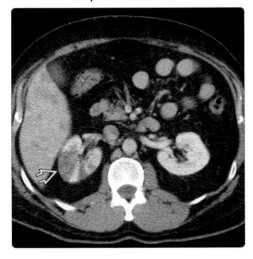

Hepatic Sarcoidosis

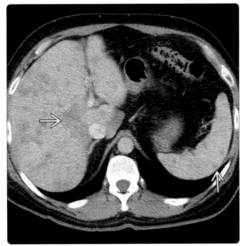

(Left) *Axial CECT in a 45-year-old man with proven sarcoidosis in the thorax, liver, and spleen shows multifocal kidney involvement ➡.* (Right) *Axial CECT in the same patient shows low-density lesions ➡ in the liver and spleen. Sections through the thorax showed extensive mediastinal and hilar lymphadenopathy.*

Hepatic Metastases

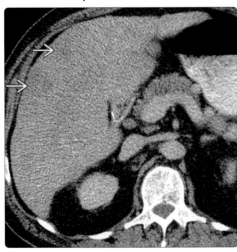

Systemic Hypervolemia

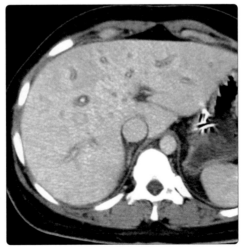

(Left) *Axial CECT in a man with melanoma and hepatic dysfunction shows diffuse low attenuation throughout the liver, suggestive of steatosis. In addition, there are several poorly defined, hypodense lesions ➡. US the next day confirmed innumerable focal, hypoechoic metastases and no evidence of steatosis.* (Right) *Axial CECT shows an enlarged, heterogeneous liver with marked perivascular edema, all due to systemic hypervolemia (overhydration with IV fluids).*

DIFFERENTIAL DIAGNOSIS

Common

- Calcified Granuloma, Liver
- Hepatic Metastases
- Hepatic Arterial Calcification
- Ethiodol-Treated Tumor, Liver

Less Common

- Hepatic Cavernous Hemangioma
- Hepatic Cysts
- Hepatic Hydatid Cyst
- Fibrolamellar Hepatocellular Carcinoma
- Cholangiocarcinoma (Peripheral, Intrahepatic)
- Hepatocellular Carcinoma
- Hepatic Adenoma
- Hepatic Opportunistic Infection
- Portal Vein Calcification
- Intrahepatic Biliary Calculi
- Pancreatobiliary Parasites
- Extrahepatic Calcifications (Mimic)

Rare but Important

- Biliary Cystadenoma or Cystadenocarcinoma
- Focal Nodular Hyperplasia
- Epithelioid Hemangioendothelioma
- Schistosomiasis, Hepatic

ESSENTIAL INFORMATION

Key Differential Diagnosis Issues

- Many more calcified hepatic lesions are evident on CT than on plain radiography
  - Due to greater sensitivity of CT for contrast differentiation
- MR is relatively insensitive to diagnosis of calcification
  - Visible only as focus of signal void due to immobile protons within calcified lesion
- Ultrasound detects calcifications as brightly echogenic foci with acoustic shadow
- Characterize pattern of calcification
  - Examples: Punctate, amorphous, eggshell, tram-track

Helpful Clues for Common Diagnoses

- **Calcified Granuloma, Liver**
  - Most common cause of hepatic calcifications
  - Histoplasmosis > tuberculosis > coccidioidomycosis, brucellosis
  - Multiple (few to dozens) small (few millimeters) punctate calcifications
  - Often present in spleen and lungs as well
  - Usually entire lesion is densely calcified
- **Hepatic Metastases**
  - Usually have faint and amorphous, rather than dense, calcification
  - Mucinous carcinomas of colon (most common), breast, ovary, or stomach
    - Other less common: Melanoma, thyroid carcinoma, neuroendocrine, chondrosarcoma, leiomyosarcoma, neuroblastoma
  - Mixture of fat and calcification seen in metastatic malignant teratoma (uncommon tumor)

- Tumors that become necrotic in response to chemotherapy are more likely to calcify
- **Hepatic Arterial Calcification**
  - Aneurysmal, eggshell, rounded, or tram-track calcification
  - Diabetic arteriopathy; long segmental calcifications of medium-sized arteries, including hepatic
- **Ethiodol-Treated Tumor, Liver**
  - Iodized poppy seed oil (Lipiodol) administered intraarterially, localizes in hepatocellular carcinoma and other tumors
  - Used as adjunct to diagnosis and therapy
  - Spherical collection within tumor
  - Usually even more dense than calcified hepatic lesions
    - Check for history of angiographic treatment; check prior scans

Helpful Clues for Less Common Diagnoses

- **Hepatic Cavernous Hemangioma**
  - Large hemangiomas often have central scar that may calcify in 10-20% cases
    - Phlebolith-like thrombi within vascular channels less common
  - Remainder of mass will show characteristic features of hemangioma
    - Peripheral nodular enhancement, progressive fill-in, isodense to blood vessels
  - Also seen in sclerosing hemangioma
- **Hepatic Cysts**
  - Cyst wall calcification uncommon
- **Hepatic Hydatid Cyst**
  - Wall and contents may calcify
    - Curvilinear or ring calcification
  - May get calcified hydatid sand in dependent portion of cyst
  - Complete wall calcification is usually sign of inactive hydatid infection
- **Fibrolamellar Hepatocellular Carcinoma**
  - Typically affects young adults
  - Uncommon tumor but usually (> 60%) has large, central scar with calcification
  - Tumor is large at presentation (> 10 cm) with heterogeneous enhancement
  - Most have lymphatic &/or other metastases (lung, bone) at time of presentation
- **Cholangiocarcinoma (Peripheral, Intrahepatic)**
  - Fibrotic mass arising from intrahepatic bile ducts
  - Causes volume loss of affected part of liver with capsular retraction
  - Calcification is uncommon feature
- **Hepatocellular Carcinoma**
  - Much more common than fibrolamellar hepatocellular carcinoma but uncommonly has calcification
  - May have punctate or irregular scar calcification
- **Hepatic Adenoma**
  - Punctate or capsular calcification seen in minority of cases
  - Other features include foci of hemorrhage and fat (more evident on MR than on CT)
- **Hepatic Opportunistic Infection**
  - Cytomegalovirus, toxoplasma, pneumocystic, etc.

- o Few to innumerable punctate calcifications
- o Seen in patients with AIDS, bone marrow or organ transplantation
- **Portal Vein Calcification**
  - o Calcification of wall due to portal hypertension
  - o Portal vein thrombus may calcify
  - o May result from bland thrombus; may follow septic thrombophlebitis
- **Intrahepatic Calculi and Biliary Parasites**
  - o Often coexist; more common in Asian populations
  - o *Clonorchis* (liver fluke) is common
  - o Calcium bilirubinate stones in recurrent pyogenic cholangitis are often calcified
  - o Fascioliasis: Liver fluke found in South and Central America
    - – Low-density nodular and branching lesions, often subcapsular; other findings: Hepatic capsule thickening, subcapsular hematoma, nodular calcifications
- **Extrahepatic Calcifications (Mimic)**

- o Calcification in pleura, peritoneum, gallbladder, kidney, etc.
- o May overlap liver and mimic hepatic calcification

Helpful Clues for Rare Diagnoses

- **Biliary Cystadenoma or Cystadenocarcinoma**
  - o Thick, fibrous capsule with rare calcification
- **Focal Nodular Hyperplasia**
  - o Calcification in central scar is extremely rare and small relative to size of entire lesion
- **Epithelioid Hemangioendothelioma**
  - o Rare malignant tumor of lower aggressiveness
  - o Typically causes multiple confluent peripheral hepatic masses
    - – Dystrophic calcifications in ~ 20%
    - – Characteristic retraction of overlying hepatic capsule
- **Schistosomiasis, Hepatic**
  - o Calcification of ova more common in *Schistosoma japonicum*; endemic in parts of Asia
  - o Causes dystrophic calcification and fibrosis in liver
    - – CT appearance: Turtle back pattern

Calcified Granuloma, Liver

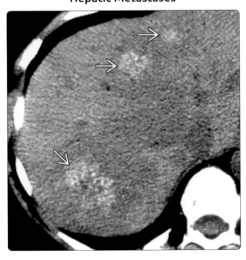

Hepatic Metastases

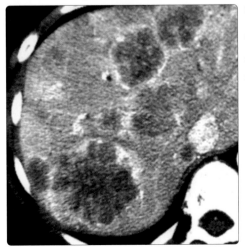

(Left) Axial NECT shows multiple small focal calcifications ➡ in the liver and spleen, which are typically healed granulomas, usually from histoplasmosis or tuberculosis. (Right) Axial NECT shows several calcified metastases ➡ from mucinous adenocarcinoma of the colon.

Hepatic Metastases

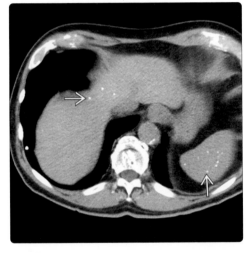

Hepatic Metastases

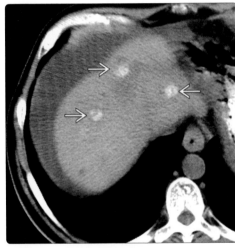

(Left) Axial NECT in a man with primary colon cancer shows faint calcification ➡ within several metastatic foci. (Right) Axial CECT in the same patient shows rim enhancement of the metastases. Note that the calcification is much less evident after contrast administration.

Hepatic Arterial Calcification

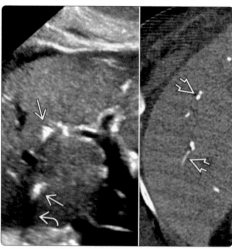

Ethiodol-Treated Tumor, Liver

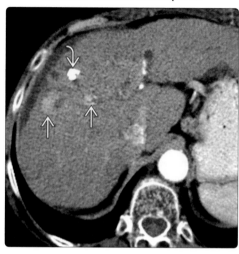

(Left) *Echogenic foci* ➡ *with posterior acoustic shadowing* ➡ *on US correspond to severe vascular calcification on NECT* ➡. *Please note that this can be mistaken for biliary or portal venous air.* (Right) *Axial CECT shows hypervascular foci of viable hepatocellular carcinoma* ➡ *on this arterial-phase CECT. The very dense focus* ➡ *is residual Lipiodol that had been given as part of intraarterial chemotherapy.*

Hepatic Cavernous Hemangioma

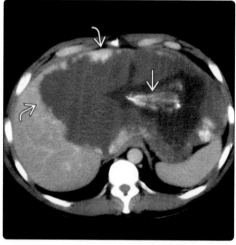

Hepatic Hydatid Cyst

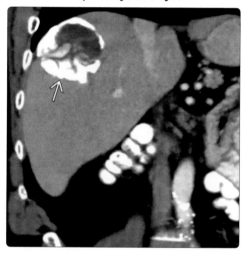

(Left) *Axial CECT shows a huge hepatic cavernous hemangioma with typical peripheral nodular enhancement* ➡. *Note the calcification* ➡ *within the large central scar.* (Right) *Cystic lesion in the liver with curvilinear ring-like calcification of wall* ➡ *is shown. This usually indicates no active infection if calcification is completely circumferential.*

Fibrolamellar Hepatocellular Carcinoma

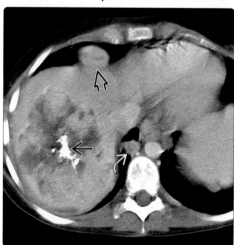

Hepatocellular Carcinoma

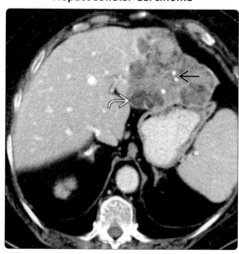

(Left) *Axial CECT shows a large mass in the right lobe in this adolescent boy. Note the calcification* ➡ *within the large, poorly enhancing scar and cardiophrenic lymphadenopathy* ➡. *Also present are lung metastases* ➡. (Right) *Axial CECT shows a heterogeneous left lobe mass that contains foci of fat density* ➡ *as well as focal calcifications* ➡. *While uncommon, these features are suggestive of hepatocellular carcinoma when seen in a mass within a cirrhotic liver.*

Hepatic Adenoma

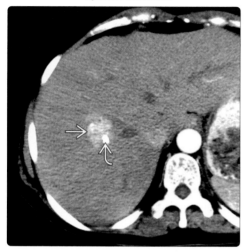

Hepatic Adenoma

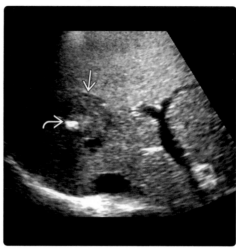

(Left) *Axial arterial-phase CECT in a young woman with hepatic adenoma shows a hypervascular mass* ➡️ *with eccentric calcification* ➡️. (Right) *Sagittal US in the same patient shows an encapsulated mass* ➡️ *with a heterogeneous echo pattern and a focus of bright signal* ➡️ *with acoustic shadowing.*

Portal Vein Calcification

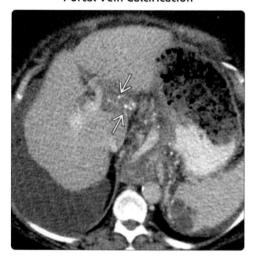

Portal Vein Calcification

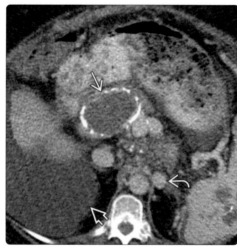

(Left) *Axial CECT in a 61-year-old woman with cirrhosis shows calcification in the porta hepatis within the walls of the portal vein* ➡️. (Right) *Axial CECT in the same patient shows eggshell calcification* ➡️ *that represents an aneurysmally dilated and thrombosed portal vein and varix. Note the other varices* ➡️, *small cirrhotic liver, and ascites* ➡️.

Intrahepatic Biliary Calculi

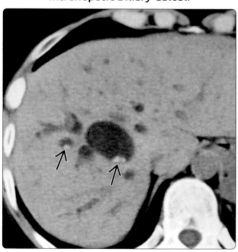

Focal Nodular Hyperplasia

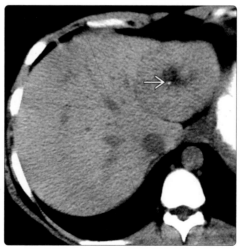

(Left) *Axial CECT shows calculi* ➡️ *within massively dilated cystic dilations of the intrahepatic ducts in a patient with Caroli disease.* (Right) *Axial NECT shows a tiny focus of calcification* ➡️ *in the central scar of an otherwise typical focal nodular hyperplasia (FNH). The mass showed bright homogeneous enhancement on arterial-phase CECT, and the calcification became less apparent. Calcification in an FNH is quite rare.*

DIFFERENTIAL DIAGNOSIS

Common

- Hepatic Pyogenic Abscess
- Hepatic Infarction
- Hepatic Tumor Following Treatment
  - Hepatocellular Carcinoma
  - Metastases and Lymphoma, Hepatic
  - Hepatic Adenoma
- Gas in Bile Ducts or Gallbladder
- Portal Venous Gas
- Hepatic Venous Gas

Less Common

- Retained Foreign Body
- Hepatic Transplantation
- Biloma
- Hepatic Amebic Abscess
- Hepatic Hydatid Cyst
- Hepatic Trauma
- Hepatic Venous Gas

ESSENTIAL INFORMATION

Key Differential Diagnosis Issues

- 5 pathways to developing gas
  - Infection by gas-forming organism
  - Infarction of liver or lesion
  - Open wound or surgical drain
  - Reflux of gas into lesion from biliary tree
  - Gas within portal veins

Helpful Clues for Common Diagnoses

- **Hepatic Pyogenic Abscess**
  - 4 major routes for bacteria to liver
    - Portal vein thrombophlebitis
      - □ Most often due to subacute diverticulitis or (less commonly) appendicitis
    - Ascending cholangitis
      - □ Usually associated with choledocholithiasis, ± incompetence of sphincter of Oddi
      - □ Surgical biliary-enteric anastomosis also predisposes to ascending cholangitis
    - Direct extension
      - □ e.g., perforated ulcer or diverticulitis of colonic hepatic flexure
    - Traumatic
      - □ Usually penetrating or iatrogenic (hepatic or biliary surgery)
  - Multiseptate or cluster of grapes appearance of abscess
  - Gas is present in ~ 20% of pyogenic abscesses
    - Gas-producing organisms (*Escherichia coli* and *Klebsiella pneumoniae* most common)
  - Present in small foci or as gas-fluid level
  - Often accompanied by transient hepatic attenuation difference (THAD) due to hyperemia and thrombophlebitis of portal vein branch
  - CT: Double target sign
    - Low-attenuation central zone (liquefied necrotic tissue/pus)
    - High-attenuation inner rim (pyogenic membrane)
    - Low-attenuation outer layer (edema of liver parenchyma)
  - Rim, capsule, and septal enhancement
    - May be multiseptate or cluster of smaller abscesses
  - MR findings
    - T1: Hypointense to hyperintense mass
    - T2: Variably hyperintense mass, high signal intensity perilesional edema
    - T1 C+: Hypointense pus in center, rim or capsule enhancement; small abscesses < 1 cm may show homogeneous enhancement
    - DWI: Restriction
- **Hepatic Infarction**
  - Uncommon due to dual blood supply
    - Usually requires interruption of both portal venous and hepatic arterial supply
  - Etiologies
    - Iatrogenic (cholecystectomy, hepatobiliary surgery, transjugular intrahepatic portosystemic shunt, Whipple)
    - Liver transplantation (hepatic artery stenosis or thrombosis)
    - Blunt trauma
    - Hypercoagulable states and vasculitis
  - Wedge-shaped, rounded, ovoid, or irregularly shaped low-attenuation areas parallel to bile ducts
  - More conspicuous after enhancement (as perfusion defects)
  - Bile lakes seen as late sequela
    - Especially in liver transplant setting
    - Hepatic artery thrombosis → biliary and hepatic necrosis
- **Hepatic Tumor Following Treatment**
  - Any treatment that results in sudden death of substantial amount of tissue (benign or malignant)
    - Chemoembolization
    - Radiofrequency or cryoablation
    - Chemotherapy, especially transarterial chemoembolization
    - Surgical ligation of hepatic arterial branch
  - Imaging, symptoms, and laboratory signs closely mimic hepatic abscess
    - Fever, leukocytosis, and pain are common
  - Presence of hepatic gas immediately following surgery does not necessarily imply infection
  - Injection of ethanol for ablation may mimic or cause intrahepatic gas
    - Ethanol is of near-gas attenuation
- **Gas in Bile Ducts or Gallbladder**
  - Many potential causes
  - Pneumobilia, incompetent sphincter of Oddi, emphysematous cholecystitis, sphincterotomy, etc.
  - Gas collects in central bile ducts near porta hepatis
- **Portal Venous Gas**
  - Mesenteric ischemia, bowel necrosis, and other causes
  - Branching pattern favoring periphery of liver
  - Look for bowel wall pneumatosis, mesenteric vascular thrombosis, and related findings

Helpful Clues for Less Common Diagnoses

- **Retained Foreign Body**

- Retained surgical sponge: Will have opaque stripe
  - Retained sponge (gossypiboma) often leads to abscess
  - Sponge is often surrounded by larger collection of fluid with enhancing rim
- Oxidized surgical gelatin (Surgicel): Used for intraoperative hemostasis
  - Multifocal gas without fluid component
  - May have linear or curvilinear collections of gas
  - Does not imply infection
- **Hepatic Transplantation**
  - Biliary gas may be expected following biliary-enteric anastomosis
  - Portal venous gas in early posttransplant period (< 9 days) is often insignificant
  - Hepatic artery thrombosis (HAT) or stenosis may cause biliary necrosis
    - Typical appearance is branching fluid collections paralleling portal triads
    - Usually no gas within these collections unless there is biliary gas (as with biliary-enteric anastomosis)
      - ☐ Bacterial superinfection of infarcted tissue may release gas
  - Less commonly, allograft parenchymal infarction may result from HAT
    - Gas may be found within hepatic allograft itself
- **Biloma**
  - Communication with bile ducts may allow gas to enter biloma
  - Infection of biloma by gas-forming organisms may release gas
  - HAT → biliary and hepatic necrosis
- **Hepatic Amebic Abscess**
  - Usually solitary
  - Often has capsule
  - Right lobe (70-80%), usually peripheral; associated right-sided atelectasis and pleural effusion
  - Uncommonly septate
  - Gas is rare unless abscess becomes superinfected with bacteria or ruptures into GI tract

- Often see THAD due to thrombophlebitis of portal vein and hyperemia of abscess capsule
- **Hepatic Hydatid Cyst**
  - Usually large
  - Multiseptate
  - Often has calcified wall
  - Rarely has gas unless superinfected or communicating with gut
  - Mother cyst contains hydatid matrix/sand + daughter cysts
  - T2 MR: Daughter cysts: Bright, increased intensity relative to matrix
  - US: Multiseptate cyst with daughter cysts and echogenic material between cysts
- **Hepatic Trauma**
  - Gas may be found in hepatic or portal veins or liver parenchyma
  - Often transient and of little significance
  - Larger areas of parenchymal gas may follow traumatic hepatic infarction
    - Due to devascularization of affected segment
- **Hepatic Venous Gas**
  - Usually iatrogenic, introduced through air in IV infusion lines
    - More common with femoral vein catheterization
    - More common with aggressive, rapid IV infusions

Hepatic Pyogenic Abscess

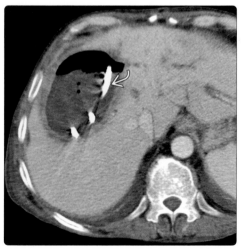

Hepatic Pyogenic Abscess

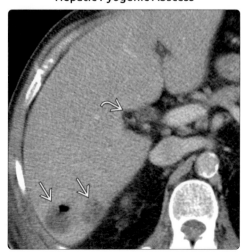

(Left) Axial CECT shows a liver abscess with fluid and gas. Note the percutaneously placed drainage catheter ➦. (Right) Axial CECT shows 2 abscesses ➥, one of which contains gas. This patient has ascending cholangitis, and gas may enter the abscesses from gas-containing ducts ➥ or result from infection itself.

(Left) *Axial CECT shows nonenhancement of the left lobe* ➡ *with portal venous gas* ➡*; infarction followed attempted resection of peripheral cholangiocarcinoma.* **(Right)** *Axial CECT shows devascularization of the right lobe from blunt trauma. The hepatic artery and veins to the right lobe were avulsed. The gas bubble* ➡ *is due to infarction, not infection.*

Hepatic Infarction

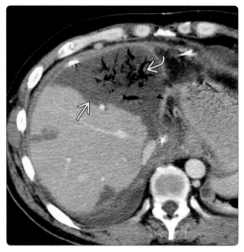

Hepatic Infarction

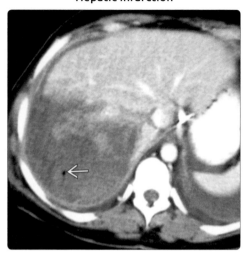

(Left) *Axial CECT in a colon cancer patient shows metastases* ➡*, some of which have been treated with radiofrequency ablation. One of these has gas within it as well as surgical clips* ➡*, the latter the result of bleeding after ablation that required intervention. Gas bubbles are not the result of infection but rather infarction of hepatic tissue (or tumor).* **(Right)** *Axial CECT shows 2 large hepatic masses* ➡ *(metastatic breast cancer). The larger lesion has gas due to tumor infarction as a result of chemotherapy; there was no infection.*

Hepatic Tumor Following Treatment

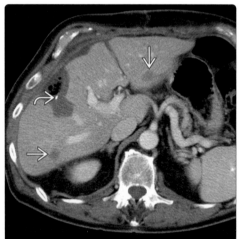

Hepatic Tumor Following Treatment

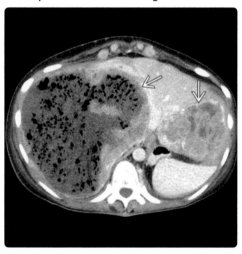

(Left) *Axial T2 MR in a 63-year-old man with pancreatic cancer and right upper quadrant pain shows fluid and air* ➡ *corresponding to T1-hyper- and hypointense signal, respectively, on T1 pre-* ➡*, arterial-* ➡*, and venous-* ➡ *phase images with absence of enhancement, representing a gas-containing abscess.* **(Right)** *Coronal CECT shows extensive bowel pneumatosis* ➡ *from ischemia and portal venous gas in the periphery of the liver* ➡*.*

Portal Venous Gas

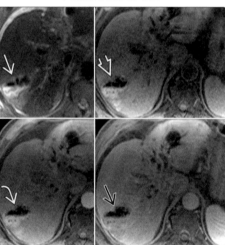

Portal Venous Gas

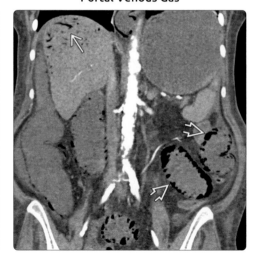

Portal Venous Gas

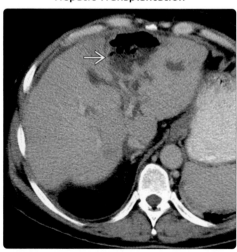

Retained Foreign Body

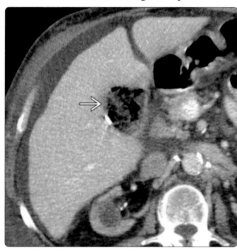

(Left) *US in a woman with cirrhosis and acute abdominal pain following a hypotensive episode shows bubbles of gas ➡ within the portal veins. CT showed pneumatosis within bowel walls and luminal distention with fluid due to bowel infarction.* **(Right)** *Axial CECT shows a surgical clip and collection of gas ➡ in or adjacent to the liver. This is oxidized surgical gelatin (Surgicel) that was used as a hemostatic device and left in place. Note the relative absence of fluid within the collection.*

Retained Foreign Body

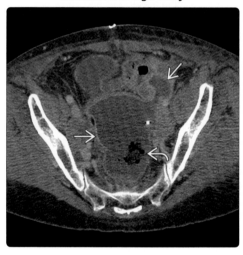

Hepatic Transplantation

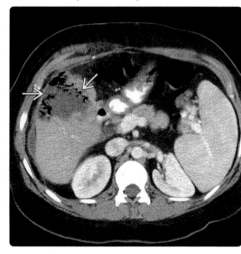

(Left) *Axial CECT shows a large postoperative abscess ➡. Within the abscess, there is a tightly packed collection of gas bubbles ➡ that represents oxidized surgical cellulose (Surgicel) that had been placed to control bleeding at surgery.* **(Right)** *Axial CECT in a patient with hepatic allograft malfunction shows a wedge-shaped collection of fluid and gas ➡, representing an infected biloma due to hepatic artery thrombosis.*

Hepatic Transplantation

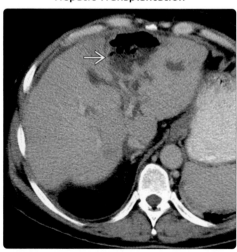

Biloma

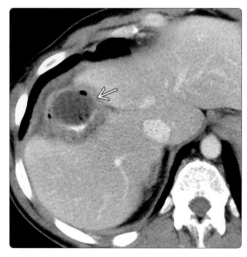

(Left) *Axial CECT in a patient with acute dysfunction of a hepatic allograft shows a collection of gas and fluid ➡ in the left hepatic lobe, strongly suggestive of an infected biloma due to hepatic artery stenosis or thrombosis. Arterial thrombosis was subsequently confirmed.* **(Right)** *Axial CECT shows a focal collection of fluid and gas ➡ that was the result of a deep liver laceration several days prior.*

DIFFERENTIAL DIAGNOSIS

Common

- Ischemic Enteritis
- Ischemic Colitis
- Pneumatosis of Intestine
- Postoperative Bowel
- Pneumobilia (Mimic)

Less Common

- Diverticulitis
- Appendicitis
- Small Bowel Obstruction
- Pancreatitis, Acute
- Abdominal Abscess
- Hepatic Infarction
- Ulcerative Colitis
- Infectious Colitis
- Caustic Gastritis

ESSENTIAL INFORMATION

Key Differential Diagnosis Issues

- Almost any cause of infection, inflammation, trauma, or ischemia of any part of GI tract, including pancreas, may result in portal venous gas
- Any cause of pneumatosis may result in portal venous gas (or free intraperitoneal gas)
  - Causes include medications (especially immunosuppressive), endoscopy, bowel anastomoses
- CT and US detect portal venous gas more commonly than radiography

Helpful Clues for Common Diagnoses

- **Ischemic Enteritis**
  - Small bowel ischemia is more likely to progress to infarction than colonic ischemia
  - Intramural pneumatosis usually accompanies portal venous gas, but these are late and ominous signs of infarction
- **Ischemic Colitis**

- Segmental colonic wall thickening in watershed distribution ± pneumatosis and portal venous gas
- May progress to infarction with portal venous gas but more likely to resolve spontaneously or evolve into stricture
- **Pneumatosis of Intestine**
  - Any cause of pneumatosis may lead to portal venous gas, including medications, bowel obstruction, or anastomosis
  - Even benign pneumatosis cystoides of colon can cause portal venous gas
- **Pneumobilia (Mimic)**
  - Gas within bile ducts may be mistaken for portal venous gas on radiography, CT, US
  - **Gas within bile ducts tends to collect more centrally within liver**
    - **Portal venous gas flows toward periphery of liver**

Helpful Clues for Less Common Diagnoses

- **Diverticulitis and Appendicitis**
  - Chronic untreated inflammation of colon, appendix, or small bowel may result in mesenteric and portal vein thrombophlebitis
  - Veins may have thickened walls, luminal gas, progress to thrombosis
  - Look for associated pyogenic liver abscess
- **Pancreatitis, Acute**
  - Especially severe or necrotizing pancreatitis, ± infection
- **Hepatic Infarction**
  - Especially if iatrogenic (e.g., hepatic artery embolization)
  - Acute death of hepatic tissue may release gas into portal veins
- **Ulcerative or Infectious Colitis**
  - Mucosal ulceration may allow intraluminal gas to enter colonic wall and mesenteric/portal veins
  - Toxic megacolon resulting from ulcerative or infectious colitis may also lead to portal venous gas

(Left) *Axial CECT in this older man with bowel infarction shows extensive intrahepatic portal venous gas* ➡ *extending out toward the periphery of the liver.* **(Right)** *Axial CECT in the same patient shows dilated small bowel (ileus) with some segments having pneumatosis* ➡. *The mesenteric vein draining the affected bowel contains gas* ➡. *High-density interloop fluid* ➡ *represents hemorrhage from the infarcted bowel.*

Ischemic Enteritis

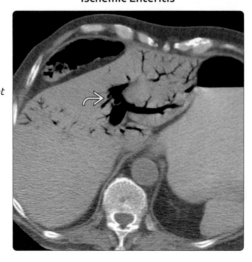

Ischemic Enteritis

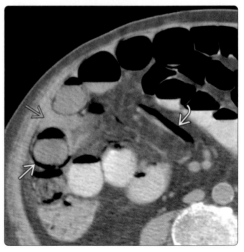

Ischemic Enteritis

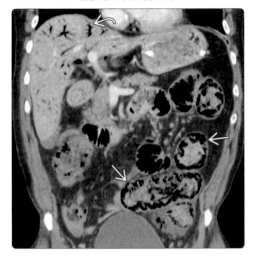

Ischemic Colitis

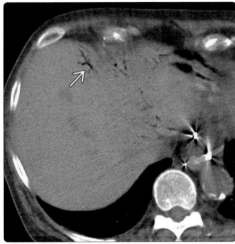

(Left) *Coronal CECT shows extensive small bowel pneumatosis* ➡ *and portal venous gas* ➡ *due to bowel ichemia.* (Right) *Axial NECT in an older man with acute onset of abdominal pain and hypotension shows gas within the peripheral branches of the portal vein* ➡.

Ischemic Colitis

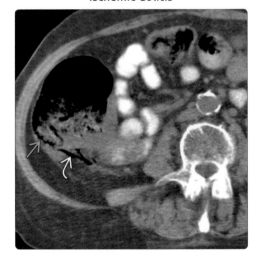

Diverticulitis

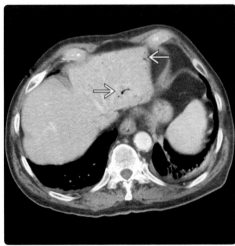

(Left) *Axial NECT in the same patient shows gas within the wall of the cecum* ➡ *and the ileocolic vein* ➡. *The infarcted colon was resected, but the patient did not survive.* (Right) *Axial CECT shows portal venous gas* ➡ *due to diverticulitis with portal vein thrombophlebitis, which resolved with antibiotics alone.*

Diverticulitis

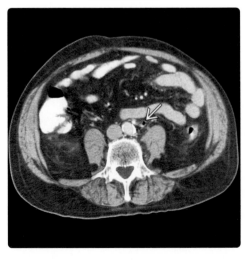

Hepatic Infarction

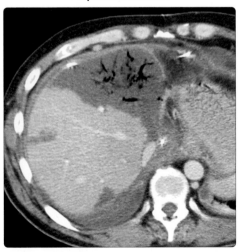

(Left) *Axial CECT in the same patient with sigmoid diverticulitis (who also had portal venous gas) shows gas in the inferior mesenteric vein* ➡. *This also resolved with antibiotics alone.* (Right) *Axial CECT shows extensive gas in the left portal veins and infarction of the left lobe following an aborted attempt to resect a left lobe tumor.*

DIFFERENTIAL DIAGNOSIS

Common

- Cirrhosis
- Focal Confluent Fibrosis
- Senescent Change
- Postsurgical (Mimic)

Less Common

- Congenital Absence of Hepatic Segments
- Liver Metastases
- Primary Sclerosing Cholangitis
- Congenital Hepatic Fibrosis
- Schistosomiasis

ESSENTIAL INFORMATION

Key Differential Diagnosis Issues

- Widened fissures: Congenital, acquired, or iatrogenic loss of hepatic parenchyma

Helpful Clues for Common Diagnoses

- **Cirrhosis**
  - Widening of fissures indicates fibrosis and volume loss; sensitive sign of cirrhosis
  - Look for enlarged caudate and signs of portal hypertension (splenomegaly, varices, ascites)
- **Focal Confluent Fibrosis**
  - Common in advanced cirrhosis
  - 90% of cases involve medial segment of left lobe &/or anterior segment of right lobe (segments 8 and 4) with sparing of caudate and lateral segments
  - Lesions are isoattenuating to adjacent liver parenchyma on venous-phase CECT (80%)
  - May show delayed, persistent enhancement like other fibrotic liver lesions
  - **Does not wash out** (↓ in enhancement) unlike hepatocellular carcinoma (HCC)
- **Senescent Change**
  - Older adults (> 70 years) often have asymptomatic volume loss of liver and widened fissures

- Do not label older patient as cirrhotic without clinical correlation
- **Postsurgical (Mimic)**
  - Liver segments may be resected, or tumors may have been ablated

Helpful Clues for Less Common Diagnoses

- **Congenital Absence of Hepatic Segments**
  - Most commonly affects anterior and medial segments
  - Look for deep gallbladder fossa, absence of signs of portal hypertension
- **Liver Metastases**
  - Some cancers (e.g., breast) induce fibrosis and volume loss de novo (pseudocirrhosis)
  - Tumor volume loss and hepatic fibrosis may result from IV or arterial chemoembolization
- **Primary Sclerosing Cholangitis**
  - Results in liver volume loss even before true cirrhosis has developed
  - Liver has rounded contours due to atrophy of peripheral segments of liver and hypertrophy of deep right and caudate lobes
  - Look for irregular dilation and strictures of bile ducts
  - Check for history of inflammatory bowel disease
- **Congenital Hepatic Fibrosis**
  - Part of spectrum of congenital fibropolycystic liver disease
  - Leads to portal hypertension; may simulate or develop into cirrhosis
  - Look for associated biliary or renal abnormalities
    - Caroli disease; recessive or dominant polycystic disease
  - Hepatic arteries are enlarged and tortuous
  - Differentiating feature of congenital hepatic fibrosis
    - Normal or ↑ medial segment vs. small medial segment in viral or alcoholic cirrhosis
- **Schistosomiasis**
  - *Saccharina japonica* causes extensive fibrosis of liver
  - Look for periportal and pericapsular septal calcifications
  - Tortoise shell appearance

(Left) *Axial CECT shows a dysmorphic liver with signs of cirrhosis (wide fissures ➡, caudate hypertrophy ➡, nodular surface ➡) and stigmata of portal hypertension (splenomegaly ➡). **(Right)** Pre- (A) and postcontrast images in a patient with cirrhosis show an area of decreased T1 signal ➡ and progressive enhancement ➡ through the arterial (B), venous (C), and delayed (D) phases, indicative of a fibrotic process that is consistent with confluent fibrosis.*

Cirrhosis

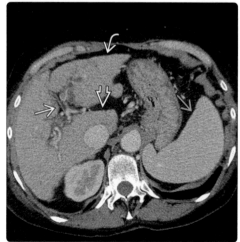

Focal Confluent Fibrosis

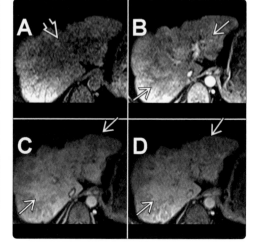

Senescent Change

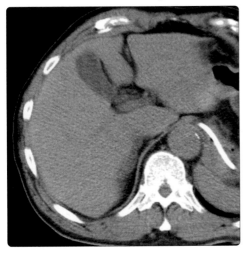

Congenital Absence of Hepatic Segments

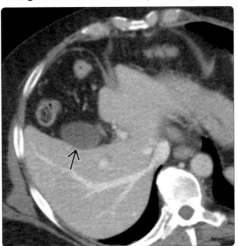

(Left) *Axial CT shows a small medial segment with the gallbladder lying deep within the liver and a relatively wide fissure for the falciform ligament. These findings would be suggestive of cirrhosis in a younger patient but may be normal, especially in older adults. This man had no clinical evidence of liver disease.* (Right) *Axial CECT shows absence of the medial segment with omental fat and colon herniating into the space between the right lobe and lateral segment. The gallbladder ⊟ marks the interlobar plane.*

Liver Metastases

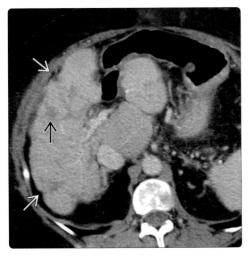

Primary Sclerosing Cholangitis

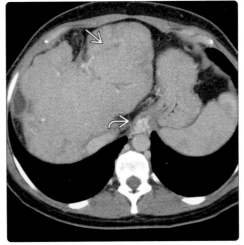

(Left) *Axial CECT in a woman with known hepatic metastases from breast cancer shows a dysmorphic liver with widened fissures, a lobulated and nodular contour ➡ that closely simulates cirrhosis. Subtle hypodense lesions ⊟ indicate widespread mets.* (Right) *Axial CECT shows a cirrhotic liver with beaded intrahepatic biliary ductal dilatation ➡ of primary sclerosing cholangitis. Liver is small with varices ➡, widened fissures, and rounded contours due to peripheral hepatic scarring and hypertrophy of the more central segments.*

Congenital Hepatic Fibrosis

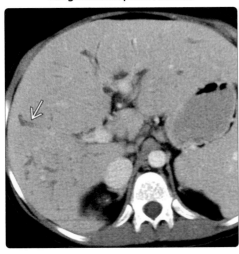

Schistosomiasis

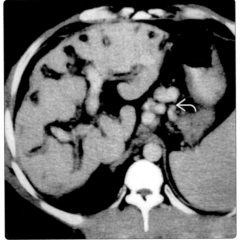

(Left) *Axial CECT shows a dysmorphic liver with widened fissures and dilated, ectatic bile ducts ➡ due to Caroli disease and congenital hepatic fibrosis.* (Right) *Axial CECT shows signs of cirrhosis and portal hypertension, including large varices ➡. Note the extraordinarily widened hepatic fissures deeply dividing the segments of the liver along the portal vein branches. This is a characteristic feature of hepatic schistosomiasis.*

DIFFERENTIAL DIAGNOSIS

Common

- Primary Sclerosing Cholangitis
- Cirrhosis (Mimic)
  - Hepatitis
  - Peribiliary Cysts
- Portal Vein Thrombophlebitis (Mimic)
  - Diverticulitis
  - Hepatic Pyogenic Abscess
- Cholangiocarcinoma, Intrahepatic or Hilar

Less Common

- Budd-Chiari Syndrome
- Primary Biliary Cholangitis
- Chemotherapy Cholangitis
- AIDS Cholangiopathy
- Fibropolycystic Liver Diseases
  - Congenital Hepatic Fibrosis
  - Caroli Disease
  - Choledochal Cyst
  - Biliary Hamartomas
- Recurrent Pyogenic Cholangitis
- Hepatic Hydatid Disease

ESSENTIAL INFORMATION

Key Differential Diagnosis Issues

- Dysmorphic liver refers to distortion and scarring of parenchyma
  - May result from inflammation, infection, ischemia, or tumor
    - Or effects of treatment for these conditions
- Distinguish among dilated ducts, periportal edema, and thrombosed portal or hepatic veins
  - Appearance will vary by modality
    - US: Dilated hepatic artery in cirrhosis may simulate dilated ducts
      - Color Doppler can resolve this issue
    - CT or MR: Periportal edema may simulate dilated ducts
      - Edema usually found surrounding vessels; bile duct lies on only one side
    - CECT: Unopacified veins may simulate ducts
      - Vessels > water attenuation
    - Cholangiography: Intrahepatic ducts may be distorted by masses or regenerating nodules, simulating cholangitis

Helpful Clues for Common Diagnoses

- Primary Sclerosing Cholangitis
  - Often results in chronic liver damage
    - In patients with primary sclerosing cholangitis (PSC)-induced end-stage cirrhosis, liver is markedly deformed (to much greater extent than with other common causes of cirrhosis)
    - Lobular contour of liver with preferential scarring of periphery
      - Sparing and hypertrophy of caudate and deep right lobe

---

    - Sometimes to degree simulating central neoplastic mass (pseudotumoral enlargement of caudate)
  - Multifocal "beaded" strictures of intra- and extrahepatic ducts with intervening sites of dilated and normal ducts
  - Pruned appearance of biliary tree develops as disease progresses with obliteration of small peripheral ducts
  - Visualization of greater than expected number of peripheral ducts on MRCP is clue to presence of peripheral intrahepatic ductal strictures
- Cirrhosis (Mimic)
  - Rarely causes ductal dilation
    - But may cause pathologic processes that simulate dilated ducts
    - Regenerating nodules may compress and distort intrahepatic ducts
  - **Peribiliary cysts** are dilated peribiliary glands; may simulate dilated ducts ± small cystic masses in portal triads
  - Periportal edema may simulate ducts
- Portal Vein Thrombophlebitis (Mimic)
  - Thrombosed portal vein branches may simulate dilated ducts on CECT or MR
    - Primary thrombosis of portal vein (hypercoagulable states)
      - Produces characteristic distortion of liver that simulates cirrhosis
  - May result from subacute diverticulitis or appendicitis
  - Thrombosed portal veins may simulate dilated ducts
  - Liver may be damaged from infection or ischemia
- Cholangiocarcinoma, Intrahepatic or Hilar
  - Arising from confluence (Klatskin) or branch ducts (intrahepatic)
  - Ducts are dilated upstream from tumor
  - Liver parenchyma shows volume loss ± visualization of tumor

Helpful Clues for Less Common Diagnoses

- Budd-Chiari Syndrome
  - Peripheral biliary ducts may get distorted and dilated due to central hepatic hypertrophy
  - Thrombosed hepatic veins may simulate dilated ducts but are more central
  - Liver is distorted with peripheral > central volume loss, scarring, hepatocellular necrosis and steatosis
- Primary Biliary Cholangitis
  - Irregular and "pruned" ducts leading to vanishing bile duct syndrome as disease progresses
  - Lace-like fibrosis, prominent lymphadenopathy, and hepatomegaly (early) along with positive antimitochondrial antibody test
- Chemotherapy Cholangitis
  - Intraarterial chemotherapy used for primary hepatocellular carcinoma or metastases
  - Liver distortion due to tumors and parenchymal scarring
  - Ducts are damaged and strictured with appearance like primary sclerosing cholangitis
- AIDS Cholangiopathy
  - Liver may be distorted by infection &/or tumor
  - Papillary stenosis with proximal common bile duct (CBD) dilation, strictures/ulcerations of CBD, and intrahepatic strictures: Unique to AIDS cholangiopathy

- **Fibropolycystic Liver Diseases**
  - Encompasses spectrum of related lesions of liver and biliary tract caused by abnormal embryologic development of ductal plates
  - Lesions may occur in isolation or in any combination; may be clinically silent
    - Or, may cause cholangitis, portal hypertension, GI bleeding, infection, etc.
  - Liver may be distorted by congenital fibrosis (simulates cirrhosis) or by scarring (especially with Caroli disease)
    - Bile ducts may be primary site of pathology (e.g., Caroli disease), coexist with primary parenchymal disease (e.g., fibrosis), or be distorted by extrinsic mass effect
  - **Congenital hepatic fibrosis**
    - Dysmorphic liver, portal hypertension
    - Enlarged and possibly supernumerary hepatic arteries
  - **Caroli disease**
    - Dilatation (usually saccular) of large intrahepatic ducts with alternating biliary strictures
    - Liver often progressively damaged by cholangitis, obstruction
  - **Choledochal cyst**
    - Fusiform or cystic dilation of intrahepatic ± extrahepatic bile duct
  - **Biliary hamartomas**
    - Multiple "cysts" of nearly uniform size, up to 15 mm; no biliary connection
      - Mimic cysts on CT and MR but are often echogenic on US
    - Liver and bile ducts are normal unless coexisting disease, such as Caroli or congenital fibrosis
- **Recurrent Pyogenic Cholangitis**
  - Usually in Asian, poorly nourished populations
  - Liver distorted by chronic infection and biliary obstruction (abscesses, cirrhosis)
  - Bile ducts enormously dilated by pus and stones
- **Hepatic Hydatid Disease**
  - Cysts may distort liver
  - Cysts may communicate with ducts, leading to cholangitis

Primary Sclerosing Cholangitis

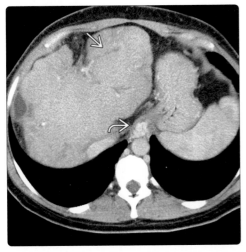

Primary Sclerosing Cholangitis

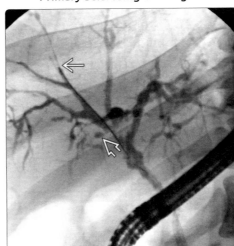

(Left) Axial CECT shows a small liver with deep scars and lobular contour, typical of cirrhosis due to primary sclerosing cholangitis (PSC). Note the irregular dilation of intrahepatic ducts ➡ and esophageal varices ➡. (Right) ERCP shows segmental strictures ➡ and "diverticula" ➡ involving the intra- and extrahepatic bile ducts, resulting in a beaded appearance of the ducts.

Primary Sclerosing Cholangitis

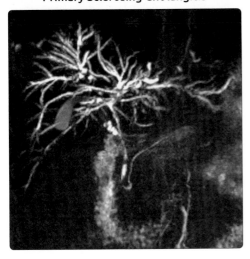

Hepatitis

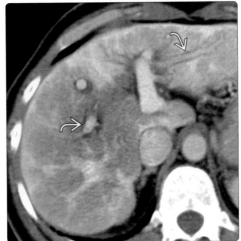

(Left) Coronal MRCP MIP in a 37-year-old man with PSC shows extensive intrahepatic strictures with alternating sites of narrowing and ductal dilatation. (Right) Axial CECT in a 47-year-old woman with autoimmune hepatitis shows evidence of periportal edema ➡ that might be mistaken for dilated bile ducts, except that the lucent band extends completely around the portal vein branches.

Peribiliary Cysts

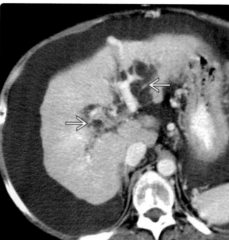

Peribiliary Cysts

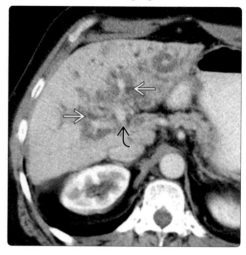

(Left) *Axial CECT in a patient with advanced cirrhosis and ascites shows saccular and spherical cystic lesions* ➡ *(peribiliary cysts) paralleling the portal triads.* **(Right)** *Axial CECT shows cirrhotic morphology of the liver with reduced size, wide fissures, and ascites noted. The portal vein branches* ➡ *are surrounded by a collar of low density, some of which probably represents periportal edema; however, there are also discrete, low-density focal lesions* ➡ *that represent periportal cysts within the bile duct walls.*

Portal Vein Thrombophlebitis (Mimic)

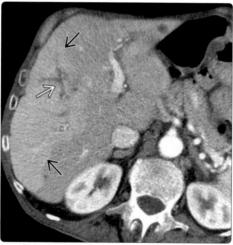

Portal Vein Thrombophlebitis (Mimic)

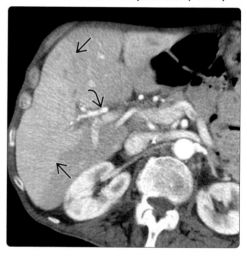

(Left) *Axial arterial-phase CECT shows hyperperfusion of the anterior right lobe of the liver* ➡ *due to thrombosis of the anterior branch of the right portal vein. The thrombosed intrahepatic branches* ➡ *might be mistaken for dilated bile ducts.* **(Right)** *Axial CECT in a patient with transient hepatic attenuation difference (THAD)* ➡ *due to thrombosis of the anterior right portal vein shows the increased size of the right hepatic artery* ➡ *that is compensating for the decreased flow through the portal vein.*

Cholangiocarcinoma, Intrahepatic or Hilar

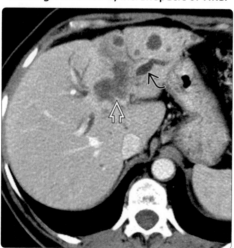

Budd-Chiari Syndrome

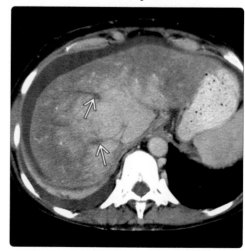

(Left) *Axial CECT shows a heterogeneous left lobe mass* ➡ *that obstructs intrahepatic ducts* ➡ *and causes volume loss of the left lobe. This was a multifocal cholangiocarcinoma.* **(Right)** *Axial CECT shows thrombosed hepatic veins* ➡ *simulating dilated ducts. Ascites, peripheral hepatic damage, and central hypertrophy are typical findings of Budd-Chiari.*

Budd-Chiari Syndrome

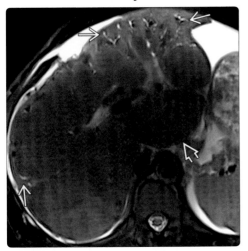

Primary Biliary Cholangitis

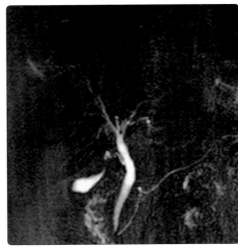

(Left) *Dilatation of the biliary tree in the periphery of the liver* ➡ *is due to caudate lobe hypertrophy* ➡ *and resulting narrowing of the biliary tree in the central liver as well as peripheral volume loss.* (Right) *Coronal MRCP in a 58-year-old woman with primary biliary cholangitis shows signs of advanced disease with decreased visualization of the peripheral intrahepatic ducts (vanishing bile duct syndrome).*

Fibropolycystic Liver Diseases

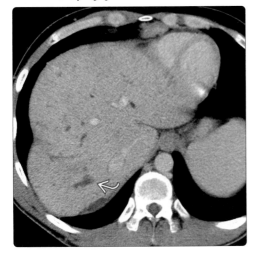

Caroli Disease

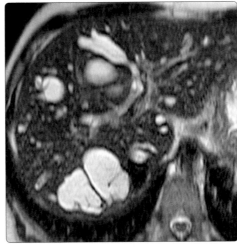

(Left) *Axial CECT shows a dysmorphic liver with irregular dilation of intrahepatic ducts* ➡. *On lower sections, hepatic arteries were enlarged, and small, cystic kidneys were noted. All findings were related to fibropolycystic disease of the liver and kidneys, including congenital hepatic fibrosis.* (Right) *Axial T2 MR shows cystic and irregular cylindrical dilation of intrahepatic bile ducts, characteristic of Caroli disease. Progressive liver failure resulted in transplantation.*

Recurrent Pyogenic Cholangitis

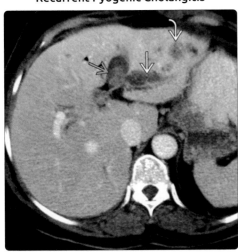

Hepatic Hydatid Disease

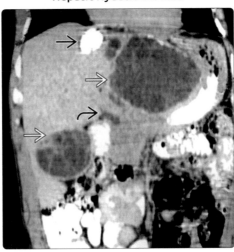

(Left) *Axial CECT shows dilated ducts* ➡ *with a large pigment calculus* ➡ *and a small liver abscess* ➡. (Right) *Coronal CECT shows 2 large, cystic masses* ➡ *with daughter cysts and a densely calcified cyst* ➡. *Bile ducts* ➡ *are dilated due to communication of one of the cysts with the ducts.*

DIFFERENTIAL DIAGNOSIS

Common

- Transient Hepatic Attenuation/Intensity Difference
- Cholecystitis
- Liver Metastases
- Hepatocellular Carcinoma
- Liver Biopsy or Trauma
- Arterioportal Shunt, Cirrhosis
- Anomalous Blood Supply

Less Common

- Hepatic Pyogenic Abscess
- Hepatic Cavernous Hemangioma
- Focal Nodular Hyperplasia
- Hepatic Arteriovenous Malformation
- Superior Vena Cava Obstruction, Abdominal Manifestations
- Portal Vein Occlusion
- Extrinsic Compression of Liver
- Hereditary Hemorrhagic Telangiectasia (Osler-Weber-Rendu)

ESSENTIAL INFORMATION

Key Differential Diagnosis Issues

- Transient hepatic attenuation or intensity differences (THAD or THID, respectively)
  - Focal areas of hepatic parenchymal enhancement visible only on arterial phase of contrast-enhanced imaging
    - Unique to liver, due to its dual blood supply
  - 3 major etiologies
    - Portal vein branch compression or occlusion
      □ Metastases
      □ Hepatocellular carcinoma (HCC)
      □ Benign masses
      □ Portal vein thrombosis
    - Arterioportal shunt or anomalous blood supply; diversion and mixing of blood (and contrast medium) from high-pressure arteries to low-pressure portal vein distribution
      □ Congenital arteriovenous fistula
      □ Post liver biopsy
      □ HCC
    - Siphoning or sump effect: Hypervascular mass or inflammatory process draws more arterial flow into segment of liver
      □ Pyogenic liver abscess
      □ Amebic abscess
      □ Focal nodular hyperplasia (FNH)
      □ HCC
      □ Hypervascular metastases

Helpful Clues for Common Diagnoses

- **Transient Hepatic Attenuation/Intensity Difference**
  - Small, wedge-shaped, subsegmental; abut liver capsule
  - Presumably due to occlusion of small portal venous branch
  - Check portal venous-phase images for subtle mass at apex of wedge-shaped THAD/THID
  - Most THAD or THID lesions are not visible on nonenhanced CT or MR

  - No corresponding signal abnormality on T2 or DWI; T2 or DWI abnormality of underlying lesion if present
  - Longstanding alterations of arterioportal supply may result in altered metabolism (e.g., focal fatty infiltration or focal sparing)
- **Cholecystitis**
  - Severe acute cholecystitis may cause inflammation and hyperemia of adjacent liver
  - Origin of hot spot or rim sign surrounding gallbladder fossa on Tc-HIDA scan
- **Liver Metastases**
  - Usually from GI tract or pancreas
  - Cause occlusion of portal vein branch, eliciting compensatory increased hepatic arterial flow to segment
  - Look for spherical mass (metastasis) at apex of triangular defect (THAD or THID)
  - Hypervascular metastases may cause THAD by occlusion of portal vein &/or by drawing more arterial flow into involved segment (sump effect)
- **Hepatocellular Carcinoma**
  - 3 mechanisms cause THAD
    - Portal vein occlusion (tumor invasion)
    - Arteriovenous shunting through tumor
    - Siphon or sump effect of hypervascular tumor
  - HCC usually heterogeneously hypervascular with washout and capsule
  - Look for cirrhotic liver
- **Liver Biopsy or Trauma**
  - Arteriovenous or arterioportal shunt is common, usually transient, result
  - Early filling of veins that drain involved segment
  - Can follow any hepatic trauma or intervention
    - Liver biopsy
    - Percutaneous transhepatic biliary drain
    - Radiofrequency ablation
- **Arterioportal Shunt, Cirrhosis**
  - Often idiopathic, very common in cirrhosis
  - Usually small, peripheral, wedge-shaped
  - No abnormality on corresponding precontrast T1 and T2 images
  - Larger, spherical, more central lesions are difficult to distinguish from HCC and other hypervascular tumors
  - Recommendation: Just follow small lesions on sequential scans
    - Often resolve spontaneously
- **Anomalous Blood Supply**
  - Anomalous hepatic venous drainage; common along falciform ligament, surrounding gallbladder fossa, and in segment IV
  - Common areas of THAD and also of focal fat &/or focal sparing

Helpful Clues for Less Common Diagnoses

- **Hepatic Pyogenic Abscess**
  - May compress portal vein and draw increased arterial flow into involved segment of liver
  - Usually multiseptate or cluster of grapes appearance
- **Hepatic Cavernous Hemangioma**
  - Any hepatic mass may compress portal vein branch, leading to THAD or THID

Focal Hyperperfusion Abnormality (THAD or THID)

- o Hemangiomas (even small) may have arterioportal shunts within mass
- **Focal Nodular Hyperplasia**
  - o Uncommonly causes THAD, due to mass effect on portal vein or hypervascularity of FNH lesion (sump effect)
  - o Uniformly and markedly hypervascular on arterial phase; isodense/-intense on nonenhanced, venous and delayed phases
- **Hepatic Arteriovenous Malformation**
  - o May be isolated anomaly or part of systemic disorder
  - o Osler-Weber-Rendu or hereditary hemorrhagic telangiectasia (HHT)
  - o Multisystemic inherited disorder with arteriovenous malformations in nose, lungs, GI tract, liver, brain
  - o Large, tortuous extrahepatic ± intrahepatic arteries with early filling and enlargement of hepatic ± portal veins
  - o Vascular masses and telangiectasias within liver
  - o Focal nodular hyperplasia in patients with HHT is 100x more prevalent than general population
- **Superior Vena Cava Obstruction, Abdominal Manifestations**
  - o Peridiaphragmatic collateral veins traverse left lobe of liver to return blood to inferior vena cava
  - o Large zone of hypervascularity without mass effect
  - o Collateral veins will be evident
  - o Pseudolesions on nuclear medicine studies
    - – e.g., "hot" accumulation of Tc-99m sulfur colloid in left lobe of liver in patients with superior vena cava obstruction
    - – "Hot" accumulation of FDG within THAD on PET/CT
- **Portal Vein Occlusion**
  - o e.g., hypercoagulable state; portal vein thrombophlebitis
    - – Thrombophlebitis often due to undiagnosed diverticulitis or appendicitis
- **Extrinsic Compression of Liver**
  - o e.g., subcapsular hematoma; may decrease portal perfusion, increase arterial flow
    - – Tends to affect periphery of liver in lentiform, rather than wedge-shaped, pattern

Transient Hepatic Attenuation/Intensity Difference

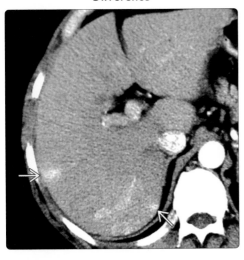

Transient Hepatic Attenuation/Intensity Difference

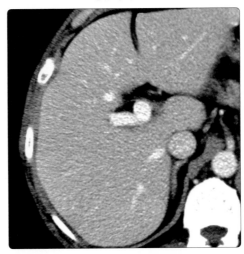

(Left) *Axial arterial-phase CECT shows several small, triangular, capsular-based foci of hyperattenuation ➡. These are typical idiopathic, benign transient hepatic attenuation differences (THADs).* (Right) *Axial portal venous-phase CECT in the same patient shows disappearance of the peripheral hyperdensities, identifying them as foci of THAD.*

Cholecystitis

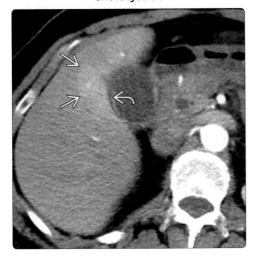

Liver Metastases

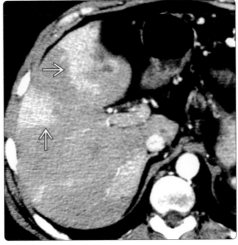

(Left) *Axial arterial-phase CECT in a patient with severe acute cholecystitis shows a distended gallbladder with a thickened wall ➡. Adjacent liver shows abnormal enhancement ➡, indicating ↑ perfusion and suggesting inflammation.* (Right) *Axial arterial-phase CECT in a patient with metastatic pancreatic carcinoma shows several wedge-shaped foci of hyperdensity ➡. The metastatic foci that are blocking the portal venous tributaries are less clearly seen.*

(Left) *Axial portal venous-phase CECT in the same patient shows disappearance of the wedge-shaped THADs but better definition of the metastases* 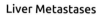 *that caused them.* (Right) *Axial arterial-phase CECT in a 60-year-old man with cirrhosis shows several foci of hepatocellular carcinoma (HCC)* ➡, *one with a wedge-shaped zone of hypervascularity* ➡ *distal to the mass that is due to portal vein branch occlusion.*

Liver Metastases

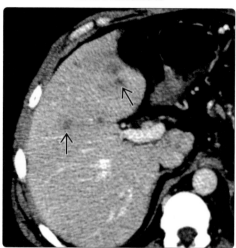

Hepatocellular Carcinoma

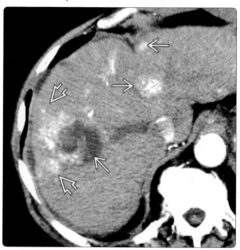

(Left) *Axial portal venous-phase CECT in the same patient shows the HCC nodules* ➡ *washing out to become hypodense to the liver. Much of the THAD zone of hyperdensity is now isodense to liver.* (Right) *Axial arterial-phase CECT in a 46-year-old man with cirrhosis shows hyperenhancement of the lateral segment* ➡ *and early opacification of the left portal vein* ➡, *the result of a percutaneous liver biopsy causing an arterioportal shunt.*

Hepatocellular Carcinoma

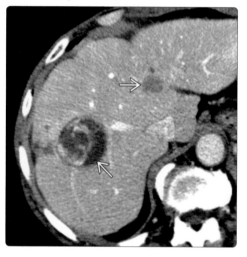

Liver Biopsy or Trauma

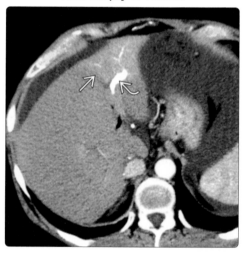

(Left) *Axial portal venous-phase CECT in the same patient shows homogeneous enhancement of the left lobe with resolution of the THAD. This iatrogenic arterioportal shunt resolved spontaneously.* (Right) *Axial T1 C+ MR in a 69-year-old man with hepatitis C virus (HCV) cirrhosis shows multiple wedge-shaped, hyperenhancing foci* ➡, *mostly in the periphery of the liver.*

Liver Biopsy or Trauma

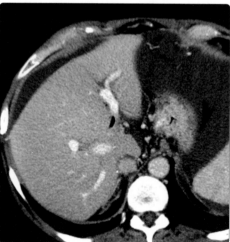

Arterioportal Shunt, Cirrhosis

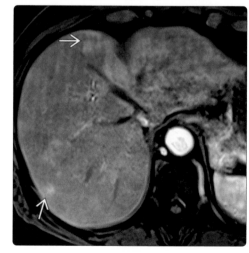

Focal Hyperperfusion Abnormality (THAD or THID)

Arterioportal Shunt, Cirrhosis

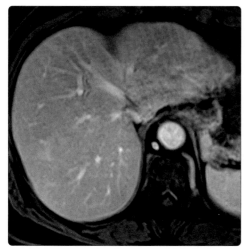

Hepatic Pyogenic Abscess

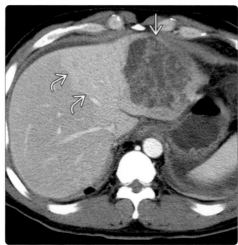

(Left) *Axial portal venous-phase T1 C+ MR in the same patient shows no corresponding areas of abnormality. T2 and DWI sequences did not show any abnormalities either. Findings are consistent with arterioportal shunts.* (Right) *Axial early venous-phase CECT in a 41-year-old woman shows a pyogenic abscess ➡ in the left lobe with a typical multiseptate appearance. The entire left lobe of the liver is hyperenhancing with a straight line demarcation ➡.*

Hepatic Pyogenic Abscess

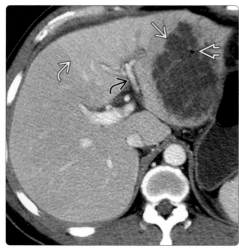

Hepatic Cavernous Hemangioma

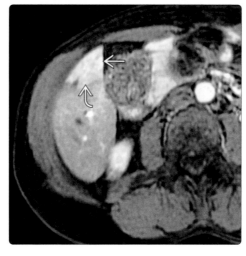

(Left) *Axial CECT in the same patient shows gas ➡ within the pyogenic abscess ➡. The hyperperfused left lobe ➡ is presumably due to the sump effect of the abscess, rather than portal vein occlusion, because the left portal vein is patent ➡.* (Right) *Axial arterial-phase T1 C+ MR in a 56-year-old woman shows a brightly enhancing lesion ➡ and surrounding region of transient hepatic hyperperfusion ➡, a transient hepatic intensity difference (THID). This was found to be a capillary hemangioma.*

Hepatic Cavernous Hemangioma

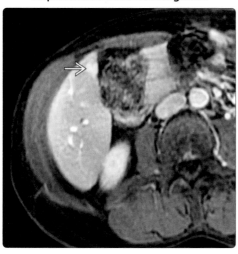

Focal Nodular Hyperplasia

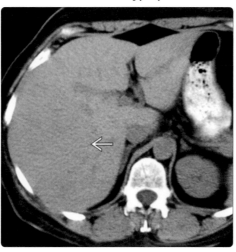

(Left) *Axial portal venous-phase T1 C+ MR in the same patient shows the small hemangioma ➡, but the THID has resolved.* (Right) *Axial NECT in a 48-year-old woman shows a subtle mass ➡ that is almost isodense to the liver.*

(Left) *Axial arterial-phase CECT in the same patient shows a large, brightly enhancing focal nodular hyperplasia (FNH)* ➡ *with ↑ density of surrounding right lobe* ➡ *due to sump effect. The FNH and background liver were almost isodense on venous and delayed phases.*

(Right) *Coronal arterial-phase CECT in a 54-year-old woman shows a tangle of enlarged vessels* ➡ *that are nearly isodense with other visible arteries (e.g., renal). Note early filling of accessory right hepatic vein* ➡. *No mass was evident on delayed phase.*

Focal Nodular Hyperplasia

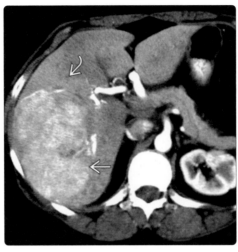

Hepatic Arteriovenous Malformation

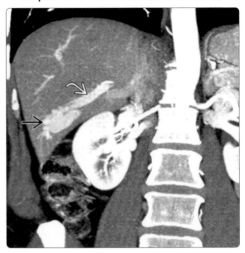

(Left) *Coronal arterial-phase CECT in the same patient shows the arteriovenous malformation* ➡ *along with hyperenhancement of the surrounding liver parenchyma.*

(Right) *Axial arterial-phase CECT in a 33-year-old woman with a chronic aortic dissection shows the aortic intimal flap* ➡ *along with an occluded superior vena cava (SVC)* ➡ *and numerous venous collaterals* ➡ *in the chest wall.*

Hepatic Arteriovenous Malformation

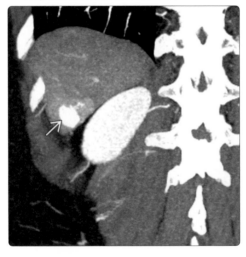

Superior Vena Cava Obstruction, Abdominal Manifestations

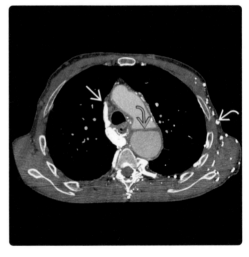

(Left) *Axial arterial-phase CECT in the same patient shows marked enhancement of the medial ("quadrate") segment* ➡ *due to collateral vessels* ➡ *traversing the liver.*

(Right) *Axial MR in a patient with hilar cholangiocarcinoma shows THID on arterial phase* ➡, *which are isointense on venous phase* ➡. *Note absence of corresponding abnormality on precontrast T1* ➡ *and T2* ➡ *MR, as it is a vascular phenomenon and likely due to thrombosed branch of portal vein.*

Superior Vena Cava Obstruction, Abdominal Manifestations

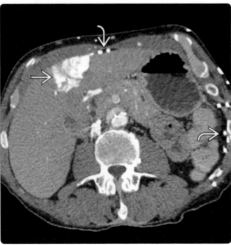

Portal Vein Occlusion

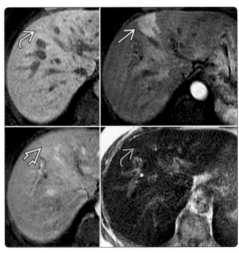

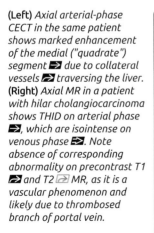
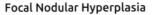

Portal Vein Occlusion

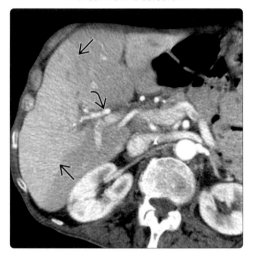

Portal Vein Occlusion

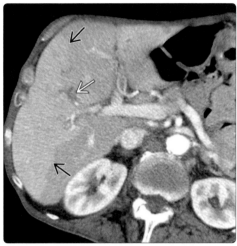

(Left) *Axial early venous-phase CECT in a 71-year-old man with liver dysfunction shows hyperperfusion of the anterior segments of the right lobe with a straight line demarcation ➯. The anterior branch of the right portal vein is occluded, and the accompanying hepatic arterial branch ➯ is enlarged.* (Right) *Axial early venous-phase CECT in the same patient shows hyperenhancement of the anterior hepatic segments ➯ and thrombosis of the anterior right portal vein ➯.*

Portal Vein Occlusion

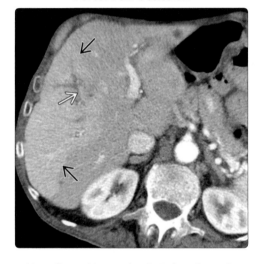

Portal Vein Occlusion

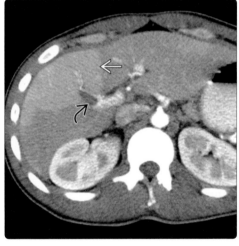

(Left) *Axial early venous-phase CECT in the same patient shows the thrombosed branches of the anterior right portal vein ➯, which might be mistaken for dilated bile ducts. The hyperenhanced right lobe ➯ is due to ↑ arterial flow delivering contrast-opacified blood, while the remainder of the liver is perfused by less opacified portal vein flow.* (Right) *Axial arterial-phase CECT shows a THAD ➯ limited to the anterior segments of the right lobe due to thrombosis of the segmental portal vein ➯.*

Hereditary Hemorrhagic Telangiectasia (Osler-Weber-Rendu)

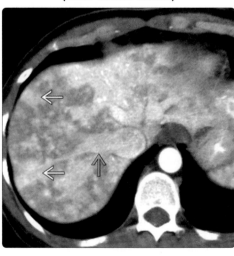

Hereditary Hemorrhagic Telangiectasia (Osler-Weber-Rendu)

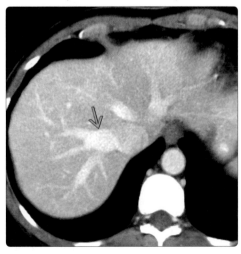

(Left) *Axial arterial-phase CECT in a middle-aged man with nosebleeds and hemoptysis shows multiple foci of ↑ hepatic enhancement ➯ and early filling of enlarged hepatic veins ➯, characteristic features of hereditary hemorrhagic telangiectasia (HHT) (Osler-Weber-Rendu syndrome).* (Right) *Axial portal venous-phase CECT in the same patient shows a homogeneous liver with only the enlarged hepatic veins ➯ as a sign of the underlying HHT.*

DIFFERENTIAL DIAGNOSIS

Common

- Dilated Bile Ducts (Mimic)
- Systemic Hypervolemia
- Passive Hepatic Congestion
- Hepatitis (Acute)
  - Hepatitis, Alcoholic
  - Hepatitis, Viral
  - Hepatic Injury From Toxins
- Cholangitis
  - Ascending Cholangitis
  - Primary Sclerosing Cholangitis
  - Recurrent Pyogenic Cholangitis
  - AIDS-Related Cholangitis
  - Chemotherapy-Induced Cholangitis
- Posttransplant Liver
  - Biliary Necrosis, Posttransplantation
  - Lymphedema, Posttransplantation
- Hepatic Trauma

Less Common

- Porta Hepatis Lymphadenopathy
- Cirrhosis
  - Peribiliary Cysts
- Portal Vein Thrombosis
- Steatosis (Fatty Liver)
- Hepatocellular Carcinoma
- Cholangiocarcinoma
- Hepatic Metastases and Lymphoma
- Hepatic Inflammatory Pseudotumor

ESSENTIAL INFORMATION

Key Differential Diagnosis Issues

- Any process that increases production of hepatic extracellular fluid, or impairs capacity for lymphatics to carry this away, will result in periportal lymphedema
  - Loose areolar tissue in portal triads is easily distended by fluid
  - Common pathway for spread of fluid
    - Fluid may be lymph, bile, or blood
- Common pitfalls
  - Mistaking periportal fluid for dilated bile ducts
  - Mistaking clotted portal vein branches for dilated ducts
- MRCP or ERCP best tool for distinguishing among etiologies for branching, nonenhancing structures

Helpful Clues for Common Diagnoses

- **Dilated Bile Ducts (Mimic)**
  - Lie on only 1 side of portal triad
  - Periportal lucency, by definition, surrounds portal triad on all sides
  - Biliary obstruction may also cause periportal edema
  - Intrahepatic bile ducts should be > 1/2 diameter of adjacent portal vein branch
- **Systemic Hypervolemia**
  - Overhydration, as in rapid fluid resuscitation of trauma patients
  - Liver produces lymph faster than lymphatics can carry it away

- Look for distention of inferior vena cava (IVC)
- **Passive Hepatic Congestion**
  - e.g., congestive heart failure, constrictive pericarditis, tricuspid valve incompetence
  - Results in periportal lymphedema
  - Look for distention and reflux of vascular contrast medium into hepatic veins and IVC on arterial-phase CECT
- **Hepatitis (Acute)**
  - Any cause (alcohol, viral, toxic)
  - Often results in striking periportal edema &/or gallbladder wall edema
    - Any or all of these may cause or simulate periportal edema
- **Cholangitis**
  - Any form (ascending, primary sclerosing, recurrent pyogenic, AIDS, chemotherapy)
  - Bile duct wall thickening, periductal edema, and possibly ductal obstruction
  - **Ascending cholangitis**
    - Caused by passage of common duct stone
    - Or other etiology for incompetence of sphincter of Oddi
    - Allows reflux of duodenal contents into common bile duct (CBD)
    - Bile duct walls appear thickened on T1 and T2 MR with progressive hyperenhancement of duct walls on T1 C+ MR
  - **Primary sclerosing cholangitis**
    - Causes irregular strictures and upstream dilation of intra- and extrahepatic ducts
      □ Multifocal "beaded" strictures of intra- and extrahepatic ducts with intervening sites of dilated and normal ducts
    - Biliary dilation may simulate or cause periportal edema
    - Bile duct wall thickening and periportal edema are often striking on US
    - Usually associated with ulcerative colitis
  - **Recurrent pyogenic cholangitis**
    - Typically encountered in malnourished patients from Asia
    - Intra- and extrahepatic bile ducts grossly distended with pus and calculi
    - Periportal edema may coexist with biliary ductal dilation
  - **AIDS-related cholangitis**
    - Caused by opportunistic infection of bile ducts
    - Imaging findings may simulate primary sclerosis cholangitis
    - Papillary stenosis with tapered narrowing of distal CBD and proximal CBD dilatation
    - Dilated intrahepatic ducts with CBD thickening and periductal hyper-/hypoechoic areas on US
    - MR/MRCP very sensitive (85-100%) and specific (92-100%)
  - **Chemotherapy-induced cholangitis**
    - Affected bile ducts may show periductal edema, mural thickening, and enhancement with adjacent fat stranding in hepatoduodenal ligament

- Usually limited to patients receiving chemotherapy through direct hepatic artery catheterization and infusion
- **Posttransplant Liver**
  - Lymphatics are severed during transplantation
    - Lymphatics reform connections, but this takes some time
    - Periportal lymphedema is common and may persist for weeks; not sign of rejection
  - Biliary necrosis may occur as complication of transplantation
    - Bile ducts receive only arterial supply; hepatic arterial stenosis or thrombosis causes biliary necrosis before hepatic infarction
    - Often takes form of intrahepatic fluid collections paralleling bile ducts; may be branching or spherical
- **Hepatic Trauma**
  - Blood may spread along portal tracts in branching pattern
    - May be mistaken for dilated bile ducts or deep parenchymal laceration
    - Periportal blood is almost never only sign of hepatic trauma; usually limited to lobe of liver with intrahepatic hematoma or laceration

Helpful Clues for Less Common Diagnoses

- **Porta Hepatis Lymphadenopathy**
  - May result in lymphedema
- **Cirrhosis**
  - May cause periportal edema &/or simulate periportal edema
    - May cause peribiliary cysts (dilated peribiliary glands)
  - May cause portal vein obstruction
    - Look for nonenhancing branching structures in expected path of portal vein branches
    - Cavernous transformation of portal vein (collaterals) may also be mistaken for edema on NECT (but enhance like other vessels on CECT)
- **Portal Vein Thrombosis**

- Portal vein branches that do not enhance on CECT are likely to be misinterpreted as dilated bile ducts or periportal edema
- Thrombosis may result from cirrhosis (portal hypertension), hypercoagulable condition, or portal vein thrombophlebitis (e.g., from diverticulitis)
- **Steatosis (Fatty Liver)**
  - May have perivascular distribution, simulate edema
    - More likely to be mistaken on CT; steatosis should not be mistaken for fluid on US or MR
  - Often appears spherical when sectioned in short axis in dome of liver
- **Hepatocellular Carcinoma**
  - May result in nonspecific lymphedema &/or invade or obstruct bile ducts or portal vein
  - Prone to invade portal vein
    - Look for distention of portal vein, enhancing tumor thrombus, contiguity with parenchymal tumor
- **Cholangiocarcinoma**
  - Peripheral or hilar
  - Possible etiologies of branching, nonenhancing structures
    - Dilated bile ducts
    - Periportal edema
    - Thickened bile duct walls
- **Hepatic Metastases and Lymphoma**
  - Any hepatic malignancy may result in excess lymphatic output, periportal edema
  - Vascular or biliary encasement by periportal hepatic mass without vascular occlusion or thrombosis may occur
- **Hepatic Inflammatory Pseudotumor**
  - Small mass in hepatic hilum appearing identical to Klatskin tumor (short-segment stricture with dilation of ducts upstream) (lymphoplasmacytic type)
  - Look for imaging, clinical, and laboratory (serum IgG4 levels) evidence of IgG4-related sclerosing disease
  - Often multisystem disorder (e.g., autoimmune pancreatitis, cholangitis, pneumonitis, etc.)

Dilated Bile Ducts (Mimic)

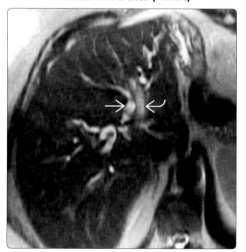

Dilated Bile Ducts (Mimic)

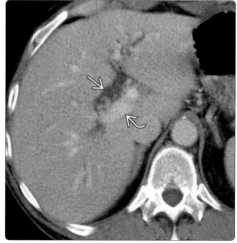

(Left) Axial T2 FS MR shows dilated intrahepatic bile ducts ➡ running parallel to, and on one side only of, the portal venous branches ➡ in a patient with an obstructing ductal stone. (Right) Axial CECT shows dilated intrahepatic bile ducts ➡ due to carcinoma of the pancreatic head. The ducts lie on only one side (usually anteromedial) of the portal vein ➡ branches.

(Left) *Axial CECT in a healthy 22-year-old woman shows a collar of low-density edema ⮕ surrounding portal venous branches caused by overhydration following motor vehicle crash. Note distended inferior vena cava (IVC), also due to hypervolemia.* **(Right)** *Axial CECT in a 78-year-old woman with congestive heart failure shows periportal edema ⮕ and a distended IVC ⮕.*

Systemic Hypervolemia

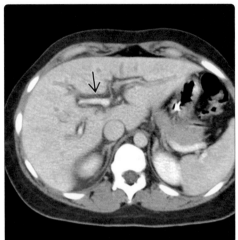

Passive Hepatic Congestion

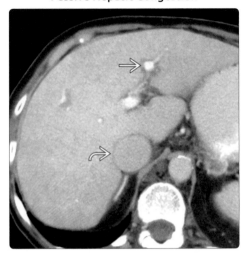

(Left) *Axial CECT in a 35-year-old man shows a collar of periportal lymphedema ⮕ and porta hepatic lymphadenopathy ⮕ due to acute viral hepatitis.* **(Right)** *Axial CECT in the same patient shows marked gallbladder wall edema ⮕ and a small amount of ascites.*

Hepatitis (Acute)

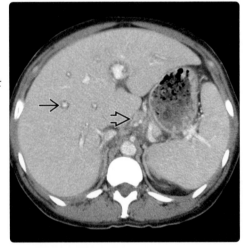

Hepatitis (Acute)

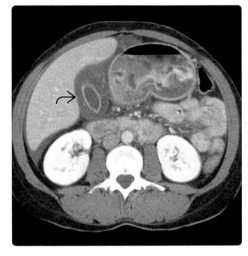

(Left) *Axial CECT shows periportal edema ⮕, mild dilation of ducts ⮕, and a pyogenic abscess ⮕, all due to ascending cholangitis following Whipple resection for pancreatic carcinoma.* **(Right)** *Axial CECT shows periportal lymphedema ⮕ and gas within mildly dilated ducts ⮕, plus a liver abscess ⮕, all due to ascending cholangitis following Whipple resection for pancreatic carcinoma.*

Ascending Cholangitis

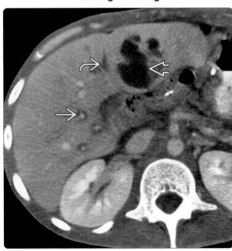

Ascending Cholangitis

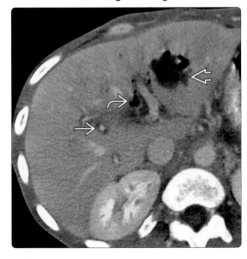

Primary Sclerosing Cholangitis

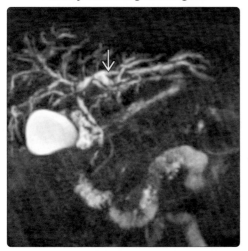

Primary Sclerosing Cholangitis

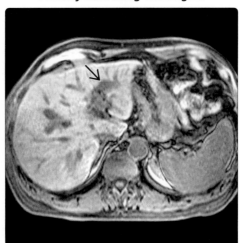

(Left) *Coronal MRCP shows irregular arborization of the intrahepatic ducts with a beaded appearance of some segments. In this 60-year-old man with ulcerative colitis and primary sclerosing cholangitis, portions of the left hepatic ducts ⮕ are more dilated than the common duct.* (Right) *Axial T1 FS MR in the same patient shows low-intensity fibrosis ⮕ paralleling the portal veins and mimicking dilated bile ducts.*

Recurrent Pyogenic Cholangitis

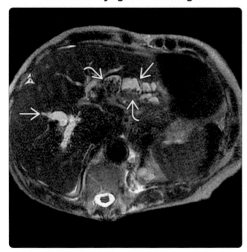

Recurrent Pyogenic Cholangitis

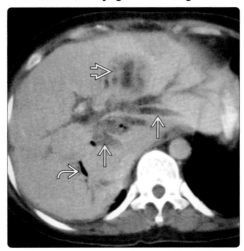

(Left) *Axial T2 FS MR in an older Asian woman shows dilated intrahepatic bile ducts ⮕ containing innumerable calculi ⮕. Recurrent pyogenic cholangitis can cause periportal edema in addition to massively dilated bile ducts.* (Right) *Axial CECT in a 45-year-old Asian woman with recurrent bouts of cholangitis and sepsis shows grossly dilated bile ducts ⮕, some of which contain gas ⮕, plus a hepatic abscess ⮕.*

AIDS-Related Cholangitis

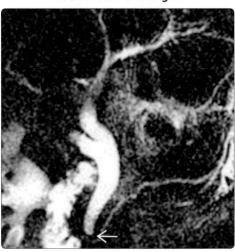

Chemotherapy-Induced Cholangitis

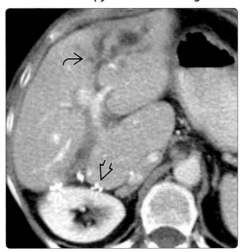

(Left) *Coronal oblique MRCP shows dilation and irregular arborization of the bile ducts and a stricture ⮕ of the distal common bile duct due to AIDS-related cholangiopathy. Similar findings could be seen with primary sclerosing cholangitis.* (Right) *Axial CECT shows surgical clips ⮕ from right hepatic lobectomy (for metastases). Irregular dilation of intrahepatic ducts ⮕ is the result of hepatic intraarterial chemotherapy.*

Biliary Necrosis, Posttransplantation

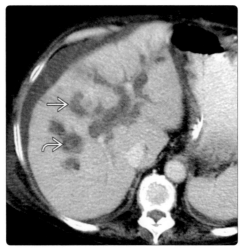

Lymphedema, Posttransplantation

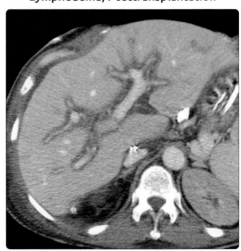

(Left) *Axial CECT shows dilated intrahepatic ducts with indistinct walls ➡ due to biliary necrosis. Intrahepatic bilomas ⇗ and ascites are also noted. These are classic signs of hepatic artery stenosis or thrombosis following liver transplantation.* **(Right)** *Axial CECT shows classic periportal edema that surrounds the portal venous branches. This is a common finding in recent liver transplant recipients and does not imply injury to the allograft.*

Hepatic Trauma

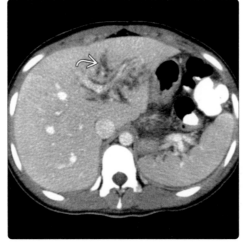

Peribiliary Cysts

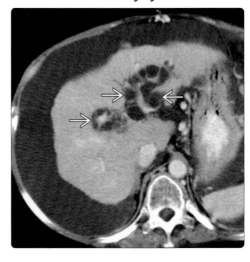

(Left) *Axial CECT in a 20-year-old woman injured in a motor vehicle crash shows the left lobe irregular laceration/hematoma with some blood ⇗ tracking along portal vein branches.* **(Right)** *Axial CECT in a 45-year-old woman with advanced cirrhosis shows cystic and tubular water-density structures ➡ that parallel the portal veins. These are biliary cysts, not dilated ducts.*

Peribiliary Cysts

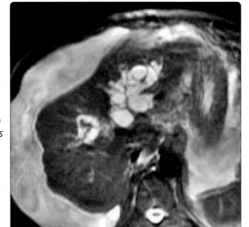

Portal Vein Thrombosis

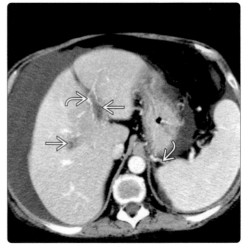

(Left) *Axial T2 FS MR in the same patient shows another view of the cystic and tubular water-intensity lesions that parallel the portal veins and mimic dilated ducts.* **(Right)** *Axial CECT shows low-density, branching structures ➡ that mimic dilated bile ducts but represent occluded portal vein branches. Note collateral veins ⇗ in this 58-year-old woman who had an autologous bone marrow transplantation prior to becoming hypercoagulable.*

Portal Vein Thrombosis

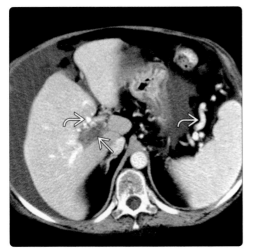

Steatosis (Fatty Liver)

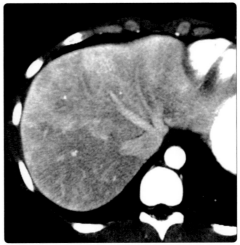

(Left) *Axial CECT in the same patient shows a thrombosed right portal vein ➡ that might be mistaken for a dilated duct. Again, note collateral veins ➡. (Right) Axial CECT shows mottled lucency in the liver, mostly in a perivascular distribution due to steatosis (fatty liver). Steatosis often favors the perivascular planes and "spares" the liver adjacent to the gallbladder fossa.*

Hepatocellular Carcinoma

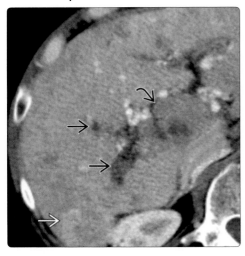

Cholangiocarcinoma

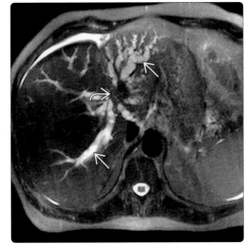

(Left) *Axial arterial-phase CECT shows an enhancing tumor thrombus ➡ distending the main portal vein. Note the thrombosed right portal vein ➡ simulating dilated ducts and the enhancing hepatocellular carcinoma ➡. (Right) Axial MRCP shows dilation of intrahepatic ducts ➡ with obstruction near the confluence of the right and left main ducts due to cholangiocarcinoma ➡. Malignant biliary obstruction may mimic or cause periportal edema.*

Hepatic Metastases and Lymphoma

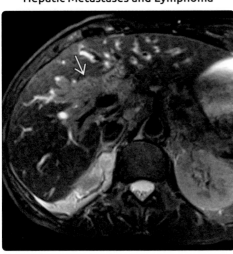

Hepatic Inflammatory Pseudotumor

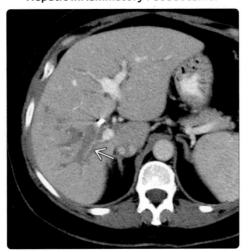

(Left) *Axial T2 FS MR in a 66-year-old man with chronic lymphocytic leukemia (CLL) shows an infiltrative mass with intermediate signal intensity in a periportal distribution ➡ without venous invasion. (Right) Axial CECT in the portal venous-parenchymal phase shows periportal hypoattenuation ➡ that encases and narrows the right portal vein. This was interpreted as cholangiocarcinoma, but surgical resection (right hepatectomy) showed only inflammatory pseudotumor of the liver and bile ducts.*

DIFFERENTIAL DIAGNOSIS

Common
- Regenerating (Cirrhotic) Nodules
- Calcified Granulomas
- Pneumobilia

Less Common
- Hepatic Metastases
- Hepatocellular Carcinoma
- Dysplastic Nodules (Cirrhosis)
- Hepatic Adenoma
- Cholangiocarcinoma (Peripheral)
- Fibrolamellar Hepatocellular Carcinoma
- Nodular Regenerative Hyperplasia
- Hepatic Sarcoidosis
- Hepatic Hematoma
- Hereditary Hemorrhagic Telangiectasia
- Portal Vein Gas
- Hepatic Portal or Venous Collaterals
- Primary Biliary Cholangitis

Rare but Important
- Peliosis Hepatis
- Hepatic Angiomyolipoma

ESSENTIAL INFORMATION

Key Differential Diagnosis Issues
- Most hepatic lesions are hyperintense on T2 MR due to excess water content
  - Includes most inflammatory and neoplastic lesions
- Lesions may be completely or partly hypointense on T2 MR
- Sources for hypointense appearance
  - Blood degradation products
    - Almost any liver lesion that undergoes necrosis or hemorrhage may show foci of hypointensity on T2 MR
  - Macromolecules
    - Smooth muscle, fibrosis, mucin, fibrinogen, keratin
  - Necrosis
    - Especially coagulative necrosis
  - Melanin
  - Calcium
  - Flowing blood
- Relative hypointensity on T2 MR
  - Lesions with fatty component
  - Depends on MR sequence used to achieve fat suppression
    - May cause signal loss from lesions that contain lipid or macroscopic fat
    - Examples
      - Some hepatocellular carcinoma (HCC)
      - Adenomas
      - Angiomyolipomas
      - Teratomas

Helpful Clues for Common Diagnoses
- **Regenerating (Cirrhotic) Nodules**
  - Usually not apparent on T1 MR
  - Hypointense on T2 MR, especially GRE
    - Due to presence of iron within these siderotic nodules

- Lesions may bloom (appear larger) on GRE MR
  - Due to increased susceptibility effects of iron
  - Usually < 1-cm diameter, hypovascular, numerous (hundreds)
- **Calcified Granulomas**
  - Common in histoplasmosis, healed TB
  - Similar lesions in spleen
  - Remainder of liver is normal
  - No mobile protons = signal void on T2 MR
- **Pneumobilia**
  - Gas in bile ducts
  - More linear distribution when seen in longitudinal section
  - Signal void in air-containing structures

Helpful Clues for Less Common Diagnoses
- **Hepatic Metastases**
  - Especially likely following therapy
  - Foci of old hemorrhage or necrosis may appear hypointense on T2 MR
    - Coagulative necrosis = hypointense on T2 MR
      - e.g., following ethanol or radiofrequency (RF) ablation
      - Appears hyperintense on T1 MR
    - Liquefactive necrosis = hyperintense on T2 MR
  - Tumors with large mucin content may appear hypointense
    - Colorectal, gastric, pancreatic, ovarian
  - Metastatic melanoma
    - Melanin within metastases may cause hypointensity on T2 MR, hyperintensity on T1 MR (opposite of usual pattern)
- **Hepatocellular Carcinoma**
  - Usually hyperintense on T2 MR
  - Potential causes for hypointense foci
    - Necrosis, old hemorrhage, iron deposits, fat on fat-saturated T2 MR
    - Lesions treated with transarterial chemoembolization (TACE) or RF ablation
- **Dysplastic Nodules (Cirrhosis)**
  - Premalignant lesions in cirrhotic liver
  - Hyperintense on T1 MR, hypointense on T2 MR (opposite of HCC)
    - Hypointensity due to iron or sinusoidal blood flow within lesions
  - Usually 1-4 cm in diameter
  - Hypovascular
  - Usually take up and retain gadoxetate (Eovist/Primovist)
- **Hepatic Adenoma**
  - Usually nearly isointense or slightly hyperintense on T2 MR
    - May have foci of hypointensity due to old hemorrhage &/or necrosis
  - Fat-suppressed T2 MR sequences may cause signal loss in adenomas with large amounts of lipid
- **Cholangiocarcinoma (Peripheral)**
  - Extensive fibrosis in tumor may account for hypointense foci
  - Associated with focal hepatic volume loss; delayed persistent enhancement
- **Fibrolamellar Hepatocellular Carcinoma**

○ Large mass with eccentric bands of scar tissue (fibrosis) and calcification that are hypointense on T2 MR
○ Affects adolescents and young adults disproportionately

- **Nodular Regenerative Hyperplasia**
  ○ Large, regenerating nodules are macroscopic or multiacinar form of nodular regenerative hyperplasia
  ○ Common in Budd-Chiari syndrome, congenital heart disease
  ○ Hypervascular nodules 1-4 cm in diameter ± halo of enhancement
  ○ Usually more numerous and greater conspicuity on T1 C+ MR
    – Few that are detectable on T2 MR are typically hypointense

- **Hepatic Sarcoidosis**
  ○ Liver often diffusely abnormal with innumerable ≤ 1-cm nodules
  ○ May be indistinguishable from cirrhosis with regenerating nodules
  ○ Look for lymphadenopathy, lung disease

- **Hepatic Hematoma**
  ○ Old hemorrhage may appear dark on T2 MR

- **Hereditary Hemorrhagic Telangiectasia**
  ○ Osler-Weber-Rendu syndrome
  ○ Large feeding hepatic arteries and draining veins with telangiectasias and arteriovenous malformations
    – Flowing blood accounts for hypointense foci
  ○ Check for history of epistaxis, family history

- **Portal Vein Gas**
  ○ Signal void in vessel due to gas
  ○ Usually due to bowel ischemia or infection
    – e.g., diverticulitis

- **Hepatic Portal or Venous Collaterals**
  ○ Portal vein thrombosis with cavernous transformation
  ○ Also increased hepatic arterial supply to compensate for decreased portal flow
    – Flowing blood accounts for foci of hypointensity
  ○ Hepatic vein occlusion with intra- or perihepatic collaterals (Budd-Chiari syndrome)

- **Primary Biliary Cholangitis**

○ Periportal halo (seen in 1/4 patients) → significant fibrosis (≥ stage II)
  – Hypointense on T2 MR due to fibrosis

Helpful Clues for Rare Diagnoses

- **Peliosis Hepatis**
  ○ Rare, associated with drugs, chronic illness
  ○ Presence of sinusoidal blood pools may account for hypointensity on T2 MR

- **Hepatic Angiomyolipoma**
  ○ Presence of smooth muscle (macromolecules) and fat may account for foci of hypointensity

Regenerating (Cirrhotic) Nodules

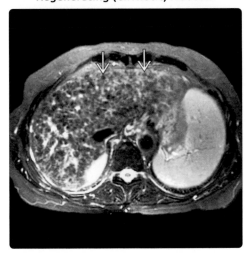

Pneumobilia

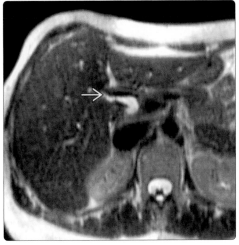

(Left) Axial T2 MR shows innumerable tiny, hypointense, regenerative nodules ➡ within a cirrhotic liver. These are usually not visible on T1 MR. (Right) Axial T2 FS MR shows a gas-fluid level within the common duct ➡ with the gas floating above the bile as a signal void.

Hepatic Metastases

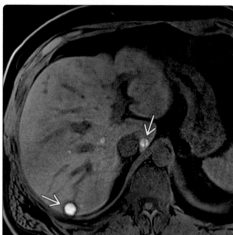

Hepatic Metastases

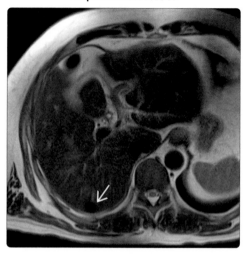

(Left) *Axial T1 FS MR in a patient with hepatic metastases from melanoma primary shows hyperintense lesions* ➡ *due to melanin content. Most metastases are hypo- or isointense to liver on T1 MR.* **(Right)** *Axial T2 HASTE MR in the same patient shows that the lesion* ➡ *is poorly visible and hypointense due to melanin content.*

Hepatocellular Carcinoma

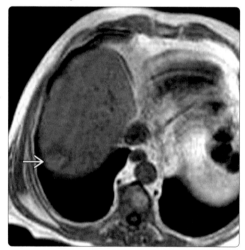

Hepatocellular Carcinoma

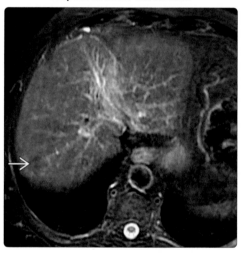

(Left) *Axial T1 MR in a man with hepatocellular carcinoma (HCC) treated with TACE shows a hyperintense mass* ➡ *due to coagulative necrosis. The lesion was avascular on contrast-enhanced MR sequences.* **(Right)** *Axial T2 MR in the same patient shows a hypointense mass* ➡ *due to coagulative necrosis. Untreated, viable HCC is usually hyperintense on T2 MR.*

Dysplastic Nodules (Cirrhosis)

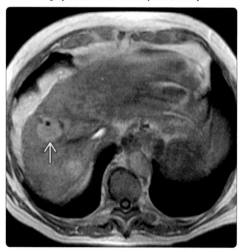

Dysplastic Nodules (Cirrhosis)

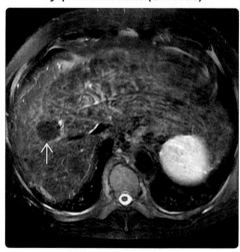

(Left) *Axial T1 MR in a man with alcoholic cirrhosis shows a hyperintense lesion* ➡ *that was not hypervascular on contrast-enhanced sequences (not shown).* **(Right)** *Axial T2 MR in the same patient shows a hypointense lesion* ➡ *that was biopsied and proven to be a dysplastic nodule. Viable HCC is usually hyperintense on T2 MR, variably intense on T1 MR, and hypervascular.*

Cholangiocarcinoma (Peripheral)

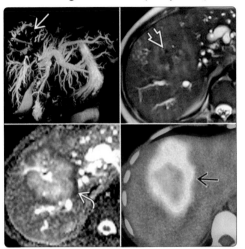

Nodular Regenerative Hyperplasia

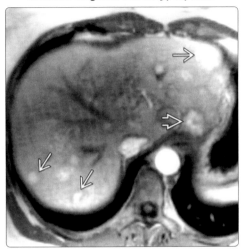

(Left) *Axial MRCP shows diffuse upstream dilation of the biliary tree from the mass ➡, which is hypointense centrally due to fibrosis ➡. There is restricted diffusion on ADC map in the periphery ➡ that corresponds to FDG-avid tumor on PET/CT ➡.* (Right) *Axial T1 C+ MR shows many hypervascular lesions ➡ within the liver of a patient with Budd-Chiari syndrome. At least 1 of the lesions ➡ has a central scar and a hypointense halo, a characteristic feature of multiacinar nodular regenerative hyperplasia (NRH).*

Nodular Regenerative Hyperplasia

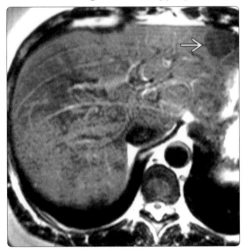

Hepatic Sarcoidosis

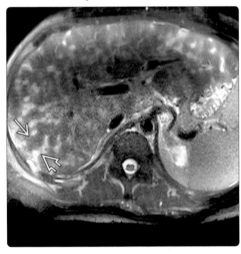

(Left) *Axial T2 MR shows one ➡ of many focal liver lesions in a patient with Budd-Chiari syndrome that proved to be multiacinar NRH. The lesion is hypointense on T2 MR, but many more lesions were apparent on T1 C+ MR.* (Right) *Axial T2 FS MR shows multiple hypointense nodules ➡ with surrounding lace-like fibrosis (hyperintense bands) ➡.*

Hereditary Hemorrhagic Telangiectasia

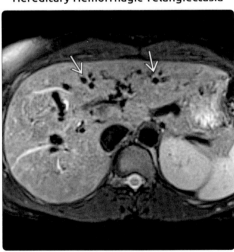

Primary Biliary Cholangitis

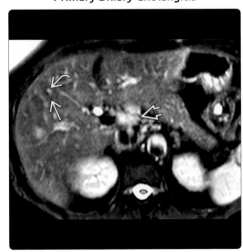

(Left) *Axial T2 FS MR in a 30-year-old woman with hereditary hemorrhagic telangiectasia shows multiple hypointense foci ➡ that represent dilated hepatic veins.* (Right) *Axial T2 FS MR in a 58-year-old woman with primary biliary cholangitis (PBC) shows periportal halo sign as hypointense areas ➡ around the portal veins ➡ and enlarged porta hepatis lymph nodes ➡.*

DIFFERENTIAL DIAGNOSIS

Common

- Steatosis (Fatty Liver)
- Hepatic Adenoma
- Hepatocellular Carcinoma
- Hemorrhagic Hepatic Cyst
- Dysplastic Nodules
- Liver Hematoma
- Hepatic Metastases

Less Common

- Hepatic Pyogenic Abscess
- Postoperative Packing Material
- Post Tumor Ablation
- HELLP Syndrome
- Focal Nodular Hyperplasia
- Nodular Regenerative Hyperplasia
- Hepatic Angiomyolipoma
- Peliosis Hepatis

Rare but Important

- Lipoma, Liver
- Liposarcoma, Liver
- Xanthoma, Liver
- Hepatic Adrenal Rest Tumor
- Hepatic Pseudolipoma
- Teratoma, Liver

ESSENTIAL INFORMATION

Key Differential Diagnosis Issues

- Only 4% of liver lesions are hyperintense on T1 MR
- Any lesion containing fat, hemorrhage, high protein content, or sinusoidal dilation may appear hyperintense on T1 MR
- Focal signal dropout on opposed-phase T1 MR indicates intra- or intercellular lipid
- Focal signal dropout on fat-suppressed images indicates macroscopic fat
- High signal on T1 MR without signal dropout on these techniques indicates presence of blood, protein, or sinusoidal dilation

Helpful Clues for Common Diagnoses

- **Steatosis (Fatty Liver)**
  - Focal fatty infiltration, can simulate mass(es)
  - Bright signal on in-phase GRE with focal signal dropout on opposed-phase T1 GRE MR is key finding
  - Presence of normal vessels coursing through "lesion" excludes neoplasm
  - Can be patchy post severe acute pancreatitis or partial or complete pancreatic resection
- **Hepatic Adenoma**
  - Heterogeneous mass with ↑ signal intensity on T1 MR due to fat &/or recent hemorrhage
  - 35-75% have evidence of fat on opposed-phase or fat-suppressed sequences
  - Lesion with these characteristics in young female without cirrhosis is almost diagnostic of adenoma
- **Hepatocellular Carcinoma**

- Only ~ 5-10% of hepatocellular carcinomas (HCCs) have MR evidence of fat content
- Small (< 1.5 cm) well-differentiated HCCs are more often associated with diffuse-type fatty change (signal suppression on opposed phase)
- Larger tumors may have macroscopic fat (lose signal on fat-suppressed sequence)
- Heterogeneous, hypervascular mass in cirrhotic liver with these features is diagnostic of HCC
- Treated HCCs are often hyperintense on T1 MR
  - In response to embolization or ablation
  - May represent hemorrhage &/or denatured proteins/coagulative necrosis
  - Effectively treated lesions will show no enhancement
- **Hemorrhagic Hepatic Cyst**
  - Will be variably bright on both T1 and T2 MR
    - Due to blood breakdown products
  - No enhancement of contents or mural nodularity
- **Dysplastic Nodules**
  - In cirrhotic liver, dysplastic nodules are considered premalignant lesions
  - Typically appear bright on T1, dark on T2 MR
    - Opposite findings of typical HCC
    - Also are hypovascular and dark on DWI MR
  - Most cirrhotic regenerating nodules are invisible on T1 MR
    - Some are hyperintense due to excess iron (siderotic nodules)
- **Liver Hematoma**
  - Due to trauma; much less frequently coagulopathy or hemolysis, elevated liver enzymes, low platelets (HELLP) syndrome
  - Subacute hemorrhage appears hyperintense on T1 MR
    - Does not lose signal with opposed-phase or fat-suppressed sequences
- **Hepatic Metastases**
  - Rarely are bright on T1 MR, except occasionally for melanoma metastases (due to melanin protein)
  - Metastases may contain fat (liposarcoma) or hemorrhage (hypervascular metastases, especially after chemotherapy)

Helpful Clues for Less Common Diagnoses

- **Hepatic Pyogenic Abscess**
  - May have bleeding within abscess to account for hyperintense portions
  - Proteinaceous debris can also be hyperintense on T1 MR
  - Rim or capsule enhancement
- **Postoperative Packing Material**
  - Omental fat is used as packing material in hepatobiliary surgeries (e.g., focal resection or radiofrequency ablation)
  - Will be bright on T1 MR but lose signal on fat-suppressed imaging sequences
- **HELLP Syndrome**
  - Complication of toxemia of pregnancy with spontaneous hepatic infarction and hemorrhage
  - Diagnosis is usually evident clinically
- **Focal Nodular Hyperplasia**
  - Presence of fat in focal nodular hyperplasia (FNH) is rare, usually patchy distribution

- Most FNH lesions are nearly isointense to normal liver on T1 and T2 MR
  - ○ May appear hyperintense in diffusely steatotic liver
  - ○ May also have bright signal on T1 MR due to sinusoidal dilation within lesion
- **Nodular Regenerative Hyperplasia**
  - ○ a.k.a. large (multiacinar) regenerative nodules
  - ○ Usually encountered as multiple small masses in liver damaged by Budd-Chiari syndrome
  - ○ 75% of lesions are bright on T1, iso- or hypointense on T2 MR
    - − ± halo of low signal on T1 MR
  - ○ Show hypervascularity persisting through arterial and venous phases
  - ○ Lesions resemble FNH on imaging and histology
- **Hepatic Angiomyolipoma**
  - ○ Benign mesenchymal tumor composed of variable amounts of smooth muscle, fat, and proliferating blood vessels
  - ○ Fatty component of tumor results in hyperintense foci on T1 MR
  - ○ Signal dropout on fat-suppressed sequence
    - − Surrounding etched artifact at interface with surrounding liver on opposed-phase images without loss of signal in lesion
  - ○ More common in patients with tuberous sclerosis complex
    - − Look for angiomyolipomas (AMLs) and cysts in kidneys
- **Peliosis Hepatis**
  - ○ Uncommon to rare benign disorder causing sinusoidal dilation and presence of multiple blood-filled lacunar spaces
  - ○ Associated with immunocompromised states, chronic illness, medications

Helpful Clues for Rare Diagnoses

- **Lipoma, Liver**
  - ○ Rare; may have similar appearance as hepatic AML
- **Liposarcoma, Liver**
  - ○ Primary tumor extremely rare

  - ○ Metastases may have fat
  - ○ Rare, as primary hepatic tumor or metastasis or local invasion from retroperitoneal tumor
- **Xanthoma, Liver**
  - ○ In Langerhans cell histiocytosis
  - ○ Multisystem disorder with rare hepatic involvement
  - ○ Uniformly hyperechoic on US, low attenuation on CT
- **Hepatic Adrenal Rest Tumor**
  - ○ Ectopic collection of adrenocortical cells
  - ○ May be functional or nonfunctional
- **Hepatic Pseudolipoma**
  - ○ Pseudolipoma of Glisson capsule; detached colonic epiploic appendix
  - ○ Typically located along hepatic dome; commonly posterior
  - ○ Contains degenerated fat enveloped by liver capsule
  - ○ Signal dropout on fat-suppressed sequence
    - − Surrounding etched artifact at interface with surrounding liver on opposed-phase images without loss of signal in lesion
- **Teratoma, Liver**
  - ○ Hepatic lesion is usually invasion or metastasis from malignant tumor outside liver

Steatosis (Fatty Liver)

Steatosis (Fatty Liver)

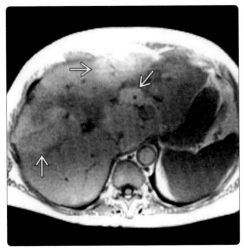

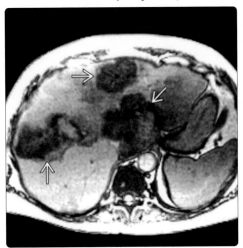

(Left) *Axial T1 MR shows a heterogeneous liver with geographic foci of high intensity ➥, representing multifocal steatosis.* (Right) *Axial opposed-phase T1 GRE MR in the same patient shows selective signal dropout from the foci of focal fatty infiltration ➥.*

Hepatic Adenoma

Hepatic Adenoma

(Left) *Axial T1 C+ MR shows a hepatic mass with central low intensity* ⤵ *and peripheral enhancement* ➡, *which was hyperintense on precontrast imaging (not shown). There was enhancement and increased signal on FS imaging, the latter due to hemorrhage within the tumor.* (Right) *Axial T2 MR shows a hepatic mass that has central low-signal contents* ⤵ *and peripheral high-signal contents* ➡, *the latter due to hemorrhage within this tumor.*

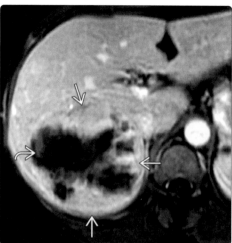

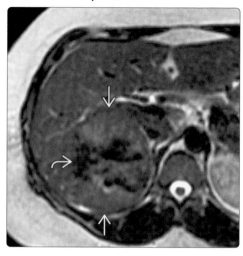

Hepatic Adenoma

Hepatic Adenoma

(Left) *Axial T1 MR in a young woman taking oral contraceptives shows 2 spherical, hyperintense lesions* ➡. *These were encapsulated and heterogeneously hypervascular on other phases of imaging.* (Right) *Axial T1 MR shows an exophytic hepatic mass* ⤵ *that is hyperintense to liver, reflecting the presence of fat within the lesion. Note also the capsule* ➡.

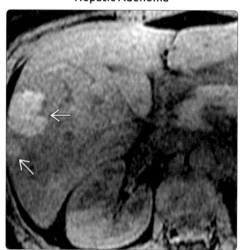

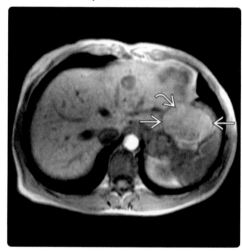

Hepatocellular Carcinoma

Hepatocellular Carcinoma

(Left) *Axial in-phase T1 MR in a 60-year-old man with cirrhosis shows a mass* ➡ *that is slightly hyperintense to background liver. On opposed-phase T1 MR, there are multiple foci of signal dropout within the mass* ⤑, *indicative of lipid content.* (Right) *Axial arterial-phase T1 C+ MR in the same patient shows a heterogeneously hypervascular mass* ➡ *within a cirrhotic liver. On delayed-phase T1 C+ MR, the mass* ⤑ *shows washout and a capsule, typical of hepatocellular carcinoma (HCC).*

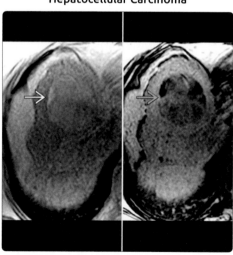

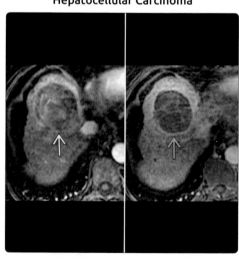

Hepatocellular Carcinoma

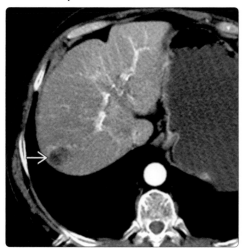

Hepatocellular Carcinoma

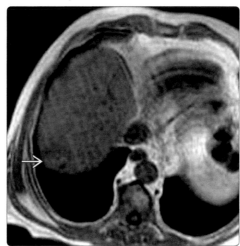

(Left) *Axial arterial-phase CECT in a 70-year-old man who had successful transarterial chemoembolization of an HCC shows no enhancement of the mass* ➡. (Right) *Axial T1 MR in a 70-year-old patient s/p transarterial chemoembolization of an HCC shows a tumor* ➡ *that is hyperintense, indicative of coagulative necrosis.*

Hemorrhagic Hepatic Cyst

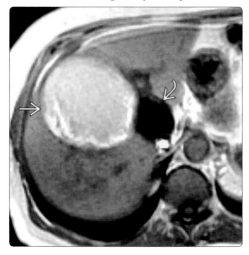

Dysplastic Nodules

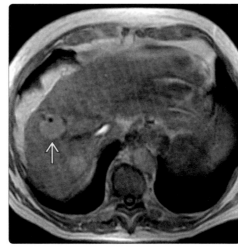

(Left) *Axial T1 MR shows a large, somewhat complex, hyperintense, hemorrhagic cystic lesion* ➡. *The smaller lesion is a typical simple cyst* ➡, *hypointense on this sequence.* (Right) *Axial T1 MR in a 50-year-old man with cirrhosis shows a focal mass* ➡ *that is hyperintense relative to the cirrhotic liver.*

Dysplastic Nodules

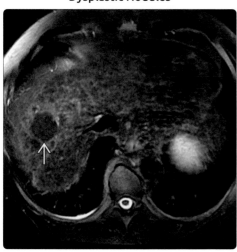

Liver Hematoma

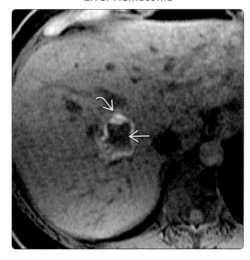

(Left) *Axial T2 FS MR in the same patient shows a mass* ➡ *that is hypointense relative to the cirrhotic liver. The mass showed minimal vascularity or enhancement and was not bright on DWI, all typical features of a dysplastic nodule.* (Right) *Axial T1 FS MR shows a focal mass* ➡ *with a bright rim* ➡, *likely representing blood from biopsy, which confirmed metastasis.*

Liver

Hepatic Metastases

Hepatic Metastases

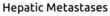

(Left) *Axial T1 MR shows multiple hyperintense masses* ➡, *typical of melanoma, due to the melanin content of these metastases. Most common hepatic metastases are hypointense on T1 MR.* (Right) *Axial T1 FS MR in a patient with colon cancer shows a focal, heterogeneously hyperintense mass* ➡, *representing metastasis.*

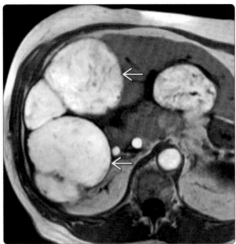

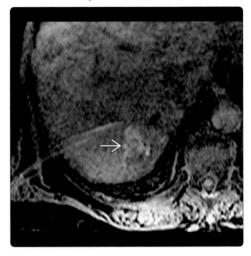

Hepatic Pyogenic Abscess

Hepatic Pyogenic Abscess

(Left) *Axial MR shows multiple pyogenic abscesses in the liver. The T1-hyperintense areas* ➡ *correspond to the T2-hypointense areas* ➡ *and are due to proteinaceous debris.* (Right) *Axial T1 MR shows a cluster of lesions in the right hepatic lobe that are mostly isointense with liver parenchyma but contain hyperintense foci* ➡, *representing hemorrhage (confirmed on needle aspiration of the abscesses).*

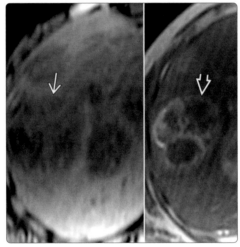

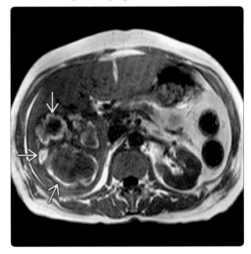

HELLP Syndrome

Focal Nodular Hyperplasia

(Left) *Axial T1 FS MR in a woman with toxemia of pregnancy shows a large, subcapsular hematoma* ➡, *part of which is hyperintense* ➡. (Right) *Axial T1 FS MR shows 2 subtle hepatic masses* ➡ *that are almost isointense to background liver, although both have some foci of hyperintensity. Both lesions showed homogeneous arterial-phase hyperenhancement and prolonged retention of gadoxetate (Eovist), diagnostic of focal nodular hyperplasia (FNH).*

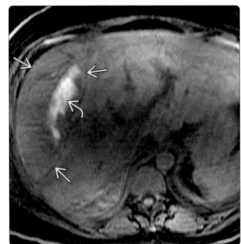

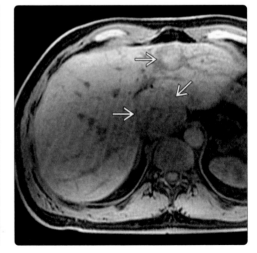

Nodular Regenerative Hyperplasia

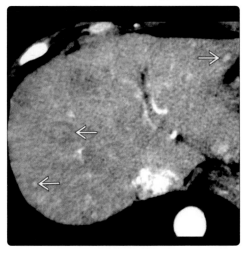

Nodular Regenerative Hyperplasia

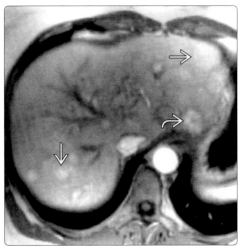

(Left) *Axial arterial-phase CECT in a woman with a hypercoagulable condition shows multiple subtle, hypervascular foci* ➡. **(Right)** *Axial T1 C+ MR in a woman with a hypercoagulable condition shows multiple lesions* ➡ *on arterial-phase contrast-enhanced MR that were also slightly hyperintense on precontrast MR. One lesion* ➡ *has a capsule and central scar, simulating FNH.*

Hepatic Angiomyolipoma

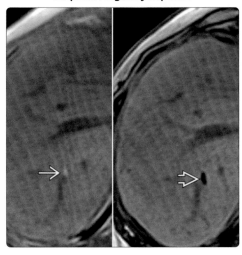

Peliosis Hepatis

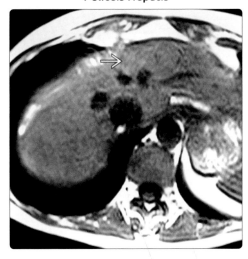

(Left) *In-phase MR in a patient with tuberous sclerosis shows a T1-bright lesion* ➡ *that drops signal on the out-of-phase image* ➡, *consistent with a hepatic angiomyolipoma secondary to the presence of fat.* **(Right)** *Axial T1 MR in a 42-year-old woman with a long history of oral contraceptive use shows a subtle mass* ➡ *that is just slightly hyperintense to liver. CT and contrast-enhanced MR showed multiple hypervascular foci that simulated metastases but proved to be peliosis hepatis.*

Liposarcoma, Liver

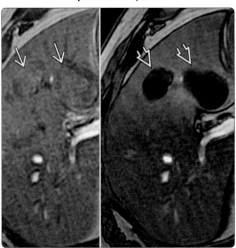

Hepatic Pseudolipoma

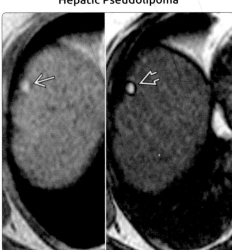

(Left) *Iso- to slightly hyperintense masses on the in-phase image* ➡ *drop signal on the out-of-phase image* ➡, *indicative of fat content in this patient with metastatic liposarcoma to the liver.* **(Right)** *Axial T1 in-phase GRE MR shows a small, hyperintense hepatic lesion* ➡. *Opposed-phase image shows peripheral etching artifact* ➡ *without decreased internal signal intensity due to macroscopic fat.*

DIFFERENTIAL DIAGNOSIS

Common

- Hepatic Metastases
- Hepatic Pyogenic Abscess
- Hepatocellular Carcinoma
- Hepatic Hematoma

Less Common

- Hepatic Adenoma
- Focal Nodular Hyperplasia
- Nodular Regenerative Hyperplasia
- Peripheral (Intrahepatic) Cholangiocarcinoma
- Hepatic Amebic Abscess

ESSENTIAL INFORMATION

Key Differential Diagnosis Issues

- Most benign hepatic masses do **not** have capsule or circumferential rim evident on MR or CT
  - Most cysts, cavernous hemangiomas, focal nodular hyperplasia
- Halo = edema or compressed liver

Helpful Clues for Common Diagnoses

- **Hepatic Metastases**
  - Most common etiology for lesions with circumferential rim on MR or CT
    - Often have peritumoral halo with double ring pattern
  - Metastases are usually heterogeneously hyperintense on T2WI
- **Hepatic Pyogenic Abscess**
  - Usually multiloculated or cluster of grapes appearance
  - Abscess contents are hyperintense with thick, perilesional edema; also bright on T2WI
  - Double target sign on CT
    - Low-attenuation central zone (liquefied necrotic tissue/pus)
    - High-attenuation inner rim (pyogenic membrane)
    - Low-attenuation outer layer (edema of liver parenchyma)

- **Hepatocellular Carcinoma**
  - In patients with cirrhosis of chronic liver injury
    - Presence of capsule in hypervascular mass with washout is diagnostic of hepatocellular carcinoma in this setting
    - Look for signs of cirrhosis, ascites, portal vein invasion
- **Hepatic Hematoma**
  - Following blunt or penetrating trauma, including iatrogenic injuries
  - Chronic hematoma may have hemosiderin in rim that is hypointense on T1WI, often hyperintense on T2WI

Helpful Clues for Less Common Diagnoses

- **Hepatic Adenoma**
  - May have thin, usually incomplete capsule that is hypointense on T2WI
  - Look for evidence of hemorrhage, fat, necrosis within mass
    - Much more evident on MR than on CT
    - e.g., MR may show lipid content by signal loss on fat-suppressed or opposed-phase GRE sequences
- **Focal Nodular Hyperplasia**
  - May have pseudocapsule of prominent draining veins
    - Hypointense on T1WI pre- and postcontrast sequences
- **Nodular Regenerative Hyperplasia**
  - In Budd-Chiari: Hypervascular nodules ± hypointense halo
  - Large regenerative nodules = macroscopic, multiacinar form of nodular regenerative hyperplasia
- **Peripheral (Intrahepatic) Cholangiocarcinoma**
  - Portal and delayed venous phase: Progressive central fill-in, washout of peripheral tumor rim (peripheral washout sign)
  - DWI: Target sign with peripheral hyperintensity due to restriction
- **Hepatic Amebic Abscess**
  - Usually 1 or few lesions
  - Contents bright on T2WI; hypointense rim but perilesional edema bright on T2WI

Hepatic Metastases

Hepatic Metastases

(Left) Axial T2 MR shows multiple hepatic metastases from colon cancer, some of which have a peritumoral halo ➡. (Right) Axial T1 C+ MR shows multiple hepatic metastases from colon cancer with a peritumoral capsule or halo ➡.

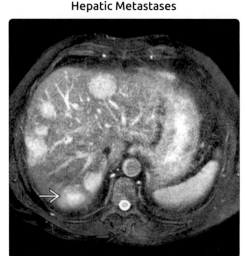

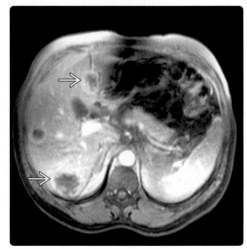

Hepatic Pyogenic Abscess

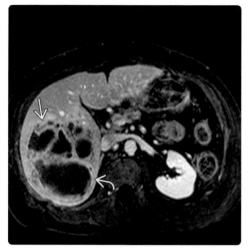

Hepatic Pyogenic Abscess

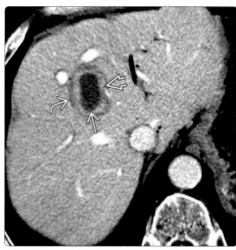

(Left) Axial T1 C+ MR shows a multiseptate mass (or cluster of adjacent masses) ➡ with contrast enhancement of its septa and the surrounding (inflamed) liver ➡. (Right) Axial CECT shows a double-target sign of an abscess. A low-attenuation central zone (pus) ➡, high-attenuation inner rim (pyogenic membrane) ➡, and low-attenuation outer layer (edema) ➡ are noted.

Hepatocellular Carcinoma

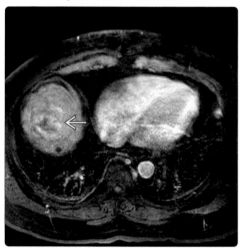

Hepatocellular Carcinoma

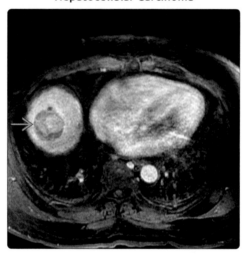

(Left) Axial arterial-phase T1 C+ MR in a 56-year-old man shows a hepatic mass ➡ with heterogeneous hypervascularity, which was also bright on T2 and DWI (not shown). (Right) Axial delayed-phase T1 C+ MR in the same patient shows washout and a capsule ➡, the 2 most characteristic features of hepatocellular carcinoma.

Hepatocellular Carcinoma

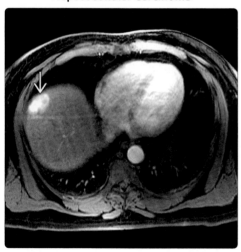

Hepatocellular Carcinoma

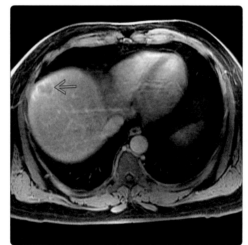

(Left) Axial arterial-phase T1 C+ MR in the same patient shows the heterogeneously hypervascular mass ➡. (Right) Axial delayed-phase T1 C+ MR in the same patient shows the mass with washout and a capsule ➡, findings diagnostic of hepatocellular carcinoma in the setting of chronic liver disease.

Hepatic Hematoma

Hepatic Hematoma

(Left) *Axial T2 MR in a young woman with recent liver transplantation shows a bright, encapsulated hepatic lesion* ➡️, *typical of subacute hematoma. The midline signal void* ➡️ *is an artifact due to metallic clips and coils.* (Right) *Axial T1 FSE MR in a young woman with perihepatic hematoma following liver transplantation shows a lesion with a bright rim or capsule* ➡️.

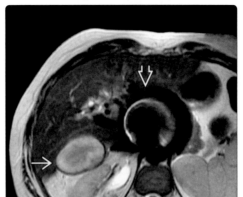
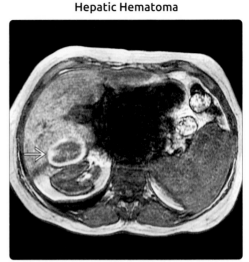

Hepatic Adenoma

Hepatic Adenoma

(Left) *Axial arterial-phase CECT in a 25-year-old woman shows a heterogeneous, hypervascular mass* ➡️ *that was substantially hypodense to the liver (not shown), likely on the basis of lipid content.* (Right) *Axial CECT in the same patient shows the hepatic mass is encapsulated* ➡️. *The hypodensity of the mass is indicative of lipid content, another typical feature of hepatic adenoma.*

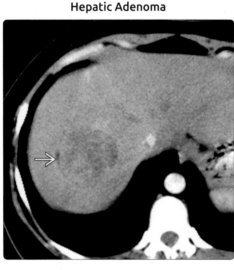
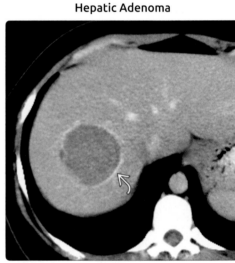

Hepatic Adenoma

Hepatic Adenoma

(Left) *Axial in-phase GRE MR in a young woman shows a hepatic mass* ➡️ *that is encapsulated and slightly hyperintense to background liver.* (Right) *Axial opposed-phase GRE T1 MR in the same patient shows selective signal loss indicative of lipid content and characteristic of hepatic adenoma.*

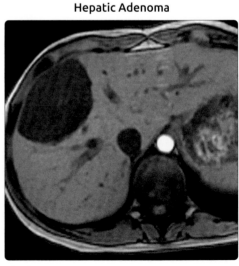

Focal Nodular Hyperplasia

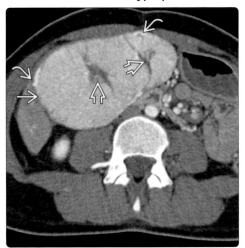

Focal Nodular Hyperplasia

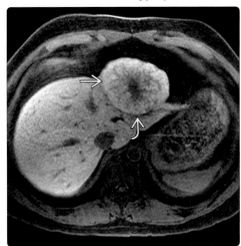

(Left) *Axial venous-phase CECT in an 18-year-old woman with a palpable abdominal wall mass shows a hypervascular mass ➡ with a central, eccentric scar ➡. Dilated veins ➡ on the surface of the mass simulate a capsule.* (Right) *Axial delayed-phase T1 C+ MR in a young man shows an exophytic mass ➡ that retains more contrast (is brighter) than background liver. Also note the central scar and a pseudocapsule ➡ that is composed mostly of dilated draining veins.*

Nodular Regenerative Hyperplasia

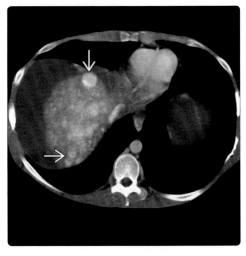

Nodular Regenerative Hyperplasia

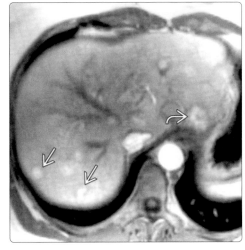

(Left) *Axial CECT in a young man with Budd-Chiari syndrome shows multiple hypervascular nodules ➡ and ascites. Some of the nodules were encapsulated and others had central scars. In this clinical setting, the findings are characteristic of the macroscopic form of nodular regenerative hyperplasia (NRH).* (Right) *Axial T1 C+ MR shows hypervascular masses in a patient with Budd-Chiari syndrome. Some of the lesions show a hypointense halo ➡ and a central scar ➡, findings typical of multiacinar NRH, or large regenerative nodules.*

Peripheral (Intrahepatic) Cholangiocarcinoma

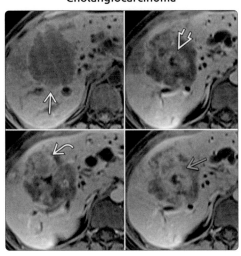

Hepatic Amebic Abscess

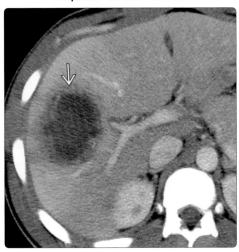

(Left) *A large mass that is hypointense on T1 MR ➡ shows progressive enhancement centrally on arterial ➡, portal venous ➡, and delayed ➡ phases due to fibrotic changes centrally (peripheral washout sign).* (Right) *Axial CECT in a young man shows a solitary mass ➡ with a shaggy wall or capsule. Note the hyperemia of the anterior segments of the right hepatic lobe, due in part to occlusion of the anterior branch of the right portal vein.*

DIFFERENTIAL DIAGNOSIS

Common

- Simple Hepatic Cysts
- Hepatic Cavernous Hemangioma
- Metastases and Lymphoma, Hepatic
- Biliary Hamartoma
- Autosomal Dominant Polycystic Disease, Liver
- Multifocal Fatty Infiltration
- Hepatic Pyogenic Abscess
- Hepatocellular Carcinoma
- Hepatic Sarcoidosis

Less Common

- Opportunistic Infection, Hepatic
- Regenerative or Dysplastic Nodules in Cirrhosis
- Hepatic Adenoma
- Hepatic Amebic Abscesses
- Hepatic Hydatid Cysts

Rare but Important

- Hepatic Angiomyolipoma
- Epithelioid Hemangioendothelioma
- Caroli Disease

ESSENTIAL INFORMATION

Key Differential Diagnosis Issues

- On portal venous and delayed-phase CECT, almost all detectable hepatic lesions are hypodense (hypoattenuating)
- In order to narrow DDx, need to characterize contents and margins of lesions
  - e.g., water density = cysts, cystic metastases, polycystic liver, biliary hamartoma
  - Neoplasms and abscesses have less distinct walls than cysts
- Very helpful to compare with NECT and arterial-phase CECT, if available
  - e.g., contents of cysts and abscesses do not enhance; all (nonnecrotic) tumors do
  - Lesion that is hyperdense on hepatic arterial phase (HAP) but becomes hypodense on portal venous phase is definitely neoplastic
- Hepatic lesions that are "too small to characterize" rarely represent metastases
- Lesions that are lower than blood density on NECT rarely represent metastases
- Look for hypervascularity surrounding lesions, solid component, nodularity, or perilesional edema

Helpful Clues for Common Diagnoses

- **Simple Hepatic Cysts**
  - Commonly are multiple and of variable size
  - Larger ones will measure water density and have sharply defined walls, no or few septa
    - Small lesions: Indistinct walls and uncertain density due to volume averaging
    - Thin CT section minimizes this problem
- **Hepatic Cavernous Hemangioma**
  - Multiple lesions are not rare

- May be innumerable and in other organs and body wall (Kasabach-Merritt syndrome)
  - CT criteria: Blood pool density on NECT; nodular peripheral enhancement, isodense to blood pool on CECT
  - Flash-filling hemangiomas may have surrounding perfusion change on arterial phase
- **Metastases and Lymphoma, Hepatic**
  - Most common cause for multiple solid, hypodense lesions in adult
  - Most common primary sites: Colorectal, pancreas, breast, lung, stomach, ocular
  - Most common histology: Adenocarcinoma, squamous cell, neuroendocrine, lymphoma, sarcoma
    - Colon cancer comprises 50% of cases of metastatic cancer
  - Almost all are hypo- or isodense to liver on portal venous and delayed imaging
    - Many will have hypervascular rim on HAP (not considered hypervascular)
  - Even hypervascular metastases washout to become hypodense on venous and delayed imaging
- **Biliary Hamartoma**
  - Usually multiple to innumerable, nearly uniform in size, < 15 mm in diameter
  - Fibrotic tissue in walls may cause nodular periphery on CECT or CEMR and echogenicity on US
    - Starry-sky appearance on MRCP
  - Biliary hamartomas are common cause of multiple "too small to characterize" lesions
- **Autosomal Dominant Polycystic Disease, Liver**
  - Innumerable cysts, many with calcified walls and higher density (blood)
  - Cysts vary in size and often distort and enlarge liver
  - Associated cysts in kidneys and other organs; family history
- **Multifocal Fatty Infiltration**
  - May closely simulate metastases
  - Often has perivascular distribution or follows fissures
    - Blood vessels traverse lesion without mass effect
  - Definitive diagnosis by in- and opposed-phase GRE MR
  - May be seen following severe acute pancreatitis or post pancreatic resection
- **Hepatic Pyogenic Abscesses**
  - Pyogenic are more common and multiple than with amebic or hydatid
  - Associated pleural effusion, atelectasis, portal vein thrombophlebitis
  - Usually multiseptate or cluster of grapes appearance
- **Hepatocellular Carcinoma**
  - Usually in cirrhotic liver or one damaged by chronic hepatitis
  - Associated signs of portal hypertension, venous invasion
  - Most lesions are heterogeneously hypervascular on arterial-phase CECT
    - Washout to hypodensity on venous and delayed imaging

Helpful Clues for Less Common Diagnoses

- **Opportunistic Infection, Hepatic**

- o Innumerable "microabscesses" in immunocompromised patients
- o *Candida* is most common organism
  - – Other fungi, tuberculosis, and other organisms are less common
- o Usually multiple to innumerable
- o Irregular margins; size from few mm to ~ 15 mm
- **Regenerative or Dysplastic Nodules in Cirrhosis**
  - o Patients with severe cirrhosis
  - o Look for arterial enhancement and washout to exclude hepatocellular carcinoma
  - o Diffuse, lace-like, thick bands of fibrosis
  - o Fatty changes: Diffuse or geographic areas of low attenuation
    - – Usually limited to alcoholic hepatitis with early cirrhosis
- **Hepatic Adenoma**
  - o Uncommon disease, but lesions are often multiple; may be innumerable (adenomatosis)
  - o Larger lesions usually heterogeneous due to presence of fat, hemorrhage, or necrosis
  - o Associated history of oral contraceptives, anabolic steroids, glycogen storage disease
    - – Obesity and steatosis predispose to multiplicity and rapid growth of adenomas
  - o MR evidence of capsule, intralesional lipid, and hemorrhage favor adenoma
- **Hepatic Amebic Abscesses**
  - o Usually in right lobe (70-80%); usually peripheral
  - o Usually isolated or no more than a few
  - o Complex fluid contents with distinct capsule
  - o Imaging and demographics suggest Dx
    - – Easily confirmed by serology

Helpful Clues for Rare Diagnoses

- **Hepatic Angiomyolipoma**
  - o Multiple lesions are seen almost exclusively in tuberous sclerosis syndrome
  - o Only 50% of hepatic angiomyolipomas have substantial fat component

- o Hepatic angiomyolipomas in kidney; cystic lesions in lungs
- **Epithelioid Hemangioendothelioma**
  - o Multiple, peripheral, confluent hepatic masses
  - o Often with target appearance and overlying hepatic capsular retraction
- **Caroli Disease**
  - o Multiple cyst-like spaces within liver that communicate with biliary tree
  - o Central dot sign = portal venous radicle wrapped by ectatic ducts

Other Essential Information

- In nononcology patient, appearance of benign lesions on CECT is often sufficiently characteristic to obviate additional evaluation
  - o Oncology patient: Most metastases have characteristic appearance and biological behavior (e.g., interval growth or regression on therapy) to not require additional imaging evaluation
- Cysts, hemangiomas, and multifocal steatosis have characteristic appearance on MR, allowing confident diagnosis
- Biliary hamartomas are markedly underdiagnosed by radiologists
  - o Comprise many "too small to characterize" lesions seen on CT

Alternative Differential Approaches

- Lesions that may be hyperdense on arterial phase but hypo- or isodense on portal venous and delayed phase
  - o Benign
    - – Adenomas, focal nodular hyperplasia (FNH), nodular regenerative hyperplasia
      - □ Different types of benign lesions may coexist (cysts, hemangiomas, FNH, adenomas)
  - o Malignant
    - – Hepatocellular carcinoma and metastases
      - □ Especially from neuroendocrine, renal, sarcoma primaries, and, occasionally, from primary tumors in ovary, choriocarcinoma, breast, melanoma

---

Simple Hepatic Cysts

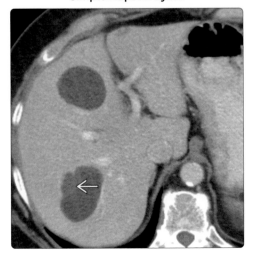

Hepatic Cavernous Hemangioma

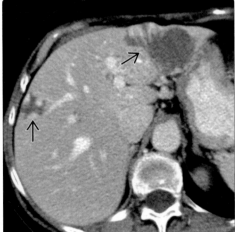

(Left) *Axial CECT shows multiple water density hepatic lesions with no discernible walls. One of the larger cysts has a thin septum ➡, but there is no nodularity of the wall.* **(Right)** *Axial CECT shows 2 hepatic masses ➡, each with characteristic peripheral nodular enhancement isodense with blood vessels.*

Metastases and Lymphoma, Hepatic

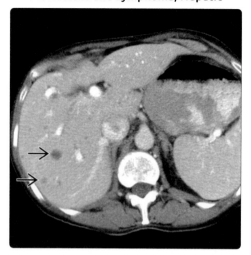

Metastases and Lymphoma, Hepatic

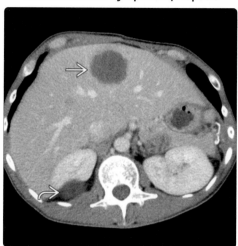

(Left) *Axial CECT in a woman with metastatic ovarian carcinoma shows multiple hypodense liver metastases ➡. The lesions are almost cystic in appearance, reflecting the cystic nature of the primary tumor.* **(Right)** *Axial CECT in a patient with metastatic squamous cell carcinoma shows 1 of several near-water density hepatic lesions ➡ that may be compared with the appearance of a simple renal cyst ➡. Indications that the hepatic lesions are not simple cysts include the subtle wall thickening and irregularity.*

Metastases and Lymphoma, Hepatic

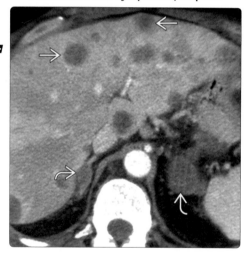

Metastases and Lymphoma, Hepatic

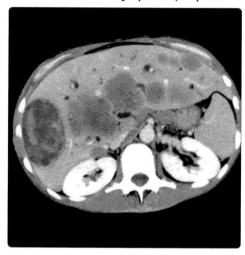

(Left) *Axial CECT in a patient with metastatic pancreatic carcinoma shows multiple hypodense liver metastases ➡ with poorly defined margins. Also note bilateral adrenal metastases ➡.* **(Right)** *Axial CECT in a patient with AIDS and hepatic lymphoma shows multiple hypodense hepatic masses.*

Biliary Hamartoma

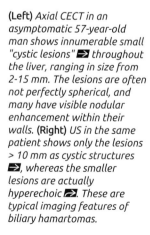

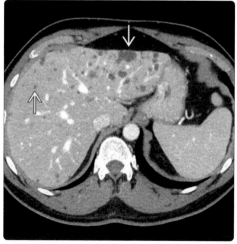

Biliary Hamartoma

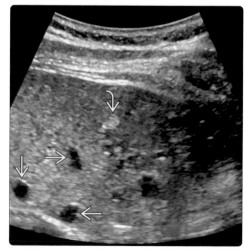

(Left) *Axial CECT in an asymptomatic 57-year-old man shows innumerable small "cystic lesions" ➡ throughout the liver, ranging in size from 2-15 mm. The lesions are often not perfectly spherical, and many have visible nodular enhancement within their walls.* **(Right)** *US in the same patient shows only the lesions > 10 mm as cystic structures ➡, whereas the smaller lesions are actually hyperechoic ➡. These are typical imaging features of biliary hamartomas.*

Autosomal Dominant Polycystic Disease, Liver

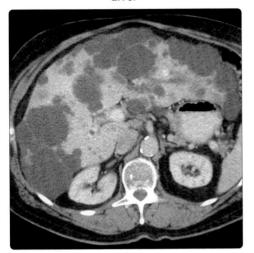

Hepatic Pyogenic Abscess

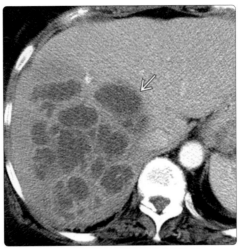

(Left) *Axial CECT shows innumerable hepatic cysts of varying size with only small cysts noted in normally functioning kidneys.* (Right) *Axial CECT in an older woman with ascending cholangitis shows a large, multiseptate mass ➡, typical for pyogenic abscess. This was confirmed and treated with percutaneous catheter placement.*

Multifocal Fatty Infiltration

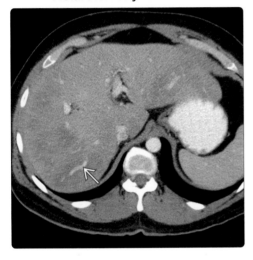

Multifocal Fatty Infiltration

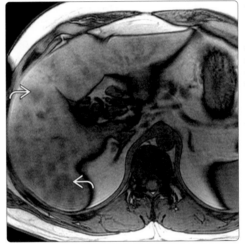

(Left) *Axial CECT in a 36-year-old man shows multifocal, hypodense lesions that predominantly lie in a perivascular distribution, surrounding hepatic vessels ➡. Note that the vessels are not narrowed or displaced by the hypodense lesions.* (Right) *Axial opposed-phase T1 GRE MR in the same patient clearly shows signal dropout from each of the perivascular foci of steatosis ➡, meaning the diagnosis can be made with confidence. Axial in-phase T1 GRE MR showed no apparent lesions.*

Hepatocellular Carcinoma

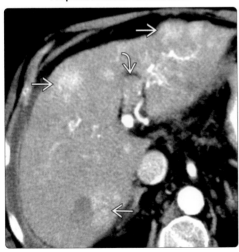

Hepatocellular Carcinoma

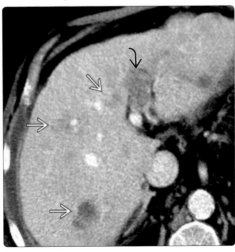

(Left) *Axial arterial-phase CECT in a 55-year-old man shows multiple hypervascular masses ➡. Also note an enhancing tumor within the left portal vein ➡.* (Right) *Axial portal venous-phase CECT in the same patient shows multiple lesions ➡ that are hypodense to the background liver, indicating tumor washout. Also note hypodense tumor ➡ within the dilated left portal vein.*

(Left) *Axial CECT shows numerous hypodense nodules or small masses in the liver and spleen ➡. On this and other sections, CT also showed upper abdominal and thoracic lymphadenopathy ➡. Biopsy confirmed sarcoidosis.* **(Right)** *Axial CECT shows innumerable small (< 2 cm), irregular hypodense lesions in this febrile, immunocompromised patient. Biopsy confirmed Candida microabscesses.*

Hepatic Sarcoidosis

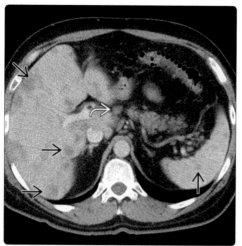

Opportunistic Infection, Hepatic

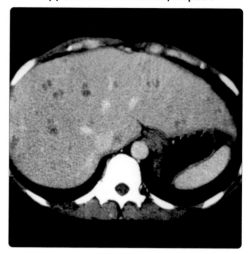

(Left) *Axial CECT in a young woman with acute leukemia and fever shows several small, spherical, hypodense hepatic lesions ➡ that have alternating concentric circles of hypodense and hyperdense rings (target sign). Biopsy confirmed Candida abscesses.* **(Right)** *Longitudinal US in the same patient shows more lesions ➡, including smaller lesions with central echogenic foci and through transmission ➡, indicative of fluid content. Thin-needle US-guided aspiration confirmed Candida infection.*

Opportunistic Infection, Hepatic

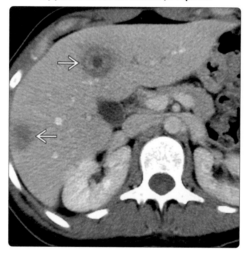

Opportunistic Infection, Hepatic

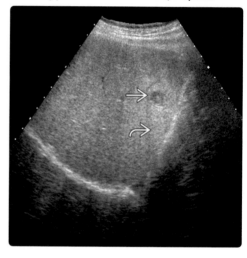

(Left) *Axial CECT shows multiple hypodense, encapsulated ➡ hepatic masses ➡. In this febrile, Hispanic immigrant, amebic abscess was considered and confirmed by serology. Amebic abscesses are rarely so numerous as in this case.* **(Right)** *Coronal CECT in a young Jordanian immigrant with fever shows 2 large, multiseptate hepatic masses ➡. Note the characteristic daughter cysts ➡ within one of the lesions.*

Hepatic Amebic Abscesses

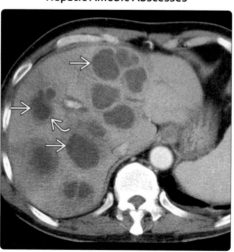

Hepatic Hydatid Cysts

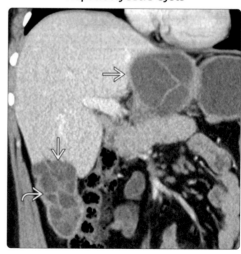

Regenerative or Dysplastic Nodules in Cirrhosis

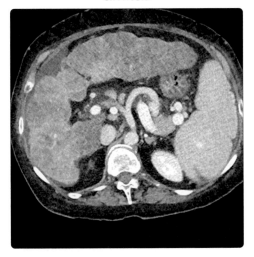

Hepatic Adenoma

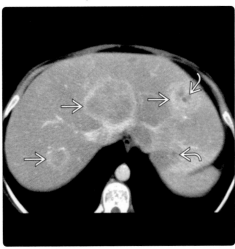

(Left) *Axial CECT in a patient with severe cirrhosis and stigmata of portal hypertension shows innumerable hypodense, regenerating/dysplastic nodules present.* (Right) *Axial CECT shows multiple hypodense but enhancing masses with encapsulation* ➡. *Very low-density foci* ➡ *suggest fat content, which was confirmed by MR within these multiple hepatic adenomas.*

Hepatic Angiomyolipoma

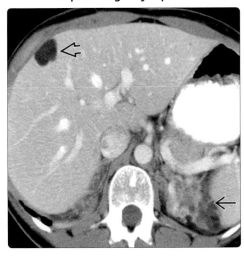

Hepatic Angiomyolipoma

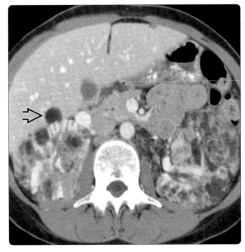

(Left) *Axial CECT shows fat density masses in the liver* ➡ *and kidneys* ➡ *in this patient with tuberous sclerosis.* (Right) *Axial CECT shows fat density masses within the liver* ➡ *and kidneys in this patient with tuberous sclerosis and angiomyolipomas.*

Epithelioid Hemangioendothelioma

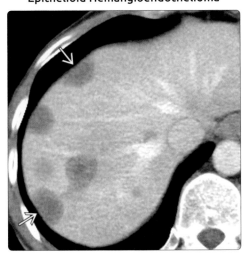

Caroli Disease

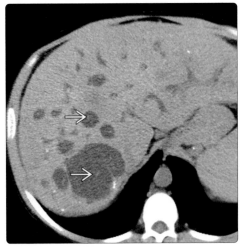

(Left) *Axial CECT shows multiple peripheral lesions with a target appearance and retraction of the overlying hepatic capsule* ➡ *and a characteristic appearance of epithelioid hemangioendothelioma.* (Right) *Axial CECT shows multiple cystic lesions in the liver. Note the central dot sign* ➡, *representing the hepatic artery enveloped by the cystic bile duct dilations.*

DIFFERENTIAL DIAGNOSIS

Common

- Cirrhotic Regenerating Nodule
- Dysplastic (Hepatic) Nodule
- Any Mass in Fatty Liver (Mimic)
- Focal Sparing in Fatty Liver
- Hepatic Metastases
- Hepatic Hematoma

Less Common

- Hemorrhage Within Hepatic Tumor
  - Hepatic Adenoma
  - Hepatocellular Carcinoma
- Calcification Within Primary Hepatic Tumor
  - Hepatic Cavernous Hemangioma
  - Fibrolamellar Carcinoma
- Hepatic Pseudotumor
  - Budd-Chiari Syndrome
  - Primary Sclerosing Cholangitis
- HELLP Syndrome

ESSENTIAL INFORMATION

Key Differential Diagnosis Issues

- Consider whether mass is abnormally dense (hyperattenuating) or whether surrounding liver is abnormally low in attenuation (e.g., steatosis)
  - Compare with spleen
  - Liver should be slightly hyperdense to spleen on NECT
- Abnormally ↑ attenuation due to variety of causes
  - Excessive iron
    - Siderotic regenerating nodules
  - Blood
    - Spontaneous hemorrhage in hepatic tumor
    - Trauma
    - Coagulopathic hemorrhage
    - **H**emolysis, **e**levated **l**iver enzymes, **l**ow **p**latelets (HELLP) syndrome
  - Calcification
    - Punctate or more amorphous calcification in hepatic tumors
    - Common in fibrolamellar carcinoma and mucinous adenocarcinoma metastases
- Mass may represent relatively normal liver surrounded by liver of abnormally low attenuation
  - Focal area of sparing in diffusely steatotic liver
    - Anatomic distribution helpful in making diagnosis
  - Hepatic pseudotumor within liver with extensive damage
    - Spared area may hypertrophy and simulate mass

Helpful Clues for Common Diagnoses

- **Cirrhotic Regenerating Nodule**
  - May be hyperattenuating due to excess iron and copper
  - Essential to recognize on NECT
    - Avoid characterizing as hypervascular because these may remain hyperattenuating on CECT
    - Regenerating nodules usually become isodense to cirrhotic liver on portal venous and delayed CECT
  - MR is good problem solver

- Regenerating nodules appear as hypointense (black) lesions on T2 and, especially, on GRE images
- T2 gradient-echo and fast low-angle shot (FLASH) images
  - Markedly hypointense (best sequence for detection)

- **Dysplastic (Hepatic) Nodule**
  - Considered precursor to hepatocellular carcinoma (HCC)
  - Usually > 2 cm in diameter; hypovascular
  - T1 MR: Hyperintense; T2 MR: Hypointense (low grade)
- **Any Mass in Fatty Liver (Mimic)**
  - Mass of soft tissue attenuation may appear hyperdense within fatty liver
  - Even water attenuation cyst may appear hyperdense within severely steatotic liver
  - Focal nodular hyperplasia (FNH) in fatty liver appears hyperdense on NECT and does not blend in on portal venous phase
    - Prolonged enhancement of entire FNH on hepatobiliary phase (delayed, ~ 20 minutes) on specific hepatobiliary MR contrast agents
- **Focal Sparing in Fatty Liver**
  - Regions of liver surrounding gallbladder fossa and medial segment (#4) are often spared from diffuse steatosis
  - Appears hyperdense on NECT
  - Hypoechoic on US compared to hyperechoic fatty liver
  - Spared area has normal intensity on MR sequences
    - Rest of fatty liver will show signal dropout on opposed-phase GRE MR
- **Hepatic Metastases**
  - Mucinous adenocarcinoma metastases (calcification)
    - Colon carcinoma most common
    - Others include ovarian cystadenocarcinoma, malignant teratoma, and osteogenic carcinoma
  - Malignant melanoma
    - Melanin within metastatic foci may appear hyperdense on NECT
    - Metastases may also appear hyperintense on T1 MR
      - Unlike most metastases that are hypo- to isointense
- **Hepatic Hematoma**
  - Clotted blood may be hyperdense to normal liver
  - Result of blunt or penetrating trauma, including liver biopsy or other interventions
  - Rarely, spontaneous hepatic bleeding due to anticoagulation

Helpful Clues for Less Common Diagnoses

- **Hemorrhage Within Hepatic Tumor**
  - Hepatic adenoma and HCC are 2 neoplasms most likely to exhibit spontaneous hemorrhage
  - Rarely seen with hypervascular metastases, primary angiosarcoma, and others
- **Calcification Within Primary Hepatic Tumor**
  - Conventional HCC
    - Calcification is rare, usually punctate
  - Fibrolamellar carcinoma
    - 2/3 have calcification in large, irregular, stellate scar
    - Lymph node and lung metastases may be present
    - Young adult
  - Adenoma

- Calcification in only ~ 5-10%, punctate
- Most common in young women on oral contraceptives
- MR often shows encapsulation, lipid content, focal hemorrhage
  - Hemangioma
    - Calcification seen in hyalinized (sclerosed) hemangioma
      □ Mild to ↓ T2 hyperintensity and ↓ to absent arterial-phase enhancement vs. typical hemangiomas, mild portal venous-phase enhancement ± centripetal fill in ± capsular retraction ± calcifications
      □ Also sometimes referred to as solitary necrotic nodule
    - May also be seen within central scar in large (> 10 cm) hemangioma with other typical features
- **Hepatic Pseudotumor**
  - In Budd-Chiari syndrome and primary sclerosing cholangitis
  - Caudate and deep right lobe are usually spared

- These areas may hypertrophy (pseudotumor), but normal attenuation is maintained
  - Central spared areas appear relatively dense compared with peripheral portions of liver that are abnormally low in density
    - Peripheral low density from necrosis, fat, and fibrosis
- **HELLP Syndrome**
  - Complication of pregnancy with toxemia and disseminated intravascular coagulation
  - Foci of infarction ± hemorrhage within liver
    - Hematoma may be intrahepatic or subcapsular
      □ Intrahepatic or subcapsular fluid collection (hematoma) on US or CT
      □ Acute: Hyperattenuating clot (24-72 hours)
      □ Chronic: ↓ attenuation after 72 hours (lysed clot)
    - May bleed into peritoneal cavity

Cirrhotic Regenerating Nodule

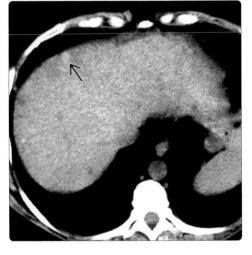

Dysplastic (Hepatic) Nodule

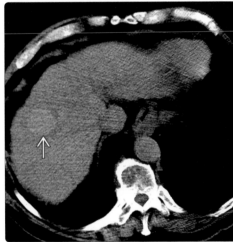

(Left) Axial NECT shows a heterogeneous, cirrhotic liver with both hypo- and hyperdense nodules. The hyperdense nodule ➡ was not visible on CECT, representing a benign, siderotic, regenerative nodule. (Right) Axial NECT in a 50-year-old man with cirrhosis shows a spherical, hyperdense nodule ➡ that showed minimal enhancement on arterial- or venous-phase CECT. The lesion was hyperintense on T1 and hypointense on T2 MR, and it retained contrast on delayed-phase imaging (not shown).

Any Mass in Fatty Liver (Mimic)

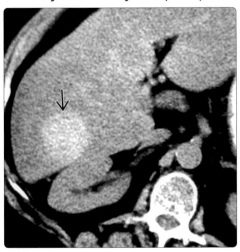

Any Mass in Fatty Liver (Mimic)

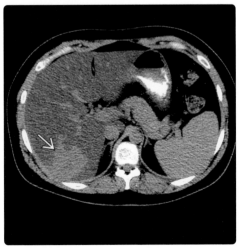

(Left) Axial NECT in a middle-aged woman shows a mass ➡ that is hyperdense to the steatotic liver and isodense to the blood pool, proven cavernous hemangioma. (Right) Axial NECT in a 37-year-old woman with focal nodular hyperplasia (FNH) in a fatty liver shows that the lesion ➡ stands out in a darker background of hepatic steatosis.

Focal Sparing in Fatty Liver

(Left) *Axial CECT shows a diffusely steatotic liver with a mass ➡ that represents an area of focal sparing (normal liver).* (Right) *Axial NECT shows several lesions ➡ that are hyperdense (partially calcified), representing metastases from mucinous adenocarcinoma of the colon.*

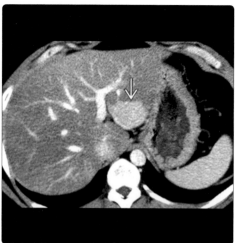

Hepatic Metastases

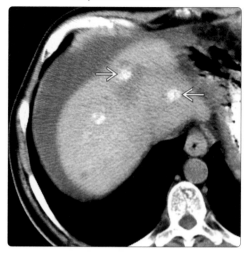

Hepatic Hematoma

(Left) *Axial NECT shows high-density clotted blood in a crescentic collection ➡ around the liver and in a deep linear collection ➡ within the liver due to a liver biopsy.* (Right) *Axial NECT shows a large, heterogeneous mass ➡ in the left lobe, representing spontaneous hemorrhage in an anticoagulated patient. There was no underlying tumor.*

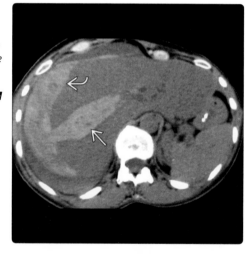

Hepatic Hematoma

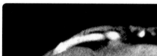

Hepatic Adenoma

(Left) *Axial NECT in a young woman shows a mass ➡ in the left lobe with hyperdense foci ➡, representing areas of hemorrhage within a hepatic adenoma.* (Right) *Axial CECT in the same patient shows enhancement ➡ of the nonnecrotic and nonhemorrhagic portions of this hepatic adenoma.*

Hepatic Adenoma

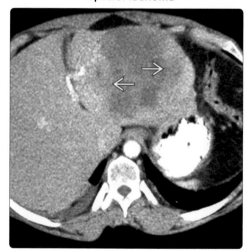

Hepatocellular Carcinoma

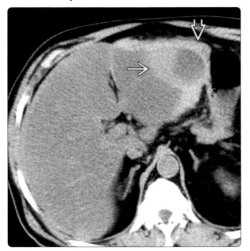

Hepatic Cavernous Hemangioma

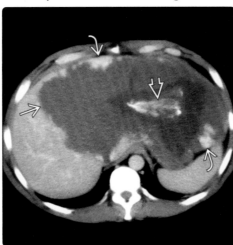

(Left) *Axial NECT shows a heterogeneous mass in the left lobe with hyperdense foci within the mass ➡ and around the liver ⇒, representing hemorrhage. CECT showed an enhancing mass, identified as hepatocellular carcinoma.* (Right) *Axial CECT shows a huge mass ➡ with peripheral nodular enhancement ➚, typical of cavernous hemangioma. A central scar ⇒ is partially calcified.*

Fibrolamellar Carcinoma

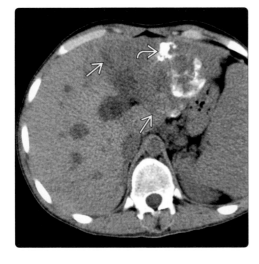

Fibrolamellar Carcinoma

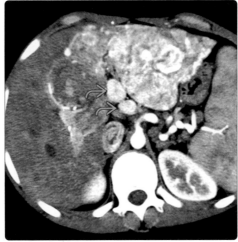

(Left) *Axial NECT in a 17-year-old boy shows a large mass ➡ in the left lobe. Note large foci of calcification ➚.* (Right) *Axial arterial-phase CECT in the same patient shows heterogeneous hypervascularity within this left lobe mass. Also note hypervascular-enhancing porta hepatis lymph node metastases ➘.*

Budd-Chiari Syndrome

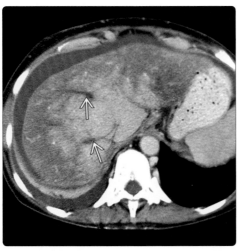

Primary Sclerosing Cholangitis

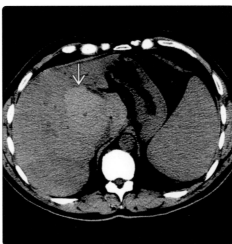

(Left) *Axial CECT shows enlargement of the caudate lobe, hyperdense to the rest of the liver, due to sparing of the caudate and peripheral atrophy and fibrosis, the characteristic pseudotumor appearance in Budd-Chiari syndrome. Thrombosed hepatic veins ➡ and ascites are noted.* (Right) *Axial NECT shows massive hypertrophy and ↑ density of the caudate lobe ➡ compared with the atrophic and hypodense peripheral portions of the liver. CECT and MR showed irregular dilation of bile ducts, characteristic of PSC.*

DIFFERENTIAL DIAGNOSIS

Common

- Steatosis (Fatty Liver)

Less Common

- Hepatitis
- Passive Hepatic Congestion
- Hepatic Infarction
- Toxic Hepatic Injury
- Hepatic Metastases and Lymphoma
- Hepatic Sarcoidosis
- Opportunistic Infections, Hepatic
- Hepatocellular Carcinoma (Infiltrative)
- Wilson Disease
- Radiation Hepatitis
- Budd-Chiari Syndrome
- Glycogen Storage Disease

ESSENTIAL INFORMATION

Key Differential Diagnosis Issues

- Look for mass effect, usually absent in steatosis, present in neoplastic etiologies

Helpful Clues for Common Diagnoses

- **Steatosis (Fatty Liver)**
  - Diffuse, geographic, or multifocal low attenuation
  - Localizes around fissures and hepatic veins
  - Blood vessels traverse low-density focus without mass effect
  - Loss of signal intensity on opposed-phase GRE MR is best sign

Helpful Clues for Less Common Diagnoses

- **Hepatitis**
  - Viral and autoimmune hepatitis usually do not alter attenuation of liver unless there is sudden, massive hepatic necrosis
    - Associated findings: Periportal edema, gallbladder wall edema

- **Passive Hepatic Congestion**
  - Dilated and early enhancement (due to reflux) of inferior vena cava (IVC) and hepatic veins
  - Heterogeneous, mottled, reticulated, mosaic hepatic parenchymal pattern (nutmeg liver)

- **Toxic Hepatic Injury**
  - Ingestion of poisonous mushrooms, carbon tetrachloride, or excess of certain medications (e.g., acetaminophen)
  - Can cause steatosis &/or necrosis

- **Hepatic Metastases and Lymphoma**
  - Lymphoma commonly causes diffuse hepatic infiltration
    - Other findings: Splenomegaly, subtle focal masses in liver and spleen, lymphadenopathy
  - Breast, lung, and melanoma are particularly likely to cause diffuse metastases

- **Hepatic Sarcoidosis**
  - Low-density, enlarged liver or innumerable small, hypodense granulomas

- **Opportunistic Infections, Hepatic**
  - Viral, mycobacterial, etc., in AIDS patients or transplant recipients
  - Usually small, discrete, hypodense or T2-hyperintense lesions representing microabscesses

- **Hepatocellular Carcinoma (Infiltrative)**
  - May simulate steatosis on NECT
  - Heterogeneity, hypervascular foci, and mass effect usually evident on CECT

- **Wilson Disease**
  - Causes low, not high, attenuation

- **Radiation Hepatitis**
  - Corresponding to field of external beam or distribution of radioactive embolic beads
  - Sharply demarcated boundary

- **Budd-Chiari Syndrome**
  - Areas of hepatocellular necrosis, usually in periphery
  - Other findings: Occlusion of IVC &/or hepatic veins, caudate hypertrophy, collateral vessels

(Left) *Axial CECT shows a geographic area of low attenuation throughout the anterior and medial segments. Note that hepatic vessels course through the low-density lesions without being displaced or occluded.* **(Right)** *Axial NECT shows crescentic areas of fatty attenuation ➡ with signal dropout on out-of-phase image ⇉. Hypervascularity in the adjacent liver on arterial phase ➡ blends in on venous phase ⇥, consistent with transient hepatic intensity difference.*

Steatosis (Fatty Liver)

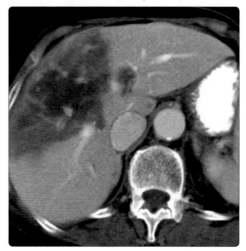

Steatosis (Fatty Liver)

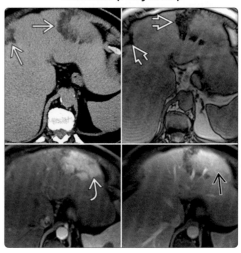

Steatosis (Fatty Liver)

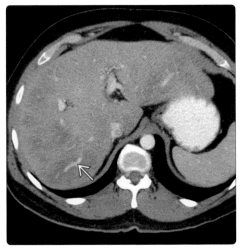

Steatosis (Fatty Liver)

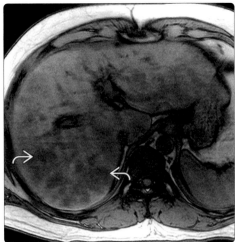

(Left) *Axial CECT shows multifocal, hypodense lesions that predominantly lie in a perivascular distribution, surrounding hepatic vessels* ➡. *The vessels are not narrowed or displaced by the hypodense lesions.* (Right) *Axial in-phase GRE MR in the same patient was normal, while opposed-phase GRE MR shows signal dropout from each perivascular foci of steatosis* ➡, *making this a confident diagnosis.*

Hepatitis

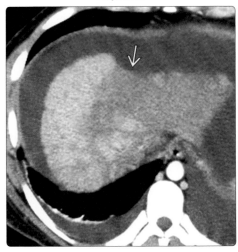

Passive Hepatic Congestion

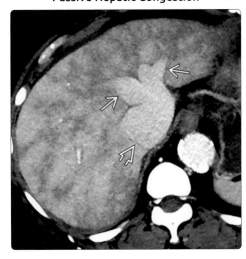

(Left) *Axial CECT shows low attenuation and volume loss of the left lobe in this patient with acute fulminant hepatitis. Note capsular retraction* ➡ *and ascites, both poor prognostic signs.* (Right) *Axial arterial-phase CECT shows early retrograde opacification of dilated hepatic veins* ➡ *and the inferior vena cava* ➡ *due to reflux of injected contrast medium through the heart, a sign of impaired antegrade hepatic venous drainage. Heterogeneous enhancement of the liver is due to passive congestion.*

Hepatic Infarction

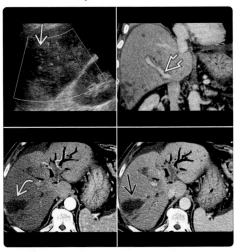

Toxic Hepatic Injury

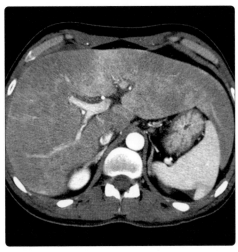

(Left) *Doppler US in a 63-year-old man with pancreatic cancer and right upper quadrant pain shows absence of flow in a hypoechoic area* ➡. *A new small filling defect in the portal vein* ➡ *and wedge-shaped areas on the arterial* ➡ *and venous* ➡ *CT phases represent infarcts.* (Right) *Axial CECT in a young man who died due to acute alcohol and acetaminophen toxicity shows diffuse hepatomegaly with heterogeneous low attenuation throughout. Periportal edema and ascites were also noted.*

Liver

(Left) *Axial CECT in a patient with melanoma and abnormal liver function tests shows diffuse low attenuation throughout the liver, suggestive of steatosis. In addition, there are several poorly defined, hypodense lesions* ➡. **(Right)** *Transverse US in the same patient confirms innumerable focal, hypoechoic metastases* ➡ *with no evidence of the diffusely ↑ echogenicity that would be expected for steatosis. This represents diffuse hepatic melanoma metastases.*

(Left) *Axial NECT shows a large, diffusely low-attenuation liver that might be misinterpreted as being due to steatosis.* **(Right)** *Axial CECT in the same patient shows innumerable focal lesions in the liver and spleen. Liver biopsy confirmed non-Hodgkin lymphoma.*

(Left) *Axial NECT in a 36-year-old man with elevated liver enzymes shows hepatomegaly and innumerable small, hypoattenuating nodules* ➡ *throughout the liver.* **(Right)** *Axial T2 FS MR in the same patient shows multiple small, hyperintense nodules.*

Hepatic Metastases and Lymphoma

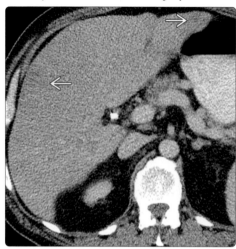

Hepatic Metastases and Lymphoma

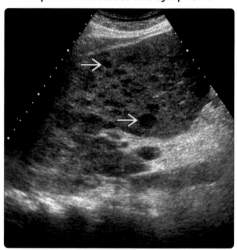

Hepatic Metastases and Lymphoma

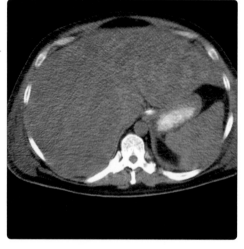

Hepatic Metastases and Lymphoma

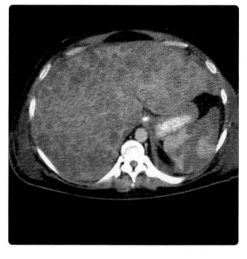

Hepatic Sarcoidosis

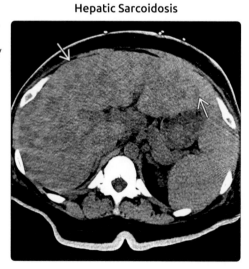

Hepatic Sarcoidosis

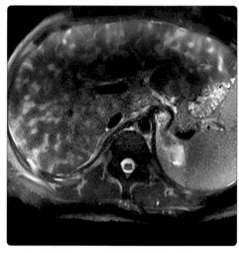

Hepatic Sarcoidosis

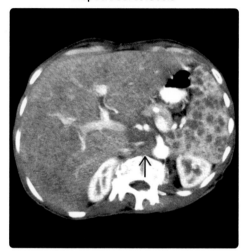

Hepatocellular Carcinoma (Infiltrative)

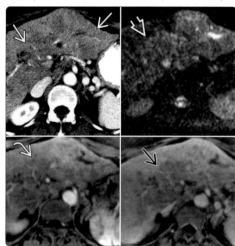

(Left) *Axial CECT shows diffuse low attenuation of the liver with subtle, very small granulomas in the liver and much larger, low-density granulomas in the spleen, + lymphadenopathy* ⮕. **(Right)** *Axial arterial-phase CT shows diffuse, hypodense areas in the liver* ⮕. *This area shows restricted diffusion on DWI MR* ⮕, *heterogeneous enhancement on arterial-phase C+ MR* ⮕, *and washout on venous-phase C+ MR* ⮕.

Wilson Disease

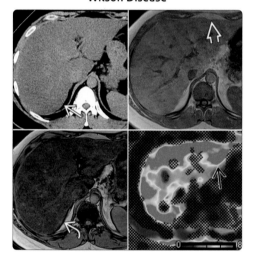

Radiation Hepatitis

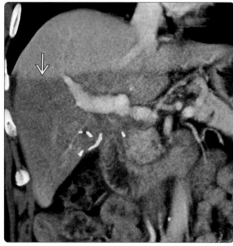

(Left) *Axial NECT shows a diffusely hypodense liver* ⮕. *Axial in-phase MR shows slight nodular contour of the liver* ⮕ *due to cirrhosis. There is signal dropout on out-of-phase MR* ⮕, *confirming severe steatosis, a common finding in the disease. MR elastogram shows ↑ stiffness in the liver, consistent with cirrhosis* ⮕. **(Right)** *Coronal CECT shows a broad zone of low attenuation through the inferior portion of the liver, sparing the superior region, with straight line demarcation* ⮕ *following radiation therapy for cholangiocarcinoma.*

Budd-Chiari Syndrome

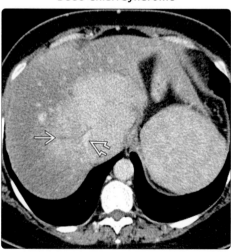

Glycogen Storage Disease

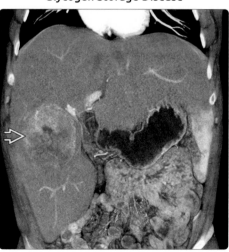

(Left) *Axial CECT shows hypertrophy of the caudate of liver, which is normal in attenuation (as compared with the spleen). The peripheral portions of the liver are ↓ in volume and attenuation due to a combination of steatosis and hepatocellular necrosis. The major hepatic veins are thrombosed* ⮕, *and the inferior vena cava is narrowed* ⮕. **(Right)** *Coronal CECT in a 28-year-old man with type IV glycogen storage disease shows liver enlargement and diffusely low attenuation. Hepatic adenoma* ⮕ *is noted.*

DIFFERENTIAL DIAGNOSIS

Common

- Focal Steatosis
- Calcified Granuloma, Liver
- Hepatic Cavernous Hemangioma
- Hepatic Metastases
- Pneumobilia
- Intrahepatic Biliary Calculi
- Hepatic Arterial Calcifications
- Pyogenic Hepatic Abscess
- Surgical Devices
- Portal Vein Gas
- Biliary Hamartomas
- Normal Anatomic Pitfalls
  - Hepatic Ligaments and Fissures
  - Diaphragmatic Leaflets

Less Common

- Hepatocellular Carcinoma
- Fibrolamellar Carcinoma
- Cholangiocarcinoma
- Hepatic Adenoma
- Amebic Hepatic Abscess
- Hepatic Hydatid Cyst
- Hepatic Infarction
- Hemangioendothelioma
- Hepatic Angiomyolipoma
- Postoperative State
- Hepatic Trauma

ESSENTIAL INFORMATION

Key Differential Diagnosis Issues

- Key question
  - Is echogenic lesion "mass" (usually spherical)?
    - Or is it linear focus [such as transjugular intrahepatic portosystemic shunt (TIPS) or gas in bile ducts]?
- There is significant overlap in US appearance of many of these entities
  - CT and MR should be considered for further evaluation of echogenic masses

Helpful Clues for Common Diagnoses

- **Focal Steatosis**
  - Typically right lobe, caudate lobe, perihilar region
    - Tends to occur along hepatic vessels
    - No mass effect with vessels running undisplaced through lesion
  - Varied appearances
    - Hyperechoic nodule, multiple confluent hyperechoic lesions
      - □ May closely simulate metastases
      - □ Or multifocal hepatocellular carcinoma (HCC)
    - Fan-shaped lobar or segmental distribution
  - CT and MR are good problem-solving tools
    - In- and opposed-phase (OOP) GRE MR is most specific
    - Signal dropout on OOP images is essentially diagnostic of lipid content
- **Calcified Granuloma, Liver**
  - Histoplasmosis, TB, etc.

- Usually small (few millimeters) and multiple
  - Spleen is also usually involved
- **Hepatic Cavernous Hemangioma**
  - Hyperechoic mass in > 2/3 of cases
    - Hemangiomas may be hypoechoic relative to steatotic liver
    - Large lesions are more heterogeneous
    - Atypical hemangiomas: Hyperechoic ring rather than uniform hyperechoic appearance
  - May have posterior acoustic enhancement (due to fluid content)
  - Giant hemangioma (> 10 cm): Lobulated, heterogeneous mass with hyperechoic border
- **Hepatic Metastases**
  - Hyperechoic metastases most commonly from GI tract (especially colon)
    - Foci of calcifications within mass may be echogenic
    - Others include vascular metastases from neuroendocrine tumors, melanoma, renal cell carcinoma, choriocarcinoma
  - Target metastases or bull's-eye patterns are seen in aggressive primary tumors
    - Bronchogenic carcinoma is classic example
- **Pneumobilia**
  - Echogenic shadowing foci in center of liver
    - Biliary gas flows toward porta hepatis
- **Intrahepatic Biliary Calculi**
  - Majority appear as highly echogenic foci with posterior acoustic shadowing
  - May have associated dilated ducts
  - More common in recurrent pyogenic cholangitis
- **Hepatic Arterial Calcifications**
  - Aneurysmal, eggshell, rounded, or tram-track calcification
  - Diabetic arteriopathy; long segmental calcifications of medium-sized arteries, including hepatic
- **Pyogenic Hepatic Abscess**
  - Gas within abscess may be echogenic
  - Most pyogenic abscesses are hypoechoic
- **Surgical Devices**
  - Clips, drains, shunts, catheters
  - Turn transducer to appreciate linear shape of device
- **Portal Vein Gas**
  - Echogenic, mobile, shadowing foci in periphery of liver
  - Gas in portal vein flows away from porta hepatis
    - Very obvious on real-time imaging
- **Biliary Hamartomas**
  - Common cause for lesions "too small to characterize"
  - Mimic cysts on CT and MR (near-water density/intensity)
  - US shows much more echogenicity and fewer cystic lesions than anticipated based on prior CT or MR
  - But may appear cystic or hyperechoic on sonography
    - Due to fibrotic foci in wall
    - Small (< 15 mm), multiple, slightly irregular in contour
- **Normal Anatomic Pitfalls**
  - Hepatic ligaments, fissures, diaphragm slips
    - Infolding of fat along these normal structures creates echogenic focus near surface of liver
    - In short-axis section, "lesions" can appear spherical and resemble masses

– Turn US beam perpendicular to show linear shape of "lesion"

Helpful Clues for Less Common Diagnoses

- **Hepatocellular Carcinoma**
  - Small lesion more likely to be hyperechoic
  - May simulate hemangioma or focal steatosis
    - Look for background of abnormal (cirrhotic) liver
    - Generally irregular hypervascularity with Doppler
  - Usually seen with HCCs containing micro- and macroscopic fat
- **Fibrolamellar Carcinoma**
  - Large, heterogeneous mass in adolescent or young adult
  - Look for central scar (may be hypo- or hyperechoic)
  - CT or MR will show hypervascularity, nodal, and other metastases in most
- **Cholangiocarcinoma**
  - Mass with ill-defined margin
    - Mostly hyperechoic (75%) and heterogeneous
  - Intrahepatic (peripheral) cholangiocarcinoma usually shows dilation of intrahepatic bile ducts "upstream" from tumor
  - CT or MR will show delayed enhancement and capsular retraction with intrahepatic cholangiocarcinoma
- **Hepatic Adenoma**
  - Fat &/or hemorrhage accounts for echogenic portions of adenomas
  - MR will show fat content and capsule in most adenomas
  - Hypervascular mass ± hemorrhage in young woman on birth control pills
- **Amebic Hepatic Abscess**
  - Usually homogeneous, hypoechoic, encapsulated, solitary
  - Hyperechoic if complicated by bacterial superinfection or fistula to bowel
- **Hepatic Hydatid Cyst**
  - Often cystic-appearing, but one may see hyperechoic foci
    - Hydatid sand, parenchymal invasion, calcified rim
- **Hemangioendothelioma**

- Infantile type: Well-defined, large hypervascular mass
- Epithelioid (adult) type: Multiple peripheral confluent masses
  - CT or MR will show multifocal masses with capsular retraction
- **Hepatic Angiomyolipoma**
  - Variable echogenicity
  - CT/MR better for showing fat, hypervascularity
- **Postoperative State**
  - Any procedure that introduces fat or gas into liver can create echogenic, shadowing lesion
    - Examples: Subsegmental resection of hepatic tumors
      □ Surgeons often place omental fat or oxidized gelatin hemostatic agents within hepatic defect
      □ Ablation (cryo- or radiofrequency) may result in gas release within necrotic tissue
- **Hepatic Trauma**
  - Intrahepatic hematoma may be hyperechoic

Alternative Differential Approaches

- **Vascular masses**
  - Cavernous hemangioma, HCC, hemangioendothelioma, some metastases
- **Fat-containing masses**
  - Focal fatty infiltration, hepatic adenoma, HCC, lipid-containing metastases, angiomyolipoma, liposarcoma, teratoma (primary or metastatic to liver)
- **Gas-containing masses**
  - Abscess, infarction, treated hepatic tumors with resulting sudden necrosis
- **Solid masses**
  - Primary liver tumors, metastases, cholangiocarcinoma
- **Masses with calcified rim**
  - Cystic masses (e.g., hydatid cyst)
  - Some cavernous hemangiomas
- **Masses with calcified scar**
  - Fibrolamellar carcinoma, cavernous hemangioma (large ones)

Focal Steatosis

Calcified Granuloma, Liver

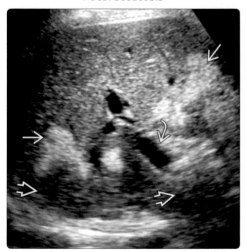
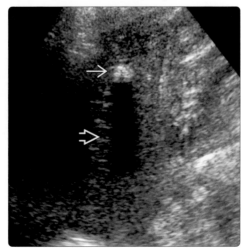

(Left) Transverse US shows multiple hyperechoic areas ➡ with posterior acoustic shadowing ⇒. Note the lack of mass effect on hepatic vessels ⤳. (Right) Axial US shows a coarsely calcified liver granuloma ➡ with posterior acoustic shadowing ⇒. Note the amorphous appearance of the calcification.

Hepatic Cavernous Hemangioma

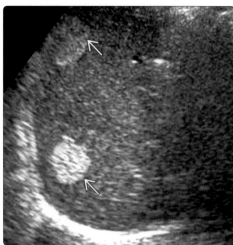

Hepatic Cavernous Hemangioma

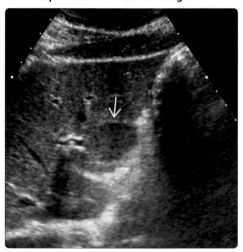

(Left) *Oblique US shows 2 hemangiomas ➡ presenting as well-defined, homogeneous, hyperechoic, rounded lesions. The appearance is typical (seen in 2/3 of hemangiomas) but nonspecific; follow-up is usually required.* (Right) *Transverse US shows an atypical hemangioma that is hypoechoic with a hyperechoic rim ➡. MR showed typical enhancement pattern of hemangioma, confirming diagnosis.*

Hepatic Metastases

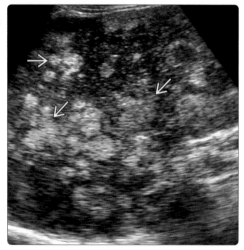

Hepatic Metastases

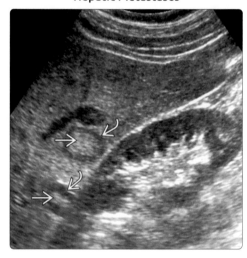

(Left) *Oblique US shows multiple echogenic metastases ➡ from a colonic primary. Other hyperechoic metastases include neuroendocrine tumor, choriocarcinoma, and melanoma.* (Right) *Longitudinal US shows target lesions in the liver representing metastases from lung carcinoma. The center ➡ is hyperechoic with a thick, hypoechoic rim ➡.*

Hepatic Metastases

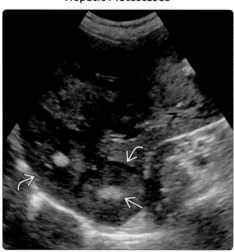

Pneumobilia

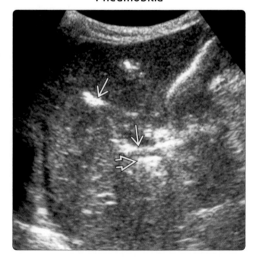

(Left) *Target lesions ➡ from metastatic squamous cell cancer (head and neck primary) have a hyperechoic center ➡ that corresponded to areas of faint calcifications on CT.* (Right) *Longitudinal US shows linear hyperechoic structures ➡, indicating pneumobilia in intrahepatic ducts. Note reverberation artifact ➡.*

Intrahepatic Biliary Calculi

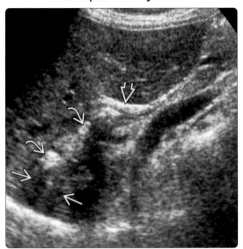

Hepatic Arterial Calcifications

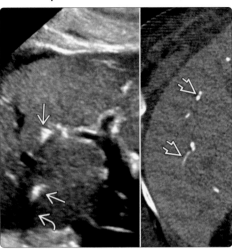

(Left) *Oblique US shows multiple intrahepatic biliary calculi in a patient with recurrent pyogenic cholangitis. The echogenic stones* ⇒ *show acoustic shadowing* ⇒. *Note also pneumobilia within an intrahepatic duct* ⇒. (Right) *Echogenic foci* ⇒ *with posterior acoustic shadowing* ⇒ *on US correspond to severe vascular calcification on NECT* ⇒. *This can be mistaken for biliary or portal venous air.*

Surgical Devices

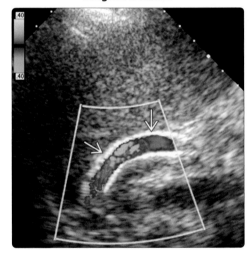

Portal Vein Gas

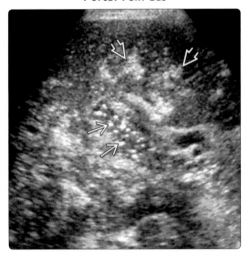

(Left) *Longitudinal color Doppler US shows color flow within a transjugular intrahepatic portosystemic shunt, indicating patency. The echogenic stent* ⇒ *does not obstruct US interrogation and has no acoustic shadow.* (Right) *Oblique US shows tiny, echogenic bubbles of gas* ⇒ *within the portal vein. There are also echogenic patches of parenchymal gas* ⇒.

Biliary Hamartomas

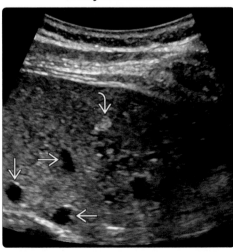

Hepatic Ligaments and Fissures

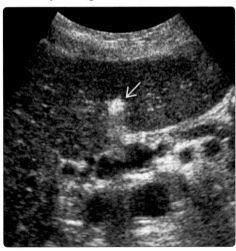

(Left) *In this patient, CT had shown innumerable small "cystic lesions" throughout the liver, ranging in size from 2-15 mm. US shows some of the lesions appearing cystic* ⇒, *while most are hyperechoic* ⇒, *typical features of biliary hamartomas.* (Right) *Transverse US shows cross section of ligamentum teres* ⇒, *which appears as a round, echogenic focus in the left lobe of the liver. Its echogenicity increases with its age. It may mimic focal echogenic hepatic tumor.*

Hepatic Ligaments and Fissures

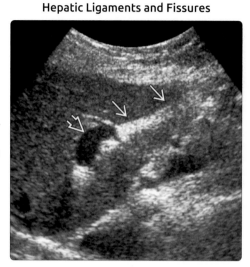

Diaphragmatic Leaflets

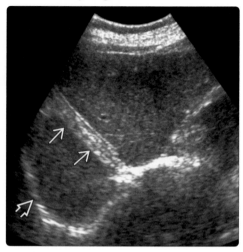

(Left) Longitudinal US in the same patient shows the ligamentum teres ➡, confirming it is not a mass. It runs from left portal vein ➡ to inferior tip of the left lobe. (Right) Oblique US shows a tubular, echogenic diaphragmatic leaflet ➡ near the dome of diaphragm ➡, which is seen in some patients when the transducer is tilted up to the most cephalad portion of the right dome of the diaphragm.

Hepatocellular Carcinoma

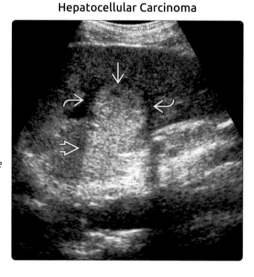

Fibrolamellar Carcinoma

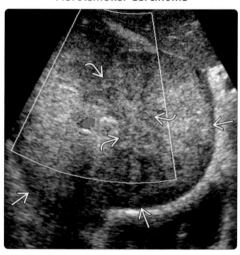

(Left) Oblique US shows a small, hyperechoic hepatocellular carcinoma (HCC) ➡, which may be homogeneous in echotexture. Posterior acoustic enhancement ➡ makes differentiation from hemangioma difficult. Note the thin, hypoechoic halo ➡, which is generally not seen in hemangiomas. (Right) Oblique color Doppler US shows a large, echogenic mass ➡ representing fibrolamellar HCC. Note the central hypoechoic scar ➡, which is typically seen in fibrolamellar HCC but is not specific.

Hepatocellular Carcinoma

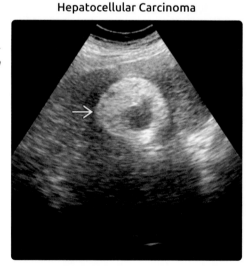

Hepatocellular Carcinoma

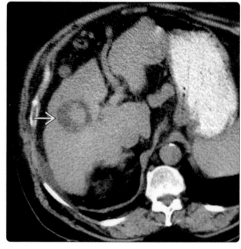

(Left) Transverse US in a 64-year-old man with cirrhosis shows an unusually echogenic mass ➡. (Right) Axial NECT in the same patient shows a mass ➡ with portions that are unusually hypodense due to the presence of fat within the tumor. While macroscopic fat was an unusual feature, the mass was also hypervascular with washout and a capsule, characteristic features of HCC.

Cholangiocarcinoma

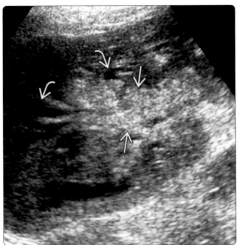

Amebic Hepatic Abscess

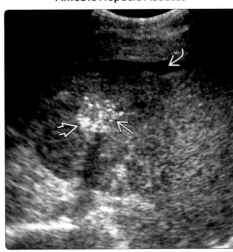

(Left) *Oblique US shows a hilar (Klatskin) tumor ➥ causing intrahepatic biliary ductal obstruction in both lobes of the liver. Note the enlarged intrahepatic ducts ➥.* (Right) *Oblique US shows a ruptured amebic abscess ➥, which has fistulized to the colon. Note the hyperechoic gas locules ➥ within the abscess and a small amount of ascites ➥.*

Hepatic Hydatid Cyst

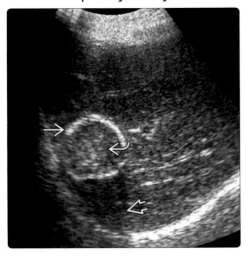

Hepatic Hydatid Cyst

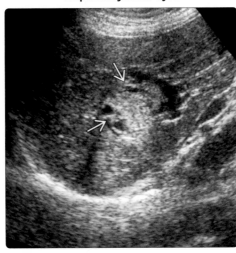

(Left) *Oblique US shows the echogenic, calcified wall ➥ of a hepatic hydatid cyst with posterior acoustic shadowing ➥. Note the echogenic content ➥, representing hydatid sand.* (Right) *Oblique US shows a hepatic echinococcus cyst with echogenic hydatid sand ➥ but no apparent calcification of the cyst wall.*

Postoperative State

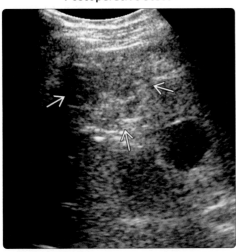

Hepatic Trauma

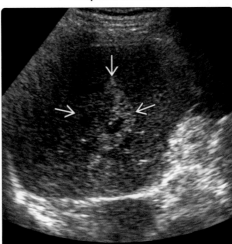

(Left) *Oblique US shows the postsurgical appearance of the liver after subsegmental resection for HCC. The resected area is packed with fat, giving it a heterogeneous appearance ➥.* (Right) *Oblique US shows a hyperechoic area of hemorrhage ➥ after hepatic trauma.*

DIFFERENTIAL DIAGNOSIS

Common

- Steatosis (Fatty Liver)
- Cirrhosis
- Hepatitis
- Metastases and Lymphoma, Hepatic
- Technical Artifact (Mimic)

Less Common

- Hepatocellular Carcinoma
- AIDS, Hepatic Involvement
- Hepatic Sarcoidosis
- Miliary Tuberculosis
- Schistosomiasis, Hepatic
- Biliary Hamartomas
- Mononucleosis
- Glycogen Storage Disease
- Wilson Disease

ESSENTIAL INFORMATION

Key Differential Diagnosis Issues

- Steatosis and cirrhosis account for most cases
- Distinguish between diffuse (widespread without discrete lesions) and multifocal (identifiable, individual, multiple lesions throughout liver)
  - Biliary hamartomas, granulomatous disease, and metastases are usually multifocal, rather than diffuse

Helpful Clues for Common Diagnoses

- **Steatosis (Fatty Liver)**
  - Diffuse increased echogenicity with acoustic shadowing
  - Liver often large with smooth contour
  - With increasing infiltration, vessels are pushed apart and hepatic veins take more curved course
  - Deeper portions of liver, vessels, and bile ducts are often poorly depicted
- **Cirrhosis**
  - Increased, irregular echogenicity + altered flow dynamics in hepatic and portal veins

- Nodular hepatic contour
- Signs of portal hypertension
  - Splenomegaly, ascites, varices
- **Hepatitis**
  - Chronic viral or acute alcoholic hepatitis causes increased echogenicity
  - Acute viral hepatitis usually causes decreased echogenicity
- **Metastases and Lymphoma, Hepatic**
  - Most are hypoechoic
  - Mucinous and vascular metastases may be hyperechoic
  - Breast and melanoma metastases may be diffuse and echogenic
- **Technical Artifact (Mimic)**
  - Improper transducer or gain setting

Helpful Clues for Less Common Diagnoses

- **Hepatocellular Carcinoma**
  - May be multifocal or diffuse
  - Usually in cirrhotic liver
- **AIDS, Hepatic Involvement**
  - Opportunistic hepatic infections (CMV, mycobacterial, etc.)
- **Hepatic Sarcoidosis**
  - Diffuse heterogeneous echo pattern
  - Granulomas may be hypoechoic nodules
  - Porta hepatis and upper abdominal lymphadenopathy usually present
- **Miliary Tuberculosis**
  - Innumerable, small echogenic granulomas
- **Schistosomiasis, Hepatic**
  - Diffuse involvement of periportal septal thickening causes increased echogenicity
- **Biliary Hamartomas**
  - When multiple or widespread
  - Multifocal rather than diffuse
  - Tiny (< 1.5-cm) echogenic nodules (due to fibrous tissue in walls)
  - Some lesions may appear more cystic
    - When fluid content exceeds nodularity

(Left) *Oblique transabdominal US shows moderate diffuse fatty infiltration with increase in echogenicity ➡, posterior acoustic shadowing ➡, and impaired definition of intrahepatic vessels ➡.*
(Right) *Transverse US of a cirrhotic liver shows increased echogenicity, coarsened architecture, and posterior acoustic shadowing ➡. Note the portal triads are not well visualized.*

Steatosis (Fatty Liver)

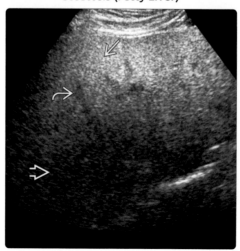

Cirrhosis

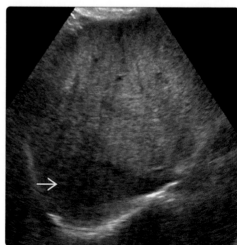

Hepatitis

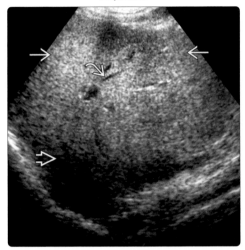

Metastases and Lymphoma, Hepatic

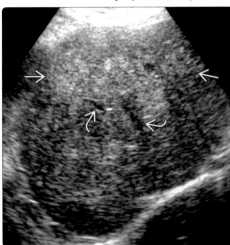

(Left) *Oblique transabdominal US in a case of acute alcoholic hepatitis shows increased echogenicity* ⮕ *and posterior shadowing* ⮕. *The hepatic veins* ⮕ *have a curved course.* (Right) *Oblique transabdominal US of diffuse infiltrative metastases shows heterogeneous increased echogenicity* ⮕ *and distortion of the vascular architecture* ⮕.

Technical Artifact (Mimic)

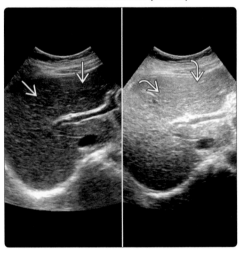

Hepatocellular Carcinoma

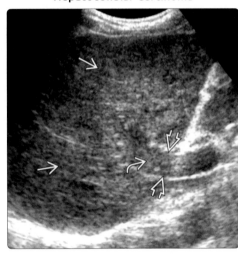

(Left) *Axial oblique US shows normal echogenicity of liver parenchyma* ⮕ *on the left. Improper gain settings can cause an artifactually increased echogenicity* ⮕, *as shown on the right.* (Right) *Oblique transabdominal US shows diffuse hepatocellular carcinoma, resulting in increased echogenicity* ⮕ *and echogenic thrombus* ⮕ *in the portal vein* ⮕. *Doppler is helpful for identifying tumor thrombus.*

Schistosomiasis, Hepatic

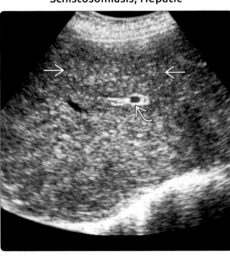

Wilson Disease

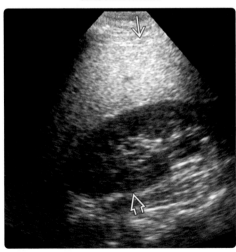

(Left) *Oblique transabdominal US shows diffuse schistosomiasis involvement of liver, resulting in periportal septal fibrosis, giving an echogenic, mottled appearance* ⮕. *Note thickened and hyperechoic portal vein walls* ⮕. (Right) *Transverse US shows a diffusely echogenic liver* ⮕ *as compared to the hypoechoic renal cortex* ⮕, *an internal reference used for diagnosis. Fatty infiltration is the earliest characteristic change in Wilson disease, which is indistinguishable from steatosis from other causes.*

DIFFERENTIAL DIAGNOSIS

Common

- Congested Liver
  - Congestive Heart Failure
  - Budd-Chiari Syndrome
- Acute Hepatitis
- Fatty Liver
- Steatohepatitis
- Fatty Cirrhosis
- Venoocclusive Disease
- Diffuse Neoplastic Infiltration
  - Infiltrative Hepatocellular Carcinoma
  - Lymphoma
  - Leukemia
  - Metastases

Less Common

- Sarcoidosis
- Glycogen Storage Disease

ESSENTIAL INFORMATION

Key Differential Diagnosis Issues

- Hepatomegaly
  - Commonly accepted to be > 15-16 cm long in midclavicular line
    - Size varies depending on sex and body size
  - Volumetric measurements are time consuming and may not be suitable for everyday practice
- Ancillary signs used to identify hepatomegaly
  - Enlargement of caudate lobe
    - Differential diagnosis of cirrhosis
  - Extension of right lobe below right kidney
    - Differential diagnosis of Riedel lobe
  - Biconvex/rounded hepatic surface contour
  - Blunted, obtuse angle; rounded, inferior tip of right lobe
- Enlargement of left lobe (normally smaller than right)
  - Considered when left lobe is present between spleen and diaphragm

Helpful Clues for Common Diagnoses

- **Congested Liver**
  - **Congestive heart failure**
    - Dilated hepatic veins and inferior vena cava (IVC)
    - Venous star appearance at IVC-hepatic vein junction (instead of "rabbit ears")
    - Dilated hepatic veins may extend to periphery of liver
    - Hepatic venous flow: Turbulent appearance and pulsatile waveform on Doppler ultrasound
    - Marked pulsatility of portal vein
    - Hypoechoic parenchyma, increased posterior enhancement, soft consistency (dynamic indentation by cardiac motion)
    - Ancillary findings: Ascites, pleural effusion, thickened visceral walls (gallbladder, bowel, stomach), splenomegaly
    - Cardiomegaly
  - **Budd-Chiari syndrome**
    - Acute phase

- Hepatomegaly and parenchymal heterogeneous echogenicity due to congestion
- Hepatic veins/IVC: Normal or distended caliber, partially/completely filled with hypoechoic material
- Absent or restricted flow in hepatic veins/IVC
- Aliasing or reversed flow in patent portions of IVC due to stenosis
- Development of small intrahepatic venous collaterals
  - Chronic phase
    - Stenotic or occluded hepatic veins/IVC
    - Compensatory hypertrophy of caudate lobe, atrophy of involved segments
    - Large regenerative nodules
- **Acute Hepatitis**
  - Diffuse decrease in echogenicity
  - Echogenicity similar to renal cortex and spleen
  - Starry-sky appearance
    - Increased echogenicity of portal triad walls against background hypoechoic liver
    - Variably seen
  - Periportal hypo-/anechoic areas due to edema
  - Marked circumferential gallbladder wall edema/thickening
    - Associated with hepatitis A virus
  - Elevated hepatic artery peak velocity on Doppler ultrasound
- **Fatty Liver**
  - Increase in size of liver and change in shape as volume of infiltration increases
    - Inferior margin of right lobe has rounded contours
    - Left lobe becomes biconvex
  - Increased echogenicity
    - Liver significantly more echogenic than kidney
    - Echogenicity may vary between segments (areas of focal fatty sparing)
  - Preservation of hepatic architecture
  - Blurred margins of hepatic veins due to increased refraction and scattering of sound
  - Vessels course through liver without distortion
    - May be spread apart secondary to expansion of liver parenchyma
  - Posterior segments of liver not clearly seen due to acoustic attenuation
  - Focal fatty sparing may simulate hypoechoic lesion
  - Soft consistency: Dynamic indentation by cardiac motion
- **Steatohepatitis**
  - Characterized by inflammation accompanying fat accumulation
    - Definitive diagnosis made by liver biopsy
  - May occur in alcoholic hepatitis and nonalcoholic steatohepatitis (NASH)
  - Etiology of NASH unknown but frequently seen in following conditions
    - Obesity
    - Diabetes
    - Hyperlipidemia
    - Drugs and toxins
  - Ultrasound findings

- Signs of fatty liver
- Firm consistency (due to inflammation) on dynamic scanning during cardiac cycle
- Irregular borders of hepatic veins due to hepatic inflammation
- Intermittent loss of visualization of hepatic veins

- **Fatty Cirrhosis**
  - Enlarged left and caudate lobes and atrophic right lobe
  - Hyperechoic but heterogeneous liver echo pattern
  - Irregular hepatic veins
  - Portal venous collaterals
  - Stiff consistency
  - Ancillary signs of portal hypertension
    - Ascites, varices, hepatofugal flow, splenomegaly

- **Venoocclusive Disease**
  - Hepatosplenomegaly and ascites
  - Periportal and gallbladder wall edema
  - Narrowing and monophasic waveform of hepatic veins due to hepatic edema
  - Slow or reversed flow in portal vein
  - Prominent hepatic arteries and elevated arterial peak systolic velocity
  - Abnormal hepatic arterial resistive index
    - < 0.55 or > 0.75 (variably seen)

- **Diffuse Neoplastic Infiltration**
  - **Infiltrative hepatocellular carcinoma**
    - Ill-defined area of markedly heterogeneous echotexture
      - Often indistinguishable from underlying cirrhosis
    - Color Doppler: Malignant portal vein thrombosis
      - Absence of normal blood flow and presence of hypoechoic thrombus extending into portal vein
      - Presence of arterialized flow in portal vein thrombus: High PPV but moderate sensitivity
  - **Lymphoma**
    - Diffuse/infiltrative form presents as innumerable subcentimeter hypoechoic foci
    - Miliary pattern
    - Periportal location

- Infiltrative pattern may be indistinguishable from normal liver
- Also look for lymphadenopathy, splenomegaly or splenic lesions, bowel wall thickening, ascites
  - **Metastases**
    - Discrete nodules and masses or infiltrative pattern
    - Lung or breast cancer: Common primary showing infiltrative pattern hepatic metastases
    - Infiltrative pattern shows heterogeneous echotexture and simulates cirrhosis

Helpful Clues for Less Common Diagnoses

- **Sarcoidosis**
  - Hepatosplenic involvement
    - Most common finding: Nonspecific hepatosplenomegaly
    - Diffuse parenchymal heterogeneous echotexture
    - Numerous small nodular pattern
    - Advanced disease may cause or simulate cirrhosis
  - Can affect almost every organ
    - Most common site: Lung
  - Upper abdominal lymphadenopathy often present
- **Glycogen Storage Disease**
  - Hepatomegaly and multiple hepatic adenomas in chronically ill young patients
  - Liver may appear diffusely echogenic
    - Indistinguishable from fatty liver
  - Requires biopsy for diagnosis

SELECTED REFERENCES

1. Chang TY et al: Utility of quantitative ultrasound in community screening for hepatic steatosis. Ultrasonics. 111:106329, 2021
2. Ferraioli G et al: Ultrasound-based techniques for the diagnosis of liver steatosis. World J Gastroenterol. 25(40):6053-62, 2019
3. Idilman IS et al: Hepatic steatosis: etiology, patterns, and quantification. Semin Ultrasound CT MR. 37(6):501-10, 2016
4. Karanjia RN et al: Hepatic steatosis and fibrosis: non-invasive assessment. World J Gastroenterol. 22(45):9880-97, 2016
5. Faraoun SA et al: Budd-Chiari syndrome: a prospective analysis of hepatic vein obstruction on ultrasonography, multidetector-row computed tomography and MR imaging. Abdom Imaging. 40(6):1500-9, 2015

Congested Liver

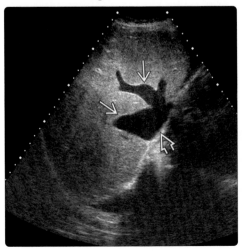

Budd-Chiari Syndrome

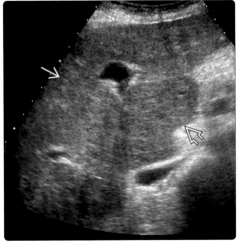

(Left) *Oblique US of the liver at the level of the hepatic venous confluence shows an enlarged liver with marked dilatation of hepatic veins ➡ and inferior vena cava (IVC) ⇉, indicating hepatic congestion in a patient with right heart failure.* **(Right)** *Transverse abdominal US in a patient with Budd-Chiari syndrome shows heterogeneous hepatic parenchymal echogenicity ➡ and hypertrophied caudate lobe ⇉. The caudate is often hypertrophied in the setting of Budd-Chiari due to its separate venous drainage into the IVC.*

(Left) *Longitudinal abdominal US in a patient with severe hepatic steatosis shows an enlarged liver, which is diffusely echogenic* ➡ *compared to the right kidney* ➡. *Note the marked attenuation of the US beam, which results in poor visualization of the diaphragm.* (Right) *Longitudinal abdominal US in a patient who presented with acute liver failure from acute alcoholic hepatitis shows a markedly enlarged liver* ➡ *extending well below the inferior renal margin.*

Fatty Liver

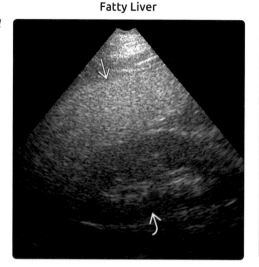

Steatohepatitis

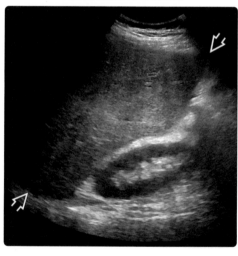

(Left) *Transverse abdominal US in a patient with venoocclusive disease shows a markedly enlarged and edematous liver resulting in narrowed hepatic veins* ➡ *and small-caliber IVC* ➡. *A small right pleural effusion is also evident* ➡. (Right) *Longitudinal abdominal US in a patient with venoocclusive disease shows marked hepatomegaly with craniocaudal length of the liver measuring 22.6 cm* ➡. *Liver extension well beyond the edge of the kidney is indicative of hepatomegaly.*

Venoocclusive Disease

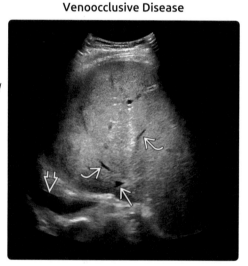

Venoocclusive Disease

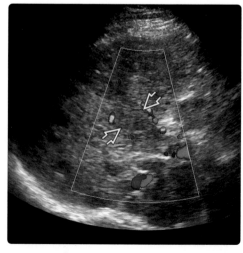

(Left) *Transverse grayscale US of the liver shows a markedly heterogeneous and enlarged liver with multiple refractive shadows* ➡ *caused by diffuse, infiltrative hepatocellular carcinoma (HCC). Focal echogenic lesion* ➡ *was shown to be a fat-containing focus of HCC.* (Right) *Transverse abdominal color Doppler US shows the right portal vein filled with echogenic material* ➡, *consistent with portal vein tumor thrombosis. Underlying liver is markedly heterogeneous because of diffuse HCC.*

Infiltrative Hepatocellular Carcinoma

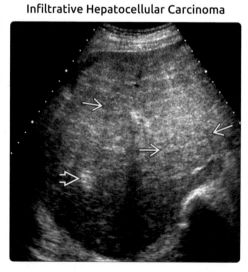

Infiltrative Hepatocellular Carcinoma

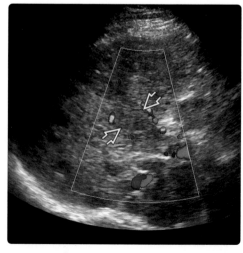

Lymphoma

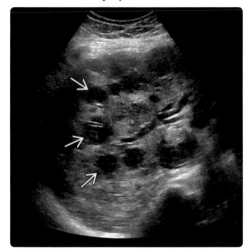

Lymphoma

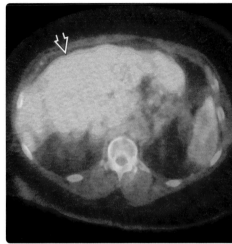

(Left) *Transverse abdominal US in a patient with lymphoma shows multiple markedly hypoechoic masses* ➡ *throughout the right lobe of the liver.* (Right) *FDG PET in the same patient shows the liver is enlarged and diffusely hypermetabolic throughout the entire liver parenchyma* ➡.

Metastases

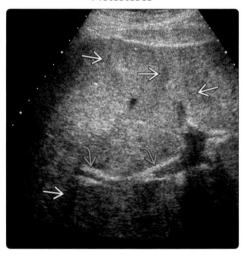

Metastases

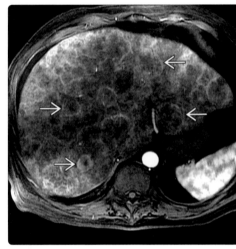

(Left) *Transverse abdominal US in a patient with hepatic metastasis from neuroendocrine tumor demonstrates enlarged and markedly heterogeneous appearance of the liver with numerous refractive shadows* ➡ *caused by underlying isoechoic metastasis. The portal veins are distorted* ➡ *by mass effect.* (Right) *T1 C+ FS MR in the same patient demonstrates that the heterogeneous liver appearance on US is due to numerous masses* ➡, *which replace virtually the entire liver parenchyma.*

Metastases

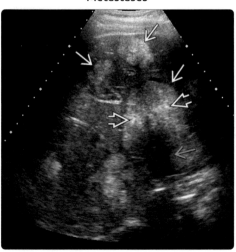

Sarcoidosis

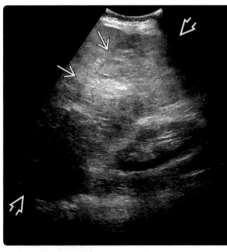

(Left) *Transverse abdominal US in a patient with colon cancer metastases in the liver shows multiple hyperechoic masses* ➡, *which enlarge the liver. Posterior acoustic shadowing* ➡ *associated with the largest mass is caused by calcifications* ➡ *in the liver metastasis.* (Right) *Transverse abdominal US in a patient with sarcoidosis shows hepatomegaly (26 cm in length)* ➡ *and heterogeneous hepatic parenchyma* ➡ *due to hepatic involvement by sarcoidosis.*

DIFFERENTIAL DIAGNOSIS

Common

- Steatosis (Fatty Liver)
- Cirrhosis
- Acute/Chronic Hepatitis
- Hepatocellular Carcinoma (Diffuse/Infiltrative)
- Infiltrative Metastasis
- Hepatic Lymphoma (Diffuse/Infiltrative)
- Biliary Hamartomas
- Technical Artifact (Mimic)

Less Common

- AIDS
- Hepatic Sarcoidosis
- Amyloidosis
- Schistosomiasis
- Glycogen Storage Disease
- Wilson Disease
- Venoocclusive Disease

ESSENTIAL INFORMATION

Key Differential Diagnosis Issues

- Diffusely increased echogenicity: Steatosis and cirrhosis account for most cases

Helpful Clues for Common Diagnoses

- **Steatosis (Fatty Liver)**
  - Diffuse increased echogenicity with acoustic attenuation
  - Liver often large with smooth contour
  - With increasing infiltration, vessels are pushed apart, and hepatic veins take more curved course
- **Cirrhosis**
  - Heterogeneous parenchymal echogenicity
  - Liver surface nodularity, volume shrinkage
  - Altered flow dynamics in hepatic vasculature
- **Acute Hepatitis**
  - Decreased parenchymal echogenicity due to edema
    - Acute alcoholic hepatitis: Increased echogenicity

  - Hepatomegaly, periportal/gallbladder edema, ascites
- **Chronic Hepatitis**
  - Increased and heterogeneous parenchymal echogenicity
- **Hepatocellular Carcinoma (Diffuse/Infiltrative)**
  - Heterogeneous liver echotexture with refractive shadows
  - May accompany portal vein tumor thrombosis
- **Infiltrative Metastasis**
  - Lung or breast primary
  - May simulate cirrhosis
- **Hepatic Lymphoma (Diffuse/Infiltrative)**
  - Hepatomegaly
  - Numerous small hypoechoic foci, miliary in pattern and periportal in location
  - May be indistinguishable from normal liver
- **Biliary Hamartomas**
  - Tiny (< 1.5-cm) echogenic nodules with comet-tail artifacts
  - Numerous tiny lesions lead to inhomogeneous and coarse liver echotexture
- **Technical Artifact (Mimic)**
  - Improper transducer or gain setting

Helpful Clues for Less Common Diagnoses

- **AIDS**
  - Microabscesses from opportunistic infection (cytomegalovirus, mycobacterium, etc.)
- **Hepatic Sarcoidosis**
  - Diffuse heterogeneous echo pattern
  - Granulomas seen as hypoechoic nodules
- **Schistosomiasis**
  - Increased echogenicity caused by diffuse periportal septal thickening
- **Amyloidosis**
  - Hepatomegaly
  - Heterogeneous parenchymal echogenicity

SELECTED REFERENCES

1. Ghadimi M et al: Advances in imaging of diffuse parenchymal liver disease. J Clin Gastroenterol. 54(8):682-95, 2020

Steatosis (Fatty Liver)

Cirrhosis

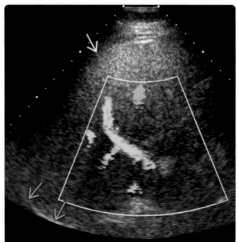

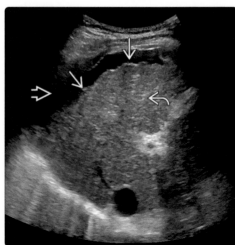

(Left) Transverse abdominal color Doppler US shows diffuse steatosis of the liver as evidenced by increased hepatic parenchymal echogenicity ➡ as well as marked attenuation of the US beam in deeper portions of the liver, resulting in poor visualization of the diaphragm ➡. (Right) Transverse abdominal US in a patient with cirrhosis shows a small liver with hepatic surface nodularity ➡ and heterogeneous parenchymal echogenicity ➡. Perihepatic ascites ➡ suggests hepatic decompensation.

Acute/Chronic Hepatitis

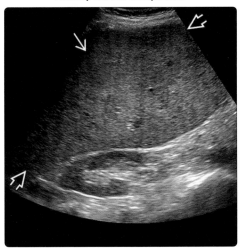

Hepatocellular Carcinoma (Diffuse/Infiltrative)

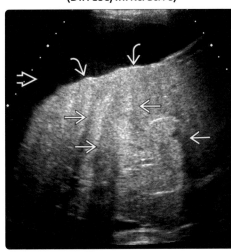

(Left) *Longitudinal abdominal US in a patient who presented with acute liver failure from acute alcoholic hepatitis shows marked hepatomegaly ➡ and slightly echogenic liver parenchyma ➡.* (Right) *Transverse abdominal US shows diffusely increased hepatic parenchymal echogenicity with multiple refractive shadows ➡ caused by diffuse, infiltrative hepatocellular carcinoma. Hepatic surface nodularity ➡ and ascites ➡ indicate underlying cirrhosis.*

Infiltrative Metastasis

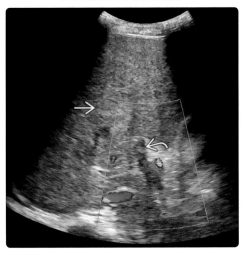

Biliary Hamartomas

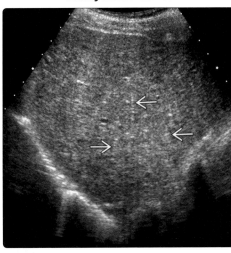

(Left) *Abdominal color Doppler US in a patient with renal cell carcinoma shows diffusely heterogeneous liver echogenicity caused by diffuse hepatic metastases ➡. Main portal vein is filled with hypoechoic material and shows no blood flow, suggesting thrombosis ➡.* (Right) *Oblique abdominal US shows diffuse and coarse liver parenchymal echotexture with multiple echogenic foci, some with associated comet-tail artifacts ➡, in a patient with numerous biliary hamartomas.*

Hepatic Sarcoidosis

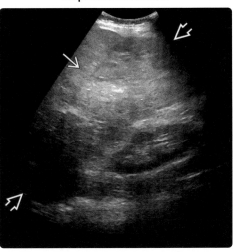

Amyloidosis

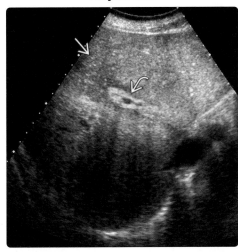

(Left) *Longitudinal abdominal US in a patient with sarcoidosis shows hepatomegaly (26-cm length) ➡ and heterogeneous liver parenchymal echogenicity ➡ due to hepatic involvement of sarcoidosis.* (Right) *Transverse abdominal US in a patient with amyloidosis shows heterogeneous and coarse liver echotexture ➡ and periportal edema ➡ due to hepatic involvement of amyloidosis.*

DIFFERENTIAL DIAGNOSIS

Common

- Hepatic Cyst
- Polycystic Liver Disease
- Pyogenic Hepatic Abscess
- Hepatic Metastases
- Recent Hepatic Hemorrhage
- Biloma
- Vessels
- Peribiliary Cyst
- Biliary Hamartoma
- Dilated Bile Ducts

Less Common

- Biliary Cystadenoma/Cystadenocarcinoma
- Hepatic Echinococcal Cyst
- Amebic Abscess
- Hepatic Lymphoma
- Ciliated Hepatic Foregut Cyst

Rare but Important

- Caroli Disease

ESSENTIAL INFORMATION

Key Differential Diagnosis Issues

- Lesions have few to no echoes within them
- Termed "simple"
  - When unilocular with no internal septa and not lobulated or irregular in contour
- Anechoic lesions tend to be round or oval-shaped with smooth contour on all surfaces
- Degree of posterior acoustic enhancement or shadowing and thickness of wall help limit differential diagnoses
- CEUS may help characterize solid components

Helpful Clues for Common Diagnoses

- **Hepatic Cyst**
  - Anechoic
  - Smooth borders but occasionally lobulated
  - Thin or imperceptible wall with no mural nodule
  - Well-defined back wall
  - Posterior acoustic enhancement
  - Often subcapsular and may bulge liver contour
  - Does not communicate with each other or bile ducts
  - No internal or mural vascularity but may distort adjacent vessels
  - May have internal echoes or septations after hemorrhage or infection
  - 1 or 2 thin septa may be seen
- **Polycystic Liver Disease**
  - May have concomitant autosomal dominant polycystic kidney disease
    - May make diagnosis of polycystic liver disease easier
    - Less likely to have pancreatic cysts as well
  - Individual cysts look identical to simple hepatic cysts
  - Number of cysts increases with age
  - When numerous and sizable, liver architecture is distorted, making diagnosis easier
  - Some cysts may be complicated by hemorrhage

- Become hyperechoic or contain debris or septa
- **Pyogenic Hepatic Abscess**
  - Anechoic (50%), hyperechoic (25%), hypoechoic (25%)
  - Small or microabscesses closely simulate small cysts
    - May have internal echogenic debris when large
  - Variable in shape with thin or thick walls
  - Borders range from well defined to irregular
  - Tendency to cluster
    - Group of small, pyogenic abscesses coalesce into single large cavity
  - May have adjacent hepatic parenchymal edema
    - Appears hypoechoic with coarse echo pattern ± vascularity
    - Vascularity may be seen in thick-walled portion
  - Diagnosis based on combination of clinical and sonographic features
- **Hepatic Metastases**
  - Anechoic hepatic metastasis
    - Suggests low degree of differentiation and high-grade malignancy
  - Usually no posterior acoustic enhancement
  - May have debris, mural nodularity, &/or thick septations
  - May have irregular margins and contour
  - Wall vascularity
  - Most common etiologies: Ovarian primary, sarcomas, GI stromal tumors (treated with Gleevec may mimic simple cyst), squamous cell metastases, and mucinous adenocarcinoma
- **Recent Hepatic Hemorrhage**
  - May be due to direct trauma, coagulopathy, or surgery/biopsy
  - Initially traumatic hematoma is usually echogenic
    - Becomes anechoic after few days
    - May have pseudowall of compressed liver parenchyma
  - Contour may be smooth or irregular
  - May be secondary hemorrhage into preexisting mass
    - Adenoma, hepatocellular carcinoma, metastasis, etc.
    - Usually not completely anechoic
- **Biloma**
  - Almost always secondary to trauma
    - Difficult to differentiate from traumatic hematoma
      - Hematomas show debris, septations over time
      - Bilomas remain anechoic
  - Round or oval in shape
  - Fluid content may be anechoic with posterior acoustic enhancement
    - Suggests fresh biloma
  - Thin capsule wall usually not discernible
  - Larger lesions may compress adjacent liver surface/architecture
  - Communicates with biliary tree
  - No vascularity within lesion
- **Vessels**
  - Portal veins: Venectasia, varicosities, collaterals from portal hypertension, aneurysms
  - Hepatic veins: Venectasia, Budd-Chiari, etc.
  - Hepatic arteries: Aneurysms, shunts, vascular malformation
  - Use of color Doppler

- – Confirm vascular nature and vessel type
- **Peribiliary Cyst**
  - Well-defined, cystic lesions of round/oval/tubular shape along portal triads
  - Usually multiple; discrete or confluent configuration
  - Smooth and thin walls without internal echoes
  - Variable size from 2 mm to 2 cm
  - No communication with biliary tree
- **Biliary Hamartoma**
  - Numerous small, hypo-/hyperechoic foci uniformly distributed throughout liver
    - – Leads to inhomogeneous and coarse appearance of liver echotexture
  - Multiple echogenic foci often associated with comet-tail artifacts
  - Typically smaller lesions appear as echogenic foci while larger lesions appear cystic
    - – Extent of echogenic foci on US is greater than anticipated
    - – Small lesions are too small to resolve sonographically
  - Color Doppler US: Twinkling artifact may be associated with echogenic foci
- **Dilated Bile Ducts**
  - May simulate anechoic nodules when viewed on cross section
  - Follow periportal distribution
    - – Long-axis orientation with hepatic artery/portal vein provide clues to its nature

Helpful Clues for Less Common Diagnoses

- **Biliary Cystadenoma/Cystadenocarcinoma**
  - Well-defined, multiloculated, anechoic or hypoechoic mass
  - Highly echogenic septa
  - May see internal echoes with complex fluid, calcifications, mural/septal nodules, or papillary projections
    - – More commonly associated with biliary cystadenocarcinoma
  - Color Doppler: Septal vascularity

- Most commonly seen in middle-aged women
- **Hepatic Echinococcal Cyst**
  - May be solitary or multiple
  - Large, well-defined, cystic liver mass with numerous peripheral daughter cysts
  - Cyst-within-cyst appearance
  - Floating membrane within cyst
  - Layered cyst wall is diagnostic
    - – Thickness reduces posterior acoustic enhancement
    - – ± calcification
- **Amebic Abscess**
  - Sharply demarcated, round or ovoid mass
  - Hypoechoic with low-level internal echoes
  - May see internal septa or wall nodularity
  - May see posterior acoustic enhancement
- **Hepatic Lymphoma**
  - May be irregular or round/oval in shape
  - ± posterior acoustic enhancement, pseudocystic appearance
  - Extrahepatic signs, such as lymphadenopathy, splenomegaly (± splenic infiltration)
- **Ciliated Hepatic Foregut Cyst**
  - Unilocular subcapsular solitary cyst located in segment 4a

Helpful Clues for Rare Diagnoses

- **Caroli Disease**
  - Central dot sign: Portal radicles within dilated intrahepatic bile ducts on color Doppler US

Technical Issues

- Important to make sure that gain settings are correct
- Gallbladder or inferior vena cava can be used as internal references for gain settings
  - These anatomic structures should normally look anechoic

SELECTED REFERENCES

1. Bartolotta TV et al: Focal liver lesions in cirrhosis: role of contrast-enhanced ultrasonography. World J Radiol. 14(4):70-81, 2022

Hepatic Cyst

Polycystic Liver Disease

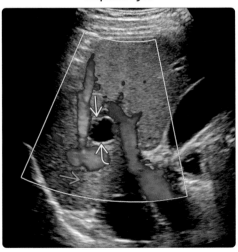

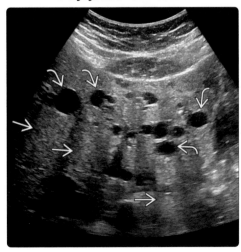

(**Left**) *Transverse color Doppler US shows a well-defined, round hepatic cyst with no internal vascularity ➡, well-defined back wall ➡, and posterior acoustic enhancement ➡, confirming the cystic nature of the lesion.* (**Right**) *Transverse US shows numerous cysts ➡ throughout the liver in a patient with polycystic liver disease. Posterior acoustic enhancement ➡ is associated with each of the cysts, confirming the cystic nature of these lesions.*

Pyogenic Hepatic Abscess

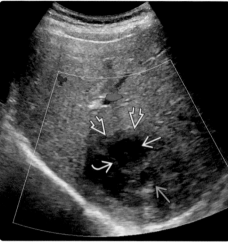

Biloma

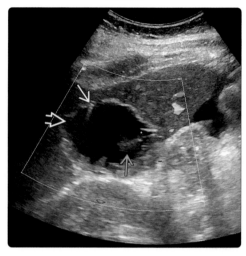

(Left) *Oblique color Doppler US shows a centrally cystic hepatic abscess ➡ with surrounding hypoechoic hepatic parenchyma ➡ in the right lobe of the liver. Central internal septations ➡ and echogenic debris ➡ are seen within the hepatic abscess.* (Right) *Transverse color Doppler US of the liver shows a biloma ➡ in a resection cavity with peripheral echogenic foci ➡ and ringdown artifact related to surgical clips. A small amount of internal debris is seen in the periphery of the biloma ➡.*

Vessels

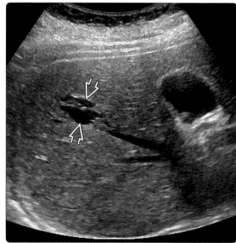

Vessels

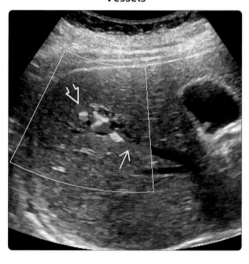

(Left) *Transverse US of the liver shows 2 adjacent well-defined, tubular-shaped, anechoic lesions ➡ in the right lobe of the liver.* (Right) *Color Doppler US in the same patient shows the lesion as a vascular structure ➡, which drains into the middle hepatic vein ➡. Color Doppler US should always be used to evaluate anechoic-appearing lesions as they may in fact be vascular, as in this case of a spontaneous intrahepatic portosystemic shunt.*

Biliary Cystadenoma/Cystadenocarcinoma

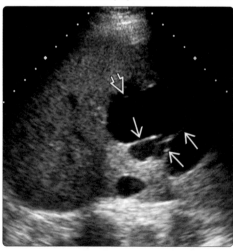

Hepatic Echinococcal Cyst

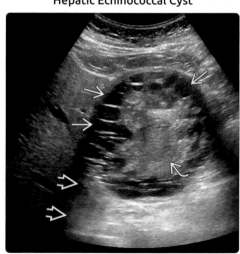

(Left) *Transverse US of the liver shows a biliary cystadenoma with sonographic imaging appearance of a complex cyst ➡ with multiple septations ➡. Most biliary cystadenomas are seen in middle-aged women.* (Right) *Transverse US shows an echinococcal cyst containing multiple peripheral daughter cysts ➡ and central heterogeneous content ➡ in the left lobe of the liver. Associated posterior acoustic enhancement ➡ is seen.*

Peribiliary Cyst

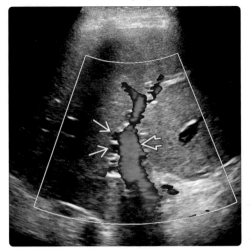

Biliary Hamartoma

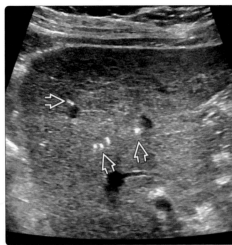

(Left) *Color Doppler US shows peribiliary cysts ➡ located adjacent to the portal vein ⇉. Peribiliary cysts should not be confused with biliary ductal dilatation, which would have a more tubular and continuous appearance adjacent to the portal vein.* (Right) *Transverse US of the liver shows multiple tiny, echogenic foci ➡ with comet-tail artifacts generated from biliary hamartomas.*

Amebic Abscess

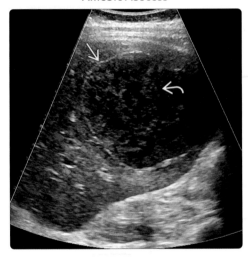

Hepatic Lymphoma

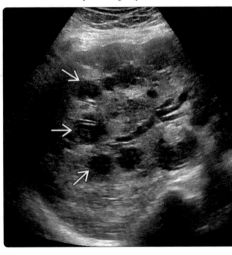

(Left) *Sagittal US of the liver shows a large, well-demarcated, encapsulated, hypoechoic amebic abscess ➡. The contents are heterogeneous due to floating debris ➡. No vascularity is seen within the abscess.* (Right) *Transverse US in a patient with lymphoma shows multiple markedly hypoechoic nodules ➡ throughout the right lobe of the liver, which have a pseudocystic appearance.*

Hepatic Metastases

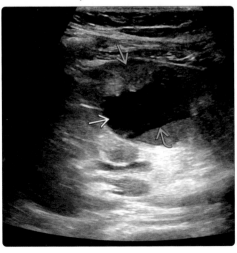

Ciliated Hepatic Foregut Cyst

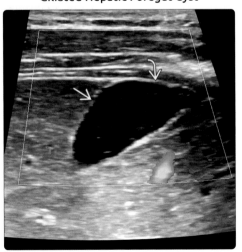

(Left) *Transverse US of cystic liver metastasis in a patient with metastatic cervical cancer shows a central cystic area ➡ as well as an echogenic soft tissue rim ➡ and layering debris ➡ within the dependent portion of the mass.* (Right) *Oblique color Doppler US in a patient with a ciliated hepatic foregut cyst shows a well-defined, ovoid, subcapsular cystic mass ➡ in segment IV of the liver ⇉. Internal content of the cystic lesion is relatively homogeneous, and no vascularity is seen.*

DIFFERENTIAL DIAGNOSIS

Common

- Complicated Benign Hepatic Cyst
- Hepatic Metastases
- Infection
  - Pyogenic Hepatic Abscess
  - Amebic Hepatic Abscess
  - Fungal Hepatic Abscess
- Focal Fatty Sparing
- Hepatocellular Carcinoma
- Infected Biloma

Less Common

- Hepatic Lymphoma
- Hepatic Adenoma
- Focal Nodular Hyperplasia
- Atypical Hemangioma
- Hepatic Hematoma
- Abnormal Bile Ducts
- Abnormal Vessels

ESSENTIAL INFORMATION

Key Differential Diagnosis Issues

- Lesions of lower echogenicity than liver parenchyma (compared to purely anechoic lesions)
  - Some low-level internal echogenicity
  - Solid lesion vs. complex cystic lesion

Helpful Clues for Common Diagnoses

- **Complicated Benign Hepatic Cyst**
  - Superimposed hemorrhage or infection in hepatic cyst
  - Septation/thickened wall ± mural calcification
  - Posterior acoustic enhancement
  - Solid appearance
    - If internal debris (clots or fibrin strands) dispersed within cyst
  - Fluid-debris level
    - If debris settles under influence of gravity
  - No mural nodule
  - Color Doppler US
    - Absence of internal or mural vascularity
    - Adjacent vessels distorted by large cyst
  - CEUS
    - No enhancement
- **Hepatic Metastases**
  - Hypoechoic metastases tend to be numerous and small
    - Larger lesions tend to have heterogeneous echogenicity
  - May have irregular or ill-defined borders
  - Hypoechogenicity
    - May reflect poor cellular differentiation and active growth
  - Suggest hypovascular and hypercellular tumor origin
    - Lung, breast, lymphoma
  - No posterior acoustic enhancement
  - Causes architectural distortion
    - If large or numerous
  - Color Doppler US may show no vascularity
    - Most are hypovascular

- Difficult to differentiate from lymphoma without history of known primary lesion
- **Pyogenic Hepatic Abscess**
  - Cystic mass with irregular border and debris
  - Posterior acoustic enhancement
  - Multiple thick or thin septations
  - Mural nodularity and vascularity
  - Adjacent parenchyma may be coarse and hypoechoic due to inflammation
  - Cluster sign: Coalescence of group of abscesses
  - May contain gas within abscess
    - Reverberation artifact or air-fluid level
  - Changes to anechoic when center becomes necrotic as center enlarges
  - Periportal distribution suggests dissemination along biliary tree
  - Random distribution suggests hematogenous spread
- **Amebic Hepatic Abscess**
  - Solitary, peripheral, round or ovoid mass
  - Abuts liver capsule, under diaphragm
  - More likely to be round or oval-shaped than pyogenic abscess
  - Hypoechoic with fine internal echoes
    - More common in amebic than pyogenic abscess
  - Internal septa may be present
  - Posterior acoustic enhancement
  - No vascularity seen in wall or septa of abscess
  - Subdiaphragmatic rupture in presence of adjacent hepatic abscess
    - Suggests amebic nature of abscess
- **Focal Fatty Sparing**
  - Normal liver echogenicity is slightly greater than that of kidney or spleen
  - Geographic hypoechoic area within echogenic liver
  - Due to direct drainage of hepatic flow into systemic circulation
  - Typical locations
    - Gallbladder fossa
      - Drained by cystic vein
    - Inferior aspect of segment 4b
      - Drained by aberrant gastric vein
    - Anterior to bifurcation of portal vein
      - Drained by aberrant gastric vein
    - Around hepatic veins
  - No architectural distortion
    - Vessels course through mass undistorted
    - No mass effect
  - Does not cross segments
- **Hepatocellular Carcinoma**
  - Hypoechoic: Most common US appearance of hepatocellular carcinoma
    - Solid tumor
    - May be surrounded by thin, hypoechoic halo (capsule)
  - Background cirrhotic liver
  - Associated signs of portal hypertension
    - Ascites, splenomegaly, portosystemic collaterals
  - Color Doppler US
    - Irregular hypervascularity
    - Portal vein thrombus with arterial neovascularity
  - CEUS

- o Heterogeneous hyperenhancement in arterial phase followed by early washout in portal venous phase and marked washout within 120 s
- **Infected Biloma**
  - o Fluid collection within liver, close to biliary tree, or in gallbladder fossa
  - o Debris or septa suggest infected biloma
  - o Color Doppler US
    - – No vascularity within lesion
    - – Adjacent hepatic parenchyma may demonstrate reactive hypervascularity

Helpful Clues for Less Common Diagnoses

- **Hepatic Lymphoma**
  - o Hypoechoic mass with irregular margins
  - o Marked hypoechogenicity
    - – Probably due to high cellular density and lack of background stroma
  - o Large/conglomerate masses may appear to contain septa and mimic abscesses
    - – May have pseudocystic appearance
  - o Other sites of involvement commonly seen
    - – Lymphadenopathy, splenomegaly ± focal splenic lesions provide clues to diagnosis
- **Hepatic Adenoma**
  - o Only slightly hypoechoic compared to normal liver parenchyma
    - – May be isoechoic
  - o May have hypoechoic rim
  - o Complications: Hemorrhage, central necrosis, and rupture may be present
  - o Color Doppler US shows distinct venous vascularity at borders
- **Focal Nodular Hyperplasia**
  - o Usually homogeneous and isoechoic to liver
    - – Occasionally hypoechoic or hyperechoic
  - o Central hypoechoic stellate scar with radiating fibrous septa
  - o Mass effect
    - – Displacement of normal hepatic vessels and ducts

- o Color Doppler: Hypervascularity
    - – Spoke-wheel pattern
      - □ Large central feeding artery with multiple small vessels radiating peripherally
    - – Large draining veins at tumor margin
    - – Hemorrhage is rare
- **Atypical Hemangioma**
  - o < 10% of hemangiomas are hypoechoic to liver parenchyma
    - – Usually with hyperechoic rim
    - – Typical atypical appearance
  - o May appear hypoechoic in fatty liver
    - – Due to background hyperechoic liver
  - o Hypoechoic areas within large lesions
    - – May represent necrosis, hemorrhage, scar, or vessels
  - o Smooth, well-defined borders
  - o May see posterior acoustic enhancement
  - o No visible color Doppler flow on US
    - – Flow too slow to be detected
    - – May be detected with power Doppler
- **Hepatic Hematoma**
  - o Echogenicity evolves over time
    - – Initially: Echogenic
    - – After 4-5 days: Hypoechoic
    - – After 1-4 weeks: Internal echoes and septations
- **Abnormal Bile Ducts**
  - o Dilated duct with sludge or tumor
  - o Interrogate in perpendicular plane to show its tubular nature
- **Abnormal Vessels**
  - o Dilated portal or hepatic vein with hypoechoic thrombus
  - o Interrogate in perpendicular plane to show its tubular nature

SELECTED REFERENCES

1. Yang J et al: Profiling hepatocellular carcinoma aggressiveness with contrast-enhanced ultrasound and gadoxetate disodium-enhanced MRI: an intra-individual comparative study based on the Liver Imaging Reporting and Data System. Eur J Radiol. ePub, 2022

Complicated Benign Hepatic Cyst

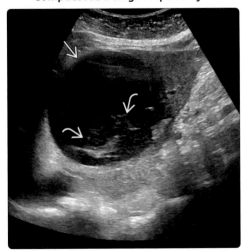

Hepatic Metastases

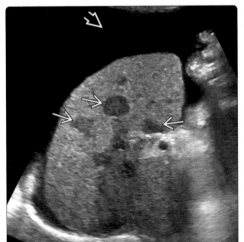

(Left) Longitudinal oblique US shows a complicated liver cyst ➡ with internal layering debris ➡ from hemorrhage. Depending on age and amount internal hemorrhage, the degree of echogenicity in complicated cysts may vary. (Right) Oblique US in a patient with breast cancer shows multiple well-defined, hypoechoic metastatic lesions ➡ in the liver. A large amount of ascites ➡ is present.

Hepatic Metastases

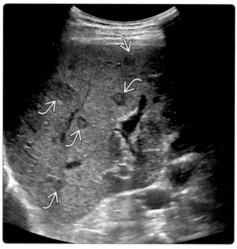

Pyogenic Hepatic Abscess

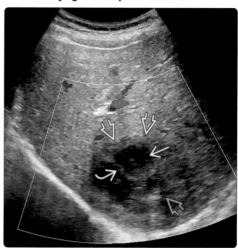

(Left) *Transverse US in a patient with colon cancer shows multiple small, hypoechoic metastatic nodules in the right lobe of the liver* ➜. **(Right)** *Oblique color Doppler US shows a centrally cystic hepatic pyogenic abscess* ➜ *with surrounding hypoechoic hepatic parenchyma* ➜ *in the right lobe of the liver. Internal septations* ➜ *and echogenic debris* ➭ *are seen within the abscess.*

Amebic Hepatic Abscess

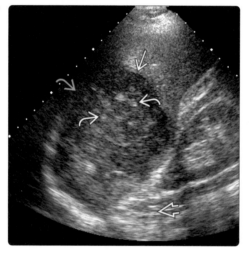

Fungal Hepatic Abscess

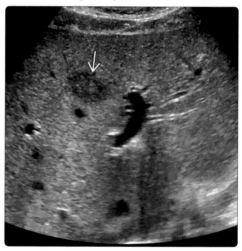

(Left) *Longitudinal US shows a large, round, hypoechoic amebic abscess in the right lobe of the liver* ➜ *abutting the liver capsule* ➭. *Internal contents are hypoechoic with heterogeneously echogenic scattered foci* ➜. *Mild posterior acoustic enhancement* ➭ *is seen.* **(Right)** *Transverse US shows a hypoechoic fungal abscess* ➜ *in segment 4 of the liver.*

Focal Fatty Sparing

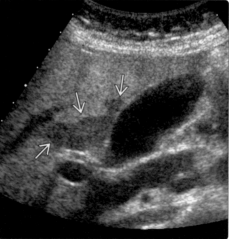

Hepatocellular Carcinoma

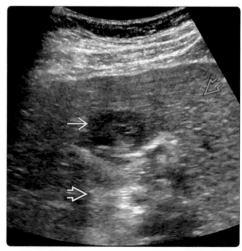

(Left) *Longitudinal US shows focal fatty sparing adjacent to the gallbladder fossa as a geographic area of decreased echogenicity* ➜ *in an otherwise echogenic liver due to diffuse steatosis. Liver adjacent to the gallbladder fossa is a typical location for fatty sparing.* **(Right)** *Transverse US shows a hypoechoic hepatocellular carcinoma* ➜. *Posterior acoustic enhancement* ➭ *is seen. Underlying liver shows heterogeneous echotexture* ➭, *indicating background cirrhosis.*

Infected Biloma

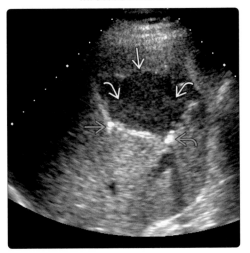

Hepatic Lymphoma

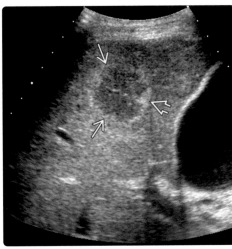

(Left) *Oblique US shows a biloma* ➡ *after surgical removal of a liver mass. Low-level internal echoes* ➡ *suggest infected bile. Peripheral surgical suture with ring-down artifact* ➡ *and clip with posterior shadowing* ➡ *are seen along the cut liver edge.* (Right) *Transverse US in a patient with hepatic lymphoma shows a well-defined, hypoechoic mass* ➡ *with a thin, hyperechoic rim* ➡ *in segment 5 of the liver.*

Hepatic Lymphoma

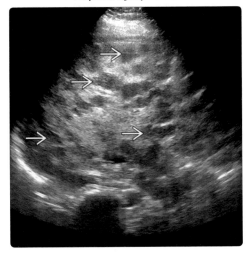

Hepatic Adenoma

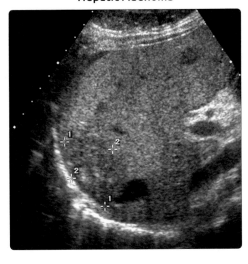

(Left) *Transverse US in a patient with hepatic lymphoma shows multiple hypoechoic nodules* ➡ *throughout the liver, consistent with diffuse hepatic involvement of lymphoma.* (Right) *Longitudinal US shows a heterogeneous, slightly hypoechoic hepatic adenoma (calipers) abutting the dome of the liver.*

Focal Nodular Hyperplasia

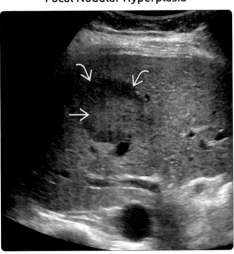

Atypical Hemangioma

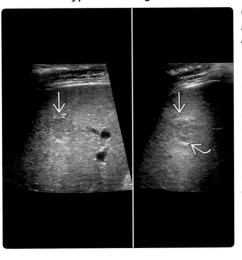

(Left) *Transverse US shows predominantly hypoechoic focal nodular hyperplasia (FNH)* ➡ *with an isoechoic center* ➡ *in the right lobe of the liver. In contrast to this case, most FNHs are isoechoic to background liver, making sonographic identification often challenging and earning the moniker "stealth lesion."* (Right) *Transverse US shows a hypoechoic hemangioma* ➡ *with a thin, hyperechoic rim* ➡ *in the right lobe of the liver, which is a "typical atypical" US finding of hepatic hemangioma.*

DIFFERENTIAL DIAGNOSIS

Common

- Focal Steatosis
- Hepatic Cavernous Hemangioma
- Hepatic Metastases
- Pyogenic Hepatic Abscess
- Normal Anatomic Pitfalls
  - Hepatic Ligaments and Fissures
  - Diaphragmatic Leaflets
  - Refractile Artifact
- Hepatocellular Carcinoma

Less Common

- Cholangiocarcinoma (Intrahepatic)
- Hepatic Adenoma
- Fibrolamellar Carcinoma
- Amebic Hepatic Abscess
- Hepatic Angiomyolipoma
- Biliary Hamartoma
- Hepatic Hydatid/*Echinococcus* Cyst
- Hepatic Epithelioid Hemangioendothelioma
- Hepatic Lipoma

ESSENTIAL INFORMATION

Key Differential Diagnosis Issues

- Is echogenic lesion mass or echogenic focus?
  - Mass: Usually spherical
  - Echogenic focus: Often linear, such as surgical device, pneumobilia, portal vein gas, etc.
- Significant overlap in appearance of many echogenic masses
  - Contrast-enhanced biphasic CT or multiphasic MR may be needed for further characterization

Helpful Clues for Common Diagnoses

- **Focal Steatosis**
  - Presence of normal vessels coursing through "lesion" excludes neoplasm
  - Varied appearances
    - Hyperechoic nodule/confluent hyperechoic lesions
      - □ May simulate metastases
    - Fan-shaped lobar/segmental distribution
  - CT or MR are good problem-solving tools
- **Hepatic Cavernous Hemangioma**
  - Typically homogeneously hyperechoic
    - Probably due to slow blood flow rather than multiple interfaces
    - Smooth or lobulated, well-defined borders
    - May have acoustic enhancement
  - Echogenicity may vary
    - Echogenicity may change over time during imaging
    - Direction and angle of insonation may alter echogenic appearance
    - May appear hypoechoic in underlying fatty liver
    - Large lesions more heterogeneous
- **Hepatic Metastases**
  - Hyperechoic metastases: Most commonly from GI tract (especially colon)
  - Vascular metastases

- Neuroendocrine tumors, melanoma, choriocarcinoma, renal cell carcinoma
  - Target or bull's-eye appearance
    - Iso- or hyperechoic metastatic nodule with hypoechoic rim or halo
    - Usually from aggressive primary tumors
    - Classic example: Bronchogenic carcinoma
  - Calcified metastasis
    - Markedly echogenic interface with acoustic shadowing or diffuse, small, echogenic foci
    - Mucinous primary: Colon, ovary, breast
    - Calcific/ossific primary: Osteosarcoma, chondrosarcoma, neuroblastoma, malignant teratoma
    - Treated metastasis
- **Pyogenic Hepatic Abscess**
  - Echogenicity of abscess
    - Anechoic (50%), hyperechoic (25%), or hypoechoic (25%)
    - Early lesions tend to be echogenic and poorly demarcated
    - May evolve into well-defined, nearly anechoic lesions
  - Cluster sign
    - Cluster of small, pyogenic abscesses coalesce into single large cavity
  - Fluid level or debris, internal septa
  - Abscess wall: Hypoechoic or mildly echogenic
  - Gas within abscess: Bright, echogenic foci with posterior reverberation artifact
- **Normal Anatomic Pitfalls**
  - **Hepatic ligaments and fissures, diaphragmatic leaflets**
    - Infolding of fat along these normal structures creates echogenic focus near surface of liver
    - In short-axis section, "lesions" can appear spherical and resemble masses
    - Turn US beam perpendicular to show linear shape of "lesion"
  - **Refractile artifact**
    - Lateral edge shadows at junction of vessels or gallbladder neck
- **Hepatocellular Carcinoma**
  - Hyperechoic appearance indicates fatty metamorphosis/hypervascularity
    - Simulates hemangioma or focal steatosis
      - □ Look for background cirrhotic liver, portal vein thrombosis, risk factors (hepatitis B, C, alcohol)
      - □ Generally irregular intratumoral vascularity
  - Small lesions more likely to be hyperechoic

Helpful Clues for Less Common Diagnoses

- **Cholangiocarcinoma (Intrahepatic)**
  - Heterogeneous mass with ill-defined margin and satellite nodules
    - Mostly hyperechoic (75%); iso-/hypoechoic (14%)
  - Isolated intrahepatic ductal dilatation upstream to mass without extrahepatic duct dilatation
- **Hepatic Adenoma**
  - Young woman with oral contraceptive use
  - Heterogeneous and hypervascular mass with hemorrhage
  - Complex, hyper-/hypoechoic mass with anechoic areas
    - Due to fat, hemorrhage, necrosis, or calcification

- Well-defined border, round or lobulated
- **Fibrolamellar Carcinoma**
  - Large, heterogeneous mass in adolescent or young adult
  - Well-defined and partially or completely encapsulated mass
  - Prominent central fibrous scar (hypo- or hyperechoic)
    - Calcification within scar common
  - Intratumoral necrosis/hemorrhage
  - Background cirrhosis or hepatitis in < 5% of patients
- **Amebic Hepatic Abscess**
  - Usually homogeneous and hypoechoic
    - Hyperechoic if complicated by bacterial superinfection or bowel fistula
  - Low-level internal echoes due to debris
  - Peripheral location: Abuts liver capsule, under diaphragm
- **Hepatic Angiomyolipoma**
  - Homo-/heterogeneous, echogenic mass
    - Hyperechoic due to fat
  - May be hypoechoic if muscle, vascular elements, or hemorrhage predominate
- **Biliary Hamartoma**
  - Numerous small, hypo-/hyperechoic foci uniformly distributed throughout liver
    - Small (< 15 mm), multiple, slightly irregular in contour
    - When small, appear hyperechoic due to inability to resolve tiny cysts
    - Leads to inhomogeneous and coarse appearance of liver echotexture
  - Multiple echogenic foci
    - Often with associated comet-tail artifacts
  - Typically smaller lesions appear as echogenic foci, whereas larger lesions appear cystic
    - Extent of echogenic foci on US is greater than anticipated, based on comparison CT or MR
    - Mimic cysts on CT and MR (near-water density/intensity)
- **Hepatic Hydatid/*Echinococcus* Cyst**
  - Membranes ± daughter cysts in complex, heterogeneous mass
  - Anechoic cyst with internal debris, hydatid sand

- *Echinococcus multilocularis*
  - Single or multiple echogenic lesions
  - Irregular, necrotic areas and microcalcifications
  - Infiltrative, solid masses
  - Invasion of inferior vena cava and diaphragm
- **Hepatic Epithelioid Hemangioendothelioma**
  - Variable echogenicity pattern
    - Predominantly hypoechoic
    - Hyper-/isoechoic lesions; may have peripheral hypoechoic rim
  - Often associated with adjacent retracted capsule
- **Hepatic Lipoma**
  - Extremely uncommon lesion
  - Contain mature adipose tissue

Alternative Differential Approaches

- Vascular masses
  - Cavernous hemangioma, hepatocellular carcinoma (HCC), hemangioendothelioma, angiosarcoma
- Fat-containing masses
  - Focal fatty infiltration, hepatic adenoma, HCC, lipid-containing metastases, angiomyolipoma, lipoma, liposarcoma, teratoma (primary or metastatic to liver)
- Gas-containing masses
  - Abscess, infarction, treated hepatic tumors with resulting sudden necrosis
- Solid masses
  - Primary liver tumors, metastases, cholangiocarcinoma
- Masses with calcified rim
  - Chronic cystic masses
- Masses with calcified scar
  - Fibrolamellar, HCC, cavernous hemangioma (large ones)

SELECTED REFERENCES

1. Brookmeyer CE et al: Multimodality imaging after liver transplant: top 10 important complications. Radiographics. 42(3):702-21, 2022
2. Metra BM et al: Beyond the liver function tests: a radiologist's guide to the liver blood tests. Radiographics. 42(1):125-42, 2022

Focal Steatosis

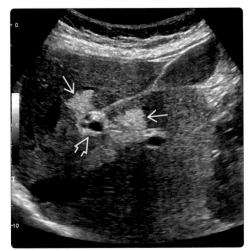

Hepatic Cavernous Hemangioma

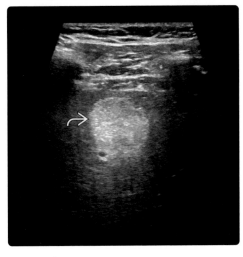

(Left) *Abdominal US shows focal fat deposition as geographic areas of increased echogenicity* ➡ *around portal vein* ➡. *The lesion shows no mass effect and vessels run through the lesion, features that are helpful in the diagnosis of focal steatosis.* **(Right)** *Transverse high-frequency US of the liver shows a well-defined, homogeneously echogenic cavernous hemangioma* ➡.

(Left) *Transverse US of the right lobe of the liver shows a typical hemangioma ➤, which is homogeneously echogenic with well-defined margins.* (Right) *Transverse US in a patient with mucinous colon cancer shows multiple large, hyperechoic metastases ➤ in the liver containing diffuse, echogenic foci ➤ related to subtle calcifications that exhibit posterior acoustic shadowing ➤. Masses distort and compress the right portal vein ➤.*

Hepatic Cavernous Hemangioma

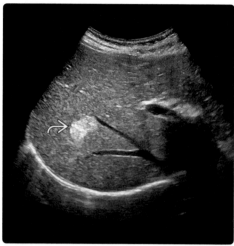

Hepatic Metastases

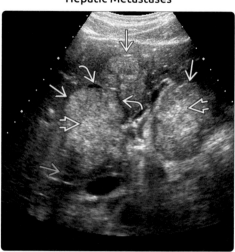

(Left) *Transverse US in a patient with carcinoid tumor shows a round, homogeneously hyperechoic metastasis in the right lobe of the liver ➤.* (Right) *Oblique US in a patient with melanoma shows a large, heterogeneously hyperechoic metastasis ➤ in the liver abutting the hepatic capsule. Thin, hypoechoic peritumoral halo is present ➤, a finding often seen with hepatic metastases.*

Hepatic Metastases

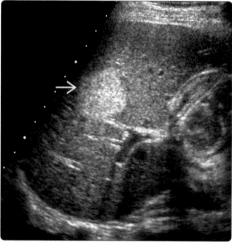

Hepatic Metastases

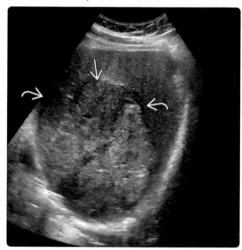

(Left) *Oblique US in a patient with liposarcoma shows a round, homogeneously hyperechoic metastasis along the margin of the right lobe of the liver ➤.* (Right) *Longitudinal US in a patient with bladder cancer shows multiple ill-defined, hyperechoic metastases in the liver ➤.*

Hepatic Metastases

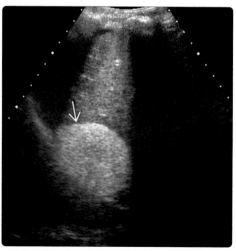

Hepatic Metastases

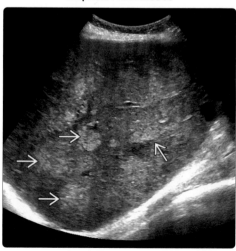

Hepatic Ligaments and Fissures

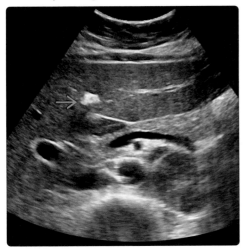

Hepatocellular Carcinoma

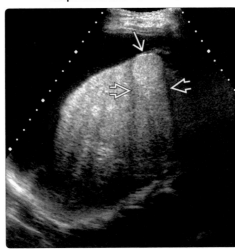

(Left) Transverse US of the left lobe of the liver shows an echogenic falciform ligament ➡. The falciform ligament attaches the liver to the anterior body wall and often contains fat, which appears echogenic. (Right) Oblique US shows a hyperechoic hepatocellular carcinoma in the subcapsular portion of the liver ➡. Lateral edge shadowing and posterior acoustic enhancement ➡ are seen.

Hepatic Adenoma

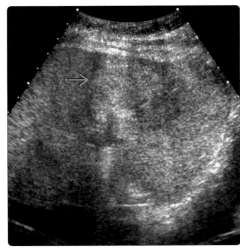

Hepatic Angiomyolipoma

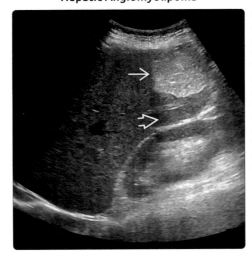

(Left) Transverse US of the left lobe of the liver in a 22-year-old woman shows an echogenic, solid mass ➡, which was proven to be hepatic adenoma. (Right) Longitudinal US shows a well-defined, homogeneously hyperechoic angiomyolipoma in the liver ➡. Slight posterior acoustic enhancement ➡ is seen associated with the angiomyolipoma (AML).

Hepatic Angiomyolipoma

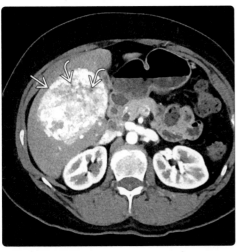

Hepatic Lipoma

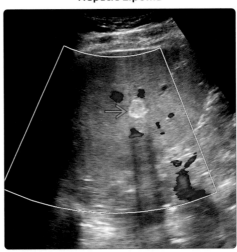

(Left) Axial arterial-phase CECT in the same patient shows the large, hypervascular AML in the right lobe of liver ➡. The mass contains tiny, hypodense foci ➡ indicating fatty components. (Right) Color Doppler US shows a well-defined, uniformly echogenic, avascular mass ➡ in the liver, found to be intrahepatic lipoma.

DIFFERENTIAL DIAGNOSIS

Common

- Hepatic Metastases
- Hepatocellular Carcinoma
- Hepatic Lymphoma
- Hepatic Adenoma
- Fungal Hepatic Abscess
- Amebic Hepatic Abscess
- Pyogenic Hepatic Abscess

Less Common

- Hepatic Atypical Hemangioma
- Hepatic Hematoma

Rare but Important

- Sarcoidosis
- Kaposi Sarcoma

ESSENTIAL INFORMATION

Key Differential Diagnosis Issues

- Target sign: Echogenic center surrounded by hypoechoic rim
  - a.k.a. bull's-eye lesions
  - Malignancy far outnumbers other causes
- Reverse target: Hypoechoic core with hyperechoic rim

Helpful Clues for Common Diagnoses

- **Hepatic Metastases**
  - Solid central tumor with hypoechoic halo
    - Halo most likely related to compressed hepatic tissue along with zone of cancer cell proliferation
  - Alternating layers of hyper- and hypoechoic tissue
  - Usually from aggressive primary tumors
    - Classic example: Bronchogenic carcinoma
- **Hepatocellular Carcinoma**
  - Background of cirrhosis, portal hypertension, ascites
  - Rare for cirrhotic livers to develop metastases from nonhepatic primary

- Any mass in cirrhotic liver is more likely hepatocellular carcinoma than metastasis
- **Hepatic Lymphoma**
  - Vast majority are uniformly hypoechoic
  - Splenomegaly or splenic lesions, lymphadenopathy, thickened bowel wall provide clues toward diagnosis
- **Hepatic Adenoma**
  - Usually isoechoic or slightly hypoechoic
  - Complications, such as hemorrhage, central necrosis, make center echogenic
  - Occasional hypoechoic rim forms target-like appearance
- **Fungal Hepatic Abscess**
  - Often multiple lesions
  - Typically in immunocompromised patient
- **Amebic Hepatic Abscess**
  - Iso- to mildly hyperechoic center with hypoechoic halo
  - Abuts liver capsule
  - Mostly in right lobe
- **Pyogenic Hepatic Abscess**
  - Central hyperechoic inflammatory nodule surrounded by hypoechoic halo of fibrosis
  - Cluster sign: Cluster of small pyogenic abscesses that coalesce into single large cavity
  - Lobulated or irregular contour

Helpful Clues for Less Common Diagnoses

- **Hepatic Atypical Hemangioma**
  - Hypoechoic center with thick or thin, hyperechoic rim
    - "Typical atypical" appearance (up to 40%)
    - Hypoechogenicity seems to be related to predominant fibrous stroma
- **Hepatic Hematoma**
  - May have laceration tract leading to hepatic surface
  - Multiple organs involved if traumatic cause

SELECTED REFERENCES

1. Metra BM et al: Beyond the liver function tests: a radiologist's guide to the liver blood tests. Radiographics. 42(1):125-42, 2022

Hepatic Metastases

Hepatic Metastases

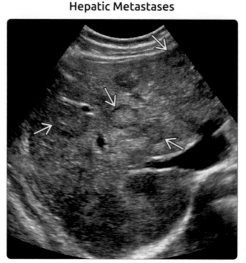
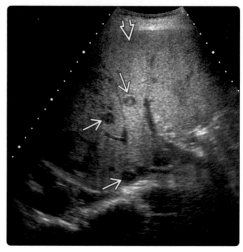

(Left) Transverse US in a patient with breast cancer metastases to the liver shows that the metastases have a classic target appearance ⬅ in which rounded, echogenic lesions are surrounded by a hypoechoic rim. (Right) Transverse US in a patient with sarcoma metastases to the liver shows multiple small hepatic metastases with a target appearance ⬅ in which echogenic, rounded lesions are surrounded by a hypoechoic rim. Background liver shows diffuse steatosis ⬅.

Hepatic Metastases

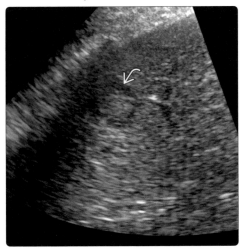

Hepatocellular Carcinoma

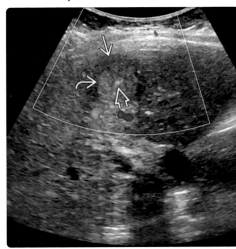

(Left) Transverse US in a patient with lung cancer metastases to the liver shows a hepatic metastasis with a target appearance in which an isoechoic lesion is surrounded by a hypoechoic rim ➔. (Right) Transverse color Doppler US of the liver shows a hyperechoic hepatocellular carcinoma ➔ with a hypoechoic halo ➔, which creates a target appearance. Detectable internal vascularity ➔ within the tumor is seen.

Hepatic Lymphoma

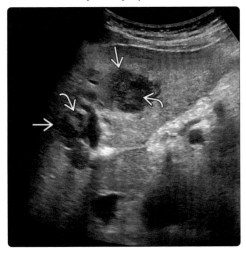

Fungal Hepatic Abscess

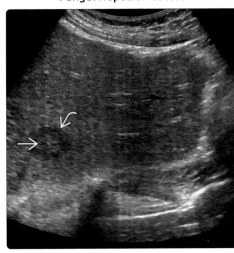

(Left) Transverse US in a patient with lymphoma shows several hypoechoic masses with central echogenic cores ➔ surrounded by a hypoechoic rim ➔. (Right) Longitudinal US of the liver shows a fungal abscess that has an echogenic center ➔ surrounded by a hypoechoic rim ➔, which creates a target appearance.

Pyogenic Hepatic Abscess

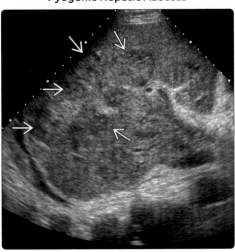

Hepatic Atypical Hemangioma

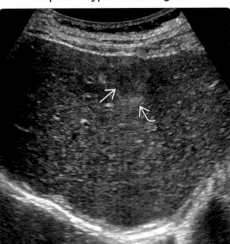

(Left) Transverse US shows multiple hepatic abscesses ➔ that appear as isoechoic masses surrounded by thin, hypoechoic rims. (Right) Longitudinal US of the liver shows an atypical hemangioma with reverse-target appearance, which is a hypoechoic mass ➔ surrounded by hyperechoic rim ➔.

DIFFERENTIAL DIAGNOSIS

Common

- Hepatic Cysts
- Hepatic Metastases
- Hepatic Steatosis (Multifocal)
- Hepatic Hemangioma
- Hepatic Lymphoma (Discrete Form)
- Cirrhosis With Regenerative/Dysplastic Nodules
- Hepatocellular Carcinoma
- Pyogenic Hepatic Abscess
- Hepatic Microabscesses
- Cholangitis
- Vessels

Less Common

- Hepatic *Echinococcus* Cyst
- Hepatic Hematoma
- Biliary Hamartoma (von Meyenburg Complexes)

Rare but Important

- Caroli Disease

ESSENTIAL INFORMATION

Helpful Clues for Common Diagnoses

- **Hepatic Cysts**
  - Uncomplicated simple cyst
    - Anechoic, rounded
    - Smooth or lobulated borders
    - Posterior acoustic enhancement
    - Thin or nondetectable wall
    - No septation/mural nodule/wall calcification
  - Hemorrhagic or infected cyst
    - Internal debris (clots or fibrin strands)
    - Septations/thickened wall, ± calcification
  - Autosomal dominant polycystic liver disease
    - Numerous cysts
    - Anechoic or with debris due to hemorrhage or infection
    - Calcification of some cyst walls
    - May have barely perceptible septations
    - No mural nodularity
    - Liver often distorted by innumerable cysts
    - Look for presence of renal cysts (adult polycystic kidney disease)
  - Do not demonstrate saccular configuration
    - vs. Caroli disease
  - Not associated with biliary duct dilatation
    - vs. hydatid cysts or Caroli disease
- **Hepatic Metastases**
  - Hypoechoic necrotic metastases
    - Usually from hypovascular tumors
    - Simulate cysts or abscesses
    - Abnormal intratumoral vascularity contains debris, mural nodules, or septa
  - Hyperechoic metastases
    - Simulate hemangioma or focal steatosis
    - Distort vessels and bile ducts
    - Vascular metastasis; from neuroendocrine tumors, choriocarcinoma, renal cell carcinoma, melanoma

- Target metastatic lesions
  - Solid, echogenic mass with hypoechoic rim or halo
  - Usually from aggressive primary tumors
- Cystic metastasis
  - May demonstrate posterior acoustic enhancement
  - Mural nodules, thick walls, fluid-fluid levels, internal septa, or debris
- Calcified metastasis
  - Markedly echogenic interface with acoustic shadowing or diffuse, small, echogenic foci
  - Treated metastasis
- **Hepatic Steatosis (Multifocal)**
  - Focal fatty infiltration
    - Location: Right lobe, caudate lobe, perihilar
    - Hyperechoic area
  - Focal fatty sparing
    - Location: Gallbladder bed, segment IV anterior to portal bifurcation
    - Hypoechoic areas within echogenic liver
  - Geographic or fan-shaped
  - In some cases, may appear as multiple echogenic nodules throughout liver
  - No mass effect
  - Vessels run undisplaced through lesion
- **Hepatic Hemangioma**
  - Well-defined margins
  - Hyperechoic mass, typically homogeneous
  - Posterior acoustic enhancement
  - Atypical features
    - Hypoechoic ± hyperechoic rim
    - Heterogeneous, calcification, irregular borders
- **Hepatic Lymphoma (Discrete Form)**
  - Well-defined nodules or masses
  - Hypoechoic or anechoic
    - Low echogenicity due to high cellular density
  - Large/conglomerate masses may appear to contain septa
    - Mimic abscesses
  - Background vascular architecture ± distortion
  - More common in immunocompromised patients
    - e.g., AIDS patients and organ transplant recipients
- **Cirrhosis With Regenerative/Dysplastic Nodules**
  - Coarse echo pattern, increased parenchymal echogenicity, other signs of cirrhosis
  - Regenerating nodules (siderotic)
    - Iso-/hypoechoic nodules (regenerating nodules)
    - Hyperechoic rim (surrounding fibrosis)
  - Dysplastic nodules
    - Hypoechoic nodule > 1 cm diameter
    - Smooth or irregular borders
    - Difficult to differentiate from small hepatocellular carcinoma
      - □ Should be further investigated with CECT or MR
- **Hepatocellular Carcinoma**
  - Most commonly hypoechoic
    - Less commonly hyperechoic or isoechoic to liver
  - Irregular hypervascularity within mass
  - Cirrhotic background liver
  - May see portal vein invasion or tumor thrombosis
- **Pyogenic Hepatic Abscess**

- ○ Cluster sign
  - – Cluster of small abscesses coalesce into single septated cavity
- ○ Complex cyst with septa and debris
- ○ ± ill-defined borders
- ○ Mural nodularity and vascularity
- ○ May contain gas within abscess
  - – Seen as echogenic foci of air or air-fluid level
- ○ Adjacent parenchyma may be coarse and hypoechoic
- ○ Color Doppler may show hypervascularity in inflamed surrounding liver parenchyma
- **Hepatic Microabscesses**
  - ○ Multiple, small, hypo-/iso-/hyperechoic lesions
  - ○ Central hypoechoic area of necrosis within hyperechoic lesion
  - ○ Target sign
    - – Central hyperechoic inflammation surrounded by hypoechoic "halo" of fibrosis
  - ○ Similar lesions may be found in spleen
- **Cholangitis**
  - ○ Circumferential bile duct wall thickening
  - ○ Dilatation of intra- and extrahepatic ducts
  - ○ Periportal hypo-/hyperechogenicity
    - – Due to periductal edema/inflammation
  - ○ Ascending cholangitis
    - – Obstructing calculus in extrahepatic duct
  - ○ Recurrent pyogenic cholangitis
    - – Biliary calculi: Cast-like and often fill duct lumen
    - – Atrophy of affected lobe/segment
- **Vessels**
  - ○ Portal veins: Venectasia, varicosities, collaterals from portal hypertension, aneurysm
  - ○ Hepatic veins: Venectasia, Budd-Chiari syndrome
  - ○ Hepatic arteries: Aneurysms, shunts, vascular malformation
  - ○ Use color Doppler to confirm vascular nature

Helpful Clues for Less Common Diagnoses

- **Hepatic *Echinococcus* Cyst**
  - ○ Large, well-defined, hypoechoic masses

- ○ Numerous peripheral daughter cysts
- ○ Intrahepatic duct dilatation may be seen
- ○ May show curvilinear or ring-like pericyst calcification
- **Hepatic Hematoma**
  - ○ Round, hyper-/hypoechoic foci
  - ○ Echogenicity evolves over time
    - – Echogenic initially
    - – Hypoechoic after 4-5 days
    - – Internal echoes and septations after 1-4 weeks
  - ○ Ancillary signs: Subcapsular hematoma, hemoperitoneum, renal or splenic laceration
- **Biliary Hamartoma (von Meyenburg Complexes)**
  - ○ Numerous small, hypo-/hyperechoic foci uniformly distributed throughout liver
    - – Leads to inhomogeneous and coarse appearance of liver echotexture
  - ○ Multiple echogenic foci
    - – Often with associated comet-tail artifacts
  - ○ Typically smaller lesions appear as echogenic foci, whereas larger lesions appear cystic
    - – Often extent of echogenic foci on US is greater than anticipated, based on comparison CT or MR

Helpful Clues for Rare Diagnoses

- **Caroli Disease**
  - ○ Hypoechoic masses
  - ○ Saccular or fusiform shape
  - ○ Central dot sign
    - – Small portal venous branches partially or completely surrounded by dilated ducts
  - ○ Intraductal calculi common and appear as echogenic nodules with dense posterior acoustic shadowing
  - ○ Communication between cysts and biliary tree may be difficult to demonstrate on US
  - ○ Areas of hepatic fibrosis associated with areas of heterogeneous echotexture (and variable echogenicity)

Hepatic Cysts

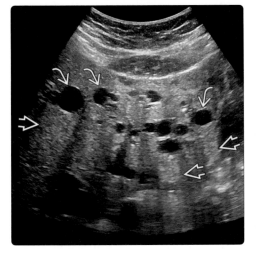

Hepatic Metastases

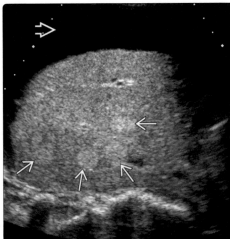

(Left) Transverse US shows innumerable cysts ⇗ throughout the liver in a patient with polycystic liver disease. Posterior acoustic enhancement ⇒ is seen associated with each cyst. (Right) Transverse US in a patient with carcinoid metastases to the liver shows multiple round, homogeneous, hyperechoic metastatic nodules in the liver ⇒. A large amount of perihepatic ascites ⇛ is seen.

(Left) *Transverse US in a patient with mucinous colon cancer shows multiple large, hyperechoic metastases ➡ containing diffuse, echogenic foci ➡ related to subtle calcifications. Note posterior acoustic shadowing caused by the calcifications ➡. (Right) Transverse US in a patient with pancreatic cancer shows numerous small, hypoechoic metastases ➡ throughout the liver. The background liver is echogenic from hepatic steatosis, a common finding in the setting of chemotherapy.*

Hepatic Metastases

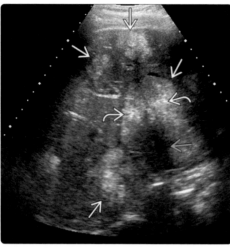

Hepatic Metastases

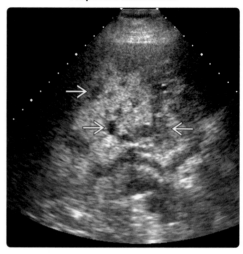

(Left) *Oblique US shows multifocal fat deposition, which appears as geographic areas of increased echogenicity ➡ around the portal vein ➡. The lesion shows no mass effect, and vessels run through the lesion, characteristic features of fatty infiltration. (Right) Transverse US in a patient with multiple hepatic hemangiomas shows 2 well-defined, homogeneously hyperechoic hemangiomas ➡ in the right lobe of the liver.*

Hepatic Steatosis (Multifocal)

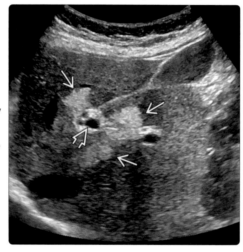

Hepatic Hemangioma

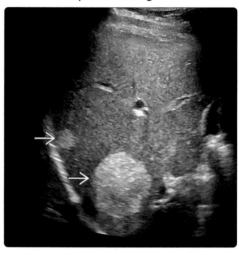

(Left) *Transverse US shows 2 well-defined, homogeneously hyperechoic hemangiomas ➡ in the liver. Hemangiomas in the liver are often multiple. (Right) Transverse US in a patient with lymphoma shows multiple hypoechoic masses ➡ throughout the liver. Lesions are markedly hypoechoic, resulting in a pseudocystic appearance characteristic of lymphoma.*

Hepatic Hemangioma

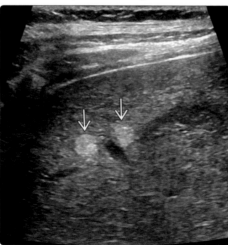

Hepatic Lymphoma (Discrete Form)

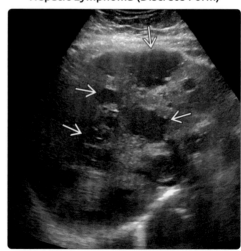

Cirrhosis With Regenerative/Dysplastic Nodules

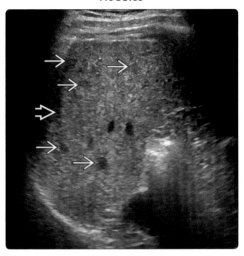

Hepatocellular Carcinoma

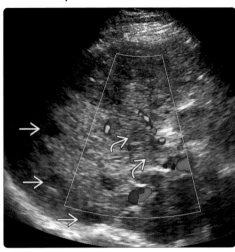

(Left) *Transverse US in a patient with hepatitis B shows numerous small, hypoechoic nodules in the liver ➡, indicating regenerative or dysplastic nodules. Coarse and heterogeneous echogenicity of liver parenchyma is consistent with underlying cirrhosis ➡.* (Right) *Transverse US shows multifocal, hypoechoic hepatocellular carcinomas ➡ throughout the liver. The right portal vein is thrombosed and filled with echogenic material that was found to represent tumor thrombus ➡.*

Pyogenic Hepatic Abscess

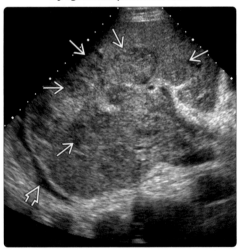

Hepatic Microabscesses

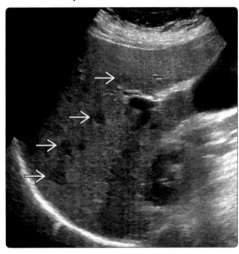

(Left) *Transverse US shows multiple hepatic abscesses ➡ in the liver, seen as ill-defined, isoechoic masses surrounded by thin, hypoechoic rims. A small amount of perihepatic ascites ➡ is present as well.* (Right) *Longitudinal US shows multiple small, hypoechoic fungal microabscesses ➡ in the right lobe of the liver.*

Hepatic *Echinococcus* Cyst

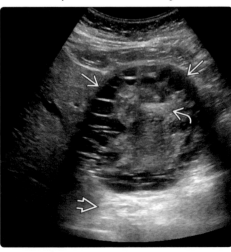

Caroli Disease

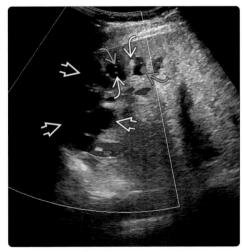

(Left) *Transverse US shows an echinococcal cyst containing multiple peripheral daughter cysts ➡ and heterogeneous material centrally ➡. Note the associated posterior acoustic enhancement ➡.* (Right) *Oblique US in a young patient with Caroli disease shows multiple dilated intrahepatic ducts ➡. Echogenic portal radicles ➡ are surrounded by dilated ducts. Some of the portal radicles within dilated ducts show color flow ➡, which creates the central dot sign appearance.*

DIFFERENTIAL DIAGNOSIS

Common

- Focal Nodular Hyperplasia
- Fibrolamellar Carcinoma
- Hepatocellular Carcinoma
- Hepatic Adenoma
- Hepatic Metastases

Less Common

- Atypical Hemangioma
- Hepatic *Echinococcus* Cyst

ESSENTIAL INFORMATION

Helpful Clues for Common Diagnoses

- **Focal Nodular Hyperplasia**
  - Mass: Typically homogeneous and isoechoic to liver
    - Occasionally hypoechoic or hyperechoic
  - Central scar: Typically hypoechoic (18% hyperechoic)
    - Contains central feeding artery
  - Color Doppler: Spoke-wheel pattern
    - Prominent central feeding artery with multiple small vessels radiating peripherally
    - Large draining veins at tumor margins
- **Fibrolamellar Carcinoma**
  - Presents in otherwise healthy young adults
    - Background cirrhosis or hepatitis in < 5% of patients
  - Large, well-defined, partially/completely encapsulated mass
  - Prominent central fibrous scar
  - Calcification within scar common
  - Intralesional necrosis/hemorrhage
  - Vascular, biliary, and nodal invasion may be present
- **Hepatocellular Carcinoma**
  - Background cirrhosis ± signs of portal hypertension
  - Central tumor necrosis/fibrosis produces apparent central scar
  - Color Doppler may show irregular tumor hypervascularity or tumor thrombus in portal vein

- **Hepatic Adenoma**
  - Well-defined, round or mildly lobulated contour
  - Hypo-/iso-/hyperechoic mass
  - Central fat, hemorrhage, necrosis, and calcification
    - May simulate central scar
  - Color Doppler shows hypervascular tumor supplied by hepatic artery
- **Hepatic Metastases**
  - Necrotic or treated metastases with necrotic center may simulate central scar
  - Necrotic center may be lined with irregular walls and contain debris
  - Color Doppler may not show vascularity as many metastases are hypovascular

Helpful Clues for Less Common Diagnoses

- **Atypical Hemangioma**
  - Hypoechoic center with hyperechoic rim may simulate central scar
    - "Typical atypical" hemangioma (up to 40%)
  - Posterior acoustic enhancement
  - No visible color Doppler flow in center of lesion
    - Flow too slow to be sonographically detected
- **Hepatic *Echinococcus* Cyst**
  - Honeycombed cyst
    - Multiple septations between daughter cysts in mother cyst
  - Spoke-wheel appearance of septa simulating central scar

SELECTED REFERENCES

1. Dong Y et al: Imaging features of fibrolamellar hepatocellular carcinoma with contrast-enhanced ultrasound. Ultraschall Med. 42(3):306-13, 2021
2. Busireddy KK et al: Multiple focal nodular hyperplasia: MRI features. Clin Imaging. 49:89-96, 2018
3. Han SB et al: Hepatocellular carcinoma with central scar on gadoxetic acid-enhanced and diffusion-weighted magnetic resonance imaging. Acta Radiol. 59(4):393-401, 2018
4. Kong WT et al: Contrast-enhanced ultrasound in combination with color doppler ultrasound can improve the diagnostic performance of focal nodular hyperplasia and hepatocellular adenoma. Ultrasound Med Biol. 41(4):944-51, 2015

Focal Nodular Hyperplasia

Focal Nodular Hyperplasia

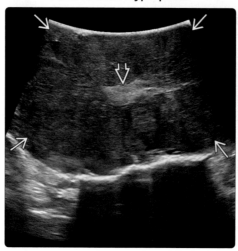

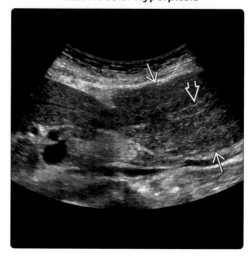

(Left) Intraoperative US using a high-frequency transducer shows hypoechoic focal nodular hyperplasia (FNH) in the liver ➡ with a hyperechoic central scar ➡. (Right) Transverse US shows a pedunculated FNH ➡ with a slightly hyperechoic central scar ➡ arising from the lateral segment of the left lobe of the liver.

Hepatic Mass With Central Scar

Focal Nodular Hyperplasia

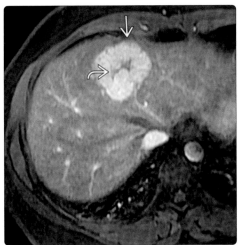

Focal Nodular Hyperplasia

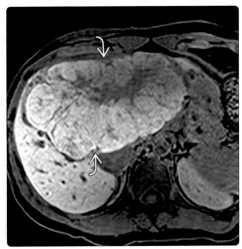

(Left) *Axial arterial-phase T1 C+ MR shows an avidly enhancing hepatic mass* ➡️ *with a lobulated contour and central hypoenhancing scar* ⇗ *, typical for FNH.* (Right) *Axial T1 MR shows a large mass* ➡️ *, which retains contrast on delayed hepatobiliary phase, confirming FNH.*

Fibrolamellar Carcinoma

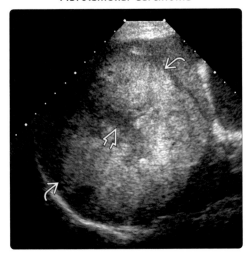

Hepatocellular Carcinoma

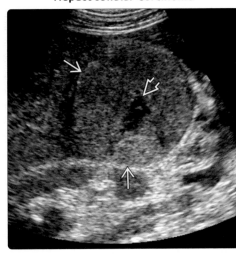

(Left) *Transverse US of the liver shows a large, predominantly echogenic mass* ➡️ *with a thick, hypoechoic central scar* ⇗ *, proven to be fibrolamellar carcinoma.* (Right) *Transverse US of the liver shows a large, lobulated, heterogeneous hepatocellular carcinoma* ➡️ *in the right lobe with a central avascular, hypoechoic scar* ➡️ *.*

Hepatic Metastases

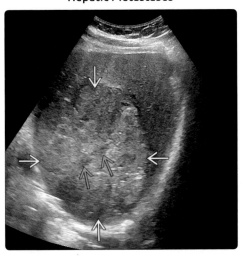

Atypical Hemangioma

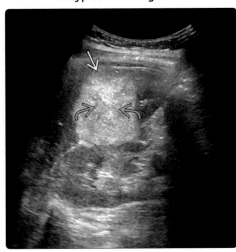

(Left) *Oblique US in a patient with melanoma shows a large, heterogeneous, hyperechoic metastasis* ➡️ *in the right lobe of the liver. Central hypoechoic areas simulate a central scar* ➡️ *.* (Right) *Longitudinal US shows a hyperechoic hemangioma of the liver* ➡️ *. The ill-defined hypoechoic area in the center* ➡️ *simulates a central scar.*

DIFFERENTIAL DIAGNOSIS

Common

- Ascending Cholangitis
- Cavernous Transformation of Portal Vein
- Portosystemic Collaterals
- Hepatic Trauma
- Acute Viral Hepatitis
- Fatty Sparing, Liver
- Diffuse/Infiltrative Hepatic Lymphoma
- Pneumobilia
- Choledocholithiasis
- Metastases

Less Common

- Peribiliary Cyst
- Hepatic Schistosomiasis
- Recurrent Pyogenic Cholangitis
- Iatrogenic Material
- Caroli Disease
- Hepatic Artery Calcification
- Cystic Duct Remnant

ESSENTIAL INFORMATION

Helpful Clues for Common Diagnoses

- **Ascending Cholangitis**
  - Periportal hypo- or hyperechogenicity adjacent to dilated intrahepatic ducts
    - Due to periductal edema/inflammation
  - Dilatation of intrahepatic bile ducts
  - Purulent bile/sludge as intraluminal echogenic material in dilated ducts
  - Circumferential thickening of bile duct wall
  - Obstructing stone in common bile duct
- **Cavernous Transformation of Portal Vein**
  - Collateralization due to portal vein occlusion
  - Usually in subacute or chronic portal vein obstruction
  - Serpiginous tubular channels along expected course of portal vein
  - Color Doppler US shows hepatopetal flow
  - Signs of portal vein occlusion
    - Acute: Enlarged portal vein
    - Chronic: Small/imperceptible portal vein
    - Color Doppler US: Lack of flow in portal vein
- **Portosystemic Collaterals**
  - Serpiginous hypoechoic channels in or around portal triad
  - Location
    - Intrahepatic: Portal-to-portal veins, portal-to-hepatic veins, portal-to-systemic veins
    - Paraumbilical vein (recanalization)
    - Gastroesophageal: Coronary and right gastric, left gastric and splenogastric
    - Lienorenal/mesenteric/retroperitoneal
  - Color Doppler US
    - Hepatofugal flow in vessels (opposite to cavernous transformation)
    - Extent of collaterals
  - Background changes of cirrhosis/portal hypertension/portal vein thrombosis

- **Hepatic Trauma**
  - Lesions are commonly located in segments VI, VII, and VIII
  - Echogenicity evolves over time
    - Initially echogenic
    - Becomes hypoechoic after 4-5 days
    - Internal echoes with septa may develop after 1-4 weeks
  - Hematoma tracking along portal triad
    - Linear, focal, or diffuse periportal lesion
  - Ancillary signs of trauma
    - Subcapsular hematoma; hemoperitoneum, renal, or splenic laceration/hematoma
  - Better evaluated by MDCT
- **Acute Viral Hepatitis**
  - Increased echogenicity of fat in periportal tissues, ligamentum venosum, and falciform ligament
  - Hepatomegaly with diffuse decrease in echogenicity
  - Starry-sky appearance
    - Increased echogenicity of portal triad walls against background of hypoechoic liver
  - Periportal hypo-/anechoic area
    - Due to hydropic swelling of hepatocytes
- **Fatty Sparing, Liver**
  - Focal, hypoechoic area within otherwise echogenic liver
  - No mass effect: Vessels run undisplaced through lesion
  - Due to direct drainage of hepatic blood into systemic circulation
  - Typical location
    - Next to gallbladder: Drained by cystic vein
    - Segment IV/anterior to portal bifurcation: Drained by aberrant gastric vein
- **Diffuse/Infiltrative Hepatic Lymphoma**
  - Subcentimeter periportal hypoechoic foci, miliary in pattern
  - Other evidence of lymphoma
    - Lymphadenopathy, splenomegaly/splenic lesions, bowel wall thickening, ascites
- **Pneumobilia**
  - Highly echogenic, linear foci in portal triad
  - Rises to nondependent portion of liver (left lobe if patient lying supine)
  - Change in position of gas with change in patient position
  - Posterior acoustic shadowing
  - Reverberation artifact deep to lesion
  - Causes
    - Recent passage of stone from or instrumentation of biliary tree
    - Choledochoenteric fistula
    - Biliary infection by gas-forming organism
- **Choledocholithiasis**
  - Multiple echogenic foci along portal triad
  - Posterior acoustic shadowing
    - Small (< 5-mm) or soft, pigmented stones may not produce posterior shadowing
  - Large stones may cause biliary obstruction, resulting in focal bile duct dilatation
- **Metastases**
  - May be located anywhere in liver
  - Usually multiple

Helpful Clues for Less Common Diagnoses

- **Peribiliary Cyst**
  - Well-defined, small, cystic structures adjacent to portal triads
  - More common in cirrhotic patients
  - Usually multiple
  - No communication with biliary tree
- **Hepatic Schistosomiasis**
  - Periportal fibrosis
    - Most severe at porta hepatis
    - Widened portal tracts
    - Clay pipestem fibrosis
      - Hyperechoic and thickened walls of portal venules
    - Bull's-eye lesion
      - Anechoic portal vein surrounded by echogenic mantle of fibrous tissue
  - Mosaic pattern
    - Network of echogenic septa outlining polygonal areas of normal-appearing liver
    - Represents complete septal fibrosis
      - Inflammation and fibrosis in reaction to embolized eggs
    - May be discontinuous and appear mottled, nodular, or sieve-like
      - Partial septal fibrosis or calcification
- **Recurrent Pyogenic Cholangitis**
  - Lateral segment of left lobe and posterior segment of right lobe more commonly involved
  - Early disease with active biliary sepsis
    - Periportal hypo- or hyperechogenicity due to periductal edema/inflammation
    - Biliary duct wall thickening due to edema
    - Floating echoes within dilated ducts due to inflammatory debris
  - Late-stage disease
    - Severe atrophy of affected segment/lobe, biliary cirrhosis
    - Crowded, stone-filled ducts
      - May appear as single heterogeneous mass
    - Stones may form casts of duct
- **Iatrogenic Material**
  - Shunt, stent, embolization material, drainage tube, staples, etc.
  - Echogenic material with strong reflective surface or smooth outline
- **Caroli Disease**
  - Anechoic masses: Saccular or fusiform shape
  - Central dot sign
    - Small portal venous branches partially/completely surrounded by dilated ducts
- **Hepatic Artery Calcification**
  - Branching, linear, echogenic structures along portal triads
  - Often marked calcifications of splenic artery and other smaller arteries
  - Risk factors
    - Longstanding diabetes
    - Chronic renal failure
    - Conditions that predispose to heavy vascular calcifications
- **Cystic Duct Remnant**
  - History of prior cholecystectomy
  - Remnant cystic duct may be dilated

SELECTED REFERENCES

1. Sharbidre K et al: Imaging of fibropolycystic liver disease. Abdom Radiol (NY). 47(7):2356-70, 2022
2. Pötter-Lang S et al: Modern imaging of cholangitis. Br J Radiol. 94(1125):20210417, 2021
3. Ramanathan S et al: Unveiling the unreal: comprehensive imaging review of hepatic pseudolesions. Clin Imaging. 80:439-53, 2021
4. Matsubara T et al: Peribiliary glands: development, dysfunction, related conditions and imaging findings. Abdom Radiol (NY). 45(2):416-36, 2020
5. Sokal A et al: Acute cholangitis: diagnosis and management. J Visc Surg. 156(6):515-25, 2019
6. Shin SW et al: Usefulness of B-mode and doppler sonography for the diagnosis of severe acute viral hepatitis A. J Clin Ultrasound. 43(6):384-92, 2015
7. Spârchez Z et al: Role of contrast enhanced ultrasound in the assessment of biliary duct disease. Med Ultrason. 16(1):41-7, 2014
8. Trenker C et al: Contrast-enhanced ultrasound (CEUS) in hepatic lymphoma: retrospective evaluation in 38 cases. Ultraschall Med. 35(2):142-8, 2014

Ascending Cholangitis

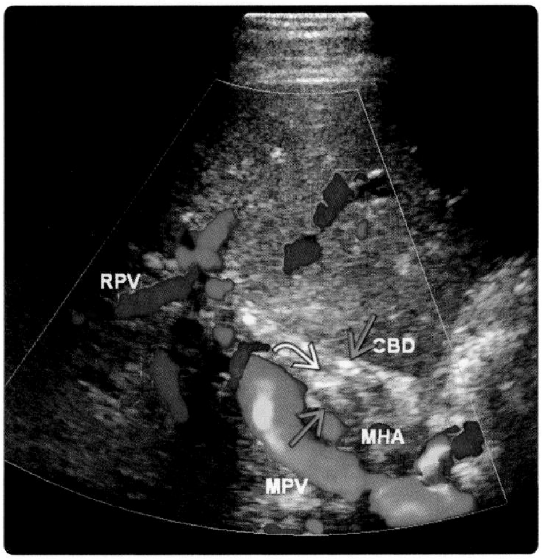

Cavernous Transformation of Portal Vein

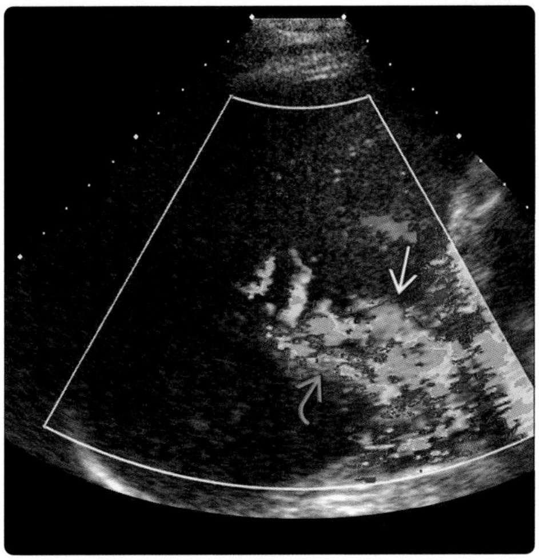

(Left) *Transverse color Doppler US in a patient with ascending cholangitis shows circumferential wall thickening of the common bile duct ➔ as well as echogenic debris ➔ within the lumen.* **(Right)** *Color Doppler US shows collateralized flow ➔ in the porta hepatis in a patient with chronic portal vein thrombosis ➔. Signal is heterogeneous because portal vein collaterals are tortuous, resulting in vessels directed toward as well as away from the transducer.*

(Left) *Transverse color Doppler US shows an intrahepatic portosystemic shunt between the right portal vein and right hepatic vein ➡️, which appears as an entangled, vascular structure that drains into the right hepatic vein ⇨. (Right) Transverse color Doppler US in a patient with hepatic cirrhosis shows a recanalized paraumbilical vein ➡️ arising from the left portal vein ⇨ and traveling anteriorly along the falciform ligament toward the inferior epigastric vein.*

Portosystemic Collaterals

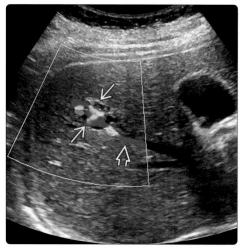

Portosystemic Collaterals

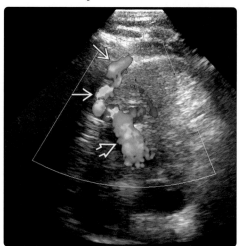

(Left) *Transverse color Doppler US in a patient with lymphoma involving the liver shows multiple markedly hypoechoic masses ➡️ in a periportal distribution (right anterior portal vein ⇨). Lesions are predominantly hypovascular, a characteristic imaging appearance of lymphoma. (Right) Transverse US shows linear, bright hyperechoic foci ➡️ caused by pneumobilia along the expected course of the biliary tree.*

Diffuse/Infiltrative Hepatic Lymphoma

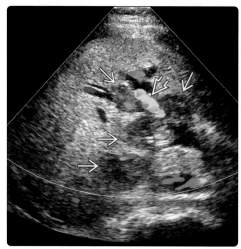

Pneumobilia

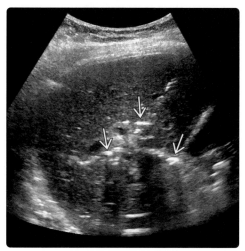

(Left) *Longitudinal color Doppler US shows multiple echogenic stones ➡️ within the common bile duct, causing upstream biliary ductal dilation ⇨. Color Doppler is helpful to distinguish avascular ducts from adjacent vasculature. (Right) Transverse color Doppler US in a patient with ovarian cancer shows an ill-defined, hypoechoic metastasis ➡️ that infiltrates the left periportal region, occluding the left portal vein, which should normally be present in this region.*

Choledocholithiasis

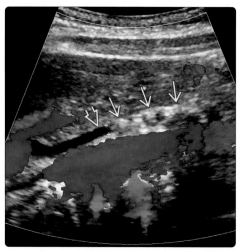

Metastases

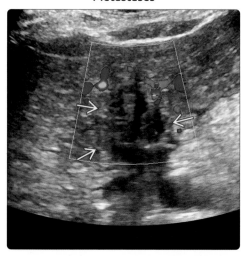

Peribiliary Cyst

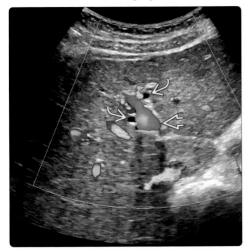

Hepatic Schistosomiasis

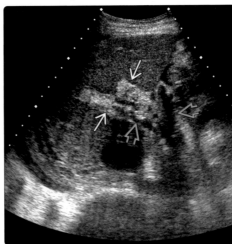

(Left) *Transverse color Doppler US shows several small, well-defined peribiliary cysts* ⇗ *along the left portal vein* ⇒. **(Right)** *Transverse US in a patient with hepatic schistosomiasis shows a thick, echogenic mantle of fibrotic tissue* ⇒ *in the periportal area, encasing the portal veins* ⇗. *(Courtesy W. Chong, MD.)*

Recurrent Pyogenic Cholangitis

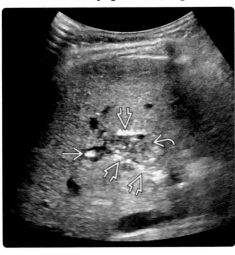

Recurrent Pyogenic Cholangitis

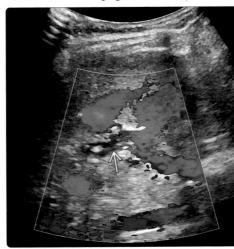

(Left) *Transverse US in a patient with recurrent pyogenic cholangitis shows echogenic intrahepatic stones* ⇒ *and sludge* ⇗ *within moderately dilated intrahepatic biliary ducts. Note the periductal hyperechogenicity* ⇒ *related to periductal inflammation.* **(Right)** *Color Doppler US in the same patient shows no flow within the dilated intrahepatic duct* ⇒, *confirming the findings are indeed in the biliary tree rather than the portal or hepatic arterial system.*

Hepatic Artery Calcification

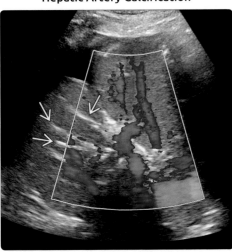

Cystic Duct Remnant

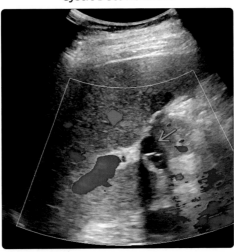

(Left) *Transverse color Doppler US shows multifocal linear, branching, echogenic structures* ⇒ *that are hepatic artery calcifications related to end-stage renal disease.* **(Right)** *Longitudinal color Doppler US in a patient s/p cholecystectomy shows a cystic duct remnant* ⇒ *appearing as a round, cystic lesion in the region of the porta hepatis.*

DIFFERENTIAL DIAGNOSIS

Common

- Cirrhosis
- Subcapsular Hepatic Neoplasm
- Hepatic Metastasis
- Infiltrative Hepatocellular Carcinoma
- Postsurgical Hepatic Resection

Less Common

- Hepatic Rupture
- Schistosomiasis

ESSENTIAL INFORMATION

Helpful Clues for Common Diagnoses

- **Cirrhosis**
  - Nodular surface contour
    - Micronodular (< 1 cm in diameter): Due to alcoholism
    - Macronodular: Due to viral hepatitis
  - Hypertrophy of caudate lobe and lateral segment of left lobe
  - Atrophy of right lobe and medial segment of left lobe
  - Widening of fissures
  - Coarse/nodular/heterogeneous parenchymal echotexture
- **Subcapsular Hepatic Neoplasm**
  - Primary or secondary subcapsular neoplasm may distort surface contour when large or numerous
  - Lesions cause architectural distortion of liver parenchyma
- **Hepatic Metastasis**
  - Commonly due to gastric, ovarian, breast, or pancreatic primary
  - Treated metastases (e.g., from breast) may shrink and fibrose, simulating nodular contour of cirrhotic liver
- **Infiltrative Hepatocellular Carcinoma**
  - Margins of tumor often indistinct
  - May see refractive shadows emanating from hepatic parenchyma

- Portal triads may be effaced or invaded
- Often associated with tumor thrombus in portal vein or hepatic vein (less common)
- **Postsurgical Hepatic Resection**
  - Combination of surgical defect and surrounding scarring causes irregularity of contour
  - Surgical material ± fat in surgical defect causes further heterogeneity of surgical site

Helpful Clues for Less Common Diagnoses

- **Hepatic Rupture**
  - Echogenic blood clot on surface of liver
  - May see breach of hepatic capsule or irregularity of capsular surface if underlying lesion is hepatocellular carcinoma
  - Hemoperitoneum may be present
    - More echogenic than ascites
  - Underlying cause
    - Large or exophytic hepatocellular carcinoma or other tumor
    - Spontaneous hepatic rupture associated with HELLP (hemolysis, elevated liver enzymes, and low platelets) syndrome
      - Thought to be secondary to endothelial dysfunction and thrombotic microangiopathy
- **Schistosomiasis**
  - Irregular/notched, liver surface
  - Echogenic periportal fibrotic bands (most severe at porta hepatis)
  - Mosaic pattern: Network of echogenic septa outlining polygonal areas of normal-appearing liver
    - Represents complete septal fibrosis (inflammation and fibrosis as reaction to embolized eggs)

SELECTED REFERENCES

1. Campos-Murguía A et al: Clinical assessment and management of liver fibrosis in non-alcoholic fatty liver disease. World J Gastroenterol. 26(39):5919-43, 2020
2. Castera L et al: Noninvasive assessment of liver disease in patients with nonalcoholic fatty liver disease. Gastroenterology. 156(5):1264-81.e4, 2019

Cirrhosis

Cirrhosis

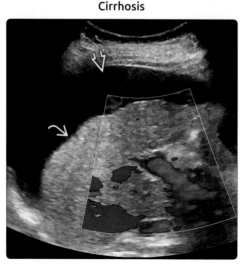

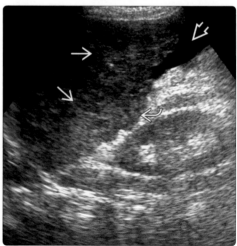

(Left) Transverse color Doppler US in a patient with cirrhosis shows a nodular and irregular liver surface ➡. A large amount of simple ascites ➡ is consistent with portal hypertension related to underlying liver disease. (Right) Grayscale US of liver shows macronodular cirrhosis with multiple solid, isoechoic nodules ➡. The liver margins appear nodular ➡ with overall shrunken liver parenchyma, and there is immediately adjacent ascites ➡ related to portal hypertension.

Subcapsular Hepatic Neoplasm

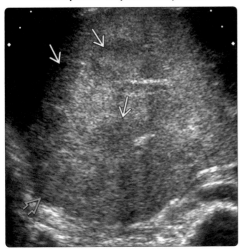

Subcapsular Hepatic Neoplasm

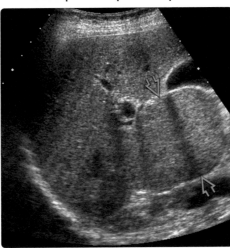

(Left) *Transverse grayscale US of the liver shows an isoechoic liver metastasis ⇨ from breast cancer that bulges and slightly distorts the liver surface. Multiple other subtle hypoechoic breast cancer metastases are seen throughout the rest of the liver ➡.* **(Right)** *Transverse grayscale US of the liver shows a large isoechoic mass in the caudate lobe of the liver, which creates a rounded bulge upon the hepatic surface in this area. This mass was a focal nodular hyperplasia ⇨.*

Hepatic Metastasis

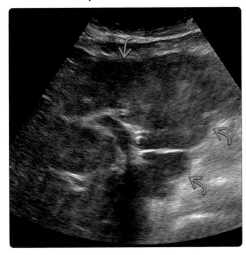

Infiltrative Hepatocellular Carcinoma

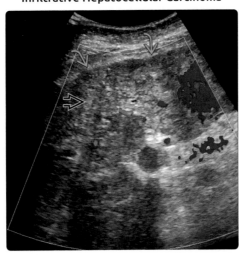

(Left) *Transverse grayscale US of the left lobe of the liver in a patient with breast cancer shows markedly irregular and nodular liver surface due to diffuse hepatic involvement with metastases ➚.* **(Right)** *Transverse color Doppler US in a patient with infiltrative hepatocellular carcinoma throughout the liver shows the infiltrative tumor causes both markedly heterogeneous echotexture ⇨ as well as irregular hepatic surface ➚.*

Hepatic Rupture

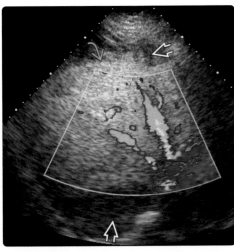

Schistosomiasis

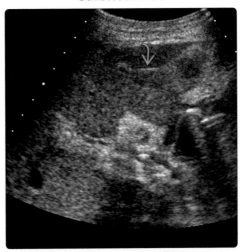

(Left) *Transverse color Doppler US in a patient with liver rupture from HELLP syndrome shows a large amount of perihepatic and subcapsular blood ➡, which causes the liver margin ➚ to appear irregular. Acute blood can be so echogenic that the liver margin can be obscured by the blood.* **(Right)** *Transverse grayscale US of a patient with schistosomiasis and periportal fibrosis, as well as hepatic capsular irregularity ➚, is shown. (Courtesy W. Chong, MD.)*

DIFFERENTIAL DIAGNOSIS

Common

- Portal Hypertension
- Portosystemic Collaterals
- Bland Portal Vein Thrombosis
- Portal Vein Tumor Thrombus
- Pulsatile Portal Vein

Less Common

- Portal Vein Gas

ESSENTIAL INFORMATION

Helpful Clues for Common Diagnoses

- **Portal Hypertension**
  - Decreased portal vein mean velocity (< 16 cm/s)
  - Portal venous pressure ≥ 10 mm Hg more than inferior vena cava pressure
  - Hepatofugal portal vein flow in severe portal hypertension
  - Absent (aphasic) portal venous flow due to stagnation
    - Lack of respiratory phasicity
    - Severe portal hypertension
  - Development of portosystemic shunts
  - Background cirrhosis, splenomegaly, ascites, thickened bowel wall
- **Portosystemic Collaterals**
  - Common locations
    - Inferior hepatic margin via gastroepiploic vein
    - Gastroesophageal junction via left gastric vein
    - Anterior abdominal wall via ligamentum teres (recanalized paraumbilical vein)
    - Lienorenal ligament via lienorenal collaterals
  - Color Doppler shows low-velocity hepatofugal flow
- **Bland Portal Vein Thrombosis**
  - Echogenic material within portal vein (acute thrombosis)
  - Poor visualization of portal vein (chronic thrombosis)
  - Cavernous transformation of portal vein in chronic thrombosis

- Color Doppler US: Interrupted/irregular flow in portal vein
- Signs of liver dysfunction or portal hypertension
  - Cirrhosis, ascites, splenomegaly, portosystemic collaterals
- **Portal Vein Tumor Thrombus**
  - Majority arise from hepatocellular carcinoma
  - Echogenic material within portal vein
  - Suspect tumor thrombus in case of adjacent hepatic malignancy
  - Color Doppler US may show tumor neovascularity within thrombus
- **Pulsatile Portal Vein**
  - Normal portal vein waveform
    - Hepatopetal and mildly phasic (gentle undulation)
  - Increased pulsatility (pulsatile waveform)
    - When there is large difference between peak systolic velocity and end-diastolic velocity
      - Tricuspid regurgitation
      - Right-sided congestive heart failure
      - Arterioportal shunting in cirrhosis
      - Arteriovenous fistula in hereditary hemorrhagic telangiectasia

Helpful Clues for Less Common Diagnoses

- **Portal Vein Gas**
  - Highly reflective foci (gas) travels within portal vein
  - Poorly defined, highly reflective parenchymal foci
  - Gas moves to periphery of liver (as opposed to biliary gas, which moves toward liver hilum)
  - High-intensity transient signals (HITS) with spectral Doppler
    - Strong transient spikes superimposed on portal venous flow pattern

SELECTED REFERENCES

1. Senzolo M et al: Current knowledge and management of portal vein thrombosis in cirrhosis. J Hepatol. 75(2):442-53, 2021
2. Daneshmand A et al: Portal venous gas: different aetiologies and their respective outcomes. ANZ J Surg. 90(5):767-71, 2020

Portal Hypertension

Portosystemic Collaterals

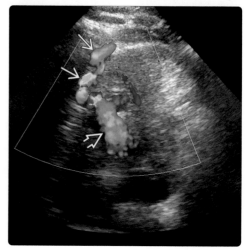

(Left) *Spectral Doppler US of the liver in a patient with portal hypertension shows retrograde (hepatofugal) flow in the portal vein ➡, a finding that appears blue on color Doppler US and is displayed below the baseline on the spectral waveform ➡. **(Right)** Transverse color Doppler US in a patient with hepatic cirrhosis shows a recanalized paraumbilical vein ➡ arising from the left portal vein ➡ and traveling anteriorly along the falciform ligament toward the inferior epigastric vein.*

Bland Portal Vein Thrombosis

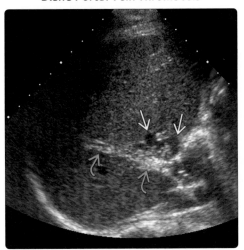

Bland Portal Vein Thrombosis

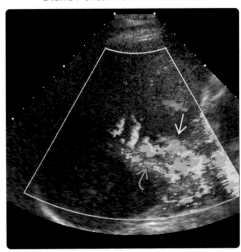

(Left) *Transverse US shows an echogenic, chronically thrombosed main portal vein ⊿ and adjacent collateralized flow ➡, indicating cavernous transformation of the portal vein.* (Right) *Color Doppler US in the same patient shows collateralized flow ➡ in the porta hepatis. Note chronic portal vein thrombosis ⊿. Color Doppler signal is heterogeneous because portal vein collaterals are tortuous, resulting in vessels directed toward as well as away from the transducer.*

Portal Vein Tumor Thrombus

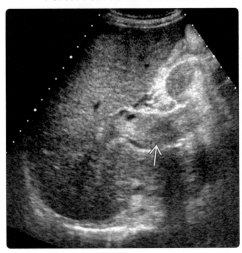

Portal Vein Tumor Thrombus

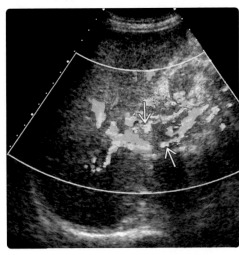

(Left) *Transverse US of the liver in a patient with hepatocellular carcinoma shows an expansile, echogenic tumor thrombus in the main portal vein ➡.* (Right) *Color Doppler US in the same patient shows multiple small feeding vessels ➡ in the tumor thrombus with a dot-dash pattern. Tumor thrombus in the setting of hepatocellular carcinoma is almost always associated with infiltrative tumor and carries a poor prognosis.*

Pulsatile Portal Vein

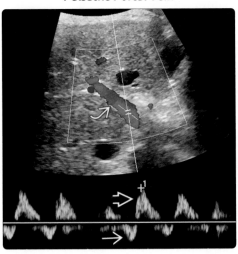

Portal Vein Gas

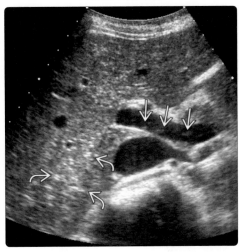

(Left) *Spectral Doppler US in a patient with right heart failure shows a pulsatile waveform with flow above ➡ and below ➡ baseline in the main portal vein ⊿. The waveform is characterized as predominantly antegrade, pulsatile, and biphasic/bidirectional.* (Right) *Oblique US of the liver shows several echogenic foci in the main portal vein ➡ representing gas bubbles. Bright, echogenic patches ➡ in the liver parenchyma more peripherally represent intraparenchymal portal venous gas.*

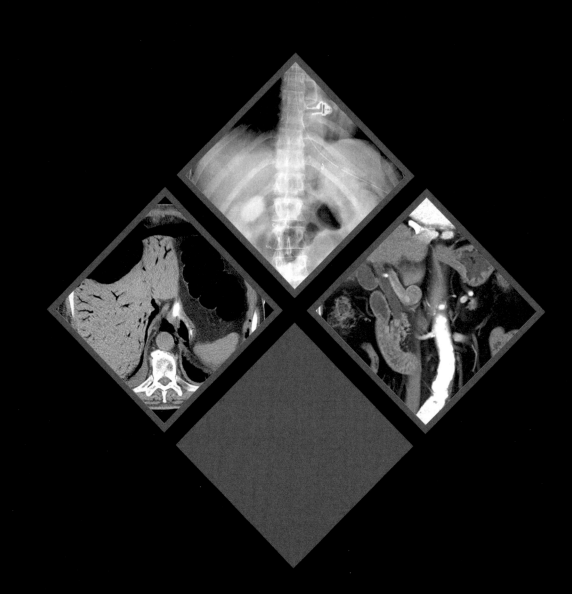
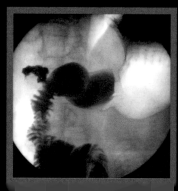
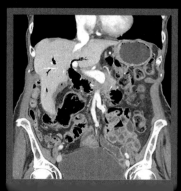
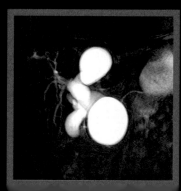

SECTION 10
Gallbladder

Generic Imaging Patterns

Distended Gallbladder   366
Gas in Bile Ducts or Gallbladder   368
Focal Gallbladder Wall Thickening   372
Diffuse Gallbladder Wall Thickening   374

Modality-Specific Imaging Findings

Computed Tomography

High-Attenuation (Hyperdense) Bile in Gallbladder   378

Ultrasound

Hyperechoic Gallbladder Wall   380
Echogenic Material in Gallbladder   382
Dilated Gallbladder   384
Intrahepatic and Extrahepatic Duct Dilatation   388

Clinically Based Differentials

Right Upper Quadrant Pain   390

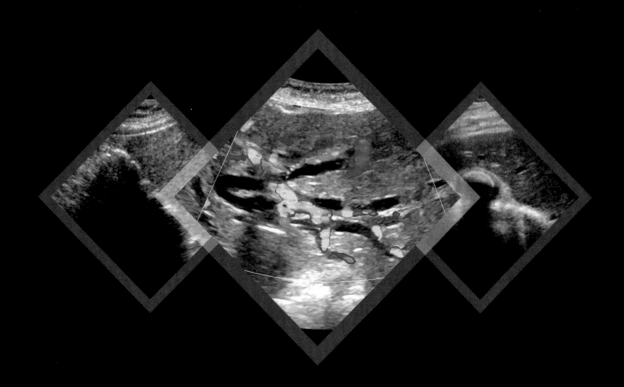

DIFFERENTIAL DIAGNOSIS

Common

- Decreased Vagal Stimulation
  - Postvagotomy State
  - Anticholinergic Medications
  - Diabetes Mellitus
- Decreased Cholecystokinin Secretion
  - Hyperalimentation
  - Prolonged Fasting
- Obstructed Flow of Bile
  - Calculous Cholecystitis
  - Choledocholithiasis
  - Pancreatic Ductal Adenocarcinoma
- Inflammation of Gallbladder by Intrinsic or Adjacent Process
- Acalculous Cholecystitis

Less Common

- Gallbladder Hydrops
- Gallbladder Empyema
- Choledochal Cyst (Mimic)

ESSENTIAL INFORMATION

Key Differential Diagnosis Issues

- No absolute size criteria, but gallbladder (GB) considered distended when > 5 cm in diameter or 10 cm in length
- GB contracts and empties in response to vagal stimulation and cholecystokinin (secreted in response to fatty foods)
  - Vagal stimulation causes GB contraction; cholecystokinin causes GB contraction, relaxation of sphincter of Oddi
- Normal emptying requires patent cystic duct and CBD

Helpful Clues for Common Diagnoses

- Causes can be divided into 5 major categories
  - **Decreased Vagal Stimulation**
    - Vagotomy, anticholinergic medicines, or diabetic neuropathy can reduce vagal stimulation and result in GB distention
  - **Decreased Cholecystokinin Secretion**
    - Prolonged fasting, hyperalimentation, and low-fat (and high-alcohol) diet result in diminished cholecystokinin secretion and consequent GB distention
  - **Obstructed Flow of Bile**
    - Cystic/common duct calculus, tumors of GB, bile ducts, ampulla, or pancreas, or CBD strictures resulting from chronic pancreatitis can obstruct bile flow from GB, resulting in distention
    - Courvoisier sign: Distention of GB with painless jaundice raises concern for malignant obstruction
    - Calculous cholecystitis often presents with distended GB due to obstruction of cystic duct by stone
  - **Inflammation of Gallbladder by Intrinsic or Adjacent Process**
    - AIDS cholangiopathy, hepatitis, pancreatitis, or perforated duodenal ulcer may cause secondary GB inflammation and distention
  - **Acalculous Cholecystitis**
    - Most often diagnosed in critically ill or ICU patients (particularly when not eating)
    - Distended GB with wall thickening, pericholecystic fluid, and positive sonographic Murphy sign

Helpful Clues for Less Common Diagnoses

- **Gallbladder Hydrops**
  - Distended GB with simple fluid contents resulting from chronic obstruction (usually due to stones)
  - No wall thickening, pericholecystic fluid, or Murphy sign
  - May result in right upper quadrant pain without fever
- **Gallbladder Empyema**
  - Distended GB filled with infected material (pus) due to acute cholecystitis with intraluminal infection
  - Usually associated with other features of cholecystitis (wall thickening, pericholecystic fluid, etc.)
  - Fluid within GB appears complex with internal debris
- **Choledochal Cyst (Mimic)**
  - Choledochal cysts may extend into porta hepatis and mimic GB
  - Other upper abdominal cysts (hepatic, renal, pancreatic) can also theoretically mimic appearance of GB

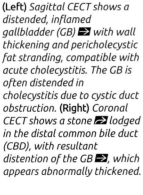

(Left) Sagittal CECT shows a distended, inflamed gallbladder (GB) ➦ with wall thickening and pericholecystic fat stranding, compatible with acute cholecystitis. The GB is often distended in cholecystitis due to cystic duct obstruction. (Right) Coronal CECT shows a stone ➥ lodged in the distal common bile duct (CBD), with resultant distention of the GB ➦, which appears abnormally thickened.

Calculous Cholecystitis

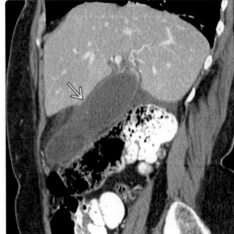

Choledocholithiasis

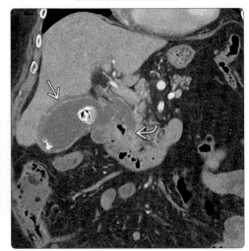

Pancreatic Ductal Adenocarcinoma

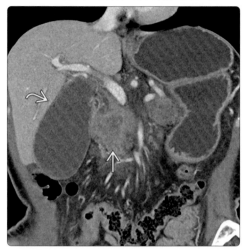

Other Obstructing Tumors

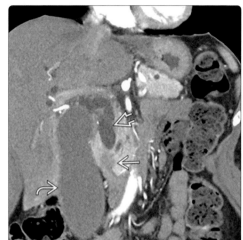

(Left) *Coronal CECT shows a large, infiltrating pancreatic mass ➡ obstructing the biliary tree and resulting in distention of the GB ➡ (Courvoisier sign).* (Right) *Coronal CECT shows a hypodense ampullary mass ➡ resulting in biliary obstruction ➡ and GB distention ➡, representing an ampullary carcinoma.*

Inflammation of Gallbladder by Intrinsic or Adjacent Process

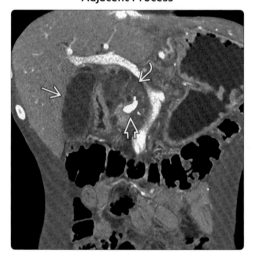

Inflammation of Gallbladder by Intrinsic or Adjacent Process

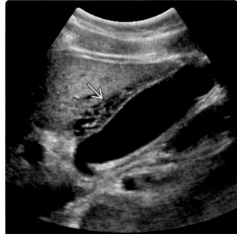

(Left) *Coronal CECT shows a large, hypodense mass ➡ with internal calcification ➡ resulting in biliary obstruction and GB distention ➡. In this case, these findings represent a chronic fibrocalcific mass related to chronic pancreatitis.* (Right) *Sagittal US shows marked GB wall edema ➡ and GB distention in a patient with acute viral hepatitis.*

Gallbladder Hydrops

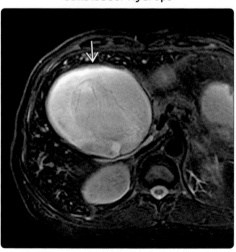

Choledochal Cyst (Mimic)

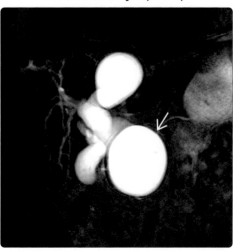

(Left) *Axial T2 FS MR shows a massively distended GB ➡ with some internal debris and sludge. The patient had no clinical signs of infection, suggesting GB hydrops.* (Right) *Coronal MRCP MIP shows a type IV choledochal cyst with dilatation of the intrahepatic and extrahepatic ducts. The large cystic component involving the extrahepatic CBD ➡ projects into the porta hepatis and could be confused for a distended GB.*

DIFFERENTIAL DIAGNOSIS

Common

- Biliary Sphincterotomy or Stent Placement
- Choledocholithiasis
- Patulous Sphincter of Oddi
- Surgical Biliary-Enteric Anastomosis
- Portal Vein Gas (Mimic)
- Hepatic Artery Calcification (Mimic)
- Biliary Instrumentation

Less Common

- Emphysematous Cholecystitis
- Gas Within Gallstones
- Biliary-Enteric Fistula (Including Gallstone Ileus)
- Duodenal Ulcer
- Inflammation Near Ampulla
- Cholangitis, Chemotherapy Induced
- Biliary Infection
  - Recurrent Pyogenic Cholangitis
- Ampullary and Periampullary Tumors

Rare but Important

- Bile Sump Syndrome
- Bronchobiliary Fistula
- Trauma
- Transarterial Hepatic Chemoembolization

ESSENTIAL INFORMATION

Key Differential Diagnosis Issues

- Gas in biliary system (pneumobilia or aerobilia) is sequelae of abnormal sphincter of Oddi function or communication between biliary tree and bowel
  - In most (but not all) cases, pneumobilia is incidental imaging finding of little significance, most often attributable to prior surgery or biliary intervention
  - Pneumobilia should be carefully distinguished from portal venous gas, since although most causes of pneumobilia are benign, portal venous gas almost always heralds presence of critical illness/ischemia
  - Large amounts of pneumobilia can reflux into gallbladder lumen itself and should not be confused with emphysematous cholecystitis
- Gas in biliary system is usually much more evident on CT than on other imaging modalities
  - Pneumobilia not uncommonly visualized on US as brightly echogenic, branching reflector (± "dirty" posterior acoustic shadowing)
  - Pneumobilia typically low signal on MR and can sometimes be confused for low-signal gallstones

Helpful Clues for Common Diagnoses

- **Biliary Sphincterotomy or Stent Placement**
  - Entails cutting muscles of sphincter of Oddi (usually during ERCP) for variety of indications, including stone removal, treating strictures, placing biliary stents, treating duct leaks, etc.
  - Allows reflux of gas from duodenal lumen into bile ducts and is very common cause of pneumobilia
    - Concurrent placement of biliary stent results in greater degrees of pneumobilia

- **Choledocholithiasis**
  - Passage of stones may lead to scarring and distortion of sphincter of Oddi, which leads to incompetence, allowing reflux of duodenal gas into bile duct
- **Patulous Sphincter of Oddi**
  - May occur spontaneously, especially in older adults, but resultant pneumobilia is usually quite minimal
  - Can also be related to prior bouts of pancreatitis (resulting in scarring of sphincter) or secondary to certain medications
- **Surgical Biliary-Enteric Anastomosis**
  - Bile duct is anastomosed to loop of bowel (usually jejunal Roux loop), allowing direct reflux of bowel gas into biliary tree
  - May be seen in setting of liver transplantation, Whipple procedure, and many other hepatobiliary surgeries
- **Portal Vein Gas (Mimic)**
  - May be mistaken for biliary gas
  - Pneumobilia collects near porta hepatis **centrally**, while portal venous gas collects in **periphery** of liver
  - Portal venous gas appears mobile with small bubbles on US, while pneumobilia is less mobile with larger collections of gas
- **Hepatic Artery Calcification (Mimic)**
  - Uncommon except with chronic renal failure but can be mistaken for biliary or portal venous gas on US
- **Biliary Instrumentation**
  - Any recent biliary instrumentation can introduce gas into biliary tree, including ERCP, percutaneous transhepatic cholangiograms, percutaneous biliary stent procedures, cholecystostomy tube placement, etc.

Helpful Clues for Less Common Diagnoses

- **Emphysematous Cholecystitis**
  - Rare complication due to gallbladder infection with gas-forming organism (usually *Clostridium perfringens*)
    - Gas in gallbladder wall or lumen may reflux into biliary tree, although this is relatively uncommon
  - Most commonly occurs in older adult or diabetic patients
  - US demonstrates echogenic reflectors in gallbladder wall or lumen with "dirty" posterior acoustic shadowing
- **Gas Within Gallstones**
  - Gas-fissuring within gallstones is incidental finding and does not imply infection or complication
  - Often has Mercedes-Benz appearance with branching or chevron pattern of gas within stone
- **Duodenal Diverticulum**
  - Periampullary diverticulum may lead to sphincter of Oddi dysfunction, allowing reflux of gas
- **Biliary-Enteric Fistula (Including Gallstone Ileus)**
  - Gallstone ileus is bowel obstruction caused by impaction of gallstone within bowel (usually terminal ileum)
    - Occurs when large gallstone erodes through adherent walls of inflamed gallbladder and duodenum (usually via cholecystoduodenal fistula)
    - Results in Rigler triad of findings, including pneumobilia, small bowel obstruction, and gallstone
  - Biliary-enteric fistulas can rarely result from other causes, including peptic ulcer disease, hepatic arterial chemotherapy [with ischemia of gallbladder/duodenum, trauma, and right upper quadrant malignancies (such as cholangiocarcinoma, gallbladder cancer, etc.)]

- **Inflammation Near Ampulla**
  - Any periampullary inflammation may result in incompetence of sphincter of Oddi with reflux of gas
  - Can be complication of any surrounding inflammatory process, including ulcer, pancreatitis, duodenitis, etc.
- **Biliary Infection**
  - May result in pneumobilia due to gas-forming infection or by resulting in incompetent sphincter of Oddi
  - Gas-containing liver abscess may communicate with biliary tree and lead to pneumobilia
  - Recurrent pyogenic cholangitis frequently demonstrates pneumobilia, most often due to stone passage through sphincter of Oddi, but rarely due to gas-forming infection
- **Ampullary and Periampullary Tumors**
  - Any benign or malignant tumor arising in ampullary or periampullary region may lead to sphincter incompetence with gas reflux
  - Malignant tumors may also result in spontaneous biliary-enteric fistula

Helpful Clues for Rare Diagnoses

- **Bile Sump Syndrome**
  - After side-to-side choledochoduodenostomy (performed to improve bile drainage), sphincter of Oddi dysfunction may lead to distal common bile duct serving as reservoir for static bile and stones
  - Bile sump syndrome occurs when distal common bile duct accumulates stones, bile, and debris, and becomes nidus for cholangitis
  - Associated with pneumobilia
- **Bronchobiliary Fistula**
  - Extremely rare condition, which is most often caused by hepatic/subphrenic abscesses or sequelae of hepatic intervention (liver resection, ablation, TACE)
  - Patients present with chronic cough and biliptysis
  - Imaging may show communication between biliary tree and bronchial tree with frequent large-volume pneumobilia
- **Transarterial Hepatic Chemoembolization**
  - Rare cause of spontaneous biliary-enteric fistulas (usually cholecystoduodenal fistula)

Biliary Sphincterotomy or Stent Placement

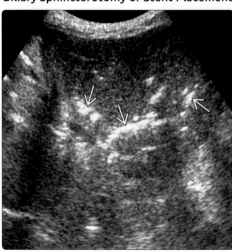

Biliary Sphincterotomy or Stent Placement

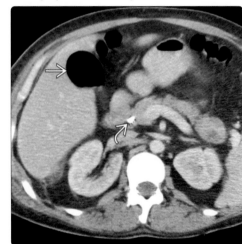

(Left) Axial NECT shows pneumobilia, predominantly located in the central, larger bile ducts ➡ within the nondependent portions of the liver. (Right) Axial CECT performed shortly after the placement of a biliary stent ➡ shows extensive gaseous distention of the gallbladder lumen ➡. Placement of a biliary stent can lead to greater degrees of pneumobilia compared to sphincterotomy alone.

Biliary Sphincterotomy or Stent Placement

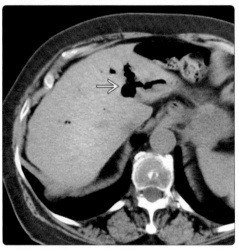

Biliary Sphincterotomy or Stent Placement

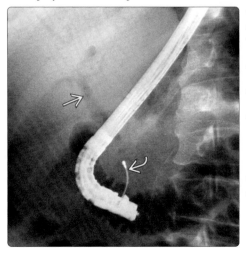

(Left) Transverse US in a patient with history of sphincterotomy shows the classic appearance of pneumobilia with branching echogenic reflectors ➡ following the expected course of the bile ducts, predominantly in the central aspect of the liver. (Right) Oblique ERCP shows gas in the bile ducts ➡ and the endoscope with a sphincterotomy device ➡ in place.

(Left) *Axial CECT shows gas in the bile ducts ➡, clearly separate from the contrast-opacified portal veins ▱. Stones were found within the common bile duct on MRCP.* **(Right)** *Frontal radiograph shows the classic appearance of pneumobilia with a branching gas pattern ➡ limited to the porta hepatis. The patient had undergone prior small bowel and liver transplantation with biliary-enteric anastomosis.*

Choledocholithiasis

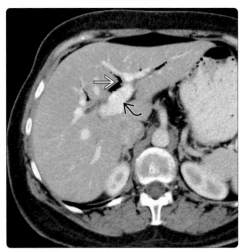

Surgical Biliary-Enteric Anastomosis

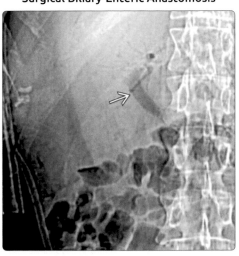

(Left) *Coronal CECT in a patient status post Whipple procedure nicely shows the hepaticojejunostomy with gas tracking from the right upper quadrant small bowel loop ➡ into the biliary tree ➡. The hepaticojejunal anastomosis is often best appreciated in the coronal plane.* **(Right)** *Coronal CECT shows gas ➡ outlining the central bile ducts in a patient status post hepaticojejunostomy as part of a Whipple procedure.*

Surgical Biliary-Enteric Anastomosis

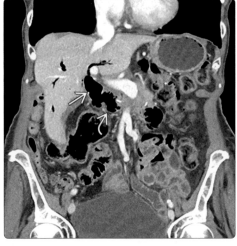

Surgical Biliary-Enteric Anastomosis

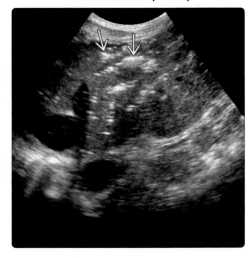

(Left) *Axial NECT shows extensive portal venous gas ➡ at the periphery of the liver in a patient with mesenteric ischemia. Unlike most cases of pneumobilia, portal venous gas is a critical imaging finding, which should raise concern for ischemia.* **(Right)** *Transverse US in a patient with bowel ischemia shows the characteristic appearance of portal venous gas with ill-defined, mobile, small echogenic reflectors ➡ primarily located at the periphery of the liver.*

Portal Vein Gas (Mimic)

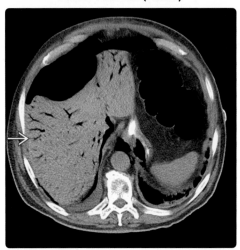

Portal Vein Gas (Mimic)

Hepatic Artery Calcification (Mimic)

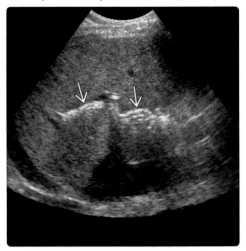

Emphysematous Cholecystitis

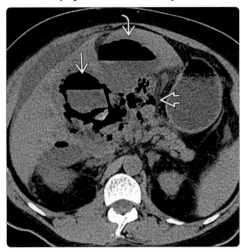

(Left) *Sagittal US in a patient with renal failure shows extensive linear, echogenic reflectors* ➡ *with posterior acoustic shadowing branching in the central liver. CT showed that these represented extensive hepatic artery calcifications.* (Right) *Axial NECT shows gas within the gallbladder lumen* ➡ *and wall due to emphysematous cholecystitis in a diabetic patient. Note the gas tracking from the gallbladder medially* ➡ *as well as the adjacent collection of gas and fluid* ➡ *secondary to perforation.*

Gas Within Gallstones

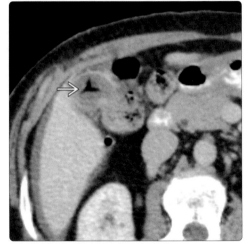

Biliary-Enteric Fistula (Including Gallstone Ileus)

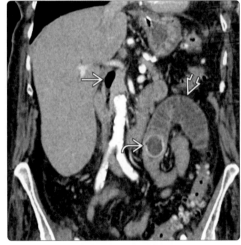

(Left) *Axial CECT shows a classic Mercedes-Benz-shaped gas fissure* ➡ *within a gallstone. This is an incidental finding, which should not be confused with emphysematous cholecystitis.* (Right) *Coronal CECT shows the classic features of a gallstone ileus, including a large gallstone* ➡ *impacted in the small bowel, obstruction and dilatation of the more proximal small bowel* ➡, *and biliary gas nicely filling the common bile duct* ➡.

Biliary-Enteric Fistula (Including Gallstone Ileus)

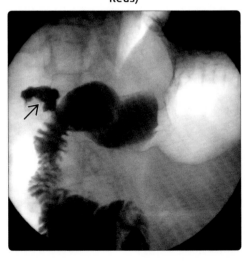

Recurrent Pyogenic Cholangitis

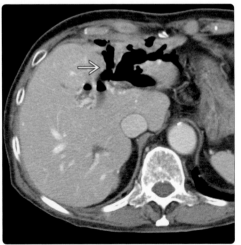

(Left) *Frontal upper GI in a patient with gallstone ileus nicely shows filling of the gallbladder* ➡ *via a cholecystoduodenal fistula.* (Right) *Axial CECT shows gross dilation and distortion of the bile ducts* ➡, *which are filled with gas and pus. The left lobe is affected more than the right and shows parenchymal atrophy as a result of chronic infection. These findings are classic for recurrent pyogenic cholangitis.*

DIFFERENTIAL DIAGNOSIS

Common

- Hyperplastic Cholecystoses
- Gallbladder Carcinoma

Less Common

- Xanthogranulomatous Cholecystitis
- Porcelain Gallbladder
- Gallbladder Metastases and Lymphoma
- Gallbladder Wall Polyps
- Intramural Hematoma, Gallbladder

ESSENTIAL INFORMATION

Key Differential Diagnosis Issues

- Normal gallbladder (GB) wall measures ≤ 3 mm and appears as thin, echogenic line on US and is barely perceptible on CT
- Significant overlap in imaging appearance of GB carcinoma, xanthogranulomatous cholecystitis, and large polyps, but cholecystectomy should be recommended in suspicious cases to exclude malignancy

Helpful Clues for Common Diagnoses

- **Hyperplastic Cholecystoses**
  - Adenomyomatosis results in GB wall thickening due to formation of intramural diverticula (Rokitansky-Aschoff sinuses) with smooth muscle and epithelial proliferation
  - Can demonstrate focal or segmental forms
    - Focal form most common at fundus and may appear mass-like with internal cystic spaces, intramural echogenic foci, and comet-tail/twinkling artifacts
    - Segmental form may cause annular thickening or strictures of GB resulting in hourglass appearance
  - Diagnosis easily made on MR, which demonstrates T2-bright cystic spaces (string of beads appearance)
- **Gallbladder Carcinoma**
  - May present with discrete polyploid mass, focal or diffuse wall thickening, or mass replacing GB

- Wall thickening tends to be irregular and nodular, often with other suspicious features (e.g., invasion of adjacent liver, bulky local lymphadenopathy, metastases)
    - Usually associated with color flow vascularity on US and heterogeneous enhancement on CT/MR
  - Eccentric, nodular, or mass-like GB wall thickening distinguishes GB carcinoma from simple cholecystitis

Helpful Clues for Less Common Diagnoses

- **Xanthogranulomatous Cholecystitis**
  - Focal or diffuse wall thickening with low-attenuation intramural bands/nodules and pericholecystic fluid
  - Low-attenuation bands/nodules (representing foamy cell infiltrate) may show signal loss on out-of-phase MR
  - Imaging features often indistinguishable from GB carcinoma, and definitive diagnosis only after resection
- **Porcelain Gallbladder**
  - Calcifications in GB wall can be diffuse or segmental, as well as either thin or thick/irregular
  - Debatable association with GB carcinoma, although focal calcification possibly associated with higher risk than diffuse calcification
  - Presence of discrete soft tissue adjacent to calcification should raise concern for carcinoma
- **Gallbladder Metastases and Lymphoma**
  - Metastases to GB uncommon, but melanoma is most common primary tumor (enhancing nodule/mass)
    - Usually in setting of widespread metastatic disease
  - Lymphoma of GB almost always secondary involvement (primary GB lymphoma incredibly rare)
    - Higher-grade lymphomas present as larger masses
- **Gallbladder Wall Polyps**
  - Inflammatory or neoplastic polyps may arise in GB wall
  - Size is biggest predictor of malignancy, as 100% of polyps ≥ 2 cm are malignant
  - Polyps ≥ 10 mm generally treated with cholecystectomy, while serial follow-up utilized for smaller polyps
- **Intramural Hematoma, Gallbladder**
  - Uncommon result of trauma with GB injury
  - Usually associated with blood in GB lumen/hemobilia

Hyperplastic Cholecystoses

Hyperplastic Cholecystoses

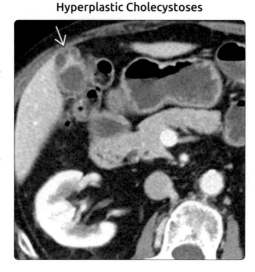
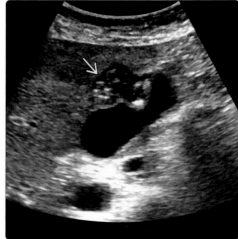

(Left) *Axial CECT shows multiple cystic spaces* ⇨ *at the gallbladder fundus, characteristic of focal adenomyomatosis.* (Right) *US shows a focal, heterogeneously echogenic mass* ⇨ *in the gallbladder that proved to be focal adenomyomatosis. Note the multiple internal echogenic foci within the mass, some of which are associated with comet-tail artifact.*

Gallbladder Carcinoma

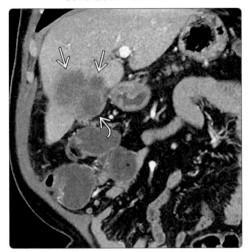

Gallbladder Carcinoma

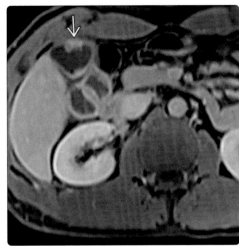

(Left) *Coronal CECT shows a soft tissue density mass* ➜ *arising from the gallbladder* ➜ *with direct invasion of the liver, a classic appearance for gallbladder cancer.* (Right) *Axial T1 C+ FS MR shows focal, nodular thickening* ➜ *from the gallbladder fundus, found to represent gallbladder carcinoma at surgical resection. Focal, nodular, or irregular gallbladder thickening should raise suspicion for malignancy.*

Xanthogranulomatous Cholecystitis

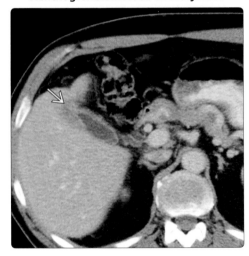

Porcelain Gallbladder

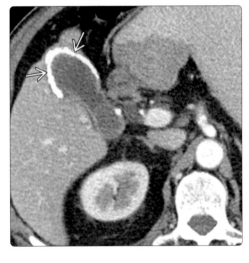

(Left) *Axial CECT shows a focally thickened wall* ➜ *of the gallbladder fundus. There is an indistinct border with the liver, initially thought to be suspicious for carcinoma but found to represent xanthogranulomatous cholecystitis at resection.* (Right) *Axial CECT shows focal, thick calcification* ➜ *of the gallbladder fundus, compatible with porcelain gallbladder. The association between porcelain gallbladder and gallbladder cancer is now considered debatable.*

Gallbladder Metastases and Lymphoma

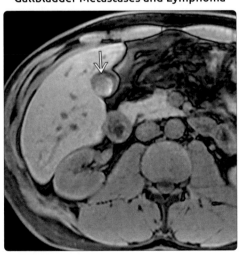

Gallbladder Wall Polyps

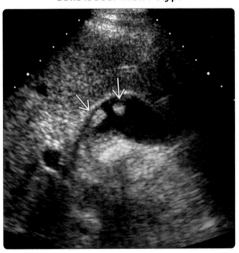

(Left) *Axial T1 FS MR shows an intrinsically hyperintense mass* ➜ *in the gallbladder, representing a metastasis from the patient's known melanoma. Melanoma metastases can be T1 hyperintense on MR due to melanin content.* (Right) *US shows 2 distinct polyps* ➜ *arising from the gallbladder wall. The management of gallbladder polyps is based on size, with polyps measuring ≥ 10 mm typically requiring cholecystectomy.*

DIFFERENTIAL DIAGNOSIS

Common

- Acute Calculous Cholecystitis
- Chronic Cholecystitis
- Hyperplastic Cholecystosis (Adenomyomatosis)
- Wall Thickening Due To Systemic Diseases
  - Congestive Heart Failure
  - Renal Failure
  - Hepatic Cirrhosis
  - Hypoalbuminemia
- Acute Hepatitis
- Acute Pancreatitis

Less Common

- Acute Acalculous Cholecystitis
- Perforated Peptic Ulcer
- Gallbladder Carcinoma
- Gallbladder Metastases
- Lymphoma
- AIDS-Related Cholangiopathy
- Gallbladder Varices

Rare but Important

- Xanthogranulomatous Cholecystitis
- Dengue Fever

ESSENTIAL INFORMATION

Key Differential Diagnosis Issues

- Clinical information is essential to derive differential diagnosis
- Presence of sepsis and right upper quadrant (RUQ) pain favor acute cholecystitis
- Presence of known systemic diseases: Congestive heart failure, renal failure, and hypoalbuminemia are important considerations
- Presence of regional disease: Acute hepatitis or pancreatitis, cirrhosis affecting gallbladder (GB) wall
- Known malignancy

Helpful Clues for Common Diagnoses

- **Acute Calculous Cholecystitis**
  - Clinical: RUQ pain, fever, positive Murphy sign
  - Acute GB inflammation secondary to calculus obstructing cystic duct
  - Gallstones ± impaction in GB neck
  - Diffuse GB wall thickening (3 mm)
    - Striated appearance: Alternating bright and dark bands within thick GB wall
    - GB wall lucency halo sign: Sonolucent middle layer due to edema
  - Distended GB (GB hydrops)
  - Positive sonographic Murphy sign
  - Presence of pericholecystic fluid
  - Complicated cholecystitis
    - Gangrenous cholecystitis
      - □ Asymmetric wall thickening
      - □ Marked wall irregularities
      - □ Intraluminal membranes
    - GB perforation

- □ Defect in GB wall
- □ Pericholecystic abscess or extraluminal stones
  - Emphysematous cholecystitis
    - □ Gas in GB wall/lumen
  - Empyema of GB
    - □ Intraluminal echoes, purulent exudate/debris
- **Chronic Cholecystitis**
  - Mostly asymptomatic
  - Diffuse GB wall thickening
    - Mean thickness ~ 5 mm
    - Smooth/irregular contour
  - Contracted GB
    - GB lumen may be obliterated in severe cases
  - Presence of gallstones in nearly all cases
- **Hyperplastic Cholecystosis (Adenomyomatosis)**
  - Adenomyomatosis of GB
  - Clinically asymptomatic, usually incidental US finding
  - Focal or diffuse GB wall thickening
  - Tiny, echogenic foci in GB wall producing comet-tail artifacts
  - Presence of cystic spaces within GB wall
  - Fundal adenomyomatosis: Smooth thickening or focal mass in fundal region ± ring down artifact
  - Hourglass GB: Narrowing of mid portion of GB
- **Wall Thickening Due To Systemic Diseases**
  - Clinical correlation is key to explain presence of GB wall thickening
  - Appearance of wall thickening is nonspecific
  - Other ancillary US findings
    - **Congestive heart failure**: Engorged hepatic veins and IVC; hypoechoic liver echo pattern
    - **Renal failure**: Small kidneys with increased parenchymal echogenicity
    - **Hepatic cirrhosis**: Coarse liver echo pattern, irregular/nodular liver contour, signs of portal hypertension (e.g., ascites, splenomegaly, varices)
    - **Hypoalbuminemia**: Presence of ascites, diffuse bowel wall thickening
- **Acute Hepatitis**
  - Clinical history: General malaise, vomiting, deranged liver function test with hepatitic pattern
  - Hepatomegaly with diffuse decrease in echogenicity
  - Starry-sky appearance: Increased echogenicity of portal triad walls against hypoechoic liver parenchyma
  - Periportal hypo-/anechoic area
  - GB lumen less dilated than in acute cholecystitis
- **Acute Pancreatitis**
  - Spread of inflammation to GB fossa
  - Nonspecific GB wall thickening
  - Diffuse/focal, swollen, hypoechoic pancreas

Helpful Clues for Less Common Diagnoses

- **Acute Acalculous Cholecystitis**
  - More commonly seen in critically ill patients (e.g., post major surgery, severe trauma, sepsis, etc.)
  - US features are similar to acute calculous cholecystitis except for absence of impacted gallstone
    - GB wall thickening: Hypoechoic, layered/striated appearance
    - GB distention: Often filled with sludge

- – Positive sonographic Murphy sign
- – Pericholecystic fluid
- **Perforated Peptic Ulcer**
  - ○ Penetrating ulcer in duodenal wall causes sympathetic GB wall thickening
  - ○ Presence of extraluminal fluid/gas
- **Gallbladder Carcinoma**
  - ○ Asymmetric or irregular GB wall thickening
  - ○ Mass replacing GB with locally advanced tumor
  - ○ Presence of gallstones
  - ○ Invasion of adjacent structures (e.g., liver, duodenum)
  - ○ Regional nodal and liver metastases
- **Gallbladder Metastases**
  - ○ Immobile, polypoid mass (usually > 1.5 cm) ± adjacent GB wall thickening
    - – Melanoma classically described as hyperechoic without acoustic shadowing
  - ○ May be contiguous spread from adjacent tumors, such as hepatocellular carcinoma, cholangiocarcinoma, or colon cancer
- **Lymphoma**
  - ○ Rare involvement of GB by secondary lymphoma
  - ○ Nonspecific diffuse GB wall thickening
  - ○ Presence of intraabdominal lymphomatous lymph nodes
- **AIDS-Related Cholangiopathy**
  - ○ Biliary inflammatory lesions caused by AIDS-related opportunistic infections leading to biliary stricture/obstruction or cholecystitis
  - ○ Diffuse GB wall thickening
  - ○ Bile duct wall thickening/inflammation
    - – Periductal hyper-/hypoechoic areas
  - ○ Focal biliary stricture and dilatation
- **Gallbladder Varices**
  - ○ Usually seen in portal hypertension or cavernous transformation of main portal vein
  - ○ Tubular structures in GB wall readily confirmed with color/power Doppler and pulsed Doppler

Helpful Clues for Rare Diagnoses

- **Xanthogranulomatous Cholecystitis**

- ○ Rare form of chronic cholecystitis
- ○ Diffuse, irregular wall thickening; may appear infiltrative; mimics GB carcinoma
- **Dengue Fever**
  - ○ Rash, fever, headache, and joint pains after travel to endemic area
  - ○ GB wall thickening from acute viral hepatic infection leading to hepatic failure

Other Essential Information

- Fever, leucocytosis, liver function tests

Alternative Differential Approaches

- Etiology of GB wall thickening
  - ○ Inflammatory conditions
    - – Acute calculous cholecystitis
    - – Acute acalculous cholecystitis
    - – Chronic cholecystitis
    - – AIDS-related cholangiopathy
    - – Secondary causes: Acute hepatitis, perforated peptic ulcer, pancreatitis
  - ○ Systemic diseases
    - – Congestive heart failure
    - – Renal failure
    - – Liver cirrhosis
    - – Hypoalbuminemia
  - ○ Neoplastic infiltration
    - – GB carcinoma
    - – Leukemic/lymphomatous infiltration

SELECTED REFERENCES

1. Gallaher JR et al: Acute cholecystitis: a review. JAMA. 327(10):965-75, 2022
2. Runde R et al: The gallbladder: what's new in 2022? Abdom Radiol (NY). ePub, 2022

Acute Calculous Cholecystitis

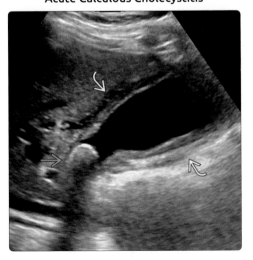

Chronic Cholecystitis

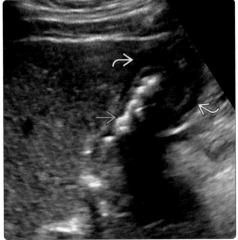

(Left) *Longitudinal oblique US of acute calculous cholecystitis shows an impacted stone ➡ in the gallbladder neck. There is diffuse edema and thickening of the gallbladder wall ➡.* **(Right)** *Longitudinal US shows a poorly distended, diffusely thickened ➡ gallbladder in a patient with chronic cholecystitis secondary to gallstones ➡.*

Hyperplastic Cholecystosis (Adenomyomatosis)

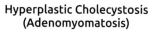
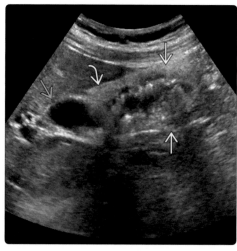

Congestive Heart Failure

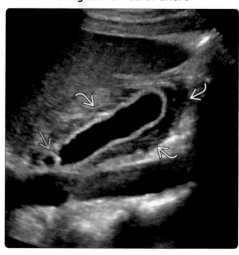

(Left) *Longitudinal US in a patient with segmental adenomyomatosis shows diffuse thickening of the gallbladder wall in the fundus ➡ with multiple small, echogenic foci. There is a transition zone ➡ (waisting) in the body with normal wall thickness in the neck ➡.*
(Right) *Longitudinal oblique US shows diffuse gallbladder wall edema secondary to heart failure. There is striated wall thickening ➡ and a fold in the gallbladder neck ➡.*

Hepatic Cirrhosis

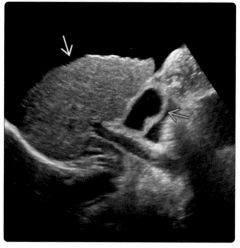

Acute Pancreatitis

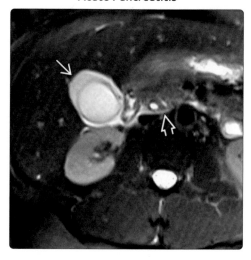

(Left) *Longitudinal oblique US through the liver and gallbladder shows a nodular cirrhotic liver ➡ surrounded by ascites. The gallbladder wall ➡ is mildly uniformly thickened. There were no stones.* **(Right)** *Axial T2 MR in a patient with acute pancreatitis shows peripancreatic fluid ➡ as well as diffuse gallbladder wall edema and thickening ➡.*

Acute Hepatitis

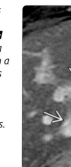
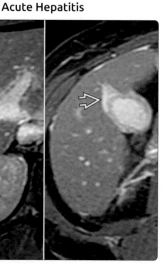

Acute Hepatitis

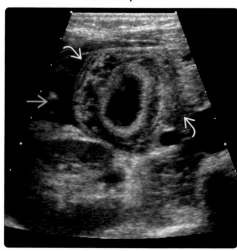

(Left) *Axial T2 FS MR shows periportal edema as linear areas of increased signal ➡ and gallbladder wall edema ➡.* **(Right)** *Transverse US in a patient with acute hepatitis and fulminant liver failure shows that the gallbladder wall is circumferentially thickened ➡ with striations. Ascites ➡ is noted.*

Gallbladder Carcinoma

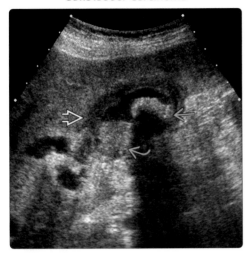

Gallbladder Carcinoma

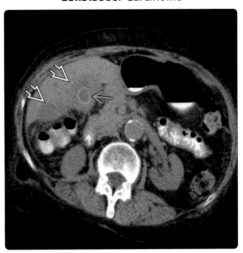

(Left) *Transverse US of gallbladder carcinoma shows a shadowing stone ➡ with sludge ➡. The gallbladder wall is thick and indistinct with loss of echogenicity ➡ at its interface with the liver.* (Right) *Axial NECT in the same patient shows a gallstone ➡. The gallbladder wall is thick and hypodense with infiltration of the adjacent liver ➡.*

Gallbladder Metastases

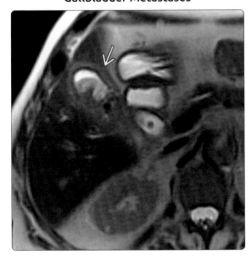

AIDS-Related Cholangiopathy

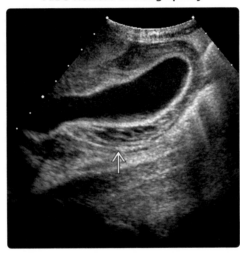

(Left) *Axial T2 HASTE MR in a patient with Klatskin cholangiocarcinoma shows progressive local spread to the gallbladder resulting in circumferential wall thickening ➡.* (Right) *Longitudinal oblique US in a patient with HIV/AIDS shows a thick-walled gallbladder without gallstones. There are linear strands in the edematous wall ➡ compatible with striated edema.*

Gallbladder Varices

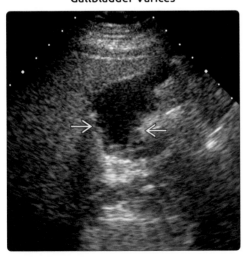

Gallbladder Varices

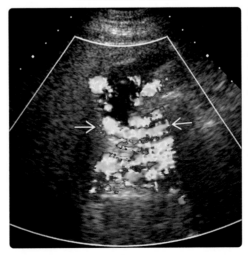

(Left) *Transverse US in a patient with cavernous transformation of the main portal vein secondary to pancreatitis shows small cystic spaces in the wall of the gallbladder neck and body ➡.* (Right) *Transverse color Doppler US in the same patient shows multiple collateral veins ➡ in the gallbladder wall and around the porta hepatis.*

DIFFERENTIAL DIAGNOSIS

Common

- Vicarious Excretion of Contrast
- Layering of Small Gallstones
- Intraluminal Contrast After Cholangiography
- Biliary Stent
- Gallbladder Sludge

Less Common

- Biliary or Hepatic Trauma
- Milk of Calcium Bile
- Biliary-Enteric Fistula or Anastomosis
- Porcelain Gallbladder (Mimic)
- Gallbladder Carcinoma (Mimic)
- Hemorrhagic Cholecystitis

ESSENTIAL INFORMATION

Key Differential Diagnosis Issues

- Most common causes of high-density bile are iatrogenic (e.g., vicarious excretion, cholangiography, stents)

Helpful Clues for Common Diagnoses

- **Vicarious Excretion of Contrast**
  - Excretion of intravenous contrast by organs other than kidneys, including hepatobiliary excretion
  - Given sensitivity of CT, contrast in gallbladder (GB) on day after contrast administration is normal, although visualization of contrast in GB on radiographs suggests ↓ renal function
- **Layering of Small Gallstones**
  - Using wide window level on CT may allow visualization of discrete stones, although may not always be possible to distinguish from other causes of hyperdense bile
  - Not always high density, as noncalcified stones can be difficult to distinguish from surrounding low-density bile
- **Intraluminal Contrast After Cholangiography**
  - High-density contrast may be seen in GB and biliary tree after ERCP or transhepatic cholangiogram
- **Biliary Stent**

- May allow reflux of enteric contrast material and gas into GB and biliary tree
- **Gallbladder Sludge**
  - Layering high-density material within GB lumen, which appears echogenic on US
  - May or may not have attenuation > bile on CT (depending on concentration of cholesterol crystals)
  - Associated with rapid weight loss, TPN, critical illness, and certain medications

Helpful Clues for Less Common Diagnoses

- **Biliary or Hepatic Trauma**
  - Injury to bile ducts, GB, or adjacent liver can result in hemobilia (including high-density blood in GB)
  - Hemobilia should prompt careful search for posttraumatic pseudoaneurysm, liver laceration adjacent to bile ducts, or GB injury
- **Milk of Calcium Bile**
  - High-density calcium carbonate precipitate within bile resulting from chronic cystic duct obstruction and biliary stasis (including chronic TPN)
  - High-attenuation bile (> 150 HU on NECT) in GB, which can extend into cystic duct or CBD
- **Biliary-Enteric Fistula or Anastomosis**
  - May allow reflux of enteric contrast and gas into GB and bile ducts
  - Spontaneous cholecystenteric fistulas are rare, but can result from gallstone ileus, trauma, tumor, or peptic ulcer disease
- **Porcelain Gallbladder (Mimic)**
  - Typically wall of GB is calcified (and hyperdense), rather than intraluminal bile itself
- **Gallbladder Carcinoma (Mimic)**
  - Usually focal, hypodense wall thickening or discrete soft tissue density mass, but enhancing tumor can theoretically mimic high-density intraluminal bile
  - Tumors often associated with gallstones
- **Hemorrhagic Cholecystitis**
  - Rare form of complicated cholecystitis that can be associated with blood in GB lumen or bile ducts (± active contrast extravasation)

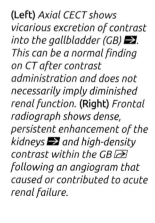

(Left) *Axial CECT shows vicarious excretion of contrast into the gallbladder (GB) ➡. This can be a normal finding on CT after contrast administration and does not necessarily imply diminished renal function.* (Right) *Frontal radiograph shows dense, persistent enhancement of the kidneys ➡ and high-density contrast within the GB ➡ following an angiogram that caused or contributed to acute renal failure.*

Vicarious Excretion of Contrast

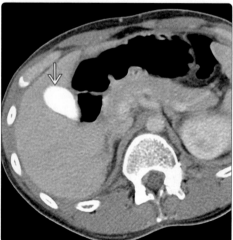

Vicarious Excretion of Contrast

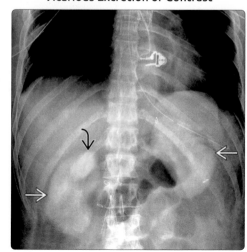

Layering of Small Gallstones

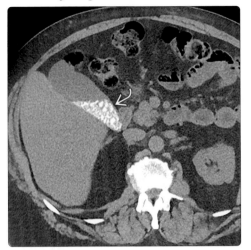

Intraluminal Contrast After Cholangiography

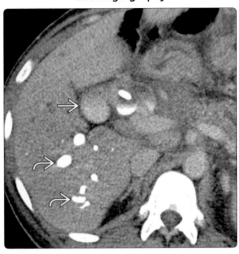

(Left) *Axial CECT shows high-density stones* ➥ *layering within the GB, juxtaposed against the normal low-density bile above.* (Right) *Axial CECT after a cholangiogram shows residual high-density contrast within the right hepatic lobe ducts* ➥ *as well as contrast within the GB* ➥. *Contrast can normally be seen in the biliary system if CT is performed immediately after a cholangiogram.*

Biliary or Hepatic Trauma

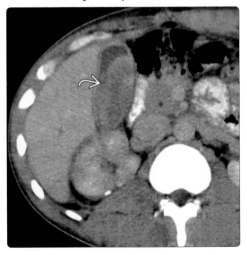

Milk of Calcium Bile

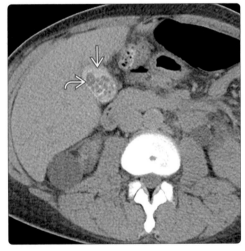

(Left) *Axial NECT in a trauma patient shows high-density clotted blood* ➥ *within the GB lumen, either due to to direct injury to the GB or passage of blood into the GB lumen through the cystic duct.* (Right) *Axial NECT shows high-density milk of calcium bile* ➥ *outlining multiple lower density gallstones* ➥ *in the gallbladder.*

Porcelain Gallbladder (Mimic)

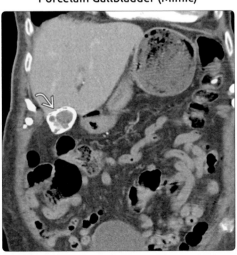

Hemorrhagic Cholecystitis

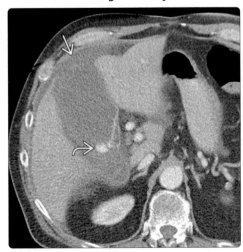

(Left) *Coronal CECT shows extensive, thick calcification* ➥ *involving nearly the entirety of the GB wall, compatible with porcelain GB.* (Right) *Axial CECT shows a distended GB in a septic patient with surrounding fat stranding, edema, and small fluid* ➥, *as well as active extravasation of contrast within the GB lumen* ➥, *compatible with hemorrhagic cholecystitis.*

DIFFERENTIAL DIAGNOSIS

Common

- Large Gallstone
- Porcelain Gallbladder
- Contracted Gallbladder With Gallstones
- Gas-Filled Duodenal Bulb

Less Common

- Hyperplastic Cholecystosis/Adenomyomatosis
- Adherent Gallstones
- Emphysematous Cholecystitis
- Gallbladder Fistula
- Iatrogenic

ESSENTIAL INFORMATION

Key Differential Diagnosis Issues

- Differentiate gas-filled duodenum from abnormal gallbladder by location and repositioning patient
- Duodenum may be mistaken for gallbladder post cholecystectomy
  - Relevant surgical history is key
  - Look for cholecystectomy scars if no history is available
  - Correlate with other imaging
- Gas in gallbladder may be surgical emergency
  - If unclear, confirm with CT

Helpful Clues for Common Diagnoses

- **Large Gallstone**
  - Strong acoustic impedance at wall-stone interface with posterior shadowing
  - Wall-echo-shadow appearance (optimize technique)
  - Mobile on changing patient's position unless stone is very large and gallbladder is contracted around it
- **Porcelain Gallbladder**
  - Diffuse gallbladder wall calcification
    - Echogenic, curvilinear line in gallbladder fossa
    - Dense posterior acoustic shadowing
  - Segmental form: Interrupted echogenic line on anterior wall

- Or multiple separate coarse, echogenic foci/clumps in wall with posterior acoustic shadowing
- **Contracted Gallbladder With Gallstones**
  - Multiple closely packed, echogenic stones without bile mimic echogenic gallbladder wall
  - Thickened gallbladder wall
  - Gallstones may not move on changing patient's position if gallbladder is severely contracted
- **Gas-Filled Duodenal Bulb**
  - Observe peristalsis
  - Reposition patient to move gas or have patient drink water to confirm

Helpful Clues for Less Common Diagnoses

- **Hyperplastic Cholecystosis/Adenomyomatosis**
  - Focal, diffuse or segmental gallbladder wall thickening
  - Tiny, echogenic foci in gallbladder wall with characteristic comet-tail artifacts
  - Segmental form: Transition from normal to thick wall in midgallbladder producing hourglass gallbladder
- **Adherent Gallstones**
  - Not curvilinear in configuration or mobile
- **Emphysematous Cholecystitis**
  - Complicated form of acute cholecystitis
  - Clinical evidence of fulminant biliary sepsis is usually present
  - Gas in gallbladder wall/lumen
    - Echogenic crescent in gallbladder with reverberation artifacts ("dirty" shadowing)
  - More common in diabetes and immunosuppressed patients
- **Gallbladder Fistula**
  - Spontaneous fistula from erosion of gallstone into duodenum: Gallstone ileus
  - Fistula to gallbladder from adjacent bowel malignancy
- **Iatrogenic**
  - Known history of intervention, such as endoscopic retrograde cholangiopancreatography or biliary stent
  - Gas in gallbladder without signs of cholecystitis

Large Gallstone

Porcelain Gallbladder

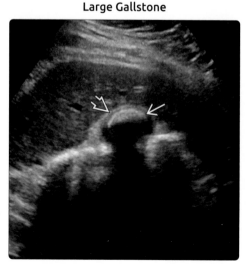
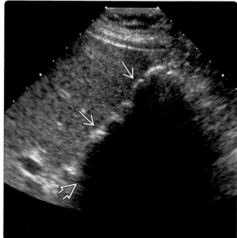

(Left) Transverse oblique US shows a large, curved, echogenic structure ➡ within the gallbladder casting a dense posterior acoustic shadow. The gallbladder wall ➡ is seen separately. This is the wall-echo-shadow sign, which differentiates a large gallstone from a porcelain gallbladder. (Right) Oblique transabdominal US shows curvilinear echogenicity ➡ in the gallbladder wall casting dense posterior acoustic shadowing ➡. Absence of the wall-echo-shadow sign suggests porcelain gallbladder.

Porcelain Gallbladder

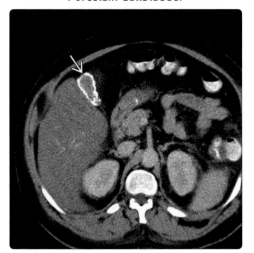

Contracted Gallbladder With Gallstones

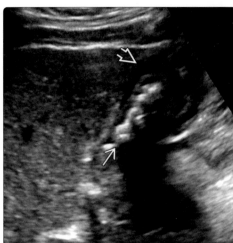

(Left) *Axial CECT in the same patient confirms the thin, diffuse gallbladder wall calcification* ➘ *in a contracted gallbladder.* **(Right)** *Oblique transabdominal US shows numerous small, shadowing, echogenic gallstones* ➘ *filling a contracted gallbladder* ➘. *The gallbladder wall is thick, suggesting chronic cholecystitis.*

Gas-Filled Duodenal Bulb

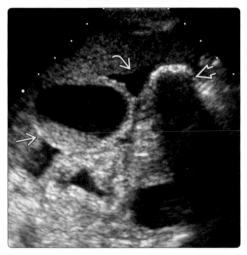

Hyperplastic Cholecystosis/Adenomyomatosis

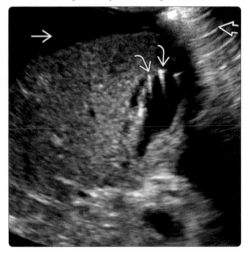

(Left) *Transverse US shows the duodenal bulb containing gas* ➘. *The gallbladder contains sludge* ➘ *in this patient with ascites* ➘ *and cirrhosis. The duodenum may be mistaken for a gallbladder.* **(Right)** *Transverse oblique US shows multiple areas of a comet-tail artifact* ➘ *emanating from the thick wall of the gallbladder. Reverberation artifact is noted from the bowel* ➘, *and there is ascites* ➘ *in this patient with chronic liver disease.*

Emphysematous Cholecystitis

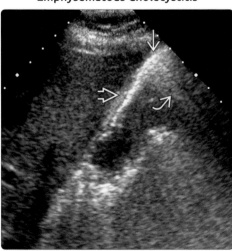

Iatrogenic

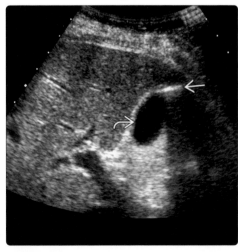

(Left) *Longitudinal US shows the gallbladder fundus in a diabetic patient with fever and right upper quadrant pain. A linear bright echo* ➘ *within a thick wall* ➘ *produces "dirty" shadowing* ➘ *that is highly suggestive of gas. This was confirmed with CT. Surgery was performed for emphysematous cholecystitis.* **(Right)** *Transverse oblique US shows a bright, linear echo with "dirty" shadowing* ➘ *representing gas in the gallbladder fundus post ERCP. The gallbladder* ➘ *was normal.*

DIFFERENTIAL DIAGNOSIS

Common
- Cholelithiasis
- Sludge/Sludge Ball/Echogenic Bile

Less Common
- Blood Clot
- Complicated Cholecystitis
- Gas Within Gallbladder Lumen
- Drainage Catheter
- Tumor
- Parasitic Infestation

ESSENTIAL INFORMATION

Helpful Clues for Common Diagnoses
- **Cholelithiasis**
  - Highly reflective intraluminal structure within gallbladder lumen
  - Posterior acoustic shadowing
  - Gravity-dependent and mobile
  - Variants
    - Bright echoes with acoustic shadowing in gallbladder fossa representing gallbladder packed with stones
    - Nonshadowing gallstones, usually small (< 5 mm)
    - Double-arc shadow sign or wall-echo-shadow (WES) sign
    - Immobile adherent/impacted gallstones
  - Complication: Acute calculous cholecystitis
    - Gallbladder distention and wall thickening, sonographic Murphy sign, pericholecystic fluid
- **Sludge/Sludge Ball/Echogenic Bile**
  - Amorphous, mid- to high-level echoes within gallbladder with lack of shadowing
  - Sediment in dependent portion
  - Mobile on changing patient's position without posterior acoustic shadowing
  - Sludge ball: Aggregate with well-defined, round contour; moves slowly

- Can be isoechoic to liver, resulting in "hepatization" of gallbladder

Helpful Clues for Less Common Diagnoses
- **Blood Clot**
  - Echogenic/mixed echoes or blood fluid level within gallbladder
  - Occasionally retractile, conforming to gallbladder shape
  - Post trauma, surgery, or hepatobiliary intervention; associated with gastrointestinal bleed
- **Complicated Cholecystitis**
  - Gangrenous cholecystitis: Intraluminal echogenic debris and membranes
    - Asymmetric wall thickening, marked wall irregularities
  - Emphysematous cholecystitis: Gas in gallbladder wall and lumen
  - Gallbladder empyema
    - Distended, pus-filled gallbladder with echogenic contents and no shadowing
- **Gas Within Gallbladder Lumen**
  - Iatrogenic from interventional procedure or endoscopy
  - Secondary to fistula with bowel as in gallstone ileus
    - Small bowel obstruction and pneumobilia, CT more definitive
- **Drainage Catheter**
  - History of percutaneous or endoscopic drainage
  - Tubular, parallel echogenic lines, ± pig-tail loop, man-made configuration
- **Tumor**
  - Primary cancers involve wall ± endoluminal mass, stones, and extension to liver
  - Hematogenous metastases most commonly from melanoma
    - Multiple > single broad-based, hypoechoic, polypoid lesions, ± wall thickening
  - Look for color Doppler flow in mass, confirm with spectral Doppler
- **Parasitic Infestation**
  - Tubular, parallel echogenic lines

(Left) Longitudinal decubitus US of the gallbladder shows a fundal curvilinear echo ➜ with a strong acoustic shadow ⬈. Note the normal wall with no cholecystitis. (Right) Transverse decubitus US of the gallbladder shows a thick wall ➡, shadowing stones ➜, and sludge ⬈ in a patient with acute cholecystitis.

Cholelithiasis

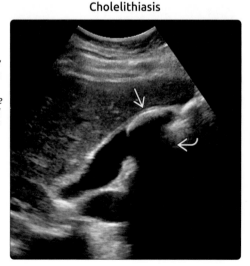

Cholelithiasis

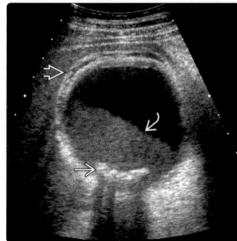

Sludge/Sludge Ball/Echogenic Bile

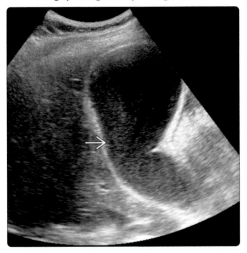

Sludge/Sludge Ball/Echogenic Bile

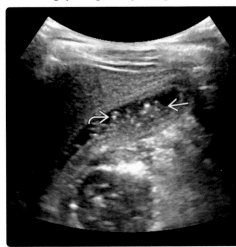

(Left) *Transverse US of the right upper quadrant shows a markedly distended, sludge-filled gallbladder ➡ in a patient with acalculous cholecystitis. Although the wall was not thick, the patient was treated with percutaneous drainage.* **(Right)** *Longitudinal decubitus US of a nondistended gallbladder shows intraluminal echoes from small, nonshadowing sludge balls ➡. Some display the comet-tail artifact ➡.*

Complicated Cholecystitis

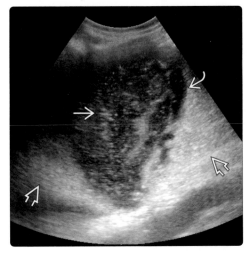

Complicated Cholecystitis

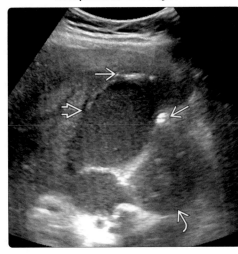

(Left) *Transverse US of the gallbladder fossa shows the gallbladder lumen to be filled with membranes ➡ with no wall. There is pericholecystic fluid ➡ and echogenic fat ➡ in this diabetic patient with gangrenous cholecystitis.* **(Right)** *Transverse US shows a distended gallbladder with intraluminal sludge, discontinuous wall ➡, pericholecystic abscess ➡, and gas in the wall ➡ from emphysematous cholecystitis.*

Drainage Catheter

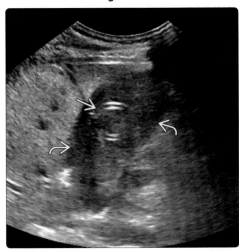

Tumor

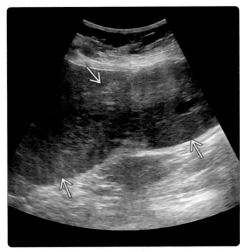

(Left) *Transverse US following percutaneous drainage for acalculous cholecystitis is shown. The pig-tail catheter ➡ is looped in the gallbladder lumen, which contains sludge ➡. The wall is indistinct.* **(Right)** *Longitudinal US shows a markedly distended gallbladder (15 cm) with low-level intraluminal echoes ➡. The lumen was filled with necrotic adenocarcinoma with muscle invasion in the neck only.*

DIFFERENTIAL DIAGNOSIS

Common

- Physiologic Dilatation
- Acute Calculous Cholecystitis
- Acute Acalculous Cholecystitis

Less Common

- Mucocele/Hydrops
- Drugs
- Post Vagotomy
- Choledochal Cyst
- Gallbladder Carcinoma
- Gallbladder Hemorrhage
- Acute Hemorrhagic Cholecystitis
- Other Causes of Cholecystitis
  - Obstruction Post Biliary Stenting
  - Ischemia Post Transarterial Hepatic Chemoembolization or in Setting of Severe Hypotension or Sepsis
  - Infectious Cholecystitis ± Empyema

Rare but Important

- Mucin-Producing Gallbladder Carcinoma
- Gallbladder Torsion/Volvulus
- Systemic Lupus Erythematosus
- Henoch-Schönlein Purpura

ESSENTIAL INFORMATION

Key Differential Diagnosis Issues

- Determine whether gallbladder is obstructed
  - Look for intrinsic lesion, such as stone, polyp, or mass
  - Look for extrinsic mass, collection, or inflammation
- Differentiate acute surgical from nonsurgical gallbladder distention
- Look for secondary signs of inflammation
  - Wall thickness, pericholecystic fluid, or inflamed fat
- Correlate with patient history, signs, and laboratory results

Helpful Clues for Common Diagnoses

- **Physiologic Dilatation**
  - Distended > 5 x 5 x 10 cm
  - Otherwise normal-appearing gallbladder
  - Secondary to
    - Prolonged fasting
    - Postoperative state
    - Total parenteral nutrition
    - Post vagotomy
- **Acute Calculous Cholecystitis**
  - Distention with
    - Gallstones
    - Wall thickening due to edema
    - Pericholecystic fluid
  - Presence of sonographic Murphy sign is key for diagnosis of acute cholecystitis
- **Acute Acalculous Cholecystitis**
  - Distention without gallstones
  - Sludge, wall thickening of gallbladder
  - Ill patient with sepsis, post surgery or trauma
  - Increased risk of wall necrosis and gangrene

- Difficult diagnosis as sonographic Murphy sign may not be elicited in obtunded or sedated patients
- Confirm with HIDA
- Or diagnostic/therapeutic percutaneous cholecystotomy

Helpful Clues for Less Common Diagnoses

- **Mucocele/Hydrops**
  - Distended gallbladder filled with watery mucoid material
  - GB wall usually normal in thickness (< 3 mm)
  - Sonographic Murphy sign negative
  - Secondary to gallbladder outlet obstruction
    - Obstructing polyp or stone
    - Obstructing masses, such as pancreaticobiliary and ampullary carcinoma
    - Acute or chronic pancreatitis
  - Courvoisier sign
    - Distended, nontender, palpable gallbladder in setting of jaundice is rarely due to obstructing gallstones
      - □ Stones are associated with chronic inflammation and lack of gallbladder distensibility
      - □ Or they produce acute obstruction with less gallbladder distention
    - Neoplasms, such as pancreatic carcinoma, are more likely as they produce chronic, lower grade obstruction
- **Drugs**
  - Various drugs may decrease gallbladder contraction
    - Including atropine, somatostatin, arginine, nifedipine, progesterone, trimebutine, loperamide, and ondansetron
- **Post Vagotomy**
  - Gallbladder volumes increase after vagotomy secondary to vagal denervation
  - Predisposes to gallstone formation
- **Choledochal Cyst**
  - Large cyst may compress or obstruct gallbladder or mimic distended gallbladder
  - Associated with biliary dilatation
  - Can be confirmed with MRCP or ERCP
- **Gallbladder Carcinoma**
  - Typically thick, irregular wall or solid tumor in lumen
  - Extension into liver
  - Gallstones typically present
  - Mucin-producing variant may produce distended, mucin-filled gallbladder
    - Smaller mural/polypoid mass
- **Gallbladder Hemorrhage**
  - Mobile internal echoes
  - Increasing echogenic luminal content over time if active bleeding
  - Retracting clot
  - Post hepatobiliary intervention or biopsy
  - Post trauma or surgery
  - Secondary to neoplasms, anticoagulation or bleeding disorder
  - Post aneurysm rupture
  - Present with
    - Pain
    - Jaundice
    - Hemobilia

- – Hematemesis
- – Hematochezia
- **Acute Hemorrhagic Cholecystitis**
  - o Intraluminal hemorrhage with signs of acute cholecystitis
  - o Underlying
    - – Atherosclerosis
    - – Diabetes
    - – Bleeding diathesis
    - – Anticoagulation therapy
- **Other Causes of Cholecystitis**
  - o Following metal bile duct stent placed for malignant biliary stricture
    - – Cholecystitis from cystic duct obstruction
  - o Ischemic cholecystitis
    - – Following transarterial hepatic chemoembolization for liver malignancy
    - – Following prolonged hypotension post trauma, hemorrhage, or sepsis
  - o Infectious cholecystitis ± empyema
    - – US findings similar to acute acalculous cholecystitis
    - – Markedly distended gallbladder with echogenic pus in lumen
    - – Sonographic Murphy sign often positive
    - – Gallbladder wall appears thickened
    - – Bacteria
      - □ *Salmonella typhi*: Acute and chronic infection
      - □ *Escherichia coli, Klebsiella, Staphylococcus* species
      - □ Leptospirosis
    - – Viral
      - □ Hepatitis A and B viruses, CMV, dengue virus
    - – Diagnoses made by clinical picture and laboratory tests
    - – Hydatid
      - □ In endemic regions
      - □ Intraluminal gallbladder membranes or cysts
      - □ Curvilinear calcifications
      - □ Typically associated with liver cysts
    - – Ascariasis
      - □ Intraluminal living or dead worms

- □ Obstructed cystic duct causing cholecystitis
- – Malaria
  - □ Can cause acalculous cholecystitis

Helpful Clues for Rare Diagnoses

- **Gallbladder Torsion/Volvulus**
  - o Older, thin women with wandering gallbladder
  - o Features of cholecystitis but difficult preoperative diagnosis
  - o Markedly dilated gallbladder
  - o May be displaced from normal location
  - o Twisting of cystic duct and artery
    - – Whirl sign on color Doppler US
- **Systemic Lupus Erythematosus**
  - o Acalculous cholecystitis due to vasculitis of gallbladder wall and bile ducts
  - o Treated nonsurgically with corticosteroids
- **Henoch-Schönlein Purpura**
  - o Associated with gallbladder hydrops or acalculous cholecystitis
  - o Characteristic skin rash

SELECTED REFERENCES

1. Jones MW et al: Gallbladder mucocele. StatPearls, 2022
2. Murtaza Khomusi M et al: Prevalence of empyema or mucocele or other histological diagnoses in patients undergoing cholecystectomy with diagnosis of chronic cholecystitis. Cureus. 14(4):e23773, 2022
3. Sharma R et al: Gallbladder hydrops. Cureus. 13(9):e18159, 2021
4. Amarnath S et al: Spontaneous perforation of an acalculous hydropic gallbladder in a diabetic patient with neuropathy: an underdiagnosed entity. Gastroenterology Res. 12(6):315-9, 2019

Physiologic Dilatation

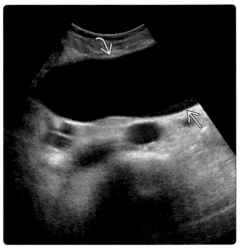

Physiologic Dilatation

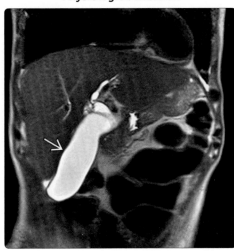

(Left) Transverse oblique US in a ventilated patient on total parenteral nutrition shows that the gallbladder is distended ⇗ with minimal sludge ⇥. There is no wall thickening. (Right) Coronal T2 HASTE MR shows a dilated gallbladder ⇗ with no stones or signs of inflammation.

Acute Calculous Cholecystitis

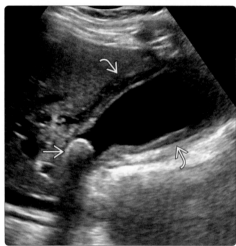

Acute Calculous Cholecystitis

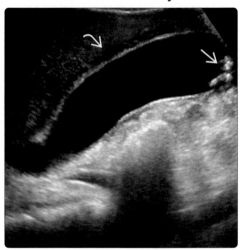

(Left) *Longitudinal oblique US shows an obstructing stone in the neck of the gallbladder ➡, which is distended with diffuse, hypoechoic wall thickening ➡ in this patient with acute calculous cholecystitis.* **(Right)** *Longitudinal oblique US shows a distended gallbladder with fundal stones ➡ and wall thickening ➡. This patient had a positive Murphy sign, consistent with acute calculous cholecystitis.*

Acute Calculous Cholecystitis

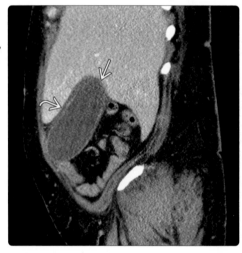

Acute Acalculous Cholecystitis

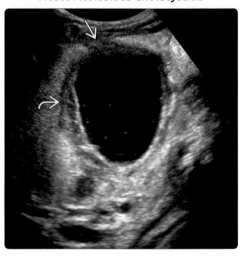

(Left) *Sagittal CECT in the same patient shows a distended gallbladder ➡ with diffuse wall thickening ➡. The stones were not visible.* **(Right)** *Transverse US shows a gangrenous gallbladder with no stones. The wall is edematous ➡ with a focal defect anteriorly ➡. A pericholecystic abscess had developed (not shown).*

Mucocele/Hydrops

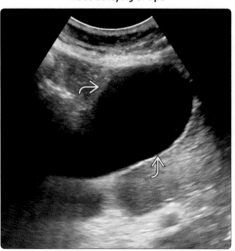

Mucocele/Hydrops

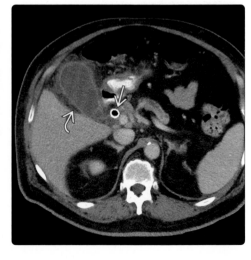

(Left) *Longitudinal oblique US in a patient with obstructive jaundice from a pancreatic head carcinoma shows a distended but otherwise normal gallbladder ➡ (Courvoisier sign).* **(Right)** *Axial CECT in the same patient after placement of a metal bile duct stent ➡ to relieve biliary obstruction shows edema of the gallbladder wall and pericholecystic stranding ➡ from acute cholecystitis, which later perforated.*

Mucocele/Hydrops

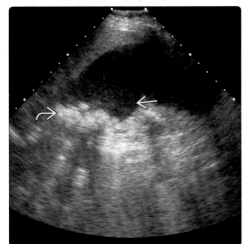

Mucocele/Hydrops

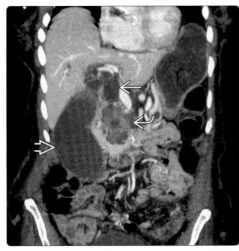

(Left) *Longitudinal oblique US in an older patient with jaundice shows a dilated gallbladder with stones* ➡ *and sludge* ➡. *The wall was normal. The common bile duct was dilated secondary to a pancreatic lesion.* (Right) *Coronal CECT in the same patient better shows the multicystic serous cystadenoma in the head of pancreas* ➡, *obstructing the bile duct* ➡ *and causing gallbladder distention* ➡.

Gallbladder Carcinoma

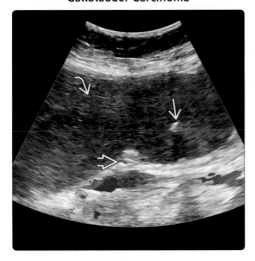

Gallbladder Carcinoma

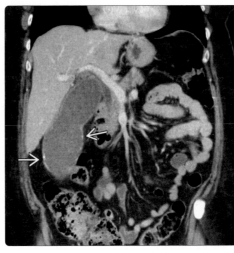

(Left) *Oblique color Doppler US shows a distended gallbladder filled with avascular, low-level echoes* ➡ *with one small stone* ➡. *The posterior wall is irregular* ➡. *The lumen was filled with necrotic adenocarcinoma.* (Right) *Coronal CECT shows a dilated gallbladder with low-density contents. There is subtle wall calcification* ➡ *and internal heterogeneity. This was largely necrotic adenocarcinoma with a small, invasive tumor in the gallbladder neck.*

Acute Hemorrhagic Cholecystitis

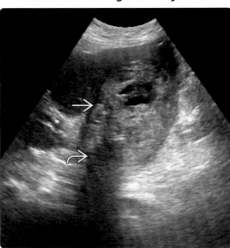

Acute Hemorrhagic Cholecystitis

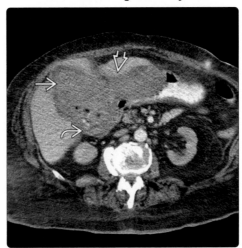

(Left) *Longitudinal oblique US shows a markedly abnormal gallbladder filled with bright echoes* ➡ *in a patient with a dropping hematocrit and signs of infection. Shadowing is noted* ➡, *but the stone is indistinct.* (Right) *Axial CECT in the same patient shows a perforated gallbladder with gallstones* ➡ *and luminal hemorrhage* ➡. *There is an adjacent hematoma* ➡. *Active bleeding was treated by embolization.*

DIFFERENTIAL DIAGNOSIS

Common

- Choledocholithiasis
- Ascending Cholangitis
- Recurrent Pyogenic Cholangitis
- Pancreatic Ductal Carcinoma
- Cholangiocarcinoma
- Choledochal Cyst

Less Common

- Sludge
- Periampullary Tumor
- Sclerosing Cholangitis
- Parasitic Infestation
- AIDS-Related Cholangiopathy
- Biliary Intraductal Papillary Mucinous Neoplasm

ESSENTIAL INFORMATION

Helpful Clues for Common Diagnoses

- **Choledocholithiasis**
  - Most common location is in common bile duct (CBD)
  - Round, echogenic focus with marked posterior acoustic shadowing
- **Ascending Cholangitis**
  - Imaging may reveal biliary duct wall thickening, intraluminal debris, or obstructing biliary stone
  - Periportal inflammatory hypo-/hyperechogenicity may be seen
- **Recurrent Pyogenic Cholangitis**
  - Bacterial colonization of brown pigment stones in both intrahepatic and extrahepatic bile ducts
  - Densely packed intrahepatic stones
  - Atrophy of involved lobe/segment of liver in later stages
- **Pancreatic Ductal Carcinoma**
  - Ill-defined, solid mass in pancreatic head
  - Pancreatic duct dilatation that abruptly tapers at point of pancreatic carcinoma
  - Vascular encasement ± regional nodal/liver metastases

- **Cholangiocarcinoma**
  - Extrahepatic cholangiocarcinoma involves biliary ducts in hepatoduodenal ligament
    - Intra- and extrahepatic biliary dilatation
    - May see irregular soft tissue thickening of extrahepatic bile duct or polypoidal mass within CBD
    - May present as periampullary mass in pancreatic head
  - Intrahepatic cholangiocarcinoma: Ill-defined, infiltrative, iso-/hyperechoic mass, often with capsular retraction
- **Choledochal Cyst**
  - Congenital biliary malformation characterized by fusiform duct dilatation
  - Most commonly involves CBD
  - Cystic extrahepatic mass separated from gallbladder and communicating with common hepatic duct or intrahepatic ducts
  - Fusiform dilatation of extra- ± intrahepatic bile ducts
  - Abrupt change in caliber at junction of dilated segment to normal ducts

Helpful Clues for Less Common Diagnoses

- **Sclerosing Cholangitis**
  - Autoimmune disease that causes multiple intra- and extrahepatic biliary strictures with dilatation
- **Biliary Intraductal Papillary Mucinous Neoplasm**
  - Ductal intraluminal mass with frond-like papillary projections
  - Hypersecretion of mucin as well as anatomic obstruction leads to markedly dilated intra- and extrahepatic biliary ducts

SELECTED REFERENCES

1. Chiow SM et al: Imaging mimickers of cholangiocarcinoma: a pictorial review. Abdom Radiol (NY). 47(3):981-97, 2022
2. Madhusudhan KS et al: IgG4-related sclerosing cholangitis: a clinical and imaging review. AJR Am J Roentgenol. 213(6):1221-31, 2019
3. Kwan KEL et al: Recurrent pyogenic cholangitis: a review of imaging findings and clinical management. Abdom Radiol (NY). 42(1):46-56, 2017
4. Oliveira IS et al: Cholangiocarcinoma: classification, diagnosis, staging, imaging features, and management. Abdom Radiol (NY). 42(6):1637-49, 2017

Choledocholithiasis

Ascending Cholangitis

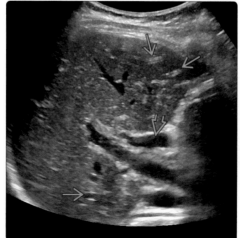
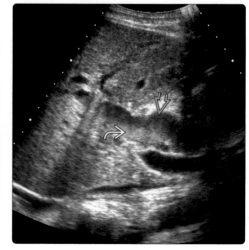

(Left) Longitudinal oblique US of the liver shows mild biliary ductal dilatation of the common bile duct ⊡ as well as mildly prominent intrahepatic biliary ducts creating subtle double ducts ⊡. The cause of mild biliary ductal dilatation was an obstructing stone in the common bile duct (not shown). (Right) Longitudinal oblique US of the liver shows a markedly dilated common duct ⊡ with layering debris ⊡ in a patient with ascending cholangitis.

Recurrent Pyogenic Cholangitis

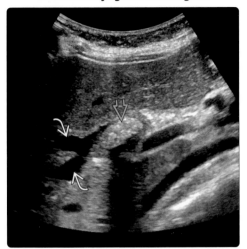

Cholangiocarcinoma

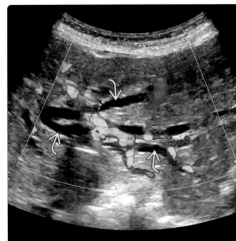

(Left) *Longitudinal oblique US of the liver shows a large intrahepatic stone* ⇨ *causing upstream biliary ductal dilatation* ➡ *in a patient with recurrent pyogenic cholangitis.* (Right) *Transverse color Doppler US of the left lobe of the liver shows moderate biliary ductal dilatation* ➡ *caused by an obstructing central cholangiocarcinoma.*

Cholangiocarcinoma

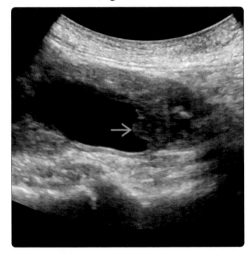

Choledochal Cyst

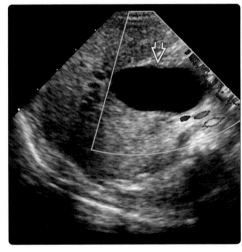

(Left) *Longitudinal oblique US of the common bile duct shows an obstructing soft tissue mass* ⇨, *which was proven to represent an intraluminal cholangiocarcinoma.* (Right) *Longitudinal color Doppler US of the right upper quadrant in a 2-month-old shows a dilated, tubular structure* ➡ *without internal color flow vascularity, which was found to be a type I choledochal cyst.*

Biliary Intraductal Papillary Mucinous Neoplasm

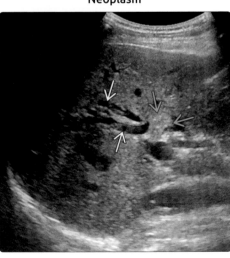

Biliary Intraductal Papillary Mucinous Neoplasm

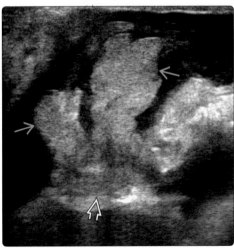

(Left) *Transverse US of the liver shows moderate intrahepatic ductal dilatation* ➡, *which was caused by a biliary intraductal papillary mucinous neoplasm* ⇨. *Biliary ductal dilatation was seen both proximal as well as distal to the lesion due to copious mucin production.* (Right) *Intraoperative US in the same patient shows the biliary intraductal papillary neoplasm has frond-like projections* ⇨ *into the biliary tree. The point where the biliary IPMN arises from the biliary duct wall* ➡ *is evident.*

DIFFERENTIAL DIAGNOSIS

Common

- Acute Cholecystitis
- Gallstones
  - Cholelithiasis
  - Choledocholithiasis
- Acute Hepatitis
- Hepatic Steatosis (Fatty Liver)
- Ascending Cholangitis
- Acute Pancreatitis
- Duodenal Ulcer
- Nephrolithiasis
- Ascending Urinary Tract Infection

Less Common

- Acute Colitis
- Appendicitis
- Omental Infarct
- Epiploic Appendagitis
- Hepatic Pyogenic Abscess
- Passive Hepatic Congestion
- Diverticulitis
- Pyelonephritis
- Thoracic Infection or Inflammation
- Hepatic Tumor

ESSENTIAL INFORMATION

Key Differential Diagnosis Issues

- Hepatobiliary etiologies (e.g., cholecystitis, hepatitis, cholelithiasis, choledocholithiasis) are most common causes of right upper quadrant (RUQ) pain
- In most cases, when patients present with classic signs and symptoms of gallbladder-related disease, US serves as best 1st-line screening modality
- Although CT lacks sensitivity and specificity for gallbladder-related disorders, it is superior modality for many other entities in differential diagnosis and may be required if US does not provide firm diagnosis
- MR/MRCP is best noninvasive imaging modality for evaluation of biliary tree (particularly for biliary stones)

Helpful Clues for Common Diagnoses

- **Acute Cholecystitis**
  - 90-95% of patients with cholecystitis have gallstones, with acute calculous cholecystitis far more common than acalculous cholecystitis
  - Patients present with fever, RUQ pain, and elevated WBC
  - US remains best diagnostic modality with imaging features including GB wall thickening, gallstones, sonographic Murphy sign, pericholecystic fluid, and wall hyperemia (on color Doppler)
  - Important complications include gangrenous cholecystitis, emphysematous cholecystitis, hemorrhagic cholecystitis, and perforation
- **Gallstones (Cholelithiasis and Choledocholithiasis)**
  - Patients may present with biliary colic (dull RUQ pain with radiation to back or right shoulder)

- US and MR have superior sensitivity for stones compared to CT (~ 80%) with CT often missing pure cholesterol stones, which are isodense to bile
- US is best initial imaging modality, but given that distal CBD is often obscured by bowel gas on US, MRCP is much better for identifying stones in common bile duct

- **Acute Hepatitis**
  - Any cause of hepatitis (alcohol, viral, toxic) may result in liver swelling that stretches liver capsule and causes RUQ pain
  - All imaging modalities are usually normal in setting of acute hepatitis, but in severe cases, enlarged liver may appear abnormally low density on CT or hypoechoic on US with prominent portal triads (starry-sky appearance)
  - Marked reactive gallbladder wall thickening is common ancillary feature

- **Hepatic Steatosis (Fatty Liver)**
  - Usually asymptomatic, although acute fatty infiltration may stretch liver capsule and cause pain
  - Most common definitions of steatosis include liver lower in attenuation than spleen on NECT or absolute attenuation of liver on NECT < 40 HU
  - MR with chemical shift imaging is most sensitive modality for diagnosing steatosis

- **Ascending Cholangitis**
  - Pyogenic infection of biliary tree due to biliary obstruction (most often due to distal obstructing stone)
  - Biliary dilatation with thickened, hyperenhancing bile duct walls, debris within duct lumen, and heterogeneous liver enhancement (most often on arterial-phase images)
    - Frequent association with pyogenic liver abscesses (25%)
  - Other forms of cholangitis (e.g., primary sclerosing and recurrent pyogenic cholangitis) may also cause acute RUQ pain

- **Acute Pancreatitis**
  - Enlarged, edematous pancreas (with loss of normal fatty lobulation) with peripancreatic fat stranding, free fluid, and inflammation (± parenchymal necrosis ± peripancreatic fluid collections)
  - Vast majority of cases secondary to alcohol abuse or gallstones
  - While primarily centered in midabdomen, inflammation frequently spreads laterally toward gallbladder and right colon, explaining frequent presentation with RUQ pain

- **Duodenal Ulcer**
  - Most likely to be symptomatic when penetrating or perforated
  - Look for thickened duodenum with adjacent extraluminal gas or enteric contrast media (although < 50% of patients have ectopic gas/contrast)
  - Inflammation centered around duodenum in anterior pararenal space, but may spread laterally to involve adjacent structures (e.g., colon, gallbladder)

- **Nephrolithiasis**
  - Nonobstructing intrarenal stones (best visualized on NECT) or stones in right ureter may cause RUQ pain

- **Ascending Urinary Tract Infection**
  - Right-sided ascending urinary tract infections may manifest with urothelial thickening/enhancement in ureter and intrarenal collecting system, periureteral fat stranding, and mild pelvocaliectasis

Helpful Clues for Less Common Diagnoses

- **Acute Colitis**
  - Any form of acute colitis (e.g., pseudomembranous, infectious, ulcerative, ischemic) that affects ascending colon can cause RUQ pain
  - Colonic wall thickening and submucosal edema with pericolonic fat stranding and inflammation
- **Appendicitis**
  - While more often presenting with right lower quadrant (RLQ) pain, tip of appendix may extend upward to RUQ and cause upper abdominal pain
  - Dilated, thickened appendix with periappendiceal fat stranding and free fluid (± ectopic gas or fluid collections in cases with rupture)
- **Omental Infarct**
  - Omental fat necrosis caused by disruption of arterial blood supply
  - Most cases are located in right abdomen adjacent to ascending colon and can present with RLQ or RUQ pain
    - Usually no evidence of other constitutional symptoms or elevated WBC
  - Ill-defined fat stranding or discrete, encapsulated, fat-containing mass in omentum (± whorled pattern of vessels leading to infarct)
- **Epiploic Appendagitis**
  - Primary thrombosis or torsion of epiploic appendage
  - Can occur anywhere, but much more common in left lower quadrant adjacent to descending/sigmoid colon
  - Similar in appearance to omental infarct with small, fat-containing mass abutting colon with adjacent fat stranding (± central dot sign)
- **Hepatic Pyogenic Abscess**
  - Can be associated with variety of causes, including recent surgery, cholangitis, septic thrombophlebitis (related to GI tract infections), etc.
  - Multiloculated cluster of thick-walled fluid collections in liver with surrounding low-density parenchymal edema (± internal gas)
  - Patients usually symptomatic with pain, fever, and elevated WBC

- **Passive Hepatic Congestion**
  - Although usually asymptomatic, enlargement and edema of liver may stretch capsule and cause RUQ pain
  - Enlarged, edematous liver may demonstrate mosaic or nutmeg pattern of heterogeneous enhancement
  - Often other ancillary findings of right heart dysfunction, including cardiomegaly (with relative enlargement of right heart), dilatation of hepatic veins and IVC, and retrograde opacification of IVC/hepatic veins on arterial-phase imaging
- **Diverticulitis**
  - Right-sided diverticulitis is uncommon in Western world but much more common in certain ethnic groups (especially Asian populations)
  - Findings similar to diverticulitis elsewhere with multiple diverticula (including at least 1 focally inflamed diverticulum), colonic wall thickening, and pericolonic fat stranding (± ectopic gas or fluid collections)
- **Pyelonephritis**
  - Infection of right kidney can result in RUQ pain
    - Patients typically febrile with flank tenderness and elevated WBC
  - Enlarged kidney with asymmetric perinephric stranding and striated or wedge-shaped areas of diminished enhancement on CECT (particularly in delayed nephrographic phase)
- **Thoracic Infection or Inflammation**
  - Any inflammatory process in right lower lung can cause RUQ pain, including pneumonia, pulmonary embolus, pulmonary infarct, pleural effusion, empyema, myocardial infarct, or pericarditis
  - Lung bases should be carefully evaluated in any patient presenting with RUQ pain
- **Hepatic Tumor**
  - Any tumor that is large or exophytic can stretch hepatic capsule and cause pain (even benign lesions, such as giant hemangioma or large cyst)
  - Hepatocellular carcinoma and hepatic adenoma, in particular, are prone to spontaneous bleeding or rupture through liver capsule with hemoperitoneum

Acute Cholecystitis

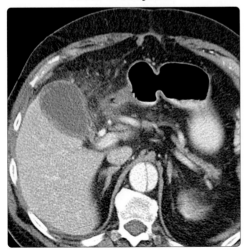

Acute Cholecystitis

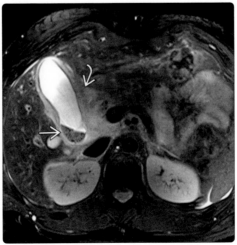

(Left) Axial CECT shows a thick-walled gallbladder with surrounding inflammation, compatible with acute cholecystitis. (Right) Axial T2 FS MR shows a thick-walled gallbladder with layering gallstones ➡, wall-thickening, and surrounding edema ➡, compatible with acute cholecystitis.

Choledocholithiasis

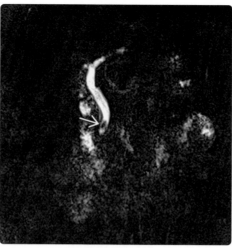

Choledocholithiasis

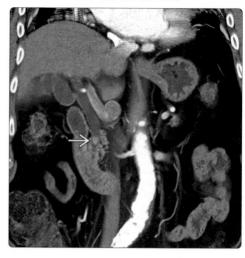

(Left) *Coronal MRCP MIP shows a low-signal stone* ⮕ *in the distal common bile duct (CBD) causing proximal biliary obstruction. MR is the best noninvasive modality for the evaluation of extrahepatic bile duct stones.* (Right) *Coronal CECT with volume-rendering shows a calcified stone* ⮕ *in the distal CBD causing mild proximal obstruction. The sensitivity of CT for gallstones is better than commonly thought, approaching 80%.*

Acute Hepatitis

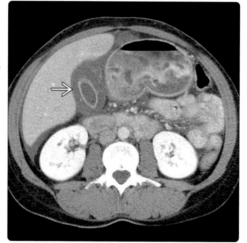

Hepatic Steatosis (Fatty Liver)

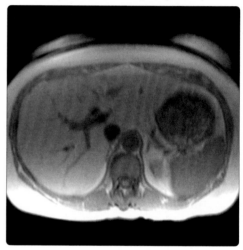

(Left) *Axial CECT shows marked thickening of the GB wall* ⮕ *and ascites in this patient with acute viral hepatitis who presented with symptoms of acute right upper quadrant (RUQ) pain. While the liver often appears normal on imaging in acute hepatitis, dramatic GB wall thickening is a common feature.* (Right) *Axial in-phase GRE MR shows homogeneous signal throughout the liver.*

Hepatic Steatosis (Fatty Liver)

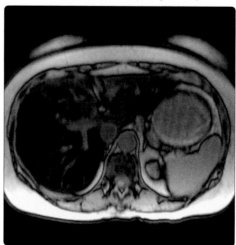

Ascending Cholangitis

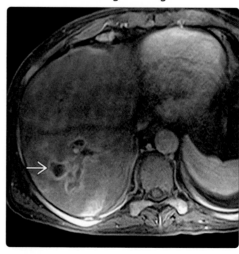

(Left) *Axial GRE opposed-phase MR in the same patient shows diffuse signal loss throughout the liver, compatible with diffuse hepatic steatosis. MR with chemical shift imaging is the most sensitive imaging modality for steatosis.* (Right) *Axial T1 C+ FS MR after liver transplant in a patient with fever shows dilated peripheral intrahepatic ducts* ⮕ *in the right hepatic lobe with wall thickening and hyperenhancement, compatible with ascending cholangitis.*

Acute Pancreatitis

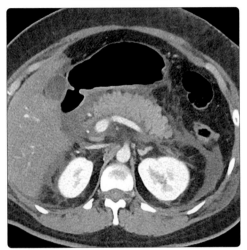

Duodenal Ulcer

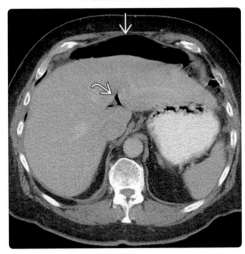

(Left) *Axial CECT shows peripancreatic fluid and infiltration of the peripancreatic fat planes in a patient with acute pancreatitis.* (Right) *Axial CECT shows extraluminal gas ➡ under the diaphragm and in the porta hepatis ➡ from a perforated duodenal ulcer.*

Duodenal Ulcer

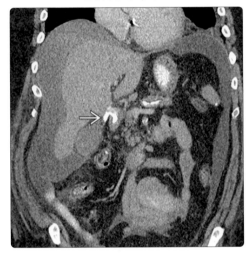

Pseudomembranous Colitis

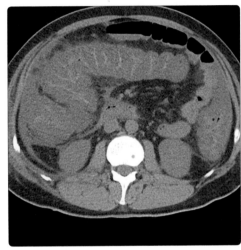

(Left) *Coronal CECT shows direct extravasation of enteric contrast ➡ from a perforated duodenal ulcer in this patient with extensive ascites and extraluminal air (not shown).* (Right) *Axial CECT shows marked thickening of the colonic wall, including the hepatic flexure and transverse colon, representing acute infectious pseudomembranous colitis.*

Infectious Colitis

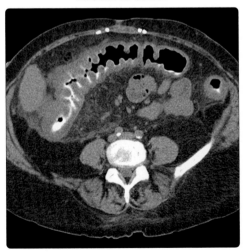

Appendicitis

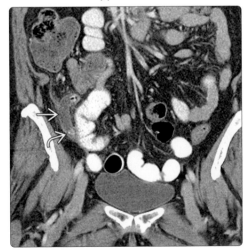

(Left) *Axial CECT shows infectious colitis in a patient with mural edema and wall thickening throughout the transverse colon and hepatic flexure.* (Right) *Coronal CECT shows a dilated appendix ➡ with mucosal enhancement, wall thickening, and a tiny appendicolith ➡, as well adjacent fat-stranding and inflammation, compatible with acute uncomplicated appendicitis.*

(Left) *Axial CECT in a patient with right abdominal pain and fever shows a thick-walled, hyperemic, dilated appendix* ➡️ *with an adjacent collection of gas and fluid* ➡️*, compatible with perforated appendicitis.* (Right) *Axial CECT in a patient presenting with RUQ pain shows an encapsulated, fat-containing mass* ➡️ *in the anterior omentum, a classic appearance for omental infarct.*

Appendicitis

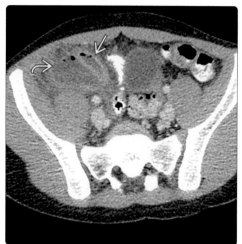

Omental Infarct

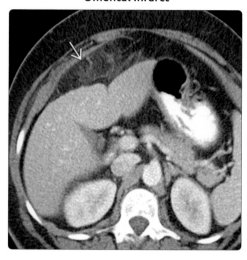

(Left) *Axial CECT shows a small, fat-containing mass* ➡️ *abutting the sigmoid colon with adjacent stranding and inflammation, a characteristic appearance for epiploic appendagitis.* (Right) *Coronal CECT shows a large, multiloculated cystic liver mass* ➡️ *with a thick, peripheral rind of enhancement, compatible with liver abscess in this patient with abdominal pain and fever.*

Epiploic Appendagitis

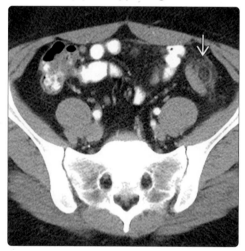

Hepatic Pyogenic Abscess

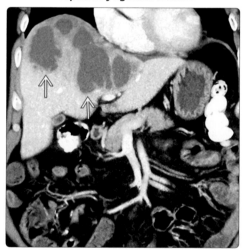

(Left) *Axial CECT shows a thick-walled cystic mass* ➡️ *in the right hepatic lobe with subtle surrounding low-density parenchymal edema, compatible with large liver abscess.* (Right) *Axial CECT in a patient with cardiac dysfunction shows the classic heterogeneous nutmeg enhancement of the liver, suggestive of passive hepatic congestion. Note the presence of other signs of volume overload, including ascites and mild anasarca.*

Hepatic Pyogenic Abscess

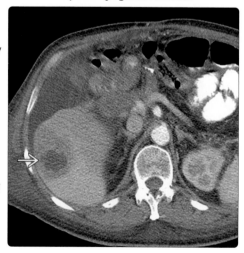

Passive Hepatic Congestion

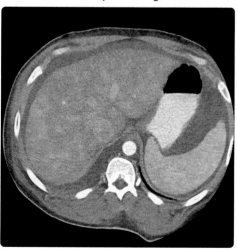

Diverticulitis

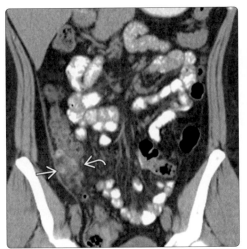

Diverticulitis

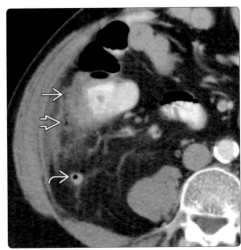

(Left) *Coronal CECT in a patient with right abdominal pain shows thickening of the right colon* ➔ *and its adjacent facia with several cecal diverticula* ➔, *compatible with acute cecal diverticulitis.* (Right) *Axial CECT shows mural thickening and extensive adjacent inflammatory change* ➔ *around the ascending colon with a small bubble of ectopic gas* ➔. *Note the normal appendix* ➔. *These findings were secondary to cecal diverticulitis.*

Pyelonephritis

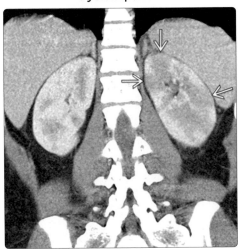

Hepatic Cavernous Hemangioma

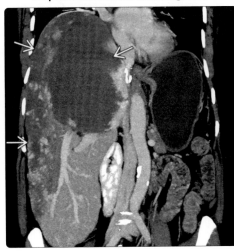

(Left) *Coronal CECT shows multiple wedge-shaped areas of low attenuation* ➔ *within the left kidney, along with subtle asymmetric perinephric edema, compatible with acute pyelonephritis.* (Right) *Coronal CECT shows multiple giant hemangiomas* ➔ *throughout the liver, demonstrating peripheral nodular enhancement. Even benign liver lesions, such as hemangiomas or cysts, can cause pain when they are very large as a result of stretching the liver capsule.*

Hepatocellular Carcinoma

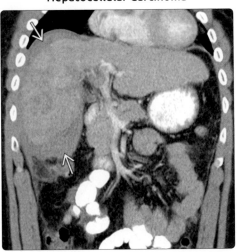

Hepatic Adenoma

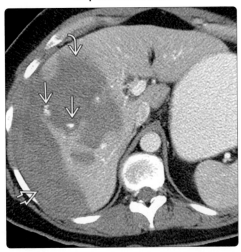

(Left) *Coronal CECT shows an infiltrative tumor throughout the right hepatic lobe with adjacent perihepatic hematoma* ➔, *compatible with bleeding infiltrative hepatocellular carcinoma.* (Right) *Axial CECT shows a right hepatic lobe mass* ➔ *with multiple foci of internal active extravasation* ➔ *and directly contiguous perihepatic hematoma* ➔. *This was found to represent a hepatic adenoma with hemorrhage.*

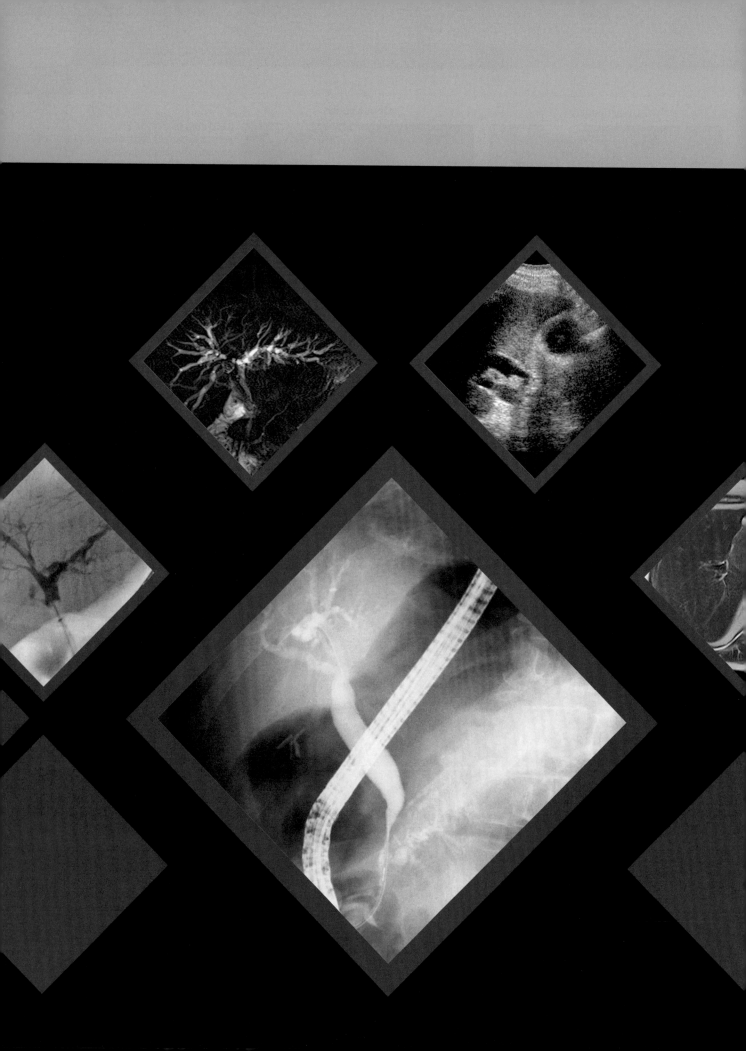

SECTION 11
Biliary Tract

Generic Imaging Patterns

Dilated Common Bile Duct 398
Asymmetric Dilation of Intrahepatic Bile Ducts 404
Biliary Strictures, Multiple 408

Modality-Specific Imaging Findings

Magnetic Resonance Imaging

Hypointense Lesion in Biliary Tree (MRCP) 412

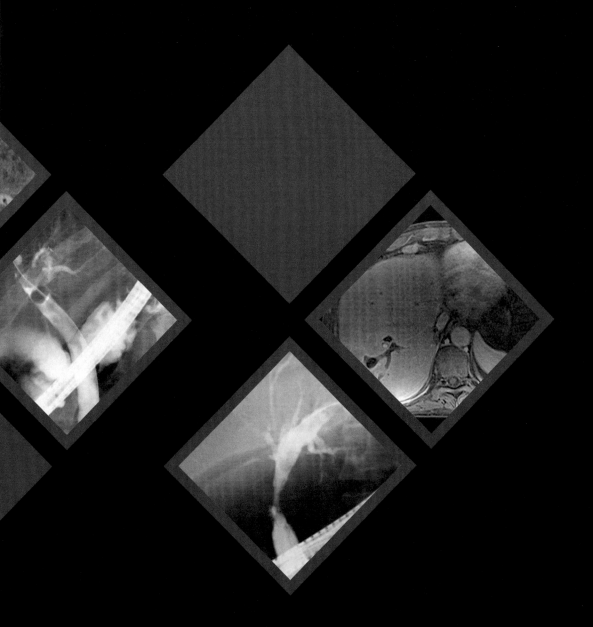

DIFFERENTIAL DIAGNOSIS

Common

- Choledocholithiasis
- Postcholecystectomy Dilatation of Common Bile Duct
- Senescent and Postoperative Dilatation
- Pancreatic Ductal Adenocarcinoma
- Chronic Pancreatitis

Less Common

- Other Ampullary, Periampullary, and Pancreatic Neoplasms
  ○ Distal Common Bile Duct Cholangiocarcinoma
  ○ Ampullary Tumors
  ○ Periampullary Duodenal Adenocarcinoma
  ○ Mucinous Pancreatic Cystic Tumors
    – Mucinous Cystic Neoplasm
    – Intraductal Papillary Mucinous Neoplasm
- Gallbladder Carcinoma
- Primary Sclerosing Cholangitis
- Pancreatic Pseudocyst
- AIDS Cholangiopathy
- Recurrent Pyogenic Cholangitis
- Biliary Trauma
- Small Bowel Obstruction
- Choledochal Cyst

Rare but Important

- Other Pancreatic Masses
- Biliary Intraductal Papillary Mucinous Neoplasm
- Pancreatobiliary Parasites

ESSENTIAL INFORMATION

Key Differential Diagnosis Issues

- When common bile duct (CBD) is only borderline enlarged, decision to pursue further testing will depend on presence of clinical and biochemical markers of biliary obstruction
  ○ Presence of elevated bilirubin (direct and indirect), alkaline phosphatase, and transaminases should raise concern for CBD obstruction
  ○ **Painful** jaundice suggests acute or subacute obstruction, usually on basis of gallstones or cholangitis
  ○ **Painless** jaundice suggests chronic obstruction, and should raise concern for malignant obstruction or longstanding inflammatory obstruction, such as primary sclerosing cholangitis (PSC)
- Size thresholds for CBD are controversial, but size should generally be < 6 mm (+ 1 mm for each decade over 60 years)
  ○ Some suggest size up to 1 cm may be within normal limits after cholecystectomy, although this is controversial
- Presence of intrahepatic and extrahepatic biliary dilatation generally more concerning for distal obstruction than dilated CBD alone

Helpful Clues for Common Diagnoses

- **Choledocholithiasis**
  ○ CT sensitivity for stones is ~ 80% with "pure" cholesterol stones often missed due to isodensity with bile
    – Gallstones on CT are variable in density, ranging from soft tissue density to calcified

- Stones can be very difficult to perceive in CBD on CT, particularly when CBD is not dilated
  ○ Stones (usually) appear as signal void on all MR pulse sequences, with T2 most sensitive
    – Some pigment stones are rarely hyperintense on T1
    – MR is clearly best modality for identification of CBD stones, although impacted stones in ampulla can still be difficult to perceive in some cases
  ○ Gallstones appear echogenic on US, but distal CBD usually poorly evaluated due to overlying bowel gas
  ○ Patients with CBD stones almost always have GB stones
- **Senescent and Postoperative Dilatation**
  ○ It is generally accepted (although not without debate) that CBD seems to increase in diameter with advanced age and following cholecystectomy
    – CBD dilatation especially common if CBD was dilated prior to cholecystectomy
- **Pancreatic Ductal Adenocarcinoma**
  ○ Most common cause of painless jaundice
  ○ Poorly marginated, hypodense mass centered in pancreatic head resulting in abrupt narrowing of distal CBD and pancreatic duct (double-duct sign) with upstream pancreatic atrophy
  ○ Often infiltrates posteriorly to encase mesenteric vasculature
- **Chronic Pancreatitis**
  ○ May produce smooth, tapered narrowing and stricture of distal CBD as it traverses pancreatic head
  ○ Other stigmata include dilated, beaded pancreatic duct with parenchymal/intraductal calcifications
  ○ Can result in focal fibroinflammatory mass in pancreatic head, which may be difficult to distinguish from pancreatic cancer

Helpful Clues for Less Common Diagnoses

- **Other Ampullary, Periampullary, and Pancreatic Neoplasms**
  ○ **Distal Common Bile Duct Cholangiocarcinoma**
    – Only 20% of extrahepatic bile duct cholangiocarcinomas arise in distal 1/3 of duct, but 95% of these lesions result in CBD obstruction
    – May present as ill-defined soft tissue mass or as discrete duct wall thickening with hyperenhancement
    – Does not typically obstruct pancreatic duct or cause pancreatic atrophy
  ○ **Ampullary Tumors**
    – Encompass wide range of histologic tumor types, including ampullary adenoma, ampullary carcinoma, and ampullary carcinoid
    – Tumor typically small and not uncommonly difficult to definitively visualize
    – May present as discrete nodule at ampulla or subtle wall thickening of medial duodenal wall at ampulla
    – Almost always obstructs CBD, but only obstructs pancreatic duct in ~ 50% and does not usually cause pancreatic atrophy
  ○ **Periampullary Duodenal Adenocarcinoma**
    – Distinction between ampullary carcinoma and periampullary duodenal adenocarcinoma may not be possible on imaging
    – Frequent obstruction of distal CBD but pancreatic atrophy or pancreatic ductal obstruction uncommon

- o **Mucinous Pancreatic Cystic Tumors**
  - Majority of mucinous cystic neoplasms (MCNs) and intraductal papillary mucinous neoplasms (IPMNs) do not cause CBD obstruction
  - IAP consensus guidelines for management of IPMN/MCN suggest presence of CBD obstruction/jaundice is high-risk feature that should prompt concern for invasive malignancy
  - MCN usually appears as unilocular cyst (± thick wall or mural nodularity), while IPMN presents as cystic lesion that communicates with pancreatic duct
  - MCN more often located in tail segment, while IPMN most common in head
- **Gallbladder Carcinoma**
  - Frequently causes CBD obstruction as result of either direct tumor extension or metastatic lymphadenopathy
  - More typically obstructs mid- or proximal CBD (rather than distal CBD) with intrahepatic biliary dilatation predominating over CBD dilatation
- **Primary Sclerosing Cholangitis**
  - Much more likely to cause strictures of CBD and intrahepatic ducts rather than impressive dilation
  - Prominent dilation of CBD or intrahepatic ducts as result of dominant CBD stricture is unusual and should raise concern for superimposed cholangiocarcinoma
- **Pancreatic Pseudocyst**
  - Pseudocysts arising in pancreatic head may cause CBD obstruction due to extrinsic mass effect
  - Obstruction in this setting may not be cured by draining pseudocyst, as CBD obstruction is often actually caused by coexisting fibrotic stricture of intrapancreatic CBD
- **AIDS Cholangiopathy**
  - Now uncommon diagnosis due to widespread utilization of HAART for HIV/AIDS
  - Can result in multiple intrahepatic and extrahepatic ductal strictures that are very similar to PSC
  - Classically results in papillary stenosis and CBD dilatation with distal CBD narrowing usually smooth and tapered
- **Recurrent Pyogenic Cholangitis**
  - Almost always diagnosed in patients from Southeast Asia

- o Results in biliary dilatation that disproportionately affects extrahepatic duct and central intrahepatic ducts (with frequent intraductal stones and purulent debris)
- **Biliary Trauma**
  - CBD injury can result in stricture or transection of duct with proximal biliary dilatation
  - Usually iatrogenic (especially during cholecystectomy or other biliary surgeries) rather than truly trauma-related
  - Usually abrupt narrowing of CBD ± adjacent biloma
- **Small Bowel Obstruction**
  - Obstruction of duodenum or Roux loop can result in increased intraluminal pressures that may impair biliary drainage and cause proximal biliary dilatation
- **Choledochal Cyst**
  - Type I choledochal cyst results in isolated fusiform CBD dilation, while type IV choledochal cyst results in cystic dilatation of intrahepatic and extrahepatic bile duct

Helpful Clues for Rare Diagnoses

- **Other Pancreatic Masses**
  - Range of other pancreatic tumors can theoretically cause CBD obstruction, particularly when large
  - Pancreatic neuroendocrine tumors and serous cystadenomas do not typically cause CBD or pancreatic duct obstruction, although very large tumors can obstruct CBD due to mass effect
  - Lymphoma of pancreas does not usually cause pancreatic or biliary ductal obstruction
- **Biliary Intraductal Papillary Mucinous Neoplasm**
  - Mucin-producing neoplasm arising from biliary mucosa
  - Can result in localized or diffuse massive dilatation of bile ducts as result of distension with mucin (± visible intraductal mural nodularity or soft tissue)
- **Pancreaticobiliary Parasites**
  - Uncommon in Western world, but parasites can involve biliary tree, resulting in ductal dilatation and strictures
  - Ascariasis can involve any portion of biliary tree, while fascioliasis preferentially involves extrahepatic duct and large intrahepatic ducts
  - Parasite may be visible within duct as filling defect

Choledocholithiasis

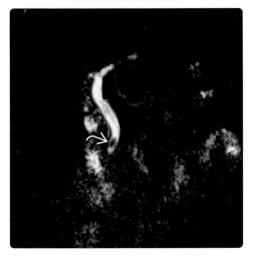

Choledocholithiasis

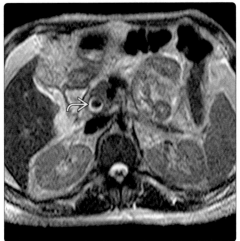

(Left) Coronal MRCP shows a low-signal stone ⏩ in the distal common bile duct (CBD). Although there are some rare exceptions, gallstones typically appear low signal on all MR pulse sequences. (Right) Axial T2 HASTE MR shows a low-signal filling defect ⏩ within the distal CBD, compatible with choledocholithiasis.

Choledocholithiasis

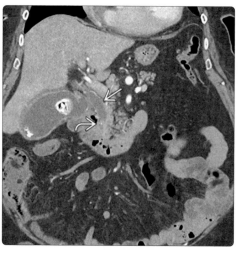

Choledocholithiasis

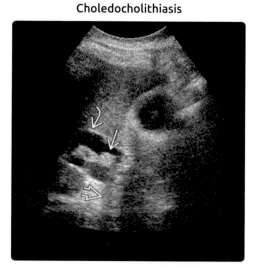

(Left) *Coronal CECT shows a mildly dilated CBD* ➡ *secondary to an obstructing stone* ➡ *in the distal CBD.* (Right) *US shows a mildly dilated CBD* ➡ *secondary to a gallstone* ➡ *with posterior acoustic shadowing* ➡. *US is often relatively insensitive for choledocholithiasis due to overlying bowel gas.*

Postcholecystectomy Dilatation of Common Bile Duct

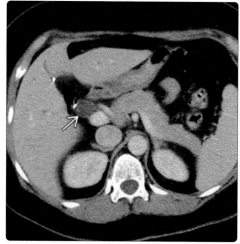

Pancreatic Ductal Adenocarcinoma

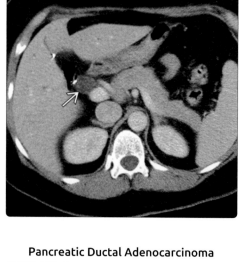

(Left) *Axial CECT shows mild dilatation of the common duct* ➡ *in a patient status post cholecystectomy. There were no signs or symptoms of biliary obstruction, and these findings were attributed to her prior cholecystectomy.* (Right) *Coronal CECT shows a hypodense mass* ➡ *in the pancreatic head, resulting in obstruction and dilatation of the CBD* ➡, *representing a pancreatic adenocarcinoma.*

Pancreatic Ductal Adenocarcinoma

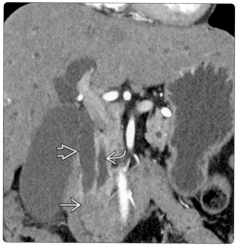

Pancreatic Ductal Adenocarcinoma

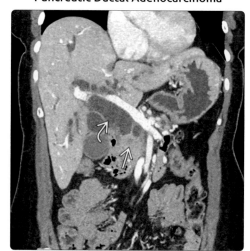

(Left) *Coronal CECT shows a double-duct sign secondary to a pancreatic head adenocarcinoma* ➡ *with dilatation of the biliary* ➡ *and pancreatic* ➡ *ducts.* (Right) *Coronal CECT shows a subtle, low-density mass* ➡ *in the pancreatic head, representing known pancreatic adenocarcinoma, resulting in obstruction and severe dilatation of the CBD* ➡ *and biliary tree.*

Pancreatic Ductal Adenocarcinoma

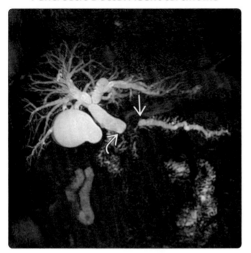

Chronic Pancreatitis

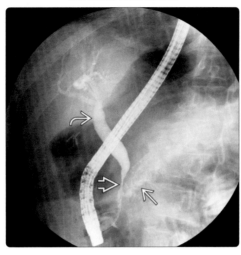

(Left) *Coronal MRCP in a patient with pancreatic adenocarcinoma shows a classic double-duct sign with abrupt narrowing of the distal CBD* ➡ *and pancreatic duct* ➡ *due to the patient's malignancy.* (Right) *Face down frontal oblique ERCP in a patient with chronic pancreatitis shows long, smooth tapering of the distal CBD* ➡ *as a result of a distal stricture, with mild associated proximal CBD dilatation* ➡. *In addition, the pancreatic duct* ➡ *appears beaded and very irregular.*

Chronic Pancreatitis

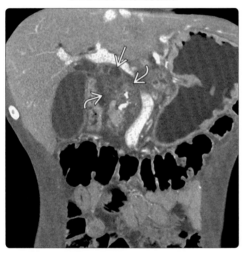

Distal Common Bile Duct Cholangiocarcinoma

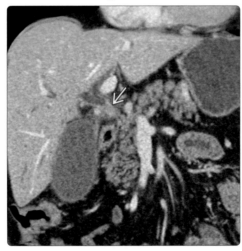

(Left) *Coronal CECT shows a partially calcified, hypodense mass in the pancreatic head, representing a focal fibroinflammatory mass* ➡ *related to known chronic pancreatitis. There is mild resultant CBD dilatation* ➡. (Right) *Coronal CECT shows subtle, focal wall thickening and enhancement in the distal CBD* ➡, *representing a distal CBD cholangiocarcinoma.*

Distal Common Bile Duct Cholangiocarcinoma

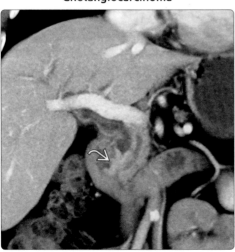

Ampullary Tumors

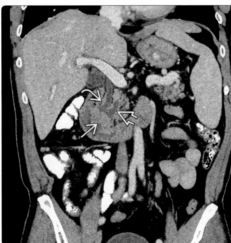

(Left) *Coronal volume-rendered CECT shows an abrupt stricture of the distal CBD* ➡ *with associated enhancement. This stricture was found to be malignant, representing cholangiocarcinoma.* (Right) *Coronal CECT shows a soft tissue mass* ➡ *at the ampulla resulting in obstruction of the CBD* ➡ *and pancreatic duct* ➡, *found to represent an ampullary carcinoma at resection.*

Ampullary Tumors

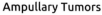

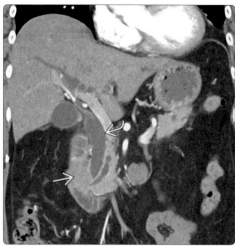

Periampullary Duodenal Adenocarcinoma

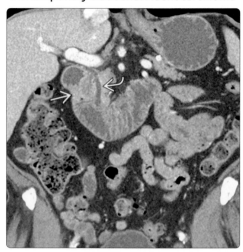

(Left) *Coronal CECT shows severe CBD dilatation ⟶ with abrupt narrowing near the ampulla due to a soft tissue mass ⟶ at the ampulla, representing an ampullary carcinoma.* (Right) *Coronal CECT shows an annular, constricting mass ⟶ of the duodenum, representing duodenal carcinoma, with involvement of the ampulla and resultant mild biliary dilatation ⟶.*

Periampullary Duodenal Adenocarcinoma

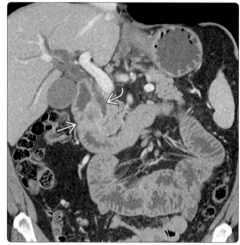

Gallbladder Carcinoma

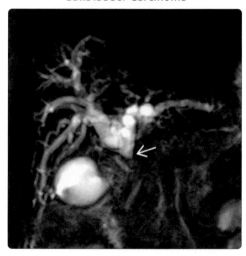

(Left) *Coronal CECT shows mass-like thickening ⟶ of the medial duodenum near the ampulla, resulting in obstruction of the CBD ⟶. This was found to be a periampullary duodenal adenocarcinoma at resection.* (Right) *Coronal MRCP MIP shows abrupt obstruction of the proximal CBD ⟶ near the confluence of ducts due to infiltrative gallbladder cancer.*

Pancreatic Pseudocyst

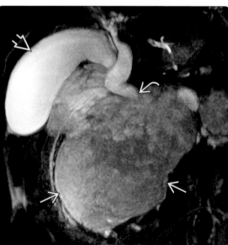

AIDS Cholangiopathy

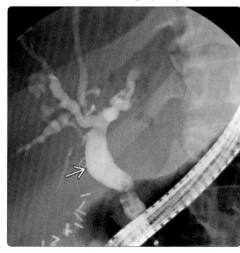

(Left) *Coronal MRCP MIP shows obstruction of the CBD ⟶ by a large pseudocyst ⟶. Note the distension of the gallbladder ⟶ secondary to biliary obstruction. The patient underwent a successful surgical procedure with enteric cyst drainage into the duodenum.* (Right) *ERCP shows diffuse dilatation of the CBD ⟶, as well as irregularity of the intrahepatic ducts, compatible with the patient's known AIDS cholangiopathy.*

Recurrent Pyogenic Cholangitis

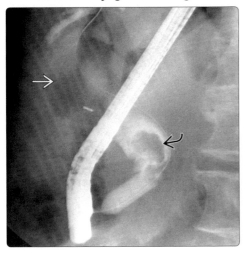

Recurrent Pyogenic Cholangitis

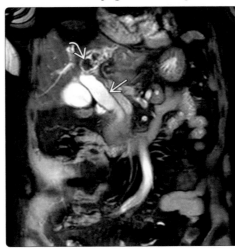

(Left) Face down frontal oblique ERCP shows a massively dilated CBD with large stones within the CBD ➔, compatible with the patient's history of recurrent pyogenic cholangitis. There is also a large amount of gas ➔ within the ducts. (Right) Coronal FIESTA MR shows severe dilatation of the CBD ➔, along with dilatation of the left hepatic lobe ducts, which are filled with multiple T2-hypointense stones ➔. These findings are compatible with recurrent pyogenic cholangitis.

Choledochal Cyst

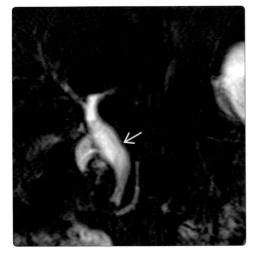

Choledochal Cyst

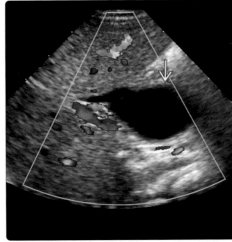

(Left) Coronal MRCP MIP shows diffuse, fusiform dilation of the extrahepatic common duct ➔, a type I choledochal cyst in the Todani classification. (Right) Color Doppler US in a young child shows a type I choledochal cyst with fusiform dilatation of the CBD ➔.

Choledochal Cyst

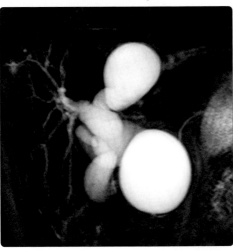

Biliary Intraductal Papillary Mucinous Neoplasm

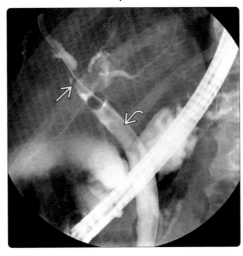

(Left) Coronal MRCP MIP shows extensive cystic dilatation of the intrahepatic and extrahepatic bile ducts, compatible with a type IV choledochal cyst. (Right) Frontal ERCP shows diffuse dilatation of the CBD with a discrete mass within the proximal CBD ➔. There is also heterogeneous filling of the CBD with contrast ➔, likely as a result of mucin. These findings were found to represent a biliary intraductal papillary mucinous neoplasm.

DIFFERENTIAL DIAGNOSIS

Common
- Primary Sclerosing Cholangitis
- Malignant Obstruction
  - Cholangiocarcinoma
  - Gallbladder Carcinoma
  - Liver Tumors
  - Periportal Lymphadenopathy
- Ascending Cholangitis

Less Common
- AIDS Cholangiopathy
- Recurrent Pyogenic Cholangitis
- Pancreato-Biliary Parasites
- Hepatic Hydatid Cyst
- Chemotherapy Cholangitis
- Biliary Intraductal Papillary Mucinous Neoplasm
- IgG4-Related Sclerosing Cholangitis
- Ischemic Cholangitis
- Caroli Disease
- Mirizzi Syndrome
- Hepatolithiasis (Intraductal Stones)

ESSENTIAL INFORMATION

Key Differential Diagnosis Issues
- Disproportionate dilatation of intrahepatic bile ducts (relative to extrahepatic duct) most often due to either one of several forms of cholangitis or obstructing mass
- Presence of significant isolated intrahepatic biliary dilatation (whether diffuse, lobar, or segmental) should always prompt careful evaluation for obstructing mass or malignant stricture
- Many different forms of cholangitis may appear similar radiographically, requiring correlation with clinical history or biopsy to make more specific diagnosis

Helpful Clues for Common Diagnoses
- **Primary Sclerosing Cholangitis**
  - Immune-mediated form of cholangitis resulting in fibrosis, inflammation, and strictures of bile ducts
  - Beaded strictures with intervening sites of normal or dilated ducts
    - Usually involves both intrahepatic and extrahepatic ducts, but isolated or disproportionate involvement of intrahepatic ducts can occur
      - Main right and left ducts are often most severely involved
    - Chronic involvement can result in unique form of cirrhosis with rounded, lobulated contour of liver with peripheral atrophy and severe hypertrophy of caudate/central liver (pseudotumoral enlargement)
  - Most often diagnosed in young men (30-40 years of age) with strong association with ulcerative colitis and autoimmune diseases
- **Malignant Obstruction**
  - **Cholangiocarcinoma**
    - Tumors arising either at liver hilum/confluence of ducts (i.e., Klatskin tumor) or peripherally in liver itself can result in proximal intrahepatic biliary dilatation

- Tumors classically demonstrate prominent delayed enhancement on multiphase imaging (CT or MR)
  - Liver peripheral to tumor may demonstrate atrophy or capsular retraction
  - Tumor may appear as discrete mass, subtle asymmetric soft tissue along margin of duct, or focal duct wall thickening and enhancement
- **Gallbladder Carcinoma**
  - Frequently extends to involve proximal extrahepatic duct or hepatic duct confluence, producing intrahepatic biliary dilatation
  - May be difficult on imaging to confidently differentiate gallbladder carcinoma from hilar cholangiocarcinoma
  - Frequently associated with liver metastases, bulky lymphadenopathy, and carcinomatosis
- **Liver Tumors**
  - Any tumor involving liver or liver hilum (e.g., HCC, metastases, lymphoma, etc.) can theoretically invade and obstruct intrahepatic ducts
  - Even benign masses, when large, may displace and dilate ducts due to extrinsic mass effect
  - Most metastases do not cause biliary dilatation, but colorectal cancers have higher propensity to do so as result of intrabiliary growth
  - HCC involvement of bile ducts is rare but when present is considered marker of aggressive disease
- **Periportal Lymphadenopathy**
  - Can obstruct proximal extrahepatic duct due to extrinsic compression and result in intrahepatic biliary dilatation
- **Ascending Cholangitis**
  - Acute pyogenic infection due to biliary obstruction, most often on basis of distal obstructing stone or reflux of bowel contents (e.g., biliary-enteric anastomosis)
  - Biliary dilatation proximal to site of obstruction with evidence of bile duct wall thickening and enhancement
    - Often associated with heterogeneous liver enhancement, particularly on arterial-phase images
  - Results in inflammatory bile duct strictures with abnormal biliary tree arborization and branching

Helpful Clues for Less Common Diagnoses
- **AIDS Cholangiopathy**
  - Increasingly uncommon entity (due to widespread utilization of HAART) seen in late-stage AIDS patients (usually CD4 < 100 mm³)
    - Inflammation of biliary tree caused by opportunistic infection
  - Beaded strictures of intrahepatic or extrahepatic ducts that may closely resemble primary sclerosing cholangitis
    - Strictures may be associated with bile duct wall thickening and enhancement on CT/MR
    - Gallbladder not uncommonly involved with wall thickening and surrounding inflammation
  - Classically associated with papillary stenosis [tapered narrowing of distal common bile duct (CBD)]
- **Recurrent Pyogenic Cholangitis**
  - Disease almost always diagnosed in patients living in or immigrating from Southeast Asia, likely related to parasitic or bacterial infection of biliary tree

- Results in significant dilatation of bile ducts, which frequently demonstrate internal stones
- Tends to involve extrahepatic and central intrahepatic ducts preferentially and may be localized to one portion of liver (especially left hepatic lobe)
  - Involved portions of liver often demonstrate parenchymal atrophy
- **Pancreato-Biliary Parasites**
  - Parasites (such as ascariasis, clonorchiasis, or fascioliasis) can involve biliary tree and result in biliary dilatation
    - Distribution of biliary involvement will depend on parasite type (e.g., clonorchiasis involves small, peripheral intrahepatic ducts)
  - Parasite may be seen within dilated duct as filling defect
- **Hepatic Hydatid Cyst**
  - Endemic in sheep-raising countries (Mediterranean, Africa, South America)
  - Can cause biliary dilatation if hepatic echinococcal cyst communicates with bile duct or ruptures into biliary tree
  - Direct communication between hydatid cyst and bile duct may rarely be directly visualized with wall defect in cyst leading into adjacent dilated bile duct
- **Chemotherapy Cholangitis**
  - Form of cholangitis resulting from intraarterial chemotherapy (such as transarterial chemoembolization)
  - Imaging features similar to PSC, including multifocal biliary strictures
  - Distribution of strictures based on hepatic arterial supply to bile ducts with preferential involvement of proximal extrahepatic bile duct and biliary confluence
- **Biliary Intraductal Papillary Mucinous Neoplasm**
  - Mucin-producing neoplasm arising from biliary mucosa, which is analogous to pancreatic IPMN
  - Results in severely dilated bile ducts filled with mucin ± enhancing mural nodularity or discrete intraductal mass
  - Can involve ducts diffusely or be localized
  - Typically older patients from East Asia who present with jaundice and repetitive bouts of cholangitis
- **IgG4-Related Sclerosing Cholangitis**

- Entity characterized by lymphoplasmacytic infiltration of biliary tree
  - Often associated with IgG4-related sclerosing disease in other organs (especially autoimmune pancreatitis)
- Strictures most commonly seen in distal CBD but can be seen anywhere in biliary tree
  - Involved bile ducts appear thickened and hyperenhancing
- Look for other stigmata of IgG4-related sclerosing disease, including findings of autoimmune pancreatitis (such enlargement of pancreas, low-density halo, etc.)
- **Ischemic Cholangitis**
  - Entity most often seen in setting of liver transplant resulting either from hepatic artery compromise (stenosis or thrombosis) or other microangiopathic/immunologic injuries
  - Multiple intrahepatic and extrahepatic strictures that may not be distinguishable from PSC without clinical history (including beaded appearance of biliary tree)
    - Tendency to involve middle 1/2 of CBD and hepatic duct confluence
    - Often associated with hyperdense (or T1-hyperintense) cast material filling bile ducts
- **Caroli Disease**
  - Congenital cystic dilatation of intrahepatic ducts with normal-caliber extrahepatic bile duct
  - Cystic dilatation of intrahepatic ducts can be focal, segmental, or diffuse with frequent intraductal stones
  - Associated with central dot sign due to enhancing portal radicle at center or periphery of dilated duct
- **Mirizzi Syndrome**
  - Obstruction of proximal extrahepatic bile duct due to gallstone impacted within cystic duct or gallbladder neck
  - Results in dilatation of intrahepatic bile ducts and proximal extrahepatic duct
- **Hepatolithiasis (Intraductal Stones)**
  - Extremely rare in Western world but higher incidence in East Asia
  - Parasitic infection (including recurrent pyogenic cholangitis) and diet play major role in development

Primary Sclerosing Cholangitis

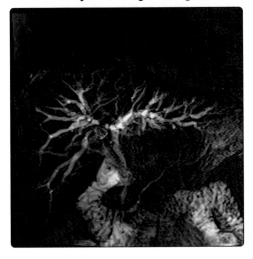

Primary Sclerosing Cholangitis

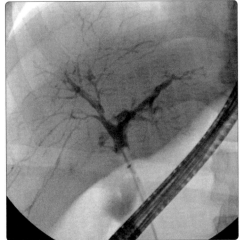

(Left) Coronal MRCP MIP in a patient with primary sclerosing cholangitis (PSC) shows mild, diffuse intrahepatic biliary ductal dilatation with the ducts showing a subtle beaded morphology. (Right) Frontal ERCP cholangiogram shows the characteristic features of PSC, including mild, diffuse biliary dilatation and classic beaded appearance of the ducts (with alternating sites of dilated, narrowed, or normal ducts).

Cholangiocarcinoma

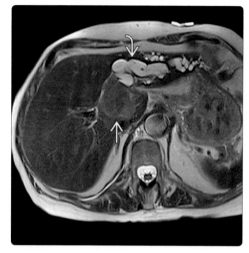

Cholangiocarcinoma

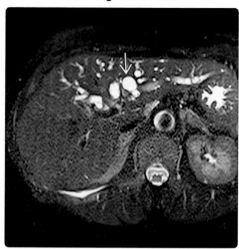

(Left) *Axial T2 MR shows a large, obstructing mass* ➡ *with intermediate hyperintensity resulting in asymmetric dilatation of the left hepatic ducts* ➡*, representing a cholangiocarcinoma.* (Right) *Axial CECT shows severe dilatation of the intrahepatic bile ducts* ➡ *in the left hepatic lobe. Although a discrete obstructing mass is difficult to identify on imaging, this was ultimately found to be an obstructing cholangiocarcinoma.*

Gallbladder Carcinoma

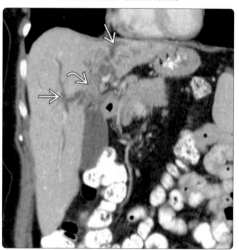

Liver Tumors

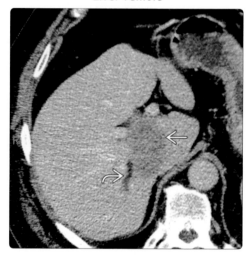

(Left) *Coronal CECT shows an infiltrative mass* ➡ *extending from the gallbladder neck to involve the confluence of ducts and result in intrahepatic biliary dilatation* ➡*. In cases such as this, differentiating a gallbladder carcinoma from a hilar cholangiocarcinoma can be difficult, but this was found to be a gallbladder carcinoma.* (Right) *Axial CECT shows a hypodense mass* ➡ *that causes obstruction of the right posterior hepatic duct* ➡*. The mass represented a metastasis from the patient's primary pancreatic cancer.*

Ascending Cholangitis

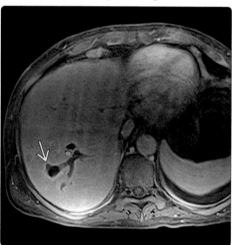

AIDS Cholangiopathy

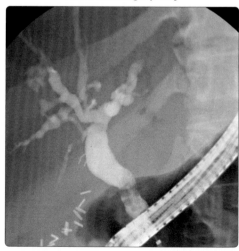

(Left) *Axial T1 C+ MR in a liver transplant patient with ascending cholangitis shows focally dilated ducts* ➡ *in the right hepatic lobe with wall thickening and hyperenhancement.* (Right) *Frontal ERCP cholangiogram in an AIDS patient with low CD4 count shows diffuse, irregular, beaded biliary dilatation, found to represent AIDS cholangiopathy.*

AIDS Cholangiopathy

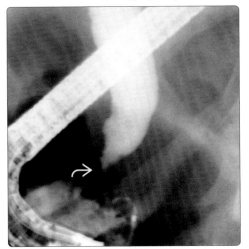

Recurrent Pyogenic Cholangitis

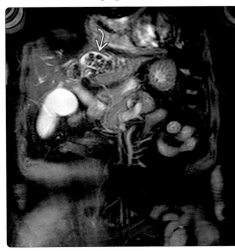

(Left) *Frontal ERCP cholangiogram in a patient with AIDS shows a grossly dilated CBD with a distal CBD structure* ➦, *typical findings of AIDS cholangiopathy with papillary stenosis.* (Right) *Coronal T2 FS MR in a patient who had immigrated from East Asia shows severely dilated bile ducts in the left hepatic lobe filled with hypointense stones* ➦, *a classic appearance for recurrent pyogenic cholangitis.*

IgG4-Related Sclerosing Cholangitis

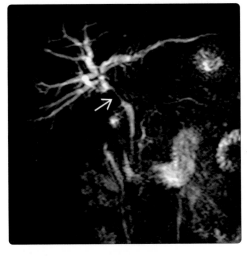

Ischemic Cholangitis

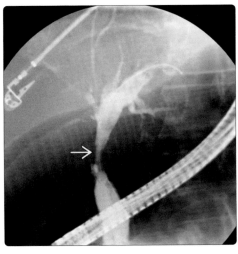

(Left) *Coronal MRCP MIP* ➦ *shows a dominant stricture* ➦ *in the proximal extrahepatic duct, found to be a manifestation of IgG4-cholangiopathy in this patient with evidence of retroperitoneal fibrosis (also thought to be IgG4 related).* (Right) *Frontal ERCP cholangiogram in a liver transplant patient with known hepatic artery stenosis shows a dominant biliary stricture* ➦ *in the proximal to mid CBD with associated intrahepatic biliary dilatation, compatible with ischemic cholangiopathy.*

Biliary Intraductal Papillary Mucinous Neoplasm

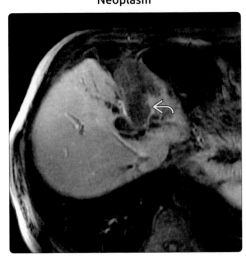

Caroli Disease

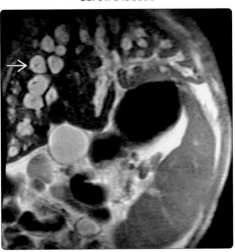

(Left) *Axial T1 C+ MR shows massive dilation of the left intrahepatic ducts* ➦ *without any obstructing mass or stricture. These findings were found to be secondary to biliary IPMN.* (Right) *Coronal T2 MR shows extensive cystic dilatation of the intrahepatic bile ducts with a few of the dilated ducts demonstrating a characteristic central dot sign* ➦. *This constellation of imaging features is classic for Caroli disease.*

DIFFERENTIAL DIAGNOSIS

Common
- Primary Sclerosing Cholangitis
- Ascending Cholangitis
- Posttransplant Liver and Ischemic Cholangiopathy
- Cirrhosis (Mimic)

Less Common
- AIDS Cholangiopathy
- Cholangiocarcinoma
- Recurrent Pyogenic Cholangitis
- Caroli Disease
- Chemotherapy Cholangitis
- Hepatic Metastases (Mimic)
- Pancreatobiliary Parasites
- Autoimmune (IgG4) Cholangitis
- Radiation Therapy
- Portal Biliopathy

Rare but Important
- Sarcoidosis
- Eosinophilic Cholangitis

ESSENTIAL INFORMATION

Key Differential Diagnosis Issues
- Sclerosing cholangitis is general term for disorders which result in fibrosis and stricturing of biliary tree
  - Most common cause is idiopathic form: **Primary sclerosing cholangitis (PSC)**
  - Many other secondary causes generally grouped together as "secondary" sclerosing cholangitis
- Most common causes of multiple biliary strictures have significant overlap in imaging appearance, making correlation with clinical history critical for diagnosis
- Multiple biliary strictures are typically benign, although development of new or dominant stricture can herald development of superimposed cholangiocarcinoma (particularly in PSC patients)
- MR/MRCP is best noninvasive modality for demonstrating distribution, length, and morphology of strictures

Helpful Clues for Common Diagnoses
- **Primary Sclerosing Cholangitis**
  - Immune-mediated disorder resulting in inflammation and fibrosis of intrahepatic and extrahepatic ducts, most often diagnosed in young male patients (30-40 years of age)
  - Multifocal beaded strictures with intervening sites of normal or dilated ducts
    - Active inflammation associated with bile duct wall thickening and enhancement on CECT and MR
    - Chronically results in pruned appearance of biliary tree
  - Chronic inflammation can result in cirrhotic liver with massive enlargement of central liver (pseudotumoral hypertrophy), atrophy of peripheral liver, and rounded/lobulated hepatic contour
    - Periphery of liver may be hypodense on CECT and mildly T2 hyperintense on MR due to fibrosis
  - Strong association with inflammatory bowel disease and other autoimmune diseases

- Any new dominant stricture should raise concern for superimposed cholangiocarcinoma
- **Ascending Cholangitis**
  - Pyogenic infection of biliary tree due to biliary obstruction
  - Dilated bile ducts with wall thickening, hyperenhancement of duct wall, and patchy heterogeneous hepatic enhancement (particularly on arterial phase)
    - May be associated with debris within bile duct, liver abscesses, or portal vein thrombosis
  - Results in strictures of biliary tree, as well as abnormal arborization pattern of intrahepatic ducts
    - Biliary tree may communicate with hepatic abscesses
- **Posttransplant Liver and Ischemic Cholangiopathy**
  - Nonanastomotic strictures may develop in transplant liver due to hepatic artery thrombosis/stenosis or immunologic injury (prolonged warm/cold ischemic time, blood antigen incompatibility, etc.)
    - Beaded strictures of biliary tree (similar to PSC) with predominant involvement of middle 1/3 of CBD and hepatic duct confluence
    - Often associated with bile duct "casts" filling dilated bile ducts (hyperdense on CT, hyperintense on T1 MR)
  - Biliary strictures in transplant liver may also develop at anastomotic site or due to cholangitis
- **Cirrhosis (Mimic)**
  - Regenerating nodules and fibrosis can distort and compress ducts due to mass effect, mimicking strictures

Helpful Clues for Less Common Diagnoses
- **AIDS Cholangiopathy**
  - Opportunistic infections of biliary tree in AIDS patients with very low CD4 counts (usually < 100 cells/mm³)
    - Now uncommon due to widespread HAART
  - Tapered, smooth narrowing of distal CBD (papillary stenosis) with long segment extrahepatic duct strictures and beaded strictures of intrahepatic ducts (like PSC)
  - May be associated with concomitant gallbladder wall thickening due to acalculous cholecystitis
- **Cholangiocarcinoma**
  - May present as discrete mass (i.e., mass-forming cholangiocarcinoma), focal wall thickening (i.e., periductal infiltrating), or intraductal nodule
  - Tumor classically characterized by increasing delayed enhancement due to fibrotic nature of tumor
  - Tumor often narrows or obstructs biliary tree with upstream biliary dilatation
    - May produce multiple strictures due to single large mass obstructing biliary tree in several locations or due to satellite lesions/metastases
- **Recurrent Pyogenic Cholangitis**
  - Occurs almost always in patients either living in or originally from Southeast Asia, likely due to parasitic infection of biliary tree
  - Dilatation of intrahepatic and extrahepatic ducts with multiple intrahepatic strictures, abnormal intrahepatic duct arborization, and stones throughout biliary tree
    - Can affect localized portions of liver, especially left hepatic lobe and right posterior lobe
    - Chronic disease can result in atrophy of affected portions of liver

- Duct dilation and intraductal stones tend to be more prominent than biliary strictures
- **Caroli Disease**
  - Congenital multifocal saccular dilatation of large intrahepatic ducts with alternating biliary strictures
    - Appears as multiple cysts throughout liver, which communicate with biliary tree
    - Characteristic central dot sign on CECT or MR with enhancing portal radicle surrounded by dilated duct
  - Caroli **syndrome** also associated with hepatic fibrosis and portal hypertension
  - Commonly associated with polycystic hepatorenal syndrome, hepatic fibrosis, and medullary sponge kidney
  - Usually known diagnosis presenting in childhood or early adulthood due to cholangitis or liver dysfunction
- **Chemotherapy Cholangitis**
  - Iatrogenic cholangitis related to intraarterial chemotherapy or transarterial chemoembolization for hepatic malignancies
  - Results in biliary strictures, which tend to involve proximal extrahepatic duct and biliary confluence more commonly that peripheral intrahepatic ducts
    - Necrosis of peripheral ducts can result in biloma or abscess formation
  - Duct strictures result from direct toxic effect of drug or due to occlusion of peribiliary vascular plexus with resultant ischemic cholangiopathy
- **Hepatic Metastases (Mimic)**
  - Masses may distort and narrow bile ducts due to mass effect, simulating strictures
- **Pancreatobiliary Parasites**
  - Parasites can cause strictures &/or biliary dilation with parasite often visible as filling defect within duct
    - Sites of involvement within biliary tree depend on individual parasite (e.g., clonorchiasis typically involves peripheral intrahepatic ducts)
- **Autoimmune (IgG4) Cholangitis**
  - Can result in strictures anywhere in biliary tree, but most commonly involves CBD
    - Smooth, long strictures without irregularity

- Can rarely appear mass-like and mimic tumor (**inflammatory pseudotumor**)
  - Involved bile duct segments demonstrate wall thickening and hyperenhancement on CT/MR
  - Frequently associated with other manifestations of IgG4-related sclerosing disease (e.g., autoimmune pancreatitis, retroperitoneal fibrosis, etc.)
- **Radiation Therapy**
  - When liver is included in radiation portal, can acutely result in radiation-induced hepatitis, and chronically may produce biliary strictures
  - Biliary stigmata typically take many years to become apparent (often > 10 years)
  - Distribution depends on portions of liver exposed to radiation
- **Portal Biliopathy**
  - Refers to abnormalities of bile ducts and gallbladder in patients with portal hypertension
  - Most commonly results in CBD strictures, but can result in pruning/strictures of intrahepatic ducts as well
    - Filling defects within ducts may actually represent venous collaterals protruding into duct lumen
  - Likely related to ischemic bile duct injury with biliary abnormalities most commonly present in patients with portal vein occlusion and cavernous transformation

Helpful Clues for Rare Diagnoses
- **Sarcoidosis**
  - Systemic sarcoidosis frequently involves liver (95%) but clinically significant in only small minority (5-15%)
  - Sarcoidosis can involve either intrahepatic or extrahepatic ducts and can mimic PSC
  - "Pruned" biliary tree due to granulomas in duct wall and fibrous adhesions from surrounding lymph nodes
- **Eosinophilic Cholangitis**
  - Rare form of cholangiopathy due eosinophilic infiltration of biliary tree with resultant strictures
  - Can range from focal stricture to multiple strictures
  - Can be difficult diagnosis to make with only subset of cases associated with peripheral eosinophilia
  - Responds well to steroid treatment

Primary Sclerosing Cholangitis

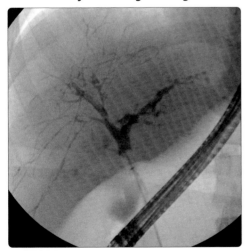

Primary Sclerosing Cholangitis

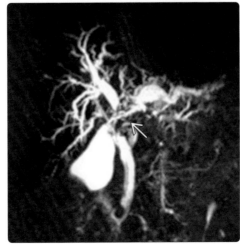

(Left) ERCP in a young male patient shows the characteristic appearance of primary sclerosing cholangitis (PSC) with extensive beaded strictures throughout the intrahepatic biliary tree. (Right) Coronal MRCP MIP shows extensive beading and irregularity of the biliary tree, compatible PSC. Note the dominant stricture ⊟➔ involving the proximal common duct and the central right and left hepatic ducts.

Biliary Strictures, Multiple

Primary Sclerosing Cholangitis

Ascending Cholangitis

(Left) *Axial CECT in the same patient shows an infiltrating, hypodense mass* ➥ *accounting for the dominant stricture, representing cholangiocarcinoma, which should always be considered with dominant or new strictures in PSC patients.* **(Right)** *Axial arterial-phase T1 C+ MR in a patient with cholangitis shows diffusely heterogeneous parenchymal enhancement and dilated bile ducts in the right lobe, which communicate with small abscesses* ➥.

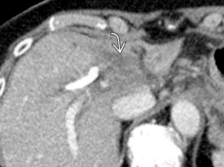
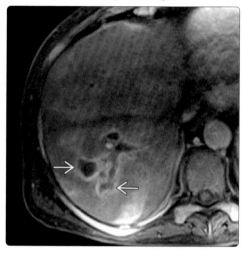

Posttransplant Liver and Ischemic Cholangiopathy

Posttransplant Liver and Ischemic Cholangiopathy

(Left) *Cholangiogram in a liver transplant patient with severe hepatic artery stenosis shows extensive strictures and irregularity of the biliary tree, representing ischemic cholangitis.* **(Right)** *Axial T1 MR in a liver transplant patient with hepatic artery thrombosis shows diffuse biliary dilatation due to ischemic cholangiopathy with hyperintense cast material* ➥ *filling the central bile ducts.*

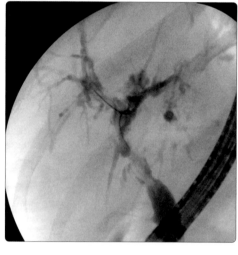
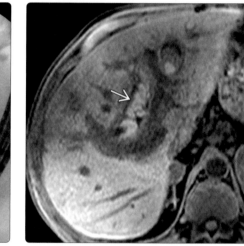

AIDS Cholangiopathy

AIDS Cholangiopathy

(Left) *ERCP in a patient with AIDS shows extensive beading, irregularity, and strictures of the intrahepatic ducts, as well as dilatation of the common bile duct (CBD), found to represent AIDS cholangiopathy.* **(Right)** *ERCP shows multiple strictures of the intrahepatic ducts, as well as dilatation of the CBD, found to represent AIDS cholangiopathy. The findings in this case are not easily distinguishable from PSC.*

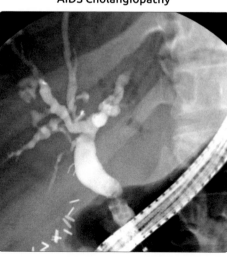
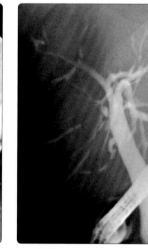

Cholangiocarcinoma

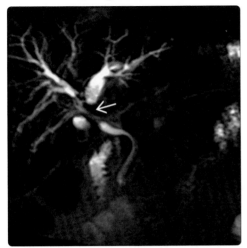

Recurrent Pyogenic Cholangitis

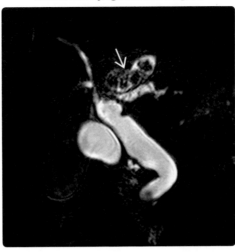

(Left) *Coronal MRCP MIP shows a large stricture ➡ involving the CBD and central right/left hepatic ducts secondary to a large cholangiocarcinoma.* (Right) *Coronal MRCP MIP in an Asian patient shows localized dilatation of the left hepatic lobe ducts ➡ with multiple low-signal stones filling the dilated ducts, compatible with recurrent pyogenic cholangitis.*

Caroli Disease

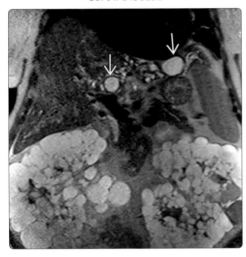

Chemotherapy Cholangitis

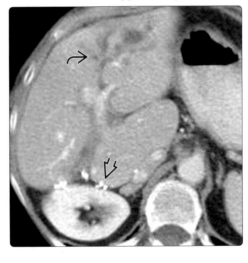

(Left) *Coronal T2 MR shows extensive enlargement of both kidneys with innumerable cysts, compatible with autosomal dominant polycystic disease. There are multiple cysts ➡ in the left hepatic lobe communicating with dilated bile ducts, compatible with Caroli disease.* (Right) *Axial CECT shows surgical clips ➡ from right hepatic lobectomy for metastases. Irregular dilation of the intrahepatic ducts ➡ in this case was the result of hepatic intraarterial chemotherapy.*

Autoimmune (IgG4) Cholangitis

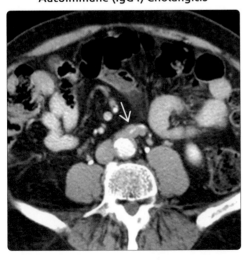

Autoimmune (IgG4) Cholangitis

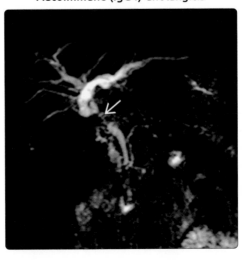

(Left) *Axial CECT shows soft tissue ➡ infiltrating along the course of the inferior mesenteric artery, found to represent retroperitoneal fibrosis (RPF).* (Right) *Coronal MRCP MIP in the same patient shows a stricture ➡ of the proximal common duct with mild upstream intrahepatic biliary dilatation. This was found to represent IgG4 cholangiopathy, which is often associated with other autoimmune diseases, such as RPF.*

DIFFERENTIAL DIAGNOSIS

Common

- Choledocholithiasis
- Pneumobilia
- Susceptibility Artifact (Mimic)
- Contraction of Sphincter of Oddi (Mimic)
- Respiratory Motion Artifact (Mimic)
- Hemobilia
- Portal Vein Gas (Mimic)
- Flow Artifact (Mimic)
- Pulsatile Vascular Compression (Mimic)
- Cystic Duct Insertion (Mimic)

ESSENTIAL INFORMATION

Key Differential Diagnosis Issues

- While MR is most sensitive modality for identifying stones in extrahepatic bile duct, knowledge of common artifacts and pitfalls is critical to avoid misinterpretation
- Optimally, any potential abnormality should be seen on more than 1 pulse sequence to confirm its veracity
- Always be certain to look at thin-section source 3D MRCP images; relying on MIP reconstructions alone increases risk of interpretation error

Helpful Clues for Common Diagnoses

- **Choledocholithiasis**
  - Most common cause of hypointense (signal void) intraductal filling defect on MR
  - Gallstones are typically low signal on all MR pulse sequences, although some pigment stones may rarely demonstrate high T1 signal
  - Typically multiple with stones also usually present in gallbladder
- **Pneumobilia**
  - Gas bubbles appear low signal on all pulse sequences but float ventrally with air-fluid levels on axial images
  - Be very cognizant of this pitfall in patients who have undergone prior biliary-enteric anastomosis, sphincterotomy, or other biliary intervention

- **Susceptibility Artifact (Mimic)**
  - Any metallic foreign body (e.g., surgical clip, coil, stent) or gas-filled structure (e.g., gas in stomach/duodenum) may produce signal void, which might mimic stone
  - Signal void due to susceptibility generally increases in size on in-phase GRE (which accentuate susceptibility artifacts) compared to opposed-phase
  - New titanium surgical clips cause less artifact
- **Contraction of Sphincter of Oddi (Mimic)**
  - Contraction of sphincter with distal narrowing may mimic stone or stricture in distal common bile duct
  - Pitfall can be avoided by acquiring several sequential 2D thick-slab MRCP acquisitions to visualize opening of sphincter of Oddi
- **Respiratory Motion Artifact (Mimic)**
  - Suboptimal breath holds may result in signal loss that might theoretically mimic filling defect
- **Hemobilia**
  - Can produce low-signal filling defect; generally occurs due to trauma, intervention, or biliary/hepatic tumors
- **Portal Vein Gas (Mimic)**
  - Particularly on axial images, gas in portal venous system might be be mistaken for pneumobilia or stones
- **Flow Artifact (Mimic)**
  - Very common cause of pseudo-filling defect, particularly on any sequence relying on single-shot fast spin-echo technique (usually HASTE in abdomen)
  - Filling defect in center of duct (rather than layering dependently) and not present on other sequences
- **Pulsatile Vascular Compression (Mimic)**
  - Arteries (e.g., hepatic, cystic, and gastroduodenal) can compress biliary tree during systole, simulating stricture or filling defect
  - Band of signal loss, rather than discrete filling defect
  - Most commonly seen across common hepatic duct or left hepatic duct due to right hepatic artery
- **Cystic Duct Insertion (Mimic)**
  - When cystic duct is large, redundant, or tortuous, it could mimic presence of filling defect at its site of insertion on common hepatic duct

(Left) Coronal MRCP shows the typical appearance of choledocholithiasis as a hypointense focus ➡ within the dilated common duct. (Right) Coronal T2 HASTE MR shows a gallstone ➡ in the distal common bile duct. This stone was less conspicuous on dedicated 3D MRCP images, stressing the importance of using all available imaging sequences when searching for common bile duct stones.

Choledocholithiasis

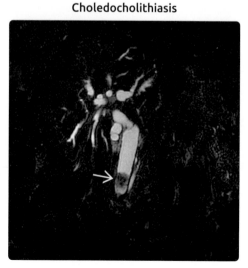

Choledocholithiasis

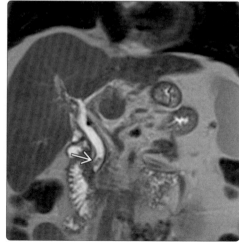

Pneumobilia

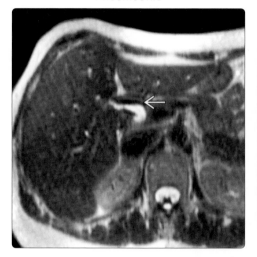

Pneumobilia

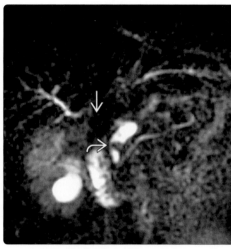

(Left) *Axial T2 MR shows an air-fluid level within the bile ducts as a signal void* ➦ *with a linear interface with the high-signal bile in the dependent position of the bile duct.* (Right) *Coronal oblique MRCP shows a focal defect in the bile duct that represents a stone* ➥*, but also a broad signal void in the more proximal duct* ➦ *due to pneumobilia.*

Susceptibility Artifact (Mimic)

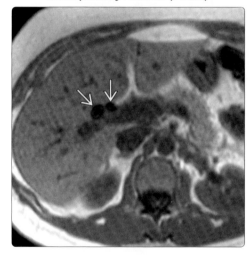

Flow Artifact (Mimic)

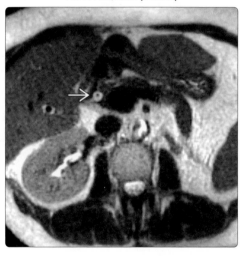

(Left) *Axial in-phase GRE MR shows 2 hypointense lesions in the porta hepatis caused by cholecystectomy clips* ➥*. These signal voids result from susceptibility artifact.* (Right) *Axial T2 HASTE MR shows a signal void* ➥ *in the center of the bile duct that was not present on coronal or MRCP sequences. This is a typical flow artifact. As in this case, flow artifacts are much more common with single-shot fast spin-echo technique.*

Pulsatile Vascular Compression (Mimic)

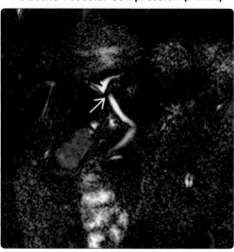

Pulsatile Vascular Compression (Mimic)

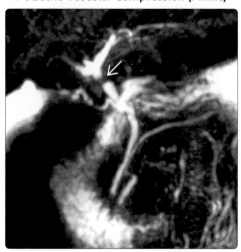

(Left) *Coronal MRCP MIP shows a band-like signal void* ➦ *extending across the proximal common hepatic duct, a classic appearance and location for vascular pulsation artifact.* (Right) *Coronal MRCP shows a signal void* ➥ *in the common hepatic duct due to compression by the hepatic artery that crosses the duct at this level.*

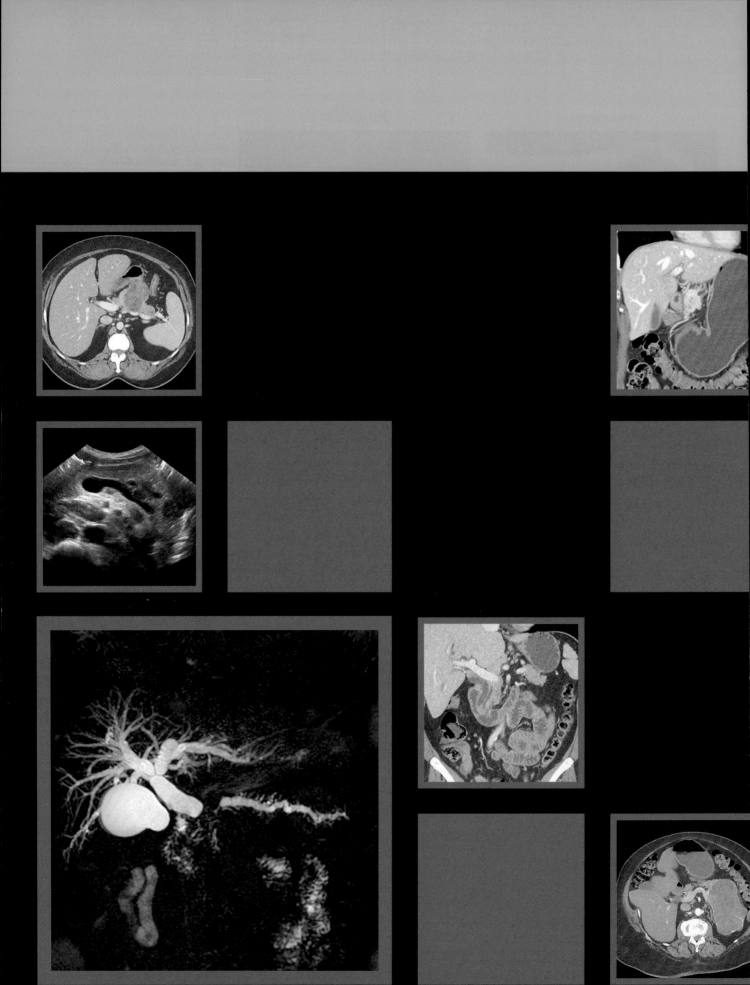

SECTION 12
Pancreas

Generic Imaging Patterns

Hypovascular Pancreatic Mass	416
Hypervascular Pancreatic Mass	422
Cystic Pancreatic Mass	426
Atrophy or Fatty Replacement of Pancreas	432
Dilated Pancreatic Duct	434
Infiltration of Peripancreatic Fat Planes	438
Pancreatic Calcifications	444

Modality-Specific Imaging Findings

Ultrasound

Cystic Pancreatic Lesion	448
Solid Pancreatic Lesion	452
Pancreatic Duct Dilatation	456

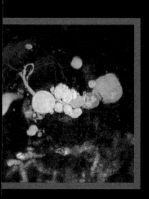

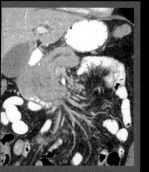

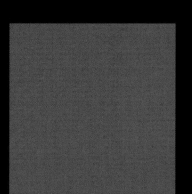

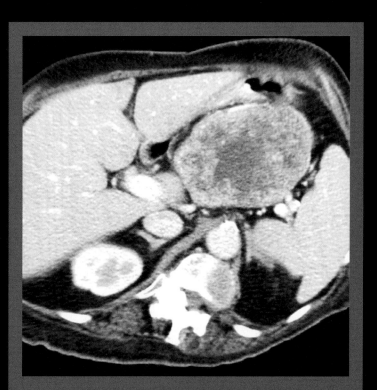

DIFFERENTIAL DIAGNOSIS

Common

- Pancreatic Ductal Adenocarcinoma
- Chronic Pancreatitis
- Normal Anatomic Variants of Pancreas (Mimic)
- Mucinous Cystic Neoplasm
- Peripancreatic Lymphadenopathy (Mimic)
- Unopacified Bowel (Mimic)
- Duodenal Diverticulum (Mimic)

Less Common

- Pancreatic Serous Cystadenoma
- Ampullary Carcinoma
- Pancreatic Metastases and Lymphoma
- Cholangiocarcinoma
- Pancreatic Neuroendocrine Tumor
- Solid Pseudopapillary Neoplasm
- Acute Pancreatitis
- Autoimmune Pancreatitis
- Groove Pancreatitis
- Agenesis of Dorsal Pancreas
- Adjacent Masses (Mimic)
  - Duodenal Carcinoma
  - Gastric Tumors
    - Gastrointestinal Stromal Tumor
  - Carcinoid Tumor
  - Desmoid Tumor
  - Retroperitoneal Sarcoma
  - Retroperitoneal Lymphoma
  - Peripancreatic Vascular Lesions
  - Adrenal Mass
    - Adrenal Carcinoma
    - Pheochromocytoma

Rare but Important

- Schwannoma
- Giant Cell Carcinoma
- Acinar Cell Carcinoma

ESSENTIAL INFORMATION

Key Differential Diagnosis Issues

- Masses that arise from structures adjacent to pancreas may simulate pancreatic mass (e.g., duodenum, adrenal, etc.)
- Pancreatitis may be very difficult to differentiate from ductal adenocarcinoma, including chronic pancreatitis (CP), focal autoimmune pancreatitis, and groove pancreatitis
- Pancreatic adenocarcinoma is most common solid hypovascular pancreatic mass
  - Pancreatic duct obstruction and parenchymal atrophy are very common with ductal adenocarcinoma but less common with other entities in differential diagnosis

Helpful Clues for Common Diagnoses

- **Pancreatic Ductal Adenocarcinoma**
  - Hypodense, poorly marginated mass with tendency to extend posteriorly and involve mesenteric vasculature
  - Usually causes pancreatic duct and biliary obstruction with upstream parenchymal atrophy

- MR: Typically T1 hypointense (compared to high T1 signal of pancreas), variable signal on T2, and hypoenhancing on T1 C+ (with delayed enhancement)
- Commonly metastasizes to liver, peritoneum, and lung
- **Chronic Pancreatitis**
  - May produce fibroinflammatory mass in pancreatic head, appearing identical to ductal adenocarcinoma
    - Can result in double-duct sign similar to malignancy with pancreatic duct and biliary obstruction
    - May require biopsy or imaging surveillance to exclude malignancy
  - Other features of CP include dilated pancreatic duct and parenchymal/intraductal calcifications
  - Gland often appears diffusely atrophic (particularly body) with ↓ T1 signal and ↓ arterial enhancement on MR (with ↑ delayed enhancement)
- **Normal Anatomic Variants of Pancreas (Mimic)**
  - Pancreatic head can appear lobulated and enlarged but probably normal if enhancement is identical to rest of gland with no ductal obstruction
  - Asymmetric fatty infiltration of pancreatic head
    - Most commonly in anterior pancreatic head due to embryologic development of dorsal/ventral pancreas
    - May mimic hypodense mass on CT but sharply demarcated from normal density posterior head and not associated with mass effect or ductal obstruction
    - MR can confirm diagnosis easily with signal loss within "mass" on out-of-phase images
- **Mucinous Cystic Neoplasm**
  - Most often seen in middle-aged women and usually located in pancreatic tail
  - Typically cystic in appearance, but complex mucinous cystic neoplasm with invasive malignancy may show substantial soft tissue component and may mimic solid mass
  - No pancreatic duct communication or obstruction
- **Peripancreatic Lymphadenopathy (Mimic)**
  - Lymphadenopathy abutting pancreas may mimic pancreatic mass, especially metastatic lymphadenopathy from upper abdominal primary tumors
  - Gallbladder cancer classically results in bulky peripancreatic adenopathy and biliary obstruction, which can be mistaken for pancreatic cancer
- **Unopacified Bowel (Mimic)**
  - Collapsed duodenum/jejunum may mimic mass
- **Duodenal Diverticulum (Mimic)**
  - Diverticulum can abut pancreas and mimic hypodense mass (particularly when filled with fluid or debris)

Helpful Clues for Less Common Diagnoses

- **Pancreatic Serous Cystadenoma**
  - Lesions with preponderance of septations can appear solid without apparent microcystic component
    - Lesions can appear hypovascular or hypervascular
  - Lesions appear well circumscribed with lobulated contour and peripheral vascularity ± central calcification
- **Ampullary Carcinoma**
  - May not be easily distinguishable from pancreatic head adenocarcinoma
  - Can produce double-duct sign, although pancreatic duct only obstructed in ~ 50%

○ Usually does not cause upstream pancreatic atrophy
- **Pancreatic Metastases and Lymphoma**
  ○ Melanoma, lung, and breast are most common hypovascular metastases to pancreas
    – Lack of ductal obstruction and presence of primary tumor should suggest correct diagnosis
  ○ Primary lymphoma of pancreas is very rare, but pancreas can be secondarily involved in generalized lymphoma
    – Vessels surrounded by tumor without attenuation or narrowing (unlike ductal adenocarcinoma)
    – Bulky lymphadenopathy almost always present
- **Cholangiocarcinoma**
  ○ May not be easily distinguishable from pancreatic head adenocarcinoma or ampullary carcinoma
  ○ Obstructs bile duct but usually no pancreatic ductal obstruction or pancreatic atrophy
  ○ Can present as discrete mass or as focal common bile duct (CBD) wall thickening
- **Pancreatic Neuroendocrine Tumor**
  ○ Usually hypervascular but rarely hypovascular
  ○ Tumors may calcify or invade mesenteric veins, features uncommon with ductal adenocarcinoma
  ○ Does not typically obstruct pancreatic duct or CBD
- **Solid Pseudopapillary Neoplasm**
  ○ Typically well circumscribed, solid, and hypovascular but can demonstrate cystic component ± internal hemorrhage
  ○ Almost always diagnosed in young female patients
- **Acute Pancreatitis**
  ○ Focal inflammation or necrosis can be mass-like and mimic tumor
  ○ Tumor typically infiltrates posteriorly into retroperitoneum, whereas pancreatitis almost always infiltrates anteriorly into mesentery
  ○ Presence of dilated pancreatic duct or CBD should raise concern for malignancy
  ○ Pancreatic cancer can rarely (~ 5%) present with pancreatitis, so equivocal cases may require short-interval follow-up or endoscopic US
- **Autoimmune Pancreatitis**

○ Most often presents with diffuse pancreatic involvement, including sausage-like enlargement of pancreas, hypodense halo around pancreas, and lack of peripancreatic inflammation
○ Can rarely present as focal "mass"
○ Does not usually obstruct pancreatic duct or CBD, although IgG4 cholangiopathy can cause biliary dilatation
- **Groove Pancreatitis**
  ○ Form of CP that results in sheet-like, curvilinear soft tissue thickening (± cystic change) in pancreaticoduodenal groove
  ○ Can result in mild pancreatic or biliary ductal dilatation
  ○ Difficult to differentiate from pancreatic or duodenal malignancy and may require surgery for diagnosis
- **Agenesis of Dorsal Pancreas**
  ○ Pancreatic head may be hypertrophied (mimicking mass), while absent body/tail may be mistaken for atrophy upstream from mass
  ○ May also mimic mass on ERCP, as injection of ventral duct ends abruptly at head
- **Adjacent Masses (Mimic)**
  ○ **Duodenal Carcinoma**
    – Can be difficult to differentiate from pancreatic adenocarcinoma but does not usually cause pancreatic duct obstruction or parenchymal atrophy

Helpful Clues for Rare Diagnoses
- **Schwannoma**
  ○ Well-circumscribed, homogeneous mass (± cystic change)
  ○ Variable enhancement but most often mildly hypervascular (mimicking neuroendocrine tumor)
- **Giant Cell Carcinoma**
  ○ Large, heterogeneous, hypodense mass most often arising from pancreatic body/tail
- **Acinar Cell Carcinoma**
  ○ Large, well-circumscribed mass with cystic/necrotic degeneration and frequent exophytic component
  ○ Does not usually cause pancreatic duct or CBD dilatation
  ○ More often confused with neuroendocrine tumors due to well-circumscribed margins and enhancement

Pancreatic Ductal Adenocarcinoma

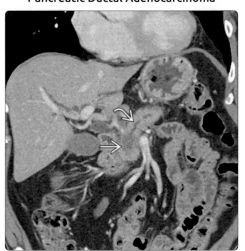

Pancreatic Ductal Adenocarcinoma

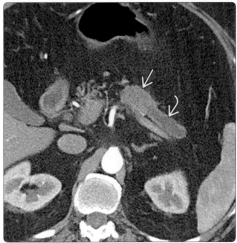

(Left) *Coronal CECT demonstrates an ill-defined, hypodense mass* ➡ *in the pancreatic head with upstream pancreatic ductal dilatation* ➡*, a classic appearance for pancreatic adenocarcinoma.* **(Right)** *Axial CECT demonstrates a hypodense mass* ➡ *in the pancreatic body with a markedly atrophic upstream pancreas and upstream pancreatic ductal dilatation* ➡*, representing pancreatic adenocarcinoma.*

Hypovascular Pancreatic Mass

Chronic Pancreatitis

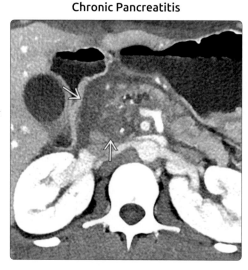

Chronic Pancreatitis

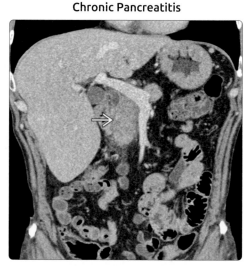

(Left) *Axial CECT demonstrates a large, hypodense mass* ➡ *in the pancreatic head with multiple internal calcifications, compatible with a fibroinflammatory mass related to chronic pancreatitis (CP). Close surveillance or biopsy may be necessary to exclude malignancy.* **(Right)** *Coronal CECT demonstrates mass-like enlargement* ➡ *of the pancreatic head/uncinate. Although thought to be a pancreatic adenocarcinoma, this was ultimately proven to be a fibroinflammatory mass related to CP.*

Normal Anatomic Variants of Pancreas (Mimic)

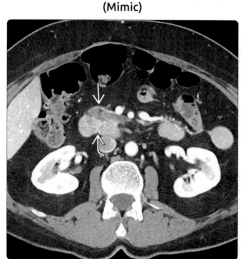

Mucinous Cystic Neoplasm

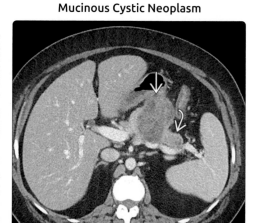

(Left) *Axial CECT demonstrates the characteristic appearance of focal fatty infiltration of the dorsal anlage. Note the low-density area in the anterior head* ➡ *(without ductal dilatation) clearly demarcated from the normal-appearing posterior head* ➡. **(Right)** *Axial CECT demonstrates a mucinous cystic neoplasm (MCN) with malignant degeneration. The mass* ➡ *itself appears predominantly solid with upstream pancreatic atrophy* ➡, *features strongly suggestive of malignancy.*

Peripancreatic Lymphadenopathy (Mimic)

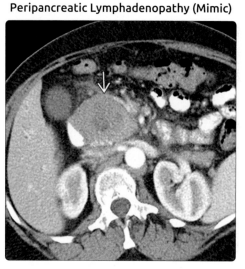

Pancreatic Serous Cystadenoma

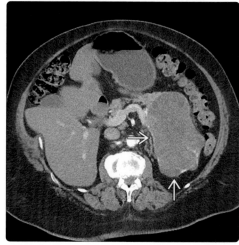

(Left) *Axial CECT demonstrates a large lymph node mass* ➡ *near the pancreatic head in a patient with lymphoma, a finding that could theoretically be confused for a primary pancreatic mass.* **(Right)** *Axial CECT demonstrates a lobulated, well-circumscribed mass* ➡ *arising from the pancreatic tail. The mass appears relatively solid with some subtle internal cystic components. This represents a serous cystadenoma, which can appear solid when septations predominate over cystic components.*

Hypovascular Pancreatic Mass

Ampullary Carcinoma

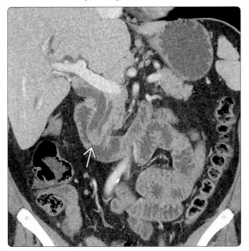

Pancreatic Metastases and Lymphoma

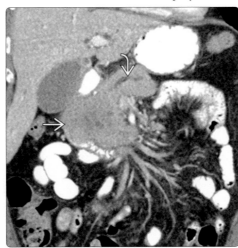

(Left) Coronal CECT demonstrates a mass ➡ centered near the ampulla, found to be an ampullary carcinoma at resection. (Right) Coronal CECT demonstrates a hypodense mass ➡ in the pancreatic head, resulting in mild obstruction of the pancreatic duct ⤵. This is an unusual case of pancreatic lymphoma, which does not usually obstruct the common bile duct (CBD) or pancreatic duct and is usually associated with more significant lymphadenopathy.

Pancreatic Metastases and Lymphoma

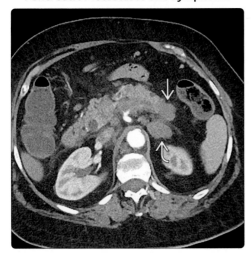

Pancreatic Metastases and Lymphoma

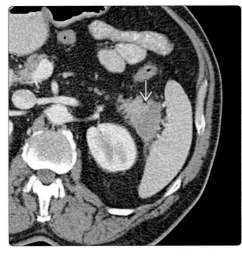

(Left) Axial CECT demonstrates an ill-defined mass in the pancreatic tail ➡ along with a left adrenal mass ⤵, both of which represent metastases from the patient's known breast cancer. (Right) Axial CECT demonstrates an infiltrative hypodense mass ➡ in the pancreatic tail. While pancreatic adenocarcinoma could appear virtually identical, this lesion represents a metastasis from the patient's lung cancer.

Pancreatic Metastases and Lymphoma

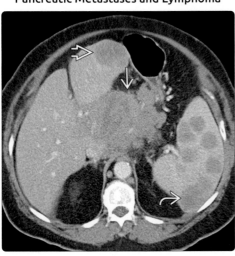

Cholangiocarcinoma

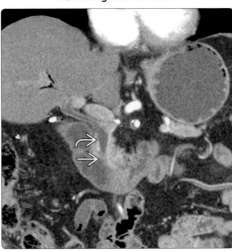

(Left) Axial CECT shows an infiltrative hypodense mass that infiltrates the pancreas ➡, along with additional lesions in the liver ⤵ and spleen ⤵, representing manifestations of the patient's non-Hodgkin lymphoma. (Right) Coronal CECT demonstrates a subtle hypodense mass ➡ obstructing distal CBD ⤵, found to be distal cholangiocarcinoma (CCA) at resection. Distal CCA can sometimes be difficult to differentiate from pancreatic head adenocarcinoma or ampullary carcinoma.

Solid Pseudopapillary Neoplasm

Acute Pancreatitis

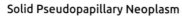
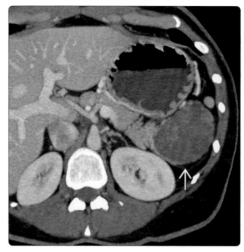
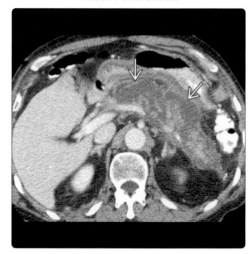

(Left) *Axial volume-rendered CECT in a young female patient demonstrates a well-circumscribed, hypodense mass* ⮕ *in the pancreatic tail with some internal heterogeneity, representing a solid pseudopapillary tumor.* (Right) *Axial CECT shows a heterogeneous, hypodense, mass-like enlargement* ⮕ *of the pancreas due to necrotizing pancreatitis. Such patients are invariably very ill with metabolic derangements that help to distinguish them from patients with an infiltrating carcinoma of the pancreas.*

Autoimmune Pancreatitis

Autoimmune Pancreatitis

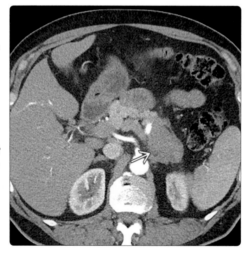
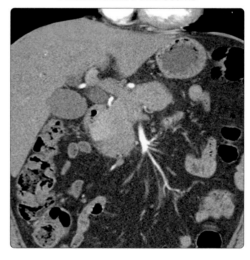

(Left) *Axial CECT demonstrates a focal hypodense mass* ⮕ *in the pancreatic tail. While virtually indistinguishable from an adenocarcinoma on imaging, this was found to be focal autoimmune pancreatitis at resection.* (Right) *Coronal CECT shows mass-like enlargement of the pancreas, particularly conspicuous in the pancreatic head and uncinate. The presence of an elevated serum IgG4 and resolution of all imaging findings with steroid medication confirmed the diagnosis of autoimmune pancreatitis.*

Groove Pancreatitis

Groove Pancreatitis

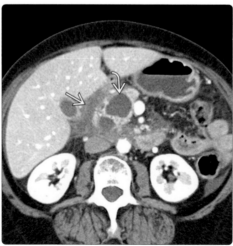
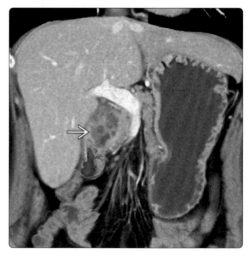

(Left) *Axial CECT demonstrates a hypodense, sheet-like mass* ⮕ *in groove between the pancreatic head and 2nd portion of duodenum, along with several cysts* ⮕ *in the pancreatic head and in the groove itself. These findings are classic for groove pancreatitis.* (Right) *Coronal volume-rendered CECT demonstrates sheet-like soft tissue* ⮕ *centered in the pancreaticoduodenal groove with internal cystic foci. Virtually impossible to differentiate from malignancy, this was found to be groove pancreatitis at resection.*

Duodenal Carcinoma

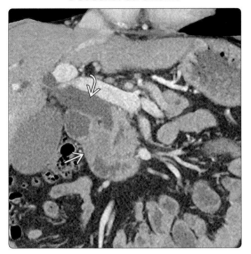

Gastrointestinal Stromal Tumor

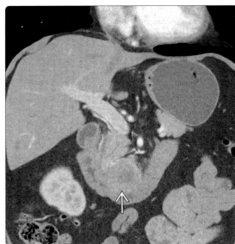

(Left) Coronal CECT demonstrates an annular constricting mass ➡ in the duodenum resulting in mild CBD dilatation ➡, found to be a duodenal adenocarcinoma at resection. (Right) Coronal CECT demonstrates a mildly enhancing mass ➡ centered between the duodenum and pancreatic head, mimicking a primary pancreatic mass. This was found to be a duodenal gastrointestinal stromal tumor at resection.

Retroperitoneal Sarcoma

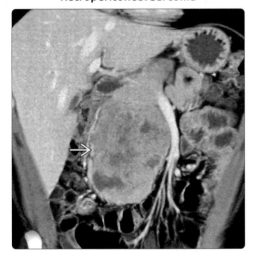

Adrenal Carcinoma

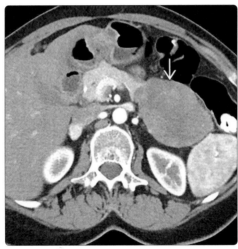

(Left) Coronal CECT demonstrates a large, mixed solid/cystic mass ➡ in the retroperitoneum, abutting the pancreatic head but with an intervening fat plane. In cases like this with large masses, the site of origin can be difficult to determine, but this was a primary retroperitoneal sarcoma arising from the IVC. (Right) Axial CECT shows a large, hypodense mass ➡ centered near pancreatic tail. While originally thought to be a primary pancreatic mass, this was found at resection to be an adrenal carcinoma abutting the pancreas.

Pheochromocytoma

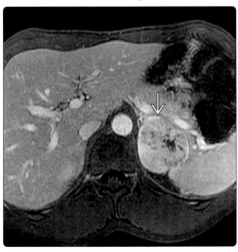

Acinar Cell Carcinoma

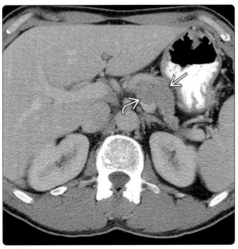

(Left) Axial T1 C+ MR shows a heterogeneous left upper quadrant mass ➡ with internal heterogeneity and enhancement, representing a large adrenal pheochromocytoma. (Right) Axial CECT demonstrates a hypodense mass ➡ in the pancreatic tail with immediately contiguous tumor thrombus in the splenic vein ➡, representing a surgically proven acinar cell carcinoma.

DIFFERENTIAL DIAGNOSIS

Common

- Pancreatic Neuroendocrine Tumor

Less Common

- Pancreatic Metastases
- Pancreatic Serous Cystadenoma
- Accessory Spleen (Mimic)
- Peripancreatic Vascular Abnormalities
- Retroperitoneal Paraganglioma (Mimic)
- Adrenal Pheochromocytoma (Mimic)
- Renal Cell Carcinoma (Mimic)
- Gastrointestinal Stromal Tumor (Mimic)
- Carcinoid Tumor (Mimic)
- Splenic Tumors (Mimic)
- Pancreatic Solid and Pseudopapillary Neoplasm

Rare but Important

- Acinar Cell Carcinoma
- Pancreatic Schwannoma
- Solitary Fibrous Tumor

ESSENTIAL INFORMATION

Key Differential Diagnosis Issues

- Differentiate pancreatic masses from lesions originating from adjacent organs (stomach, spleen, adrenal, kidney)
  - Look for fat plane separating mass and pancreas
    - Multiplanar reformations often helpful for identifying true origin of lesion
  - Confident distinction between pancreatic and peripancreatic masses not always possible, although prospective distinction may not alter surgical treatment
- Vast majority of hypervascular lesions truly arising from pancreas itself represent neuroendocrine tumors
  - Consider possibility of neuroendocrine tumor strongly in patients with predisposing syndromes, including MEN1, von Hippel-Lindau, and tuberous sclerosis
- While pancreatic neuroendocrine tumors are more common, always consider metastases in patients with history of renal cell carcinoma (RCC) or prior nephrectomy
  - RCC can metastasize to pancreas many years after initial surgical resection of renal tumor
- Always consider possibility of benign accessory spleen when confronted with hypervascular lesion near pancreatic tail, and recommend nuclear medicine study (Tc-99m heat-denatured RBC study) in equivocal cases

Helpful Clues for Common Diagnoses

- **Pancreatic Neuroendocrine Tumor**
  - Can be benign or malignant but much better prognosis compared to pancreatic adenocarcinoma
  - Now divided into syndromic and nonsyndromic tumors depending on whether lesion produces clinical syndrome due to hormone secretion
    - Syndromic tumors (such as insulinomas, gastrinomas, glucagonomas, etc.) tend to be smaller (< 3 cm) at presentation
    - Nonsyndromic tumors are often larger and more heterogeneous/aggressive in appearance with more frequent necrosis, cystic change, and calcification

- Well-circumscribed, hypervascular mass with noninfiltrative margins and frequent internal calcifications (either central or diffuse)
  - Usually avidly vascular and typically most conspicuous on arterial phase but can (in atypical cases) be more evident on venous phase or appear hypodense
  - Cystic/necrotic degeneration and internal calcification (central or diffuse) more common with larger tumors
    □ Tumors can rarely appear primarily cystic (with peripheral mural enhancement) and mimic other cystic pancreatic neoplasms
  - Most often no biliary or pancreatic ductal obstruction unless lesion is large or in rare cases where tumors secrete hormones (such as serotonin) that result in ductal stricture
  - May invade (rather than encase) mesenteric veins with resultant tumor thrombus (extremely uncommon in pancreatic adenocarcinoma), which probably increases risk for development of liver metastases
  - Metastases (most often liver and lymph nodes) have similar imaging characteristics to primary tumor
    □ Liver metastases may be very hyperintense (mimicking cysts or hemangiomas) and demonstrate internal fluid-fluid levels on T2 MR

Helpful Clues for Less Common Diagnoses

- **Pancreatic Metastases**
  - RCC is most common source of hypervascular metastases to pancreas, indistinguishable from neuroendocrine tumors in absence of history
  - Patients may present with pancreatic metastases from RCC many years (median: 11) after nephrectomy
  - RCC metastases appear as hypervascular lesions, which can be solitary or multiple, usually do not obstruct pancreatic or biliary ducts, and do not typically result in upstream parenchymal atrophy
  - Isolated RCC metastasis to pancreas may be amenable to surgical resection
- **Pancreatic Serous Cystadenoma**
  - Classic microcystic or sponge lesion is mass with multiple internal enhancing septations, multiple (> 6) small internal cystic spaces, and central calcification
  - Lesions with extensive internal septations that predominate over cystic spaces may appear solid and avidly enhancing (i.e., solid serous adenoma) without appreciable cystic component
    - May have central scar with calcification (similar to classic microcystic serous cystadenoma)
    - Does not usually obstruct pancreatic or biliary ducts
    - Often associated with considerable neovascularity, including hypertrophied feeding vessels "draped" around margins of mass
    - MR might better demonstrate internal cystic component or microcystic architecture in some cases
- **Accessory Spleen (Mimic)**
  - Benign ectopic splenic tissue of congenital origin usually located near splenic hilum
  - Pancreatic tail is 2nd most common location for splenules (20% of cases)
    - Usually located < 3 cm from pancreatic tail

○ Diagnosis usually easier with multiphase imaging, as splenule should follow enhancement pattern of normal spleen on all phases
  – Arterial phase often most valuable, as splenules demonstrate serpiginous differential enhancement of red and white pulp (similar to normal spleen)
  – Follow signal of normal spleen on all MR sequences
  – Tc-99m sulfur colloid or Tc-99m heat-denatured RBC scans utilized for differentiation in difficult cases

- **Peripancreatic Vascular Abnormalities**
  ○ Aneurysms or pseudoaneurysms (particularly those arising from splenic artery, gastroduodenal artery, or pancreaticoduodenal arcade) may mimic vascular mass
    – Should follow blood pool on all phases and communicate with adjacent vasculature
    – Pseudoaneurysms in these vessels often sequelae of prior pancreatitis (or more rarely from prior trauma)
  ○ Large splenic or portal vein abutting pancreas or varices may superficially mimic pancreatic mass
- **Retroperitoneal Paraganglioma (Mimic)**
  ○ Neuroendocrine tumors arising from autonomic nervous system usually in young to middle-aged patients
  ○ Avidly enhancing retroperitoneal mass that may abut pancreas and mimic primary pancreatic mass
- **Adrenal Pheochromocytoma (Mimic)**
  ○ Pheochromocytoma arising from left adrenal gland may abut pancreatic tail and mimic pancreatic mass
  ○ Lesions avidly enhance and classically demonstrate Hounsfield attenuation > 100 on arterial-phase images
- **Renal Cell Carcinoma (Mimic)**
  ○ Masses (especially clear cell variant of RCC) arising from upper pole of left kidney may simulate pancreatic mass
- **Gastrointestinal Stromal Tumor (Mimic)**
  ○ GIST arising from stomach or duodenum may simulate mass in pancreatic body or head
  ○ Variable enhancement, but some lesions can appear markedly vascular and hyperenhancing
- **Carcinoid Tumor (Mimic)**
  ○ Lesion arising from duodenum/ampulla or mesenteric metastasis abutting pancreas may mimic pancreatic mass

○ Usually avidly vascular with frequent hypervascular locoregional lymphadenopathy
- **Splenic Tumors (Mimic)**
  ○ Hemangioma, angiosarcoma, or hypervascular metastases to splenic hilum could simulate mass in pancreatic tail
- **Pancreatic Solid and Pseudopapillary Neoplasm**
  ○ Encapsulated, solid mass almost always diagnosed in young female patients
  ○ Solid, encapsulated, well-circumscribed mass with frequent peripheral or internal calcification and variable internal cystic and hemorrhagic components
  ○ Almost never overtly hypervascular like pancreatic neuroendocrine tumors, although well-circumscribed morphology of these tumors can lead to these lesions being mistaken for neuroendocrine tumors

Helpful Clues for Rare Diagnoses

- **Acinar Cell Carcinoma**
  ○ Very rare pancreatic tumor that may be associated with hypersecretion of lipase and unique clinical syndrome (skin rashes, arthralgias, fevers, and fat necrosis)
  ○ Typically large, well-defined mass with enhancing capsule and tendency to exophytically extend from pancreas (usually without pancreatic or biliary ductal obstruction)
  ○ Variable enhancement (may be hypovascular or hypervascular) with frequent internal hemorrhage, necrosis, and cystic degeneration
- **Pancreatic Schwannoma**
  ○ Rare, typically benign mass that may be of pancreatic or peripancreatic origin
  ○ Well-circumscribed and often mildly hypervascular (albeit less vascular than neuroendocrine tumors)
- **Solitary Fibrous Tumor**
  ○ Rare, usually benign tumor that appears large, exophytic, and hypervascular
  ○ May demonstrate calcification, cystic change, or necrosis
  ○ Indistinguishable from pancreatic neuroendocrine tumor

Pancreatic Neuroendocrine Tumor

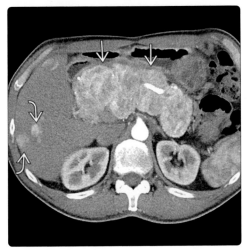

Pancreatic Neuroendocrine Tumor

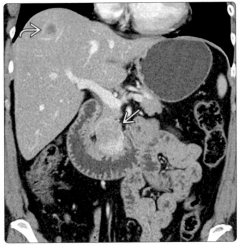

(Left) Axial arterial-phase CECT shows a massive, hypervascular mass ➡ involving nearly the entirety of the pancreas, representing a large neuroendocrine tumor. Note the presence of similar hypervascular metastases in the liver ➡. (Right) Axial CECT shows an enhancing mass ➡ between the pancreas and duodenum, found to represent a pancreatic neuroendocrine tumor at resection. Note the presence of an avidly enhancing liver metastasis ➡ as well.

(Left) *Coronal arterial-phase CECT shows an avidly enhancing pancreatic neuroendocrine tumor ➡. The pancreatic duct ➡ is obstructed by the mass, an unusual feature for neuroendocrine tumors.* (Right) *Axial arterial-phase CECT shows a markedly hypervascular mass ➡ arising from the pancreatic body, compatible with a neuroendocrine tumor. Note the upstream atrophy ➡ of the pancreas, a relatively unusual feature for neuroendocrine tumors.*

Pancreatic Neuroendocrine Tumor
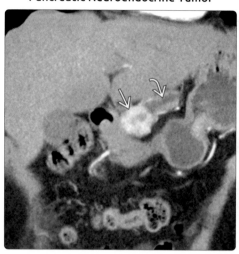

Pancreatic Neuroendocrine Tumor
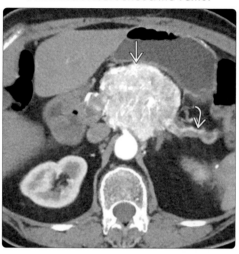

(Left) *Axial CECT shows an avidly enhancing neuroendocrine tumor ➡ in the pancreatic head. These lesions are almost always most conspicuous in the arterial phase of enhancement.* (Right) *Coronal T2 HASTE MR in the same patient shows the hyperintense mass ➡. Neuroendocrine tumors on MR imaging tend to be T1 hypointense and T2 hyperintense with similar enhancement characteristics on postcontrast images compared to CT.*

Pancreatic Neuroendocrine Tumor
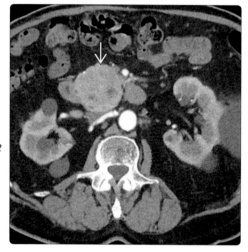

Pancreatic Neuroendocrine Tumor
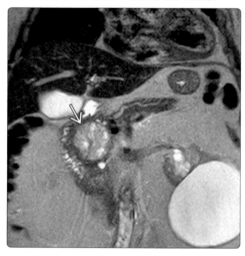

(Left) *Axial arterial-phase CECT shows a hypervascular mass ➡ arising from the pancreatic head. Indistinguishable from neuroendocrine tumor, this was found to be a solid serous cystadenoma at resection.* (Right) *Axial CECT shows an enhancing "mass" ➡ near the pancreatic tail with identical enhancement to the spleen. This was unfortunately resected under the belief that it represented a pancreatic neuroendocrine tumor but was found to represent a benign splenule at resection.*

Pancreatic Serous Cystadenoma
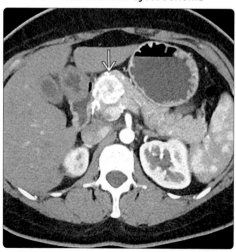

Accessory Spleen (Mimic)
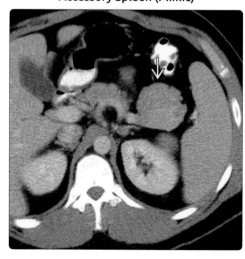

Retroperitoneal Paraganglioma (Mimic)

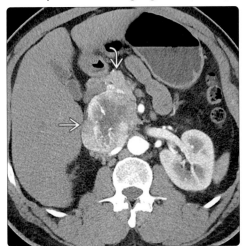

Renal Cell Carcinoma (Mimic)

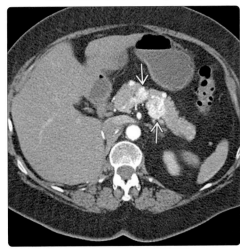

(Left) *Axial CECT shows a hypervascular mass* ➡ *in the retroperitoneum. Note that the mass abuts the pancreas* ➡ *but does not appear to be arising from the pancreas itself. This was found to be a paraganglioma at resection.* (Right) *Axial arterial-phase CECT shows multiple hypervascular lesions in the pancreas* ➡. *While these could represent multiple neuroendocrine tumors, absence of the right kidney (not shown) suggests the correct diagnosis of metastatic renal cell carcinoma (RCC).*

Renal Cell Carcinoma (Mimic)

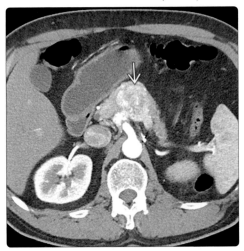

Gastrointestinal Stromal Tumor (Mimic)

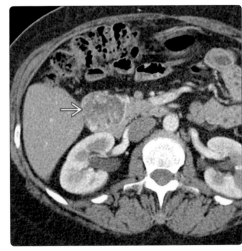

(Left) *Axial arterial-phase CECT shows a large, hypervascular mass* ➡ *in the pancreatic head. The clue to the diagnosis in this case is the absent left kidney, suggesting a metastasis from RCC.* (Right) *Axial CECT shows a hypervascular mass* ➡ *near the pancreatic head. While the mass does abut the pancreas, this was found to be a duodenal gastrointestinal stromal tumor (GIST) at resection.*

Carcinoid Tumor (Mimic)

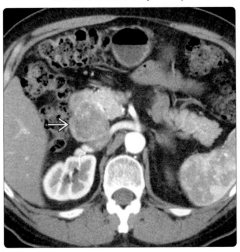

Acinar Cell Carcinoma

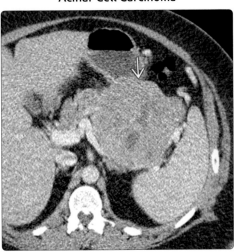

(Left) *Axial CECT shows a hypervascular mass* ➡ *abutting the pancreatic head. On careful examination, the mass arises from the duodenum (not the pancreas) and was found to be a duodenal carcinoid tumor at resection.* (Right) *Axial CECT shows a large, enhancing mass* ➡ *in the pancreatic tail. While a neuroendocrine tumor was prospectively thought to be most likely, this was found to represent a rare acinar cell carcinoma at resection.*

DIFFERENTIAL DIAGNOSIS

Common

- Intraductal Papillary Mucinous Neoplasm
- Pancreatic Pseudocyst
- Pancreatic Serous Cystadenoma
- Mucinous Cystic Neoplasm
- Lesser Sac Ascites (Mimic)
- Duodenal Diverticulum (Mimic)

Less Common

- Solid Pseudopapillary Neoplasm
- Pancreatic Neuroendocrine Tumor
- Pancreatic Ductal Adenocarcinoma
- Nonneoplastic Pancreatic Cysts
  - Autosomal Dominant Polycystic Disease
  - Cystic Fibrosis
  - von Hippel-Lindau Disease
- Lymphoepithelial Cyst
- Pseudoaneurysm (Mimic)
- Portal Vein Aneurysm (Mimic)
- Metastases and Lymphoma
- Gastrointestinal Stromal Tumor (Mimic)
- Choledochal Cyst (Mimic)

Rare but Important

- Hydatid Cyst
- Retroperitoneal Teratoma
- Duodenal Duplication Cyst

ESSENTIAL INFORMATION

Key Differential Diagnosis Issues

- Pancreatic cystic lesions are increasingly being discovered incidentally due to widespread use of CT and MR
- In many (but not all) cases, making specific diagnosis based on imaging alone may not be possible
  - Clinical history, demographics, and imaging must be used in conjunction to narrow differential diagnosis
    - Age and sex (e.g., young woman: Solid pseudopapillary neoplasm)
    - History of prior pancreatitis or imaging stigmata of chronic pancreatitis (suggestive of pseudocyst)
    - Location of lesion [e.g., body/tail for mucinous cystic neoplasm (MCN)]
    - Communication with pancreatic duct [favors intraductal papillary mucinous neoplasm (IPMN)]
    - Calcification within lesion (e.g., central calcification in serous cystadenoma)
    - Mural nodularity (worrisome for invasive malignancy)
  - Endoscopic US now routinely used in lesions judged to be at high risk based on CT/MR, providing high-resolution images of internal cyst architecture, facilitating cyst aspiration
- Pseudocysts are uncommon in absence of clear history of pancreatitis, and all cystic masses should therefore be considered potential neoplasms

Helpful Clues for Common Diagnoses

- **Intraductal Papillary Mucinous Neoplasm**
  - Most common in older men (50-70 years)

- Side-branch IPMN: Well-defined cystic lesion communicating with main pancreatic duct (MPD), which can be unilocular, multilocular, or tubular
  - Identifying communication of cyst with MPD is key to diagnosis and can be easier on MR
  - Mural nodularity suggests invasive malignancy; dilatation of MPD suggests main duct involvement
  - Often multiple with presence of multiple pancreatic cysts strongly suggesting multifocal IPMN
- Main-duct IPMN: Dilated (either segmental or diffuse), tortuous main pancreatic duct, which may demonstrate internal mural nodularity or calcification
  - ↑ risk of malignancy compared with side-branch IPMN
- Combined-type IPMN: Cystic lesion in communication with dilated main pancreatic duct

- **Pancreatic Pseudocyst**
  - Uncommon in absence of known history of pancreatitis or imaging features of chronic pancreatitis
  - Usually well-defined cystic lesion with clearly demarcated wall (± peripheral calcification)
  - Lesions adjacent to pancreas may demonstrate residual communication with pancreatic duct
  - May have internal septations but should not demonstrate mural nodularity or soft tissue component

- **Pancreatic Serous Cystadenoma**
  - Benign pancreatic tumor, which is most common in older women and is almost always incidentally identified
    - Most common in pancreatic head
  - 3 primary morphologic patterns
    - **Microcystic adenoma**: Honeycomb pattern with many (> 6) small (< 2 cm) internal cysts, enhancing septations, and central scar with calcification
    - **Macrocystic serous cystadenoma**: Oligocystic variant with few (or no) internal septations
      - □ Difficult to distinguish from MCN
    - **"Solid" serous adenoma**: Internal septations predominate over cystic component, producing apparently solid, hypervascular mass
  - Easier diagnosis on MR, which better delineates internal septations and microcystic morphology

- **Mucinous Cystic Neoplasm**
  - Almost always occurs in middle-aged women (99%)
  - "Macrocystic" lesion, which is either unilocular or composed of few (< 6) large (> 2 cm) locules
    - Most common in body or tail segments; may have calcification at periphery or in septations; thick wall, mural nodularity, or thick septations raise suspicion for malignancy
  - No communication with pancreatic duct (unlike IPMN)

- **Lesser Sac Ascites (Mimic)**
  - Most commonly seen in setting of acute pancreatitis, gastric ulcer, peritonitis, or peritoneal carcinomatosis; nonloculated fluid without definable wall bounded only by ligamentous margins of lesser sac

- **Duodenal Diverticulum (Mimic)**
  - Fluid-filled diverticulum arising from 2nd or 3rd portions of duodenum may simulate pancreatic head cyst, particularly when completely filled with fluid (without gas or enteric contrast)

Helpful Clues for Less Common Diagnoses

- **Solid Pseudopapillary Neoplasm (SPEN)**

- o Almost always in young women < 35 years of age
- o Well-defined, encapsulated mass, which is most often solid but can demonstrate variable internal cystic components and internal hemorrhage
  - – Frequent peripheral or central calcification (~ 50%); internal hemorrhage very characteristic and usually easiest to appreciate on MR
- **Pancreatic Neuroendocrine Tumor (PNET)**
  - o Some tumors can appear nearly completely cystic and can closely mimic other pancreatic cystic neoplasms
    - – Presence of mural nodularity or peripheral rim of hypervascularity on arterial-phase images should strongly suggest this diagnosis
  - o Larger tumors more likely to demonstrate cystic or necrotic degeneration
- **Pancreatic Ductal Adenocarcinoma**
  - o Very rarely cystic, although hypovascular or necrotic tumors may simulate cystic mass
  - o Tumors arising from underlying IPMN or MCN may demonstrate associated cystic component
- **Nonneoplastic Pancreatic Cysts**
  - o Relatively rare in absence of predisposing syndrome and in such cases may not be easily distinguished from pancreatic cystic neoplasms
    - – Usually simple in appearance without mural nodularity or other suspicious imaging features; do not typically communicate with pancreatic duct
  - o Most common predisposing syndromes include
    - – **Autosomal dominant polycystic disease**: Multiple asymptomatic cysts in pancreas and other organs (kidneys, liver)
    - – **Cystic fibrosis**: Pancreas can demonstrate 1 or multiple cysts (usually later in disease course)
    - – **von Hippel-Lindau disease**: Pancreas can demonstrate small, simple pancreatic cysts, as well as increased prevalence of serous cystadenoma
- **Lymphoepithelial Cyst**
  - o Rare benign cysts, which typically occur in older men
  - o Classically described as being complex in appearance with internal loculations and calcification

- – May demonstrate internal macroscopic or microscopic fat (usually easier to appreciate on MR)
  - o Usually appear extrapancreatic (abutting pancreas) or exophytic
- **Pseudoaneurysm (Mimic)**
  - o Thrombosed pseudoaneurysm arising from splenic or gastroduodenal artery can mimic cystic pancreatic mass (particularly when no residual internal flow)
- **Portal Vein Aneurysm (Mimic)**
  - o Portal vein can be markedly dilated, usually due to portal hypertension, and thrombosis of portal vein can theoretically simulate cystic mass in pancreas
- **Metastases and Lymphoma**
  - o Lymphoma is rarely truly cystic (in absence of treatment), although hypodense lymph nodes abutting pancreas can superficially mimic cystic lesion; metastases to pancreas or adjacent lymph nodes may appear cystic depending on primary tumor type
- **Gastrointestinal Stromal Tumor (Mimic)**
  - o Lesions arising exophytically from stomach or duodenum may simulate pancreatic mass; can appear cystic, necrotic
- **Choledochal Cyst (Mimic)**
  - o Cystic dilation of common bile duct (CBD) can simulate cystic pancreatic lesion, including fusiform dilatation of CBD itself or diverticulum arising from CBD; cystic lesion should be in contiguity with CBD, often easier to appreciate on MR/MRCP, not CT

Helpful Clues for Rare Diagnoses

- **Hydatid Cyst**
  - o Very rare diagnosis, even in endemic areas, although similar imaging features to hydatid cysts elsewhere; cystic mass, which may demonstrate multiple internal cysts (daughter cysts), serpiginous internal bands (water lily sign), or peripheral/internal calcification
- **Retroperitoneal Teratoma**
  - o Mature teratomas may appear primarily cystic but often demonstrate macroscopic fat or calcification
- **Duodenal Duplication Cyst**
  - o Most often arise along medial wall of 2nd/3rd duodenum, potentially mimicking pancreatic head cyst

---

Intraductal Papillary Mucinous Neoplasm

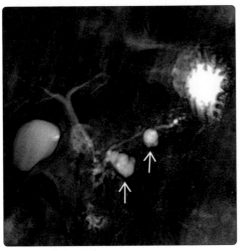

Intraductal Papillary Mucinous Neoplasm

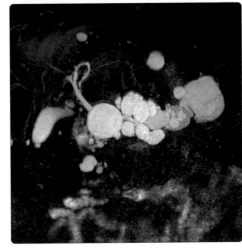

(Left) Coronal MRCP MIP demonstrates 2 cystic lesions ➡ directly communicating with the pancreatic duct in the head and tail, compatible with side-branch intraductal papillary mucinous neoplasms (IPMNs). MRCP is the best radiologic modality to demonstrate communication of a cyst with the pancreatic duct. (Right) Coronal MRCP MIP demonstrates innumerable pancreatic cysts replacing the entire pancreas, compatible with multifocal IPMNs. Multiplicity is a common feature of IPMN.

Intraductal Papillary Mucinous Neoplasm

Intraductal Papillary Mucinous Neoplasm

(Left) *Coronal CECT demonstrates a complex cystic lesion* ➡ *in the pancreatic head/uncinate with a cluster of grapes morphology.* (Right) *Coronal MRCP in the same patient demonstrates communication of the complex cystic lesion* ➡ *with the adjacent main pancreatic duct, a very typical imaging appearance for side-branch IPMN.*

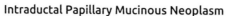
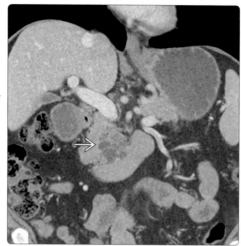
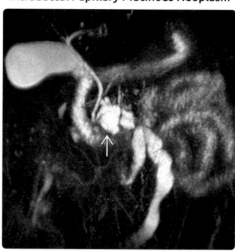

Pancreatic Pseudocyst

Pancreatic Pseudocyst

(Left) *Axial CECT in a patient with a known history of pancreatitis demonstrates a large cyst* ➡ *in the pancreatic tail. While a cystic neoplasm is certainly a possibility based on imaging alone, the patient's history allowed the correct diagnosis of a pseudocyst.* (Right) *Axial T2 FS MR in a patient with a history of recurrent pancreatitis demonstrates a pseudocyst* ➡ *in the pancreatic head with apparent communication* ➡ *with the pancreatic duct.*

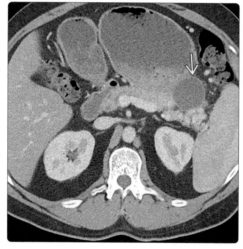
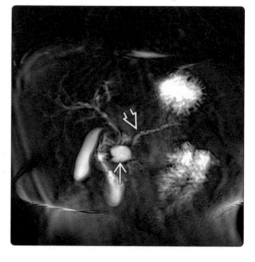

Pancreatic Serous Cystadenoma

Pancreatic Serous Cystadenoma

(Left) *Axial CECT demonstrates classic microcystic serous cystadenoma* ➡ *of the pancreas with innumerable internal tiny cystic components, enhancing septations, lobulated contour, and peripheral vascularity.* (Right) *Axial T2 FS MR demonstrates classic serous cystadenoma* ➡. *As seen in this case, the internal microcystic architecture of these lesions is almost always better assessed on MR.*

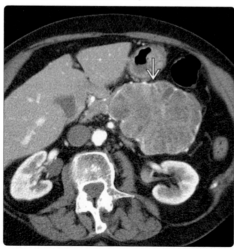
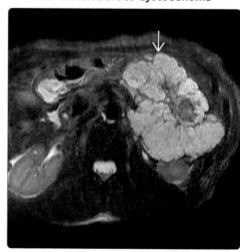

Mucinous Cystic Neoplasm

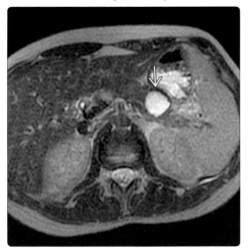

Mucinous Cystic Neoplasm

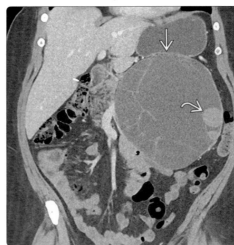

(Left) *Axial T2 MR demonstrates simple-appearing mucinous cystic neoplasm (MCN)* ➜ *in the pancreatic tail. As seen in this case, these lesions usually arise in the pancreatic tail and typically occur in middle-aged women.* (Right) *Coronal CECT show a large, complex cystic mass* ➜ *arising from the pancreatic tail with extensive internal septations and mural nodularity* ➚, *representing an MCN with invasive malignancy.*

Duodenal Diverticulum (Mimic)

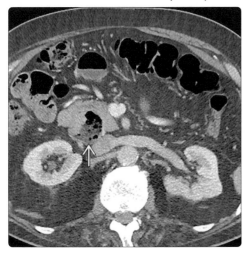

Solid Pseudopapillary Neoplasm

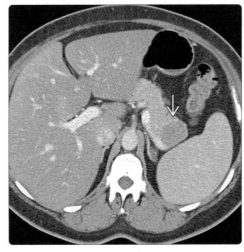

(Left) *Axial CECT demonstrates classic duodenal diverticulum* ➜ *filled with fluid and gas invaginating directly into the pancreatic head. When filled with fluid, diverticula can mimic a pancreatic cystic lesion.* (Right) *Axial CECT in a young woman demonstrates a homogeneous, hypodense lesion* ➜ *in the pancreatic tail found to be a solid pseudopapillary neoplasm (SPEN) at surgical resection, always a primary consideration when confronted with a pancreatic cyst in a young woman.*

Solid Pseudopapillary Neoplasm

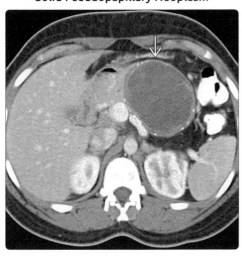

Pancreatic Neuroendocrine Tumor

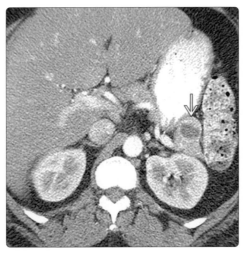

(Left) *Axial CECT shows a large, complex cystic mass* ➜ *arising from the pancreatic tail in a young woman, found to be a SPEN at resection. SPENs can demonstrate either peripheral or internal calcification, internal hemorrhage, and a combination of cystic and solid components.* (Right) *Axial CECT in the arterial phase demonstrates a cystic lesion* ➜ *in the pancreatic body with hypervascular solid component, a feature strongly suggestive of a cystic neuroendocrine tumor.*

(Left) *Axial T1 C+ MR demonstrates a cystic lesion* ⇨ *arising from the pancreatic tail. Note the subtle rim of enhancement around the margins of the cyst, a feature that allows the correct diagnosis of a cystic neuroendocrine tumor.* **(Right)** *Axial CECT demonstrates a pancreatic ductal carcinoma* ⇨ *with solid and cystic components. While pancreatic adenocarcinoma is rarely ever truly cystic, it can simulate a cystic mass due to internal necrosis or in cases when it arises from a cystic neoplasm (such as IPMN or MCN).*

Pancreatic Neuroendocrine Tumor

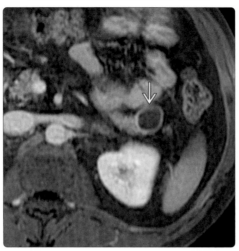

Pancreatic Ductal Adenocarcinoma

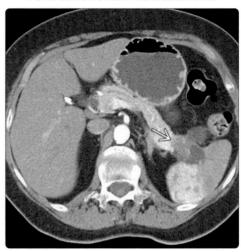

(Left) *Axial CECT in a patient with autosomal dominant polycystic kidney disease demonstrates cystic enlargement of both kidneys, as well as 1 cyst in the pancreas* ⇨*, likely due to the patient's syndrome.* **(Right)** *Axial CECT demonstrates a simple cyst* ⇨ *in the pancreatic head in a patient with cystic fibrosis (CF). Nonneoplastic simple cysts are a known feature of CF, most often in the later stages of the disorder.*

Autosomal Dominant Polycystic Disease

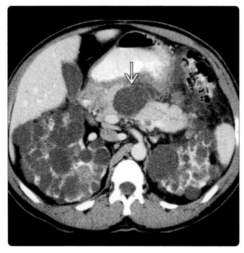

Cystic Fibrosis

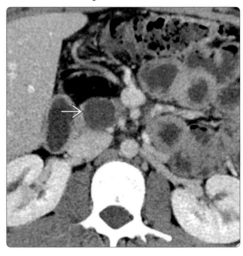

(Left) *Axial T2 MR demonstrates innumerable pancreatic cysts in a patient with von Hippel-Lindau disease.* **(Right)** *Axial CECT demonstrates a cystic lesion* ⇨ *abutting the pancreatic neck without evidence of internal mural nodularity or septa. This was found to be a lymphoepithelial cyst. These lesions can often appear to be extrapancreatic or exophytic.*

von Hippel-Lindau Disease

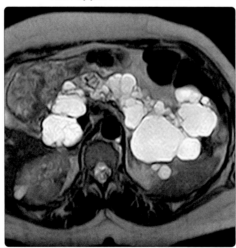

Lymphoepithelial Cyst

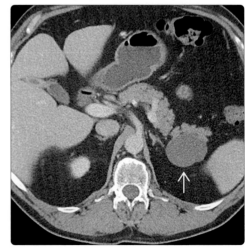

Lymphoepithelial Cyst

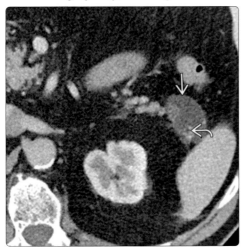

Pseudoaneurysm (Mimic)

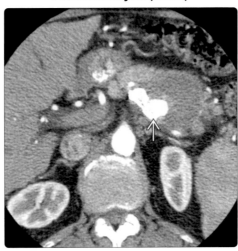

(Left) Axial CECT demonstrates a complex cyst ➡ abutting the pancreatic tail with internal mural nodularity and a subtle focus of macroscopic fat ➡. This lesion was found to be a lymphoepithelial cyst at resection. (Right) Axial CECT demonstrates a splenic artery pseudoaneurysm with enhancement ➡ of a portion of the pseudoaneurysm sac. The thrombosed portion of the aneurysm sac could superficially resemble a pancreatic cyst.

Choledochal Cyst (Mimic)

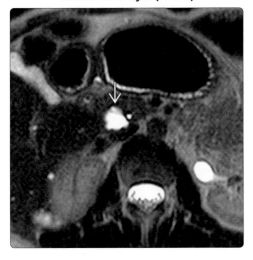

Choledochal Cyst (Mimic)

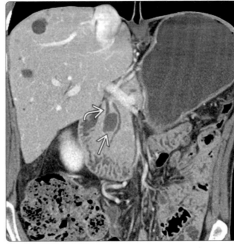

(Left) Axial T2 MR demonstrates a cystic lesion ➡ in the pancreatic head that superficially appears to be of pancreatic origin. (Right) Coronal CECT in the same patient better demonstrates that the cystic lesion seen on CT is actually a diverticulum ➡ arising from the common bile duct ➡, compatible with a choledochal cyst.

Hydatid Cyst

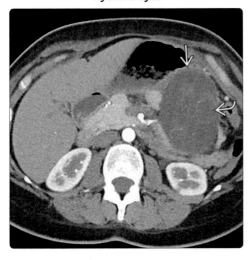

Hydatid Cyst

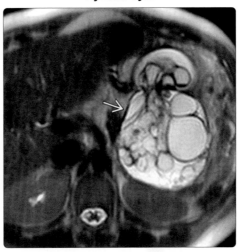

(Left) Axial CECT in a recent immigrant demonstrates a complex cystic lesion ➡ in the pancreatic tail with internal septations and subtle internal daughter cysts ➡. This was found to be an echinococcal cyst at resection. (Right) Axial T2 MR in the same patient better demonstrates the markedly complex internal architecture of this lesion ➡ with extensive internal septations and daughter cysts. The internal morphology of these lesions is often easier to appreciate on MR compared to CT.

DIFFERENTIAL DIAGNOSIS

Common

- Chronic Pancreatitis
- Senescent Change
- Obesity
- Diabetes Mellitus
- Cystic Fibrosis, Pancreas
- Cushing Syndrome and Steroid Medications

Less Common

- Asymmetric Fatty Infiltration (Normal Variant)
- Lipomatous Pseudohypertrophy
- Shwachman-Diamond Syndrome
- Agenesis of Dorsal Pancreas

ESSENTIAL INFORMATION

Key Differential Diagnosis Issues

- Fatty infiltration and atrophy do not necessarily imply pathologic condition
- Differentiate benign **diffuse** pancreatic atrophy from **upstream** pancreatic atrophy in setting of obstructed pancreatic duct (which raises concern for malignancy)
  - Pancreatic adenocarcinoma often obstructs pancreatic duct and results in severe atrophy of pancreas **upstream** from site of obstruction
  - Malignant atrophy not associated with fatty infiltration

Helpful Clues for Common Diagnoses

- **Chronic Pancreatitis**
  - Typically associated with parenchymal atrophy that is most apparent in body/tail
  - Other CT features include parenchymal/intraductal calcifications, dilated pancreatic duct, and pseudocysts
  - MR findings more sensitive for early chronic pancreatitis (CP), including ↓ T1 parenchymal signal, ↓ arterial phase enhancement, ↑ delayed enhancement, and duct side-branch ectasia
- **Senescent Change**

- Atrophy and fatty infiltration with mild pancreatic ductal dilation are normal findings in older patients
  - Can mimic CP, as older patients may also demonstrate small parenchymal calcifications, ↓ parenchymal T1 signal, and ↓ enhancement on MR
- **Obesity**
  - Particularly common in patients with type II diabetes
- **Cystic Fibrosis, Pancreas**
  - Commonly results in complete fatty replacement of pancreas (often by end of teenage years)
  - May also be associated with small pancreatic cysts
- **Cushing Syndrome and Steroid Medications**
  - Hypercortisolism (including cases secondary to steroid medications) can result in pancreatic fatty atrophy
  - Steroid medications more likely to result in fatty infiltration at higher doses for prolonged time periods

Helpful Clues for Less Common Diagnoses

- **Asymmetric Fatty Infiltration (Normal Variant)**
  - Focal accumulation of fat in anterior pancreatic head due to embryologic development of dorsal/ventral pancreas
  - Low-density area in anterior head of pancreas sharply demarcated from normal density posterior head
  - May simulate hypodense mass but should not demonstrate mass effect or ductal dilatation
- **Lipomatous Pseudohypertrophy**
  - Focal or diffuse enlargement of pancreas with fatty replacement (but preserved exocrine function)
  - Unknown etiology, but possibly potentiated by cirrhosis, viral infection, or abnormal metabolism
- **Shwachman-Diamond Syndrome**
  - Rare disorder characterized by pancreatic exocrine insufficiency, bone marrow dysfunction, and dwarfism
  - Can produce fatty infiltration similar to cystic fibrosis
  - Enlarged gland in early stages that gradually atrophies
  - No pancreatic calcifications or cysts (unlike cystic fibrosis)
- **Agenesis of Dorsal Pancreas**
  - Pancreatic head and uncinate are normal in appearance, while body and tail segments are either absent (complete agenesis) or truncated (partial agenesis)

(Left) *Axial CECT shows diffuse atrophy of the pancreas ➡, along with several pancreatic calcifications, findings that are virtually diagnostic of chronic pancreatitis.* **(Right)** *Axial NECT shows extensive fatty infiltration of the pancreas ➡ in an asymptomatic 80-year-old woman with no clinical evidence of pancreatic disease.*

Chronic Pancreatitis

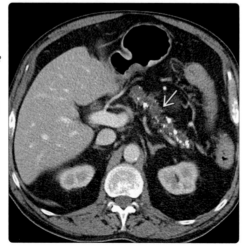

Senescent Change

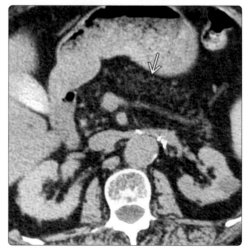

Cystic Fibrosis, Pancreas

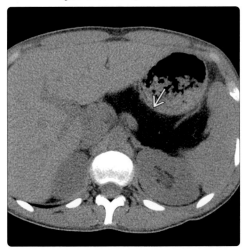

Asymmetric Fatty Infiltration (Normal Variant)

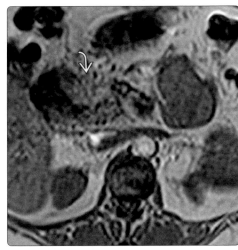

(Left) *Axial NECT in a patient with cystic fibrosis shows diffuse fatty replacement ⮞ of the pancreas. This finding is present in many cystic fibrosis patients by their late teenage years.* (Right) *Axial in-phase GRE MR shows homogeneous high signal in the entire pancreatic head ⮞.*

Asymmetric Fatty Infiltration (Normal Variant)

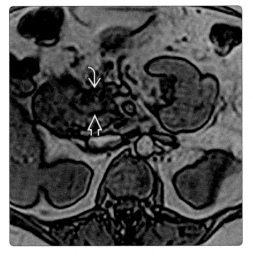

Lipomatous Pseudohypertrophy

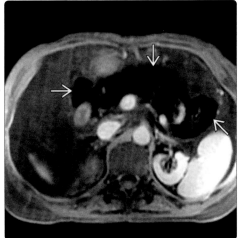

(Left) *Axial out-of-phase GRE MR in the same patient shows focal signal dropout in the anterior pancreatic head ⮞, characteristic of focal fatty infiltration. Note that the posterior pancreatic head ⮞ does not lose signal. MR is the best modality to confirm this diagnosis.* (Right) *Axial T1 C+ FS MR shows lipomatous pseudohypertrophy of the pancreas ⮞, likely attributable to chronic alcohol abuse and cirrhosis in this patient.*

Agenesis of Dorsal Pancreas

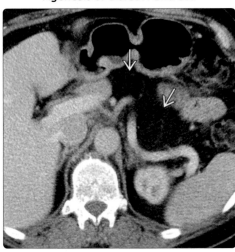

Agenesis of Dorsal Pancreas

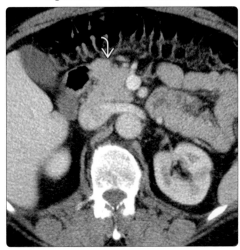

(Left) *Axial CECT incidentally shows absence of the pancreatic body and tail with fat attenuation ⮞ in place of the normal pancreatic parenchyma.* (Right) *Axial CECT in the same patient shows a normal appearance of the pancreatic head ⮞. This constellation of findings is compatible with agenesis of the dorsal pancreas.*

DIFFERENTIAL DIAGNOSIS

Common

- Pancreatic Ductal Adenocarcinoma
- Chronic Pancreatitis
- Senescent Change, Pancreas
- Intraductal Papillary Mucinous Neoplasm
- Pancreatic Divisum

Less Common

- Ampullary Carcinoma
- Duodenal Adenocarcinoma
- Pancreatic Neuroendocrine Tumor
- Choledocholithiasis
- Autoimmune Pancreatitis

ESSENTIAL INFORMATION

Key Differential Diagnosis Issues

- Normal pancreatic duct measures 3 mm in head, 2 mm in body, and 1 mm in tail
  - Normal duct should taper gradually toward body and tail
- Unexplained dilatation of pancreatic duct (in absence of clear stigmata of chronic pancreatitis) should raise concern for occult obstructing mass
  - Additional imaging features, which increase suspicion for obstructing mass
    - Abrupt or irregular narrowing of pancreatic duct
    - Pancreatic atrophy upstream from stricture
    - Double-duct sign [i.e., dilatation of both common bile duct (CBD) and pancreatic duct], which carries higher risk of malignancy compared to isolated dilatation of pancreatic duct alone
    - Locoregional lymphadenopathy or metastatic disease
  - In cases with such features, even if discrete obstructing mass is not visualized, endoscopic US may be necessary to exclude small occult obstructing lesion
- Pancreatic adenocarcinoma is, by far, most common tumor to obstruct pancreatic duct
  - Neuroendocrine tumors, lymphoma, metastases to pancreas, and focal autoimmune pancreatitis do not typically cause pancreatic ductal obstruction

Helpful Clues for Common Diagnoses

- **Pancreatic Ductal Adenocarcinoma**
  - Hypoenhancing, poorly marginated, infiltrative mass arising from pancreas
    - Tumors tend to be hypointense on T1 MR (nicely juxtaposed against hyperintense normal pancreas), have variable signal on T2 MR, and are hypoenhancing on T1 C+ MR
  - Mass results in abrupt narrowing of pancreatic duct with upstream ductal dilatation and parenchymal atrophy
    - CBD typically obstructed when tumor located in pancreatic head
    - Some tumors located in uncinate may not result in pancreatic or biliary ductal obstruction
  - Tumor commonly infiltrates posteriorly into retroperitoneum with frequent vascular encasement and narrowing

- 5% of all pancreatic adenocarcinomas are isodense to normal pancreas on CT, and secondary signs (dilated ducts, parenchymal atrophy) may be only clue to presence of subtle tumor
    - Endoscopic US may be necessary to identify these isodense lesions as well as very small masses, which are not discretely seen on CT
  - Bulky lymphadenopathy uncommon, but metastases most frequent to liver, peritoneum, and lungs
- **Chronic Pancreatitis**
  - Dilated, beaded pancreatic duct with multiple sites of stricture and associated diffuse pancreatic atrophy
    - Chronic pancreatitis is most common cause of benign pancreatic duct strictures, although benign strictures can also be seen in setting of prior trauma or surgery
  - Pancreatic parenchymal and intraductal calcifications virtually diagnostic of chronic pancreatitis
    - Intraductal stones/calcifications can obstruct pancreatic duct
  - Pseudocysts may be present and may demonstrate communication with pancreatic duct on MRCP
  - Focal fibroinflammatory mass (usually in pancreatic head) due to chronic pancreatitis can be very difficult (or impossible) to distinguish from malignancy
  - MR more sensitive (compared to CT) for early changes of chronic pancreatitis, including ectasia of pancreatic duct side branches, loss of normal T1 parenchymal signal, lack of duct distension with secretin, and ↓ exocrine function with secretin
    - Parenchyma may demonstrate diminished arterial-phase enhancement with increased delayed enhancement due to fibrosis
  - **Groove pancreatitis**, unusual form of chronic pancreatitis resulting in curvilinear soft tissue in pancreaticoduodenal groove, can also result in dilatation of upstream pancreatic duct and CBD
- **Senescent Change, Pancreas**
  - Mild pancreatic parenchymal atrophy and mild dilation of pancreatic duct are normal findings in older patients and should not be misinterpreted as pathologic enlargement
    - No published consensus on what duct diameter constitutes "mild" degree of dilatation
    - Even in cases of senescent dilatation, pancreatic duct should still taper normally toward body and tail (without any abrupt ductal cut-off)
    - No evidence of pancreatic duct strictures or intraductal stones
  - Older patients may demonstrate tiny foci of calcification, diminished parenchymal signal on T1 MR, and parenchymal hypoenhancement on T1 C+ MR, which can mimic chronic pancreatitis
  - Moderate or severe degrees of pancreatic ductal dilatation, particularly with evidence of abrupt ductal obstruction/cut-off, are not normal in older patients and should prompt further evaluation
- **Intraductal Papillary Mucinous Neoplasm**
  - Main duct or combined-type intraductal papillary mucinous neoplasm (IPMN) may result in diffuse or segmental dilatation of main pancreatic duct
    - Main pancreatic duct usually measures ≥ 5 mm
    - Amorphous calcifications may be seen within duct

- Pancreas often atrophic overlying dilated segments of duct
- Intraductal nodularity or soft tissue suggests presence of invasive malignancy
- Presence of discrete cyst communicating with dilated pancreatic duct suggests combined-type IPMN
  - Dilated duct may result in bulging of papilla of Vater into duodenum, and mucin may be seen extruding from ampulla on endoscopy
- **Pancreatic Divisum**
  - Anatomic variant of pancreatic ductal anatomy with dominant dorsal duct entering minor papilla, short ventral duct entering major papilla, and no communication between dorsal and ventral ducts
  - Dorsal pancreatic duct is commonly mildly dilated with loss of normal tapering toward pancreatic tail, likely due to functional stenosis or poor drainage of pancreatic secretions at minor papilla
    - Dilated duct may also be attributable to chronic pancreatitis due to association between divisum and pancreatitis
  - While diagnosis can be suggested based on CT, divisum easiest to appreciate on MRCP

Helpful Clues for Less Common Diagnoses

- **Ampullary Carcinoma**
  - Tumors arising from ampulla of Vater can be indistinguishable on imaging from pancreatic head adenocarcinoma or duodenal adenocarcinoma
  - Ampullary carcinoma encompasses several different histologic tumor types, each with variable prognosis
  - Lesions almost always obstruct CBD, but only ~ 50% of lesions obstruct pancreatic duct
  - Even lesions that obstruct pancreatic duct do not typically cause pancreatic parenchymal atrophy (unlike pancreatic adenocarcinoma)
- **Duodenal Adenocarcinoma**
  - Paraampullary duodenal adenocarcinomas involving ampulla may be difficult to distinguish from pancreatic head adenocarcinoma, although pancreatic atrophy and pancreatic ductal obstruction are uncommon

  - Look for tumor centered in duodenal wall or within lumen of duodenum
  - Other duodenal tumors (such as villous adenoma, carcinoid) can theoretically result in ductal obstruction
  - Duodenal adenocarcinoma has superior prognosis compared to ampullary and pancreatic adenocarcinoma
- **Pancreatic Neuroendocrine Tumor**
  - Well-circumscribed hypervascular tumor, which is typically best visualized on arterial-phase images
  - Neuroendocrine tumors do not typically cause pancreatic duct obstruction
  - Large tumors can obstruct pancreatic duct due to mass effect, and some small tumors have been shown to secrete hormones (especially serotonin) that may cause ductal stricture and obstruction
- **Choledocholithiasis**
  - Stone lodged in distal common channel can obstruct both pancreatic duct and CBD
  - Stones lodged in this location typically far easier to identify on MR compared to CT, although even MR can struggle with stones lodged in ampulla
    - Gallstones typically demonstrate low signal on all pulse sequences
  - May cause "gallstone pancreatitis" with edema and inflammation of pancreatic head
    - Correlate with history of sudden onset of pain and elevated pancreatic enzymes
- **Autoimmune Pancreatitis**
  - Diffuse form characterized by sausage-like enlargement of the pancreas with thin, peripancreatic, hypodense halo (which can demonstrate delayed enhancement), while focal form can present as focal mass mimicking primary pancreatic malignancy
  - Can result in focal (often multifocal) or diffuse pancreatic ductal narrowing, sometimes with mild pancreatic ductal dilatation upstream from these sites of narrowing
  - Faintly visible and narrowed pancreatic duct traversing pancreatic mass (duct-penetrating sign) can be seen with focal forms of autoimmune pancreatitis

Pancreatic Ductal Adenocarcinoma

Pancreatic Ductal Adenocarcinoma

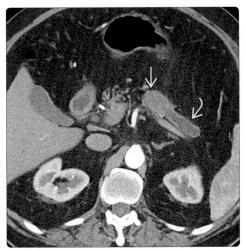

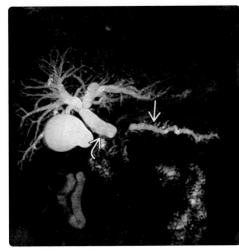

(Left) *Axial CECT shows a hypodense soft tissue mass ➡ in the pancreatic body causing abrupt obstruction of the dilated pancreatic duct ➡ along with marked upstream parenchymal atrophy, classic for pancreatic adenocarcinoma.* **(Right)** *Coronal MRCP shows the classic double-duct sign of pancreatic head adenocarcinoma with obstruction and dilatation of both the pancreatic ➡ and common bile ducts ➡.*

Pancreatic Ductal Adenocarcinoma

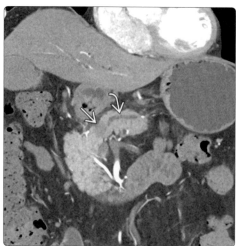

Chronic Pancreatitis

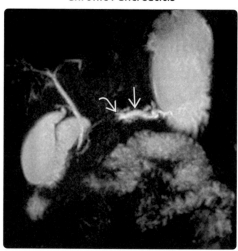

(Left) *Coronal CECT shows a subtle, hypodense mass* ➡ *in the pancreatic head causing dilatation of the pancreatic duct* ➡*, characteristic features of pancreatic adenocarcinoma.* (Right) *Coronal MRCP shows dilatation* ➡ *of the pancreatic duct in the body/tail segment, a focal stricture* ➡ *of the duct in the body, and ectasia of duct side branches. These findings were found to be secondary to chronic pancreatitis.*

Chronic Pancreatitis

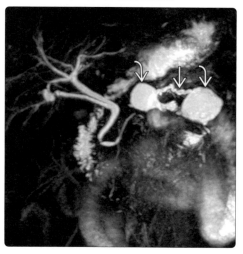

Chronic Pancreatitis

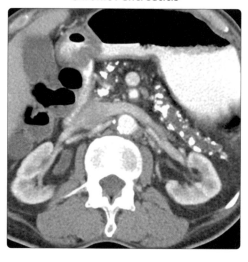

(Left) *Coronal MRCP with MIP reconstruction shows dilatation and beading of the pancreatic duct* ➡ *in the body/tail. At least 2 fluid collections* ➡ *appear to communicate with the pancreatic duct. This constellation of findings represents chronic pancreatitis with pseudocysts.* (Right) *Axial CECT shows an atrophic pancreas with a diffusely dilated pancreatic duct and multiple parenchymal/intraductal calcifications, features that are diagnostic of chronic pancreatitis.*

Intraductal Papillary Mucinous Neoplasm

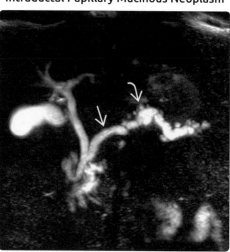

Intraductal Papillary Mucinous Neoplasm

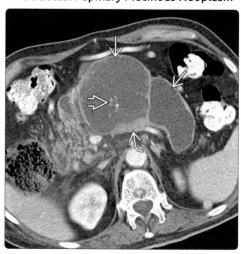

(Left) *Coronal MRCP with MIP reconstruction shows a diffusely dilated pancreatic duct* ➡ *with multiple dilated side branches* ➡*, found to represent a main-duct intraductal papillary mucinous neoplasm (IPMN) at surgery.* (Right) *Axial CECT shows a massively dilated main pancreatic duct* ➡ *with some internal calcifications* ➡ *and mural soft tissue* ➡*, confirmed to represent a main-duct IPMN at surgery.*

Pancreatic Divisum

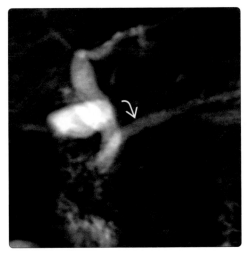

Ampullary Carcinoma

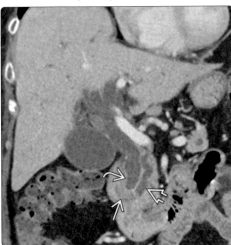

(Left) *Coronal MRCP with MIP reconstruction shows the main pancreatic duct ➘ crossing behind the common bile duct to enter the minor papilla, compatible with pancreatic divisum. As in this case, divisum can be associated with mild pancreatic ductal dilatation.* (Right) *Coronal CECT shows a mass ➡ centered at the ampulla obstructing both the common bile duct ➘ and pancreatic duct ➡. This was found to be an ampullary carcinoma at surgery.*

Ampullary Carcinoma

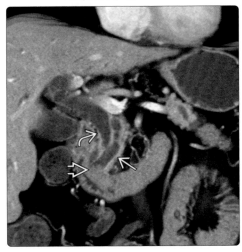

Duodenal Adenocarcinoma

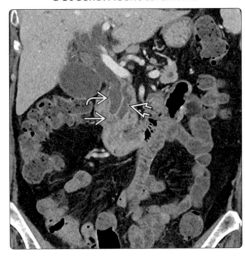

(Left) *Coronal volume-rendered CECT shows the double-duct sign with dilatation of both the common bile duct ➘ and pancreatic duct ➡. Subtle nodular tissue near the ampulla ➡ represents an obstructing ampullary carcinoma.* (Right) *Coronal CECT shows a soft tissue mass ➡ centered in the duodenum obstructing both the common bile duct ➘ and pancreatic duct ➡. This was found to be a paraampullary duodenal adenocarcinoma, which more commonly obstructs the common bile duct than the pancreatic duct.*

Pancreatic Neuroendocrine Tumor

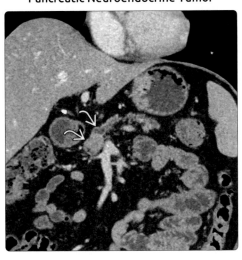

Pancreatic Neuroendocrine Tumor

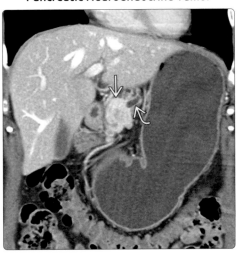

(Left) *Coronal CECT shows an enhancing mass resulting in dilatation of the pancreatic duct ➘ and resulting in upstream atrophy. Neuroendocrine tumors only rarely cause ductal obstruction due to large size/mass effect or secretion of hormones causing ductal stricture.* (Right) *Coronal CECT shows a hypervascular mass ➡ in the pancreatic head, representing a small neuroendocrine tumor. The ductal dilatation ➘ and atrophy in this case are atypical features.*

DIFFERENTIAL DIAGNOSIS

Common

- Acute Pancreatitis
- Pancreatic Ductal Carcinoma
- Anasarca
- Portal Hypertension
- Traumatic Pancreatitis
- Duodenal Ulcer
- Gastric Ulcer

Less Common

- Shock Pancreas
- Sclerosing Mesenteritis
- Autoimmune Pancreatitis
- Groove Pancreatitis
- Lymphoma
- Duodenal Diverticulitis
- Diverticulitis

ESSENTIAL INFORMATION

Key Differential Diagnosis Issues

- Any inflammatory or neoplastic process originating from structures abutting pancreas may cause infiltration of peripancreatic fat planes
  - Most commonly seen due to inflammatory conditions arising in anterior pararenal space (pancreas, duodenum, ascending colon, and descending colon)
  - Utilizing multiplanar reformations can help better determine source of inflammation
- Acute pancreatitis is overwhelmingly most common cause of infiltration of peripancreatic fat planes
- Clinical history is critical in formulating diagnosis, as several entities (e.g., traumatic pancreatitis, shock pancreas) can appear virtually identical to acute pancreatitis on imaging

Helpful Clues for Common Diagnoses

- **Acute Pancreatitis**
  - Pancreas typically appears enlarged and edematous with loss of normal fatty lobulation
    - Pancreas and surrounding fat planes can appear essentially normal in mild cases
  - Inflammation (including stranding and free fluid) spreads **ventrally** into mesentery and **laterally** within anterior pararenal space
    - May result in thickening of anterior perirenal (Gerota) fascia (forms posterior border of anterior pararenal space)
    - May produce reactive wall thickening of left/right colon and duodenum
  - Look for evidence of abnormal pancreatic enhancement to suggest necrotizing pancreatitis
  - Elevated lipase levels can confirm diagnosis
- **Pancreatic Ductal Carcinoma**
  - Hypodense, poorly marginated mass that tends to infiltrate **dorsally** into retroperitoneum to involve mesenteric vasculature
  - ~ 5% of patients with pancreatic cancer may present with clinical/biochemical signs of acute pancreatitis
    - Presence of dorsal infiltration, dilated pancreatic duct, common bile duct (CBD) obstruction, parenchymal atrophy, or metastatic disease should suggest presence of underlying tumor
- **Anasarca and Portal Hypertension**
  - Any entity that results in anasarca can cause generalized edema and infiltration, including edema of mesenteric and peripancreatic fat
  - Peripancreatic infiltration from anasarca or portal hypertension may be indistinguishable from that seen with acute pancreatitis, although generalized nature of edema should suggest correct diagnosis
- **Traumatic Pancreatitis**
  - Imaging features similar to acute pancreatitis, although clinical history and presence of fracture plane through pancreas, contusion, or peripancreatic hematoma suggest correct diagnosis
    - Fluid separating pancreas from splenic vein is sensitive sign of pancreatic injury
  - May not be evident immediately, can appear at 24-48 hr
  - May be associated with fluid collection/pseudocyst if trauma results in pancreatic duct disruption
- **Duodenal Ulcer**
  - Perforated duodenal ulcer may cause infiltration of right anterior pararenal space surrounding pancreatic head/neck
  - Multiplanar reformations may better demonstrate that inflammation is centered around duodenum (rather than pancreas)
    - Extraluminal gas or enteric contrast suggests correct diagnosis but may not always be present
  - Ulcer can rarely penetrate into pancreas and cause secondary pancreatitis
- **Gastric Ulcer**
  - Most commonly perforates into lesser sac (between posterior wall of stomach and pancreas)
    - Gastric wall usually thickened with adjacent inflammation
    - Extraluminal gas and enteric contrast allow confident diagnosis but may not always be present
  - Ulcer can rarely penetrate posteriorly into body of pancreas and cause secondary pancreatitis

Helpful Clues for Less Common Diagnoses

- **Shock Pancreas**
  - Part of hypoperfusion complex, which results from severe traumatic injury or hypotension
    - Most often seen after head/spine trauma or significant blood loss
    - Often victims of blunt trauma who were hypotensive on arrival to emergency department
  - Patients have usually been fluid resuscitated prior to CT scan, but mesenteric, bowel wall, and peripancreatic edema may persist (or worsen temporarily)
    - CT findings usually resolve within 24 hr
  - Pancreas appears enlarged and edematous with heterogeneous enhancement, mimicking both acute pancreatitis and posttraumatic pancreatitis
    - May be impossible to distinguish from traumatic injury by imaging alone, but lack of fracture plane and presence of other imaging signs of shock complex make traumatic pancreatitis less likely

- Other features of shock complex include diffuse small bowel wall thickening with mucosal enhancement, hyperenhancement of kidneys and adrenal glands, and small aorta/inferior vena cava
- **Sclerosing Mesenteritis**
  - Idiopathic inflammatory and fibrotic disorder affecting mesentery (a.k.a. retractile mesenteritis, fibrosing mesenteritis, or panniculitis)
  - Imaging appearance variable depending on acuity
    - Acute mesenteritis: Left upper quadrant "misty mesentery" with fat stranding and induration, thin surrounding pseudocapsule, and prominent mesenteric lymph nodes with halo of spared surrounding fat
      - □ Infiltrated fat planes usually in jejunal mesentery (caudal to pancreas), rather than truly peripancreatic
      - □ Any other cause of "misty mesentery" can infiltrate peripancreatic fat planes as well
    - Chronic mesenteritis: Fibrotic soft tissue mass with desmoplastic reaction and calcification
- **Autoimmune Pancreatitis**
  - Can involve pancreas diffusely (most common) or focally
  - Pancreas enlarged and edematous with thin, hypodense halo (which may demonstrate delayed enhancement)
  - General paucity of peripancreatic infiltration and fat stranding compared with acute edematous or necrotizing pancreatitis
  - Pancreatic duct is normal in size or narrowed (not dilated or obstructed)
  - Often associated with other autoimmune diseases, including retroperitoneal fibrosis, IgG4 cholangiopathy, and Riedel thyroiditis
    - Bile ducts may be dilated with wall thickening and hyperenhancement (especially distal CBD) as result of concomitant IgG4 cholangiopathy
- **Groove Pancreatitis**
  - Rare form of chronic pancreatitis resulting in sheet-like, curvilinear soft tissue thickening in pancreaticoduodenal groove (between 2nd portion of duodenum and pancreatic head)

- May be associated with cysts in groove and medial wall of duodenum
  - Can be very difficult to differentiate prospectively from pancreatic head adenocarcinoma or duodenal adenocarcinoma, and most patients ultimately undergo Whipple resection to exclude malignancy
- **Lymphoma**
  - Primary pancreatic lymphoma is very rare (usually in immunocompromised or older adult patients) with most cases representing secondary lymphomatous involvement of pancreas
    - Almost always significant lymphadenopathy elsewhere and other sites of lymphomatous involvement
  - Homogeneous soft tissue mass that may infiltrate pancreas and peripancreatic fat planes, potentially mimicking acute pancreatitis on imaging (but not clinically)
  - Tumor encases peripancreatic vasculature without attenuation, narrowing, or occlusion
  - No obstruction of CBD or pancreatic duct
  - No atrophy of pancreas upstream from mass
- **Duodenal Diverticulitis**
  - Duodenal diverticulum can perforate spontaneously or after intubation, resulting in surrounding inflammation
  - Inflammation can involve pancreatic head, simulating acute pancreatitis
  - Recognizing that inflammation is centered around diverticulum and presence of extraluminal gas or enteric contrast are keys to diagnosis
  - Duodenal diverticulum (especially when large) may be predisposing factor for acute pancreatitis
- **Diverticulitis**
  - Inflammation can extend into anterior pararenal space when diverticulitis originates from ascending/descending colon
    - May spread medially within anterior pararenal space to peripancreatic region, potentially simulating acute pancreatitis

Acute Pancreatitis

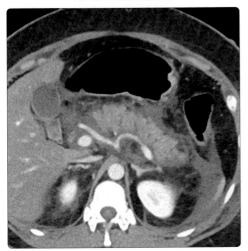

Acute Pancreatitis

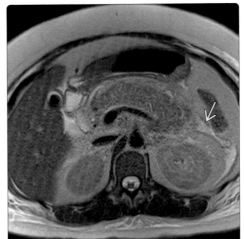

(Left) Axial CECT shows pancreatic edema with diffuse peripancreatic fat stranding and fluid, compatible with acute pancreatitis. (Right) Axial T2 MR shows enlargement of the pancreas with fluid tracking into the left anterior pararenal space ➡, compatible with acute pancreatitis.

Acute Pancreatitis

Acute Pancreatitis

(Left) *Axial CECT shows necrotizing pancreatitis with a fluid collection ➡ replacing much of the pancreatis and with only a portion of the normal pancreatic tail ➡ identified. Foci of internal gas ➡ are secondary to fluid aspiration (rather than gas-forming infection).* (Right) *Axial T2 FS MR shows edema in the pancreatic bed with a fluid collection ➡ replacing much of the pancreatic body and tail. Only a small portion of the normal pancreas ➡ is identified, compatible with acute necrotizing pancreatitis.*

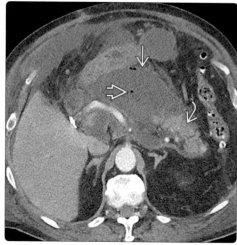

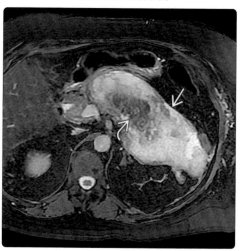

Pancreatic Ductal Carcinoma

Pancreatic Ductal Carcinoma

(Left) *Coronal CECT shows a subtle, hypodense mass ➡ in the pancreatic head resulting in dilatation of the upstream pancreatic duct ➡, representing pancreatic adenocarcinoma.* (Right) *Axial CECT shows an infiltrative mass ➡ arising from the pancreatic body with encasement of the celiac trunk ➡ and hepatic artery ➡, a classic appearance for pancreatic adenocarcinoma. Unlike pancreatitis, pancreatic adenocarcinoma infiltrates dorsally into the retroperitoneum.*

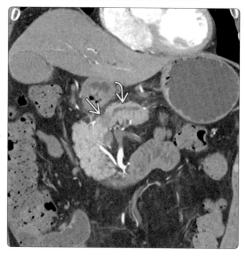

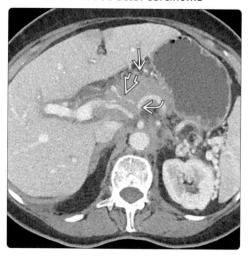

Pancreatic Ductal Carcinoma

Pancreatic Ductal Carcinoma

(Left) *Axial CECT shows diffuse tumor infiltration replacing the entire pancreas, a rare manifestation of pancreatic adenocarcinoma.* (Right) *Axial CECT shows a typical appearance of pancreatic adenocarcinoma as a hypodense mass ➡ resulting in marked atrophy ➡ of the upstream gland with upstream pancreatic ductal dilatation.*

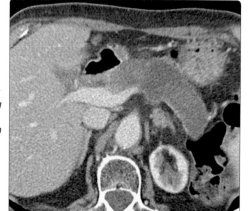

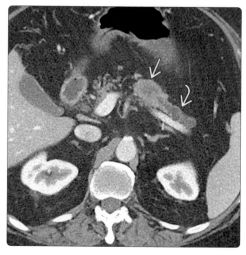

Portal Hypertension

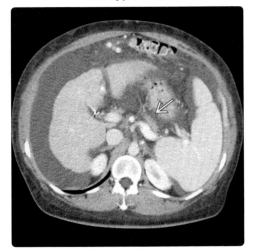

Traumatic Pancreatitis

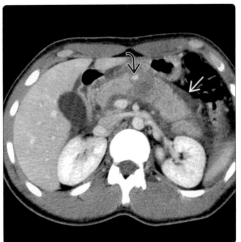

(Left) *Axial CECT shows cirrhosis with multiple stigmata of portal hypertension, including ascites, varices, and splenomegaly. In this setting, the resulting peripancreatic edema* ➡ *is impossible to distinguish from acute pancreatitis.* (Right) *Axial CECT shows a fracture plane through the pancreatic body with extensive peripancreatic edema* ➡ *and active bleeding* ⤷, *compatible with acute traumatic pancreatic injury.*

Traumatic Pancreatitis

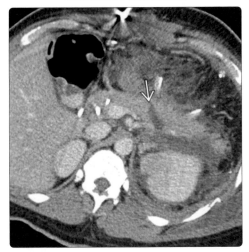

Duodenal Ulcer

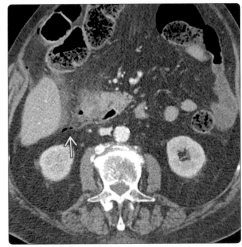

(Left) *Axial CECT after a gunshot wound to the abdomen shows a fracture plane* ➡ *through the pancreatic body with extensive peripancreatic fat stranding and fluid, compatible with posttraumatic pancreatic laceration with pancreatitis.* (Right) *Axial CECT shows inflammation adjacent to the duodenum with several foci of free air* ➡, *representing the sequelae of a perforated duodenal ulcer.*

Gastric Ulcer

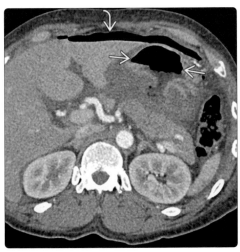

Shock Pancreas

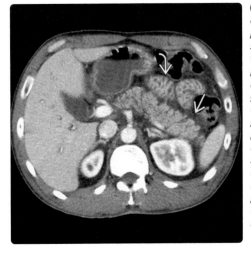

(Left) *Axial CECT shows an outpouching* ➡ *of gas and fluid projecting from the stomach with adjacent gastric wall thickening and large pneumoperitoneum* ➡, *representing perforated gastric ulcer.* (Right) *Axial CECT shows infiltration of fat planes* ➡ *around the pancreas, along with intense mucosal enhancement and submucosal edema of the entire small bowel* ➡ *(shock bowel). The pancreatic findings do not reflect direct traumatic injury, but rather, shock pancreas.*

Shock Pancreas

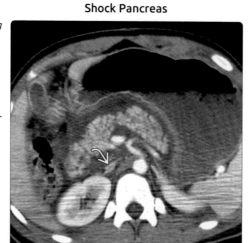

Sclerosing Mesenteritis

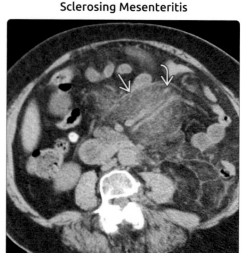

(Left) *Axial CECT in the setting of shock physiology shows marked edema/infiltration of the peripancreatic fat planes. Also note the collapsed cava sign* ➡️*, a flattened appearance of the inferior vena cava due to hypovolemia.* **(Right)** *Axial CECT shows extensive infiltration of the jejunal mesentery, caudal to the pancreas, with a thin capsule* ➡️ *and small mesenteric nodes* ➡️*, a classic appearance for sclerosing mesenteritis.*

Sclerosing Mesenteritis

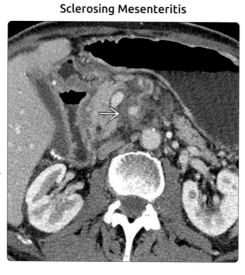

Autoimmune Pancreatitis

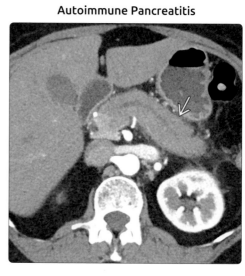

(Left) *Axial CECT shows ill-defined soft tissue* ➡️ *surrounding the superior mesenteric artery, initially thought to represent an uncinate process pancreatic adenocarcinoma. Surprisingly, this was found to represent sclerosing mesenteritis at biopsy.* **(Right)** *Axial CECT shows sausage-shaped enlargement of the pancreatic body with subtle infiltration of surrounding fat, seemingly limited by a thin capsule* ➡️*. This was found to be a manifestation of autoimmune pancreatitis.*

Autoimmune Pancreatitis

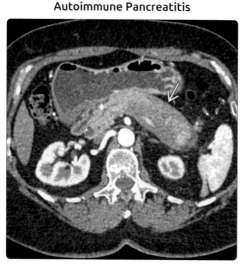

Autoimmune Pancreatitis

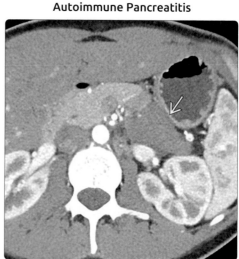

(Left) *Axial CECT shows induration* ➡️ *surrounding the pancreatic body and tail. This was found to represent autoimmune pancreatitis.* **(Right)** *Axial CECT shows a focal, hypodense mass* ➡️ *arising from the pancreatic tail. While indistinguishable on imaging from a pancreatic adenocarcinoma, this lesion resolved with steroid treatment and represents autoimmune pancreatitis.*

Groove Pancreatitis

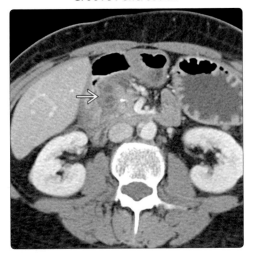

Groove Pancreatitis

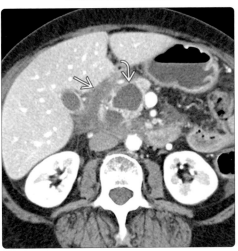

(Left) *Axial CECT shows hypodense soft tissue thickening* ➡️ *in the pancreaticoduodenal groove. Although malignancy was suspected, this was found to be groove pancreatitis at resection.* (Right) *Axial CECT shows soft tissue thickening* ➡️ *in the pancreaticoduodenal groove with several cysts* ➡️ *in the adjacent pancreatic head, representing groove pancreatitis.*

Lymphoma

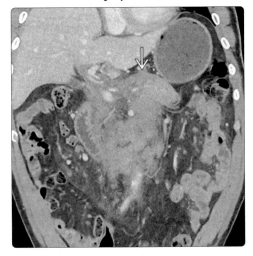

Lymphoma

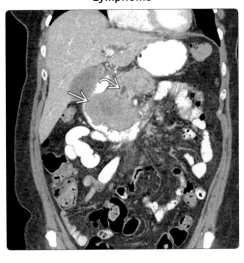

(Left) *Coronal CECT shows lymphomatous infiltration of the pancreas* ➡️*, which appears abnormally hypodense and infiltrated with extensive contiguous lymphadenopathy and soft tissue tracking downward into the mesentery.* (Right) *Coronal CECT shows a hypodense mass* ➡️ *in the pancreatic head, resulting in mild upstream pancreatic ductal dilatation* ➡️*. This was found to represent lymphoma on biopsy, although pancreatic ductal obstruction is an unusual feature.*

Lymphoma

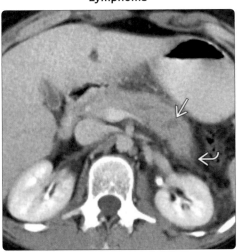

Duodenal Diverticulitis

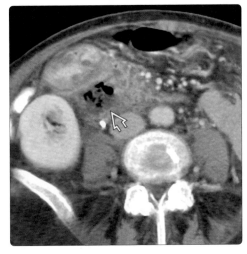

(Left) *Axial CECT shows one of several small, hypodense pancreatic masses* ➡️ *along with infiltration of the surrounding fat* ➡️*. These findings were found to represent acute lymphoblastic lymphoma with pancreatic involvement.* (Right) *Axial CECT shows extraluminal gas and fluid* ➡️ *near the 2nd portion of duodenum and pancreatic head, along with extensive inflammatory infiltration, representing the sequelae of perforated duodenal diverticulum.*

DIFFERENTIAL DIAGNOSIS

Common

- Chronic Pancreatitis
- Senescent Change, Pancreas
- Peripancreatic Vascular Lesions (Mimic)
- Choledocholithiasis (Mimic)
- Duodenal Diverticulum (Mimic)

Less Common

- Calcified Cystic or Solid Pancreatic Masses
  - Pancreatic Neuroendocrine Tumor
  - Pancreatic Serous Cystadenoma
  - Mucinous Cystic Neoplasm
  - Solid Pseudopapillary Neoplasm
  - Pancreatic Pseudocyst
  - Intraductal Papillary Mucinous Neoplasm
  - Pancreatic Metastases
- Cystic Fibrosis
- Hereditary Pancreatitis

Rare but Important

- Kwashiorkor
- Hyperparathyroidism
- Groove Pancreatitis
- Shwachman-Diamond Syndrome

ESSENTIAL INFORMATION

Key Differential Diagnosis Issues

- Parenchymal calcifications are most common with chronic pancreatitis, but scattered punctate parenchymal calcifications are not uncommon in older patients due to senescent change
- Splenic artery vascular calcifications much more common than pancreatic parenchymal calcifications and should not be misinterpreted to suggest chronic pancreatitis
- Calcifications can be seen with variety of cystic and solid pancreatic masses
  - Pancreatic adenocarcinoma almost **never** demonstrates calcification, and presence of calcification should suggest alternative diagnosis
  - Pancreatic neuroendocrine tumor is most common pancreatic solid mass to show calcification
  - Many pancreatic cystic lesions can demonstrate calcification, and pattern of calcification may help in diagnosis [e.g., central calcification in serous cystadenoma or peripheral calcification in mucinous cystic neoplsm (MCN)]

Helpful Clues for Common Diagnoses

- **Chronic Pancreatitis**
  - Pancreatic parenchymal fibrosis resulting from chronic inflammation, most often due to alcohol abuse
  - Calcifications (usually multiple) can be either parenchymal or intraductal, ranging in size from punctate to large (~ 1 cm)
    - Calcifications most commonly occur in pancreatic head (and may be clustered in that location)
    - Large intraductal stones can contribute to pancreatic ductal obstruction and dilatation

- Other CT stigmata of chronic pancreatitis include dilated, beaded pancreatic duct (± strictures), parenchymal atrophy, and pseudocysts
- Degree of pancreatic calcification related to severity of patient's fibrosis and disease
  - Calcifications most common with chronic pancreatitis due to alcohol (90% with calcification have history of alcohol abuse)

- **Senescent Change, Pancreas**
  - Older patients may demonstrate features that mimic chronic pancreatitis, including mild pancreatic ductal dilatation, parenchymal atrophy, and few punctate parenchymal calcifications
  - Typically patients over age of 70 without symptoms of pancreatic endocrine or exocrine deficiency

- **Peripancreatic Vascular Lesions (Mimic)**
  - Vascular calcifications adjacent to pancreas can mimic primary pancreatic calcification
    - Tram-track atherosclerotic calcifications of splenic artery are very common (more common than true pancreatic calcifications)
    - Aneurysms or pseudoaneurysms involving splenic artery, gastroduodenal artery, or pancreaticoduodenal arteries can demonstrate peripheral or eggshell calcification and mimic true pancreatic calcification
    - Chronic splenic vein thrombus may demonstrate calcification (or mural wall thickening with calcification)

- **Choledocholithiasis (Mimic)**
  - Calcified stone in distal common bile duct may be difficult to distinguish from pancreatic calcification
    - Often associated with proximal biliary dilatation
  - Use multiplanar reformations to localize stone to distal common bile duct

- **Duodenal Diverticulum (Mimic)**
  - High-density oral contrast (or medication) within diverticulum (when diverticulum abuts pancreas) may mimic parenchymal calcification

Helpful Clues for Less Common Diagnoses

- **Calcified Cystic or Solid Pancreatic Masses**
  - **Pancreatic neuroendocrine tumors (PNET)**
    - Internal calcifications are common and frequently coarse and irregular (central > eccentric)
      - Most common etiology for calcified, **solid** pancreatic mass
      - Small masses can rarely appear almost completely calcified
      - Nonsyndromic tumors and large masses with central necrosis more likely to develop calcification
    - Typically hypervascular tumors, which avidly enhance on arterial-phase images

  - **Pancreatic serous cystadenoma**
    - Classic appearance is microcystic adenoma: Honeycomb or sponge pattern with multiple (> 6) small (< 2 cm) internal cysts, central scar, and central calcification
    - Calcifications usually appear dystrophic in center of lesion (in scar) or as thin calcification within septation
    - Usually asymptomatic lesion found in older women ("grandmother" tumor)

- o **Mucinous cystic neoplasm (MCN)**
  - Premalignant or frankly malignant cystic tumor found most often in middle-aged women
  - Unilocular or multilocular cystic lesion classically found in pancreatic tail, which may demonstrate thick wall, septations, or mural nodularity
  - Curvilinear calcifications can be seen frequently (16%) in either cyst wall or septations
- o **Solid pseudopapillary neoplasm (SPEN)**
  - Almost always seen in young female patients
  - Usually large, solid, encapsulated mass with enhancing capsule (± cystic components)
    - □ Usually no pancreatic or biliary duct obstruction
    - □ May demonstrate internal hemorrhage
  - Calcifications are very common (~ 50%) and can be peripheral or central
- o **Pancreatic pseudocyst**
  - Chronic pseudocysts may demonstrate peripheral calcification or layering milk of calcium
  - Usually associated with clinical history or imaging stigmata of prior pancreatitis
- o **Intraductal papillary mucinous neoplasm (IPMN)**
  - Mucin-producing tumor that arises from main pancreatic duct or side branches
  - Can present as dilated pancreatic duct [main-duct intraductal papillary mucinous neoplasm (IPMN)] or cystic lesion in communication with main pancreatic duct (side-branch IPMN)
  - Side-branch IPMN can demonstrate peripheral or septal calcification in 20%
  - Main-duct IPMN can demonstrate amorphous calcifications within dilated main pancreatic duct
- o **Pancreatic metastases**
  - Metastases to pancreas are rare, but metastases from mucinous tumors of gastrointestinal tract can demonstrate calcification
- • **Cystic Fibrosis (CF)**
  - o Pancreatic findings include small parenchymal or intraductal calcifications (usually tiny or punctate), fatty replacement of pancreas, and small pancreatic cysts

- o Most common cause of pancreatic calcification in children [but seen in only minority of CF patients (~ 8%)]
  - Pancreatic calcifications in CF imply advanced pancreatic fibrosis
- • **Hereditary Pancreatitis**
  - o Autosomal dominant trait associated with several gene mutations (*PRSS1*, *SPINK1*, and *CFTR*)
  - o Results in chronic pancreatitis in unusually young patients (often < 20 years of age) with peak incidence at 5 years of age
  - o 50% develop intraductal calcifications, which are often unusually large and round in morphology
  - o Consider in presence of pancreatic calcifications or other imaging features of chronic pancreatitis in young patient

Helpful Clues for Rare Diagnoses
- • **Kwashiorkor**
  - o Clinical syndrome associated with severe malnutrition and protein deficiency
    - Virtually never diagnosed in developing world, but can be seen in developing world in areas of famine
  - o May be associated with pancreatic calcification, as well as clinical signs of pancreatic insufficiency (diabetes and steatorrhea)
- • **Hyperparathyroidism**
  - o Can be associated with pancreatic calcifications either on basis of recurrent pancreatitis or hypercalcemia
- • **Groove Pancreatitis**
  - o Unusual form of chronic pancreatitis affecting pancreaticoduodenal groove (between pancreatic head and duodenum) usually associated with alcohol abuse
  - o Characterized by thickening and cyst formation in groove, as well as parenchymal/groove calcification
- • **Shwachman-Diamond Syndrome**
  - o Autosomal recessive disorder associated with pancreatic insufficiency along with number of other skeletal and hematologic disorders (leukemia, short stature, etc.)
  - o Can result in fatty replacement of pancreas with scattered calcifications

Chronic Pancreatitis

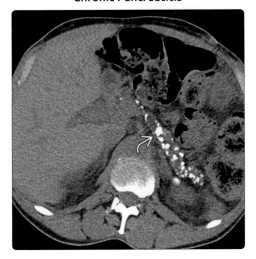

Chronic Pancreatitis

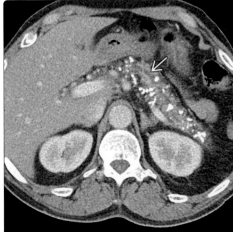

(Left) Axial NECT shows diffuse pancreatic atrophy and multiple pancreatic calcifications ⊅ in a patient with chronic pancreatitis. Chronic pancreatitis is, by far, the most common cause of pancreatic calcification. (Right) Axial CECT in a patient with chronic pancreatitis shows characteristic imaging features, including glandular atrophy, a mildly dilated pancreatic duct ⊡, and multiple calcifications.

Pancreatic Calcifications

(Left) *Axial CECT shows a rim-calcified lesion ➡ that represents a thrombosed portal vein aneurysm in a patient with cirrhosis and portal hypertension. An abnormality such as this could easily be mistaken for a calcified pancreatic cystic mass.* (Right) *Coronal NECT shows a calcified stone ➡ in the distal common bile duct (CBD). When viewed in the axial plane, a stone in this location could conceivably be confused for a pancreatic calcification.*

Peripancreatic Vascular Lesions (Mimic)

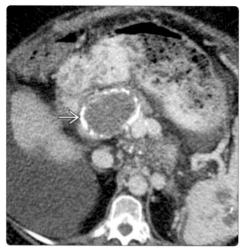

Choledocholithiasis (Mimic)

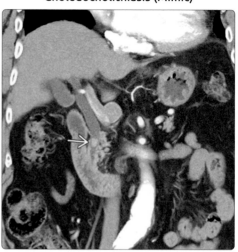

(Left) *Axial CECT shows a hypoenhancing mass ➡ in the pancreatic tail with coarse internal calcification ➡, along with innumerable poorly defined liver metastases ➡. This was found to represent neuroendocrine tumor at biopsy.* (Right) *Coronal CECT shows a mixed cystic and solid pancreatic mass with discrete multilocular cystic components ➡, along with extensive central dystrophic calcification ➡. This was confirmed at resection to represent serous cystadenoma.*

Pancreatic Neuroendocrine Tumor

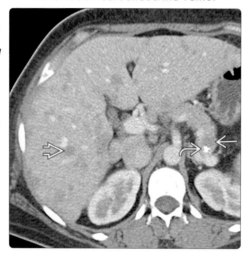

Pancreatic Serous Cystadenoma

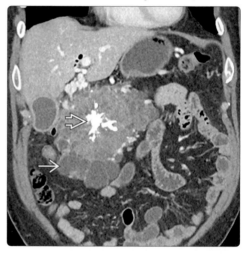

(Left) *Axial CECT shows a large, cystic mass ➡ arising from the pancreatic tail with a large central dystrophic calcification ➡.* (Right) *Axial T2 FS MR in the same patient shows the multicystic nature of the mass with a large, hypointense central scar ➡. As the imaging appearance suggests, this was confirmed at resection to represent serous cystadenoma.*

Pancreatic Serous Cystadenoma

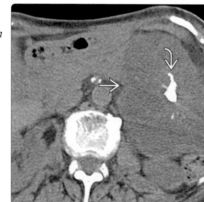

Pancreatic Serous Cystadenoma

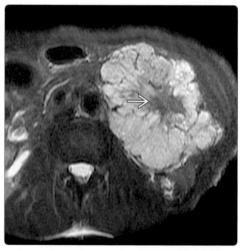

Pancreatic Calcifications

Mucinous Cystic Neoplasm

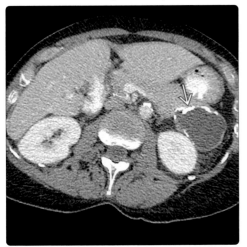

Solid Pseudopapillary Neoplasm

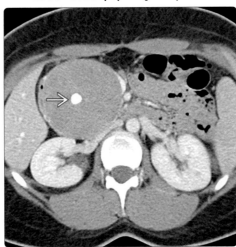

(Left) Axial CECT shows a cystic mass in the pancreatic tail with curvilinear peripheral calcification ➡, a classic pattern for a mucinous cystic neoplasm. (Right) Axial CECT in a young female patient shows a low- and intermediate-density pancreatic mass with central calcification ➡, confirmed to represent a solid pseudopapillary neoplasm (SPEN) at resection. Calcifications in SPEN can be central or peripheral.

Solid Pseudopapillary Neoplasm

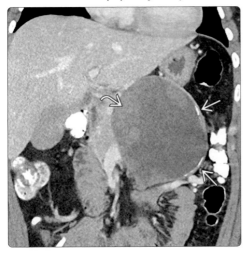

Pancreatic Pseudocyst

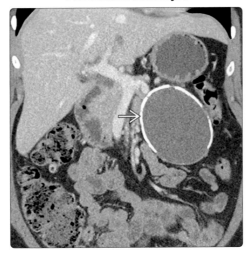

(Left) Coronal CECT in a young female patient shows a pancreatic mass with peripheral calcification ➡, confirmed to represent SPEN at resection. The higher density components ➡ could represent either soft tissue or hemorrhage (common in SPEN). (Right) Coronal CECT shows a large, cystic lesion near the pancreatic tail with extensive rim calcification ➡. Although the patient did not have a known history of pancreatitis, this was surprisingly found to represent a pseudocyst.

Intraductal Papillary Mucinous Neoplasm

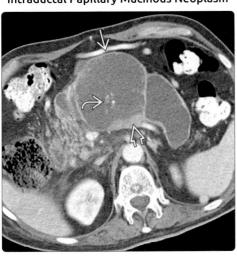

Pancreatic Metastases

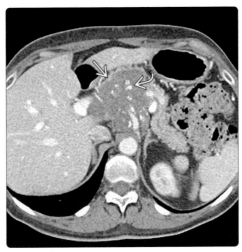

(Left) Axial CECT shows a massively dilated main pancreatic duct ➡ with subtle internal speckled calcifications ➡, as well as enhancing soft tissue ➡, compatible with a main-duct intraductal papillary mucinous neoplasm (IPMN) with invasive carcinoma. (Right) Axial CECT shows a large mass ➡ involving the pancreatic head, neck, and uncinate process with internal coarse and speckled calcification ➡. This represents an unusual metastasis to the pancreas from primary mucinous colon cancer.

DIFFERENTIAL DIAGNOSIS

Common

- Pancreatic Pseudocyst
- Serous Cystadenoma of Pancreas
- Mucinous Cystic Neoplasm
- Intraductal Papillary Mucinous Neoplasm

Less Common

- Necrotic Pancreatic Ductal Carcinoma
- Solid Pseudopapillary Neoplasm
- Cystic Pancreatic Neuroendocrine Tumor
- Congenital Cyst
- Lymphoepithelial Cyst
- Cystic Metastases

ESSENTIAL INFORMATION

Key Differential Diagnosis Issues

- US can characterize simple or macrocystic pancreatic lesions
  - Most represent pancreatic pseudocysts
- Remaining benign and malignant cystic pancreatic lesions may appear echogenic due to numerous microcystic interfaces, soft tissue components, or complex content
- CECT or CEMR is necessary to adequately characterize internal features that are not well assessed with transabdominal ultrasound
- Endoscopic ultrasound (EUS) also provides high-resolution imaging but is invasive and requires conscious sedation
  - Can be used for biopsy or fluid aspiration in indeterminate cases
- Key features that guide differential diagnosis
  - Location and size
  - Wall thickness
  - Loculation and number of locules
  - Internal septations and septal thickness
  - Presence of solid components and vascularity
  - Central scar
  - Calcification and location
  - Communication with pancreatic duct
  - Fluid characterization/presence of hemorrhage
  - Pancreatic and biliary diameter
  - Upstream pancreatic atrophy
  - Evidence of acute or chronic pancreatitis
  - Locoregional adenopathy and hepatic metastases
- Consider clinical context
  - Patient demographics, pancreatitis, obstructive symptomatology, familial syndromes

Helpful Clues for Common Diagnoses

- **Pancreatic Pseudocyst**
  - Common late complication of pancreatitis
    - Develops 4-6 weeks after onset of acute pancreatitis
    - Evolves over time, whereas neoplastic lesions persist without change
  - Generally well circumscribed, smooth walled, unilocular, and anechoic with posterior acoustic enhancement
  - May be complicated
    - Multilocular
    - Internal echoes with fluid-debris level or septations
    - Wall calcification

- But shows no vascularized soft tissue elements
- Associated with other findings of acute or chronic pancreatitis
  - Parenchymal atrophy or calcification, fat stranding on CT, ductal strictures on MR
  - Generally not seen with mucinous cystic neoplasm (MCN), primary mimic of pseudocyst

- **Serous Cystadenoma of Pancreas**
  - Benign pancreatic tumor
  - Commonly in pancreatic body and tail; 30% occur in pancreatic head
  - Typically composed of small cystic areas separated by internal septations
  - Septa coalesce to form central echogenic scar with "sunburst" calcification
  - Can mimic nonspecific solid and cystic tumor
    - Heterogeneous, echogenic appearance due to numerous interfaces
    - Intralesional color Doppler flow in fibrovascular septa
  - Characteristic honeycomb appearance on CT, MR, and EUS
  - Less commonly, may see oligocystic variant that may be indistinguishable from MCN by imaging
    - EUS-guided cyst aspiration may be helpful in making diagnosis
  - Usually seen in older women (mean age: 61 years)

- **Mucinous Cystic Neoplasm**
  - Tumors range in grade from benign with malignant potential to invasive carcinoma
  - More common location: Pancreatic body and tail
  - Anechoic or hypoechoic, thick-walled, cystic mass ± mildly thickened septa
  - Can demonstrate peripheral calcification
  - May be indistinguishable from pseudocyst
  - Lacks additional findings/history of pancreatitis
  - EUS-guided biopsy may be helpful in making diagnosis
  - Solid components or marked septal thickening suggest carcinoma
  - Almost exclusively in middle-aged women (mean age: 50 years)

- **Intraductal Papillary Mucinous Neoplasm**
  - Tumor with varying malignant potential: Branch type generally benign with low malignant potential; main duct intraductal papillary mucinous neoplasm thought to be precursor to invasive pancreatic ductal adenocarcinoma
  - Typically in head of pancreas/uncinate process
  - Main duct type: Marked pancreatic ductal dilatation
    - When diffuse, may simulate chronic pancreatitis
      - However, calcification and parenchymal atrophy are not typically seen
    - If segmental, can mimic fluid collection or mucinous cystic tumor
  - Side branch type: Collections of dilated side branches
    - Anechoic or hypoechoic cyst or collection of small, anechoic cysts
    - Look for communication with pancreatic duct, which is distinguishing feature compared to other cystic neoplasms
    - May be multifocal, whereas serous cystadenoma and MCN are typically solitary
  - Occur most frequently in older men (mean age: 65 years)

Helpful Clues for Less Common Diagnoses

- **Necrotic Pancreatic Ductal Carcinoma**
  - Most common pancreatic neoplasm
  - Malignant lesion
  - Commonly in head of pancreas
  - Typically appears as ill-defined, solid, hypoechoic mass with ductal obstruction
  - May show complex cystic areas due to tumor necrosis, side branch obstruction, or adjacent pseudocyst
    - Uncommon form of common neoplasm
  - Infiltrative appearance ± vascular invasion distinguishes this entity from other solid malignancies that may show cystic change
  - Obstructive symptomatology
- **Solid Pseudopapillary Neoplasm**
  - Tumor with low-grade malignant potential
  - Commonly in pancreatic tail
  - Large, well-defined, heterogeneous, echogenic solid and cystic mass
  - Cystic areas are secondary to tumor degeneration and vary in size and morphology
  - Prominent vascular soft tissue components
  - Often shows intratumoral hemorrhage
  - Typically seen in young women (< 35 years)
- **Cystic Pancreatic Neuroendocrine Tumor**
  - All tumors > 5 mm considered malignant
  - Typically round, solid, hypoechoic mass with internal color Doppler flow
  - Central cyst formation may occur due to tumor degeneration
    - Uncommon form of uncommon neoplasm
  - Identification of hypervascular rim can be challenging
  - Familial syndromes: Multiple endocrine neoplasia type 1, von Hippel-Lindau, neurofibromatosis type 1, and tuberous sclerosis
    - May have multiple lesions
    - Occurs in younger patients (< 40 years)
- **Congenital Cyst**
  - True epithelial lining with serous fluid
  - Consider in patients with autosomal dominant polycystic kidney disease, von Hippel-Lindau, and cystic fibrosis
    - Usually multiple; can replace entire pancreas (e.g., in cystic fibrosis)
- **Lymphoepithelial Cyst**
  - Rare, benign lesion, usually in tail of pancreas
  - Nonneoplastic, no malignant behavior
  - Macrocystic morphology, multilocular or unilocular cysts
  - May see characteristic T1 hyperintensity and low T2 signal due to keratin content
  - Almost exclusively in middle-aged to older men
- **Cystic Metastases**
  - Pancreatic metastases are uncommon
  - Can occur with renal cell carcinoma, melanoma, breast cancer, lung cancer, gastric cancer, and colorectal carcinoma

SELECTED REFERENCES

1. Aziz H et al: Comparison of society guidelines for the management and surveillance of pancreatic cysts: a review. JAMA Surg. ePub, 2022
2. Hickman K et al: Pancreatic cystic lesions and the role of contrast enhanced endoscopic ultrasound. Clin Radiol. 77(6):418-27, 2022
3. Lee LS: Updates in diagnosis and management of pancreatic cysts. World J Gastroenterol. 27(34):5700-14, 2021
4. Navarro SM et al: Incidental pancreatic cysts on cross-sectional imaging. Radiol Clin North Am. 59(4):617-29, 2021
5. Yoon JG et al: Pancreatic cystic neoplasms: a review of current recommendations for surveillance and management. Abdom Radiol (NY). 46(8):3946-62, 2021
6. Blaszczak AM et al: Endoscopic diagnosis of pancreatic cysts. Curr Opin Gastroenterol. 35(5):448-54, 2019
7. Kim YS et al: Rare nonneoplastic cysts of pancreas. Clin Endosc. 48(1):31-8, 2015
8. Goh BK et al: Are the Sendai and Fukuoka consensus guidelines for cystic mucinous neoplasms of the pancreas useful in the initial triage of all suspected pancreatic cystic neoplasms? A single-institution experience with 317 surgically-treated patients. Ann Surg Oncol. 21(6):1919-26, 2014
9. Sahani DV et al: Diagnosis and management of cystic pancreatic lesions. AJR Am J Roentgenol. 200(2):343-54, 2013
10. Megibow AJ et al: The incidental pancreatic cyst. Radiol Clin North Am. 49(2):349-59, 2011
11. Hutchins G et al: Diagnostic evaluation of pancreatic cystic malignancies. Surg Clin North Am. 90(2):399-410, 2010
12. Kalb B et al: MR imaging of cystic lesions of the pancreas. Radiographics. 29(6):1749-65, 2009

Pancreatic Pseudocyst

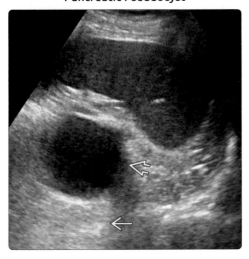

Pancreatic Pseudocyst

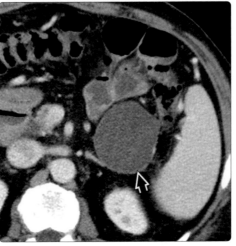

(Left) Transverse US shows a well-demarcated, anechoic lesion ⊃ with through transmission ⊃ in the tail of the pancreas, compatible with pseudocyst. (Right) Axial CECT in the same patient shows a well-demarcated, low-density cystic lesion ⊃ with a thin wall in the tail of the pancreas. Note the lack of enhancing components and marked pancreatic atrophy.

Pancreatic Pseudocyst

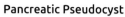

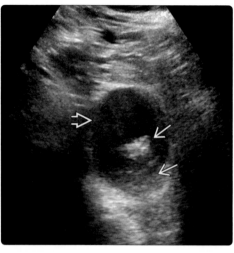

Pancreatic Pseudocyst

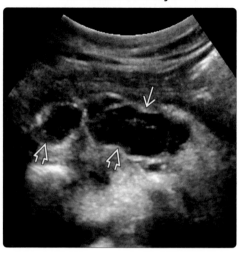

(Left) *Transverse US in the region of the pancreas shows a well-circumscribed, unilocular cystic lesion ➡ with through transmission. Note the echogenic internal contents and layering debris ➡, compatible with complex pseudocyst. (Right) Transverse US shows pancreatic ductal dilation ➡ and 2 well-circumscribed, elongated fluid collections ➡ with internal echoes in the neck and body of the pancreas, compatible with complex pseudocysts from severe pancreatitis.*

Serous Cystadenoma of Pancreas

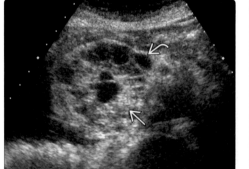

Serous Cystadenoma of Pancreas

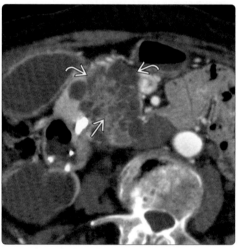

(Left) *Transverse transabdominal US shows a hyperechoic, solid-appearing mass in the head of the pancreas with small cystic components ➡ and a more echogenic center ➡. (Right) Axial CECT in the same patient better characterizes numerous small cysts ➡ within the lesion, separated by thin septa, which appear more coalescent centrally ➡.*

Serous Cystadenoma of Pancreas

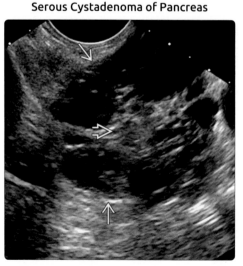

Serous Cystadenoma of Pancreas

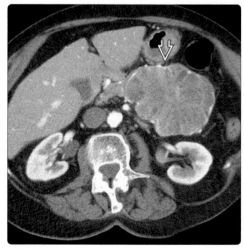

(Left) *EUS shows a multicystic mass ➡ with multiple small, internal cystic spaces representing serous cystadenoma. Echogenic components at the center ➡ represent innumerable tiny cysts separated by linear septations, resulting in a hyperechoic appearance due to highly reflective interfaces. (Right) Axial CECT shows the classic honeycomb appearance of a serous cystadenoma ➡, a microcystic lesion with thin, enhancing septa delineating small cysts.*

Cystic Pancreatic Lesion

Mucinous Cystic Neoplasm

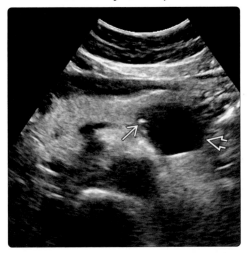

Mucinous Cystic Neoplasm

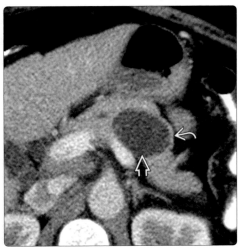

(Left) Transverse US shows a well-defined, anechoic cystic lesion ➡ in the body of the pancreas with a few hyperechoic peripheral foci ➡. (Right) Axial CECT in the same patient shows an encapsulated, oval, hypodense mass ➡ in the body of the pancreas with a thickened, enhancing cyst wall ➡. The lesion contained internal septations, not seen here.

Intraductal Papillary Mucinous Neoplasm

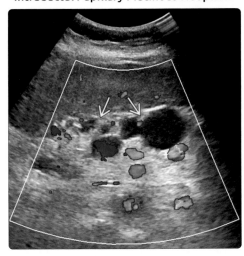

Intraductal Papillary Mucinous Neoplasm

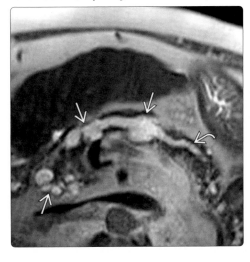

(Left) Transverse color Doppler US shows a collection of multiple small, round and oval cysts ➡ within the body of the pancreas. (Right) Axial T2 HASTE MR in the same patient better demonstrates multifocal involvement of the pancreas. Numerous T2-bright cysts ➡ are seen throughout the pancreas, several of which appear contiguous with a dilated pancreatic duct ➡, compatible with mixed, branch, and main duct intraductal papillary mucinous neoplasm.

Cystic Pancreatic Neuroendocrine Tumor

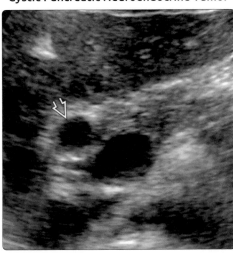

Cystic Pancreatic Neuroendocrine Tumor

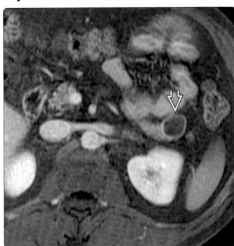

(Left) Transverse US of the pancreas shows a round, well-circumscribed cystic lesion ➡ extending exophytically from the neck of the pancreas. This was amenable to EUS-guided biopsy, which showed a cystic neuroendocrine tumor. (Right) Axial T1 C+ MR shows a round cystic lesion ➡ in the pancreatic tail with a peripheral rim of hypervascular enhancement, a typical appearance for small cystic neuroendocrine tumor.

DIFFERENTIAL DIAGNOSIS

Common

- Pancreatic Ductal Carcinoma
- Focal Acute Pancreatitis
- Chronic Pancreatitis
- Pancreatic Neuroendocrine Tumor
- Serous Cystadenoma of Pancreas
- Mucinous Cystic Neoplasm of Pancreas

Less Common

- Metastasis
- Lymphoma
- Solid Pseudopapillary Neoplasm
- Intrapancreatic Splenule

ESSENTIAL INFORMATION

Key Differential Diagnosis Issues

- Correlate with clinical information (e.g., history of pancreatitis, obstructive symptomatology)
- Pancreatic duct dilatation favors diagnosis of pancreatic ductal carcinoma
  - Biliary dilatation present as well in pancreatic head ductal carcinoma
- Other ancillary findings to look for include
  - Cystic component
  - Internal septation
  - Presence of intralesional calcification
  - Vascular encasement
  - Regional lymph node and liver metastases
- Clues to detection of small tumor
  - Focal contour irregularity
  - Subtle pancreatic duct/bile duct dilatation
- CECT or CEMR improves ability to detect and characterize solid pancreatic lesions
  - Can evaluate for vascular encasement
- Endoscopic US is invasive; however, it increases sensitivity for lesion detection and can be used to guide biopsy for diagnosis

Helpful Clues for Common Diagnoses

- **Pancreatic Ductal Carcinoma**
  - Arises from ductal epithelium of exocrine pancreas
  - Location: Head of pancreas (60-70%), body (20%), diffuse (15%), tail (5%)
  - Average size: ~ 2-3 cm
  - Pathology: Scirrhous infiltrative adenocarcinoma with dense cellularity and sparse vascularity
  - Typical US findings
    - Poorly defined, homogeneous or heterogeneous, hypoechoic mass
    - Pancreatic duct dilatation upstream from tumor with abrupt tapering at site of obstruction
    - Bile duct dilatation seen in pancreatic head tumor
    - Necrosis/cystic component is rarely seen
    - Displacement/encasement of adjacent vascular structures (e.g., superior mesenteric vessels, splenic artery, hepatic artery, gastroduodenal artery)
    - Presence of liver and regional nodal metastases
    - Ascites due to peritoneal metastases

- **Focal Acute Pancreatitis**
  - Clinical information very important for correct imaging interpretation
    - Acute onset of epigastric pain, fever, and vomiting
    - Raised serum amylase and lipase
    - Presence of underlying predisposing factors: Biliary stone, alcoholism, drugs (e.g., steroid), trauma, etc.
  - Focal, ill-defined, hypoechoic enlargement of pancreatic parenchyma
    - Heterogeneous appearance in cases with intrapancreatic necrosis/hemorrhage
  - Blurred pancreatic outline/margin
  - Presence of peripancreatic fluid collection
  - Lack of pancreatic duct dilatation
  - No parenchymal calcification
- **Chronic Pancreatitis**
  - Longstanding clinical symptoms, recurrent attacks of epigastric pain, typically radiates to back
  - Most common US features
    - Diffuse atrophy
    - Main pancreatic duct beading and side branch dilatation
    - Parenchymal and ductal calcifications
  - Can have focal involvement with mass-like appearance
  - Look for smoothly stenotic or normal main duct penetrating abnormal region on MRCP
- **Pancreatic Neuroendocrine Tumor**
  - Functioning and nonfunctioning subtypes have distinct appearances
    - Functioning tumor usually small, solid, well-circumscribed, hypo-/isoechoic mass
    - Nonfunctioning tumors tend to be larger with more heterogeneous echo pattern due to necrosis, calcification, and cystic change
    - Solid components are typically hypervascular on power Doppler US and hyperenhancing on CT and MR
  - Detection may be difficult with small functioning tumors
  - Endoscopic US detects tumors in pancreatic head and body
  - Intraoperative US is useful for tumor localization
  - Liver and regional lymph node metastases seen in 60-90% at clinical presentation
    - Hyperechoic liver metastases more suggestive of neuroendocrine tumors than ductal carcinoma
- **Serous Cystadenoma of Pancreas**
  - Commonly in pancreatic body and tail; 30% occur in pancreatic head
  - Composed of tiny cysts separated by internal septations
  - Septa coalesce to form central echogenic scar with "sunburst" calcification
  - US appearance depends on size of individual cysts
    - Slightly echogenic, solid-appearing mass (small cysts provide numerous acoustic interfaces)
    - Partly solid-appearing mass with anechoic cystic areas; cysts usually at periphery due to central scar
    - Multicystic mass with internal septations and solid component
  - Typically no pancreatic duct dilatation
    - However, large lesions in head of pancreas can behave more aggressively
  - Intralesional color Doppler flow in fibrovascular septa

- Usually seen in older women (6th decade)
- **Mucinous Cystic Neoplasm of Pancreas**
  - More common in pancreatic body and tail
  - Well-demarcated, anechoic or hypoechoic, thick-walled, cystic mass
    - Uni-/multilocular cysts separated by thick, echogenic septations
  - Solid papillary tissue protruding into tumor suggests malignancy
  - Liver metastases appear as thick-walled, cystic hepatic lesions
  - Seen almost exclusively in middle-aged women

Helpful Clues for Less Common Diagnoses

- **Metastasis**
  - Nonspecific imaging findings
  - Focal or diffuse involvement
  - Renal cell carcinoma: Most common primary; often solitary
  - Other sources: Lung, GI, breast, melanoma, ovary, liver; typically disseminated disease
- **Lymphoma**
  - Secondary lymphoma more common than primary lymphoma
    - Known clinical history of systemic lymphomatous involvement
  - Large, homogeneous, solid mass
  - Presence of peripancreatic nodal masses
  - Peripancreatic vessels displaced or stretched
- **Solid Pseudopapillary Neoplasm**
  - Most common in pancreatic tail
  - Well-demarcated, large, heterogeneous, echogenic, solid and cystic mass
  - Small, cystic areas often present due to tumor degeneration
    - Often with intratumoral hemorrhage
  - Dystrophic calcification occasionally seen
  - No pancreatic duct dilatation or calcification
  - Prominent vascular soft tissue components
    - → hypervascular pattern with color Doppler

- Liver metastases seen in ~ 4% of patients
- Typically seen in young women (< 35 years)
- **Intrapancreatic Splenule**
  - Congenital anomaly arising from aberrant splenic embryologic fusion
  - 2nd most common location for accessory spleens is in pancreatic tail
  - Appears as small, well-circumscribed, solid mass, usually at tip and not > 3 cm from tail
  - Easily mistaken for primary pancreatic mass, particularly neuroendocrine tumor
  - Follows attentuation of spleen on all phases of CT and intensity of spleen on all MR sequences
  - Confirm with Tc-99m-labeled heat-damaged red blood cells

SELECTED REFERENCES

1. Farrukh J et al: Pancreatic adenocarcinoma: imaging techniques for diagnosis and management. Br J Hosp Med (Lond). 83(5):1-12, 2022
2. Gandhi NS et al: Imaging mimics of pancreatic ductal adenocarcinoma. Abdom Radiol (NY). 43(2):273-84, 2018
3. Al-Hawary MM et al: Mimics of pancreatic ductal adenocarcinoma. Cancer Imaging. 13(3):342-9, 2013
4. Bhosale PR et al: Vascular pancreatic lesions: spectrum of imaging findings of malignant masses and mimics with pathologic correlation. Abdom Imaging. 38(4):802-17, 2013
5. Dimcevski G et al: Ultrasonography in diagnosing chronic pancreatitis: new aspects. World J Gastroenterol. 19(42):7247-57, 2013
6. Coakley FV et al: Pancreatic imaging mimics: part 1, imaging mimics of pancreatic adenocarcinoma. AJR Am J Roentgenol. 199(2):301-8, 2012
7. Raman SP et al: Pancreatic imaging mimics: part 2, pancreatic neuroendocrine tumors and their mimics. AJR Am J Roentgenol. 199(2):309-18, 2012

Pancreatic Ductal Carcinoma

Pancreatic Ductal Carcinoma

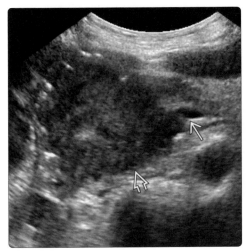

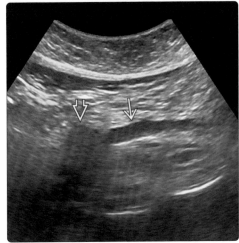

(Left) Transverse transabdominal US shows a large, infiltrative, solid, hypoechoic mass in the head of the pancreas ➡ abutting the superior mesenteric vein ➡, raising concern for vascular encasement. (Right) Transverse transabdominal US shows a poorly defined, infiltrative, hypoechoic mass ➡ in the head of the pancreas, obstructing the pancreatic duct, which is dilated upstream ➡.

Solid Pancreatic Lesion

Pancreatic Ductal Carcinoma

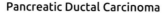

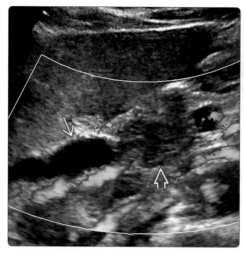

Pancreatic Ductal Carcinoma

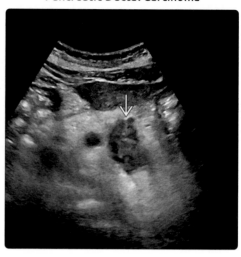

(Left) *Longitudinal oblique power Doppler US shows an ill-defined, solid, hypoechoic mass* ➥ *in the pancreatic head resulting in obstruction of the terminal portion of the common bile duct* ➥. **(Right)** *Transverse US shows a hypoechoic, irregular mass* ➥ *in the pancreatic body, representing biopsy-proven pancreatic adenocarcinoma.*

Focal Acute Pancreatitis

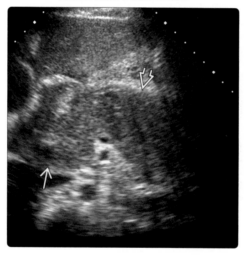

Chronic Pancreatitis

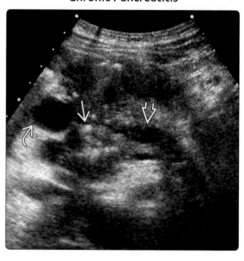

(Left) *Transverse transabdominal US shows focal enlargement* ➥ *of the distal pancreas with a homogeneous, hypoechoic appearance relative to the normal pancreas* ➥. *Note the absence of ductal dilatation.* **(Right)** *Transverse US shows parenchymal calcifications* ➥ *in the enlarged pancreatic head. Note the dilated pancreatic* ➥ *and common bile* ➥ *ducts and the pancreatic margins are indistinct.*

Pancreatic Neuroendocrine Tumor

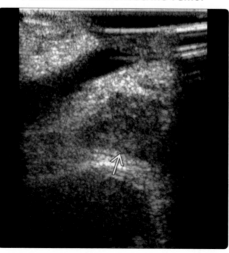

Serous Cystadenoma of Pancreas

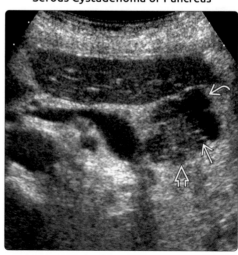

(Left) *Transverse intraoperative US shows a well-defined, hypoechoic, solid mass* ➥ *in the body of the pancreas, which was biopsy-proven pancreatic neuroendocrine tumor.* **(Right)** *Transverse transabdominal US shows a well-circumscribed, solid and cystic mass* ➥ *with peripheral loculations* ➥. *There are also tiny cystic spaces with thin, linear septations* ➥.

Serous Cystadenoma of Pancreas

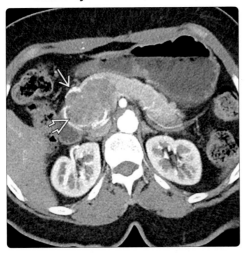

Mucinous Cystic Neoplasm of Pancreas

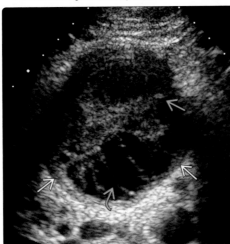

(Left) Axial CECT shows clusters of tiny cysts ⇉ separated by thin, enhancing septations in a honeycomb pattern characteristic of serous cystadenoma. Note the prominent vessels draped around the periphery of the mass ⇉. (Right) Transverse transabdominal US shows a well-circumscribed, heterogeneous, multilocular cystic mass in the pancreas with thick ➔ and thin ➔ internal septations and a thick wall ⇉.

Metastasis

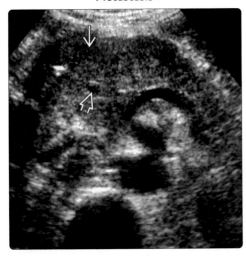

Lymphoma

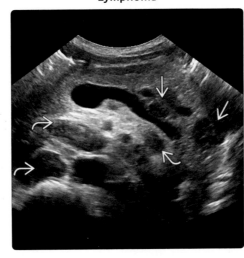

(Left) Transverse transabdominal US shows an ill-defined, solid, hypoechoic mass ➔ involving the head and body of the pancreas. The common hepatic artery is encased ⇉. Note the absence of pancreatic duct dilatation. (Right) Transverse US of the pancreas shows multiple round masses in the pancreatic tail ⇉, compatible with lymphomatous involvement. Other abnormal nodes were present in the retroperitoneum ➔ from disseminated non-Hodgkin lymphoma.

Solid Pseudopapillary Neoplasm

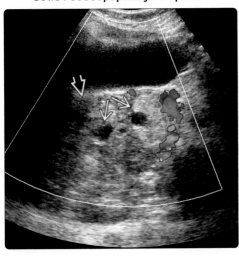

Intrapancreatic Splenule

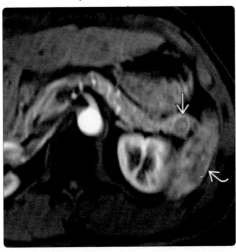

(Left) Longitudinal US shows a well-circumscribed, large, heterogeneous, echogenic, solid mass ⇉ in a 17-year-old girl. Note color Doppler flow in the periphery of the lesion and heterogeneous cystic areas of degeneration ➔. (Right) Axial T1 C+ FS MR in the arterial phase shows a small, round, well-circumscribed lesion in the tip of the tail of the pancreas ⇉. The lesion demonstrates heterogeneous enhancement, matching that of the spleen ⇉.

DIFFERENTIAL DIAGNOSIS

Common

- Chronic Pancreatitis
- Pancreatic Ductal Carcinoma
- Periampullary Tumor

Less Common

- Obstructing Distal Common Bile Duct Stone
- Intraductal Papillary Mucinous Neoplasm

ESSENTIAL INFORMATION

Key Differential Diagnosis Issues

- Pancreatic ductal dilatation: > 3 mm possibly with tortuous configuration
  - May see abrupt tapering at site of obstruction
  - Should prompt thorough search for obstructing lesion at papilla or in pancreatic head
    - US may not provide adequate visualization due to overlying bowel gas or body habitus
    - CT, MR, &/or endoscopic US should be considered
- Isolated pancreatic duct dilatation
  - Most commonly due to chronic pancreatitis
  - High possibility of pancreatic cancer if no evidence of chronic pancreatitis
  - Mild, idiopathic dilatation without tortuosity, frequently seen in older patients
- When associated with biliary duct dilatation, termed "double duct" sign
  - Etiology more likely malignant disease; most commonly pancreatic ductal adenocarcinoma
  - Obstructing common bile duct stone or benign stenosis are also possibilities if patient does not have jaundice or mass

Helpful Clues for Common Diagnoses

- **Chronic Pancreatitis**
  - Clinical history of longstanding recurrent attacks of epigastric pain; typically radiates to back
  - Atrophic pancreas with irregular outline and heterogeneous, hypo-/hyperechoic echo pattern
  - Pancreatic calcification: Intraductal and parenchymal
  - May see dilated side branches when severe
  - MR may show duct dilatation with strictures → more suggestive of chronic pancreatitis than intraductal papillary mucinous neoplasm (IPMN)
- **Pancreatic Ductal Carcinoma**
  - Causes pancreatic duct obstruction as tumor arises from ductal epithelium of exocrine pancreas
  - Irregular, ill-defined, solid, hypoechoic mass
  - Pancreatic duct dilatation upstream from tumor
  - Bile duct dilatation with tumor in pancreatic head
  - Lack of pancreatic calcification or ductal calculus
  - May see liver and regional lymph node metastases

Helpful Clues for Less Common Diagnoses

- **Obstructing Distal Common Bile Duct Stone**
  - Obstructive jaundice and epigastric pain
  - Presence of bile duct dilatation
- **Intraductal Papillary Mucinous Neoplasm**
  - Main duct type shows marked diffuse pancreatic ductal dilatation ± pancreatic atrophy
    - Calcification not typically seen and is more suggestive of chronic pancreatitis
    - Mural/intraluminal nodularity or associated soft tissue mass is suggestive of malignancy
  - Side branch duct type may show mild ductal dilatation communicating with cystic pancreatic lesion
    - Grape-like cluster of cysts with IPMN vs. unilocular cyst with chronic pancreatitis

SELECTED REFERENCES

1. Kothari K et al: Inflammatory mimickers of pancreatic adenocarcinoma. Abdom Radiol (NY). 45(5):1387-96, 2020
2. Singh VK et al: Diagnosis and management of chronic pancreatitis: a review. JAMA. 322(24):2422-34, 2019
3. Gandhi NS et al: Imaging mimics of pancreatic ductal adenocarcinoma. Abdom Radiol (NY). 43(2):273-84, 2018
4. Kim SW et al: Isolated main pancreatic duct dilatation: CT differentiation between benign and malignant causes. AJR Am J Roentgenol. 209(5):1046-55, 2017

Chronic Pancreatitis

Chronic Pancreatitis

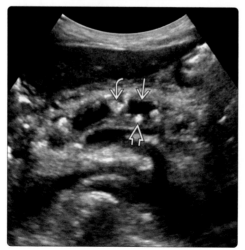

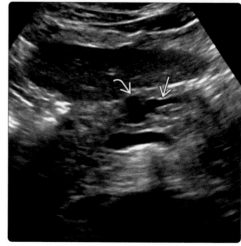

(Left) *Transverse US shows pancreatic ductal dilatation ➡ in the atrophic body of the pancreas with parenchymal ➡ and intraluminal calcifications ➡. (Right) Transverse US shows a dilated pancreatic duct ➡ communicating with a small pseudocyst ➡ in the body of the pancreas.*

Chronic Pancreatitis

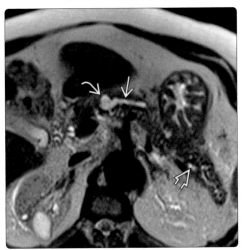

Pancreatic Ductal Carcinoma

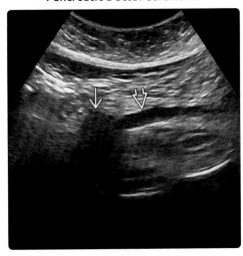

(Left) *Axial T2 HASTE MR better shows mild pancreatic ductal dilatation ➡ communicating with the small pseudocyst ➡. Note the tiny, dilated side branches ➡ in the tail of the pancreas. Pancreatic duct strictures were also seen (not shown) in this patient with a history of pancreatitis.* **(Right)** *Longitudinal US of the pancreas shows a hypoechoic mass ➡ abruptly obstructing the main pancreatic duct ➡, representing pancreatic adenocarcinoma.*

Pancreatic Ductal Carcinoma

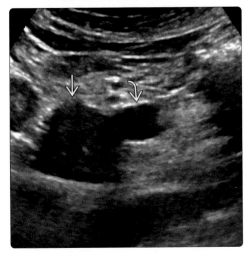

Pancreatic Ductal Carcinoma

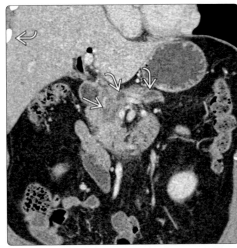

(Left) *Transverse US shows a hypoechoic mass ➡ in the pancreatic head resulting in obstruction of the pancreatic duct ➡ (which is dilated), a classic appearance for pancreatic adenocarcinoma.* **(Right)** *Coronal CECT in the same patient shows a hypodense mass ➡ in the pancreatic head with upstream pancreatic ductal dilatation ➡.*

Intraductal Papillary Mucinous Neoplasm

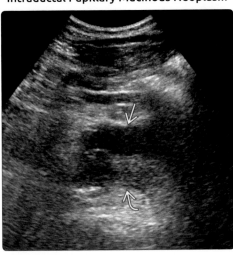

Intraductal Papillary Mucinous Neoplasm

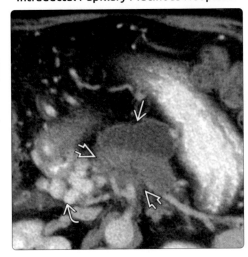

(Left) *Transverse US shows marked pancreatic ductal dilatation ➡ with low-level internal echoes and an ill-defined, hypoechoic mass posteriorly ➡.* **(Right)** *Axial CECT shows marked pancreatic ductal dilatation ➡ with an infiltrative soft tissue mass posteriorly ➡, encasing the celiac axis. Note cavernous transformation of the portal vein ➡ due to venous occlusion from the mass, which was proven by biopsy to be malignant transformation of a main duct type IPMN.*

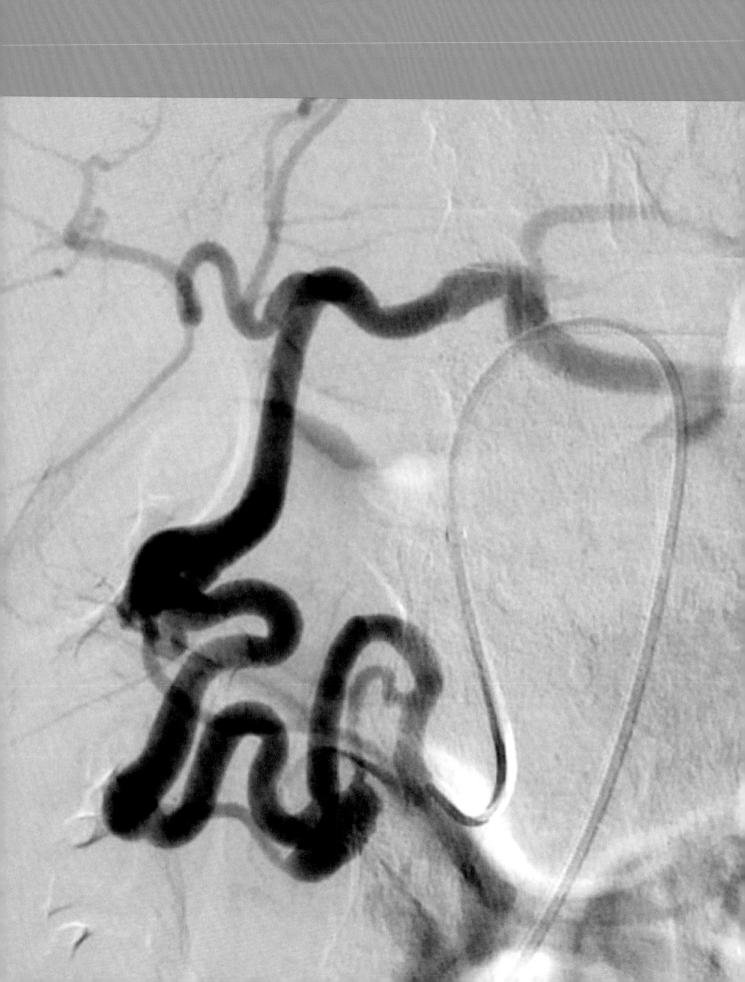

Generic Imaging Patterns

Retroperitoneal Mass, Cystic   460

Retroperitoneal Mass, Soft Tissue Density   466

Retroperitoneal Mass, Fat Containing   472

Retroperitoneal Hemorrhage   476

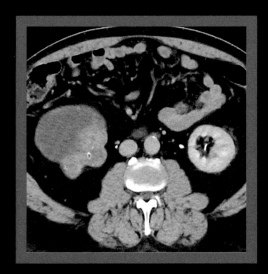

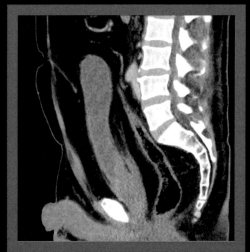

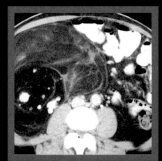

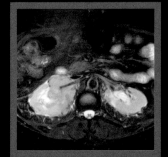

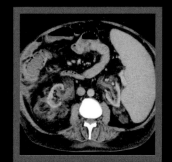

DIFFERENTIAL DIAGNOSIS

Common

- Renal Cystic Masses
  - Renal Cyst
  - Renal Cell Carcinoma (Cystic)
  - Mixed Epithelial and Stromal Tumor Family
- Pancreatic Cystic Masses
  - Pancreatitis-Related Collection
  - Mucinous Cystic Neoplasm
  - Serous Cystadenoma
  - Cystic Neuroendocrine Tumor
  - Solid and Pseudopapillary Neoplasm

Less Common

- Adrenal Cystic Masses
  - Adrenal Adenoma (Mimic)
  - Adrenal Cyst
  - Cystic Pheochromocytoma
- Urinoma
- Retroperitoneal Sarcoma (Mimic)
- Retroperitoneal Lymphocele
- Retroperitoneal Abscess
- Lymphangioma
- Neurogenic Tumor
- Retroperitoneal Seroma (Liquefied Hematoma)

Rare but Important

- Mature Cystic Teratoma
- Primary Retroperitoneal Mucinous Cystadenoma
- Cystic Retroperitoneal Mesothelioma
- Lymphangioleiomyomatosis, Retroperitoneum
- Bronchogenic Cyst
- Tailgut Cyst
- Pseudomyxoma Retroperitonei

ESSENTIAL INFORMATION

Key Differential Diagnosis Issues

- Most retroperitoneal cystic masses are easily recognized as arising from solid organs
  - Kidney
  - Pancreas
  - Adrenal
- "Cyst mass" may be fluid collection
  - Evolving hematoma
  - Seroma
  - Urinoma

Helpful Clues for Common Diagnoses

- Renal Cystic Masses
  - Renal cyst
    - By far, most common "retroperitoneal" cystic mass (> 50% of older adults)
  - Renal cell carcinoma (cystic)
    - Small percentage are cystic but usually have mural nodularity to exclude simple cyst
    - Look for claw sign to determine renal origin
  - Mixed Epithelial and Stromal Tumor Family

- Includes adult cystic nephroma (ACN) and mixed epithelial and stromal tumor (MEST), which have overlapping radiologic and pathologic features
- Complex, multicystic mass with numerous septations (± invagination into renal hilum) in postmenopausal women
- May be hard to differentiate from cystic renal cell carcinoma (Bosniak III/IV)
- Pediatric multilocular cystic nephroma (separate entity) occurs predominantly in boys 3 months to 4 years of age
- Pancreatic Cystic Masses
  - Pancreatitis-related collection
    - Pseudocyst → simple fluid; walled-off necrosis → complex with nonliquified components
    - Most common pancreatic cystic mass, especially in symptomatic patient with history of alcohol abuse or gallstones
  - Mucinous cystic neoplasm
    - Most common cystic pancreatic tumor
    - Multiseptated mass in body/tail ± mural nodularity
    - Middle-aged or older woman
  - Serous cystadenoma
    - Sponge or honeycomb appearance of well-encapsulated mass ± central scar
    - Much less common is macrocystic variant with fewer and larger cystic spaces
  - Other pancreatic cystic masses
    - Cystic neuroendocrine tumor
      - Can have internal cystic components when large
      - Some can be mostly cystic but often have solid, enhancing rim, which helps in diagnosis
    - Solid and pseudopapillary tumor
      - Young woman classically with solid and cystic mass in tail; can be very large

Helpful Clues for Less Common Diagnoses

- Adrenal Cystic Masses
  - Adrenal adenoma (mimic)
    - Lipid-rich adenoma appears near water attenuation on NECT but enhances, unlike adrenal cysts
  - Adrenal cyst
    - Water density
    - No enhancement
    - No visible wall
  - Cystic pheochromocytoma
    - Up to 1/3 have cystic components
- Urinoma
  - Perirenal or retroperitoneal collection of urine following ureteral obstruction and disruption of renal collecting system or ureter
  - Use delayed-phase imaging to look for contrast leak; can image up to several hours after administration
- Retroperitoneal Sarcoma (Mimic)
  - Necrotic tumor may mimic cystic mass
  - Myxoid components often have near water density
  - GIST can have heterogeneous, partially cystic appearance
- Retroperitoneal Lymphocele
  - Thin wall, usually unilocular; surrounding surgical clips

- o Common after pelvic node dissection/resection for prostate or bladder cancer and after retroperitoneal lymph node dissection for GYN or testicular cancer
- o Occurs in 2-18% of renal transplants
- o Can become superinfected
- **Retroperitoneal Abscess**
  - o Complex appearing, may contain gas
  - o Perirenal is most common
  - o Retroperitoneal perforation of duodenum, appendix, or diverticulitis are well-recognized sources
  - o Patient is symptomatic (fever, increased white count)
- **Lymphangioma**
  - o < 5% of lymphangiomas are abdominal
  - o Water (or less than water) density cystic mass with thin or imperceptible wall, no soft tissue
  - o Morphology: Microcystic, macrocystic, and combined variants
  - o Microcystic: Many thin septations, microlobulated borders ± calcifications
    - – Septations may be imperceptible by CT, better seen by US/MR
  - o Very soft, easily indented by adjacent vessels, does not compress adjacent organs
  - o May cross anatomic spaces
- **Neurogenic Tumor**
  - o Some may be cystic appearing (myxoid) or partially cystic
  - o Schwannoma most common retroperitoneal neurogenic tumor
  - o Ganglioneuroma often has low density on CT and appears cystic though is solid
- **Retroperitoneal Seroma (Liquefied Hematoma)**
  - o Evolving retroperitoneal hematoma (e.g., following ruptured aortic aneurysm or anticoagulation-induced hemorrhage)
  - o May become homogeneous, near water attenuation collection
  - o Compare with prior studies, history of hemorrhage

Helpful Clues for Rare Diagnoses

- **Mature Cystic Teratoma**

- o ~ 10% primary retroperitoneal location
- o Large, cystic mass in child with fat and calcification
- **Primary Retroperitoneal Mucinous Cystadenoma**
  - o Middle-aged women; rarely men
  - o Typically unilocular; not connected to ovary
  - o Enhancing nodules suggest borderline tumor or carcinoma, similar to ovary
- **Cystic Retroperitoneal Mesothelioma**
  - o Middle-aged women; ~ 50% with history of laparotomy or pelvic inflammatory disease
  - o Uni-/multilocular, benign cystic mass
- **Lymphangioleiomyomatosis, Retroperitoneum**
  - o Cystic or cystic and solid masses occur almost exclusively in women
  - o May change in size rapidly throughout day (unique to this diagnosis)
  - o Look for lung cysts, renal angiomyolipoma
- **Bronchogenic Cyst**
  - o Benign congenital cyst, which typically occurs above diaphragm
  - o Subdiaphragmatic location often on left
- **Tailgut Cyst**
  - o Found in retrorectal (presacral) space
  - o May be either unilocular or multilocular
  - o Locules tend to have different density on CT and signal intensity on MR
  - o Rarely complicated by tumor (adenocarcinoma, carcinoid)
- **Pseudomyxoma Retroperitonei**
  - o May occur in isolation without intraperitoneal disease from ruptured retrocecal appendiceal mucinous neoplasm

SELECTED REFERENCES

1. Hegazi TM et al: Retroperitoneal cystic masses: magnetic resonance imaging features. Abdom Radiol (NY). 45(2):499-511, 2020
2. Nguyen K et al: Update on MR Imaging of cystic retroperitoneal masses. Abdom Radiol (NY). 45(10):3172-83, 2020
3. Raufaste Tistet M et al: Imaging features, complications and differential diagnoses of abdominal cystic lymphangiomas. Abdom Radiol (NY). 45(11):3589-607, 2020

Renal Cyst

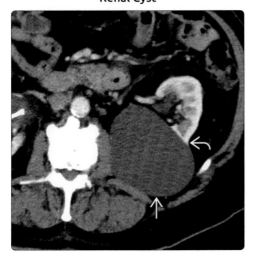

Renal Cell Carcinoma (Cystic)

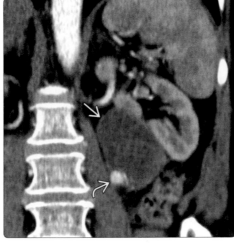

(Left) *Axial CECT shows a large, simple cyst* ➡ *in the left retroperitoneum. The claw sign* ➡ *with the renal parenchyma allows easy identification of the origin of this cyst.* (Right) *Coronal CECT shows a cystic mass* ➡ *arising from the kidney. The nodular, enhancing focus* ➡ *in the wall makes this a Bosniak IV lesion with a high likelihood of being malignant. Cystic renal cell carcinoma was found at resection.*

Renal Cell Carcinoma (Cystic)

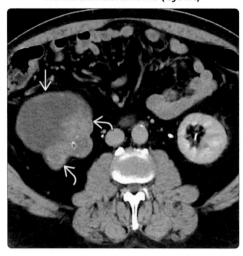

Mixed Epithelial and Stromal Tumor Family

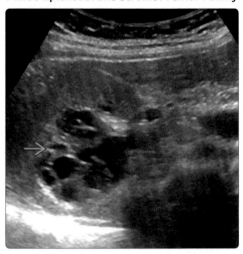

(Left) *Axial CECT shows a large, cystic mass* ➡ *arising from the lower pole of the right kidney. Note the large, solid component* ➡ *with calcification (Bosniak IV). Cystic clear cell carcinoma was found at resection.* **(Right)** *Transverse US of the right kidney shows an encapsulated, multiloculated cystic mass* ➡ *that herniates into the renal sinus, characteristic of mixed epithelial and stromal tumor.*

Mixed Epithelial and Stromal Tumor Family

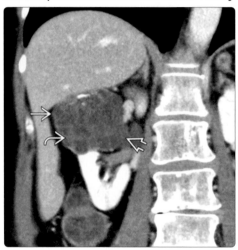

Pancreatitis-Related Collection

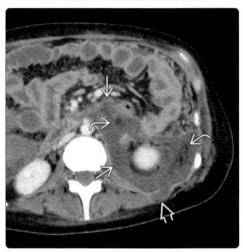

(Left) *Coronal CECT in a 64-year-old woman shows a large, complex cyst* ➡ *arising from the right kidney. Note the multiple faint septations* ➡ *and focus of calcification. The extension into the hilum* ➡ *and the age/sex of the patient are typical for this tumor.* **(Right)** *Axial CECT shows a large, rim-enhancing, cystic collection* ➡ *in the pararenal spaces surrounding the kidney. Note internal areas of nonliquified debris and fat* ➡ *, consistent with acute necrotic collection. Extension into the flank* ➡ *is also seen.*

Mucinous Cystic Neoplasm

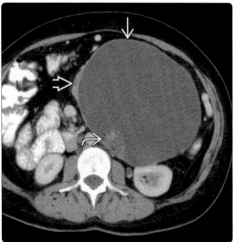

Mucinous Cystic Neoplasm

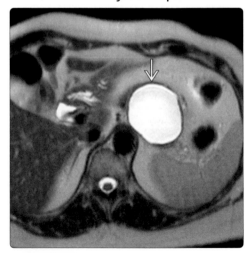

(Left) *Axial CECT in a 48-year-old woman shows a large, thin-walled, unilocular cyst* ➡ *in the left retroperitoneum. The claw sign with the pancreas tail* ➡ *helps determine origin. Note the faintly enhancing nodule* ➡ *along the posterior wall, which contained adenocarcinoma.* **(Right)** *Axial T2 MR in a 52-year-old woman shows a thin-walled, unilocular cyst* ➡ *in the pancreatic body. The patient's age and imaging findings are typical for this diagnosis.*

Serous Cystadenoma

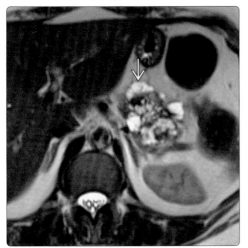

Serous Cystadenoma

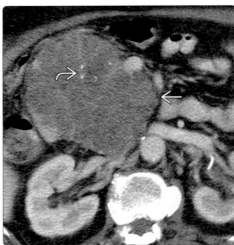

(Left) Axial T2 MR in a 78-year-old woman shows a complex cystic mass ➡ in the pancreatic tail composed of multiple tiny cysts and T2-dark septa. The patient's age and imaging findings are typical for this diagnosis. (Right) Axial CECT shows a large mass ➡ arising from the pancreatic head with a sponge or honeycomb appearance due to innumerable tiny cystic spaces. Some of the septa have focal calcifications ➹.

Cystic Neuroendocrine Tumor

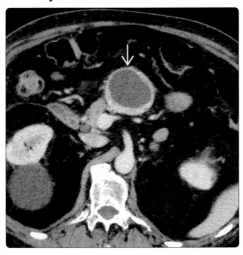

Adrenal Adenoma (Mimic)

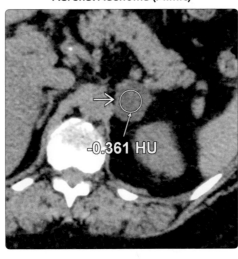

-0.361 HU

(Left) Axial CECT shows a cystic mass ➡ with a thick, enhancing wall arising from the pancreatic neck. Mucinous cystic neoplasm is a differential in this case. (Right) Axial NECT shows a water density left retroperitoneal mass ➡ arising from the adrenal gland. Postcontrast images (not shown) demonstrated enhancement. Some adenomas can mimic cysts on noncontrast imaging as they will measure near zero HU.

Adrenal Cyst

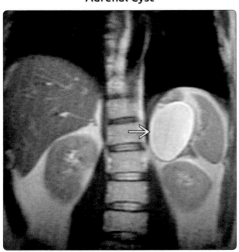

Cystic Pheochromocytoma

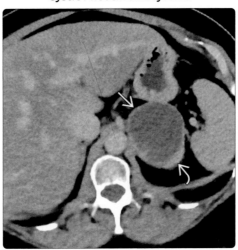

(Left) Coronal T2 MR shows a uniformly high-intensity mass ➡ in the left suprarenal region, a typical appearance for adrenal cysts. (Right) Axial CECT shows a cystic mass ➡ arising from the adrenal gland. Note the thick, enhancing wall ➹. ~ 30% of pheochromocytomas have cystic changes, and some may be largely cystic, as in this case.

(Left) *Axial CECT in a patient 2 weeks post trauma shows a rim-enhancing right retroperitoneal fluid collection* ➡ *abutting and displacing the kidney.* **(Right)** *Axial delayed-phased CECT in the same patient shows leakage of contrast-opacified urine* ➡ *into the collection, consistent with urinoma.*

Urinoma
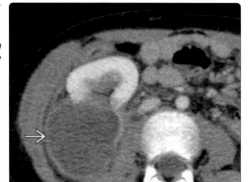

Urinoma
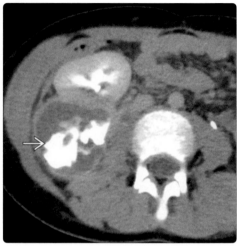

(Left) *Axial NECT shows a large, cystic right retroperitoneal and psoas muscle mass* ➡ *with a thick wall, local recurrence of dedifferentiated liposarcoma after extensive resection and IVC reconstruction* ➡. *Most retroperitoneal sarcomas are solid &/or fatty, though some may have necrotic or cystic areas.* **(Right)** *Coronal CECT shows a unilocular, thin-walled cystic mass* ➡ *extending from the pelvic sidewall to the pararenal space. This patient had recently had prostatectomy with lymph node dissection.*

Retroperitoneal Sarcoma (Mimic)
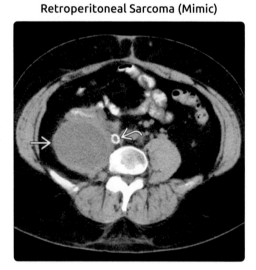

Retroperitoneal Lymphocele
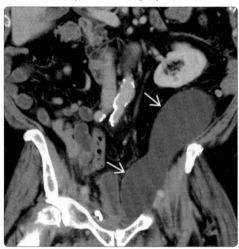

(Left) *Axial CECT shows a large, cystic, complex right retroperitoneal and psoas muscle mass* ➡ *with internal septations. Note the adjacent erosion of the lumbar endplate* ➡ *due to osteomyelitis as well as epidural abscess* ➡, *a clue to the etiology.* **(Right)** *Axial CECT shows a cystic retroperitoneal mass* ➡ *with microlobulated border and imperceptible wall, characteristic of lymphangioma. Note the lack of mass effect on the IVC or psoas muscle. A double IVC* ➡ *is also seen.*

Retroperitoneal Abscess
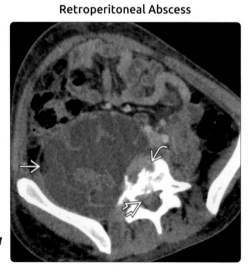

Lymphangioma
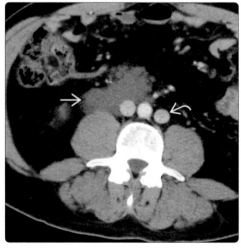

Lymphangioma

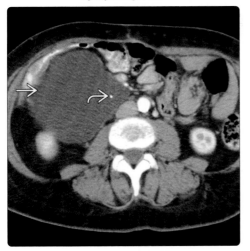

Neurogenic Tumor

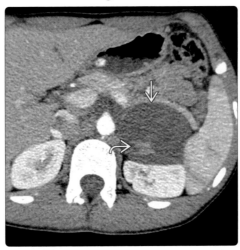

(Left) *Axial CECT shows a large, water density cyst* ➡ *that displaces abdominal and retroperitoneal structures. The presence of a small calcification* ➡ *suggests thin septa that are difficult to detect by CT.* (Right) *Axial CECT shows a left suprarenal mass* ➡, *which appears cystic, though there is a small area of possible internal enhancement* ➡. *Resection found ganglioneuroma, which are solid but can be low density and mimic a cyst on CT.*

Mature Cystic Teratoma

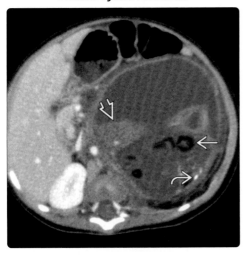

Primary Retroperitoneal Mucinous Cystadenoma

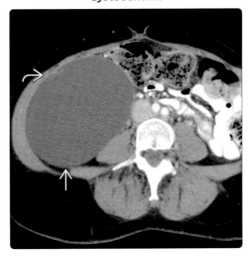

(Left) *Axial CECT in a 9-month-old girl shows a large, cystic retroperitoneal mass with mixed components, including fat* ➡, *soft tissue* ➡, *and calcification* ➡. (Right) *Axial CECT in a 53-year-old woman shows a large, cystic right retroperitoneal mass* ➡ *with a thin wall. Note the papillary-like area* ➡ *along the wall. The cyst was separate from the ovary and was benign at resection.*

Lymphangioleiomyomatosis, Retroperitoneum

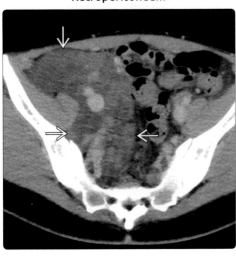

Tailgut Cyst

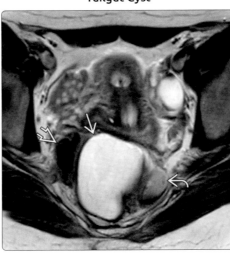

(Left) *Axial CECT in a 36-year-old woman shows a large, heterogeneous, cystic and solid right retroperitoneal mass* ➡ *extending to the pelvic sidewall and encasing (but not narrowing) vessels. The patient had lung cysts (not shown). These masses are due to lymph obstruction from smooth muscle hypertrophy.* (Right) *Axial CECT in a 29-year-old woman shows a large cyst* ➡ *between the rectum* ➡ *and coccyx. The cyst is multilocular with varying signal intensities* ➡.

DIFFERENTIAL DIAGNOSIS

Common

- Lymphoma
- Metastases
- Sarcoma
- Retroperitoneal Hemorrhage
- Infectious/Inflammatory Nodes

Less Common

- Retroperitoneal Fibrosis
- Duplications and Anomalies of Inferior Vena Cava
- Collateral Vessels and Varices
- Neurogenic Tumors
- Solitary Fibrous Tumor

Rare but Important

- Extramedullary Hematopoiesis
- Lymphangioleiomyomatosis
- Retroperitoneal Germ Cell Tumor (Primary or Within Cryptorchid Testis)

ESSENTIAL INFORMATION

Key Differential Diagnosis Issues

- Determine location and origin of mass
  - Determine if arising from retroperitoneal (RP) organ (e.g., kidney, adrenal, pancreas)
    - Look for claw sign
  - If it causes anterior displacement of RP structure [e.g., ascending or descending colon, aorta, inferior vena cava (IVC)], it is RP
    - If not arising from organ, it may be primary RP mass or metastasis
- Most RP masses are malignant
  - Lymphoma > metastases > primary sarcoma
  - Lymphoma tends to be homogeneous, solid, and enhancing; whereas metastasis and sarcoma tend to be heterogeneous with areas of necrosis
- Some lesions mimic malignancy
  - Hemorrhage, RP fibrosis, abnormal vessels, reactive lymphadenopathy
- Do not forget to look for testicular mass with scrotal US in young to middle-aged man presenting with RP mass

Helpful Clues for Common Diagnoses

- **Lymphoma**
  - Non-Hodgkin > Hodgkin for abdominal disease, especially with mesenteric nodes
  - Discrete or confluent homogeneous soft tissue masses/lymph nodes surrounding aorta and IVC
  - Confluent soft tissue mantle fills paraaortic spaces in advanced cases
    - Displacement of aorta from spine (unusual for benign etiologies)
- **Metastases**
  - Most common primary sites: GI, GU, GYN cancers
  - Testicular cancer may first present as RP mass
  - Extranodal RP metastases: Melanoma, renal cell, breast, and small cell lung cancers
    - Tend to occur in fat around kidneys
- **Sarcoma**

- Best clue: Large, heterogeneous solid (± necrotic) mass that displaces viscera
  - Liposarcoma is most common RP sarcoma
    - Most commonly, mixture of fat, hazy fat, and solid enhancing masses
  - Leiomyosarcoma is 2nd most common RP sarcoma
    - Large, encapsulated, soft tissue density mass with foci of necrosis
    - Often arises from IVC wall and can grow outward &/or inward (intraluminal)
  - Undifferentiated pleomorphic sarcoma
    - Most common soft tissue sarcoma in adults in any site (typically extremities); 3rd most common in RP
    - Nonspecific imaging; generally large and invasive
- **Retroperitoneal Hemorrhage**
  - Iatrogenic, coagulopathic, or ruptured aneurysm
  - Fluid of high density dissects along fascial planes ± involves psoas, iliacus muscles
- **Infectious/Inflammatory Nodes**
  - Mycobacterial infections, sarcoid, chronic HIV infection, lupus, reactive lymphadenopathy from chronic lower extremity infections
  - Generally multiple mildly enlarged pelvic and paraaortic lymph nodes ± abnormal enhancement/necrosis
  - History is key to diagnosis

Helpful Clues for Less Common Diagnoses

- **Retroperitoneal Fibrosis**
  - Mantle of tissue encasing lower aorta, IVC, ureters
  - Often causes ureteral obstruction and medial deviation
  - Tends to be smaller/thinner than malignant causes but biopsy often needed
- **Duplications and Anomalies of Inferior Vena Cava**
  - Left IVC can mimic RP lymphadenopathy, especially on NECT
    - Left-sided IVC joins left renal vein
  - Tubular, branching, easily recognized if followed carefully; matches blood pool enhancement
  - Azygous/hemiazygos continuation of IVC can mimic retrocrural lymphadenopathy
- **Collateral Vessels and Varices**
  - Bypassing occluded or absent IVC
  - Portal hypertension (varices often shunt to renal and gonadal veins)
- **Neurogenic Tumors**
  - Schwannoma: Most common, often paravertebral or presacral
    - ~ 3-9 cm; round, variable appearance ± cystic degeneration, calcifications
  - Paraganglioma: 2nd most common RP tumor; often located at inferior mesenteric artery (IMA) origin (organ of Zuckerkandl)
    - Avidly enhances
  - Ganglioneuroma: Well circumscribed, oval or lobulated
    - Sometimes very low density, cystic-appearing
  - Neurofibroma: Usually solitary and de novo, 10% multiple as part of neurofibromatosis type 1 (NF1)
    - Well marginated, round, homogeneous, sometimes targetoid
  - Malignant peripheral nerve sheath tumor: Rapidly enlarging, PET positive

- No reliable imaging characteristic can differentiate benign from malignant neurogenic tumors
- **Solitary Fibrous Tumor**
  o 1/3 found outside of thorax, often in extremities or retroperitoneum
    - Often presacral space displacing rectum anteriorly
  o Large, solid, avidly enhancing RP or presacral mass with dilated serpentine vessels around periphery

Helpful Clues for Rare Diagnoses

- **Extramedullary Hematopoiesis**
  o In patients with myelodysplastic conditions or hemoglobinopathies
  o Thoracic paraspinal masses most common
  o Presacral and perirenal masses may be seen in retroperitoneum
    - Other abdominal sites include liver and spleen
- **Lymphangioleiomyomatosis**
  o Cystic or cystic and solid masses occur almost exclusively in women

o May change in size rapidly throughout day (unique to this diagnosis)
o Look for lung cysts, renal angiomyolipoma (AML)

- **Retroperitoneal Germ Cell Tumor (Primary or Within Cryptorchid Testis)**
  o Primary RP germ cell tumor originates from aberrant germ cell rests
    - Nonspecific solid mass; elevated testicular cancer tumor markers
    - Differential diagnosis is undiscovered burnt-out testicular tumor metastatic to retroperitoneum
  o Cryptorchid RP testis may develop germ cell tumor (increased risk) and present late as large mass
    - Absent scrotal testis

SELECTED REFERENCES

1. Czeyda-Pommersheim F et al: Diagnostic approach to primary retroperitoneal pathologies: what the radiologist needs to know. Abdom Radiol (NY). 46(3):1062-81, 2020
2. Levy AD et al: Soft-tissue sarcomas of the abdomen and pelvis: radiologic-pathologic features, part 1-common sarcomas: From the Radiologic Pathology Archives. Radiographics. 37(2):462-83, 2017

Lymphoma

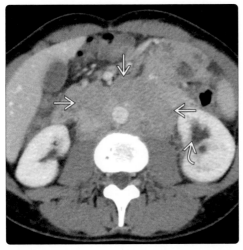

Lymphoma

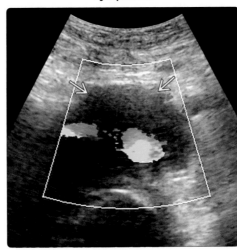

(Left) *Axial CECT shows a large, homogeneous, enhancing mass* ➡ *encasing the aorta and inferior vena cava (IVC). The mass causes mild left hydronephrosis* ➡ *as well. The appearance is typical of lymphoma.* **(Right)** *Transverse color Doppler US shows a soft tissue mass* ➡ *surrounding the aorta and IVC due to non-Hodgkin lymphoma.*

Lymphoma

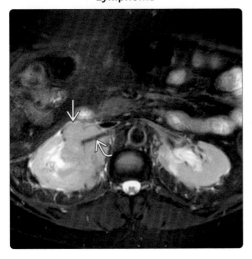

Lymphoma

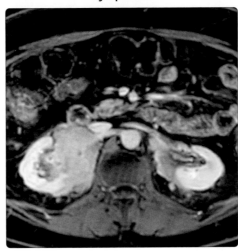

(Left) *Axial T2 FS MR shows a homogeneous, moderate-intensity right renal hilar mass* ➡ *encasing (but not narrowing) the right renal artery flow void* ➡. **(Right)** *Axial T1 C+ MR in the same patient shows homogeneous, moderate enhancement of the mass. Typically, lymphoma is solid and homogeneous, whereas other masses, such as sarcomas and metastases, may be heterogeneous and necrotic, though there is imaging overlap.*

Lymphoma

Metastases

(Left) *Axial CECT shows retroperitoneal and mesenteric adenopathy ➡ in a patient with chronic lymphocytic leukemia.* **(Right)** *Coronal CECT in a woman with ovarian cancer shows multiple enlarged lymph node masses ➡ in the paraaortic space, consistent with metastatic disease. Pelvic cancers tend to ascend upward from pelvic to paraaortic to retrocrural to thoracic and supraclavicular nodes.*

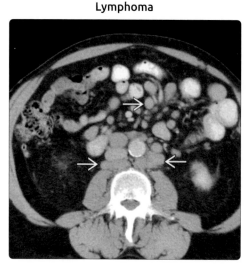

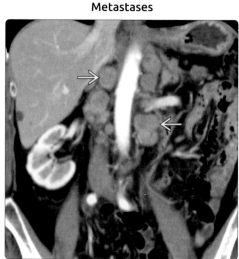

Metastases

Metastases

(Left) *Axial CECT in a 20-year-old man with flank pain shows a very large right retroperitoneal mass ➡ with nonspecific imaging features. In this patient population, testicular cancer should always be considered with a paraaortic retroperitoneal mass.* **(Right)** *Scrotal US immediately after CT in the same patient shows a vague, hypoechoic lesion ➡ in the right testis with areas of calcification ➡. Orchiectomy revealed a burnt-out germ cell tumor, and retroperitoneal biopsy showed seminoma.*

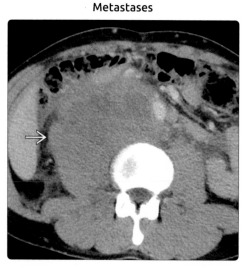

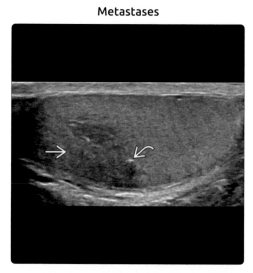

Sarcoma

Sarcoma

(Left) *Axial CECT shows a very large retroperitoneal mass with a mixture of fat ➡, low-density solid areas ➡, enhancing septa ➡, and solid enhancing areas ➡, typical of liposarcoma.* **(Right)** *Axial CECT shows a heterogeneous mass ➡ involving the IVC ➡. Resection revealed leiomyosarcoma. These commonly arise from the IVC and may be intraluminal, extraluminal, or both.*

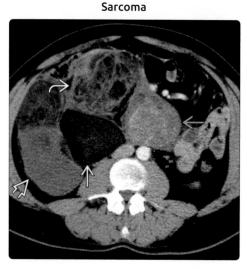

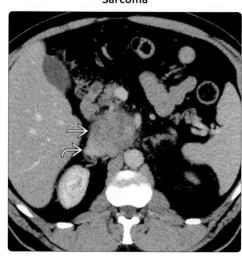

Sarcoma

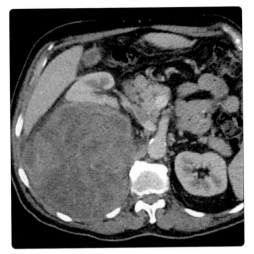

Sarcoma

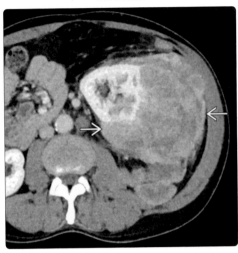

(Left) *Axial CECT shows a large, heterogeneous, solid, enhancing right retroperitoneal mass displacing the kidney anteriorly. Note the lack of claw sign, suggesting primary retroperitoneal origin. Dedifferentiated liposarcoma was found at biopsy.* (Right) *Axial CECT shows a large left retroperitoneal mass ➡ invading the kidney. Renal masses were in the differential; however, this was also a dedifferentiated liposarcoma. Some liposarcomas show no fatty elements.*

Retroperitoneal Hemorrhage

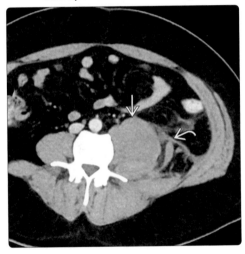

Retroperitoneal Hemorrhage

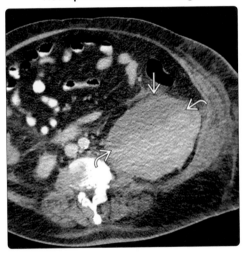

(Left) *Axial CECT in a 45-year-old man on heparin drip shows enlargement of the left psoas muscle ➡ and adjacent small posterior pararenal space hemorrhage ➡. Often, coagulopathic hemorrhage will start in the muscles and spread to the retroperitoneal spaces.* (Right) *Axial CECT shows a large left retroperitoneal mass ➡. The hematocrit level ➡ in this case is helpful to identify this as hemorrhage rather than a neoplasm.*

Infectious/Inflammatory Nodes

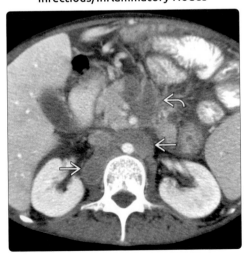

Infectious/Inflammatory Nodes

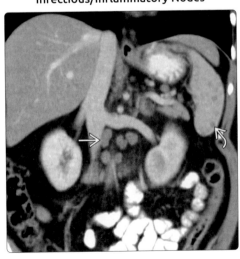

(Left) *Axial CECT in a patient with poorly controlled HIV/AIDS shows a retroperitoneal mass ➡ encasing the aorta and invading the psoas muscle. A separate central mesenteric mass ➡ is also seen. Biopsy showed Mycobacterium avium infection.* (Right) *Coronal CECT in a 54-year-old woman with a history of pulmonary sarcoid shows mildly enlarged retroperitoneal lymph nodes ➡ and multiple splenic lesions ➡, typical of abdominal sarcoid.*

Retroperitoneal Fibrosis

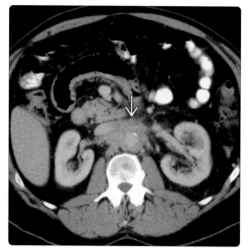

Retroperitoneal Fibrosis

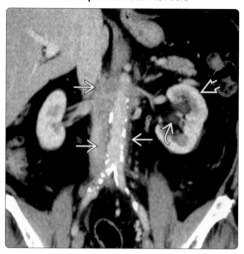

(Left) *Axial CECT shows a rind of soft tissue encasing the aorta and IVC* ➡. **(Right)** *Coronal CECT in the same patient shows the soft tissue* ➡ *extending inferiorly between the aorta and IVC as well as a delayed left nephrogram* ➡ *and mild hydronephrosis* ➡. *Primary differential is lymphoma or, rarely, metastatic disease. Biopsy is often needed to exclude malignancy and diagnose retroperitoneal fibrosis.*

Collateral Vessels and Varices

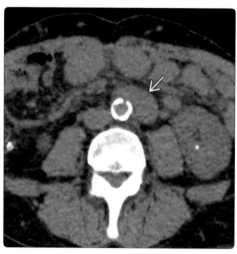

Collateral Vessels and Varices

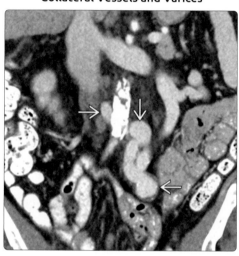

(Left) *Axial NECT shows an oval mass* ➡ *in the left paraaortic space, which was initially suspicious for a primary mass or lymphadenopathy.* **(Right)** *Coronal CECT in the same patient shows that the "mass" represents tortuous and dilated retroperitoneal varices* ➡ *related to a portosystemic shunt in the setting of cirrhosis. Reformats are useful to distinguish vessels from masses.*

Neurogenic Tumors

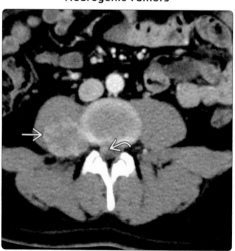

Neurogenic Tumors

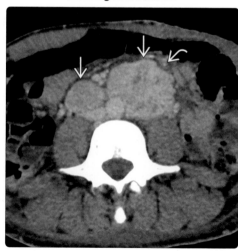

(Left) *Axial CECT in a patient with flank pain shows an avidly enhancing mass* ➡ *centered in the right psoas muscle. The appearance was nonspecific, and sarcoma was felt most likely. A small lesion was seen in the spinal canal* ➡. *Resection showed a malignant peripheral nerve sheath tumor.* **(Right)** *Axial CECT shows bilateral, avidly enhancing, solid retroperitoneal masses* ➡ *located near the inferior mesenteric artery (IMA) origin* ➡. *This patient was not hypertensive, but biopsy revealed paraganglioma.*

Neurogenic Tumors

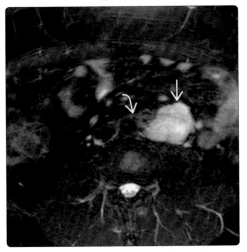

Neurogenic Tumors

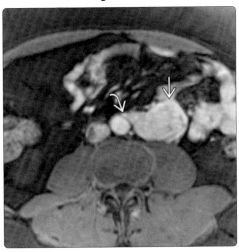

(Left) *Axial T2 FS MR in a hypertensive 47-year-old man shows a left paraaortic mass* ➔, *which is hyperintense and located near the origin of the IMA* ➔. (Right) *Axial T1 C+ MR in the same patient shows avid enhancement of the mass* ➔. *The IMA* ➔ *is again seen. The location and appearance of this lesion are typical of paraganglioma. Biochemical work-up generally helps confirm the diagnosis and avoid biopsy.*

Neurogenic Tumors

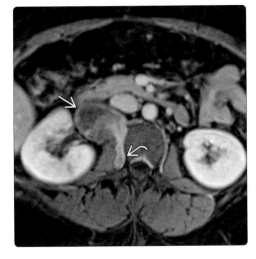

Solitary Fibrous Tumor

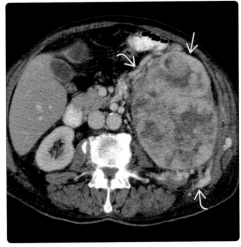

(Left) *Axial T1 C+ FS MR in an 18-year-old woman with flank pain shows a heterogeneous, enhancing mass* ➔ *in the right renal hilum. Note the tail-like extension* ➔ *toward the neuroforamen, which was a clue to the diagnosis in this case. Ganglioneuroma was found at resection.* (Right) *Axial CECT shows a very large, solid, avidly enhancing left retroperitoneal mass* ➔ *with large peritumoral vessels* ➔. *Differential included sarcoma and renal cell carcinoma; however, biopsy revealed an unexpected diagnosis of solitary fibrous tumor.*

Extramedullary Hematopoiesis

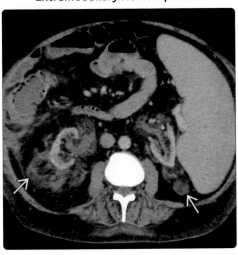

Retroperitoneal Germ Cell Tumor (Primary or Within Cryptorchid Testis)

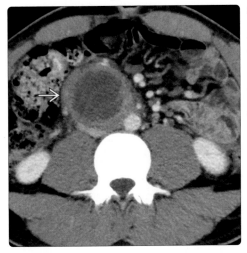

(Left) *Axial CECT in a patient with myelofibrosis shows splenomegaly and multiple bilateral perirenal masses* ➔ *with a mixture of soft tissue and fat density. Paraspinal masses were also seen in the thorax (not shown).* (Right) *Axial CECT in a 20-year-old man shows an aortocaval necrotic mass* ➔, *which is nonspecific. Scrotal US was negative. AFP was markedly elevated, and the patient was diagnosed with a primary retroperitoneal germ cell tumor.*

DIFFERENTIAL DIAGNOSIS

Common

- Liposarcoma
- Angiomyolipoma, Renal
- Adrenal Myelolipoma

Less Common

- Postsurgical Fat Necrosis
- Growing Teratoma Syndrome
- Lipoma, Retroperitoneal

Rare but Important

- Teratoma, Retroperitoneal
- Extraadrenal Myelolipoma
- Extramedullary Hematopoiesis
- Hibernoma (Brown Fat)

ESSENTIAL INFORMATION

Key Differential Diagnosis Issues

- 2 key features distinguish liposarcoma from renal angiomyolipoma (AML)
  - Liposarcoma is less vascular than AML
  - AML arises from kidney with triangular defect in cortex

Helpful Clues for Common Diagnoses

- **Liposarcoma**
  - Usually large when discovered with mixed fat and soft tissue density components as well as stranding and septa
  - Usually compresses and displaces retroperitoneal organs; invasion is uncommon
- **Angiomyolipoma, Renal**
  - Benign hamartoma composed of blood vessels, muscle, and fat
  - Large AML may simulate liposarcoma (both contain fat)
  - Renal parenchymal defect and enlarged vessels favor AML
- **Adrenal Myelolipoma**
  - Fat and soft tissue components arising from or replacing adrenal gland ± calcification

Helpful Clues for Less Common Diagnoses

- **Postsurgical Fat Necrosis**
  - Encapsulated, irregular fat in or near surgical bed (e.g., after nephrectomy)
- **Growing Teratoma Syndrome**
  - Testicular or ovarian malignant teratomas
  - Growing retroperitoneal mixed fatty density mass in patient with treated nonseminomatous germ cell tumor may represent residual teratoma (chemoresistant)
- **Lipoma, Retroperitoneal**
  - Benign lipomas are very rare in retroperitoneum; most fatty masses are liposarcoma
  - No septa, stranding, or solid component

Helpful Clues for Rare Diagnoses

- **Teratoma, Retroperitoneal**
  - Uncommon to rare as primary retroperitoneal tumor; most present in 1st decade
- **Extraadrenal Myelolipoma**
  - Classic: Mixed-density fat and soft tissue encapsulated mass in presacral space in older woman
  - Can be found anywhere in body, including perirenal and retroperitoneal locations
- **Extramedullary Hematopoiesis**
  - Occurs in myelofibrosis, leukemia, sickle cell, thalassemia, and others
  - Presacral location 2nd most common (thoracic paraspinal MC) and generally indistinguishable from extraadrenal myelolipoma
  - May contain variable amount of fat and soft tissue
- **Hibernoma (Brown Fat)**
  - Typically slightly higher attenuation than normal fat on CT
  - Highly metabolically active on FDG PET/CT

SELECTED REFERENCES

1. Fattahi N et al: Fat-containing pelvic lesions in females. Abdom Radiol (NY). 47(1):362-77, 2022

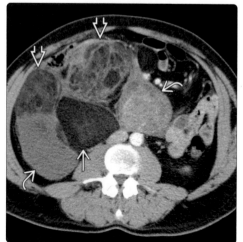

Liposarcoma

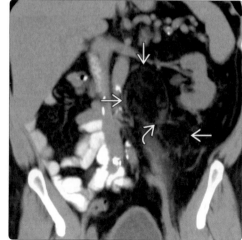

Liposarcoma

(Left) Axial CECT shows a large right retroperitoneal mass composed of multiple densities, including fat ➡, fat with septa and hazy areas ⬅, and solid masses ➡. Resection showed dedifferentiated liposarcoma. (Right) Coronal NECT shows a subtle, encapsulated left retroperitoneal mass ➡ with thin capsule and minimal hazy areas and septa internally ➡. This was a locally recurrent, well-differentiated liposarcoma.

Liposarcoma

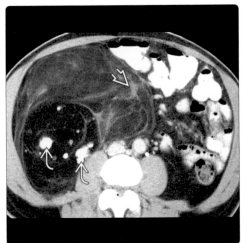

Liposarcoma

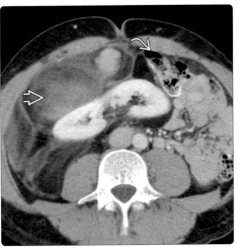

(Left) Axial CECT shows a mass that displaces the right kidney and ascending colon. The mass is mostly made up of fat density but has foci of calcification ➘, hazy areas, and soft tissue ➘ density. *(Right)* Axial CECT shows a heterogeneous mass that displaces and flattens the right kidney and displaces the ascending colon ➘. The mass is composed of fat and soft tissue ➘ elements.

Angiomyolipoma, Renal

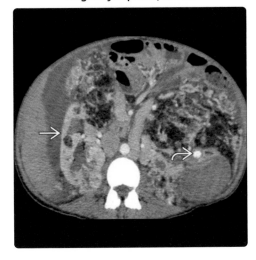

Angiomyolipoma, Renal

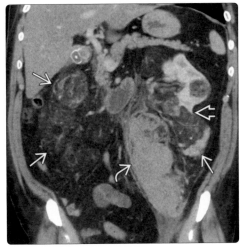

(Left) Axial CECT in a patient with tuberous sclerosis shows giant, bilateral retroperitoneal masses containing fat and intermixed enhancing soft tissue. Note that a portion of the normal right kidney ➘ is seen, and aneurysms are present ➘. *(Right)* Coronal CECT shows large, bilateral, fat-containing masses ➘ with areas of soft tissue and haziness. The left-sided mass can be seen arising from the kidney ➘ and is complicated by acute retroperitoneal hemorrhage ➘.

Angiomyolipoma, Renal

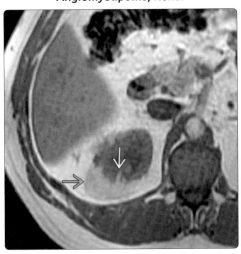

Angiomyolipoma, Renal

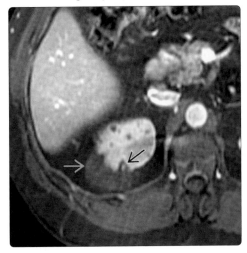

(Left) Axial T1 MR shows a lesion ➘ with signal intensity similar to fat arising from the posterior renal cortex via a small defect ➘. *(Right)* Axial T1 C+ FS MR in the same patient shows that the lesion ➘ loses signal intensity with application of fat saturation. A cortical defect (notch sign) and a feeding vessel ➘ are present.

(Left) *Axial CECT shows a large, fatty right retroperitoneal mass* ➡ *with hazy areas displacing the kidney anteriorly. Differential is broad based on this image alone.* (Right) *Coronal CECT in the same patient shows that the mass arises from the suprarenal fossa, and the normal adrenal gland is not seen. Adrenal myelolipoma was suspected and confirmed at resection.*

Adrenal Myelolipoma

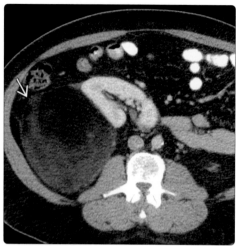

Adrenal Myelolipoma

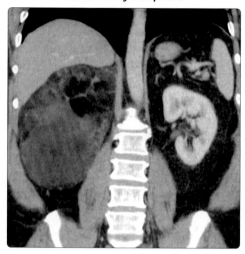

(Left) *Axial in-phase T1 MR shows a left adrenal mass* ➡ *with areas of high and intermediate signal. Axial opposed-phase T1 MR shows India ink artifact in the mass* ➡ *between the fat and soft tissue components. This is signal loss due to fat and water in the same voxel and is typical of myelolipoma.* (Right) *Axial CECT shows a large, suprarenal mass* ➡ *made up mostly of fat with large foci of calcification* ➡.

Adrenal Myelolipoma

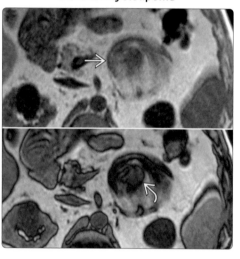

Adrenal Myelolipoma

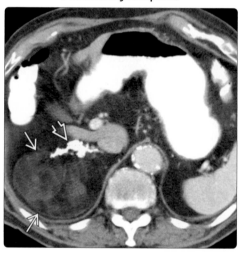

(Left) *Axial T1 MR shows a hyperintense left perirenal mass* ➡ *with a T1-dark rim. Fat-suppression images (not shown) confirmed fat contents. The patient had recently undergone partial nephrectomy, and findings are consistent with fat necrosis.* (Right) *Axial NECT shows an area of encapsulated fat* ➡ *anterior to the right kidney, adjacent to a partial nephrectomy site.*

Postsurgical Fat Necrosis

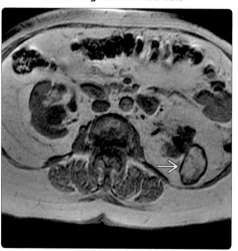

Postsurgical Fat Necrosis

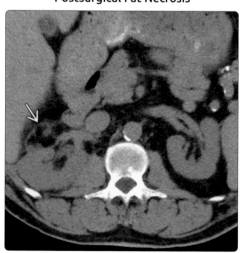

Teratoma, Retroperitoneal

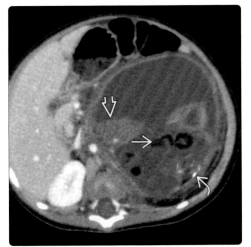

Teratoma, Retroperitoneal

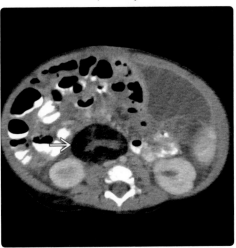

(Left) *Axial CECT in a 9-month-old girl shows a large, cystic retroperitoneal mass with mixed components including fat ➡, soft tissue ➡, and calcification ➡. (Right) Axial CECT in a 4-month-old girl shows a retroperitoneal fatty mass ➡ with a small area of central fluid.*

Extraadrenal Myelolipoma

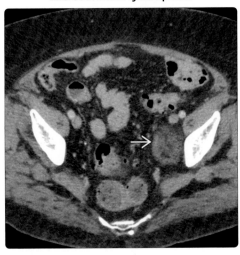

Extraadrenal Myelolipoma

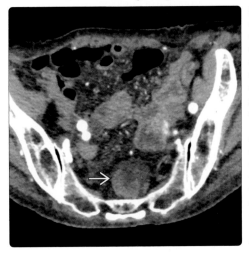

(Left) *Axial CECT in a 75-year-old woman shows a mixed fat and soft tissue mass ➡ along the left pelvic sidewall. Liposarcoma was considered as well as extraadrenal myelolipoma, which was proven upon resection. (Right) Axial CECT in an 87-year-old woman shows an incidental, mixed fat and soft tissue density, well-defined mass in the presacral space, the most common location of extraadrenal myelolipoma ➡. Extramedullary hematopoiesis could also be considered, but the patient had no predisposing condition.*

Hibernoma (Brown Fat)

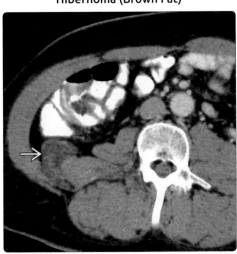

Hibernoma (Brown Fat)

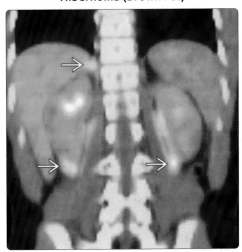

(Left) *Axial CECT shows a small right retroperitoneal mass ➡ insinuating around the quadratus muscle with mixed fat and soft tissue density. Liposarcoma was considered most likely, but this would be atypical due to its small size. Biopsy showed hibernoma. (Right) Coronal FDG PET/CT in a 12-year-old boy shows bilateral perinephric uptake ➡ with only minimally hazy fat seen on CT (not shown), consistent with brown fat.*

Retroperitoneum

DIFFERENTIAL DIAGNOSIS

Common

- Renal Trauma
- Pelvic Trauma
- Coagulopathic Hemorrhage
- Groin Arterial Puncture Site Complication
- Ruptured Abdominal Aortic Aneurysm

Less Common

- Hepatic Trauma
- Perirenal Hemorrhage
  - Renal Cell Carcinoma
  - Angiomyolipoma, Renal
  - Vasculitis
- Adrenal Hemorrhage

ESSENTIAL INFORMATION

Key Differential Diagnosis Issues

- Patient history (trauma, iatrogenic vs. spontaneous) and location of bleeding usually allows distinction of etiology

Helpful Clues for Common Diagnoses

- **Renal Trauma**
  - Perirenal hemorrhage accompanies almost all renal injuries
  - Irregular parenchymal defect ± active extravasation of blood &/or urine
- **Pelvic Trauma**
  - Extraperitoneal bleeding often extends cephalad along iliacus and psoas muscles into retroperitoneum
  - Look for active bleeding for possible intervention
- **Coagulopathic Hemorrhage**
  - Often moderate to large in size, centered in posterior pararenal space and extending to other spaces
  - Sometimes limited to rectus sheath or iliopsoas muscles
  - Classically shows hematocrit level
- **Groin Arterial Puncture Site Complication**
  - Extension from groin into retroperitoneal soft tissues of pelvis → abdomen
    - Associated with double wall and high punctures
    - Look for associated groin hematoma, pseudoaneurysm, arteriovenous fistula
- **Ruptured Abdominal Aortic Aneurysm**
  - Much more likely when aneurysm > 5 cm
  - Hematoma abuts aneurysm wall; disrupted wall calcifications, active bleeding

Helpful Clues for Less Common Diagnoses

- **Hepatic Trauma**
  - Injury to bare area of liver or inferior vena cava injury may result in retroperitoneal hemorrhage; generally extends along cava, associated with ipsilateral adrenal and renal injury
- **Perirenal Hemorrhage**
  - Renal tumors may bleed spontaneously or after trauma
    - Look for spherical mass with claw sign (parenchymal defect)
    - May be obscured by blood; follow-up imaging may be needed
    - Renal cell carcinoma most common; heterogeneous, large mass
    - Angiomyolipoma; fat component within mass
  - Vasculitis: PAN 3rd most common cause of spontaneous renal hemorrhage
  - Iatrogenic hemorrhage: Stone procedures, biopsy, ablation, partial nephrectomy
- **Adrenal Hemorrhage**
  - Common in neonates
  - May result from trauma, sepsis, shock, post partum, coagulopathy, underlying tumor or cyst, surgery
  - Bilateral hemorrhage is usually not due to direct trauma, tumor, or surgery

SELECTED REFERENCES

1. Arslan S et al: Imaging findings of spontaneous intraabdominal hemorrhage: neoplastic and non-neoplastic causes. Abdom Radiol (NY). 47(4):1473-502, 2022
2. Expert Panel on Vascular Imaging et al: ACR Appropriateness Criteria® suspected retroperitoneal bleed. J Am Coll Radiol. 18(11S):S482-7, 2021
3. Udare A et al: CT and MR imaging of acute adrenal disorders. Abdom Radiol (NY). 46(1):290-302, 2021

Renal Trauma

Renal Trauma

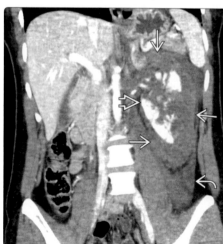
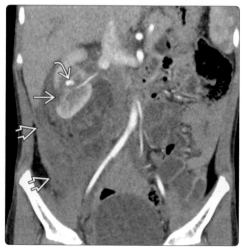

(Left) Coronal CECT in a 30-year-old woman after MVC shows a shattered left kidney ➡ with multiple lacerations and areas of devascularization, a grade V injury. Note the large perinephric space ➡ and posterior pararenal space ➡ hemorrhages. (Right) Coronal CECT in a 5-year-old boy shows a renal laceration ➡ and associated large retroperitoneal hemorrhage ➡. Note the pseudoaneurysm ➡ in the kidney, which required embolization.

Pelvic Trauma

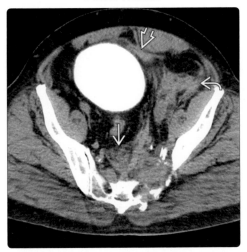

Coagulopathic Hemorrhage

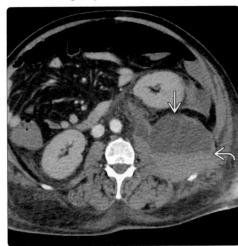

(Left) *Axial CT cystogram in a patient with extensive pelvic fractures shows presacral space hemorrhage ➡ extending along the pelvic sidewall to the posterior pararenal space ➡, displacing the bladder. Note hemorrhage in the prevesical space of Retzius ➡. These spaces communicate, and blood from the pelvis may travel upward.* (Right) *Axial CECT shows a large left posterior pararenal space hemorrhage ➡ with hematocrit level ➡, which is typical of coagulopathic bleeding.*

Coagulopathic Hemorrhage

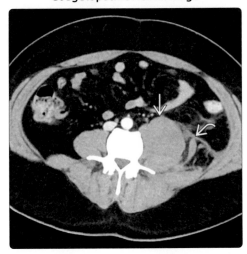

Ruptured Abdominal Aortic Aneurysm

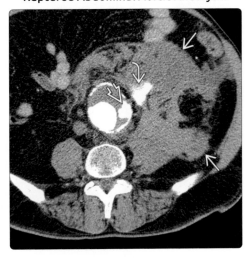

(Left) *Axial CECT in a 45-year-old man on heparin drip shows enlargement of the left psoas muscle ➡ and adjacent small posterior pararenal space hemorrhage ➡. Often, coagulopathic hemorrhage will start in the muscle and spread to the retroperitoneal spaces.* (Right) *Axial CECT in a patient with a 6-cm AAA shows a large left retroperitoneal hemorrhage ➡. Note the contrast-enhanced blood ➡ extending into the mural thrombus and the active extravasation ➡ at the site of rupture.*

Angiomyolipoma, Renal

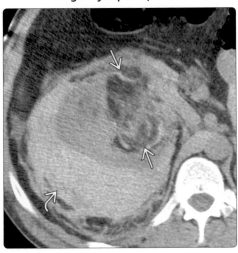

Adrenal Hemorrhage

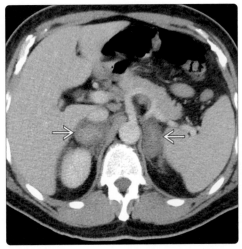

(Left) *Axial NECT shows extensive spontaneous bleeding ➡ into the perirenal space from an angiomyolipoma, which in this case is easily recognized as the heterogeneous, fat density mass ➡.* (Right) *Axial CECT in an ICU patient with COVID-19 shows bilateral adrenal masses ➡ with central hyperdensity and surrounding stranding. These findings are typical of adrenal hemorrhage, which is associated with sepsis and COVID-19 infection.*

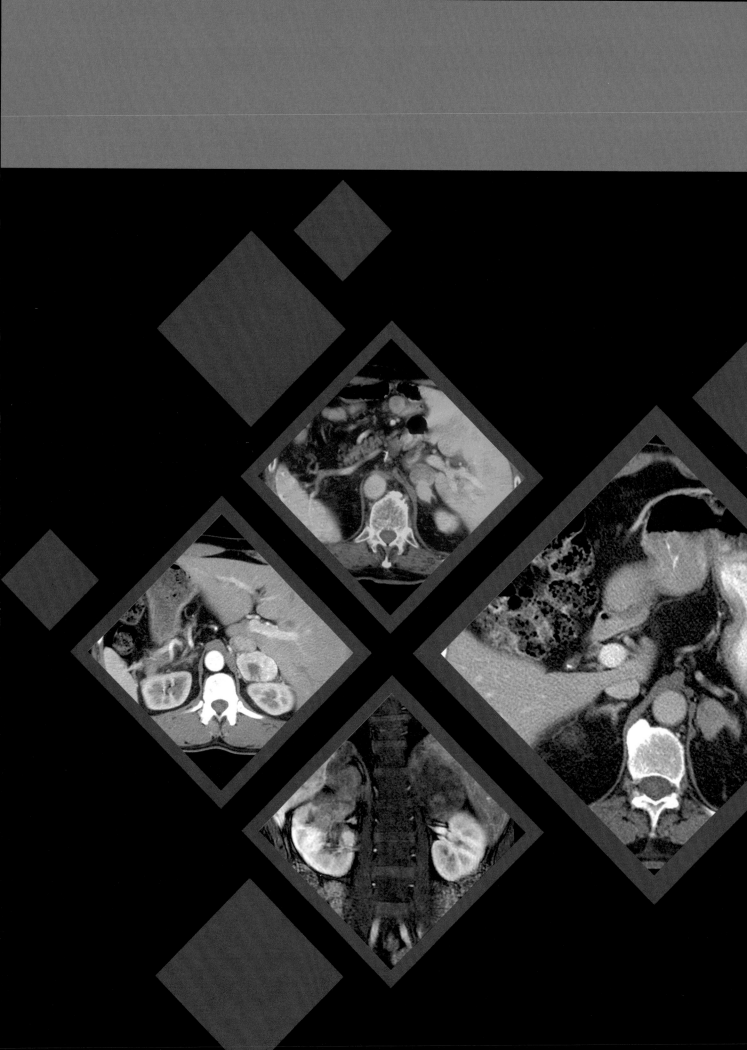

Adrenal

Generic Imaging Patterns

Adrenal Mass   480

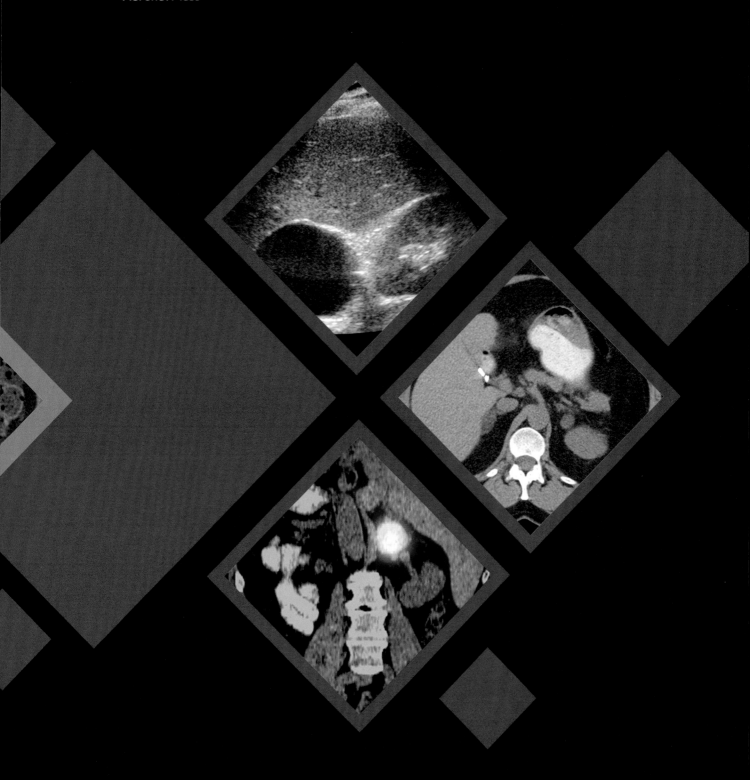

DIFFERENTIAL DIAGNOSIS

Common

- Adrenal Adenoma
- Metastases to Adrenal Gland
- Adrenal Hemorrhage
- Pheochromocytoma
- Adrenal Cyst
- Retroperitoneal Varices or Vessels (Mimic)

Less Common

- Adrenal Lymphoma
- Adrenal Myelolipoma
- Adrenal TB and Fungal Infection
- Adrenal Carcinoma
- Renal Cell Carcinoma (Mimic)
- Gastric Diverticulum (Mimic)
- Adrenal Hyperplasia
- Adrenal Ganglioneuroma

Rare but Important

- Adrenal Collision Tumor
- Adrenal Hemangioma

ESSENTIAL INFORMATION

Key Differential Diagnosis Issues

- Primary diagnostic consideration, particularly in oncologic population: Differentiate between adrenal metastasis and incidental adrenal adenoma
- Imaging-intensive approach advocated by specialty societies to confirm adenomas, though vast majority of adrenal incidentalomas are adenomas
- Combination of imaging (CT or MR) and clinical history usually allows confident diagnosis
  - CT and MR protocols geared toward identifying intracytoplasmic lipid in adenomas
  - Lipid-poor adenomas may be problematic, though washout kinetics, clinical history (malignancy), and extraadrenal findings (additional metastases) aid diagnosis
- Cushing syndrome
  - 15-25% of cases are due to autonomous adrenal adenoma
  - 80-85% of cases are due to adrenal hyperplasia
  - Adenomas usually > 2 cm
- Conn syndrome
  - 80% of cases due to adrenal adenoma
  - 20% of cases due to adrenal hyperplasia
  - Adenomas usually < 2 cm
- Addison syndrome: Adrenal insufficiency due to autoimmune disease (80% in Western countries), bilateral metastases, adrenal hemorrhage, or systemic infection
- Clinical history (hypertension) may suggest pheochromocytoma, but biochemical work-up (urine metanephrines) confirms diagnosis
- Bilateral adrenal masses: Metastases, hyperplasia, lymphoma, hemorrhage, TB, or fungal infection, pheochromocytoma (10%), adenoma (10%), or combination of 2 types of masses (e.g., adenoma on one side, myelolipoma on other)

Helpful Clues for Common Diagnoses

- **Adrenal Adenoma**
  - Well-circumscribed, round or oval, homogeneous, low-density mass on NECT
    - < 10 HU threshold: Highly specific for lipid-rich adenoma
  - Lipid-poor adenomas are best diagnosed on CT with unenhanced, enhanced, and 15-minute delayed imaging to calculate washout
    - Absolute washout: > 60%
    - Relative washout: > 40%
      - Rare false-positives: Hepatocellular carcinoma, renal cell carcinoma metastases, pheochromocytoma
  - Histology of lipid-rich adenomas characterized by intravoxel signal drop out on out-of-phase T1 MR
- **Metastasis to Adrenal Gland**
  - Primary sites include lung, breast, kidney, and melanoma
    - Cannot always be distinguished from lipid-poor adenoma by imaging alone
    - Clinical history, comparison to prior studies, and identification of additional (extraadrenal) disease aid diagnosis
    - PET/CT very useful in oncology patients; may help to identify FDG-avid adrenal metastases
- **Adrenal Hemorrhage**
  - Acute: Homogeneous, round, nonenhancing, hyperdense mass (50-90 HU)
  - Chronic: Mass with hypoattenuating center (pseudocyst), calcification
  - Unilateral: Usually due to direct trauma or iatrogenic (e.g., liver transplantation)
  - Bilateral: Usually in response to shock (postpartum; severe burns, sepsis)
- **Pheochromocytoma**
  - Well circumscribed, round, 3-5 cm in diameter (symptomatic lesions)
    - Pheochromocytoma that occurs as part of syndrome may be detected as smaller, asymptomatic mass
    - Syndromes associated with pheochromocytoma: Multiple endocrine neoplasia (types II and III), neurofibromatosis, von Hippel-Lindau, Carney syndrome, tuberous sclerosis
  - Hyperintense on T2 MR with heterogeneous, bright enhancement
  - ± hemorrhage, necrosis, calcification
  - Supporting history (e.g., hypertension, palpitations, headache) and biochemical data (urine metanephrines) drive diagnosis
- **Adrenal Cyst**
  - Well-defined, nonenhancing, water density mass ± calcification (eggshell)
    - Thin wall, septa calcification favor cyst rather than lipid-rich adenoma on NECT
  - Rarely large lesion ± internal hemorrhage
- **Retroperitoneal Varices or Vessels (Mimic)**
  - Tortuous splenic artery and varices often lie in suprarenal space
  - Contrast-enhanced CT or MR or color Doppler US can usually establish diagnosis

Helpful Clues for Less Common Diagnoses

- **Adrenal Lymphoma**
  - Non-Hodgkin lymphoma most common
  - Rounded or triangular shape; mild enhancement
  - FDG avid on PET/CT
  - Primary adrenal lymphoma is very rare; usually in presence of other sites of disease
- **Adrenal Myelolipoma**
  - Benign tumor, typically nonfunctioning
  - Macroscopic fat (> 50%) interspersed with soft tissue (myeloid elements, hemorrhage) on NECT
    - Coronal reconstructions may help determine organ of origin: Adrenal myelolipoma vs. exophytic renal angiomyelolipoma
  - Hyperintense on T1 MR with focal areas of signal loss on fat-suppressed techniques
    - Interface between fat and soft tissue elements will lose signal on opposed-phase GRE series
  - Echogenic mass on US may be indistinguishable from surrounding retroperitoneal fat unless mass effect
  - CT and MR findings are diagnostic in most cases
    - No treatment needed in most cases, though large myelolipomas may hemorrhage
    - Resection advocated for large, asymptomatic, or atypical lesions
- **Adrenal TB and Fungal Infection**
  - Acute: Heterogeneous, poorly enhancing mass(es); mild to marked enlargement of adrenal glands with preserved contour
  - Chronic: Small, calcified adrenal glands
  - Adrenal TB = most common cause of Addison syndrome (adrenal insufficiency) in developing nations
- **Adrenal Carcinoma**
  - Nonfunctioning tumors typically large (> 10 cm) at presentation
  - Functioning tumors may be smaller (< 5 cm)
  - Early invasion of IVC accounts for poor prognosis
  - ± necrosis, hemorrhage, and calcification (30%)
  - Rarely can have areas of intracytoplasmic lipid and gross fat

- **Renal Cell Carcinoma (Mimic)**
  - Large tumor from upper pole of kidney may simulate adrenal carcinoma
  - Look for claw sign (defect in renal cortex at origin of mass); coronal CT reconstruction or MR helpful to determine organ of origin
- **Gastric Diverticulum (Mimic)**
  - Rounded mass in suprarenal site
  - May contain fluid, gas, or contrast material
  - Give extra oral contrast or gas granules; place patient prone to make diagnosis
- **Adrenal Hyperplasia**
  - Adrenal glands may appear normal in shape but increased in thickness (> 10 mm) or may be nodular
  - Nodular hyperplasia can be difficult to distinguish from small adrenal adenomas or other lesions (e.g., metastases)
  - Hyperplasia or swelling may occur in response to stress, pituitary ACTH-secreting tumor (accounts for 80-85% of Cushing syndrome cases), congenital adrenal hyperplasia, or ectopic source of ACTH
- **Adrenal Ganglioneuroma**
  - Well-circumscribed lesion
  - Isodense to muscle on NECT
  - Low signal on T1 MR
  - Intermediate or high signal on T2 MR
  - Variable and heterogeneous enhancement

Helpful Clues for Rare Diagnoses

- **Adrenal Collision Tumor**
  - Coexistence of 2 contiguous but histologically distinct tumors within same adrenal gland
  - Adenoma and myelolipoma, adenoma and metastases most common combinations
- **Adrenal Hemangioma**
  - Can be large with central low attenuation (necrosis or fibrosis) ± calcification

Adrenal Adenoma

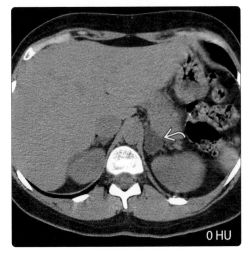

Adrenal Adenoma

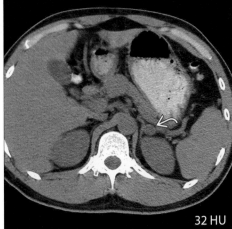

(Left) Axial NECT in a 45-year-old man shows an incidental, uniform, 2-cm, low-attenuation (0 HU) left adrenal lesion ➚. Its attenuation is characteristic of a lipid-rich adenoma. (Right) Axial NECT shows an incidental, indeterminate (32 HU) left adrenal lesion ➚. Although it is still likely a benign adenoma, a dedicated CECT was performed. Washout > 60% confirmed a lipid-poor adenoma.

Adrenal Adenoma

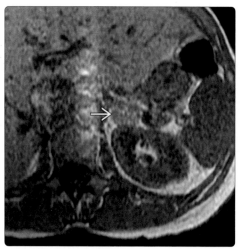

Adrenal Adenoma

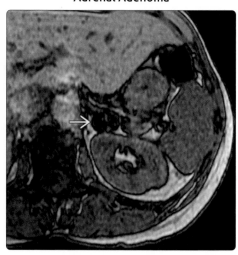

(Left) *Axial in-phase T1 MR in a 68-year-old woman with colon cancer shows a mildly heterogeneous left adrenal mass ➡.* (Right) *Axial out-of-phase T1 MR in the same patient shows diffuse signal loss in the left adrenal mass ➡, consistent with intracytoplasmic lipid in an adrenal adenoma. The mass remained stable over 4 years since incidental detection on initial surveillance imaging.*

Adrenal Adenoma

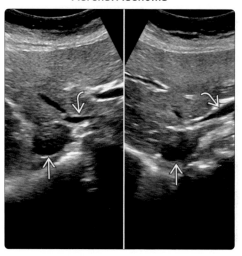

Metastases to Adrenal Gland

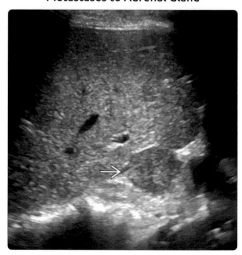

(Left) *Transverse and sagittal US in a 70-year-old woman with ↑ liver function tests show an incidental, solid right adrenal lesion ➡ posterior to the IVC ➡. The appearance on US is nonspecific; NECT confirmed a lipid-rich adenoma.* (Right) *Axial US in a patient with known lung carcinoma shows a solid right adrenal lesion ➡. Dedicated CECT showed prolonged absolute washout kinetics (< 60%). US-guided biopsy confirmed a metastasis.*

Metastases to Adrenal Gland

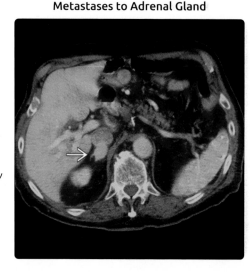

Metastases to Adrenal Gland

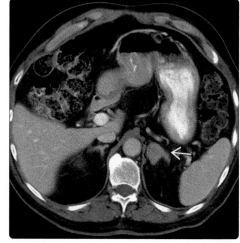

(Left) *Axial PET/CT shows an FDG-avid adrenal metastasis ➡ in a patient with esophageal carcinoma. Extraadrenal metastases typically make characterization of adrenal masses in oncology patients unnecessary, but PET may be useful for confirming solitary adrenal metastases prior to adrenalectomy.* (Right) *Axial CECT in a patient with history of lung cancer shows a new, isolated adrenal mass ➡. Although a relative washout of 42% suggests a lipid-poor adenoma, a metastasis was confirmed at adrenalectomy.*

Metastases to Adrenal Gland

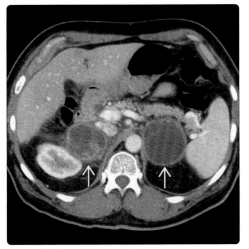

Metastases to Adrenal Gland

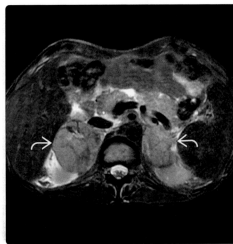

(Left) Axial CECT of a patient with back pain, lethargy, and a history of lung carcinoma shows large, necrotic adrenal metastases ➡. Lab data (↓ Na, ↑ K) and an ACTH stimulation test confirmed profound adrenal insufficiency. (Right) Axial T2 TSE MR in a 36-year-old man with malaise and adrenal insufficiency shows bulky, bilateral adrenal masses ➡.

Metastases to Adrenal Gland

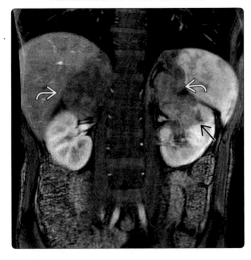

Adrenal Hemorrhage

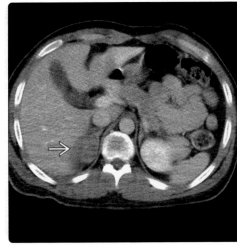

(Left) Coronal T1 C+ MR in the same patient shows mild enhancement of both masses ➡ and extension of tumor into left kidney ➡. Absence of disease elsewhere and clinical history suggested adrenal lymphoma. Biopsy confirmed diffuse B-cell lymphoma and patient was successfully treated with CHOP and Rituxan. (Right) Axial CECT in a young male patient post trauma shows right adrenal hematoma ➡. Traumatic adrenal hemorrhage is typically associated with other visceral injuries and high injury severity scores.

Adrenal Hemorrhage

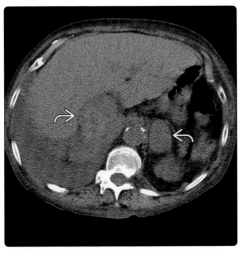

Pheochromocytoma

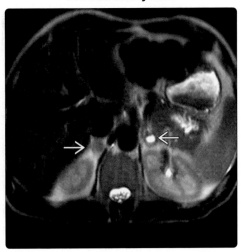

(Left) Axial NECT in a hypotensive patient with metastatic lung carcinoma shows bilateral adrenal hematomas ➡. Small adrenal metastases were seen on prior staging CT. (Right) Axial T2 MR in a man with MEN 2A syndrome and ↑ urinary metanephrines shows small, bilateral adrenal pheochromocytomas ➡. Hereditary pheochromocytomas are typically small and often bilateral.

Pheochromocytoma

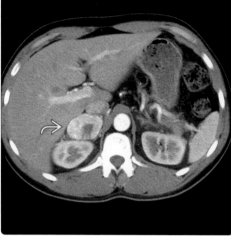

Pheochromocytoma

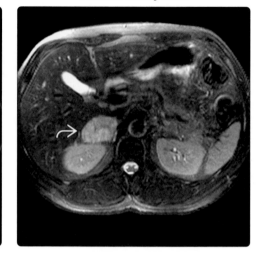

(Left) *Axial CECT in a 26-year-old man shows marked enhancement of a 4-cm right adrenal pheochromocytoma* 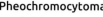. *Genetic testing, prompted by the patient's young age, confirmed an atypically large hereditary pheochromocytoma.* (Right) *Axial T2 MR in the same patient shows a slightly hyperintense right pheochromocytoma* ➔. *Marked light bulb hyperintensity was considered a characteristic feature of these lesions in the early MR literature, but this is often not the case.*

Pheochromocytoma

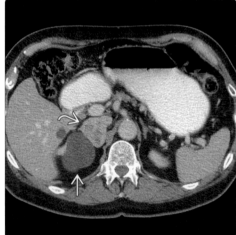

Pheochromocytoma

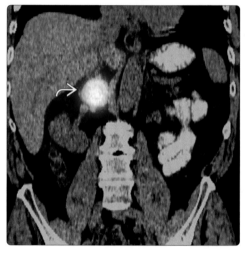

(Left) *Dedicated adrenal CT shows a vascular right adrenal mass* ➔ *with minimal washout in this older patient. Note the adjacent renal cyst* ➔. *Metanephrine evaluation was performed.* (Right) *I-123 MIBI CT-SPECT in the same patient (performed to exclude metastases) confirms a solitary 4-cm right adrenal pheochromocytoma* ➔. *Sporadic pheochromocytomas tend to occur in older patients, and classic symptoms (headache, hypertension, palpitations, sweating) may be absent.*

Adrenal Cyst

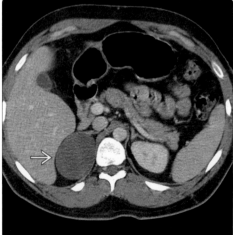

Adrenal Cyst

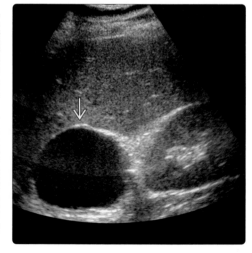

(Left) *Axial CECT shows an incidental, nonenhancing right adrenal cyst* ➔. *Differentiation of adrenal cysts from adenomas on NECT may be difficult, but septations and thin calcification favor cysts.* (Right) *Sagittal US in the same patient shows a simple suprarenal (adrenal) cyst* ➔. *Lack of cyst complexity might suggest an endothelial cyst, but pseudocysts are the most common type of adrenal cysts in surgical series.*

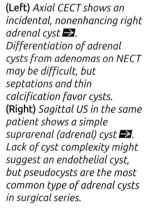
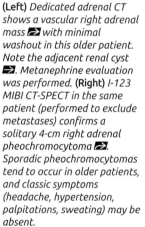

Adrenal Myelolipoma

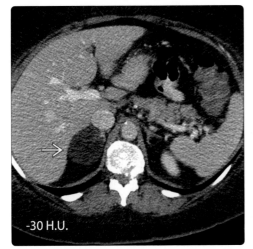

-30 H.U.

Adrenal TB and Fungal Infection

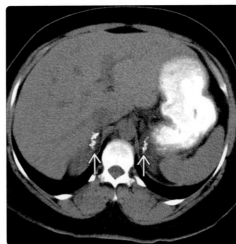

(Left) *Axial CECT shows a fat attenuation (-30 HU) adrenal lesion* ➡, *pathognomonic of adrenal myelolipoma. The differential diagnosis of large myelolipomas includes retroperitoneal liposarcomas and renal angiomyolipomas.* **(Right)** *Axial NECT shows calcified adrenals* ➡, *likely due to prior granulomatous infection. These calcifications are typically incidental, though in undeveloped countries, they may suggest adrenal tuberculosis, a common cause of adrenal insufficiency in these populations.*

Adrenal Carcinoma

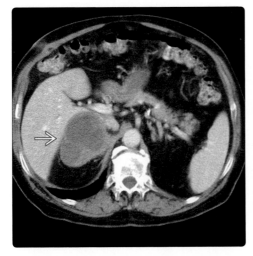

Adrenal Carcinoma

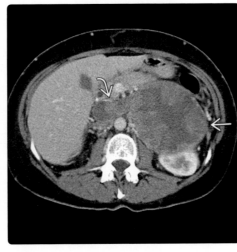

(Left) *Axial CECT in an older man with mild flank pain shows a large, heterogeneous right adrenal mass* ➡. *Resection performed after metanephrine screening confirmed adrenal carcinoma. Large, solid, unilateral adrenal masses with invasive margins should raise index of suspicion for adrenal carcinoma.* **(Right)** *Axial CECT shows a huge left adrenal carcinoma* ➡ *and tumor thrombus within the left renal vein* ➡. *These highly malignant tumors are often large at presentation and have a predilection for venous invasion.*

Adrenal Hyperplasia

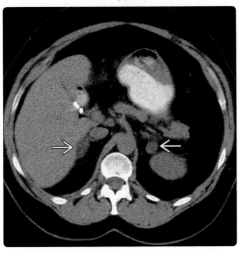

Adrenal Hyperplasia

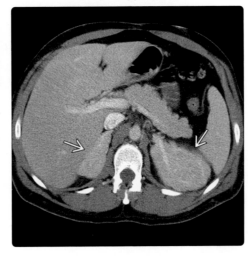

(Left) *Axial NECT in a female patient with Cushing syndrome, a suppressed ACTH, and abnormal dexamethasone suppression shows nodular adrenal glands* ➡. *ACTH-independent macronodular hyperplasia was confirmed at resection.* **(Right)** *Axial CECT shows massively enlarged adrenals* ➡, *a characteristic feature of congenital adrenal hyperplasia. This autosomal recessive disease is usually due to 21-hydroxylase deficiency, is typically diagnosed in the neonatal period, and is responsible for most adrenogenital syndromes.*

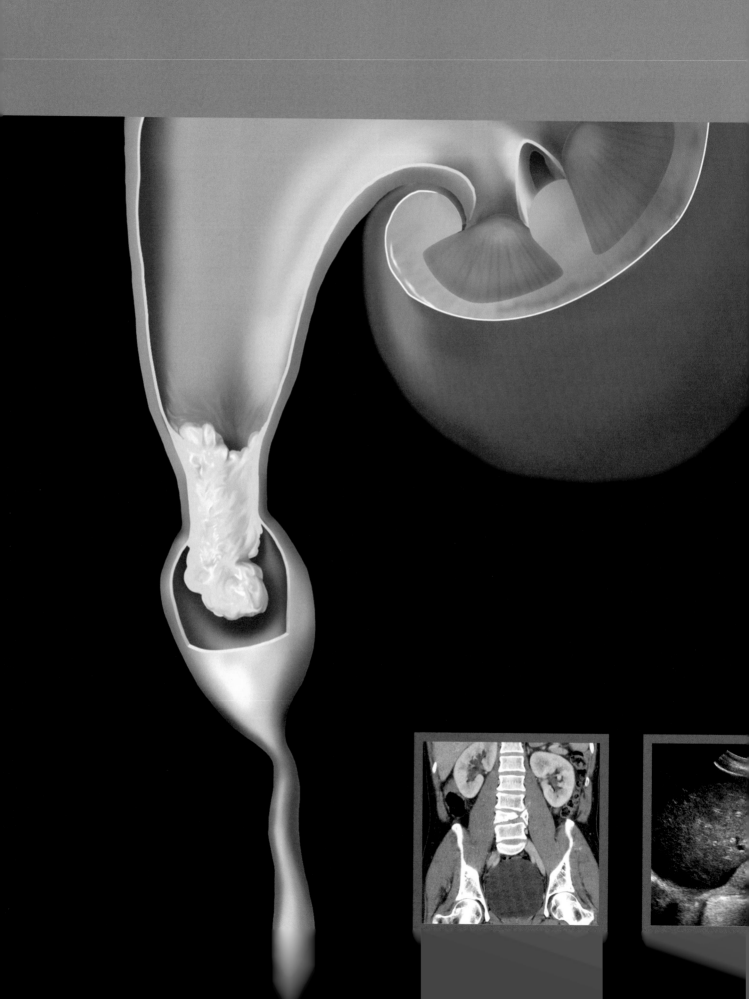

SECTION 15
Kidney

Generic Imaging Patterns

Calcifications Within Kidney 488

Congenital Renal Anomalies 492

Kidney Transplant Dysfunction 496

Solid Renal Mass 500

Cystic Renal Mass 504

Bilateral Renal Cysts 508

Infiltrative Renal Lesions 512

Perirenal and Subcapsular Mass Lesions 516

Fat-Containing Renal Mass 520

Renal Sinus Lesion 524

Gas in or Around Kidney 528

Delayed or Persistent Nephrogram 530

Wedge-Shaped or Striated Nephrogram 534

Acute Flank Pain 538

Modality-Specific Imaging Findings

Ultrasound

Enlarged Kidney 544

Small Kidney 548

Hyperechoic Kidney 552

Dilated Renal Pelvis 556

Hyperechoic Renal Mass 560

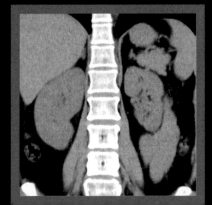
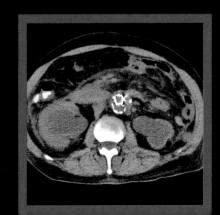
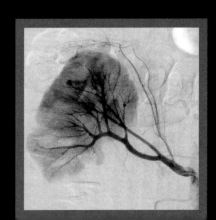

DIFFERENTIAL DIAGNOSIS

Common

- Renal Calculi
- Medullary Nephrocalcinosis
- Vascular Calcifications

Less Common

- Milk of Calcium
- Renal Cell Carcinoma
- Aneurysm
- Xanthogranulomatous Pyelonephritis

Rare but Important

- Cortical Nephrocalcinosis
- Angiomyolipoma
- Epithelioid Angiomyolipoma
- Osteosarcoma
- Oncocytoma
- Neuroendocrine Tumors
- Tuberculosis

ESSENTIAL INFORMATION

Key Differential Diagnosis Issues

- Abnormal deposition of calcium salts within tissues
- Calcifications can be broadly classified as
  - Dystrophic calcification
    - Occurs with normal levels of serum calcium and in absence of calcium metabolic derangement
    - Occurs in setting of necrosis in setting of trauma, ischemia, infarction, infection, or tumor
    - e.g., atherosclerotic disease, trauma, tumors
  - Metabolic calcification
    - Deposition of calcium salts in otherwise normal tissues
    - Occurs in patients with hypercalcemia or abnormal calcium metabolism
    - e.g., calculi, nephrocalcinosis

Helpful Clues for Common Diagnoses

- **Renal Calculi**
  - Crystallization of mineral and salt deposits in urine
  - Usually located in calyces or pelvis but may migrate to ureter or bladder
  - CT
    - Calculi are uniformly dense, except matrix and indinavir stones (rare)
    - Dense (several hundred HU) foci in calyces, renal pelvis, ureter, or bladder
    - Perinephric stranding and hydroureteronephrosis if obstructing
  - US
    - Round or ovoid, echogenic foci
    - Clean posterior acoustic shadowing
    - Twinkle artifact on color Doppler
- **Medullary Nephrocalcinosis**
  - Calcification of renal medulla due to calcium salt deposition
  - Can be caused by hyperparathyroidism, renal tubular acidosis, or medullary sponge kidney

- May lead to development of renal calculi
- CT
  - Best visualized by NECT
  - Early stages may not be seen on CT (US is superior at early detection)
  - Later stages show development of calcifications
  - Punctate to dense calcifications within medullary pyramids
- US
  - Normal echogenicity of cortex
  - Early form may show echogenic rim outlining renal medullary portions
  - Echogenic medullary portions ± shadowing
- **Vascular Calcifications**
  - Atherosclerotic calcifications within intraparenchymal renal arteries
  - Linked with diabetes and hypertension
  - Vascular distribution of calcification within kidneys
  - Linear and branching appearance

Helpful Clues for Less Common Diagnoses

- **Milk of Calcium**
  - Calyceal diverticula are congenital outpouchings of renal calyx
  - Connected to collecting system (seen on urographic phase)
  - Can be associated with layering calculi (milk of calcium)
- **Renal Cell Carcinoma**
  - Dystrophic calcification can occur within renal cell carcinomas
  - More common in papillary and chromophobe subtypes than clear cell
- **Aneurysm**
  - Renal artery aneurysms can develop peripheral calcification
  - Usually extraparenchymal, in renal hilum
  - Diagnosis can be confirmed on arterial-phase CT/MR or Doppler US
- **Xanthogranulomatous Pyelonephritis**
  - Chronic infection with replacement by lipid-laden macrophages
  - Pelvicalyceal obstruction, typically staghorn calculus
  - Diffuse, unilateral renal enlargement, cortical thinning, and dilated calyces producing bear's paw sign
  - Inflammatory tissue can invade adjacent structures

Helpful Clues for Rare Diagnoses

- **Cortical Nephrocalcinosis**
  - Can be caused by acute cortical necrosis, chronic glomerulonephritis, hypercalcemic states, ethylene glycol poisoning, sickle cell disease, or chronically rejected kidney grafts
  - US
    - Hyperechoic cortex that may or may not shadow
    - In cases of shadowing calcification, interior cortex, pyramids, and renal sinus/collecting system may not be visualized
  - CT
    - Increased density of cortex
    - May simulate appearance of corticomedullary phase on NECT

- – More chronic/severe forms appear grossly calcified
- **Angiomyolipoma**
  - Solid, heterogeneous renal cortical mass in adult with macroscopic fat is reliable sign of angiomyolipoma
  - Variable amounts of fat may be present and can be lipid-poor
  - Presence of calcification is rare; if present, suspect renal cell carcinoma
- **Epithelioid Angiomyolipoma**
  - Rare variant of angiomyolipomas
  - Considered perivascular epithelial cell tumors (PEComas)
  - Can appear aggressive with metastatic involvement
  - Can contain small foci of gross fat
  - Rarely contain calcification
- **Osteosarcoma**
  - Calcifications can be seen with osteosarcoma but are otherwise uncommon in renal sarcomas
  - Can be primary renal mass or more commonly metastatic to kidney
  - Usually show extensive calcifications
- **Oncocytoma**

- Benign renal tumor composed of eosinophilic epithelial cells arising from collecting ducts
  - Solid renal cortical mass lesion ± central stellate scar
  - Dynamic postcontrast imaging is highly variable and depends on degree of cellularity and stroma
  - Rarely contains calcifications
- **Neuroendocrine Tumors**
  - Increased risk in patients with horseshoe kidneys
  - May be completely solid or mixed solid and cystic
  - Can contain calcifications
  - Variable levels of enhancement
- **Tuberculosis**
  - Chronic infections, such as tuberculosis, can produce calcifications within kidneys
  - Active stage: Papillary destruction with echogenic masses near calyces
  - Late stage: Calcified granuloma or dense dystrophic calcification associated with shrunken kidneys

Renal Calculi

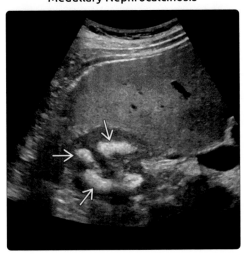

Renal Calculi

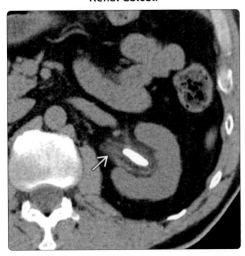

(Left) *US shows a central echogenic region* ➡ *with clean posterior acoustic shadowing* ➡*.* **(Right)** *On the corresponding NECT, this region represents a renal calculus. There is some surrounding urothelial thickening and stranding* ➡*, which could be due to inflammatory changes related to intermittent obstruction or infection.*

Medullary Nephrocalcinosis

Medullary Nephrocalcinosis

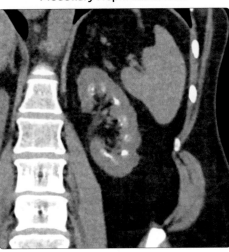

(Left) *US shows echogenic renal pyramids* ➡*.* **(Right)** *Coronal NECT in the same patient shows multiple calcifications in a medullary pyramid distribution, consistent with medullary nephrocalcinosis.*

Vascular Calcifications

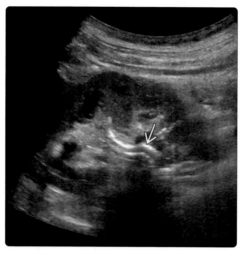

Vascular Calcifications

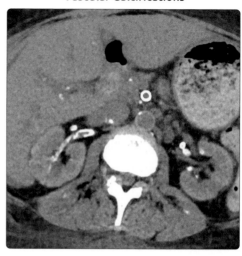

(Left) *US shows echogenic tram-track lines* ➡️*, consistent with vascular origin of the calcifications.* (Right) *Corresponding NECT in the same patient shows extensive vascular calcifications in the main renal artery with calcifications within the intraparenchymal portions of the renal artery.*

Milk of Calcium

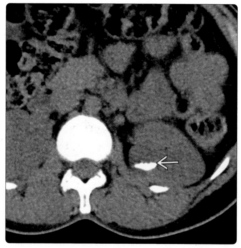

Milk of Calcium

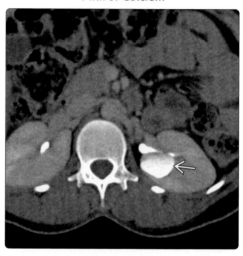

(Left) *Axial NECT shows layering, high-density material within the left kidney* ➡️*.* (Right) *Axial urographic-phase CECT shows contrast extravasating from the urinary system into the cyst containing layering, high-density material* ➡️*. This is consistent with calyceal diverticulum with milk of calcium.*

Renal Cell Carcinoma

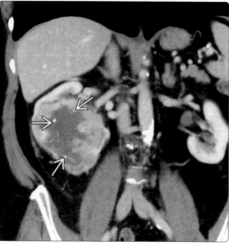

Renal Cell Carcinoma

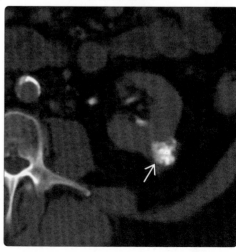

(Left) *Punctate calcifications are seen within a large, centrally necrotic right renal mass* ➡️*. The presence of calcifications was confirmed on NECT. This mass was found to be clear cell renal cell carcinoma (RCC) with dystrophic calcifications.* (Right) *Exophytic left renal mass* ➡️ *is seen involving the left kidney, which is largely replaced by calcifications. Enhancing components were difficult to ascertain given the abundance of calcifications. This was surgically removed and found to be clear cell RCC with osseous metaplasia.*

Angiomyolipoma

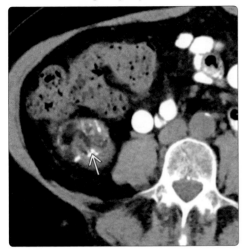

Angiomyolipoma

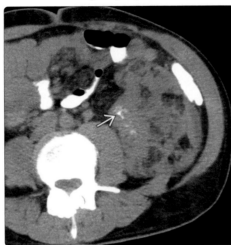

(Left) Axial NECT shows a predominantly fat-containing angiomyolipoma in the inferior pole of the right kidney. This mass originally had no calcific components but developed dystrophic peripheral calcifications after embolization ➡. (Right) Axial NECT shows a large fat and soft tissue mass ➡ arising from the left kidney. Small areas of calcification are present, which is rare in angiomyolipomas. This was surgically removed and found to be an angiomyolipoma.

Oncocytoma

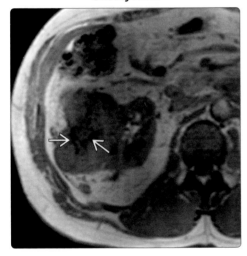

Oncocytoma

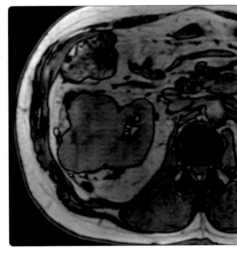

(Left) Axial in-phase MR shows a large, exophytic mass with loss of signal in the central portion ➡. Loss of signal can be seen in the setting of calcification, iron deposition, or air. (Right) Corresponding axial opposed-phase MR in the same patient shows no loss of signal within the mass.

Oncocytoma

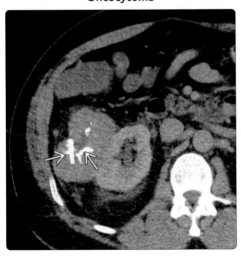

Neuroendocrine Tumors

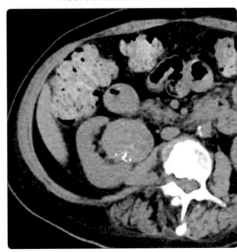

(Left) Axial CECT in the same patient shows loss of signal on in-phase MR as calcification ➡ within the central scar of this oncocytoma. (Right) Axial NECT shows a perihilar mass with small foci of calcification. This mass showed enhancement on postcontrast images and was found to be a neuroendocrine tumor.

DIFFERENTIAL DIAGNOSIS

Common

- Persistent Fetal Lobulation
- Hypertrophied Column of Bertin
- Horseshoe Kidney
- Ptotic Kidney

Less Common

- Dromedary Hump
- Renal Malrotation
- Simple Renal Ectopia
- Crossed Renal Ectopia
- Renal Agenesis
- Calyceal Diverticulum
- Ureteropelvic Junction Obstruction
- Duplex Collecting System
- Megaureter
- Ureterocele

Rare but Important

- Pancake Kidney
- Supernumerary Kidney

ESSENTIAL INFORMATION

Key Differential Diagnosis Issues

- During early development, kidneys migrate superiorly from their sacral location
- Renal hilum normally rotates to anteromedial position

Helpful Clues for Common Diagnoses

- **Persistent Fetal Lobulation**
  - Normal renal variant from persistent renal lobulation
  - More commonly seen in younger patients
  - Usually bilateral
  - Lobulated indentations occur between medullary pyramids
- **Hypertrophied Column of Bertin**
  - Normal renal variant consisting of hypertrophied cortical tissue between pyramids
  - Located in middle 1/3 of kidney
  - Can simulate mass
  - Similar imaging appearance to cortical tissue on all modalities
  - Medullary portion within hypertrophied column of Bertin can be seen (hypoechoic on US)
  - On Doppler imaging, organized linear vasculature can distinguish column of Bertin from mass
  - More common on left side
- **Horseshoe Kidney**
  - Fusion of lower poles of kidneys by isthmus
  - Isthmus composed of functional parenchyma or fibrous band
  - Isthmus fusion prevents cranial migration of kidneys at level of inferior mesenteric artery
  - Increased risk of urolithiasis and renal malignancies, including neuroendocrine tumor and urothelial carcinoma (renal cell carcinoma is most common tumor but is not at increased risk)
- **Ptotic Kidney**

- > 5 cm (~ 2 vertebral bodies) caudal displacement of kidney when moving from supine to upright position
- Based on historical IVPs, incidence may be 10-20%
- Underdiagnosed on CT and MR given nondynamic positioning; US can allow for dynamic imaging

Helpful Clues for Less Common Diagnoses

- **Dromedary Hump**
  - Focal bulge on lateral edge of left kidney caused by splenic impression
  - Can mimic mass
- **Renal Malrotation**
  - Embryologically, renal hilum is initially directed anteriorly
  - Renal hilum normally rotates to anteromedial position
  - Renal malrotation is abnormal positioning of kidney relative to hilum
    - Nonrotation: Anteriorly directed renal hilum
    - Reverse rotation: Lateral renal hilum with renal artery anterior to kidney
    - Hyperrotation: Lateral renal hilum with renal artery posterior to kidney
    - Sagittal rotation: Renal hilum rotated on sagittal plane (long axis of kidney is in axial plane)
  - Unilateral or bilateral
  - Usually asymptomatic but can be associated with uteropelvic junction obstruction, increased infection, and stone formation
- **Simple Renal Ectopia**
  - Abnormal location of kidney
  - Caused by abnormal ascension of kidney
  - Pelvic kidney is most common ectopic location but can also be rarely thoracic
  - Can be prone to poor urinary drainage and traumatic injury
- **Crossed Renal Ectopia**
  - Ectopic location of kidney on opposite side of its normal position
  - Ectopic kidney on contralateral side of its ureteral insertion
  - Can be fused (85-90%) or unfused (10-15%)
  - 4 types
    - With fusion: Both kidneys fused
    - Without fusion: Kidneys are separate
    - With solitary kidney: One kidney with ureteral insertion on contralateral side
    - Bilateral: Both kidneys located on opposite side of ureteral insertion
- **Renal Agenesis**
  - Unilateral: Bilateral renal agenesis is not compatible with life
  - Often associated with other genitourinary anomalies
    - Müllerian duct anomalies in female patients (e.g., obstructed hemivagina and ipsilateral renal anomaly)
    - Zinner syndrome: Ipsilateral seminal vesicle cysts and ejaculatory duct obstruction in male patients
  - Imaging findings
    - Ipsilateral vertical colon segment lies medial to its normal position
    - Males: Possible absence of ipsilateral vas, epididymis, testis

□ Seminal vesicle cyst is also common (may mimic ureterocele)
- Females: Possible absence or anomalies of ipsilateral part of uterus, vagina, and ovary
- Flattening of adrenal gland against psoas muscle (lying down appearance)
- Can be seen with compensatory renal hypertrophy and ureteropelvic junction obstruction and vesicoureteral reflux

- **Calyceal Diverticulum**
  o Congenital outpouching of renal calyx
  o Cystic appearance with connection to collecting system (seen on urographic phase)
  o Can be associated with layering calculi (milk of calcium)
- **Ureteropelvic Junction Obstruction**
  o Pyelocaliectasis with abrupt of ureteropelvic junction with narrowing and delayed urinary excretion
  o Congenital (most common)
    - Intrinsic stenosis due to collagen or muscle abnormality
    - Adynamic segment
    - Adhesions, bands, and crossing vessels are probably not causative
  o Acquired (scarring, vesicoureteral reflux, malignant obstruction, intraluminal lesion)
- **Duplex Collecting System**
  o Complete duplication: 2 ureters drain duplex kidney and remain separate down to bladder insertion or beyond
  o 85% of duplicated ureters obey Weigert-Meyer rule
    - Upper pole obstructed and lower refluxes
    - Upper pole ureter inserts medial and caudal to lower pole ureter
  o Location
    - Males: Insertion of ureter is always above external sphincter
      □ Insertion sites: Prostatic urethra (54%), seminal vesicles (28%), vas deferens (10%), ejaculatory duct (8%)
    - Females: Insertion is usually below sphincter, resulting in urinary incontinence

□ Insertion sites: Bladder neck and upper urethra (33%), vestibule (33%), vagina (25%), cervix and uterus (5%)
  o Incomplete duplication: 2 ureters drain duplex kidney but fuse prior to bladder insertion
- **Megaureter**
  o Encompasses spectrum of anomalies that lead to enlarged ureter (diameter > 7 mm)
  o Primary megaureter: Results from functional or anatomic abnormality at ureterovesical junction
  o Secondary megaureter: Results from abnormalities that involve bladder or urethra
- **Ureterocele**
  o Cystic dilatation of terminal ureter
    - Intravesical: Ureterocele is entirely in bladder
    - Ectopic: Insertion at bladder neck or in posterior urethra
  o Can cause obstruction to collecting system
  o ~ 80% of ureteroceles (in pediatric population) are seen in association with duplicated collecting system
  o ~ 60% of these pediatric ureteroceles have ectopic insertion
  o Adult ureteroceles are mostly intravesical and orthotopic with single ureter
  o Cobra head or spring onion appearance of distal ureter with surrounding radiolucent halo
  o Smooth, round, intravesical filling defect

Helpful Clues for Rare Diagnoses
- **Pancake Kidney**
  o Fusion of upper and lower poles of kidneys
  o Usually located anterior to aortic bifurcation
- **Supernumerary Kidney**
  o Accessory kidney is usually smaller in size
  o Most are located on left side
  o Accessory kidney may be cross-fused

Persistent Fetal Lobulation

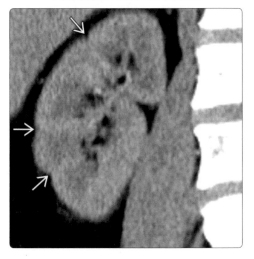

Hypertrophied Column of Bertin

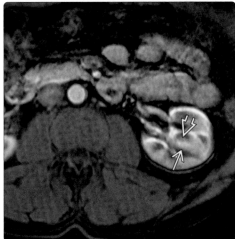

(Left) Coronal CECT shows multiple lobulations in the left kidney ➡ that occur between medullary pyramids. (Right) Axial T1 C+ FS MR shows a hypertrophied column of cortical tissue in the middle 1/3 of the left kidney ➡ with central medullary portion ➡.

Horseshoe Kidney

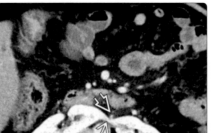

Renal Malrotation

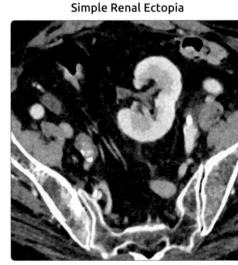

(Left) *Axial CECT shows both left and right kidneys are fused midline in the inferior poles by enhancing tissue ➡. The superior migration of the kidneys has been halted by the inferior mesenteric artery ➡.* (Right) *Coronal 3D CECT shows malrotation of the left kidney with the hilum directed anteriorly. Ureteral insertion is normal.*

Renal Malrotation

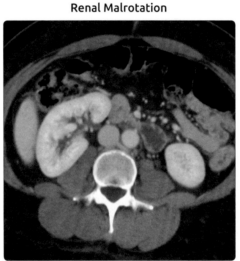

Simple Renal Ectopia

(Left) *Axial CECT shows the renal hilum of the right kidney is rotated on sagittal plane (long axis of the kidney is in the axial plane). The left kidney was normal.* (Right) *Axial CECT shows the abnormal location of the left kidney is caused by its abnormal ascension. The pelvic kidney is the most common ectopic location, as was the case in this patient.*

Crossed Renal Ectopia

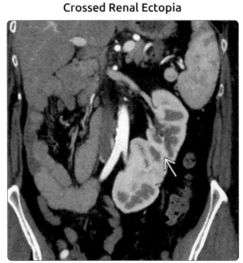

Renal Agenesis

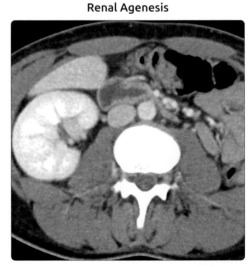

(Left) *Coronal CECT shows the ectopic location of the right kidney with fusion to the inferior pole of the left kidney ➡. There was normal ureteral insertion into the bladder.* (Right) *Axial CECT shows the right kidney is not present, consistent with agenesis. There is compensatory hypertrophy of the right kidney. This was incidentally discovered in this patient with normal renal function.*

Calyceal Diverticulum

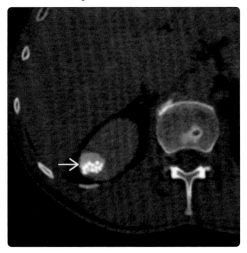

Duplex Collecting System

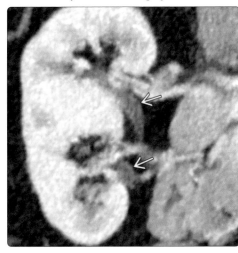

(Left) *On this urographic-phase CT, contrast enters into a diverticulum and outlines several layering calculi* ➡. (Right) *Coronal CECT shows 2 collecting systems involve the right kidney* ➡. *The ureters eventually fuse into a single ureter, consistent with a partially duplex collecting system.*

Ureteropelvic Junction Obstruction

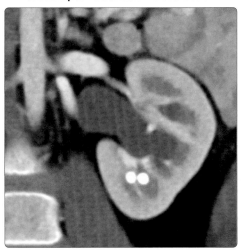

Ureteropelvic Junction Obstruction

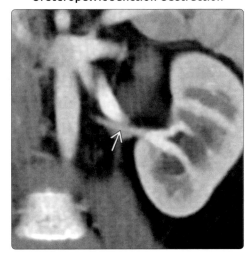

(Left) *Coronal NECT shows mild, left-sided hydronephrosis with obstruction occurring at the level of the ureteropelvic junction.* (Right) *In the same patient, a crossing renal artery is seen at the site of the ureteropelvic obstruction* ➡.

Megaureter

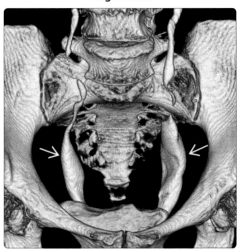

Ureterocele

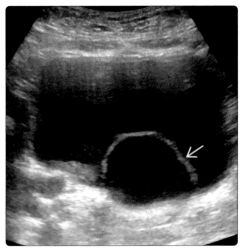

(Left) *Coronal 3D CECT shows massively dilated distal ureters are seen bilaterally* ➡. (Right) *At the site of the left ureterovesical junction, there is a cystic outpouching* ➡, *consistent with the US appearance of the cobra head sign seen with ureteroceles.*

DIFFERENTIAL DIAGNOSIS

Common

- Acute Tubular Injury
- Interstitial Fibrosis and Tubular Atrophy
- Peritransplant Collection
- Pyelonephritis
- Calcineurin Inhibitor Toxicity
- Acute Rejection

Less Common

- Transplant Renal Artery Stenosis
- Urinary Obstruction
- Venous Thrombosis

Rare but Important

- Arterial Thrombosis
- Acute Cortical Necrosis
- Compartment Syndrome
- Graft Torsion

ESSENTIAL INFORMATION

Key Differential Diagnosis Issues

- US is usually 1st-line imaging modality
- CT and MR can be useful in looking at extent of peritransplant collections and in evaluating vasculature
- Differential is influenced by timing of dysfunction relative to timing of transplant
  - Early postoperative (first 2 weeks): Rejection, renal artery/vein thrombosis, acute tubular injury, hematoma/urinoma, and compartment syndrome
  - Intermediate (1 month to 1 year): Rejection, urinary stricture, transplant renal artery stenosis, and lymphocele
  - Late (> 1 year): Interstitial fibrosis and tubular atrophy

Helpful Clues for Common Diagnoses

- **Acute Tubular Injury**
  - Kidney injury caused by damage to tubules
  - Usually caused by ischemia-reperfusion injury at time of initial transplantation
  - Reduced or absent excretion of contrast on urographic phase
  - Decreased cortical perfusion with increased resistive indices (> 0.8)
  - In severe cases, may demonstrate reversal of flow in renal artery
  - Core biopsy of kidney graft is standard for diagnosing
- **Interstitial Fibrosis and Tubular Atrophy**
  - Formerly called chronic rejection
  - Greatest cause of death-censored graft failure after 1 year
  - Due to prior episodes of rejection or other chronic insults from hypertension, calcineurin inhibitor toxicity, and infection
  - Can demonstrate cortical thinning, small kidney graft size, and increased resistive indices
  - Diagnosis made based on biopsy
- **Peritransplant Collection**
  - Hematomas, urinomas, lymphoceles, and abscesses can have considerable overlap in imaging appearance

- Hematoma: Typically within 1st week of transplantation or after intervention/biopsy
- Timing
  - Urinoma: Within 2 weeks
  - Lymphocele: 2 weeks to 6 months
  - Abscess: Weeks to any time after transplantation
- Location
  - Hematoma lateral to graft: Large collections can cause mass effect or become nidus for infection
  - Subcapsular hematoma: Can exert pressure on kidney graft (Page kidney) and cause dysfunction
  - Hematoma medial to graft: Exclude anastomotic breakdown (CTA, MRA, focused US)
  - Urinoma: Typically between graft and bladder; can be diagnosed by fluid sampling or urographic-phase CT or MR
  - Lymphocele: Can occur anywhere around graft
- Abscess: Any of above collections can get infected
- Complexity
  - Hematomas: Variable echogenicity and complexity depending on evolution of hematoma
  - Abscess: Complex, low-level echoes; may contain air (echogenic with dirty shadowing)
  - Lymphocele/urinoma: Usually simple-appearing collections
- Often requires fluid sampling to determine etiology of fluid collection
- **Pyelonephritis**
  - May be clinically silent due to immunosuppressive medications
  - Wedge-shaped areas of increased echogenicity and decreased perfusion on color Doppler
  - Urothelial thickening may be present
- **Calcineurin Inhibitor Toxicity**
  - Calcineurin inhibitors (cyclosporine and tacrolimus) are immunosuppressants used in kidney grafts
  - Can be nephrotoxic
  - Can have similar imaging features with acute tubular injury with decreased perfusion and increased resistive indices
  - Diagnosis based on combination of laboratory values, clinical history, and biopsy
- **Acute Rejection**
  - Occurs most often within first 6 months after transplantation
  - Causes inflammation of glomeruli, tubules, arteries, and interstitium
  - Classically associated with
    - Increased size of kidney graft
    - Loss of corticomedullary junction
    - Prominent hypoechoic pyramids
    - Decreased echogenicity of renal sinus
    - Increased resistive indices (> 0.8)
    - Decreased perfusion
  - Classic signs are often absent
    - Urothelial thickening is highly sensitive but not specific feature of rejection
    - May appear swollen with surrounding inflammatory changes on CT and MR
  - Diagnosis of rejection is made based on core needle biopsy of renal graft

Helpful Clues for Less Common Diagnoses

- **Transplant Renal Artery Stenosis**
  - Clinical scenario includes renal dysfunction, hypertension, and generalized/pulmonary edema
  - Arterial stenosis can occur at any part of renal artery graft or native iliac artery
  - US
    - Major features
      - Elevated velocity (> 300 cm/s)
      - Spectral broadening distal to stenosis indicating turbulent flow
      - Delayed upstroke of intraparenchymal arteries (> 0.1 s)
    - Can also present with low resistive index (< 0.6 or interval decrease from prior examinations)
  - May need confirmation by CTA or MRA in equivocal US cases or to provide vascular roadmap for invasive angiography
- **Urinary Obstruction**
  - Ureteral stricture: Narrowing of ureter usually from ischemia with development of hydronephrosis
  - Other causes of obstruction include extrinsic compression from mass/peritransplant fluid collection, calculi, fungal balls, and blood clots
  - Dilation of pyelocaliceal system and ureter to level of obstruction
  - Change in caliber of dilation of pyelocaliceal system over serial US suggests obstruction
  - Presence of debris within urine and urothelial thickening may suggest pyonephrosis
  - If dilation of pyelocaliceal system is present and bladder is full, repeat US after bladder emptying
- **Venous Thrombosis**
  - Swollen graft, increased size
  - Layering, mixed-echogenicity peritransplant hematomas can be seen
  - Thrombus can sometimes be visualized in transplant renal vein as hyperechoic filling defect
  - Increased resistive index with reversed diastolic flow (lack of venous outflow differentiates renal vein thrombosis from severe acute tubular injury)
  - Delayed and diminished perfusion after delivery of contrast

Helpful Clues for Rare Diagnoses

- **Arterial Thrombosis**
  - Normal size and appearance of graft acutely; hypoechoic, thinned cortex chronically
  - Global or segmental absent perfusion depending on extent of thrombosis
  - No true spectral Doppler signal in affected region
  - Can be confirmed with CEUS or CECT/MR
- **Acute Cortical Necrosis**
  - Isolated necrosis of renal cortex in setting of acute renal failure
  - Can be seen after severe acute tubular injury
  - Absent perfusion to renal cortex with maintained flow centrally
  - Can have normal resistive indices
  - Venous outflow from graft maintained
  - Can be confirmed with CEUS or CECT/MR
- **Compartment Syndrome**
  - If space created for kidney graft is too small, graft can become compressed
  - Decreased perfusion on color Doppler US
  - Reversal of diastolic flow in renal artery
  - Venous outflow may be patent
- **Graft Torsion**
  - Usually in patients with intraperitoneal placement of kidney graft
  - Depending on torsion degree, can lead to
    - Venous occlusion: Similar US findings to venous thrombosis
    - Combined venous and arterial occlusion: Similar US findings to arterial thrombosis
  - Kidney graft can appear enlarged and edematous

Acute Tubular Injury

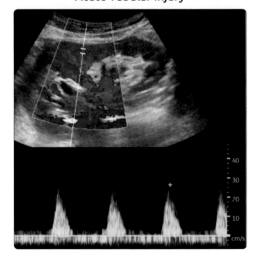

Interstitial Fibrosis and Tubular Atrophy

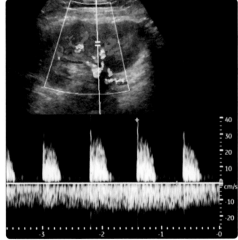

(Left) *Spectral Doppler US shows high intraparenchymal resistive indices. This patient who had a recent kidney graft with a prolonged cold ischemic time was experiencing delayed graft function. Biopsy was performed and showed acute tubular injury.* **(Right)** *Spectral Doppler US shows elevated resistive indices, and biopsy revealed underlying fibrosis. This patient was 10 years post transplantation and had experienced a slow, gradual decline in glomerular filtration rate.*

Peritransplant Collection

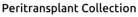

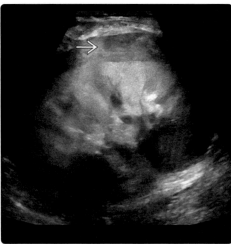

Peritransplant Collection

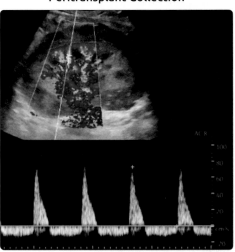

(Left) *Longitudinal US shows a large, subcapsular, heterogeneous collection* ➡️ *in this patient with decreasing urine production and perigraft pain.* (Right) *Spectral Doppler US of the intraparenchymal arteries shows reversal of diastolic flow from the subcapsular collection, consistent with Page kidney.*

Peritransplant Collection

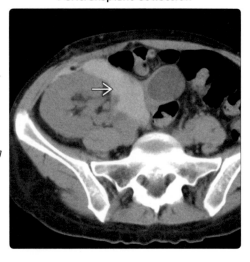

Pyelonephritis

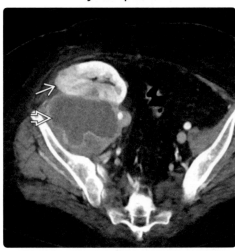

(Left) *Axial NECT shows a high-density fluid collection medial to the kidney graft* ➡️. *CT from the day prior was performed with IV contrast, and the collection at that time was simple fluid density. The high-density material was from urinary extravasation of contrast in this urinoma.* (Right) *Axial CECT shows wedge-shaped, hypoenhancing regions in this right lower quadrant kidney graft, consistent with pyelonephritis* ➡️. *A rim-enhancing fluid collection is seen posterior to the graft involving the right iliacus muscle* ➡️.

Acute Rejection

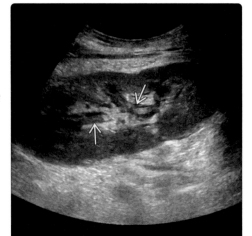

Acute Rejection

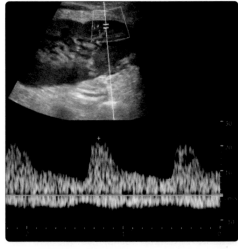

(Left) *In this patient with a kidney graft and renal dysfunction, US shows a thickened urothelium in an otherwise normal kidney* ➡️. (Right) *In the same patient, the resistive indices were normal. Biopsy revealed acute cellular rejection. Urothelial thickening can often be the only abnormal US finding in patients with rejection.*

Transplant Renal Artery Stenosis

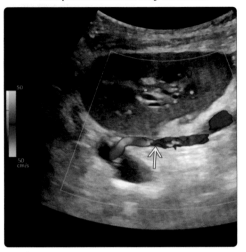

Transplant Renal Artery Stenosis

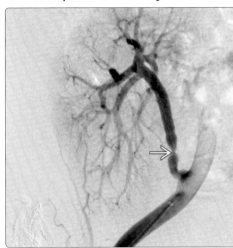

(Left) *In this patient with uncontrolled hypertension, color Doppler US shows an area of aliasing involving the graft main renal artery* ➡. *This corresponded with an area of elevated velocity.* (Right) *Angiography in the same patient shows main renal artery stenosis* ➡ *of 75%. The patient was treated with stent placement.*

Urinary Obstruction

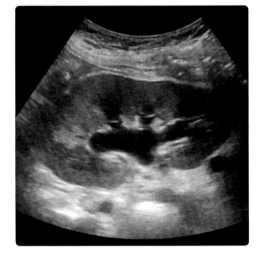

Urinary Obstruction

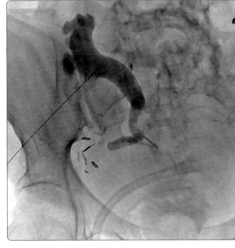

(Left) *Longitudinal US in a patient with renal dysfunction shows increasing hydronephrosis compared with prior examinations.* (Right) *In the same patient, a nephrostomy was placed, and an antegrade nephrostogram show a dilated collecting system and ureter. Contrast did not spontaneously fill the urinary bladder, consistent with distal ureteral stricture.*

Venous Thrombosis

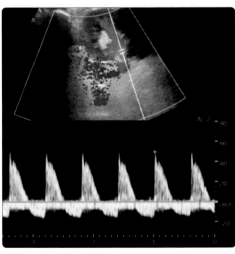

Arterial Thrombosis

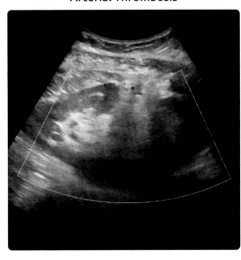

(Left) *After kidney transplantation, this patient experienced pain over the kidney graft with absent urinary output. Reversal of flow is seen in diastole within the renal artery without a visible renal vein. The patient was taken to the operative room where an occlusive venous thrombus was seen.* (Right) *In this patient with no urinary output after transplantation, US shows absent flow throughout the kidney graft. The patient was taken to the operative room and had an occlusive thrombus in the renal artery.*

DIFFERENTIAL DIAGNOSIS

Common

- Renal Cell Carcinoma
- Angiomyolipoma
- Oncocytoma
- Urothelial Carcinoma

Less Common

- Lymphoma/Leukemia
- Sarcomas
- Metastases
- Papillary Adenoma

Rare but Important

- Epithelioid Angiomyolipoma
- Metanephric Adenoma
- Neuroendocrine Tumors
- Leiomyoma
- Juxtaglomerular Cell Tumor
- Renomedullary Interstitial Cell Tumor
- IgG4-Related Kidney Disease

ESSENTIAL INFORMATION

Key Differential Diagnosis Issues

- Solid renal masses can be benign or malignant
- Presence of gross fat within lesion is only way of confidently excluding malignant lesion
- Usually require surgical excision, biopsy, or close follow-up if small or if poor surgical candidate

Helpful Clues for Common Diagnoses

- **Renal Cell Carcinoma**
  - Subtypes: Clear cell (75%), papillary (10%), chromophobe cell (5%), others (10%)
  - Unilateral > bilateral
  - If multiple or bilateral, consider syndromes (von Hippel-Lindau) or increased risk factors (acquired cystic disease)
  - Imaging
    - Clear cell subtype: Hypervascular tumors
    - Papillary and chromophobe subtypes: Hypovascular
    - Renal medullary and collecting duct carcinomas are located more centrally in kidney; renal medullary carcinoma is associated with sickle cell trait
    - Usually solid mass but may have infiltrative features
    - May invade renal vein and extend into inferior vena cava
    - May contain calcifications
    - Clear cell renal cell carcinoma (RCC) can lose signal on out of phase images
    - Very rarely may contain tiny foci of gross fat
    - ± metastases (nodes, adrenal glands, pancreas, liver, lungs, bones)
- **Angiomyolipoma**
  - Most common benign renal neoplasm
  - 90% are unilateral and solitary
  - 10% are multiple and bilateral; usually due to tuberous sclerosis complex
  - Solid, heterogeneous, renal cortical mass in adult with macroscopic fat is reliable sign of angiomyolipoma
    - Variable amounts of fat may be present

- ~ 5% of AMLs contain minimal fat (lipid-poor) and cannot be reliably diagnosed by imaging
  - Lipid-poor AMLs are often hyperdense on NECT
  - Rarely invades renal vein
  - Presence of calcification is rare; if present, suspect RCC
  - Hemorrhage more likely in large AMLs (≥ 4 cm)
- **Oncocytoma**
  - 2nd most common benign renal neoplasm
  - Benign renal tumor composed of eosinophilic epithelial cells arising from collecting ducts
  - Solid renal cortical mass lesion ± central stellate scar
  - Dynamic postcontrast imaging is highly variable and depends on degree of cellularity and stroma
  - Absence of malignant features
    - No invasion of vessels, perinephric fat, or collecting system
    - No lymphadenopathy or metastases
  - Birt-Hogg-Dubé syndrome syndrome
    - Rare autosomal dominant disorder with multisystem epithelial neoplasms
    - Multiple RCCs, renal oncocytomas, and lung cysts
- **Urothelial Carcinoma**
  - 8% of urothelial carcinomas occur at level of kidney
  - Extrarenal part of renal pelvis more common than infundibulocalyceal
  - Solid mass in collecting system that may efface renal sinus fat and invade into renal parenchyma
  - Rare calcifications (2% of renal pelvis urothelial carcinoma)
  - Usually hypoenhancing
  - ± metastases (nodes, retroperitoneum, lungs, bones)
  - May have synchronous or metachronous involvement (survey entire urothelial tract)

Helpful Clues for Less Common Diagnoses

- **Lymphoma/Leukemia**
  - Lymphomatous involvement is more common with non-Hodgkin lymphoma types (B-cell, Burkitt lymphoma)
  - Lymphoma is almost always associated with extrarenal lymphadenopathy (primary renal lymphoma is rare)
  - May be associated with splenomegaly
  - May present as multiple well-circumscribed masses or as infiltrative process
  - Usually bilateral process
  - May extend into pelvis and encase ureters and vessels
  - Soft tissue mass displaces rather than compresses or invades ureters and vessels
  - May invade adjacent organs
  - Kidney may be enlarged
  - Can lead to renal dysfunction
- **Sarcomas**
  - Subtypes include leiomyosarcoma, angiosarcoma, rhabdomyosarcoma, osteosarcoma, synovial, and Ewing
  - Leiomyosarcoma is most common sarcoma of kidney
  - Rhabdomyosarcoma and angiosarcoma are more likely to be infiltrative
  - Usually arise from capsule or renal sinus
  - Calcifications can be seen with osteosarcoma but are otherwise uncommon in renal sarcomas
- **Metastases**

- o Metastatic involvement of kidney is unlikely to be sole site of metastatic disease
- o Most commonly from lung, colorectal, stomach, and breast primaries
- o May have homogeneous or heterogeneous enhancement
- o Renal vein involvement is uncommon
- **Papillary Adenoma**
  - o Similar to papillary RCC type 1 but lacks pseudocapsule and measures ≤ 15 mm
  - o Usually incidentally noted on nephrectomy as often too small to visualize by imaging
  - o Possibly precursor to papillary RCCs but most do not progress
  - o Do not have ability to metastasize

Helpful Clues for Rare Diagnoses

- **Epithelioid Angiomyolipoma**
  - o Rare variant of angiomyolipomas
  - o Considered perivascular epithelial cell tumors (PEComas)
  - o Can appear aggressive with metastatic involvement
    - – Can contain small foci of gross fat
    - – Typically exophytic
    - – Rarely contain calcification
    - – Can hemorrhage
- **Metanephric Adenoma**
  - o Benign, epithelial renal neoplasm
  - o Arises in renal medulla
  - o US
    - – Variable echogenicity
  - o CT
    - – Rare calcifications
    - – Well circumscribed
    - – NECT: Typically hyperattenuating
    - – CECT: Mild, delayed enhancement
  - o MR
    - – T1: Low signal
    - – T2: Isointense to slightly hyperintense signal
- **Neuroendocrine Tumors**
  - o More common in patients with horseshoe kidneys

- o May be completely solid or mixed solid and cystic
- o Can contain calcifications
- o Variable levels of enhancement
- **Leiomyoma**
  - o Benign tumor, usually involving capsule
  - o Well-circumscribed, homogeneous enhancement
- **Juxtaglomerular Cell Tumor**
  - o Benign tumor
  - o Usually occurs in young adults, female predominance
  - o Clinically: Poorly controlled hypertension, hypokalemia, and hyperaldosteronism from tumor renin secretion
  - o Well-circumscribed, cortically based tumors
  - o Homogeneous mass with hypoenhancement
- **Renomedullary Interstitial Cell Tumor**
  - o Benign tumor
  - o Previously called medullary fibroma and renal hamartoma
  - o Arise from renomedullary interstitial cells; located in renal pyramids
  - o Usually subcentimeter and difficult to see by imaging; common on autopsy studies
  - o Typically nonenhancing or mildly enhancing masses
- **IgG4-Related Kidney Disease**
  - o Immune-mediated systemic disease that can involve most organs
  - o Isolated IgG4-related kidney disease is uncommon; typically associated with pancreatic &/or biliary involvement
  - o Can have discrete masses or be infiltrative
  - o Mild, progressive enhancement
  - o Typically T2 hypointense and T1 isointense on MR
  - o May resolve after steroid treatment

SELECTED REFERENCES

1. Heller MT et al: Multiparametric MR for solid renal mass characterization. Magn Reson Imaging Clin N Am. 28(3):457-69, 2020
2. Sasaguri K et al: CT and MR imaging for solid renal mass characterization. Eur J Radiol. 99:40-54, 2018
3. Ward RD et al: 2017 AUA renal mass and localized renal cancer guidelines: imaging implications. Radiographics. 38(7):2021-33, 2018

Renal Cell Carcinoma

Renal Cell Carcinoma

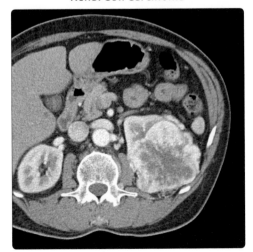

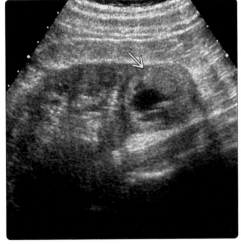

(Left) Axial CECT shows a large, heterogeneous, avidly enhancing mass involving the left kidney extending into the perinephric space. This was surgically removed and proven to be clear cell renal cell carcinoma. (Right) Long axis US shows a rounded, predominantly echogenic lesion involving the inferior pole of the kidney ➡ with mixed solid and cystic components. This patient underwent a partial nephrectomy for clear cell renal cell carcinoma.

Renal Cell Carcinoma

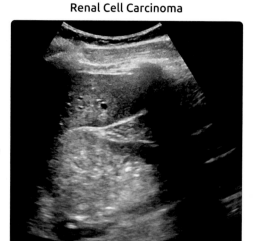

Renal Cell Carcinoma

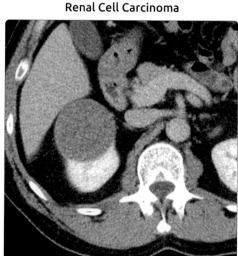

(Left) *Horizontal long axis US shows a predominantly echogenic mass involving the upper pole of the kidney with fairly homogeneous internal components. While echogenic lesions on US may represent angiomyolipomas, those > 1 cm should be further evaluated with CT or MR.* **(Right)** *Axial CECT in the same patient shows there is a homogeneous, mildly enhancing renal mass, which was resected and found to be papillary renal cell carcinoma.*

Renal Cell Carcinoma

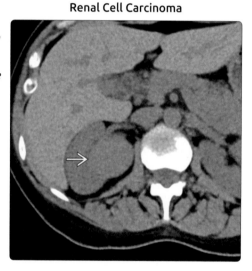

Renal Cell Carcinoma

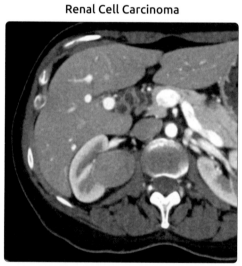

(Left) *An incidental mass was discovered on US, which led to further imaging by CT. Axial NECT shows a mildly hyperdense mass involving the left kidney centrally ➡.* **(Right)** *The same lesion was mildly enhancing on CECT. This was proven to be chromophobe renal cell carcinoma.*

Angiomyolipoma

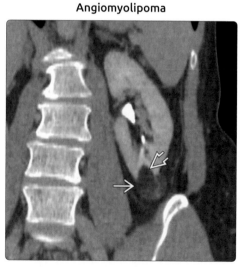

Oncocytoma

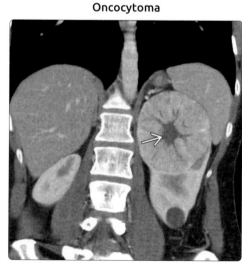

(Left) *Coronal CECT shows a predominantly fat-containing mass which extends from the inferior pole of the left kidney ➡. The lesion shows a wedge-shaped emanation from the cortex, the so-called ice cream cone sign ➡. The imaging features are diagnostic of an angiomyolipoma.* **(Right)** *Coronal CECT shows a well-circumscribed mass which arises from the superior pole of the left kidney. This mass has a central stellate scar ➡. On biopsy, this was found to be an oncocytoma.*

Urothelial Carcinoma

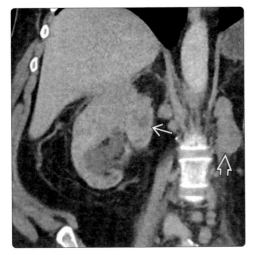

Lymphoma/Leukemia

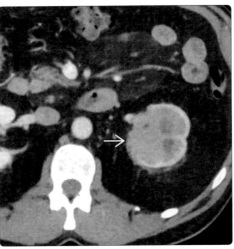

(Left) *Coronal CECT shows a well-defined, infiltrative mass involving the hilar region and the superior pole of the right kidney ➡. Numerous enlarged retroperitoneal lymph nodes are present ➡. This was proven to be urothelial carcinoma.* (Right) *Infiltrative soft tissue mass ➡ involves the hilum of the left kidney extending into the medullary portions. This was biopsy-proven to be lymphomatous involvement of the left kidney.*

Sarcomas

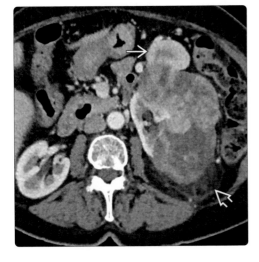

Epithelioid Angiomyolipoma

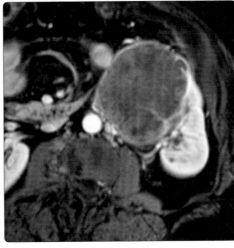

(Left) *Axial CECT shows a large, heterogeneous mass involving the left kidney with both solid ➡ and fat-containing ➡ portions. This was surgically removed and proven to be renal liposarcoma.* (Right) *Axial CEMR shows a well-circumscribed mass involving the medial aspect of the left kidney. No gross fat was detected; however, the diagnosis was epithelioid angiomyolipoma, which can have imaging features similar to a renal call carcinoma.*

Metanephric Adenoma

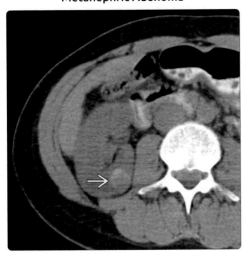

Neuroendocrine Tumors

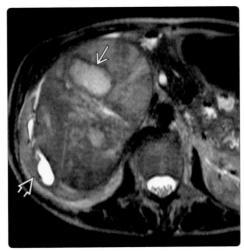

(Left) *Axial NECT shows a rounded, hyperdense lesion involving the right kidney ➡ that had minimal enhancement after contrast administration. This was found to be a benign metanephric adenoma.* (Right) *Axial T2 MR shows a large, heterogeneous mass involving the right kidney with necrotic components ➡. Mild enhancement was seen on postcontrast sequences, exerting significant effect on the right kidney ➡. This was found to be a renal neuroendocrine tumor.*

DIFFERENTIAL DIAGNOSIS

Common

- Bosniak I/II Cysts
- Peripelvic Cysts
- Renal Abscess

Less Common

- Cystic Renal Cell Carcinoma
- Trauma, Renal
- Focal Hydronephrosis

Rare but Important

- Mixed Epithelial and Stromal Tumor Family
- Multiloculated Cystic Renal Neoplasm of Low Malignant Potential
- Localized Cystic Renal Disease
- Multicystic Renal Dysplasia

ESSENTIAL INFORMATION

Key Differential Diagnosis Issues

- Both benign and malignant lesions can appear as cystic renal masses
- Cystic lesions are classified by CT and MR according to Bosniak classification, which risk stratifies cystic renal masses
  - Bosniak I: Benign simple renal cyst requiring no follow-up
  - Bosniak II: Benign (or "likely benign") renal cyst (or "mass") requiring no follow-up
  - Bosniak IIF: Large majority benign; follow-up at 6 months and then annually for 5 years
  - Bosniak III: Intermediate probability of malignancy; urologic consultation should be considered
  - Bosniak IV: Large majority malignant; urologic consultation should be considered
  - Cyst: Bosniak I or Bosniak II lesions deemed cysts
  - Cystic mass: Any other cystic lesion
- CT and MR are modalities that are amenable to Bosniak classification
  - CECT
    - Bosniak I
      - Cystic lesion that is homogeneous and fluid density (-9-20 HU)
      - Walls smooth and thin (≤ 2 mm)
      - No septations or calcifications
    - Bosniak II
      - Walls smooth and thin (≤ 2 mm) with few (1-3) septations; may have calcifications
      - Homogeneous lesion that is > 20 HU but nonenhancing (< 10 HU difference between pre- and postcontrast images); may have calcifications
      - Homogeneous lesions 21-30 HU on portal venous phase imaging
      - Homogeneous lesions too small to characterize (typically < 1 cm)
    - Bosniak IIF
      - Lesions with smooth, minimally thickened (2-4 mm) walls
      - Lesions with any smooth, minimally thickened (2-4 mm) septa

      - Lesions with many (≥ 4) smooth, thin (≤ 2 mm) septa
    - Bosniak III
      - Lesions with any thick (> 4 mm) enhancing wall or septation
      - Lesions with any irregular walls or septations
    - Bosniak IV
      - Lesions with any enhancing nodule
      - Nodule defined as ≥ 4 mm, obtusely margined, convex protrusion or any convex protrusion with acute margins
  - MR similar to CT regarding homogeneity, walls, and septations; HU replaced with T1 and T2 signal characteristics
- US
  - Not currently used in Bosniak classification
  - Can be useful in assessing hyperdense cysts on NECT
  - CEUS has high sensitivity for identifying vascular flow within cystic lesion

Helpful Clues for Common Diagnoses

- **Bosniak I/II Cysts**
  - Benign fluid contents of simple fluid or proteinaceous/hemorrhagic material
  - Extremely common; increased size and prevalence with age
  - US characteristics of cyst
    - Defined as anechoic structures with well-defined back wall and posterior acoustic enhancement; no enhancement on CEUS
    - Tiny cysts can appear as echogenic foci
  - CT characteristics of cyst
    - Density < 20 HU on NECT and < 30 HU on portal venous phase
    - Hyperdense cysts (hemorrhagic or proteinaceous) are either cysts with > 70 HU on NECT or < 10 HU on postcontrast images
  - On MR, simple cysts are T2 hyperintense and T1 hypointense; proteinaceous/hemorrhagic cysts can by T1 hyperintense but without enhancement
  - Ensure no solid/enhancing components
- **Peripelvic Cysts**
  - Asymptomatic benign cysts located in renal sinus that originate from lymphatics
  - Usually multiple and bilateral
  - Can simulate renal sinus cystic mass
  - Can also be confused with hydronephrosis
  - Peripelvic cysts do not connect with one another
  - Urographic-phase CT or MR will separate collecting system peripelvic cysts
- **Renal Abscess**
  - Usually late complication of pyelonephritis
  - May be associated with renal enlargement
  - Urothelial thickening may be present
  - US
    - Debris within bladder may be seen
    - Complex cyst containing low-level echoes
  - CT/MR
    - Inflammatory stranding around bladder and infected kidney

– Usually has shaggy, enhancing wall and infiltration of perirenal fat
- Clinical history and needle aspiration are keys to diagnosis

Helpful Clues for Less Common Diagnoses

- **Cystic Renal Cell Carcinoma**
  - Up to 15% of renal cell cacinomas (RCCs) have cystic component
  - Cystic component may be from intrinsic unilocular or multilocular cystic growth, cystic necrosis, or origination of RCC from epithelium of simple cyst
  - Thickened wall/septal enhancement is important in distinguishing RCC from other benign complex cysts
  - Clear cell, papillary, clear cell papillary, acquired cystic disease, and tubulocystic subtypes of RCC are more likely to be cystic
  - Multiple RCCs in association with cysts can be seen in acquired cystic disease (small kidneys) and von Hippel-Lindau disease
- **Trauma, Renal**
  - Evolving renal hematoma or urinoma may simulate cystic mass
- **Focal Hydronephrosis**
  - Obstructed calyx or infundibulum (e.g., TB, urothelial cell carcinoma)
  - Duplicated collecting system with obstruction of ureter from upper pole moiety
  - May be mistaken for upper pole renal cystic mass

Helpful Clues for Rare Diagnoses

- **Mixed Epithelial and Stromal Tumor Family**
  - Both adult cystic nephroma and mixed epithelial stromal tumor (MEST) have overlapping radiologic and pathologic features
  - Solitary, unilateral, well-circumscribed, fluid-filled mass with septations
    – Septations may be thin or thick and nodular
  - Heterogeneous, delayed, minimal septal enhancement
  - May herniate into renal pelvis, leading to obstruction of collecting system

- **Multiloculated Cystic Renal Neoplasm of Low Malignant Potential**
  - Benign cystic lesion previously known as multilocular cystic RCC
  - Tumor composed entirely of cysts with septa composed of nonexpansile, small groups of clear cells
  - Similar genetic profile of tumor to clear cell RCC but with no progression or metastatic potential
- **Localized Cystic Renal Disease**
  - Acquired condition characterized by multiple cysts involving portion separated by normal renal parenchyma
  - Affected side is usually functional
- **Multicystic Renal Dysplasia**
  - Sporadic disorder that can be unilateral or bilateral
  - Affected kidney is usually enlarged, irregular in contour, with multiple cysts of variable sizes
  - Can be associated with ureteropelvic junction obstruction, ureteral agenesis
  - Affected side is usually nonfunctional
  - Can simulate complex cystic neoplasm
  - Renal failure can result in cases of bilateral disease

SELECTED REFERENCES

1. Schieda N et al: Bosniak classification of cystic renal masses, version 2019: a pictorial guide to clinical use. Radiographics. 41(3):814-88, 2021
2. Magnelli LL et al: A MEST up classification? Review of the re-classification of mixed epithelial and stromal tumor and adult cystic nephroma for the abdominal radiologist. Abdom Radiol (NY). 46(2):696-702, 2021
3. Smith AD et al: Approach to renal cystic masses and the role of radiology. Radiol Clin North Am. 58(5):897-907, 2020
4. Narayanasamy S et al: Contemporary update on imaging of cystic renal masses with histopathological correlation and emphasis on patient management. Clin Radiol. 74(2):83-94, 2019
5. Silverman SG et al: Bosniak classification of cystic renal masses, version 2019: an update proposal and needs assessment. Radiology. 292(2):475-88, 2019
6. Wood CG 3rd et al: CT and MR imaging for evaluation of cystic renal lesions and diseases. Radiographics. 35(1):125-41, 2015

Bosniak I/II Cysts

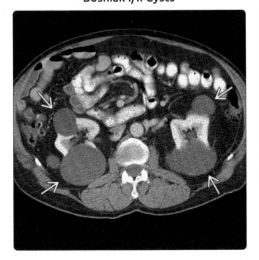

Bosniak I/II Cysts

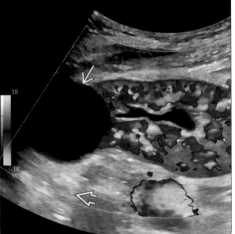

(Left) *Axial CECT in a 62-year-old man with abdominal pain shows multiple simple, exophytic renal cortical cysts ➡. Features of Bosniak I cysts include water attenuation and lack of an enhancing wall, septa, or calcifications.* **(Right)** *Although US is not included in the Bosniak classification, this lesion shows features of a simple cyst: Anechoic, well-defined back wall ➡, posterior acoustic enhancement ➡, and lack of vascular flow on Doppler imaging.*

Cystic Renal Mass

Bosniak I/II Cysts

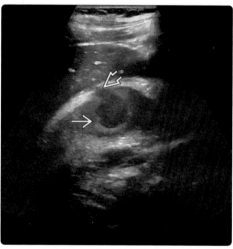

Peripelvic Cysts

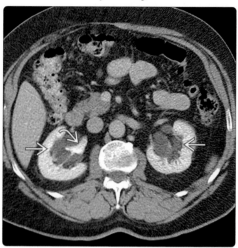

(Left) *Axial T1 MR shows a lesion in the right kidney with homogeneous high signal intensity. The lesion was hypointense with no enhancement on T2 MR and hyperdense on NECT (not shown). Imaging features are consistent with hemorrhagic cyst (Bosniak II).* **(Right)** *Axial CECT shows bilateral peripelvic cysts* ➡. *Note compression of opacified right renal pelvis* ➡. *Care should be taken to differentiate noncommunicating peripelvic cysts from hydronephrosis on US. Excretory phase CECT may be confirmatory.*

Renal Abscess

Cystic Renal Cell Carcinoma

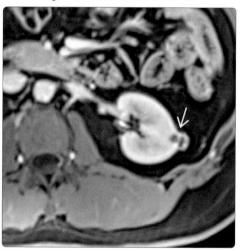

(Left) *US shows an irregular, cystic mass involving the right kidney* ➡ *with a thickened, mildly echogenic rim. A portion of this cystic mass extends to the renal capsule* ➡. *After aspiration, this was found to be an abscess.* **(Right)** *Axial CECT shows a small, complex, exophytic cystic mass involving the left kidney* ➡. *The septation shows enhancement. This was surgically removed and proven to be cystic clear cell renal cell carcinoma.*

Cystic Renal Cell Carcinoma

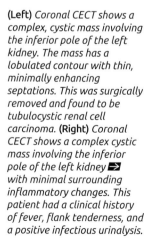

Focal Hydronephrosis

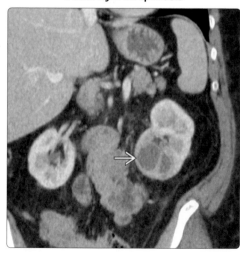

(Left) *Coronal CECT shows a complex, cystic mass involving the inferior pole of the left kidney. The mass has a lobulated contour with thin, minimally enhancing septations. This was surgically removed and found to be tubulocystic renal cell carcinoma.* **(Right)** *Coronal CECT shows a complex cystic mass involving the inferior pole of the left kidney* ➡ *with minimal surrounding inflammatory changes. This patient had a clinical history of fever, flank tenderness, and a positive infectious urinalysis.*

Mixed Epithelial and Stromal Tumor Family

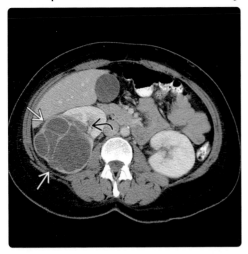

Mixed Epithelial and Stromal Tumor Family

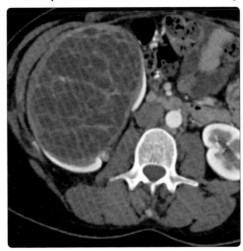

(Left) Axial CECT in a middle-aged woman with flank pain shows a complex, encapsulated cystic lesion ➡ that invaginates into the renal hilum ⤵. Enhancing, thick septa indicate a Bosniak III cyst. Adult cystic nephroma was confirmed at resection. (Right) Axial CECT shows a large, complex, cystic mass involving the right kidney with thin, minimally enhancing septations. The left kidney was normal. This was surgically removed and proven to be adult cystic nephroma (tumor in MEST family).

Mixed Epithelial and Stromal Tumor Family

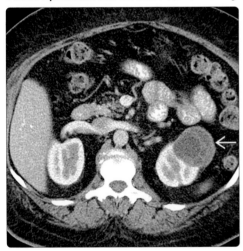

Multiloculated Cystic Renal Neoplasm of Low Malignant Potential

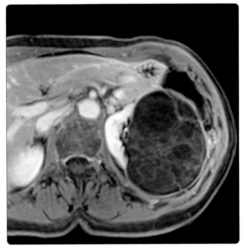

(Left) Axial CECT in a perimenopausal woman shows a complex, exophytic, cystic lesion ➡. Thick, enhancing septa indicate a Bosniak III cyst. Partial nephrectomy confirmed mixed epithelial and stromal tumor. (Right) Axial CEMR shows a complex, cystic mass involving the left kidney with multiple minimally enhancing, thin septations. This was surgically removed and proven to be multiloculated cystic renal neoplasm of low malignant potential.

Multiloculated Cystic Renal Neoplasm of Low Malignant Potential

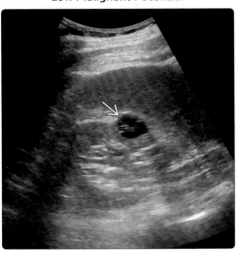

Localized Cystic Renal Disease

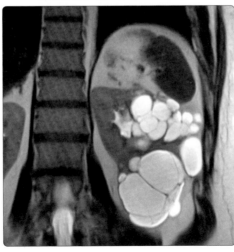

(Left) US shows an exophytic, complex, cystic mass involving the right kidney with a few thin septations ➡. No appreciable signal was seen on color Doppler imaging. This was surgically resected and proven to be multiloculated cystic renal neoplasm of low malignant potential. (Right) Axial T2 MR shows multiple cysts involving the interpolar and lower pole of the left kidney separated by normal renal parenchyma. The right kidney was normal. This patient had no clinical evidence of renal dysfunction.

DIFFERENTIAL DIAGNOSIS

Common

- Simple Renal Cysts
- Acquired Cystic Kidney Disease
- Peripelvic Cysts
- Autosomal Dominant Polycystic Disease, Kidney
- Abscesses

Less Common

- Lithium Nephropathy
- Tuberous Sclerosis
- von Hippel-Lindau Disease
- Multicystic Renal Dysplasia

Rare but Important

- Medullary Cystic Disease
- Glomerulocystic Disease

ESSENTIAL INFORMATION

Key Differential Diagnosis Issues

- Consider kidney size, number of cysts, cyst size, and location of cysts (cortical, medullary, peripelvic) as well as medication history (lithium) and renal function to narrow differential
- US characteristics of cyst
  - Defined as anechoic structures with well-defined back wall and posterior acoustic enhancement without flow on color Doppler or CEUS
  - Tiny cysts can appear as echogenic foci
- CT characteristics of cyst
  - Density < 20 HU on NECT and < 30 HU on portal venous phase
  - Hyperdense cysts (hemorrhagic or proteinaceous) are either cysts with > 70 HU on NECT or < 10 HU enhancement on postcontrast images
- On MR, simple cysts are T2 hyperintense and T1 hypointense; proteinaceous/hemorrhagic cysts can by T1 hyperintense but without enhancement
- Ensure no solid/enhancing components

Helpful Clues for Common Diagnoses

- **Simple Renal Cysts**
  - Usually asymptomatic
  - Commonly seen; increase in size and number with increasing age
  - Classification according to Bosniak system, especially when they demonstrate atypical features
  - Rarely can hemorrhage, become infected, or rupture
- **Acquired Cystic Kidney Disease**
  - Atrophic kidneys (small, thinned cortex)
  - ≥ 3 cysts per kidney in patients with end-stage renal disease (ESRD) and no history of hereditary cystic disease
  - Imaging features of renal cysts
    - Multiple; located in both cortex and medulla
    - Variable size; up to several centimeters
  - Kidney size
    - Small, atrophic
    - Cysts and kidneys may become larger
  - Patients have increased risk of developing renal cell carcinoma

- **Peripelvic Cysts**
  - Asymptomatic benign cysts located in renal sinus that originate from lymphatics
  - Usually multiple and bilateral
  - Can be confused with hydronephrosis
    - Peripelvic cysts do not connect with one another
    - Urographic-phased CT or MR will show separate collecting system peripelvic cysts
- **Autosomal Dominant Polycystic Disease, Kidney**
  - Enlarged kidneys that are increasingly replaced by numerous cysts
    - Multiple and of variable size
    - Number and size of cysts increase over time
  - Causes progressive renal failure
  - Diagnosis based on at-risk individuals and US findings (Pei-Levine criteria)
    - 15-39 years of age: ≥ 3 renal cysts total
    - 40-59 years of age: ≥ 2 cysts in each kidney
    - ≥ 60 years of age: ≥ 4 cysts in each kidney
  - Can be associated with hepatic, pancreatic, and splenic cysts
  - CT/MR can have role in renal volume, which can provide prognostic information
- **Abscesses**
  - Usually late complication of pyelonephritis
  - May be associated with renal enlargement
  - Urothelial thickening may be present
  - US
    - Debris within bladder may be seen
    - Complex cyst containing low-level echoes
  - CT/MR
    - Inflammatory stranding around bladder and infected kidney
    - Usually has shaggy, enhancing wall and infiltration of perirenal fat
  - Clinical history and needle aspiration are keys to diagnosis

Helpful Clues for Less Common Diagnoses

- **Lithium Nephropathy**
  - Lithium ingestion can lead to structured kidney damage, which can cause renal failure
  - Imaging features of renal cysts
    - Multiple, bilateral
    - Microcysts (1-2 mm)
    - Location: Cortex and medulla
    - On US, tiny cysts can appear as echogenic foci
  - Kidney size
    - Normal to small
  - Diagnosis based on biopsy and clinical history
- **Tuberous Sclerosis**
  - Autosomal dominant genetic disorder characterized by growth of hamartomous tumors
  - Multiple variable-sized cysts
  - Ancillary imaging features
    - Kidneys: Hamartomas = angiomyolipomas (often multiple and bilateral)
    - Hamartomatous tumors in brain, lung, heart, and skin
- **von Hippel-Lindau Disease**

o Hereditary, autosomal dominant disease with multiorgan, benign and malignant neoplasms
o Imaging features of renal cysts
  – Multiple and of various size
  – ~ 60% of patients have renal cysts
o Ancillary imaging features
  – Renal cell carcinoma
    □ Present in 25-45% of patients
    □ Histology: Clear cell type; location: Bilateral in 75% of cases
  – Pancreas: Cysts, serous microcystic adenomas, neuroendocrine (islet cell) tumors
  – Adrenal: Pheochromocytoma (often recurrent, multiple)
  – CNS: Hemangioblastomas of cerebellum, brainstem, spinal cord
● **Multicystic Renal Dysplasia**
o Sporadic disorder that can be unilateral or bilateral
o Affected kidney is usually enlarged, irregular in contour with multiple cysts of variable sizes

o Can be associated with ureteropelvic junction obstruction, ureteral agenesis
o Can simulate complex cystic neoplasm
o Renal failure can result in cases of bilateral disease

Helpful Clues for Rare Diagnoses
● **Medullary Cystic Disease**
o Caused by nephronophthisis (NPNH) and autosomal dominant tubulointerstitial kidney disease (ADTKP)
o Younger patient population
  – ESRD < 30 years with NPNH and 16-50 years depending on mutation of ADTKP
o Progressive renal atrophy, secondary glomerulosclerosis, and medullary cyst formation
o Cysts, usually small, seen at corticomedullary junction
o Small to normal-sized kidneys
● **Glomerulocystic Disease**
o Very rare condition associated with renal failure
o Usually affects children and young adults
o Tiny cysts in renal cortex that arise from proximal convoluted tubules and Bowman space

Simple Renal Cysts

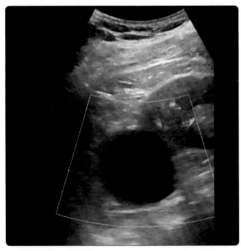

Simple Renal Cysts

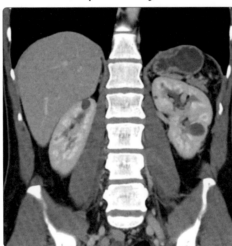

(Left) *Transverse color Doppler US shows features of a classic cyst include an anechoic, well-defined back wall, posterior acoustic enhancement, and lack of vascular flow.* **(Right)** *Coronal CECT shows several bilateral simple cysts. Bilateral simple renal cysts are common and usually incidental with no associated renal dysfunction. Cysts are more common in older patient populations.*

Simple Renal Cysts

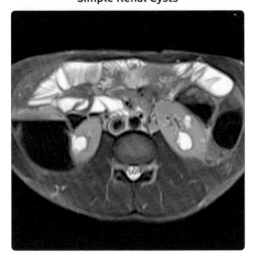

Acquired Cystic Kidney Disease

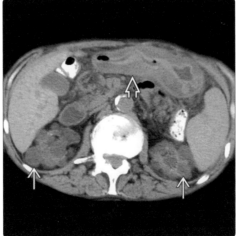

(Left) *Axial T2 FS MR shows incidentally noted, bilateral cysts. This patient had no evidence of renal dysfunction.* **(Right)** *Axial NECT shows small kidneys with numerous small cysts ➡. Gastric wall ⇒ is thickened due to gastritis induced by immunosuppressive therapy in this patient who had a renal transplant following years of dialysis therapy.*

Kidney

Acquired Cystic Kidney Disease

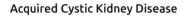

(Left) *Coronal T2 MR in a patient with end-stage renal disease shows atrophic kidneys with multiple simple cysts* ➡. *The imaging findings and clinical scenario were consistent with acquired cystic kidney disease.* **(Right)** *Coronal T2 MR in a 25-year-old man with autosomal dominant polycystic kidney disease (ADPKD) shows enlarged kidneys replaced by numerous cysts* ➡ *of varying size and signal intensity.*

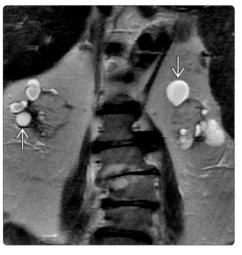

Autosomal Dominant Polycystic Disease, Kidney

(Left) *Axial NECT shows massive enlargement of both kidneys with numerous cysts of varying size and attenuation, some of which have internal hemorrhage* ➡. *This patient had renal dysfunction and was diagnosed with ADPKD.* **(Right)** *Axial NECT shows innumerable cysts of varying size and attenuation in the kidneys* ➡ *and liver* ➡. *Liver cysts are the most common extrarenal manifestation in patients with ADPKD.*

Autosomal Dominant Polycystic Disease, Kidney

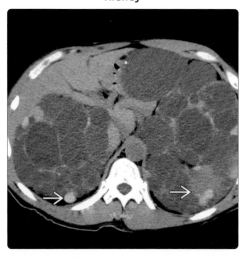

Autosomal Dominant Polycystic Disease, Kidney

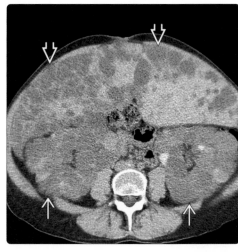

(Left) *Axial CECT shows numerous small cysts* ➡, *mostly in the cortex, in this 62-year-old man with preserved renal function and presumed type 2 ADPKD.* **(Right)** *Axial CECT shows multiple ill-defined, hypodense collections in both kidneys. There is some perinephric stranding involving the left kidney* ➡. *Urinalysis and clinical features were consistent with pyelonephritis with multiple abscesses.*

Autosomal Dominant Polycystic Disease, Kidney

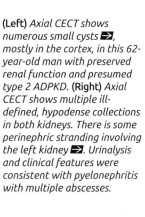 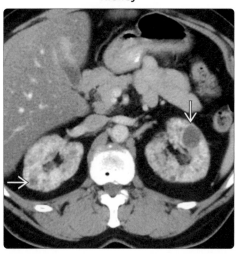

Abscesses

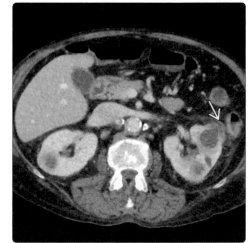

von Hippel-Lindau Disease

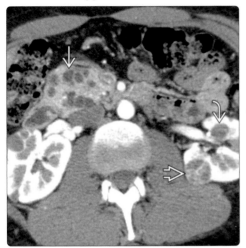

von Hippel-Lindau Disease

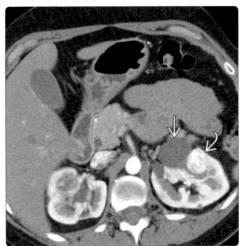

(Left) *Axial CECT shows multiple cysts in the pancreas ⇒ and kidneys ⇒ as well as one of several solid, enhancing masses ⇒ (renal cell carcinoma). These are classic features of von Hippel-Lindau syndrome.* (Right) *Axial CECT shows multiple renal cysts ⇒ and a solid, enhancing mass ⇒ (renal cell carcinoma) in this patient with von Hippel-Lindau disease.*

Lithium Nephropathy

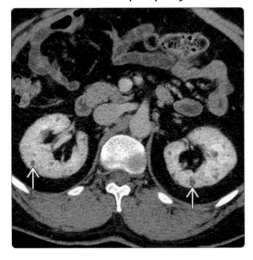

Lithium Nephropathy

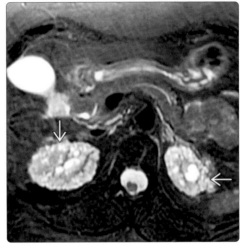

(Left) *Axial CECT shows numerous, bilateral microcysts ⇒ in normal-sized kidneys. This patient had bipolar disorder and was treated with lithium. Biopsy confirmed lithium nephropathy.* (Right) *Axial T2 MR shows numerous tiny cysts ⇒ throughout the cortex and medulla of both kidneys in a 69-year-old woman receiving long-term lithium therapy for bipolar disorder. The kidneys are diminished in size and function.*

Medullary Cystic Disease

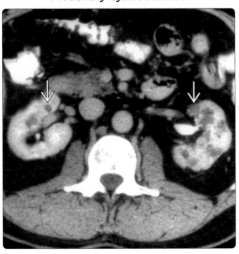

Glomerulocystic Disease

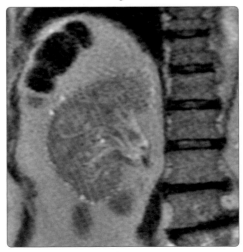

(Left) *Axial CECT shows multiple medullary and cortical cysts ⇒ in a patient with progressive renal failure, anemia, and salt-wasting nephropathy, all of which are typical imaging and clinical features of medullary cystic disease.* (Right) *Coronal T2 MR shows multiple tiny cysts peripherally within the kidneys in this patient with renal dysfunction. Biopsy was consistent with glomerulocystic disease.*

DIFFERENTIAL DIAGNOSIS

Common
- Renal Cell Carcinoma
- Urothelial Carcinoma
- Acute Pyelonephritis

Less Common
- Renal Lymphoma
- Renal Leukemia
- Renal Metastasis
- Squamous Cell Carcinoma
- Xanthogranulomatous Pyelonephritis

Rare but Important
- IgG4-Related Kidney Disease
- Renal Sarcoma
- Renal Plasmacytoma
- Renal Sarcoidosis
- Radiation Therapy

ESSENTIAL INFORMATION

Key Differential Diagnosis Issues
- Most renal masses are well-circumscribed and expansile, usually spherical in shape, and often exophytic
- Infiltrative renal lesions demonstrate interstitial infiltration, using planes of normal renal architecture for growth
- Infiltrative lesions have poorly defined margins between mass and normal renal parenchyma
- Renal masses can demonstrate mixed well-circumscribed and infiltrative patterns
- Infiltrative masses are usually hypoenhancing to renal parenchyma on venous or nephrographic phases
- Infiltrative masses include neoplastic, inflammatory, and infectious processes
- Infiltrative neoplasms are usually more aggressive with poorer outcomes

Helpful Clues for Common Diagnoses
- **Renal Cell Carcinoma**
  - Most common infiltrating mass [others may tend to be more infiltrative, but renal cell carcinoma (RCC) RCC is most common]
  - 6% of RCCs are infiltrative
  - May have mixed, well-defined mass and infiltrative features
  - Sarcomatoid or rhabdoid features within common subtypes of RCC (clear cell, papillary, chromophobe) are more likely to manifest as infiltrative
  - Infiltrative RCCs have heterogeneous enhancement, typically hypoenhancing
  - Renal vein invasion is highly suggestive of RCC
  - Renal medullary carcinoma subtype of RCC
    - Usually presents as infiltrative mass that arises from medulla and is therefore centrally located
    - Presents at younger age (median: 21 years)
    - Associated with sickle cell trait
    - Highly aggressive and often presents with metastatic disease
  - Collecting duct carcinoma subtype of RCC also arises centrally

- **Urothelial Carcinoma**
  - Invasive urothelial carcinoma (UC) arises from urothelial lining of renal pelvis
  - Older patient population (60-70 years) with male predominance
  - Expands from renal pelvis into parenchyma
  - Preserves reniform shape more than RCC
  - Hypoenhancing
  - May show more clear infiltration/involvement of urothelium
  - Can be multifocal (other urothelial lesions in ipsilateral or contralateral ureter or bladder)
  - Renal vein invasion is rare
- **Acute Pyelonephritis**
  - Striated or wedge-shaped areas of decreased enhancement
  - More common in young women; patients usually present with high fever and bacteria in urine
  - May have renal enlargement
  - Can be unilateral or bilateral
  - Clinical diagnosis based on symptoms (pain/fever) and urinalysis
  - Renal or perinephric abscess can develop and can appear mass-like or as complex fluid collections
  - Perinephric fat stranding can be seen
  - Usually resolve or scar down on follow-up after antibiotic treatment

Helpful Clues for Less Common Diagnoses
- **Renal Lymphoma**
  - Most common with non-Hodgkin lymphoma types (B-cell, Burkitt lymphoma)
  - Almost always associated with extrarenal lymphadenopathy (primary renal lymphoma is rare)
  - May be associated with splenomegaly
  - May present as multiple well-circumscribed masses or less commonly as infiltrative
  - Usually bilateral process
  - May extend into pelvis and encase ureters and vessels, but because it is soft tumor, these usually maintain patent
  - May invade adjacent structures/organs
  - Kidney may be enlarged
  - Can lead to renal failure
- **Renal Leukemia**
  - Most common with acute lymphoblastic leukemia
  - Leukemic infiltration of kidney is common but is commonly occult by imaging
  - Usually bilateral process
  - Most commonly manifest as hypoattenuating lesions in enlarged kidney
  - Can be wedge-shaped
  - Kidney may be enlarged
- **Renal Metastasis**
  - When metastasis to kidney is present, it is unlikely to be sole site
  - Most commonly from lung, colorectal, stomach and breast primaries
  - Most are distinct masses but can be infiltrative
  - Infiltrative metastases are usually solid or necrotic and rarely have calcifications

- o May have homogeneous or heterogeneous enhancement
- o Renal vein involvement is uncommon
- **Squamous Cell Carcinoma**
  - o Less common urothelial neoplasm with similar features to UC
  - o Associated with renal calculi
- **Xanthogranulomatous Pyelonephritis**
  - o Chronic inflammatory process in which renal tissue is replaced by lipid-laden macrophages
  - o Caused by chronic urinary obstruction (staghorn calculus)
  - o F > M
  - o Usually diffuse but can be focal
  - o Renal enlargement
  - o Inflammatory tissue can invade into adjacent structures

Helpful Clues for Rare Diagnoses

- **IgG4-Related Kidney Disease**
  - o Immune-mediated systemic disease that can involve most organs
  - o Isolated IgG4-related kidney disease is uncommon; typically associated with pancreatic &/or biliary involvement
  - o Can have discrete masses or be infiltrative
  - o Mild progressive enhancement
  - o Typically T2 hypointense and T1 isointense
  - o May resolve after steroid treatment
- **Renal Sarcoma**
  - o Subtypes include leiomyosarcoma, angiosarcoma, hemangiopericytoma, rhabdomyosarcoma, fibrosarcoma, osteosarcoma
  - o Leiomyosarcoma is most common sarcoma of kidney, but rhabdomyosarcoma and angiosarcoma are more likely to be infiltrative
  - o Usually arise from capsule or renal sinus
  - o Calcifications can be seen with osteosarcoma but are otherwise uncommon in renal sarcomas
- **Renal Plasmacytoma**
  - o Plasmacytomas are solitary tumors that are composed of neoplastic proliferation of plasma cells

- o Extramedullary plasmacytomas are rare
- o Infiltrative mass that extends into perirenal fat
- **Renal Sarcoidosis**
  - o Systemic disorder characterized by noncaseating granulomas
  - o Rarely involves kidneys
  - o Poorly enhances
- **Radiation Therapy**
  - o Decreased enhancement along path of treatment with involved areas of atrophy
  - o Geographic margin and history of radiation treatment to area

SELECTED REFERENCES

1. Sweet DE et al: Infiltrative renal malignancies: imaging features, prognostic implications, and mimics. Radiographics. 41(2):487-508, 2021
2. Ballard DH et al: CT imaging spectrum of infiltrative renal diseases. Abdom Radiol (NY). 42(11):2700-9, 2017

Renal Cell Carcinoma

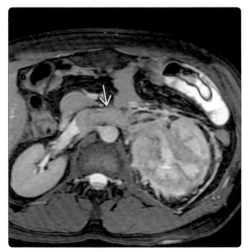

Renal Cell Carcinoma

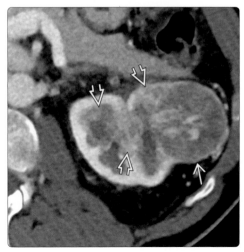

(Left) *Axial T1 C+ FS MR shows an infiltrating renal mass involving the entire left kidney that extends into and expands the left renal vein and inferior vena cava ➡. The presence of tumor thrombus favors renal cell carcinoma, which was the diagnosis in this case.* (Right) *Axial CECT shows mixed well-defined ➡ and infiltrative ➡ components to this mass, which was proven to be clear cell renal cell carcinoma with sarcomatoid features.*

Urothelial Carcinoma

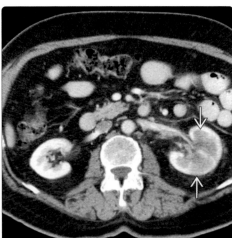

Urothelial Carcinoma

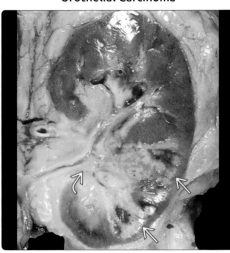

(Left) *Axial CECT shows infiltration and enlargement of the medullary portions of the left kidney* ➡ *by urothelial carcinoma.* **(Right)** *Gross photograph of the resected left kidney in the same patient shows tumor along the surface of the inferior pole of the collecting system* ➡ *with infiltration of the medullary portion of the lower pole* ➡ *and sparing of the cortex.*

Acute Pyelonephritis

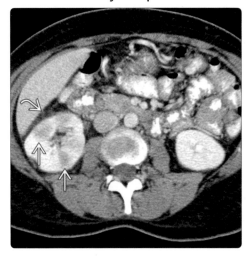

Renal Metastasis

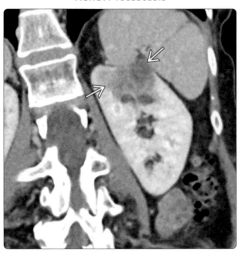

(Left) *Axial CECT shows an enlarged right kidney with striated nephrogram pattern* ➡, *characteristic (but not diagnostic) of acute pyelonephritis. Note perinephric fat infiltration* ➡. **(Right)** *Coronal CECT shows a mass involving the upper pole of the left kidney that is hypoenhancing with ill-defined, infiltrative margins* ➡. *This patient had a history of lung cancer, and this represented metastasis to the kidney.*

Xanthogranulomatous Pyelonephritis

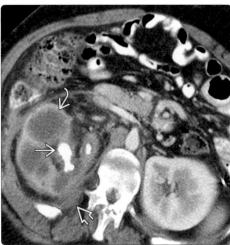

Renal Lymphoma

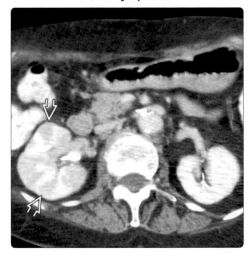

(Left) *Axial CECT shows an enlarged and nonfunctioning right kidney with an obstructing calculus* ➡. *Low-density xanthomatous inflammation* ➡ *replaces the renal parenchyma and spreads to the perirenal space* ➡. **(Right)** *Axial CECT shows an enlarged, heterogeneously enhancing right kidney* ➡ *in an older woman with no urinary tract infection. This case was biopsy-proven lymphoma of the kidney. The imaging features simulate pyelonephritis.*

Renal Lymphoma

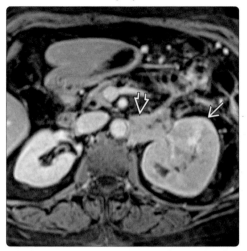

Renal Lymphoma

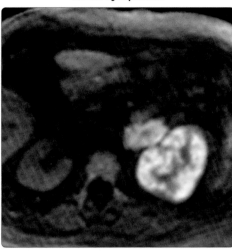

(Left) *Axial T1 C+ FS MR shows an infiltrative, hypoenhancing mass involving the entire left kidney, leading to nephromegaly ➡. Note the periaortic lymphadenopathy ➡.* **(Right)** *Axial DWI MR in the same patient shows the infiltrative left renal mass and lymphadenopathy with restricted diffusion, which is commonly seen in infiltrative renal masses, such as lymphoma.*

Renal Leukemia

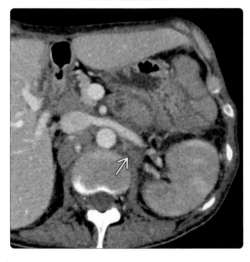

IgG4-Related Kidney Disease

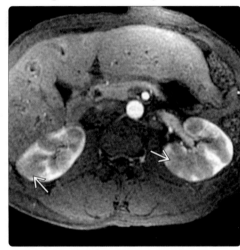

(Left) *Axial CECT shows a diffusely infiltrated left kidney with less enhancement than would normally be expected. Note the additional small retroperitoneal lymph nodes ➡. This was biopsy proven to represent leukemic infiltration.* **(Right)** *Axial T1 C+ FS MR in this patient with primary sclerosing cholangitis shows multiple infiltrating, wedge-shaped, hypoenhancing lesions in the kidneys ➡. This patient had IgG4-related kidney disease, which responded to steroid treatment.*

Renal Sarcoma

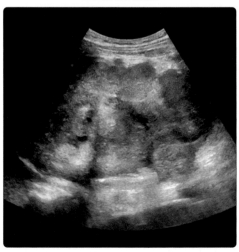

Renal Sarcoma

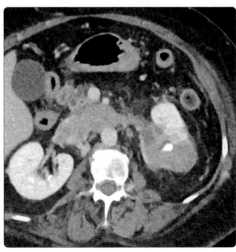

(Left) *Longitudinal US shows an infiltrative, expanded mass that involves the entirety of the right kidney. This was biopsy proven to be undifferentiated pleomorphic sarcoma.* **(Right)** *Axial CECT shows an infiltrative, hypovascular mass that involves the posterior left kidney, extending into the renal vein and inferior vena cava. Although imaging features may suggest renal cell carcinoma, this was proven to be extraosseous Ewing sarcoma.*

DIFFERENTIAL DIAGNOSIS

Common

- Renal Cell Carcinoma
- Angiomyolipoma
- Lymphoma
- Perirenal Abscess
- Perirenal and Subcapsular Hemorrhage

Less Common

- Undifferentiated Pleomorphic Sarcoma
- Liposarcoma
- Leiomyoma
- Hemangioma
- Lymphangioma
- Retroperitoneal Fibrosis
- Accessory Spleen
- Xanthogranulomatous Pyelonephritis
- Urinoma

Rare but Important

- Leiomyosarcoma
- Erdheim-Chester Disease
- Rosai-Dorfman Disease
- Castleman Disease
- Extramedullary Hematopoiesis
- Plasma Cell Neoplasms
- Metastases

ESSENTIAL INFORMATION

Key Differential Diagnosis Issues

- 4 main patterns
  - Solitary perirenal mass: Renal cell carcinoma (RCC) with perirenal spread, undifferentiated pleomorphic sarcoma, lymphoma, Castleman disease, leiomyoma, hemangioma, and lymphangioma
  - Soft tissue rind: Lymphangioma, retroperitoneal fibrosis, extramedullary hematopoiesis, Erdheim-Chester disease, and Rosai-Dorfman disease
  - Macroscopic fat: Angiomyolipoma, liposarcoma, and extramedullary hematopoiesis
  - Multiple perirenal masses: Metastases, lymphoma, and plasma cell neoplasms
- Often unable to confidently differentiate most of these processes without biopsy

Helpful Clues for Common Diagnoses

- **Renal Cell Carcinoma**
  - RCC with perirenal spread is most common perirenal mass
  - Clear cell subtype is most common and may demonstrate hyperenhancement and be heterogeneous when large
  - Papillary and chromophobe subtypes are usually hypoenhancing and homogeneous
- **Angiomyolipoma**
  - Mesenchymal neoplasm composed of smooth muscle, blood vessels, and adipose tissues
  - Most common are lipid-rich angiomyolipomas (AMLs), which contain gross fat on CT and FS MR
  - Usually echogenic on US
  - Classically have ice cream cone shape, in which AML has pyramidal interface with apex within kidney parenchyma and exophytic bulge beyond renal capsule
  - Lipid-poor AMLs may be indistinguishable from other solid renal masses
- **Lymphoma**
  - Lymphomatous involvement can be perirenal
  - Most perirenal lymphoma also have extrarenal involvement
  - Can appear as solitary masses, multiple masses, diffuse infiltrating mass, rind-like soft-tissue thickening, or directly extend from retroperitoneal lymphadenopathy
  - Soft nature of tumor usually surrounds rather than compresses adjacent tissue
- **Perirenal Abscess**
  - Abscesses most commonly arise from ascending infection
  - Can contain gas
  - Can simulate neoplasms
  - Clinical scenario can be important
- **Perirenal and Subcapsular Hemorrhage**
  - Trauma: Blunt, penetrating, or iatrogenic
  - Spontaneous coagulopathic: Hemophilia, anticoagulation
  - Tumor: AML/RCC most common
  - Vasculitis: Polyarteritis nodosa, lupus erythematosus, other small or medium vessel arteritides
  - Ruptured aneurysm or arteriovenous fistula: Aortic or renal artery
  - Density of blood products depends on maturation of hematoma
  - Consider CTA to assess for active extravasation/contained vascular Injury
  - Can cause mass effect on kidney in subcapsular space (Page kidney)

Helpful Clues for Less Common Diagnoses

- **Undifferentiated Pleomorphic Sarcoma**
  - Most common soft tissue sarcoma
  - Previously termed malignant fibrous histiocytoma
  - Large mass with areas of necrosis and hemorrhage
  - Calcification can be present
- **Liposarcoma**
  - Most common retroperitoneal malignancy
  - May involve perinephric space
  - Most commonly containing gross fat with areas of dedifferentiation appearing as soft tissue components
- **Leiomyoma**
  - Benign mesenchymal neoplasm
  - Usually arises from renal capsule and extends into perirenal space
  - Well-circumscribed soft tissue mass
  - Larger lesions may be heterogeneous
- **Hemangioma**
  - Benign mesenchymal neoplasm
  - Most are solitary and small
  - Hyperintense on T2 MR
  - Can demonstrate avid enhancement when small and peripheral nodular enhancement when large
- **Lymphangioma**
  - Benign mesenchymal neoplasms

Perirenal and Subcapsular Mass Lesions

- o May be unilateral or bilateral
- o Typically multilocular cystic lesions in perirenal space
- **Retroperitoneal Fibrosis**
  - o Chronic inflammatory and fibrotic tissue involving retroperitoneum
  - o Soft tissue encasement of aorta and adjacent structures
  - o Can lead to urinary obstruction
  - o Can be idiopathic or part of IgG4-related disease
- **Accessory Spleen**
  - o May "migrate" along splenorenal ligament to result in perirenal mass
  - o Similar density and enhancement pattern as spleen
  - o Tc sulfur colloid scan is definitive test
- **Xanthogranulomatous Pyelonephritis**
  - o Usually infiltrates and replaces kidney and perirenal space with heterogeneous, low-density mass
    - — Low density is due to lipid-laden macrophages
    - — Attenuation is usually lower than water but higher than "pure" fat
  - o Almost always associated with large calculus obstructing renal pelvis or infundibulum
    - — Affected portion (or entire) kidney is usually nonfunctional
- **Urinoma**
  - o Due to obstruction of ureter and rupture of renal fornix
  - o Urine collects within perirenal space, usually caudal to kidney
  - o Density of "mass" depends on use of contrast media
    - — On NECT, will be near water density
    - — On CECT, pyelographic phase, should see densely opacified urine within perirenal space

Helpful Clues for Rare Diagnoses

- **Leiomyosarcoma**
  - o Aggressive mesenchymal tumor
  - o Arises from smooth muscle cells usually of inferior vena cava, renal vein, or intrarenal blood vessels
  - o Rarely can originate from capsule
  - o Tend to be heterogeneous, large tumors with necrosis/hemorrhage at presentation

- o Calcification is rare
- **Erdheim-Chester Disease**
  - o Deposition of lipid-laden histiocytes in various organs, including perirenal space
  - o Perirenal soft tissue masses, usually symmetric
  - o Lung involvement: Cystic disease and septal thickening
  - o Skeletal involvement: Metaphyseal and diaphyseal sclerosis
  - o Neurological: Dural accumulations, hypothalamic involvement, and retrobulbar masses
- **Rosai-Dorfman Disease**
  - o Histiocytosis that develops in lymph nodes, skin, and bones
  - o < 5% will have perirenal involvement
  - o Perirenal soft tissue masses, usually symmetric
  - o Most commonly associated with cervical lymphadenopathy
- **Castleman Disease**
  - o Lymphoproliferative condition
  - o Can be hyperdense on NECT
  - o Usually hypoenhancing
  - o Can appear mass-like, infiltrating, or rind-like
  - o Unicentric: Typically well-defined, homogeneous mass with soft tissue attenuation
  - o Multicentric: Splenomegaly, diffuse lymphadenopathy, and ascites
- **Extramedullary Hematopoiesis**
  - o Associated with chronic anemia, leukemia, and extensive bone tumor
  - o May infiltrate kidney and perirenal space
  - o May also see other sites
    - — Spleen, paraspinal masses, etc.
- **Plasma Cell Neoplasms**
  - o Multiple myeloma or plasmacytoma may involve perirenal space

Renal Cell Carcinoma

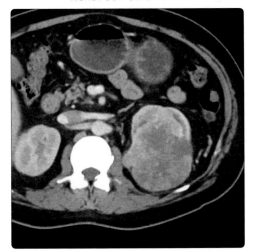

Renal Cell Carcinoma

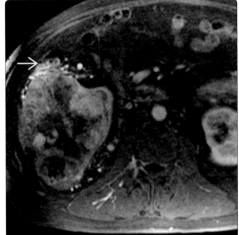

(Left) *Axial CECT shows a heterogeneous renal mass involving the posterior perirenal space. This was proven to be renal cell carcinoma.* **(Right)** *Axial T1 C+ FS MR shows a large, infiltrative, heterogeneous mass involving the right kidney that extends from the right perirenal space into the anterior right pararenal space, invading the ascending colon* ⮕.

Angiomyolipoma

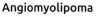

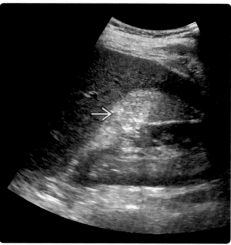

Lymphoma

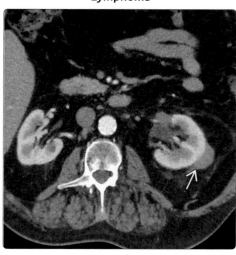

(Left) *Horizontal, long-axis US shows a large, echogenic mass that arises from the posterior aspect of the right kidney* ➡. *This was confirmed on CT to represent angiomyolipoma.* (Right) *Axial CECT shows a left perirenal mass with soft tissue attenuation* ➡. *No additional masses were seen in the abdomen or pelvis. This was biopsied and found to be primary perirenal lymphoma.*

Lymphoma

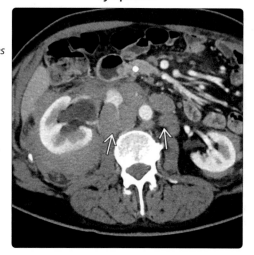

Lymphoma

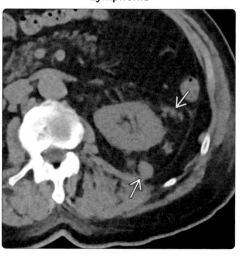

(Left) *Axial CECT shows a large soft tissue mass that involves the perirenal space. Multiple enlarged lymph nodes are also seen in the retroperitoneum* ➡. *Biopsy revealed lymphoma.* (Right) *Axial NECT shows multiple soft tissue attenuation and rounded lesions in the perirenal space* ➡. *This was biopsy-proven lymphomatous involvement.*

Perirenal Abscess

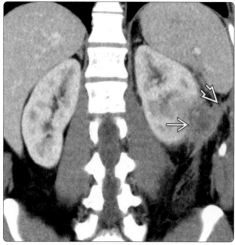

Liposarcoma

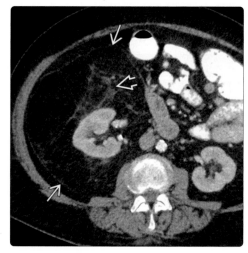

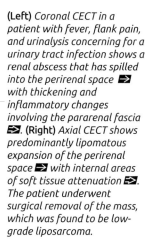

(Left) *Coronal CECT in a patient with fever, flank pain, and urinalysis concerning for a urinary tract infection shows a renal abscess that has spilled into the perirenal space* ➡ *with thickening and inflammatory changes involving the pararenal fascia* ➡. (Right) *Axial CECT shows predominantly lipomatous expansion of the perirenal space* ➡ *with internal areas of soft tissue attenuation* ➡. *The patient underwent surgical removal of the mass, which was found to be low-grade liposarcoma.*

Liposarcoma

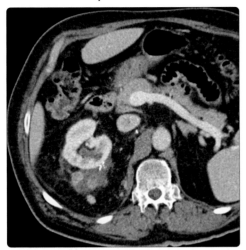

Leiomyoma

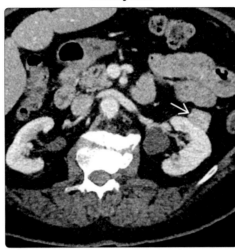

(Left) *Axial CECT shows a right perirenal mass with heterogeneous contents that have both enhancing soft tissue components and lipomatous components. This was surgically excised and found to be liposarcoma.* (Right) *Axial CECT shows a smooth mass involving the left capsular region with low-level, homogeneous enhancement* ➡. *On NECT (not shown), this mass was slightly hyperdense to the adjacent renal parenchyma. This was resected and found to be leiomyoma.*

Hemangioma

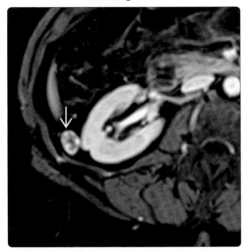

Lymphangioma

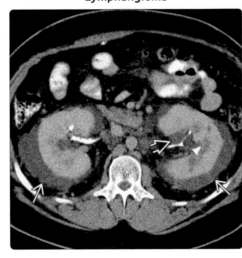

(Left) *Axial T1 C+ FS MR shows a right perirenal mass with nodular peripheral enhancement* ➡. *This lesion was T2 hyperintense and on delayed images filled in with contrast. Imaging features were diagnostic for hemangioma.* (Right) *Axial CECT shows bilateral, multilocular, cystic lesions in the perinephric spaces* ➡. *These were associated with peripelvic cysts* ➡, *and these are lymphatic in origin and usually of no clinical significance.*

Retroperitoneal Fibrosis

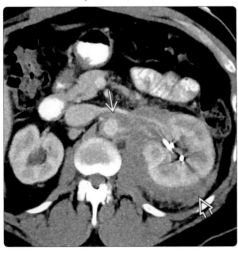

Rosai-Dorfman Disease

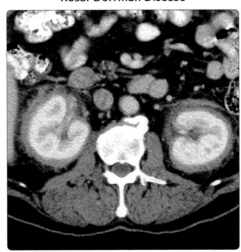

(Left) *Axial CECT shows a soft tissue mass that encases the aorta* ➡ *and left perirenal space* ➡. *A left ureteral stent was placed to treat resultant hydronephrosis from the retroperitoneal fibrosis.* (Right) *Axial CECT shows bilateral, peripelvic soft tissue rinds that encase both kidneys. This patient also had cervical lymphadenopathy, and biopsy was consistent with Rosai-Dorfman disease.*

DIFFERENTIAL DIAGNOSIS

Common
- Renal Angiomyolipoma
- Fat in Renal Scar
- Junctional Parenchymal Defect

Less Common
- Renal Cell Carcinoma
- Renal Replacement Lipomatosis

Rare but Important
- Lipoma
- Liposarcoma
- Epithelioid Angiomyolipoma
- Lipomatous Solitary Fibrous Tumor
- Oncocytoma

ESSENTIAL INFORMATION

Key Differential Diagnosis Issues
- CT fat density or loss of signal on FS MR sequences demonstrates gross fat
- Dropout of signal on opposed-phase imaging demonstrates subvoxel fat
- Echogenic lesion on US may be suggestive but is not definitive for fat
- Gross fat in renal mass most suggestive of benign angiomyolipoma
- Features that may suggest malignancy
  - Intratumoral calcifications
  - Invasion of perirenal or sinus fat
  - Large, necrotic mass with foci of fat
  - Nodal or venous invasion

Helpful Clues for Common Diagnoses
- **Renal Angiomyolipoma**
  - Most common benign mesenchymal renal tumor
    - Majority incidentally found
    - 90% single and unilateral
    - Multiple and bilaterality associated with tuberous sclerosis
  - Composed of fat, smooth muscle, and abnormal blood vessels
  - Typically homogeneous without calcifications
  - Can be diagnosed based on its gross fat content [lipid-rich vs. lipid-poor angiomyolipoma (AML)]
    - Lipid-poor AML may be difficult to distinguish from renal cell carcinoma (RCC)
  - AMLs may have angular interface between mass and parenchyma (ice cream cone shape)
  - Rarely invades renal vein but does not imply malignancy
  - Large AMLs may hemorrhage (> 4 cm)
  - US
    - Well-defined, hyperechoic mass, typically isoechoic to renal sinus fat
    - Up to 30% of small RCCs may appear hyperechoic
    - Hyperechoic lesion on US may need further evaluation by CT or MR
  - CT
    - Solid mass with macroscopic fat (< -20 HU)
    - Lipid-poor AMLs may be hyperdense on NECT and have more background enhancement than renal parenchyma
  - MR
    - Loss of signal on FS sequences as well as India ink artifact on chemical shift imaging is virtually diagnostic of AML
    - Lipid-poor AML may be T2 hypointense (similar to papillary RCC)
- **Fat in Renal Scar**
  - Defect in renal cortex after nephrectomy or infarction
  - Appearance may appear identical to AML
  - Look for prior history of surgery or atherosclerotic disease
- **Junctional Parenchymal Defect**
  - Normal variant of no clinical significance
  - Infolding of capsule and perinephric fat or outward bulging of renal sinus fat
  - Similar fat density or echogenicity as renal sinus
  - May be triangular in shape
  - At junction of upper and middle 1/3 of kidney

Helpful Clues for Less Common Diagnoses
- **Renal Cell Carcinoma**
  - Presence of fat in RCC is uncommon; it may be caused by
    - Large tumor invading renal sinus or perinephric fat
    - Lipid-producing tumoral necrosis
    - Bone metaplasia
  - Most common with clear-cell subtype
  - Small foci of fat within predominantly soft tissue mass
  - Fat-containing RCCs usually contain calcifications
  - Seen as microscopic fat on chemical shift imaging
  - Increased signal on T2 MR (although papillary RCC has decreased signal)
  - Other signs of RCC
    - Invasion of renal vein
    - Lymphadenopathy
    - Metastatic disease
- **Renal Replacement Lipomatosis**
  - Deposition of fat and inflammatory tissue in renal hilum and perirenal space
  - Can be associated with atrophy of renal parenchyma
  - Usually in response to chronic inflammation or atrophy

Helpful Clues for Rare Diagnoses
- **Lipoma**
  - Extremely rare
  - Typically arise from renal capsule
  - Well-circumscribed; composed almost entirely of macroscopic fat
- **Liposarcoma**
  - Renal liposarcomas are rare (arise from renal sinus or capsule)
  - Retroperitoneal liposarcomas (nonrenal origin) can involve kidneys
  - Imaging features vary depending on grade of tumor
    - Well-differentiated liposarcoma: Well-defined, predominantly fat-containing lesion (similar to lipoma)
    - Poorly differentiated liposarcoma: More soft tissue density components
- **Epithelioid Angiomyolipoma**

- o Rare variant of AML
- o Considered perivascular epithelial cell tumors (PEComas)
- o Can appear aggressive with metastatic involvement
  - – Can contain small foci of gross fat
  - – Typically exophytic
  - – Rarely contain calcification
  - – Can hemorrhage
- **Lipomatous Solitary Fibrous Tumor**
  - o Fat-containing variant of solitary fibrous tumor
  - o May arise from renal capsule
- **Oncocytoma**
  - o Benign renal tumor composed of eosinophilic epithelial cells arising from collecting ducts
  - o Solid renal cortical mass lesion ± central stellate scar
  - o Dynamic postcontrast imaging is highly variable and depends on degree of cellularity and stroma
  - o Rarely contains fat

SELECTED REFERENCES

1. Schieda N et al: Renal and adrenal masses containing fat at MRI: proposed nomenclature by the society of abdominal radiology disease-focused panel on renal cell carcinoma. J Magn Reson Imaging. 49(4):917-26, 2019
2. Shaaban AM et al: Fat-containing retroperitoneal lesions: imaging characteristics, localization, and differential diagnosis. Radiographics. 36(3):710-34, 2016
3. Wasser EJ et al: Renal cell carcinoma containing abundant non-calcified fat. Abdom Imaging. 38(3):598-602, 2013

Renal Angiomyolipoma

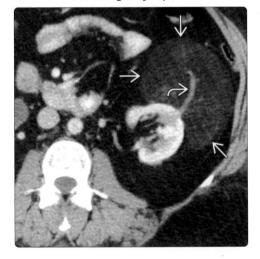

Renal Angiomyolipoma

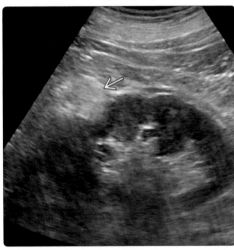

(Left) *Axial CECT shows a large, heterogeneous, fat density mass* ➡ *arising from the kidney. The prominent vascularity* ➡ *helps to identify this as an angiomyolipoma (AML) rather than a retroperitoneal liposarcoma.* **(Right)** *Longitudinal US shows an echogenic mass involving the superior pole of the kidney* ➡ *that has similar echogenicity with the surrounding perinephric fat. Given its size, this was further evaluated by CT and was diagnosed as an AML.*

Renal Angiomyolipoma

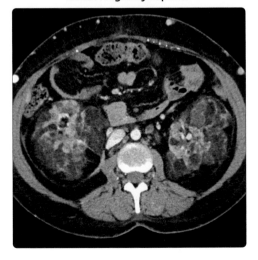

Renal Angiomyolipoma

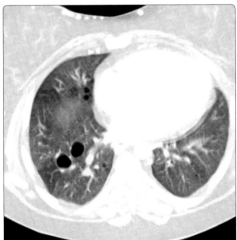

(Left) *Axial CECT shows the kidneys are largely replaced by multiple fat-containing masses. Given the multiplicity of AMLs, a diagnosis of tuberous sclerosis complex was considered.* **(Right)** *Axial CECT in the same patient shows numerous cystic spaces at the lung bases, consistent with lymphangioleiomyomatosis in a patient with tuberous sclerosis complex.*

Fat-Containing Renal Mass

Fat in Renal Scar

Fat in Renal Scar

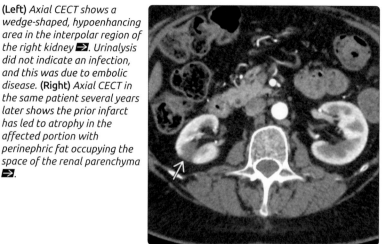

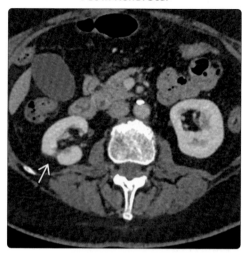

(Left) *Axial CECT shows a wedge-shaped, hypoenhancing area in the interpolar region of the right kidney* ➡. *Urinalysis did not indicate an infection, and this was due to embolic disease.* (Right) *Axial CECT in the same patient several years later shows the prior infarct has led to atrophy in the affected portion with perinephric fat occupying the space of the renal parenchyma* ➡.

Renal Cell Carcinoma

Renal Cell Carcinoma

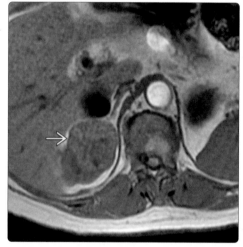

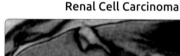

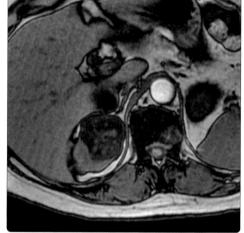

(Left) *Axial in-phase GRE MR shows a well-circumscribed mass* ➡ *involving the superior pole of the right kidney.* (Right) *Axial opposed-phase GRE MR in the same patient shows loss of signal in this renal mass diagnostic of subvoxel fat. No gross fat was identified. This was resected and found to be clear cell renal cell carcinoma.*

Renal Cell Carcinoma

Renal Cell Carcinoma

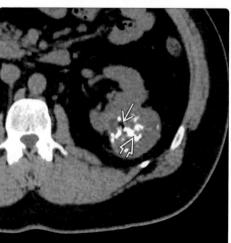

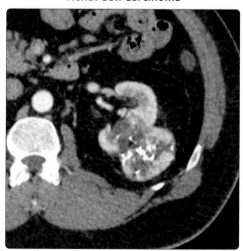

(Left) *Axial NECT shows an exophytic, well-circumscribed left renal mass with a small focus of gross fat* ➡ *with areas of stippled calcifications* ➡. *Given the presence of calcifications as well as the very small quantity of gross fat, AML could not be diagnosed.* (Right) *Axial CECT in the same patient shows an avidly enhancing lesion. This was surgically removed and found to be clear cell renal cell carcinoma.*

Renal Replacement Lipomatosis

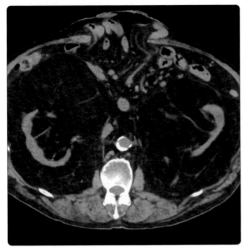

Liposarcoma

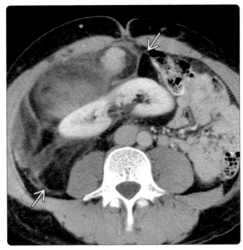

(Left) *Axial NECT shows an exuberant deposition of fat at the renal hilum and perirenal space. The native kidneys are atrophic.* (Right) *Axial CECT shows displacement and deformation of the kidney by a mass ⇥ that has mixed fat and soft tissue density. The absence of a claw sign helps to identify this as primary retroperitoneal liposarcoma rather than an AML.*

Epithelioid Angiomyolipoma

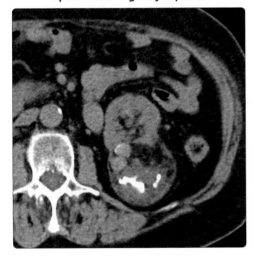

Lipomatous Solitary Fibrous Tumor

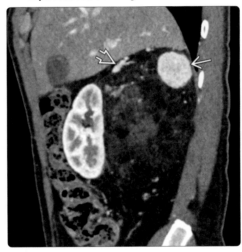

(Left) *Axial NECT shows an exophytic mass involving the left kidney with areas of gross fat, coarse calcifications, and soft tissue components. This was surgically removed and found to be epithelioid AML.* (Right) *Sagittal CECT shows a rounded, predominately fat-containing soft tissue mass ⇥ that displaces the kidney anteriorly. Large vessels ⇥ are noted. This was surgically removed and found to be lipomatous solitary fibrous tumor.*

Oncocytoma

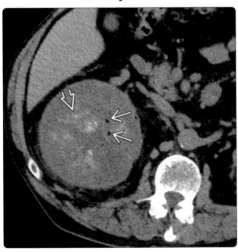

Oncocytoma

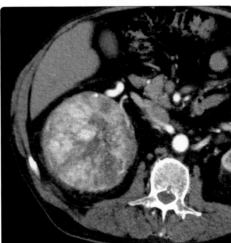

(Left) *Axial NECT shows a large, rounded renal right mass with 2 small foci of macroscopic fat ⇥ with areas of stippled calcifications ⇥. Given the small foci of fat as well as the presence of calcifications, AML could not be diagnosed.* (Right) *Axial CECT in the same patient shows a heterogeneous renal mass that was surgically removed and found to be oncocytoma.*

DIFFERENTIAL DIAGNOSIS

Common

- Urolithiasis
- Renal Sinus Cysts
- Pyelitis

Less Common

- Vascular Lesions
- Urothelial Carcinoma
- Renal Cell Carcinoma
- Renal Replacement Lipomatosis
- Xanthogranulomatous Pyelonephritis
- Lymphoma
- Angiomyolipoma
- Nerve Sheath Tumor

Rare but Important

- Neuroendocrine Tumor
- Leiomyoma
- Hemangioma
- Retroperitoneal Fibrosis
- Mixed Epithelial and Stromal Tumor Family
- Erdheim-Chester Disease
- Rosai-Dorfman Disease
- Castleman Disease
- Sarcoma

ESSENTIAL INFORMATION

Key Differential Diagnosis Issues

- Renal sinus is extension of perirenal space
- Contains multiple structures, any of which can give rise to mass lesion
  - Pelvocalyceal system (e.g., urothelial carcinoma, blood clot, fungus ball, stone)
  - Vessels [e.g., renal artery aneurysm, arteriovenous malformation (AVM), varices]
  - Lymphatics (e.g., lymphoma, lymph node metastases)
  - Nerves (e.g., neurogenic tumor)

Helpful Clues for Common Diagnoses

- **Urolithiasis**
  - Crystallization of mineral and salt deposits in urine
  - Usually located in calyces or pelvis but may migrate to ureter or bladder
  - CT
    - Calculi are uniformly dense, except matrix and indinavir stones (rare)
    - Dense (several-hundred HU) foci in calyces, renal pelvis, ureter, or bladder
    - Perinephric stranding and hydroureteronephrosis if obstructing
  - US
    - Round or ovoid, echogenic foci
    - Clean posterior acoustic shadowing
    - Twinkle artifact on color Doppler
- **Renal Sinus Cysts**
  - Peripelvic
    - Asymptomatic, benign cysts located in renal sinus that originate from lymphatics

- Often bilateral and multiple
- Usually multiple and bilateral
- Can be confused with hydronephrosis
  - Peripelvic cysts do not connect with one another
  - Urographic-phase CT or MR will show separate collecting system peripelvic cysts
  - Parapelvic
    - Renal cyst protruding into renal sinus fat
    - Usually solitary, unilateral, and spherical
    - Often found with other simple cortical cysts
- **Pyelitis**
  - Thickening of renal collecting system
  - Can be inflammatory or infectious in origin
  - Emphysematous pyelitis: Gas within collecting system caused by gas-forming bacteria

Helpful Clues for Less Common Diagnoses

- **Vascular Lesions**
  - Renal artery aneurysm/pseudoaneurysm, AVM, arteriovenous fistula (AVF), renal varices
    - Aneurysm: Look for calcification in arterial wall
    - Pseudoaneurysm and dissection usually occur in setting of trauma
      - May be seen with vasculitides, spontaneous arterial mediolysis, and infection
    - AVM/AVF
      - Look for turbulent flow on color Doppler US, premature filling of renal vein on CECT and angiography
      - AVF is usually sequela of trauma or iatrogenic injury (biopsy); AVMs are congenital/developmental abnormalities
    - Renal varices: Usually seen in setting of venous hypertension
- **Urothelial Carcinoma**
  - Irregular filling defect in renal pelvis/calyx ± infiltration of renal parenchyma
  - Often isodense to slightly hyperdense on NECT
  - Variable enhancement pattern depending on grade and growth pattern
  - Higher incidence in patients with history of urothelial cancer of bladder or ureter
- **Renal Cell Carcinoma**
  - Arises in cortex but may extend into renal sinus
  - Clear cell renal cell carcinoma is more vascular and exophytic than urothelial cancer
  - More likely to invade renal vein and inferior vena cava
- **Renal Replacement Lipomatosis**
  - Deposition of fat and inflammatory tissue in renal hilum and perirenal space
  - Can be associated with atrophy of renal parenchyma
  - Usually in response to chronic inflammation or atrophy
- **Xanthogranulomatous Pyelonephritis**
  - Low-density, fluid-filled areas in affected parenchyma (lipid-laden macrophages)
  - Kidney, or affected portion, is usually enlarged, nonfunctional, and obstructed by large staghorn calculus
  - Inflammatory tissue can invade adjacent structures
- **Lymphoma**

- o Infiltration of renal sinus ± renal parenchyma with preservation of renal shape
- o Homogeneous with mild enhancement
- o Displaces rather than compressing or invading adjacent structures (vessels, collecting system)
- o Usually occurs in presence of lymphadenopathy elsewhere
- **Angiomyolipoma**
  - o Composed mainly of fat that may blend with renal sinus fat or may mimic lipomatosis
- **Nerve Sheath Tumor**
  - o Well-circumscribed but heterogeneous masses
  - o Hyperintense on T2 MR
  - o Usually avid enhancement

Helpful Clues for Rare Diagnoses

- **Neuroendocrine Tumor**
  - o Well-circumscribed soft tissue mass
  - o Usually hypoenhancing relative to renal parenchyma
  - o Calcifications are common
- **Leiomyoma**
  - o Benign mesenchymal neoplasm
  - o Well-circumscribed soft tissue mass
  - o Larger leiomyomas may be heterogeneous
- **Hemangioma**
  - o Benign mesenchymal neoplasm
  - o Most are solitary and small
  - o Hyperintense on T2 MR
  - o Can demonstrate avid enhancement when small and peripheral nodular enhancement when large
- **Retroperitoneal Fibrosis**
  - o Chronic inflammatory and fibrotic tissue involving retroperitoneum
  - o Soft tissue encasement of aorta and adjacent structures
  - o Can lead to urinary obstruction
  - o Can be idiopathic or part of IgG4-related disease
- **Mixed Epithelial and Stromal Tumor Family**
  - o Includes adult cystic nephroma and mixed epithelial and stromal tumor

- o Solitary, unilateral, well-circumscribed, fluid-filled mass with septations
- o May herniate into renal pelvis, leading to obstruction of collecting system
- **Erdheim-Chester Disease**
  - o Deposition of lipid-laden histiocytes in various organs, including perirenal space
  - o Perirenal soft tissue masses, usually symmetric
  - o Lung involvement: Cystic disease and septal thickening
  - o Skeletal involvement: Metaphyseal and diaphyseal sclerosis
  - o Neurological: Dural accumulations, hypothalamic involvement, and retrobulbar masses
- **Rosai-Dorfman Disease**
  - o Histiocytosis that develops in lymph nodes, skin, and bones
  - o Perirenal &/or hilar soft tissue masses, usually symmetric
  - o Most commonly associated with cervical lymphadenopathy
- **Castleman Disease**
  - o Lymphoproliferative condition
  - o Can be hyperdense on NECT
  - o Usually hypoenhancing
  - o Can appear mass-like, infiltrating, or rind-like
  - o Unicentric: Typically well-defined, homogeneous mass with soft tissue attenuation
  - o Multicentric: Splenomegaly, diffuse lymphadenopathy, ascites
- **Sarcoma**
  - o Primary renal sarcoma: Rare; patients often develop metastasis before initial presentation
  - o Usually large (> 10 cm) when discovered
  - o Imaging findings are variable depending on subtype

Urolithiasis

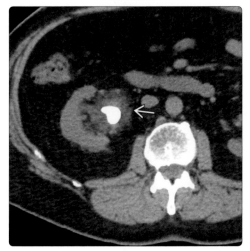

Renal Sinus Cysts

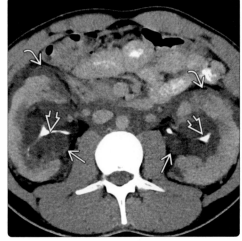

(Left) *Axial NECT shows a large right hilar renal calculus causing surrounding inflammatory changes from intermittent obstruction and urothelial irritation* ➡. *Urinalysis did not show the presence of an infection.* **(Right)** *Axial urographic-phase CT shows multiple cystic structures within the renal pelves* ➡. *Contrast within the urinary system outlines the calyces and renal pelvis* ➡. *Peripelvic cysts are lymphatic malformations and can be seen with perirenal lymphangiomatosis* ➡.

Pyelitis

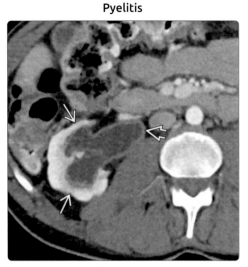

Vascular Lesions

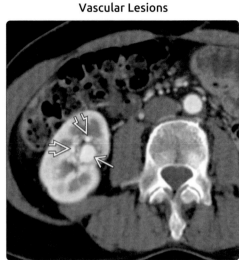

(Left) *Axial CECT in a patient with a neurogenic bladder shows areas of cortical thinning ➡ from repeated episodes of pyelonephritis as well as urothelial thickening involving the renal pelvis, consistent with pyelitis ➡, and confirmed on urinalysis.* **(Right)** *Axial CECT in a patient with hematuria shows a rounded hilar mass ➡ that has the same enhancement as the aorta. Multiple surrounding vessels are seen ➡, and early enhancement was seen within the renal vein (not shown).*

Vascular Lesions

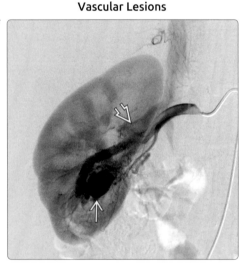

Urothelial Carcinoma

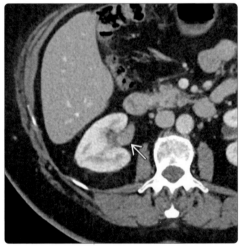

(Left) *Selective angiography of the right renal artery in the same patient shows the aneurysmal portion of the distal renal artery ➡ with numerous collateral vessels and an early draining vein ➡, as is seen with arteriovenous malformations.* **(Right)** *Axial CECT shows a hilar soft tissue density mass ➡ in a patient with hematuria.*

Urothelial Carcinoma

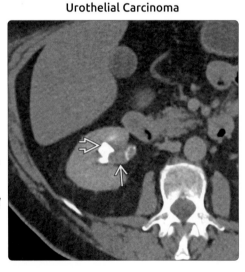

Renal Cell Carcinoma

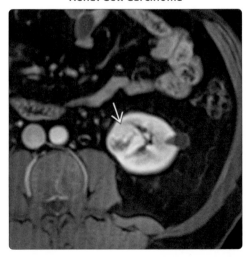

(Left) *Axial urographic-phase CT in the same patient shows the intraluminal location of this lesion ➡ with some mild associated hydronephrosis ➡. This was found to be a urothelial carcinoma.* **(Right)** *Axial CEMR shows a rounded hilar mass ➡ with similar enhancement to background renal cortex. This mass originated from the cortex but expanded into the hilum. It was surgically removed and found to be clear cell renal cell carcinoma.*

Lymphoma

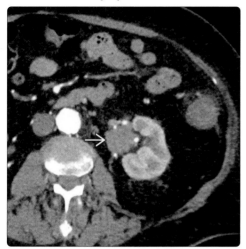

Angiomyolipoma

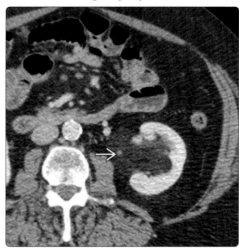

(Left) *Axial CECT shows a soft tissue mass in the hilum of the left kidney* ➡️ *with splaying of the renal arteries. This was biopsied and found to be a hilar lymphoma.* (Right) *Axial CECT shows a subtle, fat density lesion within the hilum of the left kidney with intratumoral vessels* ➡️. *This was surgically removed given its size and found to be an angiomyolipoma.*

Nerve Sheath Tumor

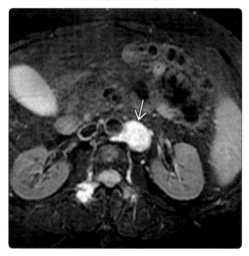

Rosai-Dorfman Disease

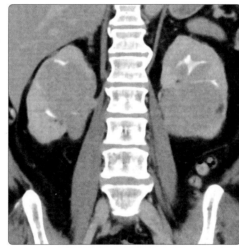

(Left) *Axial T2 MR shows an avidly hyperintense lesion near the left renal hilum* ➡️. *This was found to be a schwannoma.* (Right) *Coronal CECT shows soft tissue masses replacing the normal fat of the renal sinuses. These do not cause significant hydronephrosis. The patient also had cervical lymphadenopathy, and biopsy revealed Rosai-Dorfman disease.*

Sarcoma

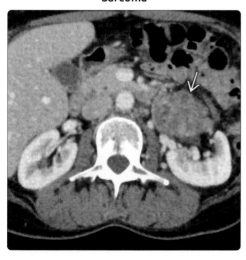

Vascular Lesions

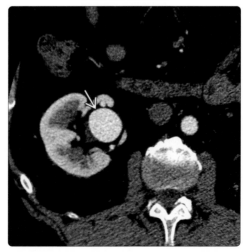

(Left) *Axial CECT shows a heterogeneous, rounded mass in the left renal hilum* ➡️. *This was biopsied and found to be a leiomyosarcoma.* (Right) *Axial CECT shows a rounded structure within the right renal hilum with enhancement similar to the aorta.* ➡️. *This showed a connection with a branch of the main renal artery and was found to be an aneurysm. These can sometimes have peripheral calcifications.*

DIFFERENTIAL DIAGNOSIS

Common

- Renal Abscess
- Emphysematous Pyelitis
- Instrumentation/Postoperative

Less Common

- Emphysematous Pyelonephritis
- Renal Infarction
- Pyonephrosis
- Xanthogranulomatous Pyelonephritis
- Extrarenal Sources

ESSENTIAL INFORMATION

Helpful Clues for Common Diagnoses

- **Renal Abscess**
  - Gas within usually spherical collection of pus
  - CECT: Thick-walled and rim-enhancing low-attenuation collection within kidney ± extension into perirenal space
  - Treatment: Usually antibiotics and percutaneous catheter drainage
- **Emphysematous Pyelitis**
  - Risk factors: Diabetes (50% of cases)
  - Gas from infection of urine; limited to renal excretory system
    - No gas in renal parenchyma
  - Prognosis/treatment: Better prognosis than emphysematous pyelonephritis; usually managed with antibiotics
- **Instrumentation/Postoperative**
  - Ureteral stent, nephrostomy, cystoscopy can introduce air into collecting system
  - Presence of gas in setting of recent renal surgery or ablation can be normal
  - Gas should resolve over time

Helpful Clues for Less Common Diagnoses

- **Emphysematous Pyelonephritis**
  - Risk factors: Diabetes (90% of cases); urinary tract obstruction
  - Necrotizing, gas-forming renal infection
  - CT: Gas in renal parenchyma
    - ± extension of gas into perirenal and pararenal space
    - ± renal or perirenal abscess
    - Presence of renal abscess has better prognosis as it implies immunologic response
  - Ultrasound: Echogenic foci in nondependent portion of renal parenchyma associated with "dirty" shadowing
  - Prognosis/treatment: Life-threatening infection that may require nephrectomy
- **Renal Infarction**
  - Sudden death of renal tissue from arterial occlusion or avulsion can release intracellular gas from infarcted tissue
    - Examples: Traumatic renal artery occlusion; renal artery embolization; radiofrequency or cryoablation
  - Does not imply infection, but clinical symptoms may be similar
- **Pyonephrosis**
  - Infected, obstructed, and dilated renal collecting system
  - Dilated renal collecting system
    - Urine attenuation may be higher than water due to presence of debris/pus
    - ± gas
- **Xanthogranulomatous Pyelonephritis**
  - Form of chronic pyelonephritis with replacement of renal parenchyma with lipid-laden macrophages
  - Usually found in setting of urinary obstruction from calculi
  - Inflammatory tissue can invade adjacent structures
- **Extrarenal Sources**
  - Retroperitoneal gas from duodenum or pancreas can extend to para- and perirenal space, preferably on right
  - Fistulation with bowel due to traumatic or iatrogenic causes
  - Pancreas: Infected necrotizing pancreatic or peripancreatic collections
  - Barotrauma

Renal Abscess

Renal Abscess

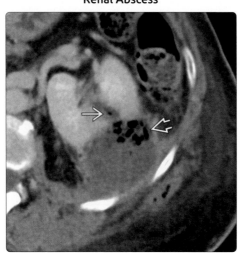

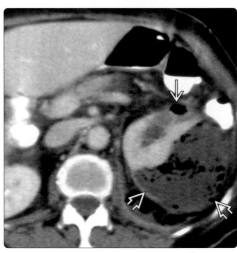

(Left) Axial CECT shows a small focus of gas and fluid within the kidney ➡ that extends into a large perirenal collection, which contains multiple foci of gas ➡. This patient had symptoms of infection and underwent a percutaneous drain of the abscess. (Right) Axial CECT shows gas ➡ and fluid within the kidney and a large perirenal fluid and gas collection ➡, compatible with abscess.

Emphysematous Pyelitis

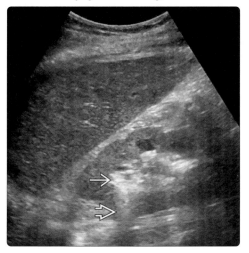

Emphysematous Pyelitis

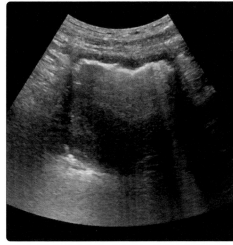

(Left) *Longitudinal US shows foci of gas within the collecting system of the right kidney, as demonstrated by echogenic foci* ➡ *with "dirty" shadowing* ➡. **(Right)** *Transverse US in the same patient shows air within the wall of the bladder, consistent with emphysematous cystitis.*

Emphysematous Pyelitis

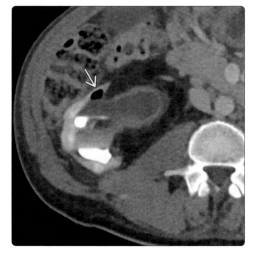

Instrumentation/Postoperative

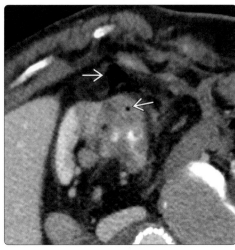

(Left) *Axial CECT shows gas within the collecting system of the right kidney* ➡. *There is urothelial thickening involving the collecting system. This patient had emphysematous pyelitis that was treated successfully with antibiotics.* **(Right)** *Axial CECT shows a renal mass, immediately post ablation, with foci of gas* ➡, *which was an expected finding. The foci of gas resolved on follow-up imaging.*

Emphysematous Pyelonephritis

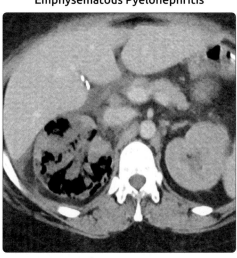

Xanthogranulomatous Pyelonephritis

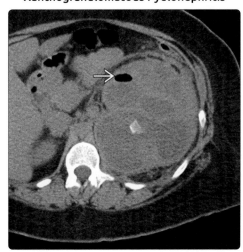

(Left) *Axial CECT shows abundant intraparenchymal gas. The patient underwent an emergent right nephrectomy and received antibiotics for Escherichia coli infection.* **(Right)** *Axial NECT shows an enlarged left kidney with surrounding perinephric stranding, a centrally obstructing renal calculus, and multiple low-attenuation, dilated calyces. This patient with xanthogranulomatous pyelonephritis developed air within one of the dilated calyces* ➡.

Delayed or Persistent Nephrogram

DIFFERENTIAL DIAGNOSIS

Common
- Urinary Obstruction
- Acute Tubular Injury
- Pyelonephritis
- Subcapsular Collection

Less Common
- Contrast-Induced Nephropathy
- Renal Vein Stenosis/Thrombosis
- Renal Artery Stenosis
- Leukemia

Rare but Important
- Infiltrative Renal Mass
- Rhabdomyolysis
- Multiple Myeloma

ESSENTIAL INFORMATION

Key Differential Diagnosis Issues
- Definition: Nephrogram that persists for > 30 min or becomes more dense after 5 min following IV or intraarterial contrast administration
- Some of these diagnoses are rarely seen since there may be increased caution of contrast use in patients with acute renal failure
- Pathophysiology: Impaired renal perfusion and impaired urine excretion and tubular transit
  - Slow inflow
    - Renal arterial stenosis (RAS), hypotension, decreased tissue compliance, hydronephrosis, pyelonephritis, acute tubular injury
  - Slow outflow
    - Renal vein thrombosis, renal vein obstruction
  - Slow urinary excretion/clearance
    - Urinary obstruction, nephron dysfunction
- Causes of unilateral delayed nephrogram
  - Renal artery/vein compromise (RAS, renal vein thrombosis), pyelonephritis, urinary obstruction, infiltrative renal mass
- Causes of segmental delayed nephrogram
  - Pyelonephritis, calyceal obstruction (stone, tumor, clot), focal injury to renal vessels, and parenchyma (contusion)

Helpful Clues for Common Diagnoses
- **Urinary Obstruction**
  - Obstructing calculus
    - Usually ureteral
      - Ureterovesical or ureteropelvic junction or at crossing of iliac vessels
    - Stone is almost always evident on CT as hyperdense focus ± dilated ureter
    - Pelvocaliectasis ± perirenal stranding
  - Obstructing tumor
    - Urothelial carcinoma
      - May obstruct renal pelvis &/or ureter
      - Dilated collecting system upstream
      - Soft tissue density mass in wall and lumen of collecting system

- More common in older patients and those with history of bladder cancer (metachronous/synchronous lesion)
  - Retroperitoneal metastases
    - Enlarged metastatic retroperitoneal lymph nodes may displace and obstruct ureters
    - Bulky retroperitoneal nodal metastases are more common with GU/GYN malignancies
    - Metastases may be to ureteral wall itself
  - Pelvic malignancies
    - May encase and obstruct intrapelvic ureters (e.g., rectal or uterine/cervical carcinoma)
  - Retroperitoneal lymphoma
    - Soft and bulky tumor; usually displaces ureters but may obstruct renal pelvis or ureter
  - Obstructing clot
    - Blood clot may obstruct renal pelvis or ureter
    - Usually occurs following trauma or biopsy; also seen with tumors
  - Renal papillary necrosis
    - Sloughed papilla may obstruct ureteropelvic junction or ureter
    - Characteristic deformities of calyces on urography
  - Ureteral stricture
    - Iatrogenic stricture is most common etiology
      - Lithotomy, ureteroscopy, ureteral catheterization, or radiation therapy
      - Also can be seen as complication of surgery to adjacent organs
    - May follow infection or inflammation of ureter itself
      - Rarely seen as sequela of adjacent inflammatory conditions (e.g., Crohn disease, diverticulitis)
  - Retroperitoneal fibrosis
    - Mantle of soft tissue that encases aorta and inferior vena cava
      - Irregular margins
      - Extending from renal vessels down to iliac bifurcation
    - Draws ureters in toward midline and encases them with fibrous tissue
    - Unilateral or bilateral ureteral obstruction
    - 2/3 are primary: Idiopathic
    - 1/3 are secondary: Medications, neoplasms
- **Acute Tubular Injury**
  - Usually causes bilateral persistent nephrograms (and acute renal failure)
  - Follows shock, placental abruption, nephrotoxic drugs
  - US: Kidney may appear echogenic with increased resistive indices
- **Pyelonephritis**
  - Diminished perfusion from decreased tissue compliance (results of tissue edema) and decreased renal function contribute to delayed nephrogram
  - Leukocytes and bacteria (pus) may plug renal tubules
  - Usually unilateral but can be bilateral
- **Subcapsular Collection**
  - May be hematoma/urinoma/abscess
  - Increased pressure on kidney can occur with large collections (Page kidney) and lead to renal dysfunction
  - Clinical scenario is important

- Consider arterial phase to look for active extravasation of contrast

Helpful Clues for Less Common Diagnoses

- **Contrast-Induced Nephropathy**
  - Much more common after arterial rather than IV administration of contrast
  - Risk is low in patients with eGFR > 30 mg/dL
  - Risk factors
    - Prior renal insufficiency, dehydration, hypertension, diabetes, heart failure, advanced age, large doses of contrast media
- **Renal Vein Stenosis/Thrombosis**
  - "Outflow" obstruction can cause decreased and delayed nephrogram
  - Can be unilateral or bilateral
  - Etiology: Dehydration (most common cause in pediatric population), nephrotic syndrome (most common cause in adults), hypercoagulable state, tumoral vascular invasion (renal cell carcinoma)
  - Intraluminal thrombus itself may be visualized on imaging
- **Renal Artery Stenosis**
  - Atherosclerosis, fibromuscular dysplasia, arteritis, dissection, embolism
  - Delayed "inflow" causes decreased perfusion and delayed nephrogram
  - Usually affected kidney is relatively small if chronic
- **Leukemia**
  - Massive tumor necrosis from chemotherapy may release uric acid into circulation
    - Can lead to calculi or plugging of tubules by uric acid
  - Masses of leukemic tissue (chloroma) may directly obstruct ureters

Helpful Clues for Rare Diagnoses

- **Infiltrative Renal Mass**
  - Infiltrative renal masses include renal cell carcinoma, lymphoma, leukemia, urothelial carcinoma, and metastases
  - Delayed nephrogram is caused by

- Hypoenhancement from infiltrative portion of tumor
- Urinary outflow obstruction: Hillar masses can obstruct urinary outflow
- Renal vein invasion: Typically with renal cell carcinoma
- **Rhabdomyolysis**
  - Death of muscle tissue may release myoglobin into circulation
  - Renal tubules can become blocked by protein plugs
- **Multiple Myeloma**
  - Renal tubules can become obstructed by myeloma protein

SELECTED REFERENCES

1. Strother MC et al: The delayed nephrogram: point-of-care quantitative measurement, validation as an indicator of obstruction, and novel use as a predictor of renal functional impairment. Eur Urol Focus. 15;S2405-4569(22)00042-6, 2022
2. Gagne SM et al: Name that nephrogram: asymmetric renal enhancement in the acute care setting. Curr Probl Diagn Radiol. 48(6):616-25, 2019
3. McDonald JS et al: Bilateral sustained nephrograms after parenteral administration of iodinated contrast material: a potential biomarker for acute kidney injury, dialysis, and mortality. Mayo Clin Proc. 93(7):867-76, 2018
4. Machida S et al: Persistent nephrogram. Intern Med. 55(24):3687-8, 2016
5. Wolin EA et al: Nephrographic and pyelographic analysis of CT urography: differential diagnosis. AJR Am J Roentgenol. 200(6):1197-203, 2013
6. Wolin EA et al: Nephrographic and pyelographic analysis of CT urography: principles, patterns, and pathophysiology. AJR Am J Roentgenol. 200(6):1210-4, 2013
7. Sidhu R et al: Imaging of renovascular disease. Semin Ultrasound CT MR. 30(4):271-88, 2009
8. Craig WD et al: Pyelonephritis: radiologic-pathologic review. Radiographics. 28(1):255-77; quiz 327-8, 2008
9. Jung DC et al: Renal papillary necrosis: review and comparison of findings at multi-detector row CT and intravenous urography. Radiographics. 26(6):1827-36, 2006
10. Tumlin J et al: Pathophysiology of contrast-induced nephropathy. Am J Cardiol. 98(6A):14K-20K, 2006
11. Kawashima A et al: Renal inflammatory disease: the current role of CT. Crit Rev Diagn Imaging. 38(5):369-415, 1997
12. Walker CP et al: Case report: rhabdomyolysis following grand mal seizures presenting as a delayed and increasingly dense nephrogram. Clin Radiol. 47(2):139-40, 1993
13. Dyer RB et al: The abnormal nephrogram. Radiographics. 6(6):1039-63, 1986

Urinary Obstruction

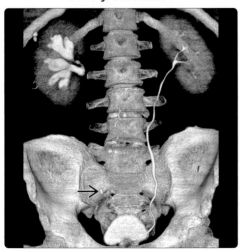

Urinary Obstruction

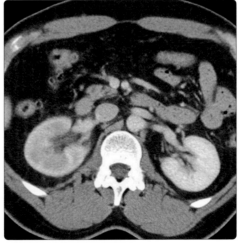

(Left) *Coronal volume-rendered delayed-phase CECT shows prompt concentration and excretion of urine from the left kidney, while the right kidney has a delayed nephrogram/pyelogram and dilated calyces due to an obstructing ureteral stone ➡.* **(Right)** *Axial CECT in a patient with obstructing right distal ureteral calculus shows a delayed right nephrogram. The right kidney is in the corticomedullary phase, while the left is in the nephrographic phase of enhancement.*

Delayed or Persistent Nephrogram

Urinary Obstruction

Urinary Obstruction

(Left) *Axial CECT in a patient with back pain shows right-sided hydronephrosis and delayed nephrogram.* (Right) *Axial CECT in the same patient shows a large, heterogeneous retroperitoneal mass at the site of right ureteral obstruction. This was biopsied and found to be leiomyosarcoma.*

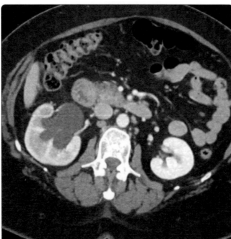

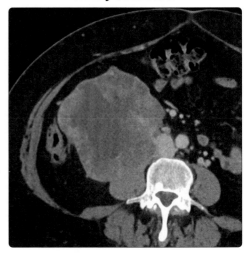

Acute Tubular Injury

Pyelonephritis

(Left) *Axial NECT shows dense, bilateral delayed nephrograms 1 day following coronary angiography in an older patient with congestive heart failure.* (Right) *Axial CECT shows a delayed right nephrogram with patchy striation and wedge-shaped defects ➡. Signs of sepsis, pyuria, and flank pain helped to confirm the diagnosis of acute pyelonephritis.*

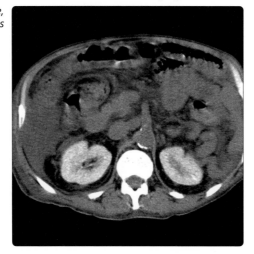

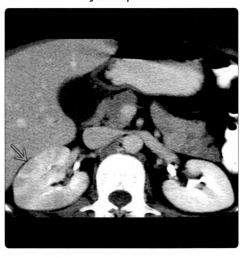

Renal Vein Stenosis/Thrombosis

Renal Vein Stenosis/Thrombosis

(Left) *Axial CECT shows a delayed nephrogram involving the left kidney with surrounding perinephric stranding ➡. Note also the filling defect within the left renal vein ➡, consistent with thrombosis in this patient with nephrotic range proteinuria.* (Right) *Axial CECT in 56-year-old woman with history of blunt trauma to the flank shows marked enlargement and decreased enhancement of the left kidney secondary to presumed traumatic thrombosis of the left renal vein ➡.*

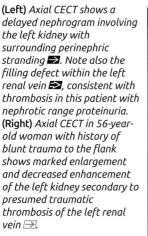
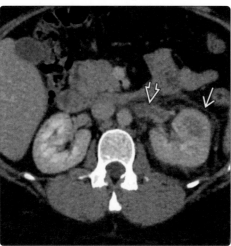

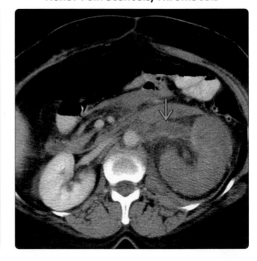

Renal Artery Stenosis

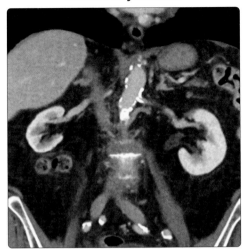

Renal Artery Stenosis

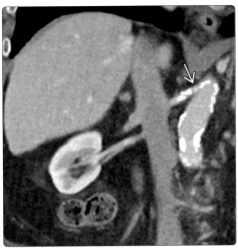

(Left) *Coronal CECT in a patient with longstanding hypertension shows that the right kidney is smaller than the left and exhibits a delayed nephrogram.* (Right) *In the same patient, the origin of the right renal artery is severely narrowed by calcified, atherosclerotic plaque* ➡.

Infiltrative Renal Mass

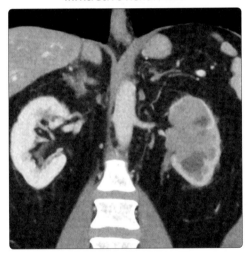

Infiltrative Renal Mass

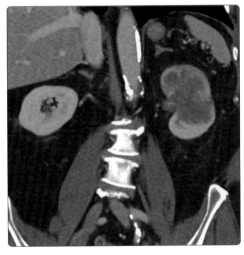

(Left) *Coronal CECT shows an infiltrative, hypoenhancing renal mass involving the hilum of the left kidney with a delayed nephrogram. This was biopsied and found to be lymphoma.* (Right) *Coronal CECT shows a delayed nephrogram involving the left kidney due to an infiltrative renal mass that extends into the hilum. The patient had primary lung adenocarcinoma, and this renal mass was metastatic disease.*

Infiltrative Renal Mass

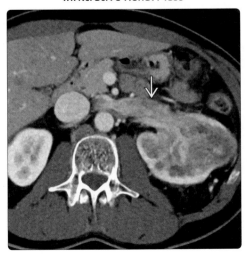

Urinary Obstruction

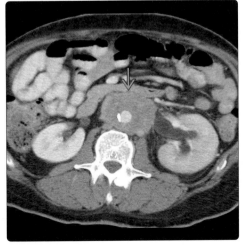

(Left) *Axial CECT of an infiltrative left renal mass relatively hypoenhancing to the renal parenchyma shows a delayed nephrogram. The mass invades and expands the left renal vein* ➡. *This was proven to be clear cell renal cell carcinoma.* (Right) *Axial CECT in 50-year-old woman with history of retroperitoneal fibrosis shows left-sided pelvocaliectasis due to obstruction of the left ureter by the fibrotic mass* ➡ *and slightly decreased enhancement of the left kidney.*

DIFFERENTIAL DIAGNOSIS

Common
- Acute Pyelonephritis
- Renal Trauma
- Acute Tubular Injury

Less Common
- Glomerulonephritis
- Renal Infarct
- Ureteral Obstruction
- Vasculitis
- Multiple Myeloma
- Rhabdomyolysis
- Infiltrative Renal Masses

Rare but Important
- Radiation Nephritis
- Renal Vein Thrombosis
- IgG4-Related Kidney Disease
- Tuberculosis

ESSENTIAL INFORMATION

Key Differential Diagnosis Issues
- Acute renal inflammatory, traumatic, infectious, or vascular diseases
- Manifests on imaging as wedge-shaped &/or striated areas of diminished enhancement on contrast-enhanced CT, MR, and US, as well as underlying changes in density, intensity, and echogenicity
- Wedge shape or striated appearance reflects pyramidal shape of renal lobule

Helpful Clues for Common Diagnoses
- **Acute Pyelonephritis**
  - Unilateral or bilateral
  - Typically bacterial from ascending infection (bladder source)
  - Can be normal sized, but severe forms can lead to diffuse enlargement
  - Wedge-shaped striations
    - NECT: Not usually seen well; may show perirenal inflammatory changes
    - CECT: Wedge-shaped areas of hypoenhancement
    - US: Wedge-shaped areas of increased echogenicity and decreased perfusion on color Doppler
  - NECT and US are not sensitive in its detection
  - Bladder may be thickened with surrounding inflammation or show echogenic debris on US
  - Pyelonephritis is clinical rather than imaging diagnosis
- **Renal Trauma**
  - Typical clinical setting: Blunt injury due to motor vehicle crash
    - Renal arterial injury usually follows rapid deceleration injury (fall or high-speed motor vehicle crash)
  - Contusion and renal hematoma may cause striated and wedge defects
  - May be associated with surrounding stranding or hematoma

  - Look for active extravasation of contrast on CECT during arterial and venous phases (vascular injury) and extravasation on urographic phase (urinoma)
- **Acute Tubular Injury**
  - Characterized by acute kidney injury from tubular epithelial injury
  - Most common cause of acute kidney injury
  - Caused by ischemia
    - Intrarenal blood vessel involvement (microscopic polyangiitis, microangiopathies) or hypotension/shock
    - Direct toxic injury: Myoglobin, hemoglobin, monoclonal light chains, bile/bilirubin, and exogenous agents (drugs, heavy metals, and organic solvents)
  - Usually evaluated by US to exclude other causes of acute kidney injury
  - US features include normal or enlarged kidney; may be echogenic
  - CECT usually shows delayed but persistent uptake of contrast within kidney with little or no excretion; can appear as wedge-shaped areas of injury

Helpful Clues for Less Common Diagnoses
- **Glomerulonephritis**
  - Inflammation and injury of glomerular tissue
    - Primary glomerulonephritis (GN): GN without accompanying condition
    - Secondary GN: GN in association with other condition or disease, such as diabetes, lupus, or drug use
    - Renal enlargement and swollen appearance due to inflammation, though less commonly can have wedge-shaped areas of involvement
    - US: Affected areas of renal cortex appear echogenic
- **Renal Infarct**
  - Typical clinical settings
    - Embolic: Cardiac valve vegetations, prior myocardial infarction, or atrial fibrillation
    - Thrombotic: Aortic &/or renal artery dissection; atherosclerosis
  - Wedge-shaped area of ischemia/infarction
  - Affected areas on US typically appear hypoechoic, especially when chronic
  - Arterial dissection or emboli may result in wedge-shaped parenchymal defects
    - Cortical scarring and volume loss over time
  - Straight line demarcation of normal/abnormal kidney suggests vascular etiology
  - Cortical rim sign
    - Preserved perfusion of subcapsular rim of tissue
    - Seen in 50% of cases; 6-8 hours after infarction
- **Ureteral Obstruction**
  - Ureteral obstruction from stone or mass prior to collecting system at level of calyx or infundibulum, or involving 1 of 2 ureters in duplicated collecting system, can lead to wedge-shaped areas
  - Will show segmental dilated calyx or infundibulum
  - Look for renal calculi, particularly on NECT, and areas of urothelial thickening on urographic phase
- **Vasculitis**
  - Polyarteritis, lupus, etc.
  - Striated and wedge-shaped lesions indistinguishable from acute pyelonephritis on imaging

- Clinical setting: Patient with known autoimmune (collagen vascular) disease
  - Episodes of symptoms referable to visceral ischemia or spontaneous hemorrhage
- **Multiple Myeloma**
  - Collecting tubules may be plugged with excreted myeloma protein
  - Imaging findings similar to acute pyelonephritis
    - Clinical presentation is very different (no fever; known or easily confirmed myeloma)
- **Rhabdomyolysis**
  - Release of massive amounts of myoglobin into serum from damaged skeletal muscle may block renal tubules
    - Clinical: May cause acute renal failure
    - Imaging: Decreased or striated nephrogram, usually bilateral
  - Clinical setting: Crush injury, muscle trauma, certain drug effects
    - Especially drug overdose with prolonged muscle hypoxia
- **Infiltrative Renal Masses**
  - Infiltrative renal masses include renal cell carcinoma, urothelial carcinoma, lymphoma, and metastases
  - Can spare architecture of normal renal parenchyma
  - Involved area is typically hypoenhancing
  - Look for renal vein extension of tumor suggestive of renal cell carcinoma

Helpful Clues for Rare Diagnoses

- **Radiation Nephritis**
  - Decreased enhancement along path of treatment with involved areas of atrophy
  - Geographic margin and history of radiation treatment to area
- **Renal Vein Thrombosis**
  - Can result from hypercoagulable state or nephrotic syndrome (most commonly with membranous GN)
  - If venous involvement involves segmental veins, wedge-shaped area of hypoperfusion can be seen on contrast-enhanced studies
  - US: Decreased echogenicity, renal vein thrombus may be difficult to visualize
  - CT: Filling defect in renal vein seen on venous phase; decreased and delayed parenchymal enhancement if occlusive
  - Unilateral (left sided more common) > bilateral
- **IgG4-Related Kidney Disease**
  - Immune-mediated systemic disease that can involve most organs
  - Isolated IgG4-related kidney disease is uncommon; typically associated with pancreatic &/or biliary involvement
  - Can have discrete masses or be infiltrative (which can appear wedge-shaped)
  - Mild progressive enhancement
  - Typically T2 hypointense and T1 isointense
  - May resolve after steroid treatment
- **Tuberculosis**
  - Results from hematogenous spread to kidneys
  - Microabscesses develop in periglomerular tissues
  - Can appear similar to pyelonephritis with hypoenhancement and renal swelling at site of infection

---

Acute Pyelonephritis

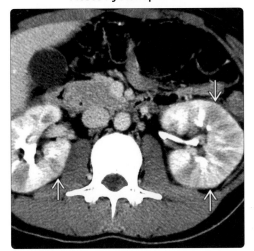

Acute Pyelonephritis

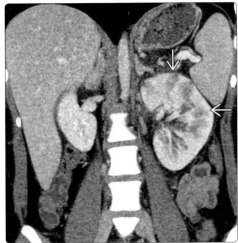

(Left) Axial CECT shows bilateral, wedge-shaped areas of renal parenchymal hypoenhancement (striated nephrograms) from pyelonephritis ➡. (Right) Coronal CECT in a 19-year-old woman presenting with weakness and nausea while in treatment for urinary tract infection reveals radiating, hypoenhancing bands ➡ of the left kidney, typical of striated nephrogram and compatible with acute pyelonephritis. The enhancement of the right kidney is normal, suggesting a unilateral process.

Acute Pyelonephritis

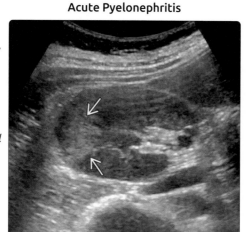

Renal Trauma

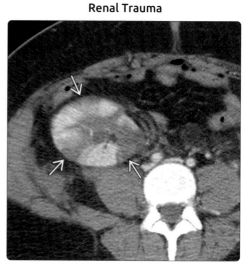

(Left) *Wedge-shaped, hyperechoic region within the interpolar region of the kidney* ➡ *is consistent with pyelonephritis. This area showed decreased perfusion on color Doppler, and the bladder showed layering debris.* (Right) *Axial CECT obtained post blunt abdominal trauma reveals striated nephrogram* ➡ *of right lower quadrant renal allograft from multiple infarcts/contusions.*

Renal Trauma

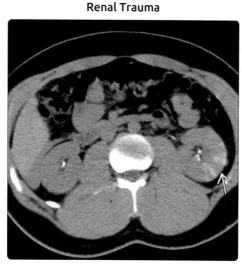

Glomerulonephritis

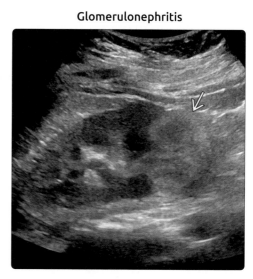

(Left) *Axial NECT shows a striated appearance* ➡ *of the left kidney due to renal contusion on this scan performed several hours after administration of IV contrast medium.* (Right) *Longitudinal US in a patient with acute kidney injury shows a focal area of increased echogenicity involving the inferior pole* ➡. *This area was targeted for biopsy and showed focal glomerulonephritis.*

Renal Infarct

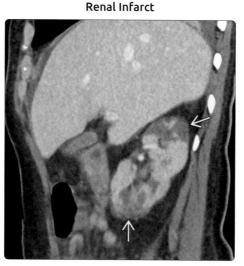

Vasculitis

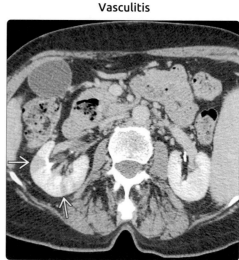

(Left) *Sagittal CECT shows multiple wedge-shaped areas of hypoenhancement involving the right kidney* ➡. *These were areas of infarction in a patient with embolic disease.* (Right) *Axial CECT shows multiple wedge-shaped and striated zones of decreased parenchymal enhancement* ➡ *in this 70-year-old woman with vasculitis due to Wegener granulomatosis.*

Metastases and Lymphoma, Renal

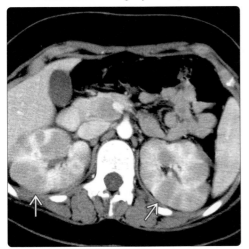

Infiltrative Renal Masses

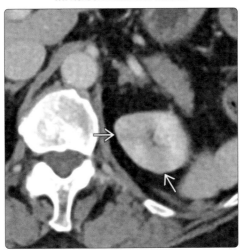

(Left) *Axial CECT shows a mottled appearance of both kidneys due to parenchymal deposits of lymphoma* ➡. *Most of the lesions have a spherical rather than wedge shape.* **(Right)** *Wedge-shaped, hypoenhancing areas involve the superior pole of the left kidney* ➡ *in a patient with hematuria. Ureteroscopy showed an infiltrative urothelial carcinoma.*

Radiation Nephritis

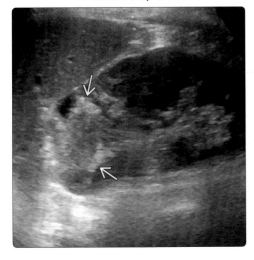

Radiation Nephritis

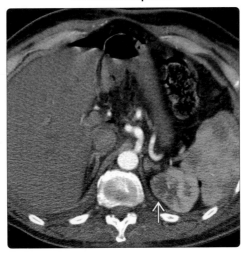

(Left) *Longitudinal US shows a wedge-shaped, hyperechoic region involving the superior pole of the left kidney* ➡. *This patient had a history of lung adenocarcinoma, and this area represented an area of metastatic involvement.* **(Right)** *Axial CECT shows decreased parenchymal enhancement and subtle volume loss in the medial portion of the left kidney* ➡ *due to radiation nephritis that followed treatment for vertebral metastasis.*

Renal Vein Thrombosis

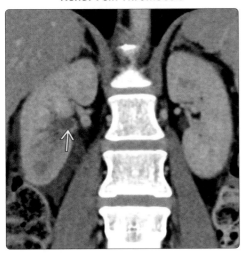

IgG4-Related Kidney Disease

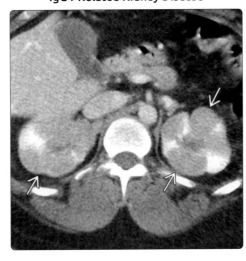

(Left) *Coronal CECT shows a wedge-shaped area of decreased perfusion in the inferior pole of the right kidney. Within the draining segmental renal vein, there is occlusive venous thrombosis* ➡. **(Right)** *Axial CECT shows multiple wedge-shaped, hypoenhancing lesions* ➡ *in both kidneys. This was biopsy-proven IgG4-related sclerosing disease.*

DIFFERENTIAL DIAGNOSIS

Common

- Obstructing Urolithiasis
- Pyelonephritis
- Renal Hemorrhage
- Ureteral Stricture
- Urinary Retention
- Retroperitoneal Hemorrhage
- Musculoskeletal Causes

Less Common

- Pyonephrosis
- Renal Cell Carcinoma
- Gynecologic Causes
- Gastrointestinal Causes
- Renal Infarction
- Adrenal Hemorrhage or Infarction
- Retroperitoneal Fibrosis
- Xanthogranulomatous Pyelonephritis

Rare but Important

- Loin Pain Hematuria Syndrome
- Nutcracker Syndrome
- Renal Ptosis

ESSENTIAL INFORMATION

Key Differential Diagnosis Issues

- Differential diagnosis is broad; however, most causes of flank pain are due to stone disease
- Alternative diagnoses are encountered at rate of ~ 3-10%

Helpful Clues for Common Diagnoses

- **Obstructing Urolithiasis**
  - Very common disease [14% of men, 6% of women (lifetime risk)]
  - Almost all stones are hyperdense at CT due to calcium
    - Matrix and indinavir stones are minimally dense (rare)
  - Obstructing stone almost always at 1 of 3 locations of relative narrowing, in order of frequency
    - Ureterovesical junction (UVJ)
    - Ureteropelvic junction (UPJ)
    - Pelvic brim (where ureter crosses over iliac vessels)
  - Obstructing stones can range in size from tiny (1 mm) to large; may be multiple stones (Steinstrasse)
  - Associated findings
    - Most ureteral stones are associated with some degree of hydronephrosis (from very mild to moderate)
      - Severe hydronephrosis is generally only seen in chronic obstruction
    - Renal enlargement, delayed nephrogram
    - Perinephric and periureteral stranding
    - Urothelial thickening around stone or soft tissue rim sign (differentiates from phlebolith)
    - Bulging ureteral orifice (UVJ stone)
    - Calyceal (forniceal) rupture
    - Infectious complications: Pyelonephritis, pyonephrosis, xanthogranulomatous pyelonephritis
  - Nonobstructing urolithiasis is often asymptomatic though may cause flank pain

- **Pyelonephritis**
  - NECT: Often occult when mild
    - Look for renal enlargement, perinephric stranding, and fascial thickening with lack of hydronephrosis or stone
  - CECT: Striated nephrogram; may be bilateral
  - Complications: Renal abscess → focal collection in parenchyma ± perinephric space
- **Renal Hemorrhage**
  - Trauma is most common etiology
    - Includes iatrogenic (stone intervention, biopsy, etc.)
  - Wunderlich syndrome: Spontaneous, nontraumatic renal hemorrhage
    - Renal mass hemorrhage is most common: Angiomyolipoma or renal cell carcinoma classically
    - Renal artery aneurysm rupture, dissection, renal vein thrombosis, ruptured bleeding cyst (particularly autosomal dominant polycystic kidney disease)
    - Vasculitis: Polyarteritis nodosa → spontaneous perinephric hemorrhage with small visceral aneurysms
- **Ureteral Stricture**
  - UPJ obstruction
    - Large renal pelvis with hydronephrosis due to narrowing at UPJ; normal distal ureter ± crossing vessel
    - Dietl crisis: Acute flank pain, nausea, vomiting ± hematuria due to intermittent hydronephrosis from UPJ obstruction
      - Imaging findings may resolve in pain-free episodes
      - Classically, school-aged children
      - UPJ obstruction may cause acute pain in adults after excessive hydration, coffee or binge drinking (so-called beer drinker's hydronephrosis) due to distention of collecting system
  - History of stones: Stricture may develop after prolonged stone impaction or stone intervention
  - Tumor: Retroperitoneal lymphadenopathy, encasement by tumors, metastatic, fibrosis
  - Iatrogenic ureteral injury: Typically post gynecologic or other pelvic surgery
  - Urothelial carcinoma: Least common location occurs in ureter
  - Fibroepithelial polyp: Elongated filling defect in ureter ± hydronephrosis
  - Endometriosis: Distal stricture
  - Other: Radiation therapy, after renal ablation, TB, malakoplakia, IgG4, vasculitis, congenital causes
- **Urinary Retention**
  - Distended bladder and bilateral hydronephrosis
- **Retroperitoneal Hemorrhage**
  - Spontaneous hemorrhage in setting of anticoagulation
  - Ruptured abdominal aortic aneurysm
- **Musculoskeletal Causes**
  - Range of acute and chronic soft tissue or bony injuries to flank and spine may present with flank pain
    - Generally, no specific imaging findings
  - 11th and 12th rib fractures or bone lesions may be detected on CT

Helpful Clues for Less Common Diagnoses

- **Pyonephrosis**

- Hydronephrosis with thickened and enhancing urothelium
- Fluid-debris level
- ± stone or other etiology of ureteral obstruction
- ± cystitis
- **Renal Cell Carcinoma**
  - Rarely presents as painful mass; typically incidental or vague symptoms
- **Gynecologic Causes**
  - Hemorrhagic cyst, ruptured cyst, torsion, pelvic inflammatory disease, ectopic pregnancy, ovarian neoplasm
- **Gastrointestinal Causes**
  - Appendicitis, diverticulitis (particularly right colon or descending colon), perforated or obstructed colon cancer
  - Cholecystitis, pancreatitis (particularly when retroperitoneal extension of necrotizing collections)
  - Omental infarction, epiploic appendagitis
- **Renal Infarction**
  - Aortic dissection, embolic disease (atrial fibrillation, left ventricular apical thrombus)
  - Ranges from tiny to large, wedge-shaped areas
  - Tends to be lower density on CECT than pyelonephritis
- **Adrenal Hemorrhage or Infarction**
  - Adrenal hemorrhage
    - Sepsis, pregnancy, trauma, masses
  - **Nonhemorrhagic adrenal infarction**
    - Rare condition seen almost exclusively in pregnant women in 3rd trimester
    - Adrenal vein thrombosis → ischemia/infarction of adrenal → enlarged, edematous, nonenhancing adrenal with surrounding stranding
- **Retroperitoneal Fibrosis**
  - Soft tissue encasing aorta/inferior vena cava pulling ureters medially with hydronephrosis
  - May extend into renal hila or rarely perinephric space
- **Xanthogranulomatous Pyelonephritis**

- Enlarged kidney with staghorn calculus and rounded, low-density lesions distending collecting system and replacing parenchyma (bear-paw kidney)
- May extend outside of kidney into flank, retroperitoneum, and organs

Helpful Clues for Rare Diagnoses

- **Loin Pain Hematuria Syndrome**
  - Unilateral or bilateral chronic flank pain and microscopic or gross hematuria
  - Typically young to middle-aged female patients
  - Diagnosis of exclusion: Lack of stones, hydronephrosis, other causes by imaging
- **Nutcracker Syndrome**
  - Symptomatic compression of left renal vein between aorta and superior mesenteric artery (SMA), resulting in vein outflow obstruction
    - Hematuria, flank pain, orthostatic proteinuria, dysmenorrhea, varicocele
  - Flattened left renal vein between SMA and aorta with beak sign and collaterals to spine, gonadal veins
    - Many patients show normal, benign compression and lack symptoms
- **Renal Ptosis**
  - Abnormal mobility of kidney in upright position with torsion/obstruction of vessels &/or collecting system
  - Best diagnosed with supine and upright IV pyelogram

SELECTED REFERENCES

1. Parmar N et al: Wunderlich syndrome: wonder what it is. Curr Probl Diagn Radiol. 51(2):270-81, 2022
2. Badawy M et al: Adrenal hemorrhage and hemorrhagic masses; diagnostic workup and imaging findings. Br J Radiol. 94(1127):20210753, 2021
3. Chagué P et al: Non-hemorrhagic adrenal infarction during pregnancy: the diagnostic imaging keys. Tomography. 7(4):533-44, 2021
4. Gopireddy DR et al: "Renal emergencies: a comprehensive pictorial review with MR imaging". Emerg Radiol. 28(2):373-88, 2021
5. Jha P et al: Imaging of flank pain: readdressing state-of-the-art. Emerg Radiol. 24(1):81-6, 2017
6. Rucker CM et al: Mimics of renal colic: alternative diagnoses at unenhanced helical CT. Radiographics. 24 Suppl 1:S11-28; discussion S28-33, 2004

Obstructing Urolithiasis

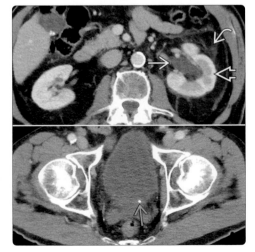

Obstructing Urolithiasis

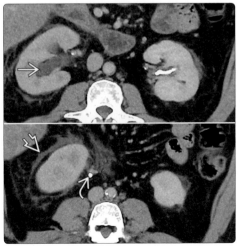

(Left) *CECT in a patient with acute severe left flank pain shows left hydronephrosis ➡, delayed nephrogram ⇉, and perinephric stranding/fluid ↗ due to a 2-mm obstructing stone ⇥ at the ureterovesical junction (UVJ), the most common location of stone obstruction.* **(Right)** *Axial CECT in a patient with right flank pain shows right hydronephrosis ➡, delayed nephrogram, and perinephric stranding ➡. An obstructing stone ↗ is seen at the ureteropelvic junction (UPJ), the 2nd most common location of stone obstruction.*

Obstructing Urolithiasis

Obstructing Urolithiasis

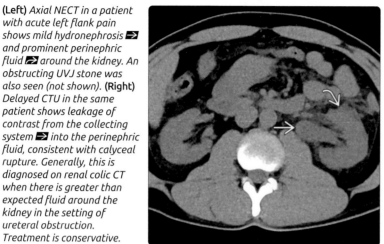

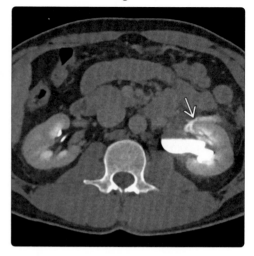

(Left) *Axial NECT in a patient with acute left flank pain shows mild hydronephrosis* ➡ *and prominent perinephric fluid* ➡ *around the kidney. An obstructing UVJ stone was also seen (not shown).* **(Right)** *Delayed CTU in the same patient shows leakage of contrast from the collecting system* ➡ *into the perinephric fluid, consistent with calyceal rupture. Generally, this is diagnosed on renal colic CT when there is greater than expected fluid around the kidney in the setting of ureteral obstruction. Treatment is conservative.*

Obstructing Urolithiasis

Obstructing Urolithiasis

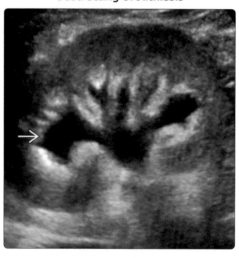

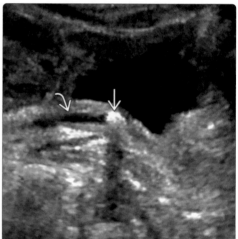

(Left) *Longitudinal US of the left kidney shows mild hydronephrosis* ➡. **(Right)** *Longitudinal US of the bladder in the same patient shows an echogenic, shadowing stone* ➡ *at the UVJ with upstream dilation of the ureter* ➡.

Obstructing Urolithiasis

Obstructing Urolithiasis

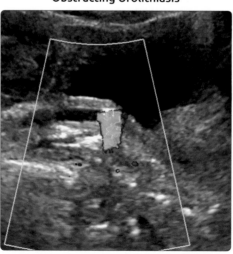

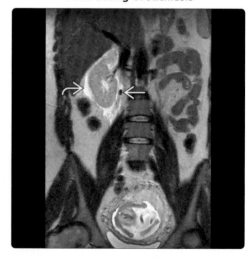

(Left) *Color Doppler US of the same patient shows twinkle artifact (alternating strong color variation), which is typical of stones and can be useful to identify on US.* **(Right)** *Coronal T2 MR in a pregnant patient at 15 weeks shows an obstructing UPJ stone* ➡. *Note the large perinephric fluid* ➡, *which helps distinguish obstruction from physiologic hydronephrosis of pregnancy.*

Pyelonephritis

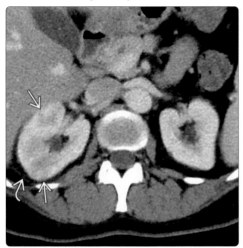

Renal Hemorrhage

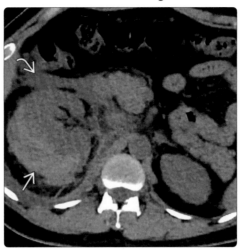

(Left) *Axial CECT shows right renal enlargement and striated nephrogram ➡, consistent with pyelonephritis. Also note the subtle perinephric fat stranding and fascial thickening ➡.* **(Right)** *Axial NECT shows a large right subcapsular hematoma ➡ and perinephric hemorrhage ➡ in a 33-year-old man who reported no trauma and therefore has spontaneous renal hemorrhage (Wunderlich syndrome). Further imaging was recommend to look for renal mass or vasculitis.*

Renal Hemorrhage

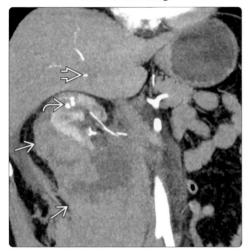

Renal Hemorrhage

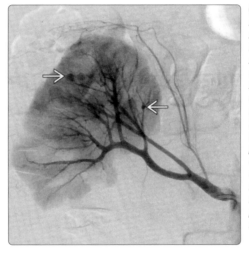

(Left) *Coronal MIP CECT in the same patient shows the large, subcapsular, and perinephric hemorrhage ➡. Note the small aneurysms ➡ in the upper pole of the kidney. Small hepatic artery aneurysms ➡ were also seen. PAN vasculitis was felt most likely.* **(Right)** *AP angiogram of the right kidney in the same patient confirms small aneurysms ➡. Findings were consistent with vasculitis and most typical of polyarteritis nodosa (PAN), which may present with spontaneous renal hemorrhage.*

Renal Hemorrhage

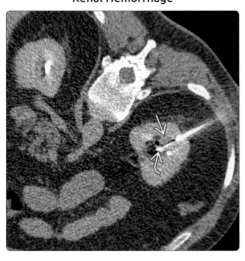

Renal Hemorrhage

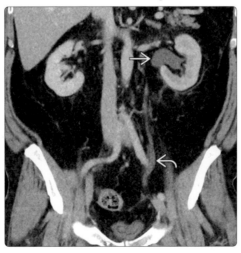

(Left) *Axial CT-guided biopsy of a small renal mass ➡ in a patient presenting with flank pain and hematuria shows the needle tip ➡ passing close to the collecting system.* **(Right)** *Coronal CECT in the same patient 2 days later is shown. Mild hydronephrosis ➡ and delayed nephrogram is seen due to small clots in the midureter ➡. Postintervention hemorrhage is commonly found in the perinephric space but may involve the collecting system and cause obstruction.*

Renal Hemorrhage

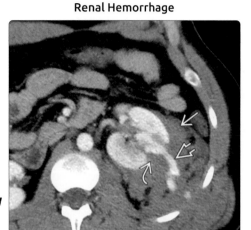

Ureteral Stricture

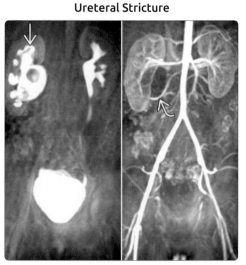

(Left) *Axial CECT in a patient who was stabbed in the flank shows a large perinephric hemorrhage* ➡ *due to a renal laceration* ➡. *Note the large-volume, active extravasation* ➡, *requiring emergent embolization.* (Right) *Coronal MR urogram in a 4-year-old girl shows moderate hydronephrosis* ➡ *and no contrast in the right ureter on delayed postcontrast image. Angiogram shows an accessory right renal artery* ➡ *crossing the UPJ and causing the obstruction.*

Ureteral Stricture

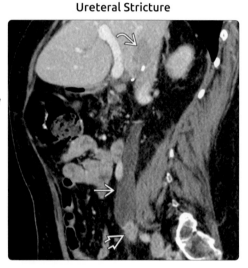

Urinary Retention

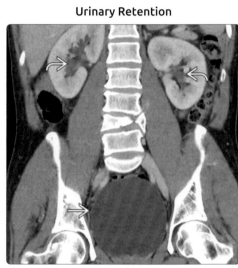

(Left) *Sagittal CECT in a patient with colon cancer shows ureter dilation* ➡ *due to a mass at the midureter* ➡, *which represented metastasis. Liver metastasis* ➡ *is also seen.* (Right) *Coronal CECT in a patient with altered mental status, history of substance abuse, and flank pain shows a distended urinary bladder* ➡ *and mild bilateral hydronephrosis* ➡. *Acute urinary retention may cause pain or be incidentally seen at CT.*

Retroperitoneal Hemorrhage

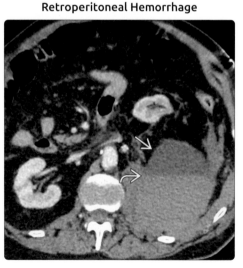

Musculoskeletal Causes

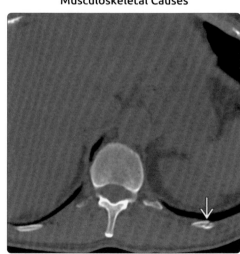

(Left) *Axial CECT shows a large, dense, left retroperitoneal fluid collection* ➡ *with hematocrit level* ➡, *displacing the kidney anteriorly. This is typical of coagulopathic hemorrhage.* (Right) *Axial NECT in a patient with left flank pain and concern for urolithiasis shows an acute 11th rib fracture* ➡ *as an alternative diagnosis.*

Pyonephrosis

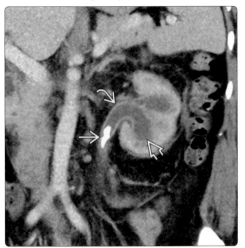

Renal Infarction

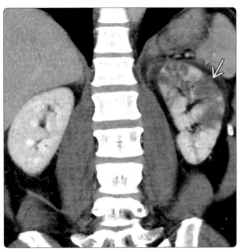

(Left) Coronal CECT in a patient presenting with flank pain and sepsis shows an obstructing UPJ stone ➡ and mild hydronephrosis ➡. Note the diffuse urothelial thickening and enhancement ➡. (Right) Coronal CECT shows multiple wedge-shaped areas of nonenhancement ➡ in this patient who had cardiomyopathy and left ventricular thrombus, which embolized. Renal infarctions tend to be lower density than pyelonephritis.

Adrenal Hemorrhage or Infarction

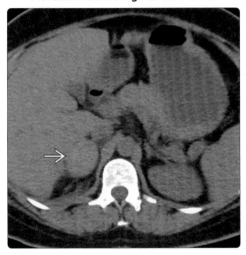

Adrenal Hemorrhage or Infarction

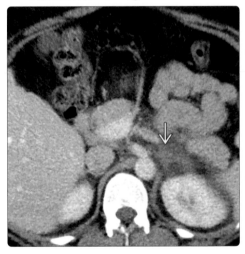

(Left) Axial NECT in a woman 1 day post partum shows a hyperdense right adrenal mass ➡ with surrounding hemorrhage, consistent with adrenal hematoma. Adrenal hemorrhage is associated with pregnancy and requires a high degree of suspicion for diagnosis. (Right) Axial CECT in a pregnant patient in the 3rd trimester shows an enlarged, thickened left adrenal gland ➡ with poor enhancement and surrounding stranding. This is typical of adrenal infarction, which classically occurs in the 3rd trimester.

Xanthogranulomatous Pyelonephritis

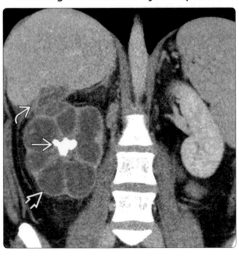

Nutcracker Syndrome

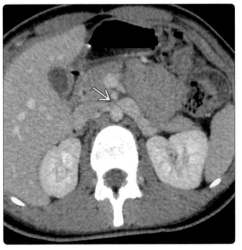

(Left) Coronal CECT shows a large staghorn calculus ➡ with large, dilated, surrounding calyces ➡ containing low-density material. XGP may extend beyond the kidneys to the flank, retroperitoneum, or other organs, as in this case with extension into the subcapsular liver ➡. (Right) Axial CECT in a 16-year-old girl with chronic flank pain and microscopic hematuria shows severe narrowing of the left renal vein ➡ between the aorta and SMA. Collaterals were also seen to the spine and gonadal vein (not shown).

DIFFERENTIAL DIAGNOSIS

Common

- Hydronephrosis
- Acute Pyelonephritis
- Acute Glomerulonephritis
- Acute Tubular Injury
- Subcapsular Fluid Collections

Less Common

- Compensatory Renal Hypertrophy
- Primary Renal Tumors, Infiltrative
- Autosomal Dominant Polycystic Kidney Disease
- Renal Fusion Anomalies
- Renal Tuberculosis

Rare but Important

- Acute Renal Vein Thrombosis
- Acute Cortical Necrosis
- HIV-Associated Nephropathy
- Multicystic Renal Dysplasia
- Xanthogranulomatous Pyelonephritis

ESSENTIAL INFORMATION

Key Differential Diagnosis Issues

- CT and MR are more accurate than US in assessing kidney size
- In adults, normal kidneys are 9-13 cm in length
- Kidney enlargement can be unilateral or bilateral depending on disease process
- Enlargement can be secondary to diffuse process or cysts/masses
- Acute causes: Obstruction, infection, inflammation
- Chronic causes: Cellular hypertrophy, abnormal protein deposition, malignancies, infection, glomerular or microvascular proliferation

Helpful Clues for Common Diagnoses

- **Hydronephrosis**
  - Dilated renal collecting system
  - Common etiologies: Calculi, ureteropelvic junction obstruction, bladder outlet obstruction, gravid uterus, and malignant compression of ureter
  - If associated with infection, must be treated emergently
  - Enlarged kidney usually seen in acute setting with preservation of renal cortical thickness
  - Can be seen with perirenal stranding on CT/MR
- **Acute Pyelonephritis**
  - Can be normal-sized, but severe forms can lead to diffuse enlargement
  - Can be unilateral or bilateral
  - Typically bacterial from ascending infection (bladder source)
  - Wedge-shaped striations
    - NECT: Not usually seen well; may show perirenal inflammatory changes
    - CECT: Wedge-shaped areas of hypoenhancement
    - US: Wedge-shaped areas of increased echogenicity and decreased perfusion on color Doppler
  - Bladder may be thickened with surrounding inflammation or show echogenic debris on US

- US and NECT are not sensitive in detecting pyelonephritis
- Pyelonephritis is clinical rather than imaging diagnosis
- **Acute Glomerulonephritis**
  - Inflammation and injury of glomerular tissue
    - Primary glomerulonephritis (GN): GN without accompanying condition
    - Secondary GN: GN in association with other condition or disease, such as diabetes, lupus, or drug use
  - Renal enlargement and swollen appearance due to inflammation
  - US: Renal cortex can appear echogenic with resultant prominent hypoechoic pyramids
  - Chronic GN: Small kidney due to renal scarring and atrophy from repeated insults
  - Diagnosis made on biopsy and clinical situation
- **Acute Tubular Injury**
  - Characterized by acute kidney injury from tubular epithelial injury
  - Most common cause of acute kidney injury
  - Caused by ischemia
    - Intrarenal blood vessel involvement (microscopic polyangiitis, microangiopathies) or hypotension/shock
    - Direct toxic injury: Myoglobin, hemoglobin, monoclonal light chains, bile/bilirubin, exogenous agents (drugs, heavy metals, organic solvents)
  - Usually evaluated by US to exclude other causes of acute kidney injury
  - US features include normal or enlarged kidney; may be echogenic
  - CECT usually shows delayed but persistent uptake of contrast within kidney with little or no excretion
- **Subcapsular Fluid Collections**
  - May represent abscess, blood, urine, and lymph
  - May mimic large renal mass, especially when fluid is isodense/isoechoic to renal parenchyma
  - Can compress renal parenchyma (Page kidney)

Helpful Clues for Less Common Diagnoses

- **Compensatory Renal Hypertrophy**
  - Associated with unilateral renal agenesis or hypoplasia
  - Solitary kidney enlarges as result of compensatory hypertrophy
  - Otherwise unremarkable kidney
- **Primary Renal Tumors, Infiltrative**
  - Infiltrative pattern of renal tumors can enlarge kidney but maintain renal architecture
  - Infiltrative renal tumors include renal cell carcinoma, urothelial carcinoma, leukemia, lymphoma, and metastatic disease
  - May be associated with lymphadenopathy or metastatic disease
  - Infiltrative component usually hypoenhancing relative to normal parenchyma
  - Should be correlated with clinical picture and may require biopsy
- **Autosomal Dominant Polycystic Kidney Disease**
  - Usually presents in adulthood
  - Innumerable simple or hemorrhagic cysts bilaterally of varying size in cortex or medulla
  - Extrarenal manifestations include hepatic cysts

- o Eventually leads to end-stage renal disease
- **Renal Fusion Anomalies**
  - o Congenital anomalies
  - o Horseshoe kidney: 2 functioning kidneys on either side of vertebral column fused at their lower poles
  - o Cross-fused renal ectopia: Ectopic kidney that crosses midline and fuses with contralateral kidney
  - o Fused pelvic kidney (pancake): Extensive medial fusion of both kidneys
- **Renal Tuberculosis**
  - o Results from hematogenous spread to kidneys
  - o Microabscesses develop in periglomerular tissues
  - o Can appear similar to pyelonephritis with hypoenhancement and renal swelling at site of infection
  - o Sites of infection can calcify chronically (putty kidney), and kidney can become small in size
  - o More common in certain parts of world

Helpful Clues for Rare Diagnoses

- **Acute Renal Vein Thrombosis**
  - o Can result from hypercoagulable state or nephrotic syndrome (most commonly with membranous GN)
  - o US: Decreased echogenicity; renal vein thrombus may be difficult to visualize
  - o CECT: Filling defect in renal vein seen on venous phase, decreased and delayed parenchymal enhancement if occlusive
  - o Unilateral (left-sided more common) > bilateral
- **Acute Cortical Necrosis**
  - o Absent cortical perfusion with maintained medullary flow
  - o Results from microvascular thrombosis with cortical infarction
  - o Caused by abruptio placentae, postpartum hemorrhage, shock, sepsis, and toxins
  - o Kidney size can be normal or increased acutely
    - US: Enlarged echogenic kidneys with hypoechoic subcapsular rim
    - CECT and CEMR: Nonenhancing outer cortex is diagnostic

- o Chronically, kidney may be decreased in size
- **HIV-Associated Nephropathy**
  - o Kidney injury caused either by virus itself or antiretroviral medications
  - o Can cause GN or tubulointerstitial/vascular nephropathies
  - o US: Hyperechoic, enlarged kidneys with decreased corticomedullary differentiation
  - o Much less common in modern era
  - o Biopsy required for diagnosis
- **Multicystic Renal Dysplasia**
  - o Sporadic disorder that can be unilateral or bilateral
  - o Affected kidney is usually enlarged, irregular in contour, with multiple cysts of variable sizes
  - o Can be associated with ureteropelvic junction obstruction, ureteral agenesis
  - o Can simulate complex cystic neoplasm
  - o Renal failure can result in cases of bilateral disease
- **Xanthogranulomatous Pyelonephritis**
  - o Chronic infection with replacement by lipid-laden macrophages
  - o Pelvicalyceal obstruction, typically staghorn calculus
  - o Diffuse unilateral renal enlargement, cortical thinning, and dilated calyces producing bear paw sign
  - o Inflammatory tissue can invade adjacent structures

SELECTED REFERENCES

1. Zulfiqar M et al: Imaging of renal infections and inflammatory disease. Radiol Clin North Am. 58(5):909-23, 2020
2. Shen CL et al: Symmetric nephromegaly. Clin Exp Nephrol. 23(3):427-8, 2019

Hydronephrosis

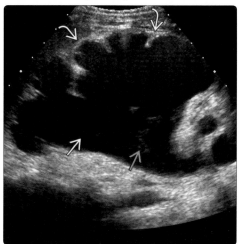

Hydronephrosis

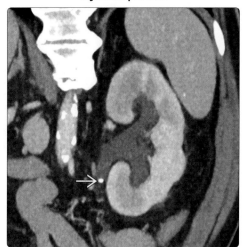

(Left) *Longitudinal US shows a markedly enlarged right kidney with severe hydronephrosis ➡, hydroureter, and cortical thinning ➡ in a patient with history of posterior urethral valves and severe reflux. Renal pelvis echoes ➡ could represent infection, blood, or cellular debris. **(Right)** Curved MPR CECT shows an enlarged left kidney (15 cm) caused by acute hydronephrosis from a proximal ureteral calculus ➡.*

(Left) *Coronal CECT shows multiple wedge-shaped areas of decreased enhancement ➡. Urothelial thickening is present ➡. The left kidney is enlarged in this patient with candidal infection of the kidneys.* (Right) *In this patient with acute kidney injury, the kidney is enlarged and edematous with increased echogenicity. Biopsy revealed acute glomerulonephritis.*

Acute Pyelonephritis

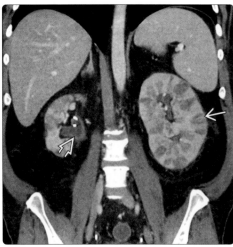

Acute Glomerulonephritis

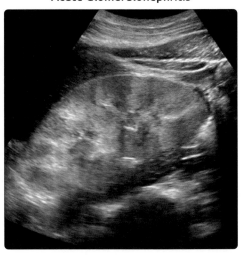

(Left) *Axial CECT shows a large, subcapsular collection involving the right kidney containing higher than simple fluid density ➡. This was a spontaneous subcapsular hematoma. There is mass effect on the kidney parenchyma ➡, consistent with Page kidney.* (Right) *Coronal CECT shows the right kidney congenitally atrophic ➡, which has led to compensatory hypertrophy of the left kidney. In this patient, renal function was normal.*

Subcapsular Fluid Collections

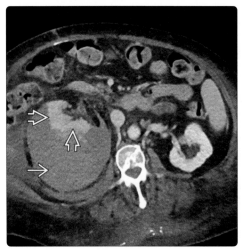

Compensatory Renal Hypertrophy

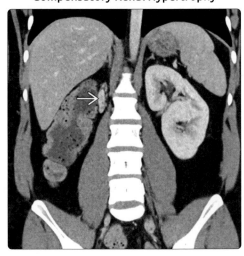

(Left) *Coronal CECT shows an infiltrative mass that expands and largely replaces the right kidney. Biopsy revealed undifferentiated pleomorphic sarcoma.* (Right) *Axial CECT shows an infiltrative mass involving the left kidney ➡, expanding Its size. There is tumor invasion of the left renal vein ➡. This was diagnosed as clear cell renal cell carcinoma.*

Primary Renal Tumors, Infiltrative

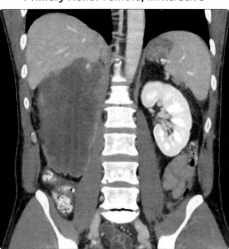

Primary Renal Tumors, Infiltrative

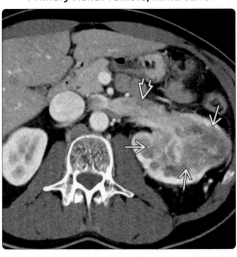

Autosomal Dominant Polycystic Kidney Disease

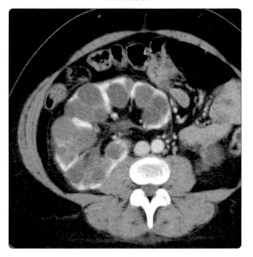

Autosomal Dominant Polycystic Kidney Disease

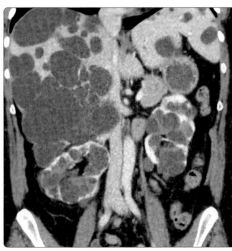

(Left) *Axial CECT shows a malrotated, enlarged right kidney with numerous cysts.* (Right) *In the same patient, the renal cysts are bilateral, and numerous cysts are present within the liver. The patient was developing renal dysfunction and diagnosed with autosomal dominant polycystic kidney disease.*

Acute Renal Vein Thrombosis

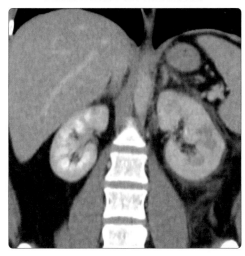

Acute Renal Vein Thrombosis

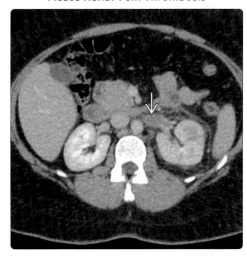

(Left) *Coronal CECT shows the left kidney is mildly enlarged compared to the right with perinephric stranding and delayed nephrogram.* (Right) *In the same patient, a filling defect is seen within the left renal vein ➡, consistent with renal vein thrombosis.*

HIV-Associated Nephropathy

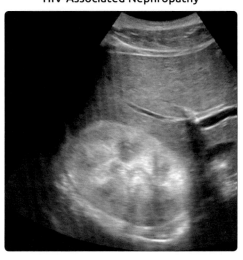

Xanthogranulomatous Pyelonephritis

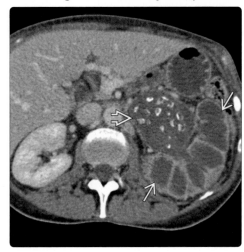

(Left) *The right kidney is enlarged, edematous, and shows increased echogenicity relative to the liver parenchyma. This patient with renal dysfunction had a biopsy consistent with HIV-associated nephropathy.* (Right) *Enlarged left kidney with dilated and enlarged calyces gives a multiloculated appearance ➡, the bear's paw sign, with a dilated renal pelvis ➡ containing numerous calculi. This patient underwent a nephrectomy that revealed xanthogranulomatous pyelonephritis.*

DIFFERENTIAL DIAGNOSIS

Common

- Chronic Diabetic Nephropathy
- Chronic Glomerulonephritis
- Chronic Hypertensive Nephropathy
- Chronic Lupus Nephritis
- Chronic Reflux Nephropathy
- Postobstructive Atrophy
- Partial Nephrectomy/Post Ablative Therapy/Post Surgery
- Chronic Renal Allograft Rejection/Chronic Allograft Nephropathy

Less Common

- Chronic HIV Nephropathy
- Multicystic Dysplastic Kidney
- Recurrent Infection
- Chronic Renal Artery Stenosis
- Chronic Renal Infarction
- Chronic Vascular Injury
- Posttraumatic Renal Atrophy
- Following Acute Cortical Necrosis or Acute Tubular Injury
- Post Chemotherapy

Rare but Important

- Chronic Radiation Nephropathy
- Chronic Nephritis (Alport Syndrome)
- Renal Cystic Dysplasia
- Medullary Cystic Disease Complex
- Tuberculous Autonephrectomy
- Renal Hypoplasia
- Supernumerary Kidney
- Chronic Lead Poisoning

ESSENTIAL INFORMATION

Key Differential Diagnosis Issues

- Renal atrophy is end result of many pathologic processes
- Causes of loss of renal parenchyma include
  - Acquired: Infection, inflammation, obstruction, reflux, trauma, necrosis/ischemia, fibrosis, surgical intervention
  - Congenital: Hypoplasia, dysplasia
- Imaging findings are not specific for cause
- Renal size and cortical thickness are useful in differentiating acute from chronic kidney disease
- Determine if abnormality is unilateral or bilateral, global or focal/multifocal
- Hydronephrosis suggests ureteral obstruction or vesicoureteral reflux
- Renal echogenicity is variable but commonly ↑ in renal parenchymal disease
- Usually not possible to determine cause of small, echogenic, scarred kidney
- Clinical history is essential for diagnosis
- Biopsy usually not indicated if kidneys are small

Helpful Clues for Common Diagnoses

- **Chronic Diabetic Nephropathy**
  - Small kidneys + ↑ cortical echogenicity
  - Corticomedullary differentiation (CMD) usually preserved, unless patient is in overt renal failure

- **Chronic Glomerulonephritis**
  - Small kidneys + smooth renal outline
  - Parenchyma remains echogenic
- **Chronic Hypertensive Nephropathy**
  - Due to progressive nephrosclerosis
  - Small kidneys + irregular cortical thinning
  - ↓ cortical vascularity due to arteriolar fibrosis and hyaline degeneration
- **Chronic Lupus Nephritis**
  - Small kidneys
  - Variable renal echogenicity and CMD
- **Chronic Reflux Nephropathy**
  - Unilateral or bilateral vesicoureteral reflux in childhood
  - May cause focal/diffuse renal scarring and atrophy
  - Cortical scars are common in upper and lower pole
  - Dilated calyces next to scar suggest diagnosis
  - Calyces and pelvis may be dilated initially but shrink as kidney atrophies
  - Focal areas of compensatory hypertrophy seen adjacent to cortical scars
  - Small kidneys + irregular renal outline
- **Postobstructive Atrophy**
  - Caused by longstanding ureteropelvic junction (UPJ), ureteric or bladder outlet obstruction
  - Results in progressive ↓ in renal blood flow and glomerular filtration
  - Small kidney with cortical thinning and variable hydronephrosis
- **Partial Nephrectomy/Post Ablative Therapy/Post Surgery**
  - Small residual kidney with preserved CMD
  - Compensatory hypertrophy of contralateral kidney may be evident
  - History is essential
- **Chronic Renal Allograft Rejection/Chronic Allograft Nephropathy**
  - Irreversible cause of renal allograft dysfunction
  - Small transplant kidney with cortical thinning and ↑ cortical echogenicity
  - ↓ color Doppler flow
  - ↓ arterial diastolic flow

Helpful Clues for Less Common Diagnoses

- **Chronic HIV Nephropathy**
  - Normal or enlarged kidneys becoming small with progressive renal failure
  - ↑ cortical echogenicity, loss of CMD and sinus fat
- **Multicystic Dysplastic Kidney**
  - Initially unilateral enlarged kidney replaced by noncommunicating cysts of varying sizes
  - Undergoes partial or complete involution in infancy
  - Later appears small and echogenic ± cysts
  - Contralateral diseases common, such as vesicoureteric reflux, UPJ obstruction, and ureteric stenosis
- **Recurrent Infection**
  - Risk factors: Calculi, urinary tract obstruction, neurogenic bladder, and urinary diversion
  - Small kidney, parenchymal scarring
  - Focal cortical thinning causing irregular outline
  - Pseudotumors from adjacent hypertrophy

- **Chronic Renal Artery Stenosis**
  - Mostly atherosclerosis affects main, interlobar, or interlobular renal arteries or arterioles
  - Progressive generalized reduction in kidney size caused by ischemia
  - Produces renal atrophy
  - Smooth contour
- **Chronic Renal Infarction**
  - Renal atrophy after acute renal infarction caused by embolism or thrombosis
  - Atrophy may be focal (segmental) or global
  - Parenchymal loss depends on distribution of occluded artery
  - Infarcted area may be contracted, producing renal scar
- **Chronic Vascular Injury**
  - Sequela of vasculitides, such as polyarteritis nodosa or ischemia from fibromuscular dysplasia
  - End result of nonspecific small echogenic kidneys
- **Posttraumatic Renal Atrophy**
  - Caused by segmental renal infarction due to renal artery thrombosis after blunt renal trauma or after embolization for bleeding
  - Contracted kidney + irregular outline
  - Collateralization may be demonstrated
- **Following Acute Cortical Necrosis or Acute Tubular Injury**
  - May be associated with cortical or medullary calcification
- **Post Chemotherapy**
  - Scarring after therapy for renal lymphoma, leukemia, or metastases

Helpful Clues for Rare Diagnoses

- **Chronic Radiation Nephropathy**
  - Occurs after renal irradiation for bone marrow transplantation
  - Begins months to years after irradiation
  - Areas of diminished perfusion may be seen
  - Small kidneys with ↑ renal echogenicity
- **Chronic Nephritis (Alport Syndrome)**
  - Chronic hereditary nephritis

- Small kidneys + smooth renal outline
- ↑ cortical echogenicity due to cortical nephrocalcinosis
- **Renal Cystic Dysplasia**
  - May be bilateral
  - Associated with posterior urethral valve, renal duplication, crossed-fused ectopia, horseshoe and pelvic kidneys
  - Unilateral small kidney with ↑ echogenicity and small cortical cysts
- **Medullary Cystic Disease Complex**
  - Inherited cystic renal disease
  - Progressive tubular atrophy with glomerulosclerosis
  - Echogenic kidneys with progressive ↓ in size
  - Multiple small medullary cysts
- **Tuberculous Autonephrectomy**
  - Calcified caseous pyonephrosis with UPJ fibrosis
  - Shrunken kidney + extensive calcification
  - Dilated calyces
- **Renal Hypoplasia**
  - At least 50% smaller than normal
  - Has fewer calyces and papillae
  - Renal function normal for its size
  - Usually unilateral
  - Differentiation from obstruction, chronic pyelonephritis, and ischemia difficult
- **Supernumerary Kidney**
  - Extremely rare, hypoplastic 3rd kidney
  - Connected to dominant kidney either completely or by loose areolar connective tissue
  - Most are caudal to orthotopic kidney
- **Chronic Lead Poisoning**
  - Bilateral, small kidneys
  - Blood level of lead useful for diagnosis

Chronic Diabetic Nephropathy

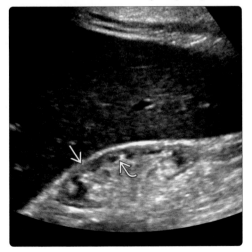

Chronic Glomerulonephritis

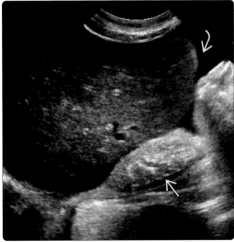

(Left) Longitudinal US of the right kidney in a patient with end-stage renal disease and diabetes shows diffuse cortical thinning ➡ with ↑ echogenicity and preserved corticomedullary differentiation ➡. (Right) Longitudinal US shows the right kidney in a patient with end-stage renal disease and cirrhosis. The kidney ➡ is small (8 cm) with ↑ echogenicity and loss of corticomedullary differentiation. Ascites and nodular liver contour ➡ are present.

(Left) *Longitudinal US shows the right kidney in a patient with end-stage renal disease. The kidney* ⮕ *is small and lobulated, a nonspecific appearance, which can be the end result of many disorders. Note the prominent perinephric fat* ⮕ *between the liver* ⮕ *and kidney.* **(Right)** *Longitudinal US of the right kidney in a 1-year-old with history of grade III-IV reflux shows an atrophic kidney* ⮕ *with no hydronephrosis. No focal scars were detected.*

Chronic Hypertensive Nephropathy

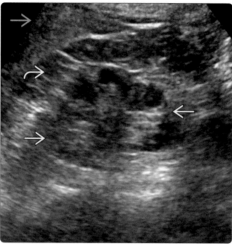

Chronic Reflux Nephropathy

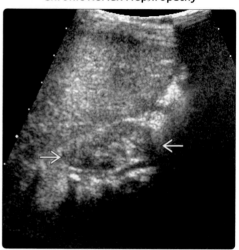

(Left) *Longitudinal US of the left kidney shows a lobulated contour with cortical loss* ⮕ *in the upper and mid to lower poles. There is mild pelvic dilatation* ⮕. **(Right)** *Coronal NECT in the same patient confirms the atrophy of the left kidney with cortical loss* ⮕. *A few tiny calcifications* ⮕ *are noted, not seen on US.*

Chronic Reflux Nephropathy

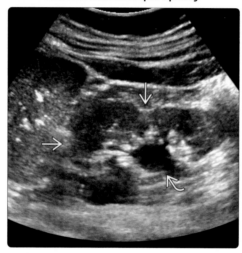

Chronic Reflux Nephropathy

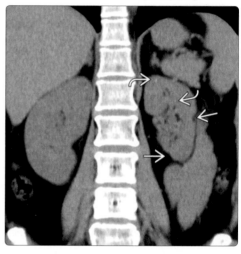

(Left) *Coronal T2 HASTE MR in the same patient performed for gallbladder disease shows calyceal dilatation under areas of cortical loss* ⮕. *MR has superior contrast resolution to CT and is less affected by body habitus than US.* **(Right)** *Longitudinal US shows the right kidney in a patient with established HIV nephropathy. The renal cortex is markedly echogenic* ⮕ *and small with loss of sinus fat.*

Chronic Reflux Nephropathy

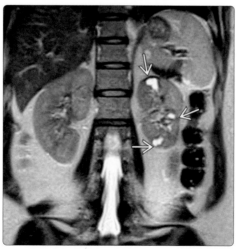

Chronic HIV Nephropathy

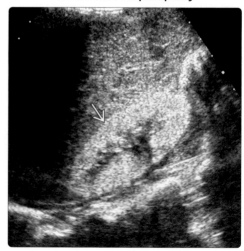

Postobstructive Atrophy

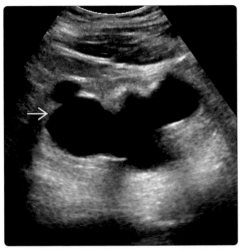

Postobstructive Atrophy

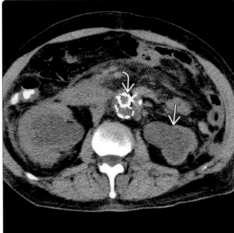

(Left) *Longitudinal US of the left kidney shows severe hydronephrosis ➡ and cortical thinning, which was secondary to chronic ureteral obstruction; however, severe reflux can also produce this appearance.* **(Right)** *Axial NECT in the same patient shows bilateral hydronephrosis with more atrophy on the left ➡ and an aortic stent graft ➡. Renal failure precluded the use of IV contrast.*

Partial Nephrectomy/Post Ablative Therapy/Post Surgery

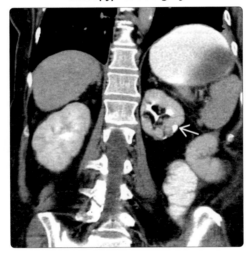

Partial Nephrectomy/Post Ablative Therapy/Post Surgery

(Left) *Longitudinal US shows the left kidney post partial nephrectomy 20 years prior. The kidney ➡ is small (6 cm) with preserved corticomedullary differentiation.* **(Right)** *Coronal CECT in the same patient shows loss of cortex overlying midpole calyces ➡ status post lower pole resection.*

Renal Hypoplasia

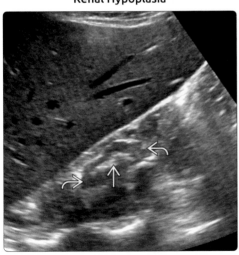

Chronic Renal Infarction

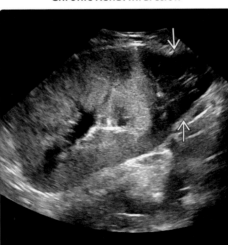

(Left) *Longitudinal US shows the liver and atrophic right kidney in a patient with testicular cancer post retroperitoneal lymph node dissection. The right kidney ➡ is very small with global cortical thinning. Renal sinus fat ➡ is preserved.* **(Right)** *Longitudinal US shows a renal transplant with scarring of the lower pole ➡, a sequela of thrombosis of a lower pole accessory artery.*

DIFFERENTIAL DIAGNOSIS

Common

- Glomerulonephritis
- Diabetic Nephropathy
- Chronic Kidney Disease
- Acute Interstitial Nephritis
- Acute Tubular Injury
- Medullary Nephrocalcinosis
- Acute Pyelonephritis
- Hypertensive Nephrosclerosis

Less Common

- Kidney Transplant Rejection
- Renal Amyloidosis
- Renal Tuberculosis

Rare but Important

- Cortical Nephrocalcinosis
- Emphysematous Pyelonephritis
- HIV-Associated Nephropathy
- Lithium Nephropathy
- Acute Cortical Necrosis

ESSENTIAL INFORMATION

Key Differential Diagnosis Issues

- ↑ renal echogenicity is most commonly diffuse and secondary to renal parenchymal disease
- Cortical echogenicity greater than liver or spleen is abnormal
- Cortical echogenicity equal to sinus fat is markedly abnormal
- Pyramids may be dark when disease is confined to cortex
- Secondary to multiple diseases
- ↑ renal echogenicity indicates abnormal kidneys but not specific to any particular disease process
- Degree of echogenicity correlates poorly with severity of renal impairment
- Renal biopsy indispensable in diagnosis of renal parenchymal disease
- Role of US
  - Determine renal size and cortical thickness
    - Differentiating acute from chronic renal insufficiency
  - Exclude ureteral obstruction
- Kidney may be enlarged, normal-sized, or small
- Differentiate from focal areas of ↑ echogenicity

Helpful Clues for Common Diagnoses

- **Glomerulonephritis**
  - Inflammation affecting glomerulus, which can be caused by several disease processes
    - Infectious: Poststreptococcal, bacterial endocarditis, viral infections (HIV, hepatitis B, C)
    - Autoimmune: Lupus, Goodpasture syndrome, IgA nephropathy
    - Vasculitis: Polyarteritis, granulomatosis with polyangiitis (Wegener granulomatosis)
    - Sclerotic conditions: Hypertension, diabetic nephropathy, focal segmental glomerulosclerosis
  - Acute: Renal enlargement and ↑ echogenicity
  - Chronic: Renal atrophy and ↑ echogenicity

  - Medullary portion typically spared from ↑ echogenicity, making them appear markedly hypoechoic
- **Diabetic Nephropathy**
  - Single most important cause of renal failure in adults
  - Diabetes involves glomerulus, interstitium, and vessels
  - Early: Normal or enlarged kidneys with preserved cortical thickness
  - Chronic: Small, echogenic kidney with thin cortex and variable corticomedullary differentiation (CMD)
  - ↑ resistive index (RI) on Doppler studies with ↑ cortical echogenicity
- **Chronic Kidney Disease**
  - Can be caused by many different etiologies, including glomerulonephritis, tubulointerstitial nephritis, and vascular disease
  - Imaging appearance: Small, echogenic kidneys
  - Kidneys may be surrounded by hypoechoic-appearing fat
- **Acute Interstitial Nephritis**
  - 2/3 caused by NSAIDs and antimicrobial medications
  - Interstitial edema and inflammatory infiltrates
  - Glomeruli are typically normal
  - Can cause enlarged, echogenic kidneys
  - Diagnosis based on biopsy
  - Treatment: Drug withdrawal and steroids
- **Acute Tubular Injury**
  - Most common cause of reversible renal failure
  - Caused by hypotension/sepsis and drug, metal, and solvent exposure
  - Deposition of cellular debris within tubules
  - Can cause appearance of echogenic, enlarged kidneys
- **Medullary Nephrocalcinosis**
  - Calcification of renal medulla due to calcium salt deposition
  - Can be caused by hyperparathyroidism, renal tubular acidosis, or medullary sponge kidney
  - Echogenic medullary portions ± shadowing
  - Early form may show echogenic rim outlining renal medullary portions
  - Normal echogenicity of cortex
  - May lead to development of renal calculi
- **Acute Pyelonephritis**
  - May be normal-sized or enlarged when severe
  - Wedge-shaped areas of ↑ echogenicity may be seen with ↓ perfusion on color Doppler US
  - Thickened urothelium and mild hydronephrosis
  - Can be associated with abscesses, which may appear as complex fluid collections or simulate solid renal masses
  - Debris may be present in bladder
- **Hypertensive Nephrosclerosis**
  - 25% of end-stage renal disease
  - Renal echogenicity depends on chronicity
  - ↑ RI with ↑ cortical echogenicity

Helpful Clues for Less Common Diagnoses

- **Kidney Transplant Rejection**
  - Kidney graft can appear echogenic, though normal echogenicity is more common
  - ± enlarged, swollen appearance of kidney graft
  - Thickened urothelium may be present
  - Usually nonelevated resistive indices

- **Renal Amyloidosis**
  - Deposition of β-sheet fibrils
  - May be primary or secondary (multiple myeloma, rheumatoid arthritis, tuberculosis, renal cell carcinoma, Hodgkin disease)
  - Acute: Kidney may be enlarged and echogenic
  - Chronic: Thinned renal cortex
  - Diagnosis based on biopsy
- **Renal Tuberculosis**
  - Calcifications typically within parenchyma
  - May demonstrate amorphous, granular, curvilinear, or mass-like morphology
  - Dense calcification with progressive atrophy in end stage (putty kidney)

Helpful Clues for Rare Diagnoses

- **Cortical Nephrocalcinosis**
  - Hyperechoic cortex that may or may not shadow
  - In cases of shadowing calcification, interior cortex, pyramids, and renal sinus/collecting system may not be visualized
  - Can be caused by acute cortical necrosis, chronic glomerulonephritis, hypercalcemic states, ethylene glycol poisoning, sickle cell disease, and chronically rejected kidney grafts
- **Emphysematous Pyelonephritis**
  - Diabetes, immunocompromise, clinical picture of sepsis
  - Gas-forming necrotizing renal infection
  - Diffuse or segmental
  - Bright echoes with posterior "dirty" shadowing
- **HIV-Associated Nephropathy**
  - Occurs more commonly in African American patients
  - Present with nephrotic syndrome and may progress rapidly to end-stage renal disease
  - Typically large, echogenic kidneys with preserved CMD
  - Later, sinus blends with cortex, and kidneys become small
  - Not as common in modern era
- **Lithium Nephropathy**
  - Innumerable tiny cysts in cortex and medulla of normal-sized kidneys
  - Cysts produce bright, punctate echoes
- **Acute Cortical Necrosis**
  - Associated with shock, sepsis, snake bites, and exposure to toxins, abruptio placentae, or postpartum hemorrhage
  - Microvascular thrombosis leading to cortical ischemia
  - Subcapsular area spared; hypoechoic rim initially
  - Rapid cortical calcification may ensue: Curvilinear/shadowing
  - Diffuse ↑ parenchymal echogenicity

SELECTED REFERENCES

1. Gupta P et al: Ultrasonographic predictors in chronic kidney disease: a hospital based case control study. J Clin Ultrasound. 49(7):715-9, 2021
2. Spiesecke P et al: Multiparametric ultrasound findings in acute kidney failure due to rare renal cortical necrosis. Sci Rep. 11(1):2060, 2021
3. Drudi FM et al: Multiparametric ultrasound in the evaluation of kidney disease in elderly. J Ultrasound. 23(2):115-26, 2020
4. Kelahan LC et al: Ultrasound assessment of acute kidney injury. Ultrasound Q. 35(2):173-80, 2019

Glomerulonephritis

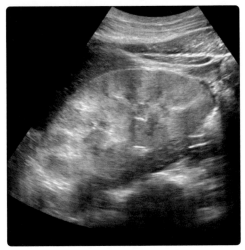

Glomerulonephritis

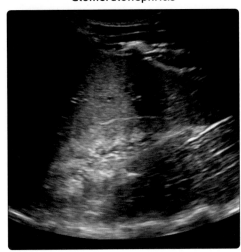

(Left) In this patient with acute kidney injury, the kidneys appear edematous with ↑ echogenicity. Biopsy revealed acute glomerulonephritis. (Right) In the same patient 2 years later, US shows a smaller, echogenic kidney, indicating chronic kidney disease from repeated episodes of glomerulonephritis.

Chronic Kidney Disease

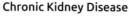
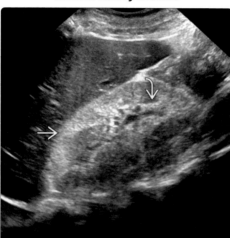

Acute Tubular Injury

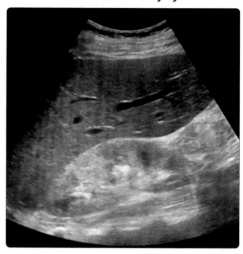

(Left) *Longitudinal US shows a normal-sized right kidney with diffuse ↑ in cortical echogenicity ➡. Pyramids are not conspicuous. The renal sinus ➡ is barely seen.* (Right) *In this patient with acute kidney injury, the kidney is normal in size but echogenic when compared with the adjacent liver parenchyma. Biopsy revealed severe acute tubular injury.*

Medullary Nephrocalcinosis

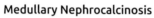
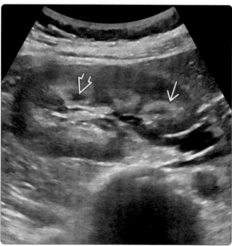

Medullary Nephrocalcinosis

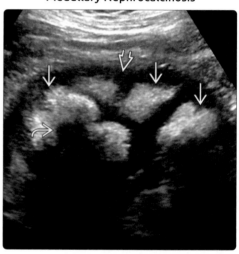

(Left) *The renal pyramids show peripheral areas of ↑ echogenicity ➡ with sparing of the most central portion of the pyramid ➡. This pattern indicates early medullary nephrocalcinosis.* (Right) *As medullary nephrocalcinosis progresses, the pyramids ➡ show some shadowing ➡. The entire medullary pyramid is echogenic. The cortex ➡ is less echogenic than the pyramids.*

Kidney Transplant Rejection

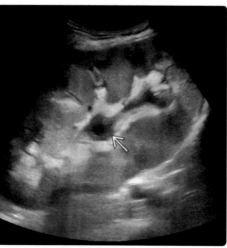

Renal Amyloidosis

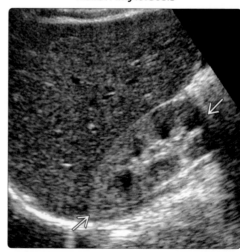

(Left) *In this patient with a kidney graft, the kidney appears edematous and echogenic. Of note, there is urothelial thickening ➡, which can be seen in the setting of kidney transplant rejection, although this finding is not specific.* (Right) *Longitudinal transabdominal US of the kidney ➡ shows a subtle ↑ in cortical echogenicity with preserved corticomedullary differentiation. Renal echogenicity may be normal in early stages of renal amyloid, despite deranged renal function.*

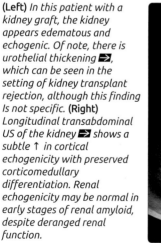

Cortical Nephrocalcinosis

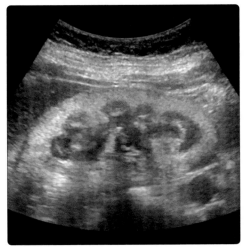

Cortical Nephrocalcinosis

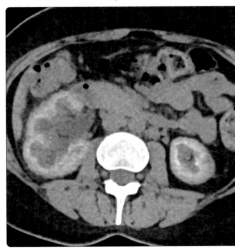

(Left) This renal cortex is markedly echogenic with sparing of the medullary pyramids. The kidney is normal in size. (Right) Axial NECT shows kidneys with ↑ density in the cortex and sparing of the medullary pyramids. This patient had cortical nephrocalcinosis from oxalosis.

Emphysematous Pyelonephritis

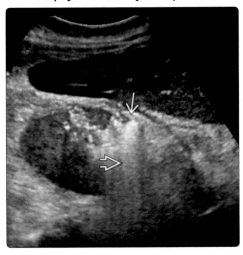

Emphysematous Pyelonephritis

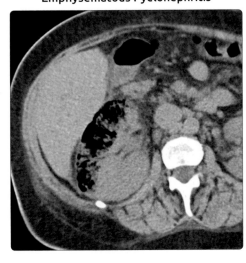

(Left) A portion of the renal parenchyma shows ↑ echogenicity ➡ with "dirty" posterior shadowing ➡, consistent with intraparenchymal air. (Right) Axial NECT in the same patient confirms parenchymal air. This patient was septic and underwent a nephrectomy for emphysematous pyelonephritis.

HIV-Associated Nephropathy

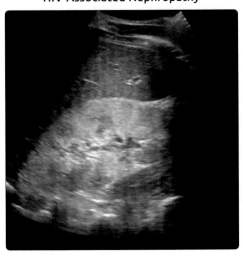

Lithium Nephropathy

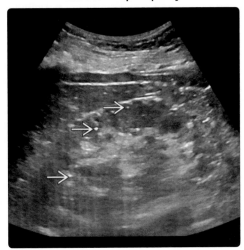

(Left) In this patient with history of HIV and acute kidney injury, US shows an enlarged, echogenic kidney. Biopsy confirmed HIV-associated nephropathy. (Right) Multiple punctate echogenic foci are seen within the kidneys ➡. This patient had a history of bipolar disorder treated with lithium. Biopsy confirmed lithium nephropathy.

DIFFERENTIAL DIAGNOSIS

Common

- Obstructed Renal Pelvis
- Reflux Into Dilated Renal Pelvis
- Extrarenal Pelvis
- Physiologic Distention of Renal Pelvis
- Parapelvic Cyst
- Prominent Renal Vessel
- Urothelial Carcinoma

Less Common

- Pyonephrosis
- Hemonephrosis
- Renal Sinus Hemorrhage
- Pararenal Fluid Collections
- Peripelvic Cyst
- Intrarenal Abscess
- Calyceal Diverticulum
- Acute Renal Vein Thrombosis

Rare but Important

- Pyelogenic Cyst
- Multilocular Cystic Nephroma
- Lucent Sinus Lipomatosis
- Renal Lymphoma
- Retroperitoneal Lymphoma
- Renal Artery Aneurysm
- Arteriovenous Malformation
- Intrarenal Varices
- Renal Lymphangiomatosis

ESSENTIAL INFORMATION

Key Differential Diagnosis Issues

- Important to differentiate between obstruction and nonobstruction
  - Follow ureter to level of obstruction to determine cause
- US is 1st-line modality for detection but other modalities, such as CT, MR, VCUG, and retrograde pyelography, may be required for definitive diagnosis
- Nuclear scintigraphy differentiates obstruction from nonobstructive dilatation

Helpful Clues for Common Diagnoses

- **Obstructed Renal Pelvis**
  - Isolated dilatation of renal pelvis is uncommon
  - Dilatation elsewhere in GU tract determined by level of obstruction
    - e.g., ureteropelvic junction obstruction manifests with pelvic dilatation and (to lesser degree) calyceal dilatation
    - Ureterovesical junction obstruction presents with hydroureter as well as pelvicalyceal dilatation
  - Determine if unilateral or bilateral
  - Level of obstruction helps narrow differential diagnosis
  - Most common cause of unilateral obstruction is stone disease
  - Other causes include bladder, ureteral or other pelvic mass, retroperitoneal mass or hemorrhage, aortic aneurysm, retroperitoneal fibrosis, iatrogenic injury
- **Reflux Into Dilated Renal Pelvis**
  - Hydroureter may be present in addition to renal pelvic dilatation
  - VCUG essential in determining reflux
    - In future, contrast-enhanced voiding urosonography may be used in place of VCUG to evaluate for reflux without use of ionizing radiation
- **Extrarenal Pelvis**
  - Common finding in neonates and often incidentally noted in other age groups
    - Renal pelvis projects medial to renal sinus
  - Appearance may simulate early obstruction, but calyces are not dilated
- **Physiologic Distention of Renal Pelvis**
  - Commonly noted when bladder is distended
    - Frequent in pregnant patients, most commonly in 3rd trimester; R > L
    - Fetal pyelectasis can result in mild pelvic dilatation in neonates, which subsequently resolves
- **Parapelvic Cyst**
  - 1-3% of renal parenchymal cysts; usually solitary
  - May be mixed picture, as parapelvic cysts can compress collecting system, resulting in true dilatation
- **Prominent Renal Vessel**
  - May mimic pelvic dilatation, but color Doppler US denotes flow
    - Always remember to use color Doppler when concerned about pelvic dilatation or cystic lesion to distinguish from vessel
- **Urothelial Carcinoma**
  - Hypoechoic mass in dilated pelvis, though usually slightly hyperechoic to renal parenchyma
  - Can mimic hemorrhage or pus
  - On color Doppler US, note internal vascularity within urothelial carcinoma

Helpful Clues for Less Common Diagnoses

- **Pyonephrosis**
  - Debris (pus) in dilated pelvicalyceal system
  - Look for presence of urothelial thickening and cause, such as stone
- **Hemonephrosis**
  - Blood within dilated pelvicalyceal system ± blood in bladder
  - Echogenicity variable depending upon age of blood products
- **Renal Sinus Hemorrhage**
  - In absence of trauma, most often secondary to anticoagulation, but can be secondary to occult neoplasm, vasculitis, or blood dyscrasia
  - Cystic lesion of variable echogenicity disrupting normal central echocomplex with mass effect upon renal pelvis and tension upon infundibula
  - Should spontaneously resolve in 3-4 weeks
- **Pararenal Fluid Collections**
  - May occur in setting of infection, obstruction, or transplantation; include urinoma, hematoma, abscess, and lymphocele near renal hilum
- **Peripelvic Cyst**
  - Lymphatic collection in renal sinus, distinct from parapelvic cyst, which is intraparenchymal
  - Often multiple and bilateral (unlike parapelvic cyst)

- **Intrarenal Abscess**
  - Hypoechoic parenchymal lesion, which may mimic collecting system dilatation
  - May also be associated with hydronephrosis and urothelial thickening
  - Most often secondary to acute pyelonephritis but relatively rare
- **Calyceal Diverticulum**
  - Typically upper pole, connects with calyx
    - Lined with transitional cell epithelium
  - May appear like simple cyst or dilated calyx
  - Prone to calculus formation and infection: Containing milk of calcium and debris
  - On excretory-phase CT/MR, VCUG, or retrograde pyelography, diagnostic filling of diverticulum with contrast
- **Acute Renal Vein Thrombosis**
  - Dilated vein with hypoechoic thrombus
    - Chronic thrombosis often shows greater internal echogenicity and organized clot along walls
  - Absent venous color Doppler flow

Helpful Clues for Rare Diagnoses

- **Pyelogenic Cyst**
  - Similar to calyceal diverticulum but communicates with pelvis rather than calyx
- **Multilocular Cystic Nephroma**
  - Encapsulated multilocular cystic renal lesion with internal septa
    - On MR/CT, note enhancement of septa
  - May herniate into renal pelvis, mimicking pelviectasis, or may cause hydronephrosis
- **Lucent Sinus Lipomatosis**
  - Very rarely, renal sinus fat may appear less echogenic than normal and mimic hydronephrosis or hypoechoic mass
    - Secondary to chronic steroid use, obesity, diabetes, renal atrophy, and inflammation
  - More evident when there is chronic kidney disease and hyperechoic kidneys

- **Renal Lymphoma**
  - Multiple forms, including hypoechoic infiltration of renal sinus
    - May mimic dilated renal pelvis or cause hydronephrosis
- **Retroperitoneal Lymphoma**
  - Retroperitoneal adenopathy may demonstrate contiguous extension into renal pelvis, mimicking dilatation of collecting system
  - Distinct from renal lymphoma
- **Renal Artery Aneurysm**
  - Pulsatile fluid-filled structure with diagnostic color/power Doppler US
  - Typically small (< 2 cm) and saccular
  - Located at bifurcation of main renal artery
- **Arteriovenous Malformation**
  - Congenital malformation, which appears hypoechoic on grayscale US
  - Color Doppler flow reveals hypervascular mass with aliasing
- **Intrarenal Varices**
  - May present as cystic renal mass
  - May mimic hydronephrosis
  - Associated with arteriovenous malformation
- **Renal Lymphangiomatosis**
  - Multiple cystic lesions in both parapelvic and perirenal areas
  - Related to lymphatic obstruction

SELECTED REFERENCES

1. Ma TL et al: Parapelvic cyst misdiagnosed as hydronephrosis. Clin Kidney J. 6(2):238-9, 2013
2. Darge K et al: Pediatric uroradiology: state of the art. Pediatr Radiol. 41(1):82-91, 2011
3. Sheth S et al: Imaging of renal lymphoma: patterns of disease with pathologic correlation. Radiographics. 26(4):1151-68, 2006
4. Browne RF et al: Transitional cell carcinoma of the upper urinary tract: spectrum of imaging findings. Radiographics. 25(6):1609-27, 2005
5. Rha SE et al: The renal sinus: pathologic spectrum and multimodality imaging approach. Radiographics. 24 Suppl 1:S117-31. Review, 2004
6. Nahm AM et al: The renal sinus cyst-the great imitator. Nephrol Dial Transplant. 15(6):913-4, 2000

Obstructed Renal Pelvis

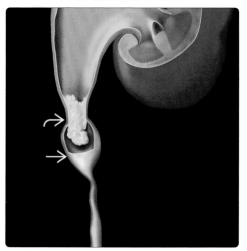

Obstructed Renal Pelvis

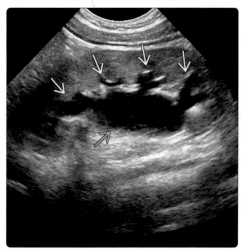

(Left) Graphic shows an obstructing polypoid tumor ➡️ at the ureteropelvic junction. The proximal ureter is dilated around the tumor, producing the goblet sign ➡️. (Right) Longitudinal US shows hydronephrosis with pelvic dilatation ➡️ to a greater degree than calyceal dilatation ➡️, consistent with ureteropelvic junction obstruction.

Reflux Into Dilated Renal Pelvis

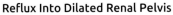

Reflux Into Dilated Renal Pelvis

(Left) *Longitudinal US of the left kidney shows pelvic ➡ and calyceal ➡ dilatation.* (Right) *VCUG evaluation in the same patient reveals left grade 4 reflux.*

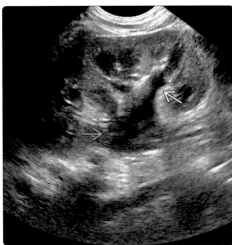

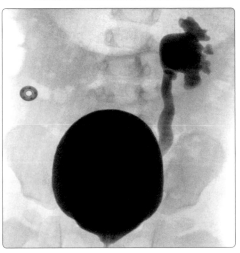

Extrarenal Pelvis

Extrarenal Pelvis

(Left) *Longitudinal color Doppler US shows an anechoic central structure in the left kidney without flow ➡ distinct from the central sinus fat ➡, representing extrarenal pelvis.* (Right) *Axial CECT in the same patient shows left extrarenal pelvis ➡.*

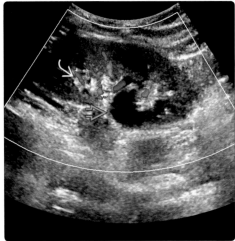

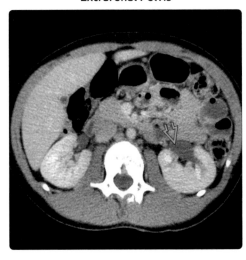

Parapelvic Cyst

Parapelvic Cyst

(Left) *Longitudinal US shows a large, anechoic structure in the upper pole and interpolar region ➡.* (Right) *Coronal CECT in the same patient shows a discrete cyst in the upper pole of the left kidney ➡ approaching the pelvis, representing parapelvic cyst.*

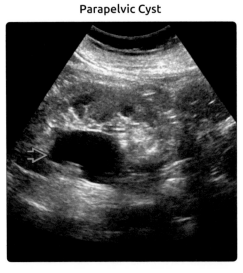

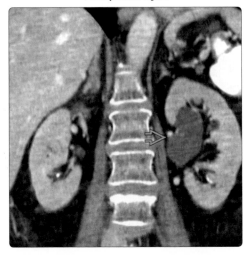

Pyonephrosis

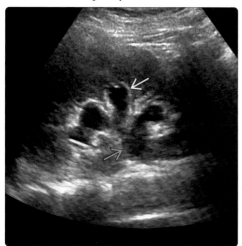

Pyonephrosis

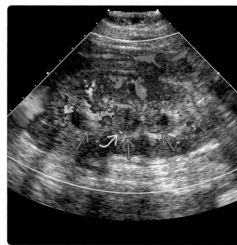

(Left) *Longitudinal US of the right kidney shows low-level echoes in the dilated renal pelvis ⮕, representing pyonephrosis. Note urothelial thickening ⮕, an ancillary finding of urinary tract infection.* (Right) *Longitudinal color Doppler US shows hypoechoic tissue filling the dilated renal collecting system ⮕ with internal color flow ⮕, distinguishing this material as neoplasm rather than avascular pus or clot.*

Calyceal Diverticulum

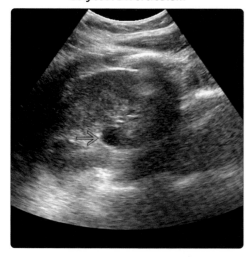

Calyceal Diverticulum

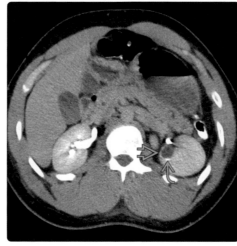

(Left) *Longitudinal US shows an anechoic structure in the interpolar region of the left kidney ⮕. Given this image alone, one might suspect pelviectasis or a simple cyst.* (Right) *Axial CECT in the same patient shows a small amount of layering contrast ⮕ within the lesion ⮕ on excretory phase, confirming calyceal diverticulum.*

Multilocular Cystic Nephroma

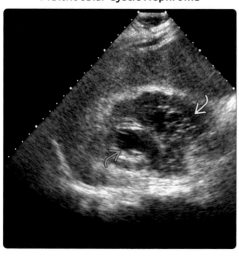

Multilocular Cystic Nephroma

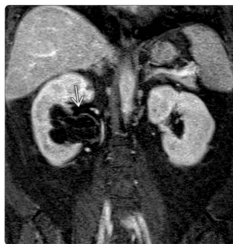

(Left) *Longitudinal US shows dilatation of the renal pelvis ⮕, which contains a cystic mass with thin internal septa ⮕.* (Right) *Coronal T1 C+ MR in the same patient shows a mass with septal enhancement ⮕ entering the renal pelvis. Histopathology confirmed multilocular cystic nephroma.*

DIFFERENTIAL DIAGNOSIS

Common

- Renal Angiomyolipoma
- Renal Cell Carcinoma

Less Common

- Fat in Renal Scar
- Renal Junctional Line/Cortical Parenchymal Defect
- Renal Calculi
- Medullary Nephrocalcinosis
- Column of Bertin
- Renal Papillary Necrosis
- Complex Cyst/Milk of Calcium Cyst
- Emphysematous Pyelonephritis
- Renal Metastases
- Acute Pyelonephritis

Rare but Important

- Xanthogranulomatous Pyelonephritis
- Tuberculosis, Urinary Tract
- Renal Oncocytoma
- Renal Trauma

ESSENTIAL INFORMATION

Key Differential Diagnosis Issues

- Same lesions that cause fat-attenuation lesions on CT and MR usually cause echogenic lesion on US
  - Echogenicity alone is not reliable indication of fat content
  - Other sources of renal echogenicity include calcification and gas
    - Lesions with calcification: Milk of calcium cyst, complex renal cysts, renal cell carcinoma (RCC)
    - Lesions with gas: Renal abscess, emphysematous pyelonephritis
- Echogenic masses ≤ 1 cm are likely angiomyolipomas (AMLs) or indolent RCCs and may not require additional imaging
- RCCs > 1 cm are more likely to be echogenic; echogenic lesions > 1 cm need more definitive characterization with CT or MR

Helpful Clues for Common Diagnoses

- **Renal Angiomyolipoma**
  - Well-defined, hyperechoic mass with echogenicity similar to renal sinus
  - Echogenicity created by high fat content and multiple vessel-tissue interfaces
  - ± posterior shadowing: Not typically seen with other masses
  - Larger tumors usually have prominent vascularity evident on color Doppler
  - US alone is not reliable in diagnosing AML; significant overlap with RCC
- **Renal Cell Carcinoma**
  - 30% of small RCCs appear as hyperechoic masses, may mimic AML
    - Presence of necrosis in mass, cystic components, internal calcifications, or anechoic rim favors RCC but large overlap

  - Larger RCC may have foci of calcification (also echogenic), rarely fat
  - Mass with calcification and fat raises concern for RCC

Helpful Clues for Less Common Diagnoses

- **Fat in Renal Scar**
  - e.g., following partial nephrectomy
    - Fat may be placed into cortical defect
    - Ablation zone post ablation may appear echogenic (fat-halo sign)
- **Renal Junctional Line/Cortical Parenchymal Defect**
  - Echogenic line at anterosuperior aspect, upper pole of right kidney, lower pole of left kidney
    - Infolding of renal capsule and fat creates hyperechoic line or mass
  - Also can see extension of renal sinus fat into same location
  - Less commonly appears as triangular focus known as parenchymal defect
- **Renal Calculi**
  - Highly echogenic with sharp posterior shadowing
  - Calculi or milk of calcium may form within calyceal diverticulum, mimic hyperechoic mass
  - Most stones show color and power Doppler twinkling artifacts
    - Useful ancillary finding in equivocal cases (though twinkling may be seen without underlying stone)
- **Medullary Nephrocalcinosis**
  - Echogenic medullary pyramids; may be peripheral echogenicity early
  - Highly echogenic renal medulla; may simulate echogenic mass
- **Column of Bertin**
  - Renal cortex protruding into renal sinus: Between upper and midcalyces
  - Typically isoechoic to cortex, though alterations in tissue orientation change acoustic reflectivity
  - Column may be echogenic when seen en face
    - Doppler may confirm cortex origin; CECT for problematic cases
- **Renal Papillary Necrosis**
  - Early stage: Echogenic ring in medulla = necrotic papillae, surrounded by rim of fluid
  - Late stage: Multiple cystic cavities in medullary pyramids ± nonshadowing echogenic sloughed papillae
  - Calcified sloughed papilla with strong acoustic shadowing simulates stone, may cause obstructive hydronephrosis
- **Complex Cyst/Milk of Calcium Cyst**
  - Bright, echogenic reflectors with ring-down artifact may be seen within septa of minimally complex renal cysts; may be ignored
  - Milk of calcium cyst: Layering calcification may create fluid/debris level
- **Emphysematous Pyelonephritis**
  - Gas within infarcted, infected parenchyma is echogenic
    - Nondependent linear echogenic lines with strong distal posterior acoustic shadowing
  - Clinically, extremely ill patient with fever, flank pain, and electrolyte imbalance

- o Different from emphysematous pyelitis where gas is limited to renal pelvis and calyces (less serious diagnosis)
- **Renal Metastases**
  - o Variable echogenicity, typically hypoperfused masses
  - o Look for metastases in other organs
  - o Most common primary tumors include lung carcinoma, breast carcinoma, contralateral RCC
- **Acute Pyelonephritis**
  - o Although pyelonephritis is common, sonographic manifestations are usually not seen
  - o When present, wedge-shaped area of increased echogenicity within parenchyma
  - o Decreased focal vascularity on Doppler US in involved portion of kidney
  - o Can be hypoechoic, related to liquefaction and abscess formation
  - o Can be multiple lesions with patchy, heterogeneous renal parenchyma
  - o Other associated features of renal inflammation: Renal enlargement, urothelial thickening of renal pelvis, and bladder debris

Helpful Clues for Rare Diagnoses

- **Xanthogranulomatous Pyelonephritis**
  - o Highly reflective central echo complex with strong shadowing corresponding to large staghorn stone
  - o Echogenicity depends on amount of debris and necrosis within masses
- **Tuberculosis, Urinary Tract**
  - o Active stage: Papillary destruction with echogenic masses near calyces
  - o Late stage: Calcified granuloma or dense dystrophic calcification associated with shrunken kidneys
- **Renal Oncocytoma**
  - o Cannot be differentiated from RCC on imaging
  - o Variable in echogenicity; may contain central scar, central necrosis, or calcification
- **Renal Trauma**
  - o Hematoma can be hyperechoic or heterogeneous during acute phase
  - o Regional distortion of corticomedullary differentiation

Renal Angiomyolipoma

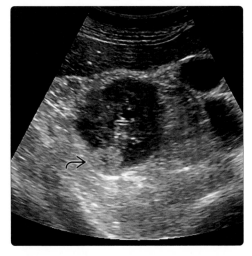

Renal Angiomyolipoma

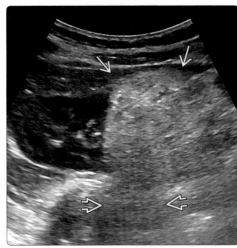

(Left) *Axial US shows a 1.3-cm, uniform, highly echogenic lesion ⤷. Although small renal lesions are likely angiomyolipomas (AMLs) (as in this case), CT confirmation is typically recommended to exclude small renal cell carcinomas (RCCs).* **(Right)** *Sagittal US shows a huge, weakly shadowing, echogenic lower pole AML ➡. Shadowing ⤳ is likely due to interspersed fat and soft tissue components. Large AMLs may hemorrhage.*

Renal Angiomyolipoma

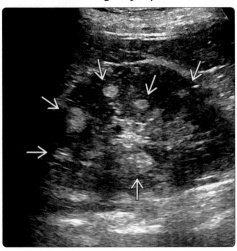

Renal Angiomyolipoma

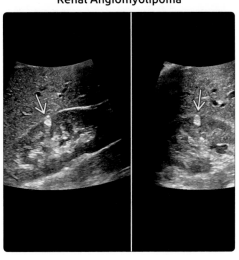

(Left) *Sagittal US shows many small, echogenic angiomyelolipomas ➡ in a patient with tuberous sclerosis.* **(Right)** *Sagittal and transverse US of the right kidney show a < 1-cm, highly echogenic renal lesion ➡. Echogenicity is greater than sinus fat. Recent work has suggested that these tiny lesions may be ignored, but current dogma is that targeted NECT confirmation of fat or US follow-up is needed.*

(Left) *Sagittal US in a 55-year-old woman with flank pain shows an echogenic right interpolar renal lesion* ➡️. *Note cystic spaces* ➡️ *and halo* ➡️. *Partial nephrectomy performed after staging CT confirmed clear cell RCC.* (Right) *Surveillance US in a patient with cirrhosis and splenomegaly* ➡️ *shows an echogenic left renal lesion* ➡️. *Sonographic features that suggest RCC include hypoechoic halo* ➡️ *and tiny cystic spaces* ➡️. *Biopsy confirmed clear cell RCC.*

Renal Cell Carcinoma

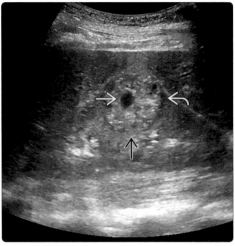

Renal Cell Carcinoma

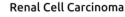
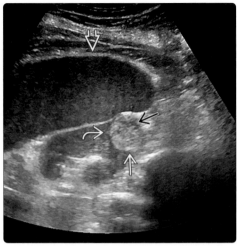

(Left) *Sagittal US in a patient with atherosclerosis and renal insufficiency shows an echogenic interpolar lesion* ➡️. *Real-time US examination and coronal CT confirmed an old renal infarct and invaginating retroperitoneal fat within a renal scar.* (Right) *Sagittal US of a young male patient with right upper quadrant pain shows a junctional cortical defect* ➡️. *This line occurs at a plane of embryologic fusion of renunculi (embryologic elements forming kidneys) and is typically seen at the upper and middle 1/3 of the kidney.*

Fat in Renal Scar

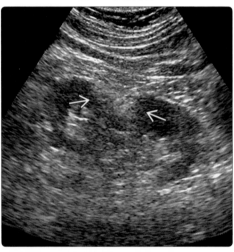

Renal Junctional Line/Cortical Parenchymal Defect

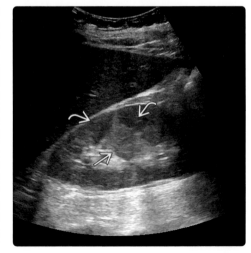

(Left) *Sagittal US of a patient with hematuria shows highly echogenic renal medulla* ➡️. *These medullary rings are thought to be due to the dilated collecting tubules of medullary sponge kidney. When viewed transversely, echogenic medulla may simulate a mass.* (Right) *Sagittal US shows a band of cortical tissue* ➡️ *separating pyramids* ➡️ *of renal medulla, a column of Bertin. When viewed en face, columns may appear echogenic. Color Doppler US or CECT may confirm normal invaginating cortex.*

Medullary Nephrocalcinosis

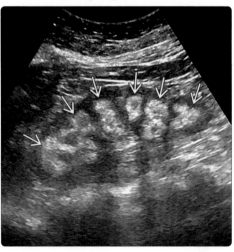

Column of Bertin

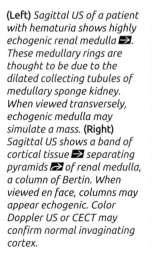

Complex Cyst/Milk of Calcium Cyst

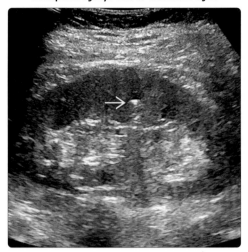

Emphysematous Pyelonephritis

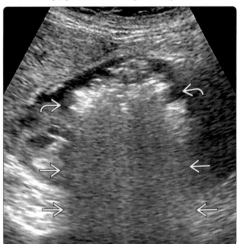

(Left) *Sagittal US in a patient with flank pain shows punctate echogenicity and a subtle posterior comet-tail artifact within the back wall of a tiny cyst ➡. Layering crystals (milk of calcium) within cysts or calyceal diverticula may be confused with calculi, though note the absence of shadowing.* (Right) *Sagittal US in a patient with diabetes and sepsis shows most of the right kidney replaced by amorphous echogenicity ➡. "Dirty" posterior shadowing ➡ is due to the gas of emphysematous pyelonephritis.*

Acute Pyelonephritis

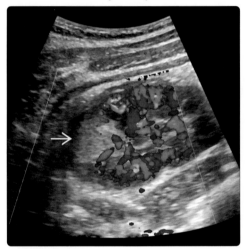

Acute Pyelonephritis

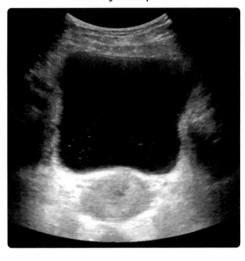

(Left) *Color Doppler US shows a wedge-shaped area of increased echogenicity involving the superior pole of the right kidney ➡, corresponding with decreased perfusion.* (Right) *In the same patient, debris is seen in the bladder, which correlates with pyuria seen on urinalysis. The patient was diagnosed with acute pyelonephritis.*

Tuberculosis, Urinary Tract

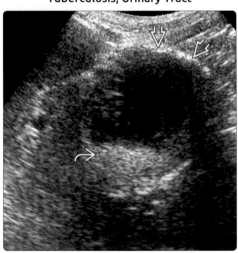

Renal Oncocytoma

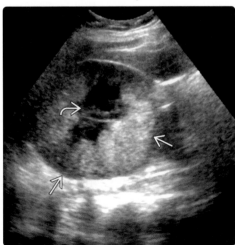

(Left) *Transverse US shows a renal tuberculosis abscess with a calcified wall ➡ and internal echogenic debris ➡. Abscess formation is secondary to stricture at the calyceal infundibulum.* (Right) *Longitudinal US shows a large, mildly hyperechoic mass ➡ within the right kidney. It has a spiculated, central hypoechoic scar ➡, which is suggestive of an oncocytoma; however, RCC cannot be excluded, and excision is required.*

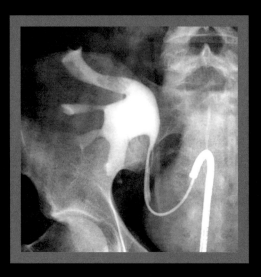

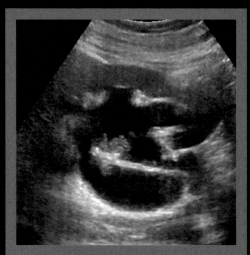

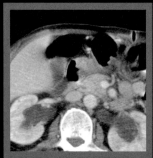

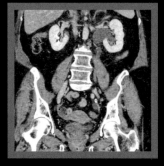

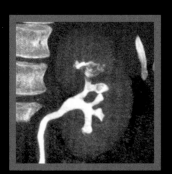

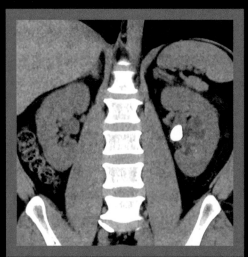

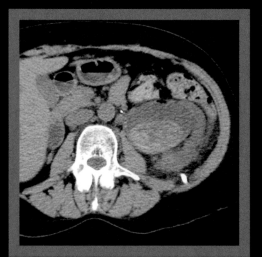

SECTION 16
Collecting System

Dilated Renal Calyces   566

Filling Defect, Renal Pelvis   570

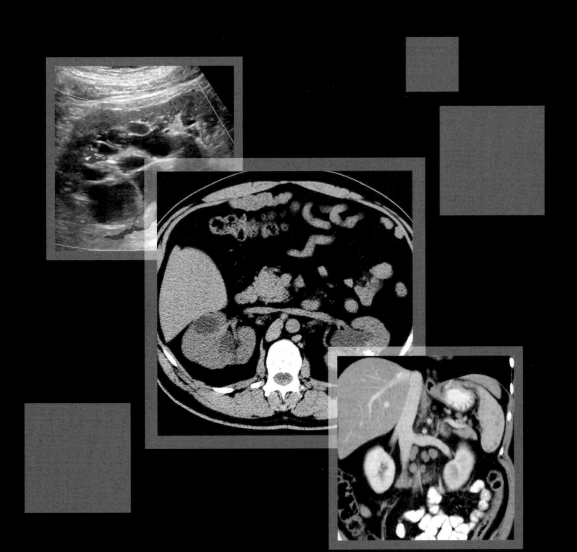

DIFFERENTIAL DIAGNOSIS

Common

- Ureteral Obstruction
  - Ureteral Stone
  - Urothelial Carcinoma
  - Retroperitoneal Fibrosis
  - Periureteral Metastases
  - Primary Pelvic Malignancy
    - Prostate Carcinoma
    - Rectal Carcinoma
    - Cervical and Endometrial Carcinoma
- Ureterectasis of Pregnancy
- Ureteral Duplication
- Distended Urinary Bladder
- Vesicoureteral Reflux
- Prominent Extrarenal Pelvis (Mimic)
- Renal Sinus Cysts (Mimic)
- Ureteropelvic Junction Obstruction
- Pyonephrosis

Less Common

- Pyelonephritis, Xanthogranulomatous
- Calyceal Diverticulum
- Renal Papillary Necrosis
- Renal Tuberculosis
- Megacalycosis, Megaureter
- Blood-Filled Renal Pelvis

ESSENTIAL INFORMATION

Key Differential Diagnosis Issues

- Determine if all calyces are dilated and in communication with dilated renal pelvis and ureter
- CT and MR are complementary to US
  - Include pyelographic (delayed)-phase-enhanced images

Helpful Clues for Common Diagnoses

- **Ureteral Obstruction**
  - Most common cause with several specific etiologies (calculi, tumor, etc.)
  - CT and MR better than US at showing etiology of ureteral obstruction
  - **Ureteral stone**
    - Dilated ureter ends at high-density intraluminal focus
  - **Urothelial carcinoma**
    - Several different imaging appearances depending on location and size (in order of frequency)
      □ Bladder cancer may obstruct ureteral orifice → hydronephrosis
      □ Large infiltrative renal mass obstructing collecting system
      □ Wall thickening or filling defect in renal pelvis > ureter
  - **Retroperitoneal fibrosis**
    - Encases and obstructs ureters through lumbar region
    - Mantle of soft tissue surrounds aorta and inferior vena cava
    - Secondary retroperitoneal fibrosis occurs due to malignancy (typically retroperitoneal lymph nodes) often after treatment

  - **Periureteral metastases**
    - Mass adjacent to ureter or within wall
    - Typical malignancies: Breast, lymphoma, melanoma
  - **Primary pelvic malignancy**
    - Dilated ureter ends in soft tissue density mass or retroperitoneal nodes that encase ureter
- **Ureterectasis of Pregnancy**
  - Due to hormonal influence + mass effect of gravid uterus
  - Affects right kidney more than left
  - May persist after pregnancy
  - May be difficult to distinguish from obstructing stone when presenting with flank pain
    - MR useful, as it will show perinephric fluid in obstruction; otherwise, low-dose CT appropriate
- **Ureteral Duplication**
  - Upper pole ureter is more often ectopic in insertion and dilated
  - Look for 2 ureters on 1 side; upper pole ureter will have delayed concentration and excretion of contrast medium if it is obstructed
  - Either ureter can be obstructed by calculi and other etiologies
- **Distended Urinary Bladder**
  - May cause back pressure and dilation of ureters and calyces
  - Reimage after emptying bladder
    - Should return to normal caliber
- **Vesicoureteral Reflux**
  - Acute or chronic dilation of ureter and calyces; scarred parenchyma
- **Prominent Extrarenal Pelvis (Mimic)**
  - Calyces and ureter not dilated
  - Common and asymptomatic
- **Renal Sinus Cysts (Mimic)**
  - Very common
  - Diagnosis is based on demonstration of lack of communication of cysts with each other or renal pelvis
  - Cysts often oval or irregular shape with discrete walls and nontypical blunted calyx shape
  - Delayed imaging on CECT usually unnecessary to distinguish renal sinus cysts from hydronephrosis, as appearance differs significantly
- **Ureteropelvic Junction Obstruction**
  - Relatively common congenital narrowing at ureteropelvic junction (UPJ) that often results in striking dilation of pelvis and calyces, especially with fluid or diuretic challenge
  - May be due to crossing vessel that compresses UPJ
  - Typically diagnosed in childhood, occasionally first diagnosed in adults
- **Pyonephrosis**
  - Hydronephrosis + infected urine; often require urgent nephrostomy
  - Diffuse urothelial thickening and enhancement is key to diagnosis (± pyelonephritis findings)
    - Stone, malignancy, and other mechanical causes of dilation usually do not show this
  - Fluid may be higher than water density on CT; fluid-debris level on US

Helpful Clues for Less Common Diagnoses

- **Pyelonephritis, Xanthogranulomatous**
  - Underlying calculi may cause hydro- or pyonephrosis
  - Xanthomatous replacement of parenchyma may be low density, mimicking caliectasis
- **Calyceal Diverticulum**
  - Outpouching from calyx may simulate focal caliectasis
  - Obstructing stone may be present at apex
- **Renal Papillary Necrosis**
  - Calyces may appear blunted and dilated due to sloughed papillae
- **Renal Tuberculosis**
  - May cause stricture of infundibula and focal hydronephrosis
  - Caseous infection of parenchyma may mimic caliectasis
- **Megacalycosis, Megaureter**
  - Rare congenital anomalies, often incidental in adult
  - Megacalycosis: Dilated calyces with renal pelvis or ureter dilation
  - Megaureter: Ureter dilation ± calyceal dilation

- Range of etiology (obstruction due to adynamic distal segment, reflux, or neither)
  - Renal function may remain normal
- **Blood-Filled Renal Pelvis**
  - Trauma or coagulopathic hemorrhage may distend renal pelvis and calyces with blood

SELECTED REFERENCES

1. Campo I et al: Magnetic resonance urography of congenital abnormalities - what the radiologist needs to know. Pediatr Radiol. 52(5):985-97, 2021
2. Houat AP et al: Congenital anomalies of the upper urinary tract: a comprehensive review. Radiographics. 42(2):462-86, 2021
3. Sweet DE et al: Infiltrative renal malignancies: imaging features, prognostic implications, and mimics. Radiographics. 41(2):487-508, 2021
4. Ali O et al: Upper urinary tract urothelial carcinoma on multidetector CT: spectrum of disease. Abdom Radiol (NY). 44(12):3874-85, 2019

Ureteral Obstruction

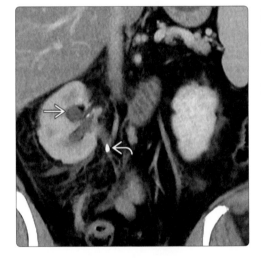

Ureteral Stone

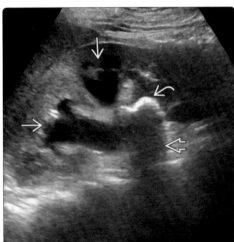

(Left) *Coronal CECT shows mild hydronephrosis ➡ due to an obstructing ureteropelvic junction (UPJ) stone ➡. This is the 2nd most common location of stone obstruction.* (Right) *Longitudinal US of the right kidney shows dilated calyces ➡ due to a large obstructing renal pelvic stone ➡. Note the posterior acoustic shadow ➡.*

Urothelial Carcinoma

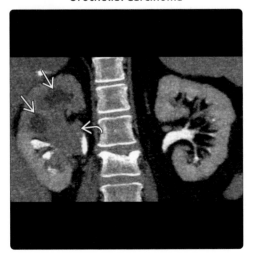

Urothelial Carcinoma

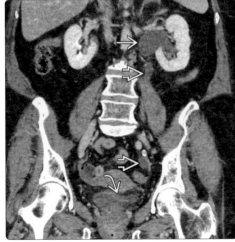

(Left) *Coronal CTU MIP image shows dilated right upper pole calyces ➡ due to obstruction by a large infiltrative mass ➡ in the renal hilum and renal pelvis, typical of urothelial carcinoma.* (Right) *Coronal CECT shows left hydronephrosis ➡ and hydroureter ➡ due to an obstructing bladder carcinoma ➡.*

(Left) *Axial CECT shows a dilated left renal pelvis and calyces ➡. Notice the thick, irregular rind of soft tissue ➡ around the aorta. Lower sections (not shown) showed ureter encasement by the fibrosis.* **(Right)** *Coronal T1 C+ FS MR shows severely dilated calyces ➡ in the left upper pole moiety of a duplicated collecting system. Other images showed a dilated ectopic ureter inserting on the vagina.*

Retroperitoneal Fibrosis

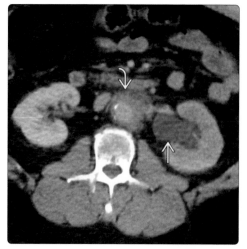

Ureteral Duplication

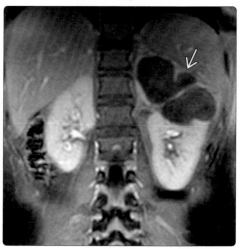

(Left) *Axial CECT shows bilateral dilation of the calyces and ureters ➡ in an 80-year-old man with benign prostatic hyperplasia (BPH) and a distended urinary bladder. These findings resolved after catheterization of the bladder.* **(Right)** *Axial CECT in the same patient shows distention of the urinary bladder ➡ due to prostatic hypertrophy.*

Distended Urinary Bladder

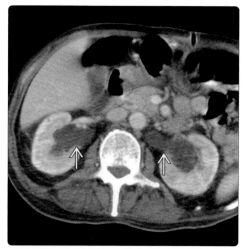

Distended Urinary Bladder

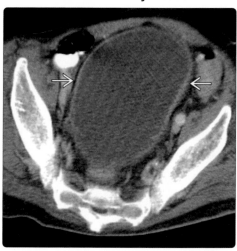

(Left) *Axial NECT shows dilated calyces ➡ bilaterally due to chronic reflux. Note the cortical calcifications ➡ associated with the cortical scarring.* **(Right)** *Axial CECT shows a dilated renal pelvis ➡ without calyceal dilation ➡. This is a normal variant, which should not be confused with hydronephrosis, that would show calyceal dilation.*

Vesicoureteral Reflux

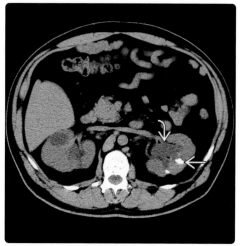

Prominent Extrarenal Pelvis (Mimic)

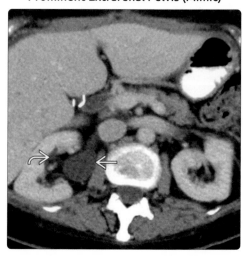

Renal Sinus Cysts (Mimic)

Renal Sinus Cysts (Mimic)

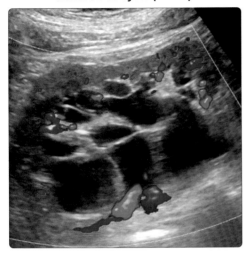

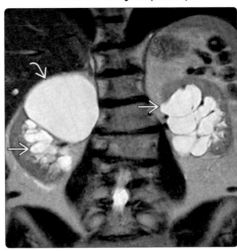

(Left) *Longitudinal color Doppler US of the kidney shows multiple large cysts in the renal pelvis. This could be confused for hydronephrosis, but notice the lack of communication between the cysts and discrete walls.* (Right) *Coronal T2 MR shows multiple large renal sinus cysts ➡. Notice the discrete wall and lack of intercommunication, which distinguishes this from hydronephrosis. A large renal cortical cyst ➡ is also seen.*

Renal Sinus Cysts (Mimic)

Ureteropelvic Junction Obstruction

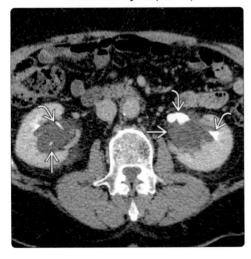

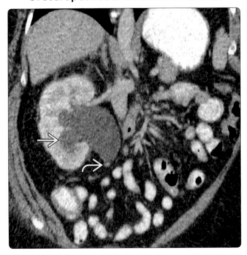

(Left) *Axial delayed CTU shows multiple large cysts ➡ in the renal sinus bilaterally. Normal, nondilated renal pelvis and calyces ➡ can be seen. Such large cysts can mimic hydronephrosis but generally have a different morphology and do not communicate.* (Right) *Double-oblique reformatted CECT shows hydronephrosis ➡ of the right kidney with delayed nephrogram. Notice the severe dilation of the renal pelvis with abrupt narrowing at the UPJ ➡.*

Pyonephrosis

Pyelonephritis, Xanthogranulomatous

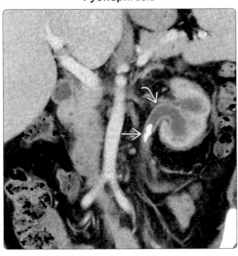

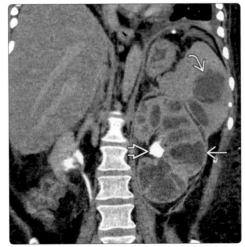

(Left) *Coronal CECT shows an obstructing UPJ stone ➡. Also notice the urothelial thickening and enhancement ➡ in this patient who presented with pyonephrosis and required urgent collecting system drainage.* (Right) *Coronal CECT shows an enlarged left kidney with markedly dilated calyces ➡ and a central, large renal stone ➡. XGP can sometimes extend beyond the kidney into other organs or the flank soft tissues, as in this case with collections in the spleen ➡. Patient required nephrectomy and splenectomy.*

DIFFERENTIAL DIAGNOSIS

Common

- Urolithiasis
- Blood Clot
  - Trauma
  - Coagulopathic Hemorrhage
  - Tumor, Pseudoaneurysm
- Urothelial Carcinoma
- Gas in Collecting System
  - Emphysematous Pyelitis/Pyelonephritis
  - Instrumentation of Kidney

Less Common

- Renal Cell Carcinoma
- Renal Papillary Necrosis
- Fungus Ball
- Papilloma

ESSENTIAL INFORMATION

Key Differential Diagnosis Issues

- Differential of stone, blood, tumor, gas is typically easy based on CT density and enhancement

Helpful Clues for Common Diagnoses

- **Urolithiasis**
  - Almost all calculi are dense on CT and are easy to distinguish from other etiologies
- **Blood Clot**
  - Almost always have gross hematuria; history of trauma (including biopsy, intervention), anticoagulation helpful
  - CT: Hyperdense filling defect (NECT: 60-80 HU); no enhancement, conforms to shape of collecting system
    - ± hydronephrosis ± reactive urothelial thickening/enhancement
  - May see concomitant bladder clot
  - If unexplained bleeding, look for underlying tumor or pseudoaneurysm if recent intervention
- **Urothelial Carcinoma**
  - Irregular or smooth filing defect with avid enhancement

  - Other patterns: Wall thickening and enhancement; diffuse, infiltrative mass
  - Renal pelvis is 2nd most common site (bladder is most common)
  - Usually seen in men > 60 years of age; history of smoking or exposure to chemical
- **Gas in Collecting System**
  - Iatrogenic: Ureteral stent, nephrostomy
  - Emphysematous pyelitis: Gas, infection limited to urine
  - Pyonephrosis: US may show layering debris or echogenic urine

Helpful Clues for Less Common Diagnoses

- **Renal Cell Carcinoma**
  - May protrude into pelvis, compressing collecting system, or directly invade collecting system
  - CT/MR: Expansile enhancing filling defect contiguous with renal mass
- **Renal Papillary Necrosis**
  - Associated with NSAIDs abuse, sickle cell disease; also seen with opportunistic infections and TB
  - Blunted calyx, sloughed papillae as filling defect in upper urinary tract
  - CTU: Ball on tee sign → collection of contrast in necrotic papilla cavity (ball) adjacent to calyx (tee)
- **Fungus Ball**
  - Classically *Candida* spp., many others described
  - Usually seen in debilitated, older patients or with chronic indwelling nephrostomy tubes
- **Papilloma**
  - Benign uroepithelial neoplasm, which typically are found around bladder neck and rarely in upper urinary tract
  - Indistinguishable from urothelial cancer

SELECTED REFERENCES

1. Shampain KL et al: Benign diseases of the urinary tract at CT and CT urography. Abdom Radiol (NY). 44(12):3811-26, 2019

Urolithiasis

Urolithiasis

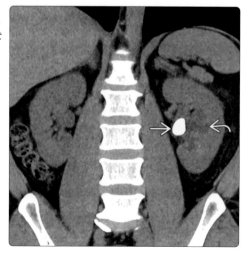

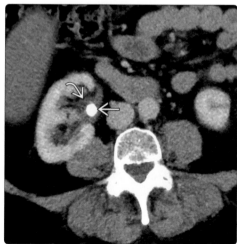

(Left) Coronal NECT shows a hyperdense filling defect ➡ in the left renal pelvis, consistent with stone. Note mild hydronephrosis ➡. (Right) Axial CECT shows a hyperdense stone ➡ in the renal pelvis. Note the surrounding urothelial thickening and enhancement ➡, which is often reactive to chronic stone disease.

Tumor, Pseudoaneurysm

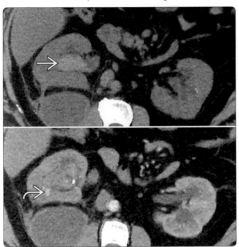

Blood Clot

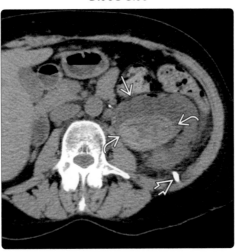

(Left) *Axial NECT in a patient who had recently undergone percutaneous nephrolithotomy shows a hyperdense filling defect ➡ conforming to the renal pelvis, consistent with clot. Axial CECT shows the small parenchymal blush ➡, which was a bleeding pseudoaneurysm.* (Right) *Axial NECT shows a markedly dilated renal pelvis ➡ due to ureter obstruction. Note the oval, hyperdense clot ➡ layering, which was a complication of nephrostomy ➡ placement.*

Trauma

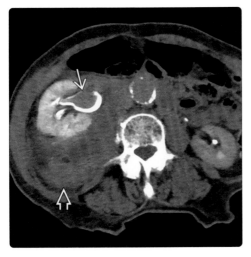

Coagulopathic Hemorrhage

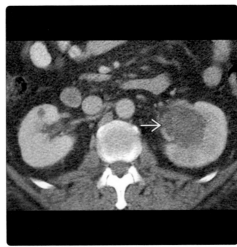

(Left) *Axial delayed-phase CECT after trauma shows a large filling defect ➡ conforming to the renal pelvis, consistent with clot. A large, perinephric hemorrhage ➡ is also seen.* (Right) *Axial CECT in a patient with a history of hematuria on anticoagulation shows heterogeneous, slightly hyperdense blood expanding the left renal pelvis ➡. Also note the delayed left nephrogram due to obstruction.*

Urothelial Carcinoma

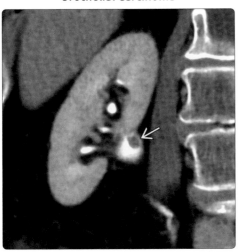

Urothelial Carcinoma

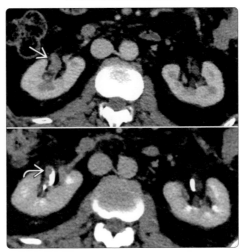

(Left) *Coronal CTU in a 69-year-old man with history of bladder cancer shows a small, round, smooth filling defect ➡ in the renal pelvis.* (Right) *Axial CECT shows an enhancing filling defect ➡ mildly expanding the right renal pelvis. Delayed phase shows irregular margins ➡.*

(Left) *Axial corticomedullary-phase CTU in a 79-year-old man with hematuria shows an enhancing mass* ➡ *in the left renal pelvis with ill-defined margins.* (Right) *Axial delayed-phase CTU in the same patient shows the mass* ➡ *filling the collecting system with a slightly irregular margin. High-grade urothelial cancer was found at biopsy.*

Urothelial Carcinoma

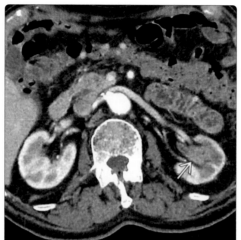

Urothelial Carcinoma

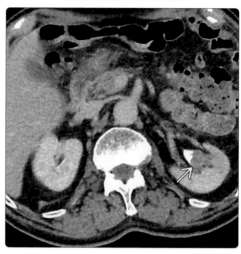

(Left) *Axial NECT shows a vague, hyperdense filling defect in the pelvis* ➡ *with hydronephrosis* ➡. *Note enhancement of the lesion* ➡. *Delayed phase shows the filling defect well* ➡. *High-grade urothelial cancer was found at biopsy. All 3 phases are helpful for diagnosing urothelial cancer on CTU.* (Right) *Retrograde pyelogram shows an irregular filling defect* ➡ *in the upper pole calyx and infundibulum of a renal allograft in a patient who had gross hematuria. The lesion was confirmed to be urothelial carcinoma.*

Urothelial Carcinoma

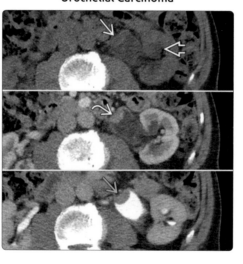

Urothelial Carcinoma

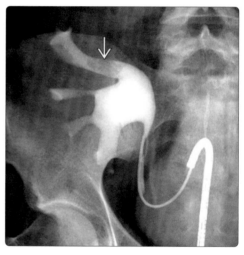

(Left) *Coronal NECT in a septic, diabetic, older patient shows gas in the renal pelvis* ➡ *and proximal ureter* ➡. *Note the extensive stranding and fluid* ➡ *around the kidney.* (Right) *Axial CECT in a patient with percutaneous nephrostomy* ➡ *shows gas* ➡ *within the left collecting system, which is iatrogenic due to instrumentation. The patient did not have signs of urinary infection.*

Emphysematous Pyelitis/Pyelonephritis

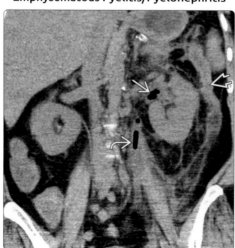

Instrumentation of Kidney

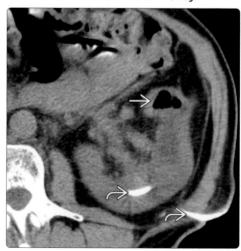

Emphysematous Pyelitis/Pyelonephritis

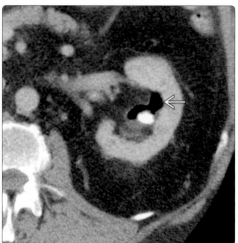

Renal Cell Carcinoma

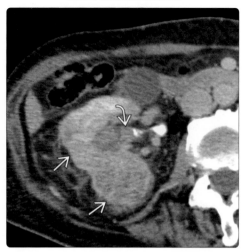

(Left) *Axial CECT in an older adult man with signs and symptoms of urinary tract infection shows gas within the renal pelvis ➡ without parenchymal gas, consistent with emphysematous pyelitis.* (Right) *Axial CTU shows a large, enhancing, exophytic renal mass ➡ most typical of renal cell carcinoma. The filling defect in the renal pelvis ➡ represents collecting system invasion, which is sometimes seen, though much less often than renal vein invasion.*

Renal Papillary Necrosis

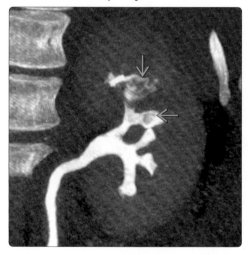

Fungus Ball

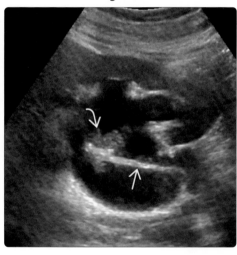

(Left) *Coronal CECT MIP shows filling defects ➡ within the upper pole calyces, representing sloughed papillae (and, possibly, hemorrhage) in this patient with a history of papillary necrosis in the setting of sickle cell disease.* (Right) *Longitudinal US in an immunocompromised patient with candiduria shows severe hydronephrosis and an ureter stent ➡. Note the echogenic filling defect ➡ in the pelvis surrounding the stent, which was a fungus ball adhered to the stent/foreign body.*

Papilloma

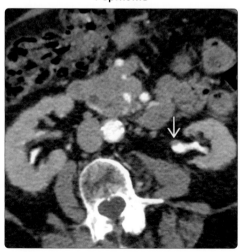

Papilloma

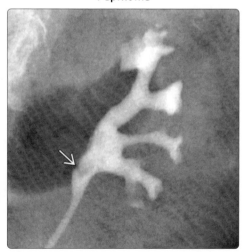

(Left) *Axial CTU in a patient with hematuria shows a tiny filling defect ➡ in the left renal pelvis. Urothelial carcinoma was suspected.* (Right) *Retrograde pyelogram in the same patient shows the tiny filling defect ➡ in the pelvis. Biopsy revealed papilloma, a benign lesion, which is rare and generally indistinguishable from urothelial carcinoma.*

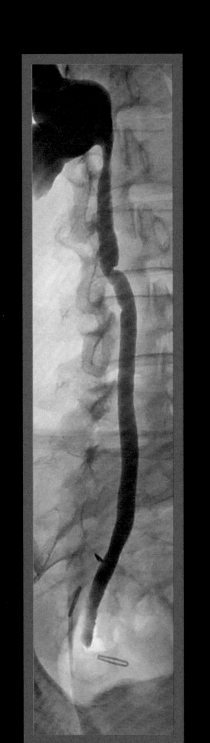
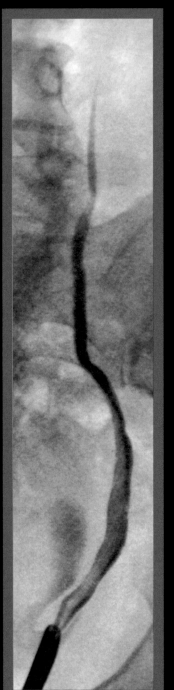
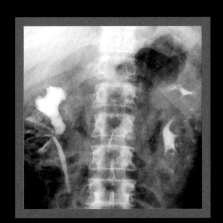
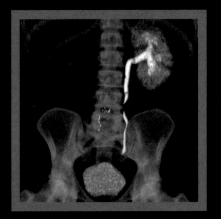
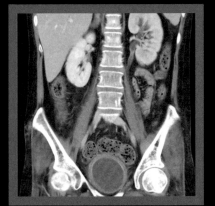

SECTION 17
Ureter

Generic Imaging Patterns

Ureteral Filling Defect or Stricture   576
Cystic Dilation of Distal Ureter   580

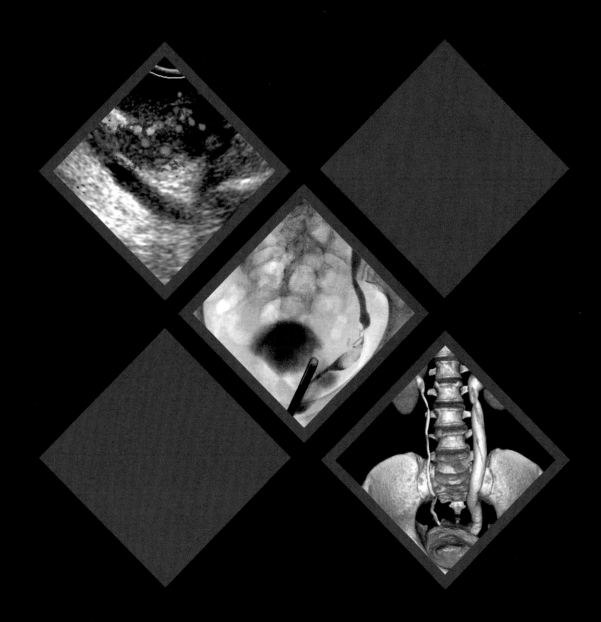

DIFFERENTIAL DIAGNOSIS

Common

- Iatrogenic and Postoperative
- Urolithiasis
- Urothelial Carcinoma
- Retroperitoneal Metastasis

Less Common

- Locally Advanced Pelvic Cancer
- Retroperitoneal Fibrosis
- Infectious Ureteritis
- Blood Clot

Rare but Important

- Endometriosis
- Sloughed Papilla
- Ureteritis Cystica
- Vascular Compression
- Ureteral Papilloma
- Ureteral Fibroepithelial Polyp
- IgG4-Related Disease
- Vasculitis
- Malakoplakia
- Congenital Midureteral Stricture

ESSENTIAL INFORMATION

Helpful Clues for Common Diagnoses

- **Iatrogenic and Postoperative**
  - Most common etiology
  - Seen after lithotomy, ureteroscopy, ureteral stents
  - Most common site of postoperative stricture is at site of anastomosis of ureter to bladder, neobladder, or ileal conduit
  - Also seen following nonurologic abdominal surgeries
    - May result from ischemic injury to ureter if retroperitoneal surgery disrupts blood supply
    - Alternatively can result from direct injury; look for adjacent clip
  - May occur at ureteropelvic junction (UPJ) or proximal ureter after nephron-sparing treatments (microwave/cryoablation or partial nephrectomy)
  - Also seen following radiation therapy for pelvic malignancy
- **Urolithiasis**
  - Almost all stones are dense at CT
  - 25% of patients with prolonged stone impaction (> 2 months) develop stricture
  - Most strictures are secondary to edema and are transient, resolving in 6-12 weeks
  - Most common location is ureterovesical junction (UVJ) > UPJ > midureter
- **Urothelial Carcinoma**
  - Intraluminal filling defect or focal wall thickening ± dilation of upstream ureter
  - More common in distal ureter (70%), presumably due to stasis
  - Rarely multiple synchronous sites of involvement (bladder, renal pelvis, contralateral ureter)
- **Retroperitoneal Metastasis**
  - May be to ureters themselves or, more commonly, to retroperitoneal nodes
  - Can encase/invade and obstruct ureters
  - Breast cancer has propensity to metastasize to ureter

Helpful Clues for Less Common Diagnoses

- **Locally Advanced Pelvic Cancer**
  - Cervical cancer: FIGO stage IIIB, hydronephrosis due to direct tumor extension to distal ureter
  - Rectal, prostate, bladder, and other GYN cancers may invade and obstruct ureter if advanced
  - Large pelvic masses can cause mass effect on ureter due to compression (at pelvic brim) rather than direct invasion
- **Retroperitoneal Fibrosis**
  - CT shows soft tissue encasing aorta and inferior vena cava of variable extent through lumbar region
  - Encases, obstructs, and medially displaces ureters
  - Majority associated with IgG4 disease
    - Look for other imaging manifestations (i.e., pancreas, biliary, renal)
- **Infectious Ureteritis**
  - TB causes multiple findings including irregularity, intraluminal filling defects, ulcerations, and strictures ("chronic granulomatous ureteritis")
    - Kidney and renal pelvis also generally involved
  - Schistosomiasis more often involves distal ureter strictures and diffuse, thin bladder calcification
    - Associated with ureteritis cystica and bladder squamous cell carcinoma
  - BK virus ureteritis occurs in hematopoietic cell transplant recipients and may show ureter wall thickening and enhancement ± structures
- **Blood Clot**
  - Patients with gross hematuria may form clots in the renal pelvis, which pass into ureter
  - Hyperdense filling defect in ureter with no enhancement
  - Other areas of blood clot in renal pelvis or bladder
  - May cause acute flank pain due to obstruction

Helpful Clues for Rare Diagnoses

- **Endometriosis**
  - Urinary tract involvement is more common in deep infiltrating endometriosis with bladder (85%) > > ureter (10%), kidney (4%), or urethra (2%)
  - Can be extrinsic (60%) involvement with ureter compression or intrinsic/invasive into ureter wall (40%)
  - History and patient's demographics are helpful clues
  - US: Hypoechoic nodule along hyperechoic walls of ureter or uterosacral ligament ± upstream dilation
  - MR: Focal ↓ T2 signal nodule along ureter
- **Sloughed Papilla**
  - Seen in setting of renal papillary necrosis
  - Usually multiple round or triangular-shaped filling defects in renal pelvis or ureter
  - Look for other findings of papillary necrosis
    - Ball-on-tee sign, lobster claw sign
- **Ureteritis Cystica**
  - Reactive proliferative changes of urothelium with formation of multiple small, subepithelial cysts in ureter wall

- Usually in proximal 1/3 of ureter
- Smooth, small nodular filling defects (2-3 mm)
- **Vascular Impression**
  - By artery, vein, or lymphatic
  - Classically occurs at UPJ and can cause UPJ obstruction
  - Look for aneurysm, collateral vessels
  - Vascular impressions are common in renal anomalies, such as ectopic or horseshoe kidney
    - Supernumerary vessels often cross and may obstruct collecting system
- **Ureteral Papilloma**
  - Usually small pedunculated mass indistinguishable from urothelial carcinoma
  - Found in bladder and less commonly UPJ and ureter
- **Ureteral Fibroepithelial Polyp**
  - Presents at younger age than urothelial carcinoma
  - Elongated, soft tissue density, intraluminal mass with smooth surface and enhancement ± hydroureter/hydronephrosis
  - May grow large and protrude into bladder
- **IgG4-Related Disease**
  - GU IgG4 disease most commonly involves kidneys in 1/3 - 1/4 of patients
  - Ureteral involvement is rare
  - 3 patterns of involvement: Polypoid mass, segmental ureter wall thickening, and periureteral fibrosis
    - All patterns can present with urinary obstruction
  - Often mimics urothelial carcinoma; look for other involved organs
- **Vasculitis**
  - Etiology: Necrotizing vasculitis, scleroderma, polyarteritis nodosa (PAN), Wegner granulomatosis, dermatomyositis, Henoch-Schönlein purpura, Churg-Strauss
  - Morphology: Short or long segment, single or multiple, unilateral or bilateral
  - CT: Ureteral wall thickening; calcification may be seen
- **Malakoplakia**
  - More common in immunosuppressed and diabetic patients

- Bladder is most frequently involved organ (40%) followed by renal parenchyma, upper urinary tract, prostate, and urethra
- Variable appearance ranging from flat plaques to nodules and masses ± ulceration
- Imaging findings overlap with urothelial cancer
- **Congenital Midureter Stricture**
  - Rare cause of congenital hydronephrosis
  - Typically short, focal stricture of midureter best diagnosed on retrograde urography

Other Essential Information

- Routine CT is able to detect and characterize ureteral strictures
  - When hydronephrosis is seen, ureter should always be followed to point of obstruction
- CT urography adds sensitivity and specificity, particularly for small and intraluminal masses
- Retrograde pyelography still essential for best depiction of intraluminal and mucosal ureteral pathologies and allows for biopsy &/or treatment
- Remember that there are normal areas of ureteral narrowing that should not be confused with stricture
  - Relative narrowing ± tortuosity at UPJ
  - Narrowing in midureter where it crosses over pelvic brim/iliac vessels
  - Narrowing at ureterovesical junction

SELECTED REFERENCES

1. Zahid M et al: Imaging of ureter: a primer for the emergency radiologist. Emerg Radiol. 28(4):815-37, 2021
2. Leonardi M et al: Endometriosis and the urinary tract: from diagnosis to surgical treatment. Diagnostics (Basel). 10(10), 2020
3. Moosavi B et al: Beyond ureterolithiasis: gamut of abnormalities affecting the ureter. Clin Imaging. 40(4):678-90, 2016
4. Potenta SE et al: CT urography for evaluation of the ureter. Radiographics. 140209, 2015

Iatrogenic and Postoperative

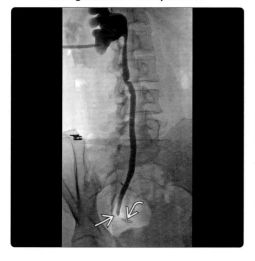

Iatrogenic and Postoperative

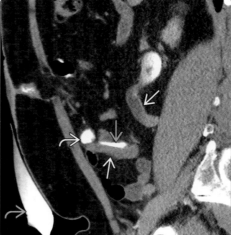

(Left) Antegrade nephrostogram in a woman post recent hysterectomy shows hydronephrosis and stricturing of the distal ureter ➡. Note the proximity of surgical clips ➡. GYN surgery is one of the most common causes of ureter injury. (Right) Sagittal CTU in a patient with an ileal loop urostomy shows a dilated and obstructed right ureter ➡ due to an anastomotic stricture at the ileal loop ➡. A normal distal left ureter ➡ containing contrast is also seen excreting into the loop and ostomy bag ➡.

Urolithiasis

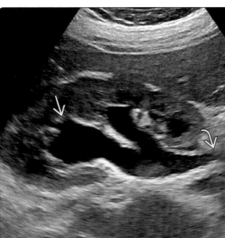

Urolithiasis

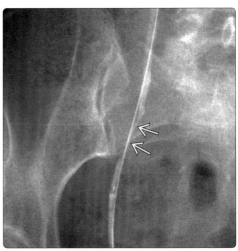

(Left) *Longitudinal US of the right kidney shows moderate hydronephrosis* ➡ *and proximal hydroureter* ⬈ *in a patient who had been treated for an impacted midureter stone several months ago. Subsequent CT (not shown) showed no recurrent obstructing stone.* (Right) *Retrograde pyelogram in the same patient, with a guidewire in the ureter, shows a focal stricture* ➡ *in the midureter that required treatment. The etiology was thought to be due to prolonged stone impaction.*

Urothelial Carcinoma

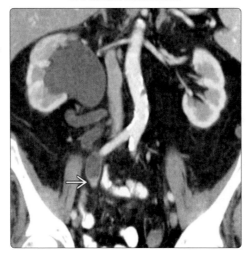

Urothelial Carcinoma

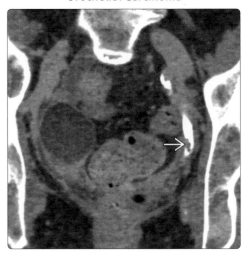

(Left) *Coronal CECT shows hydroureteronephrosis due to a midureteral stricture* ➡. *Note the focal wall thickening and enhancement of the ureter, confirmed to be urothelial carcinoma.* (Right) *Coronal CTU in a patient with bladder cancer shows an irregular intraluminal filling defect* ➡ *in the left distal ureter.*

Retroperitoneal Metastasis

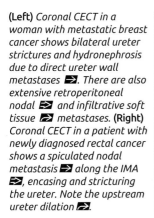

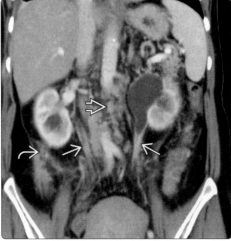

Retroperitoneal Metastasis

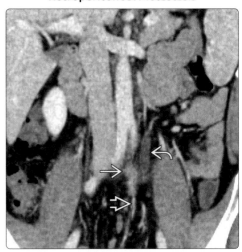

(Left) *Coronal CECT in a woman with metastatic breast cancer shows bilateral ureter strictures and hydronephrosis due to direct ureter wall metastases* ➡. *There are also extensive retroperitoneal nodal* ⬈ *and infiltrative soft tissue* ➡ *metastases.* (Right) *Coronal CECT in a patient with newly diagnosed rectal cancer shows a spiculated nodal metastasis* ➡ *along the IMA* ⬈, *encasing and stricturing the ureter. Note the upstream ureter dilation* ⬈.

Retroperitoneal Fibrosis

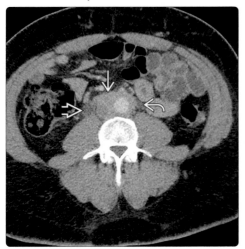

Retroperitoneal Fibrosis

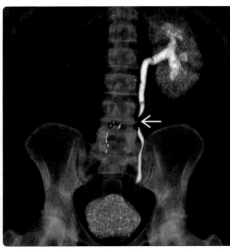

(Left) *Axial CECT shows a soft tissue rind* ➡️ *around the aorta with dilated right* ➡️ *and left* ➡️ *ureters.* (Right) *3D CTU in the same patient better shows the medialization and focal stricture of the left ureter* ➡️. *Note that the right ureter is not seen because the right kidney did not excrete contrast due to severe obstruction.*

Infectious Ureteritis

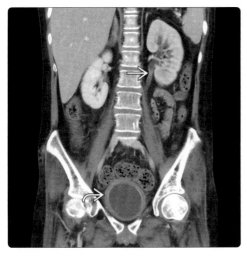

Ureteritis Cystica

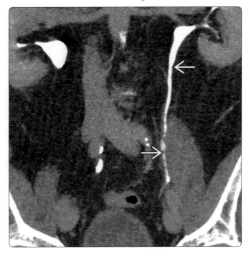

(Left) *Coronal CECT in a bone marrow transplant recipient shows proximal ureteral thickening, enhancement, and stricturing* ➡️ *with very mild upstream hydronephrosis. Note diffuse bladder wall thickening and enhancement* ➡️. *This was due to BK virus infection.* (Right) *Coronal CTU MIP shows multiple tiny, round filling defects* ➡️ *in the upper and midureter.*

Blood Clot

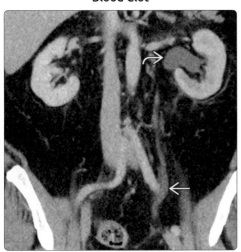

IgG4-Related Disease

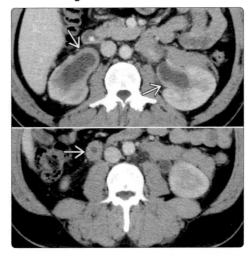

(Left) *Coronal CECT in a patient 1 day post left CT-guided renal mass biopsy, presenting with acute flank pain, shows a distended left midureter with subtle, hyperdense clot* ➡️. *Note the distended renal pelvis* ➡️ *due to obstruction.* (Right) *Axial CECT shows diffuse urothelial wall thickening* ➡️ *and enhancement resulting in stricturing and bilateral hydronephrosis. Other masses were seen in the prostate and inguinal canals, clues to a multiorgan disorder.*

DIFFERENTIAL DIAGNOSIS

Common

- Ureteral Obstruction
  - Stone, Tumor, Stricture
- Ureterocele
- Ectopic Ureter

Less Common

- Bladder Diverticulum (Mimic)
- Periureteral Cystic Lesions (Mimic)
- Congenital Megaureter

ESSENTIAL INFORMATION

Helpful Clues for Common Diagnoses

- **Ureteral Obstruction**
  - Urolithiasis > bladder tumor > ureteral tumor/stricture
  - CT and MR superior to US
- **Ureterocele**
  - Cystic dilation of distal ureter into bladder lumen
  - Classification scheme divides ureteroceles between intravesical and ectopic subtypes
    - **Intravesical**: Ureterocele is entirely in bladder
      - Cobra head or spring onion deformity of distal ureter with surrounding radiolucent halo
    - **Ectopic**: Insertion at bladder neck or in posterior urethra
      - Smooth, radiolucent intravesicular mass near bladder base
      - 80% seen in association with duplicated collecting system
  - Excretory-phase CT or MR urography are preferred imaging tools
  - Ureteroceles in adult are usually single collecting systems and orthotopic
- **Ectopic Ureter**
  - Inserts along developing mesonephric duct (precursor of trigone, epididymis, vas deferens, ejaculatory ducts, and seminal vesicles)
  - Mostly inserts outside bladder
    - Always above external sphincter in males
      - Prostatic urethra most common insertion site in male patients
    - Insertion is usually below sphincter in female patients, resulting in urinary incontinence
      - Urethra or vestibule most common insertion site in female patients
  - 80% occur in setting of duplication in pediatric population

Helpful Clues for Less Common Diagnoses

- **Bladder Diverticulum (Mimic)**
  - Usually multiple; may contain stones, debris, or tumor
  - Diverticula near ureterovesical junction may mimic ureteral dilatation (Hutch or acquired)
  - Color jet connecting to bladder very useful to distinguish diverticulum from other paravesical masses and from dilated ureter
- **Periureteral Cystic Lesions (Mimic)**
  - Seminal vesicle cyst and Gartner duct cyst may occasionally be confused with ureterocele
  - Knowing classic location of these cysts is helpful for differentiation; MR is helpful in selected cases to better delineate anatomy
- **Congenital Megaureter**
  - Megaureter: Encompasses spectrum of anomalies that lead to enlarged ureter (diameter ≥ 7 mm)
  - Primary obstructive megaureter: Functional obstruction at juxtavesical segment of ureter due to absent peristalsis

SELECTED REFERENCES

1. Campo I et al: Magnetic resonance urography of congenital abnormalities - what the radiologist needs to know. Pediatr Radiol. 52(5):985-97, 2021
2. Houat AP et al: Congenital anomalies of the upper urinary tract: a comprehensive review. Radiographics. 42(2):462-86, 2021
3. Adeb M et al: Magnetic resonance urography in evaluation of duplicated renal collecting systems. Magn Reson Imaging Clin N Am. 21(4):717-30, 2013
4. Shebel HM et al: Cysts of the lower male genitourinary tract: embryologic and anatomic considerations and differential diagnosis. Radiographics. 33(4):1125-43, 2013

Ureteral Obstruction

Ureterocele

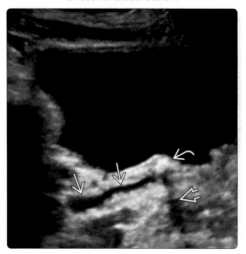 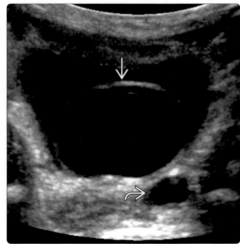

(Left) Oblique US of the bladder shows a dilated distal right ureter ➡ terminating in an echogenic stone ➡ at the ureterovesical junction. Note the posterior acoustic shadowing ➡. This is the most common location to find an obstructing stone. (Right) Transverse US in an 11-month-old girl shows a large cystic filling defect ➡ in the bladder associated with left ureter dilation ➡.

Ureterocele

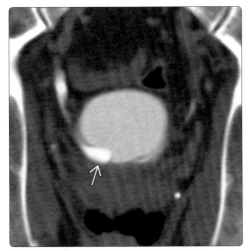

Ectopic Ureter

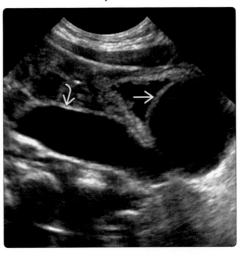

(Left) *Coronal delayed-phase CT urography shows a dilated distal ureter with a cobra head appearance* ➡ *protruding into the bladder lumen. This was an incidental intravesical ureterocele in a nonduplicated collecting system.* **(Right)** *Longitudinal US of the bladder shows a markedly dilated distal ureter* ➡ *in the setting of complete collecting system duplication. This ends in an ectopic location with an associated ureterocele* ➡.

Ectopic Ureter

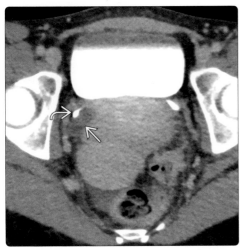

Bladder Diverticulum (Mimic)

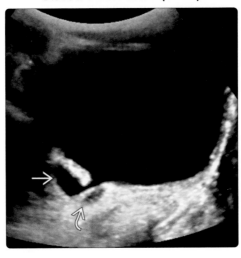

(Left) *Axial delayed-phase CT urography shows a dilated cystic structure* ➡ *posterior to the right ureter* ➡. *Other images (not shown) showed communication to a hydronephrotic upper pole renal moiety in a duplicated collecting system. This is an ectopic ureter, which inserted on the vagina.* **(Right)** *Transverse US of the bladder in a child shows a cystic lesion* ➡ *adjacent to the normal right ureter* ➡ *representing a small Hutch diverticulum. The neck of the diverticulum is well seen, which allows for confident diagnosis.*

Periureteral Cystic Lesions (Mimic)

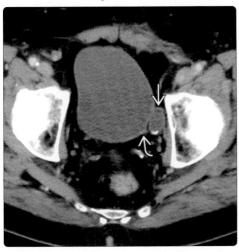

Congenital Megaureter

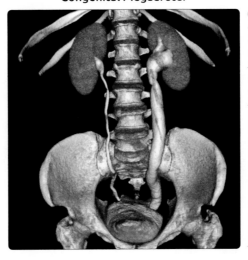

(Left) *Axial CECT shows a cystic tubular lesion* ➡ *along the posterolateral bladder wall containing a layering stone, which could be confused for the ureter. On close inspection, this is separate from the normal ureter* ➡ *and represents a bladder diverticulum.* **(Right)** *Coronal CECT shows diffuse dilation of the left ureter and calyces in a 55-year-old woman with repeated urinary tract infections and no evidence of reflux or obstruction. Note the absence of renal scarring or decreased function.*

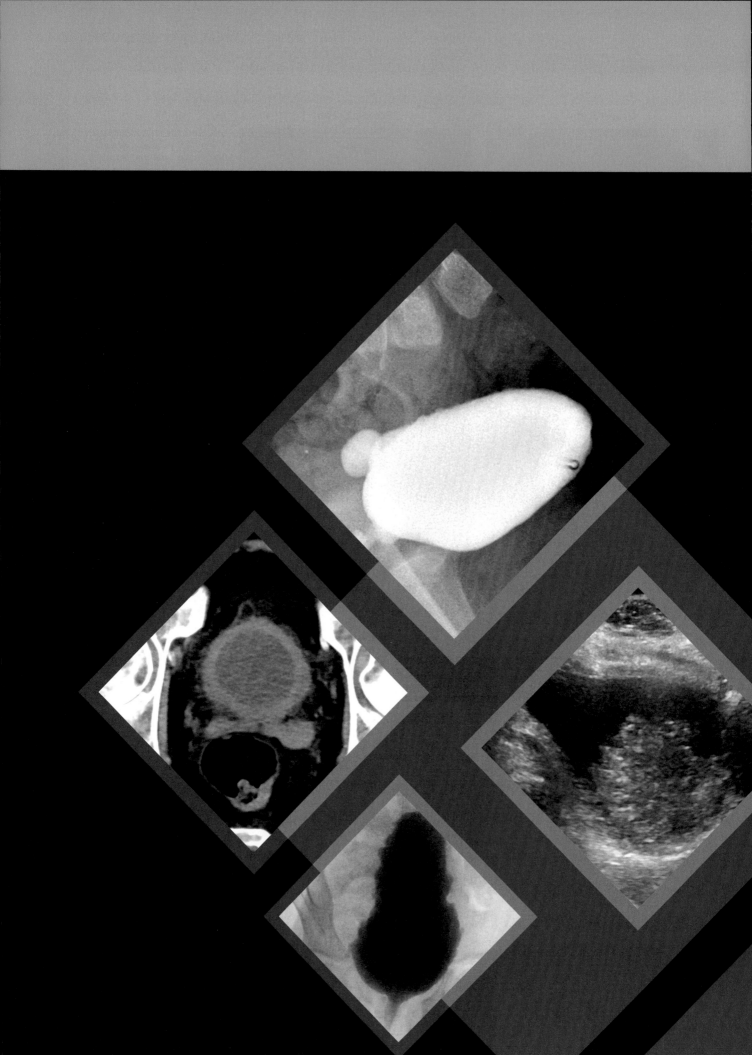

SECTION 18
Bladder

Generic Imaging Patterns

Filling Defect in Urinary Bladder — 584
Urinary Bladder Outpouching — 590
Gas Within Urinary Bladder — 592
Abnormal Bladder Wall — 594

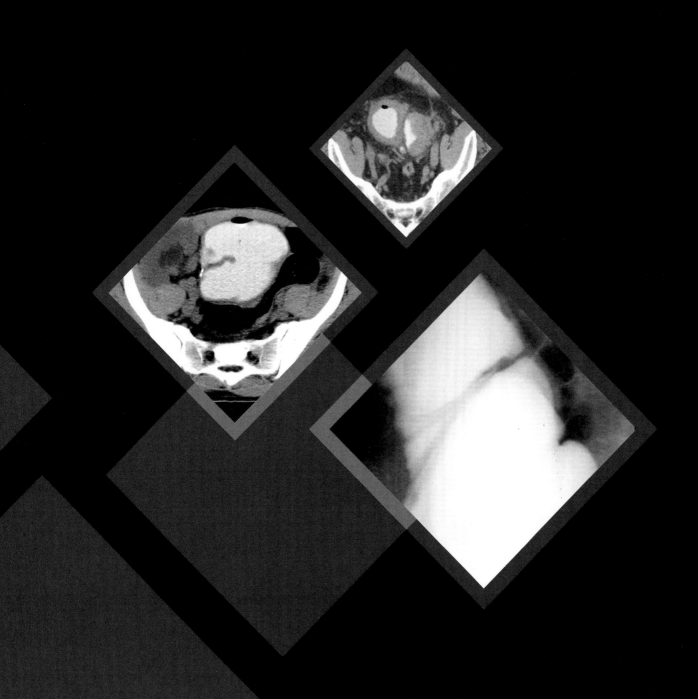

DIFFERENTIAL DIAGNOSIS

Common

- Bladder Carcinoma
- Bladder Calculi
- Blood Clot
- Diverticulitis
- Bladder Fistulas
- Extravesical Pelvic Mass
  - Benign Prostatic Hyperplasia
  - Prostate Carcinoma
  - Rectal Carcinoma
  - Cervical Carcinoma
  - Endometriosis
- Ureterocele
- Postoperative State

Less Common

- Foreign Body
- Urachal Carcinoma
- Cystitis Cystica et Glandularis
- Inverted Papilloma
- Inflammatory Myofibroblastic Pseudotumor
- Mesenchymal Neoplasms
- Metastasis and Lymphoma

ESSENTIAL INFORMATION

Key Differential Diagnosis Issues

- Mobility, location, and shape of lesion suggest diagnosis or limit differential
  - Decubitus US or prone CT can be used to see if mass is mobile (blood clot or fungus ball) and distinguish it from fixed lesion (neoplastic or inflammatory)
  - Enhancement of lesion = neoplastic or inflammatory
    - Excludes calculi, blood clot, debris
  - Chronic inflammation of bladder leads to clinical and imaging features that are difficult to distinguish from neoplastic disease
  - Cystoscopy and biopsy often necessary to differentiate neoplastic and inflammatory lesions

Helpful Clues for Common Diagnoses

- **Bladder Carcinoma**
  - Types: Urothelial carcinoma is most common; squamous cell carcinoma and adenocarcinoma are rare
  - Sessile or pedunculated soft tissue mass projecting into lumen
  - Similar to increased density to bladder wall on CECT
  - Can never exclude cancer by imaging (CTU sensitivity: 79-86%)
    - Cystoscopy is gold standard for evaluation of lower urinary tract; all patients with unexplained gross hematuria (and some patients with microscopic hematuria) require cystoscopy
- **Bladder Calculi**
  - Smooth, round or ovoid; can be spiculated (jackstone), laminated, or faceted
  - US: Mobile, echogenic, shadowing foci
  - All radiopaque on CT; most radiopaque on plain films

- Often associated with chronic bladder outlet obstruction, such as in BPH or neurogenic bladder
- May form around neglected stent or catheter (or other foreign body)

- **Blood Clot**
  - US: Mobile mass, no acoustic shadow, no internal vascularity
  - Attenuation value 50-60 HU; no enhancement on CECT
  - Variable appearance based on size and age of blood
- **Diverticulitis**
  - Commonly causes inflammatory thickening of adjacent wall of bladder
  - Abscess arising from sigmoid diverticulitis especially prone to involve bladder
  - May give rise to colovesical fistula (most common cause in industrialized countries)
- **Bladder Fistulas**
  - Gas in bladder, bladder wall thickening
  - Enterovesical: Diverticulitis most common cause
    - Other causes include Crohn disease, radiation (cystitis &/or enteritis), carcinomas of bladder, bowel, or other pelvic viscera
  - Vesicovaginal: Patient has persistent vaginal discharge
    - Cystography, CT cystogram, or enteric contrast CT are preferred modalities to show communication
- **Extravesical Pelvic Mass**
  - Any neoplastic (or inflammatory) process arising in pelvis can indent or invade bladder
    - Neoplastic: Carcinoma of prostate, rectum, cervix
    - Inflammatory: Endometriosis, pelvic abscess
  - Benign prostatic hyperplasia (BPH)
    - Protrudes into bladder base as pedunculated enlargement and can displace trigone
      - Seen in up to 27% of men
    - Median lobe hypertrophy is older terminology as it is misnomer (there is no median lobe)
      - Intravesical prostatic protrusion is currently used
    - Bladder is often trabeculated and enlarged (± diverticula) from chronic outlet obstruction
  - Prostate carcinoma
    - Mass effect of tumor may indent bladder base similar to BPH
    - Tumor may invade bladder, causing intramural or even intraluminal mass
  - Cervical carcinoma
    - FIGO stage IV invades bladder
  - Endometriosis
    - Direct implantation of endometrium, typically in uterovesical pouch
    - Contains areas of hemorrhage (inherent T1 hyperintensity on MR) and shows avid enhancement
- **Ureterocele**
  - Intravesical: Ureterocele is entirely in bladder
    - Eccentric cystic filling defect near trigone; fills with excreted contrast at CT urography
    - Cobra head or spring onion deformity of distal ureter
  - Ectopic: Insertion at bladder neck or in posterior urethra
  - High association with duplicated renal collecting system in children (in adults generally orthotopic and single ureter)

- **Postoperative State**
  - Prior transurethral bladder resection may cause focal wall thickening, mimicking mass
  - Surgeries, such as segmental cystectomy, bladder augmentation, and psoas-hitch ureterocystostomy, result in distortion of normal bladder anatomy and apparent filling defects
    - Generally, bladder is unusual in shape &/or bowel anastomoses are seen, allowing for identification of prior procedure

Helpful Clues for Less Common Diagnoses

- **Foreign Body**
  - Bladder catheter (Foley) is extremely common in hospitalized patients
  - Next most common cause is introduction during autoeroticism or child abuse
    - Pieces of catheters, hair, sutures, and other objects are reported
  - Can become nidus for calcification if chronic
- **Urachal Carcinoma**
  - Mass ± calcification extending up from dome of bladder toward umbilicus
  - Infected urachal cyst may have similar appearance
- **Cystitis Cystica et Glandularis**
  - Cystic metaplasia of von Brunn nest (invaginations of urothelium); common on autopsy studies but rarely seen at imaging
  - Thought to be due to chronic bladder irritation
  - Focal bladder mass with predilection for trigone; may have cystic foci but often indistinguishable from malignancy
- **Inverted Papilloma**
  - May arise in bladder (or ureter or renal pelvis); benign
  - Usually small, pedunculated mass indistinguishable from malignancy
- **Inflammatory Myofibroblastic Tumor**
  - Polypoid mass caused by nonneoplastic proliferation of myofibroblasts and inflammatory cells
  - Previously known as inflammatory pseudotumor

- Usual appearance is vascular, bulky mass in patient with gross hematuria; may have prominent rim enhancement
- **Mesenchymal Neoplasms**
  - Primary neoplasms of bladder deriving from nonepithelial elements
    - Leiomyoma, paraganglioma, fibroma, hemangioma, neurofibroma, plasmacytoma
  - Rare; altogether account for < 5% of bladder tumors; malignant counterparts (sarcomas) are exceedingly rare
  - Mesenchymal tumors are intramural and overlying urothelium is intact though this is difficult to evaluate on imaging
  - Imaging features of mesenchymal tumors and papillary urothelial carcinoma overlap
  - Several mesenchymal tumors have quasicharacteristic features on MR
    - Increased T1 signal in paraganglioma; decreased T2 in leiomyoma; target sign in neurofibroma
- **Metastasis and Lymphoma**
  - Focal lesion or diffuse wall thickening
  - Melanoma, breast and gastric cancer are most common
  - Lymphoma usually secondary involvement rather than primary

SELECTED REFERENCES

1. Son Y et al: Cystitis cystica et glandularis causing lower urinary tract symptoms in a 29-year-old male. Cureus. 13(8):e17144, 2021
2. Hirshberg B et al: MDCT imaging of acute bladder pathology. Curr Probl Diagn Radiol. 49(6):422-30, 2020
3. Walker SM et al: Role of mpMRI in benign prostatic hyperplasia assessment and treatment. Curr Urol Rep. 21(12):55, 2020
4. Buddha S et al: Imaging of urachal anomalies. Abdom Radiol (NY). 44(12):3978-89, 2019
5. Wentland AL et al: Bladder cancer and its mimics: a sonographic pictorial review with CT/MR and histologic correlation. Abdom Radiol (NY). 44(12):3827-42, 2019
6. Trinh TW et al: Bladder cancer diagnosis with CT urography: test characteristics and reasons for false-positive and false-negative results. Abdom Radiol (NY). 43(3):663-71, 2018
7. Didier RA et al: The duplicated collecting system of the urinary tract: embryology, imaging appearances and clinical considerations. Pediatr Radiol. 47(11):1526-38, 2017
8. Parada Villavicencio C et al: Imaging of the urachus: anomalies, complications, and mimics. Radiographics. 36(7):2049-63, 2016

Bladder Carcinoma

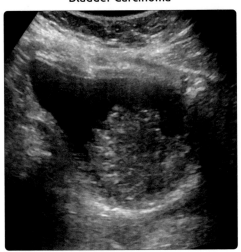

Bladder Carcinoma

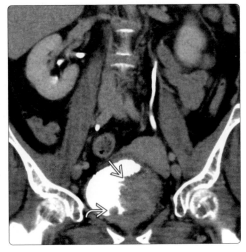

(Left) Longitudinal US of the bladder in a patient with gross hematuria shows a large mass with an irregular surface. Color Doppler showed flow, and decubitus positioning showed that the mass was immobile, suggestive of a neoplastic etiology. (Right) Coronal CTU in the same patient shows a large left bladder mass ➡ with papillary projections, typical of urothelial carcinoma. Bladder cancer can be multifocal, as in this patient with a similar smaller mass ➡.

Bladder Carcinoma

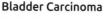

Bladder Carcinoma

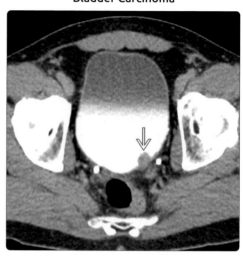

(Left) *Axial nephrographic-phase CTU in a patient with microscopic hematuria shows a small bladder mass* ➡ *with moderate enhancement compared to urine. Urothelial carcinoma often enhances, to a variable degree, greater than urine, and can be detected well in this phase, even when small.* (Right) *Axial delayed-phase CTU in the same patient shows the relative hypodense bladder mass* ➡ *compared to the enhanced urine. Careful scrutiny of the bladder wall and windowing is necessary to detect subtle bladder cancers.*

Bladder Carcinoma

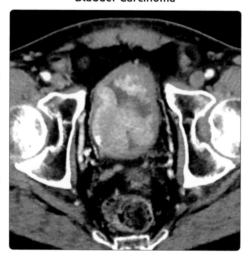

Bladder Carcinoma

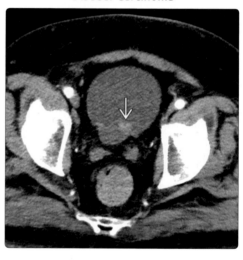

(Left) *Axial CECT shows a large bladder mass occupying the entire lumen. This is an atypical presentation of bladder cancer, which is advanced and multifocal. Avid enhancement can help distinguish this from a large clot.* (Right) *Axial CECT in a trauma patient shows a small, subtle mass* ➡ *in the left bladder trigone. Bladder cancer is sometimes found incidentally on CT as it may be clinically silent. Such patients should be referred for cystoscopy.*

Bladder Calculi

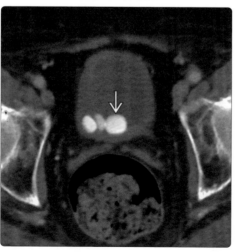

Bladder Calculi

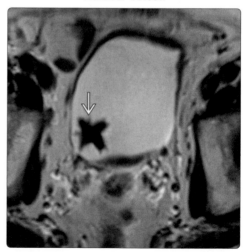

(Left) *Axial CECT shows multiple bladder stones* ➡. *Bladder stones are hyperdense and readily identified by CT. They range from small to large, may be lamellated, and are often seen in patients with chronic urine stasis, such as in benign prostatic hyperplasia (BPH).* (Right) *Axial T2 MR obtained for prostate MR shows a spiculated jackstone* ➡ *in the bladder, so called for its resemblance to the childhood toy.*

Bladder Calculi

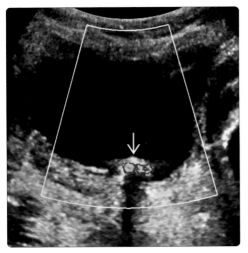

Bladder Calculi

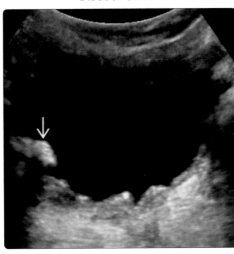

(Left) *Transverse US of the bladder shows a hyperechoic shadowing stone* ➔ *with a typical twinkle artifact, which occurs as a Doppler artifact to strong reflectors.* (Right) *Transverse US in the same patient now in the right lateral decubitus position shows that the stone* ➔ *is mobile, having moved to the right bladder wall. US (or prone CT/MR) can determine if a mass is fixed or mobile.*

Blood Clot

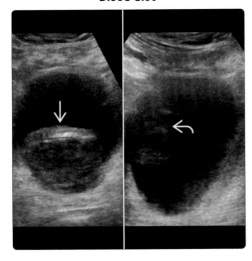

Blood Clot

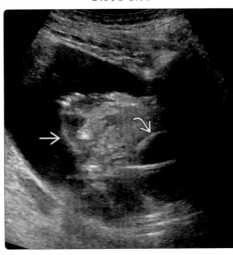

(Left) *Transverse US of the bladder in the supine position in a patient with gross hematuria shows a heterogeneous filling defect* ➔ *in the dependent bladder. The abnormality* ➔ *moves to the right wall with decubitus positioning, confirming that this is a blood clot and not a neoplasm.* (Right) *Longitudinal US shows a large, heterogeneous clot* ➔ *formed around a Foley catheter* ➔.

Blood Clot

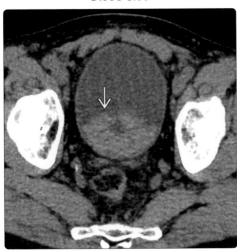

Blood Clot

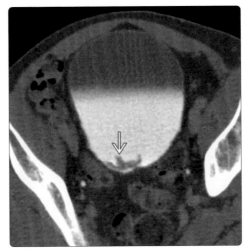

(Left) *Axial NECT in a patient with gross hematuria shows a large, hyperdense blood clot* ➔. *A clot will lack enhancement and often is heterogeneous and may have irregular, angulated margins, unlike a mass.* (Right) *Axial delayed-phase CTU shows a curvilinear filling defect* ➔ *with irregular margins, consistent with a small clot. Note that it is not attached to the wall, unlike a mass.*

Filling Defect in Urinary Bladder

Diverticulitis

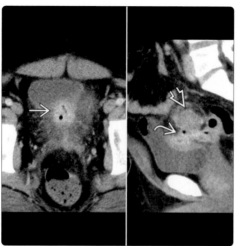

Bladder Fistulas

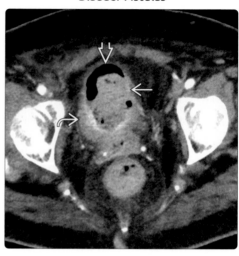

(Left) *Axial CECT shows an enhancing filling defect at the bladder dome with central gas* ➡️. *Sagittal CECT shows that this is due to fistula* ➡️ *and abscess* ➡️ *formation from perforated diverticulitis.* (Right) *Axial CECT shows a heterogeneous filling defect* ➡️ *in the bladder containing foci of gas. Also note the larger anterior bladder lumen gas* ➡️. *Bladder wall thickening and mucosal enhancement* ➡️ *is also present. In this case, the filling defect is stool secondary to a large colovesical fistula due pelvic radiation therapy.*

Benign Prostatic Hyperplasia

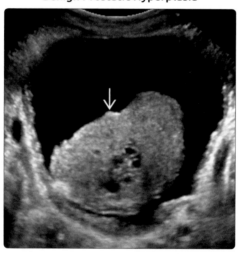

Benign Prostatic Hyperplasia

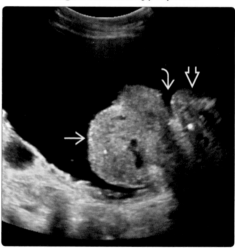

(Left) *Transverse US in a man with a urinary obstruction shows a heterogeneous bladder mass* ➡️ *near the trigone with cystic foci.* (Right) *Longitudinal US in the same patient shows that the "mass"* ➡️ *is contiguous with an enlarged and heterogeneous prostate gland* ➡️. *Notice the urethral inlet as a funnel-shaped area* ➡️. *BPH may extend into the bladder base, which is termed intravesical prostatic protrusion. The enlarged prostate can be readily identified on US by its typical location, shape, and appearance.*

Benign Prostatic Hyperplasia

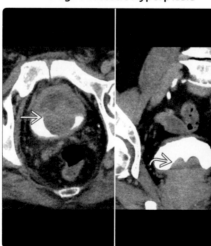

Cervical Carcinoma

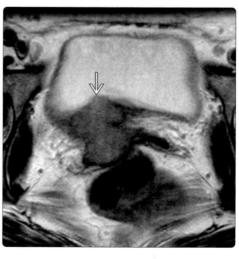

(Left) *Axial delayed-phase CTU shows a large filling defect* ➡️ *in the bladder base. Coronal image shows the smooth bilobar configuration* ➡️ *typical of intravesical prostatic protrusion of BPH. This used to be known as median lobe hypertrophy.* (Right) *Axial T2 MR in a patient with cervical cancer shows a T2-intermediate mass* ➡️ *extending from the cervix into the bladder lumen, consistent with FIGO stage IV. All types of pelvic cancers can invade the bladder when advanced and show a bladder filling defect.*

Endometriosis

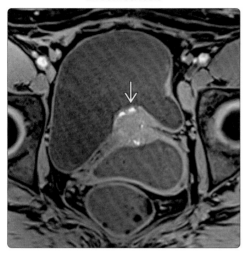

Foreign Body

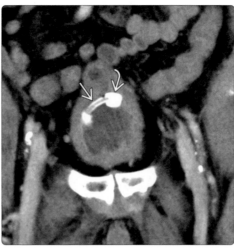

(Left) *Axial precontrast T1 MR shows a posterior bladder wall mass ➡, which also involves the anterior vaginal wall. Note the T1-hyperintense foci within. This is a classic appearance of bladder endometriosis.* **(Right)** *Coronal CECT shows a tubular filling defect ➡ in the bladder encrusted by 2 stones ➡. This was a retained catheter fragment, which had been in the bladder for years in a patient with a need for chronic catheterization.*

Urachal Carcinoma

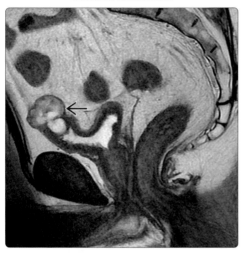

Cystitis Cystica et Glandularis

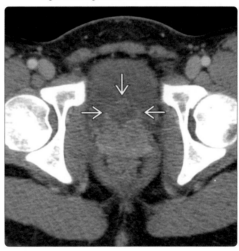

(Left) *Sagittal T2 SSFSE MR demonstrates a complex solid/cystic mass ➡ in the bladder dome. The patient underwent partial cystectomy, and pathology was consistent with urachal adenocarcinoma. These lesions often show variable increased T2 due to mucin content.* **(Right)** *Axial CECT shows a subtle bladder trigone filling defect with central cystic appearance ➡. Resection revealed cystitis cystica. This may have a cystic appearance and is commonly found at the trigone but is generally indistinguishable from malignancy.*

Inverted Papilloma

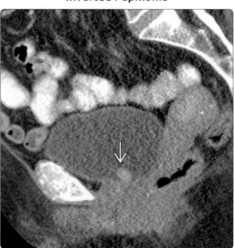

Mesenchymal Neoplasms

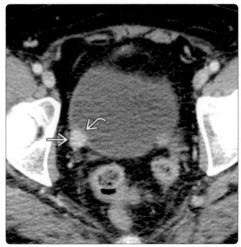

(Left) *Sagittal CECT shows a small polypoid bladder mass ➡ near the bladder neck. Resection showed inverted papilloma.* **(Right)** *Axial CECT in a 51-year-old woman shows a small, hypervascular bladder mass ➡ centered on the wall with predominant exophytic growth. There is suggestion of normal overlying urothelium ➡. While urothelial carcinoma is in the differential, this mass was a paraganglioma.*

DIFFERENTIAL DIAGNOSIS

Common

- Bladder Diverticulum
- Bladder Fistulas
- Neurogenic Bladder
- Cystocele
- Bladder Trauma
- Bladder Herniation

Less Common

- Urachal Remnant
- Postoperative Bladder
- Everted Ureterocele
- Iatrogenic

ESSENTIAL INFORMATION

Helpful Clues for Common Diagnoses

- **Bladder Diverticulum**
  - Most are acquired and secondary to bladder outlet obstruction (most common benign prostatic hyperplasia)
  - Congenital form, known as Hutch diverticulum, is rare
    - Caused by congenital weakness in detrusor muscle anterolateral to ureteral orifice
  - Usually near ureterovesical junction; can be multiple and large
  - May be complicated by stones or bladder cancer
- **Bladder Fistulas**
  - To small bowel, colon, vagina, skin
  - Secondary to inflammatory or neoplastic processes in bladder or adjacent organs
  - Look for gas in bladder, focal wall thickening, perivesical inflammatory changes, direct communication
- **Neurogenic Bladder**
  - Distended &/or thick walled bladder with trabecula and multiple diverticula or pseudodiverticula
- **Cystocele**
  - Very common in middle-aged to older women

- Posterior midline outpouching at base, best seen on sagittal imaging
- **Bladder Trauma**
  - Intraperitoneal rupture: Intraperitoneal contrast spill around bowel loops ± visualized defect at dome
  - Extraperitoneal: Flame-shaped collection of extravasated urine lateral or anterior to bladder
    - May extend to other contiguous extraperitoneal spaces (scrotum, thigh, retroperitoneum, etc.)
- **Bladder Herniation**
  - May herniate into inguinal, femoral, or obturator canals or into perineal hernia

Helpful Clues for Less Common Diagnoses

- **Urachal Remnant**
  - Midline cystic collection opening into bladder dome ± stones
  - Urachal associated adenocarcinoma often presents as heterogeneous, mucinous mass with exophytic growth
- **Postoperative Bladder**
  - Isolated loop of ileum &/or segment of colon is used to augment bladder and may appear as superior outpouching
  - Neobladder constructed out of ileum or colon may have unusual shape or outpouching
    - Loop of ileum ("chimney") often extends superiorly and is anastomosed to ureters
- **Everted Ureterocele**
  - Ureterocele may temporarily evert during voiding or bladder filling and mimic diverticulum
  - Continuous with ureter
  - If seen during VCUG, check initial images and look for intravesical ureterocele
- **Iatrogenic**
  - Site of prior suprapubic catheterization

SELECTED REFERENCES

1. Fouladi DF et al: Imaging of urinary bladder injury: the role of CT cystography. Emerg Radiol. 27(1):87-95, 2020

Bladder Diverticulum

Bladder Diverticulum

(Left) Axial CTU shows a large right posterolateral bladder diverticulum ➡ filled with contrast. Note the narrow neck ⬈. These generally occur in the setting of chronic bladder outlet obstruction, most commonly from benign prostatic hyperplasia. (Right) Axial CECT shows a posterolateral outpouching ➡ consistent with diverticulum. Note the soft tissue filling defect ⬅ in the diverticulum, an invasive urothelial carcinoma in this case.

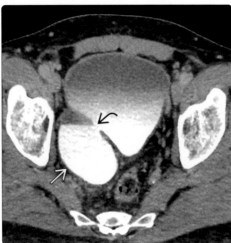

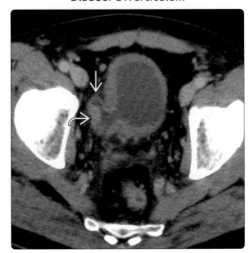

Bladder Diverticulum

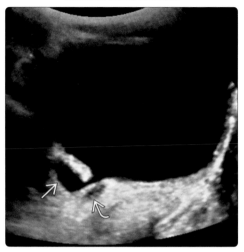

Cystocele

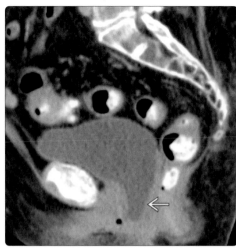

(Left) Transverse US in a 6-year-old boy with hematuria and a UTI shows a small right diverticulum ➡ with a narrow neck just anterior and lateral to a prominent right ureter ➡. This is typical of a Hutch diverticulum. (Right) Sagittal CECT shows an inferior bladder outpouching ➡ at the neck between the vagina and urethra. This is typical of cystocele and is very common in middle-aged to older women, though may only be seen with Valsalva.

Neurogenic Bladder

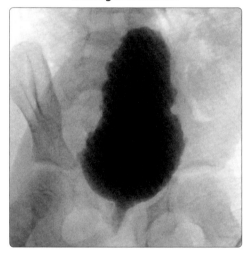

Bladder Herniation

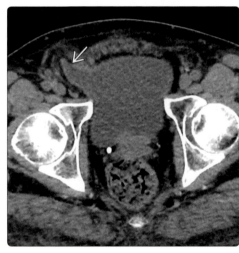

(Left) Oblique cystogram in an 11-year-old boy with a tethered spinal cord shows a pinecone-shaped bladder with trabeculation and pseudodiverticula, typical of neurogenic bladder. (Right) Axial NECT shows a right anterior bladder outpouching ➡ at the internal inguinal ring due to an inguinal hernia. The bladder can enter an inguinal, femoral, obturator, or perineal hernia.

Urachal Remnant

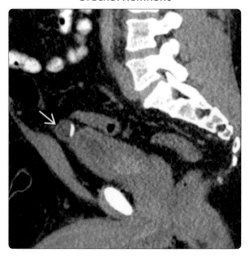

Postoperative Bladder

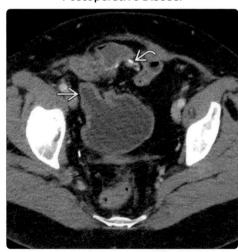

(Left) Sagittal NECT shows a cystic outpouching ➡ at the bladder dome, typical of a urachal diverticulum. The calcification represents small stones layering in the diverticulum. (Right) Axial CECT in a patient with history of bladder cancer shows an irregular outpouching ➡ at the right anterior wall. Note the small bowel staple line ➡, a clue that this is an ileal neobladder.

DIFFERENTIAL DIAGNOSIS

Common

- Iatrogenic
- Bladder Fistulas
- Cystitis

Less Common

- Emphysematous Cystitis

ESSENTIAL INFORMATION

Key Differential Diagnosis Issues

- Gas in bladder should not be automatically attributed to catheterization
  - Confirm history of recent catheterization
  - Look for evidence of bladder fistula
- Evaluate medical record for clinical signs and symptoms of infected urine or fistula
  - Dysuria, pneumaturia, heavy growth of multiple coliform bacteria from urine
- Gas bubbles suspended within urine is suggestive of complex urine consistency and should raise possibility of infection &/or fistula

Helpful Clues for Common Diagnoses

- **Iatrogenic**
  - Most common cause of bladder gas
  - Check for history of recent instrumentation
    - Foley catheter, suprapubic bladder catheter
    - Cystoscopy
  - Usually not large volume of gas
- **Bladder Fistulas**
  - Secondary to inflammatory or neoplastic process in bladder or adjacent organs
    - Colovesical fistula
      □ Diverticulitis (most common cause: 80% of cases)
      □ Look for signs of diverticulitis: Colonic wall thickening, diverticula, abscess adjacent to bladder, loss of fat plane between bowel and bladder, tethering of bladder, focal bladder wall thickening

- Enterovesical fistula
  □ Crohn disease is most common cause
- Vesicocutaneous fistula
  □ Usually due to surgical complication or trauma
- Vesicovaginal fistula
  □ Gynecologic surgery is most common cause
  - Cystography and enema can identify fistula in < 50% of cases; CT or MR has much higher sensitivity for detection of fistula itself and secondary signs
- **Cystitis**
  - Gas bubbles may be due to gas-forming organism
  - Bladder wall thickening ± mucosal hyperenhancement ± perivesical inflammatory changes
  - Usually involves entire bladder wall

Helpful Clues for Less Common Diagnoses

- **Emphysematous Cystitis**
  - Most commonly seen in patients with longstanding and poorly controlled diabetes mellitus and patients on immunosuppression
  - Due to bacterial fermentation of excessive glucose within urothelium and urine
  - Gas in bladder wall ± lumen
  - Responsible organisms are: *Escherichia coli, Enterobacter aerogenes, Klebsiella pneumonia, Proteus mirabilis*
  - More likely to become septic and die than nonemphysematous bacterial cystitis
  - Unlike other emphysematous infections, patients rarely need surgical treatment; antibiotics generally curative

SELECTED REFERENCES

1. El-Ghar MA et al: CT and MRI in urinary tract infections: a spectrum of different imaging findings. Medicina (Kaunas). 57(1):32, 2021
2. Nepal P et al: Gas where it shouldn't be! Imaging spectrum of emphysematous infections in the abdomen and pelvis. AJR Am J Roentgenol. 216(3):812-23, 2021
3. Nepal P et al: Imaging spectrum of common and rare infections affecting the lower genitourinary tract. Abdom Radiol (NY). 46(6):2665-82, 2021
4. Hirshberg B et al: MDCT imaging of acute bladder pathology. Curr Probl Diagn Radiol. 49(6):422-30, 2020
5. Yu M et al: Complicated genitourinary tract infections and mimics. Curr Probl Diagn Radiol. 46(1):74-83, 2017

Iatrogenic

Iatrogenic

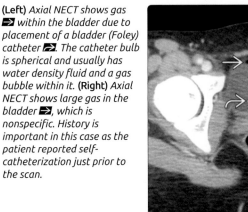 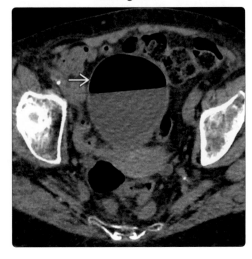

(Left) Axial NECT shows gas ⇨ within the bladder due to placement of a bladder (Foley) catheter ⇲. The catheter bulb is spherical and usually has water density fluid and a gas bubble within it. (Right) Axial NECT shows large gas in the bladder ⇨, which is nonspecific. History is important in this case as the patient reported self-catheterization just prior to the scan.

Bladder Fistulas

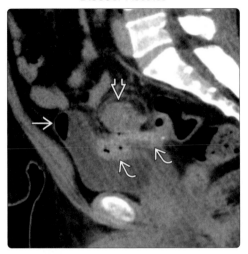

Bladder Fistulas

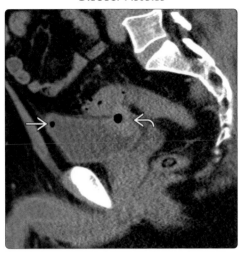

(Left) *Sagittal CECT shows luminal bladder gas ➡, sigmoid wall thickening ⮕, and a soft tissue tract ➡ extending from the sigmoid to the bladder wall. Notice gas in the tract and focal bladder wall thickening, consistent with diverticulitis-associated colovesical fistula.* (Right) *Sagittal NECT shows a tiny bubble of gas ➡ in the bladder. Notice the abnormal colon wall with diverticula and a collection containing gas ➡ between the sigmoid and bladder. Therefore, this is due to a colovesical fistula from diverticulitis.*

Cystitis

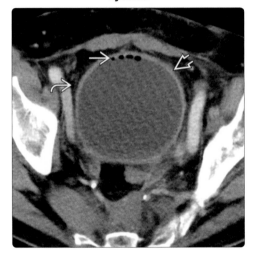

Cystitis

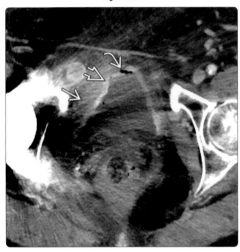

(Left) *Axial CECT in a 71-year-old man with diabetes shows several bubbles of gas in the bladder lumen ➡. Notice the bladder wall thickening ➡ and mild hyperenhancement as well as perivesical stranding ➡, consistent with acute cystitis.* (Right) *Axial CECT in an older adult patient with sepsis shows bladder wall thickening ➡ and mural hyperenhancement ➡ with tiny gas ➡ in the lumen. In some cases of cystitis, bacteria will produce gas.*

Emphysematous Cystitis

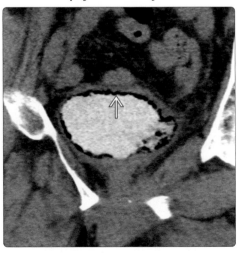

Emphysematous Cystitis

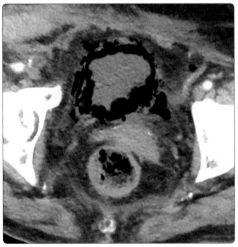

(Left) *Delayed-phase coronal CECT shows multiple bubbles of gas confined to the bladder mucosa ➡, consistent with emphysematous cystitis. This is due to gas formation by bacteria translocated into the bladder wall.* (Right) *NECT shows multiple bubbles of gas in the bladder wall and extending into the fat around the bladder. This form of cystitis is generally more severe than nonemphysematous cystitis but usually responds well to antibiotic therapy.*

DIFFERENTIAL DIAGNOSIS

Common

- Underdistended Bladder
- Normal Trigone
- Chronic Bladder Outlet Obstruction
- Bacterial Cystitis
- Chronic Cystitis
- Neurogenic Bladder
- Bladder Carcinoma
- Invasion by Pelvic Neoplasm
- Reaction to Pelvic Infection or Inflammation

Less Common

- Emphysematous Cystitis
- Bladder Wall Trauma
- Fungal or Viral Cystitis
- Tuberculous Cystitis
- Bladder Schistosomiasis
- Eosinophilic Cystitis
- Amyloid

ESSENTIAL INFORMATION

Key Differential Diagnosis Issues

- Bladder wall thickness should be evaluated ideally on distended bladder
- Mild to moderate diffuse bladder wall thickening is commonly encountered in middle age to older adults at imaging and is usually chronic
- Be aware of normal thickening of trigone
- Classify bladder wall thickening as focal or diffuse pattern
  - Focal wall thickening is more suspicious for neoplastic process as diffuse wall thickening is rarely neoplastic
- Check kidneys and ureters for hydronephrosis; check for other clues of infectious cause
- Medical history can often narrow differential diagnosis

Helpful Clues for Common Diagnoses

- **Underdistended Bladder**
  - Common cause for pseudothickening of bladder wall
- **Normal Trigone**
  - Normal mild thickening between ureteral orifices (interureteric ridge)
  - May pose diagnostic challenge in patients with prostatomegaly
- **Chronic Bladder Outlet Obstruction**
  - Classically in middle aged to older men secondary to benign prostatic hyperplasia
    - May be seen in younger men due to urethral stricture, posterior urethral valves, other obstructing causes
  - Also occurs in women less frequently due to variety of causes
    - Sphincter hyperfunction, antiincontinence surgery, urethral stricture, pelvic organ prolapse, urethral diverticula
  - Diffuse bladder wall thickening with trabeculations
  - ± diverticula, stones
- **Bacterial Cystitis**
  - Most common etiology: *Escherichia coli*

  - Transurethral seeding of bladder from perineum in women
  - Bladder outlet obstruction and urinary stasis in men
  - Usually smooth, diffuse bladder wall thickening, hyperemia, perivesical stranding
    - Debris floating or layering at US
  - Look for ascending UTI: Ureteral thickening and enhancement; pyelonephritis
- **Chronic Cystitis**
  - Chronic and recurrent bacterial cystitis
  - Associated with decreased bladder capacity and vesicoureteral reflux
  - Radiation cystitis: Sequelae of radiation therapy for pelvic malignant neoplasm (uterine, cervical, prostate, and rectal carcinoma)
    - Small-volume bladder with diffuse, irregular wall thickening
    - May be associated with obstructive hydronephrosis
    - May have fistulous communication with adjacent viscera secondary to necrosis
  - Chemotherapeutic agents induce cystitis, often causing hemorrhagic cystitis
    - Common agents: Cyclophosphamide (cytoxan), ifosfamide, bacillus Calmette-Guérin (BCG) instillation for Ca bladder
  - Interstitial cystitis: Idiopathic condition causing severe pain, urgency, and frequency
  - Recurrent bacterial infection: Malakoplakia; rare, presents with bladder mass
- **Neurogenic Bladder**
  - Bladder dysfunction caused by neurologic damage
  - Bladder appearance depends on level of lesion (e.g., round, Christmas tree, distended)
  - Often diffuse bladder thickening ± trabeculations
- **Bladder Carcinoma**
  - May uncommonly appear as focal bladder wall thickening without measurable mass
    - More common: Sessile or pedunculated soft tissue mass projecting into lumen
  - Similar to increased density to bladder wall on CECT
  - US: Focal, immobile mass ± Doppler flow
    - Scan patient in decubitus position to differentiate from mobile blood clot or debris
  - Can never exclude cancer by imaging (CT urogram sensitivity 79-86%)
    - Cystoscopy is gold standard for evaluation of lower urinary tract
  - Prominent wall thickening adjacent to mass may be clue to advanced bladder cancer
- **Invasion by Pelvic Neoplasm**
  - Common tumors
    - Male: Rectal, prostate
    - Female: Cervix, uterine, vaginal, ovarian
  - Loss of fat plane between bladder wall and adjacent pelvic neoplasm, focal wall thickening and enhancement
  - Visible intramural mass is less common
    - May be associated with fistulous communication, particularly after treatment
- **Reaction to Pelvic Infection or Inflammation**
  - Infectious or inflammatory processes adjacent to bladder may cause localized wall thickening

○ Crohn disease: Inflamed bowel or fistula formation

○ Sigmoid colonic diverticulitis: Bladder wall thickening may be reactive but should prompt careful search for fistula

Helpful Clues for Less Common Diagnoses

- **Emphysematous Cystitis**
  - ○ Infection of bladder by gas-forming bacterial or fungal organism
    - *E. coli*, *Enterobacter aerogenes*, *Klebsiella pneumonia*, *Proteus mirabilis*
    - Associated with age, diabetes, chronic kidney disease, neurogenic bladder
    - Patients more likely to become septic and die than with nonemphysematous bacterial cystitis
  - ○ CT is modality of choice as it is highly sensitive and can localize gas to wall
    - Multiple foci of air within bladder wall ± air in lumen
    - Gas trapped in lateral and posterior walls, not rising to anterior bladder lumen, allows differentiation of intraluminal gas vs. gas in bladder wall
  - ○ US: Echogenic foci within area of bladder wall thickening with "dirty" shadowing
    - May be hard to distinguish from intraluminal gas; can use decubitus imaging
  - ○ Radiographs: Curvilinear lucency in shape of bladder
  - ○ Unlike other emphysematous infections, patients rarely need surgical treatment; antibiotics generally curative
- **Bladder Wall Trauma**
  - ○ Spectrum of focal hematoma to perforation
  - ○ Often associated with pelvic fractures
  - ○ CT cystogram test of choice
- **Fungal or Viral Cystitis**
  - ○ *Candida albicans* is most common fungal organism
  - ○ May be associated with fungal ball within bladder
  - ○ Viral: BK virus hemorrhagic cystitis occurs in hematopoietic cell transplant recipients and nephropathy occurs in kidney transplant recipients
- **Tuberculous Cystitis**

○ Hematogenous spread of primary tubercular infection, usually lungs (caused by *Mycobacterium tuberculosis*)

○ Secondary to renal ± ureteric involvement

○ Earliest form of bladder tuberculous cystitis starts around ureteral orifice

○ Typically low-volume bladder with diffuse wall thickening ("thimble bladder") ± wall calcification

○ Fibrotic changes near ureteric orifice result in vesicoureteric reflux

○ Associated with localized or generalized pyonephrosis

- **Bladder Schistosomiasis**
  - ○ Infection of urinary system by parasite *Schistosoma hematobium*
  - ○ Thick-walled, fibrotic bladder
  - ○ Calcification within bladder wall is classic imaging appearance
  - ○ Small capacity bladder with inability to completely empty
  - ○ ± hydronephrosis and hydroureter due to distal ureteric stricture
  - ○ May present with bladder mass; classically squamous cell carcinoma
  - ○ Often difficult to differentiate from tuberculosis based on imaging
- **Eosinophilic Cystitis**
  - ○ Very rare; nonspecific thickening or mass
  - ○ May result in fibrosis with small capacity bladder and ureteral orifice obstruction
  - ○ Etiology often unknown; can be seen after mitomycin therapy for bladder cancer
- **Amyloid**
  - ○ Primary and secondary amyloid deposition is very rare
  - ○ Focal wall thickening or mass with nonspecific features

SELECTED REFERENCES

1. El-Ghar MA et al: CT and MRI in urinary tract infections: a spectrum of different imaging findings. Medicina (Kaunas). 57(1), 2021
2. Karaosmanoglu AD et al: Imaging findings of infectious and inflammatory diseases of the urinary system mimicking neoplastic diseases. Abdom Radiol (NY). 45(4):1110-21, 2020

Underdistended Bladder

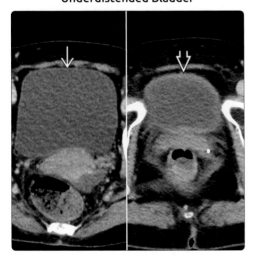

Normal Trigone

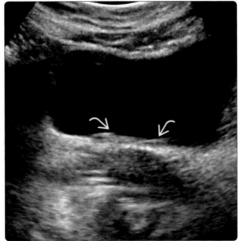

(Left) *Axial CECT shows marked changes in the bladder wall thickness related to distension. A normal thin wall is seen in the well-distended bladder ➡, whereas a thick wall is seen in the underdistended bladder ➡. Care should be taken not to overcall bladder wall thickening.* **(Right)** *Transverse transabdominal US shows focal thickening ➡ at the interureteric ridge (trigone), a normal finding.*

Chronic Bladder Outlet Obstruction

(Left) *Longitudinal US in a 77-year-old man shows a heavily trabeculated bladder wall ➡. Note the enlarged prostate gland and intravesical prostatic protrusion ➡, which is the most common cause.*
(Right) *Coronal T2 MR shows a thick bladder wall ➡ with numerous trabeculations ➡. The patient has benign prostatic hyperplasia (not shown) and chronic lower urinary tract symptoms.*

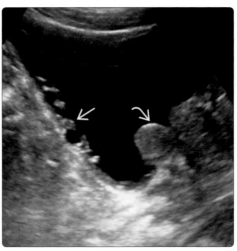

Chronic Bladder Outlet Obstruction

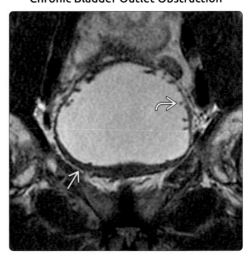

Bacterial Cystitis

(Left) *Transverse US shows diffuse bladder wall thickening ➡ with layering debris ➡ and floating echoes ➡ in a patient with a UTI.*
(Right) *Axial CECT shows diffuse bladder wall thickening and enhancement ➡ along with perivesical fat stranding ➡. These findings are typical of acute bacterial cystitis.*

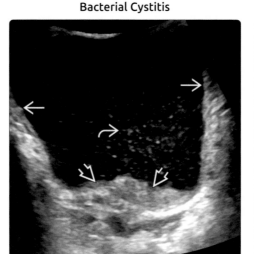

Bacterial Cystitis

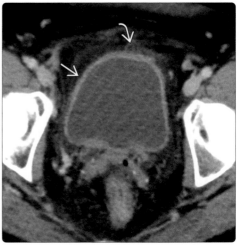

Chronic Cystitis

(Left) *Coronal CECT in a patient with treated prostate cancer shows a markedly thickened bladder wall ➡ with very small capacity and associated distal ureter strictures with bilateral hydronephrosis ➡. These are typical findings of radiation cystitis.* **(Right)** *Coronal NECT in a patient with history of bladder cancer who developed chronic BCG cystitis shows a small, thick-walled ➡ bladder with perivesical stranding. Also note bilateral hydronephrosis due to fibrosis and stricturing of the ureteral orifice.*

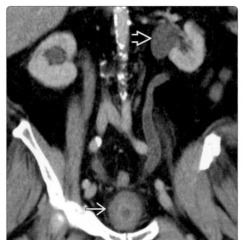

Chronic Cystitis

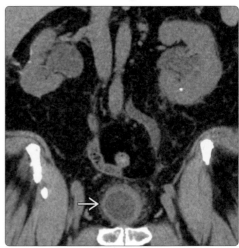

Bladder Carcinoma

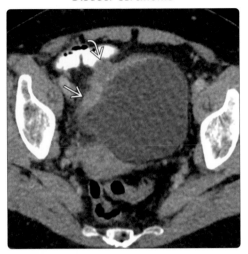

Reaction to Pelvic Infection or Inflammation

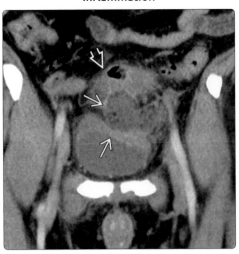

(Left) *Axial CECT shows focal, irregular bladder wall thickening ➡ of the lateral and anterior wall. Note the irregularity of the thickening with extension toward the perivesical fat ➡, a clue that this is muscle invasive bladder cancer.* (Right) *Coronal CECT shows perforated diverticulitis with early abscess formation between the sigmoid ➡ and bladder. Note the bladder wall thickening ➡ at the dome, which is reactive to the infection. This appearance could also be associated with a fistula.*

Emphysematous Cystitis

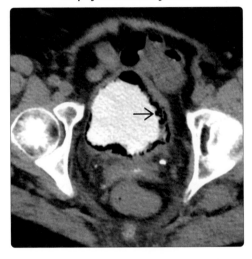

Emphysematous Cystitis

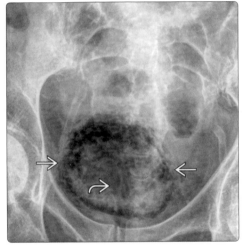

(Left) *Axial NECT shows multiple bubbly foci of gas ➡ conforming to the wall of the bladder. Contrast is present in the lumen from a prior CT, which nicely shows the location of the gas in the urothelium.* (Right) *AP radiograph of the pelvis shows mottled gas ➡ conforming to the shape of the bladder wall, consistent with emphysematous cystitis. Note that rectal gas ➡ can be seen separately, confirming that this is not stool.*

Fungal or Viral Cystitis

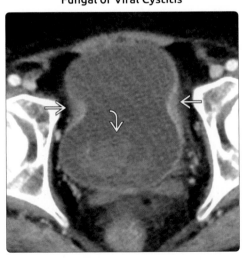

Eosinophilic Cystitis

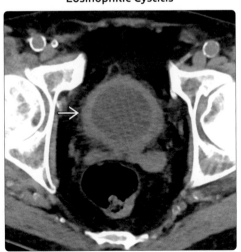

(Left) *Axial CECT in 19-year-old bone marrow transplant recipient shows BK viral hemorrhagic cystitis with areas of focal wall thickening and enhancement ➡ and dependent clot in the lumen ➡.* (Right) *Axial NECT shows marked bladder wall thickening ➡ with mild perivesical stranding. Findings are nonspecific, and the patient was subsequently diagnosed with eosinophilic cystitis by biopsy.*

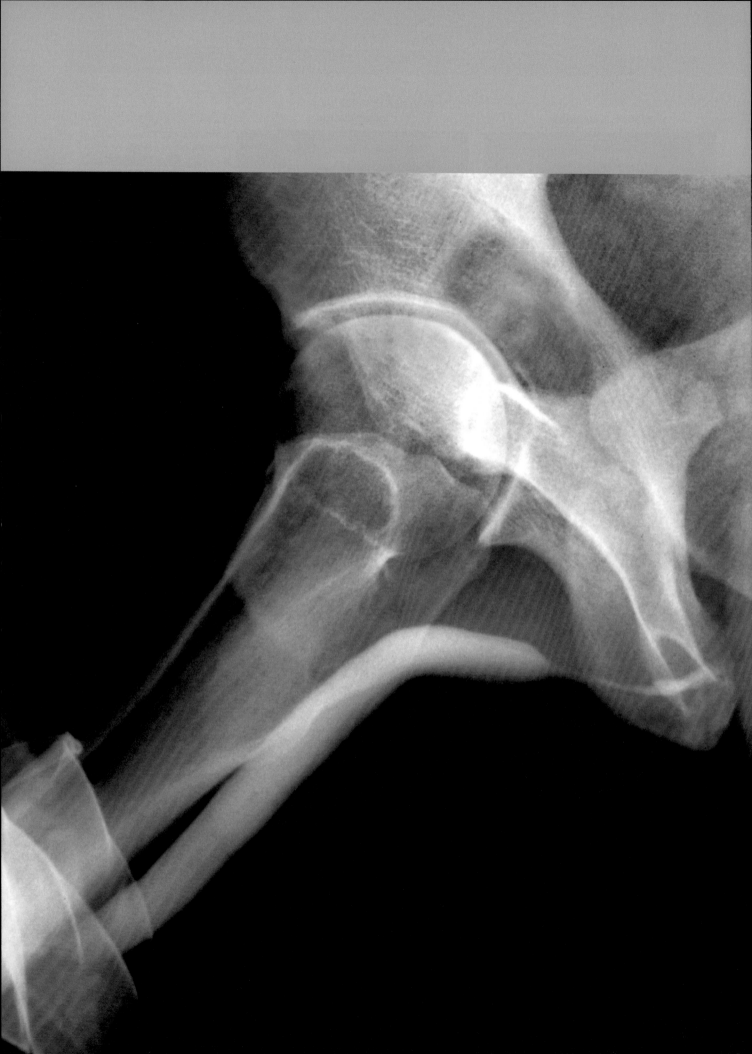

Generic Imaging Patterns

Urethral Stricture   600

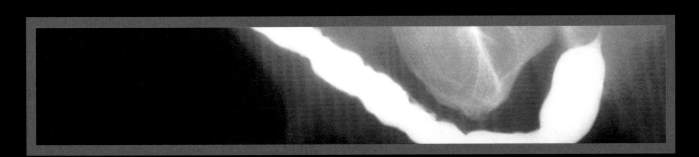

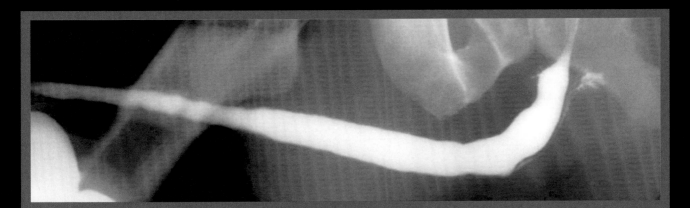

DIFFERENTIAL DIAGNOSIS

Common

- Idiopathic
- Iatrogenic Injury
- Urethral Trauma

Less Common

- Infectious
- Inflammatory Diseases
- Urethral Carcinoma

Rare but Important

- Cowper Gland Adenocarcinoma or Syringocele

ESSENTIAL INFORMATION

Key Differential Diagnosis Issues

- Presence and cause of stricture are usually evident to urologist performing cystoscopy
- Filling of glands of Littré is nonspecific but suggestive of infectious or inflammatory process
- Reflux into Cowper ducts and gland is associated with stricture but can be normal finding

Helpful Clues for Common Diagnoses

- **Idiopathic**
  - Most common cause in resource-rich countries
  - 34% of penile strictures and 64% of bulbar strictures have no identifiable cause
- **Iatrogenic injury**
  - Instrumentation: Cystoscopy, urethroplasty
  - Urethral catheterization: Repetitive or long term
  - Surgery: Transurethral resection of prostate, radical prostatectomy
  - Irradiation/ablation: Prostate or cervical cancer, cryoablation or other local prostate therapy
  - Post urethroplasty: Stricture may recur after urethroplasty
- **Urethral Trauma**
  - May be diagnosed at time of trauma or present late

- Straddle injuries, blows to perineum
- Penile fracture during intercourse
- Often solitary short-segment stricture
- Pelvic fractures often associated with posterior urethral strictures

Helpful Clues for Less Common Diagnoses

- **Infectious**
  - More common in low-resource countries, rare in high-resource countries
  - Often multifocal
  - Tuberculosis is rare, causes multiple fistulas ("watering can perineum")
- **Inflammatory Diseases**
  - Lichen sclerosus
    - Most common cause of diffuse stricture and up to 13% off all strictures
    - Long-segment anterior, sparing bulbar
  - Amyloid: Rare, focal, or diffuse stricture
- **Urethral Carcinoma**
  - Irregular narrowing ± fistula
  - Squamous cell carcinoma, urothelial carcinoma and adenocarcinoma possible depending on location and sex
  - 60% in bulbomembranous urethra

Helpful Clues for Rare Diagnoses

- **Cowper Gland Adenocarcinoma or Syringocele**
  - Syringocele: Smooth impression on bulbar urethra, classically in young boy
  - Carcinoma: Arises from Cowper glands in urogenital diaphragm and may invade/stricture urethra

SELECTED REFERENCES

1. Sheehan JL et al: The pre-operative and post-operative imaging appearances of urethral strictures and surgical techniques. Abdom Radiol (NY). 46(5):2115-26, 2021
2. Ramanathan S et al: Imaging of the adult male urethra, penile prostheses and artificial urinary sphincters. Abdom Radiol (NY). 45(7):2018-35, 2020
3. Childs DD et al: Multimodality imaging of the male urethra: trauma, infection, neoplasm, and common surgical repairs. Abdom Radiol (NY). 44(12):3935-49, 2019

Idiopathic

Iatrogenic Injury

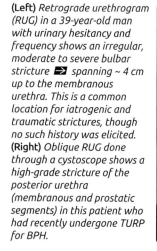
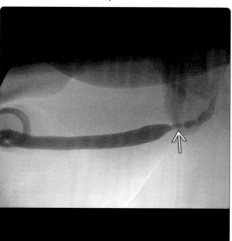
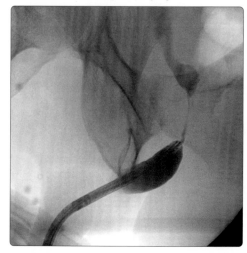

(Left) Retrograde urethrogram (RUG) in a 39-year-old man with urinary hesitancy and frequency shows an irregular, moderate to severe bulbar stricture ➡ spanning ~ 4 cm up to the membranous urethra. This is a common location for iatrogenic and traumatic strictures, though no such history was elicited. (Right) Oblique RUG done through a cystoscope shows a high-grade stricture of the posterior urethra (membranous and prostatic segments) in this patient who had recently undergone TURP for BPH.

Urethral Trauma

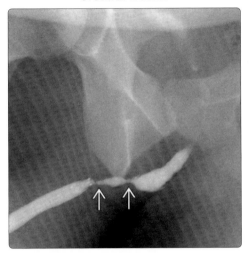

Urethral Trauma

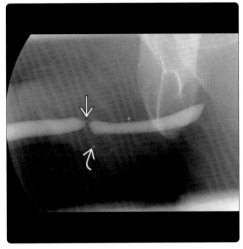

(Left) *RUG in a 26-year-old man with history of bicycle trauma 10 years prior requiring self-catheterization to void is shown. Contrast injected via cystoscope outlines a moderate-length stricture ➡ of the bulbar urethra with mild proximal dilation.* (Right) *Oblique RUG in a patient post gunshot wound to the pelvis 3 months prior shows a short-segment penile urethra stricture ➡. Notice the adjacent metallic bullet fragments ➡.*

Infectious

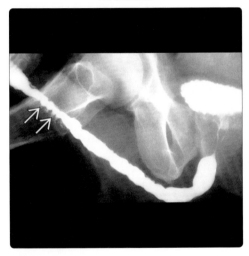

Inflammatory Diseases

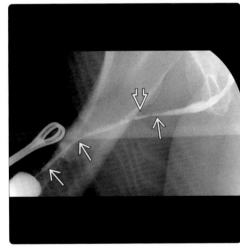

(Left) *Oblique RUG shows a long-segment irregular narrowing of the penile and bulbous urethra with filling of the glands of Littré ➡. Filling of these small submucosal mucus-secreting glands is highly associated with infectious and inflammatory etiologies.* (Right) *Oblique RUG in a patient with lichen sclerosus shows a long anterior urethral stricture ➡. This is the most common cause of a long-segment stricture. Notice glands of Littré ➡ are seen.*

Urethral Carcinoma

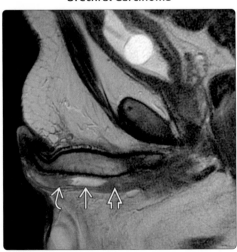

Urethral Carcinoma

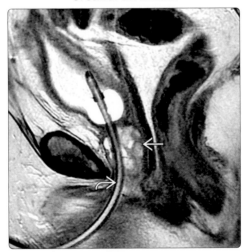

(Left) *Sagittal T2 MR shows a dilated bulbar urethra ➡ secondary to in irregular mass in the penile urethra ➡. A 2nd lesion ➡ is also seen in the more proximal bulbar urethra. Biopsy revealed adenocarcinoma.* (Right) *Coronal T2 MR shows a heterogeneous mass ➡ arising from the urethra in a 63-year-old woman. This had caused bladder outlet obstruction and dysuria; note the bladder catheter ➡.*

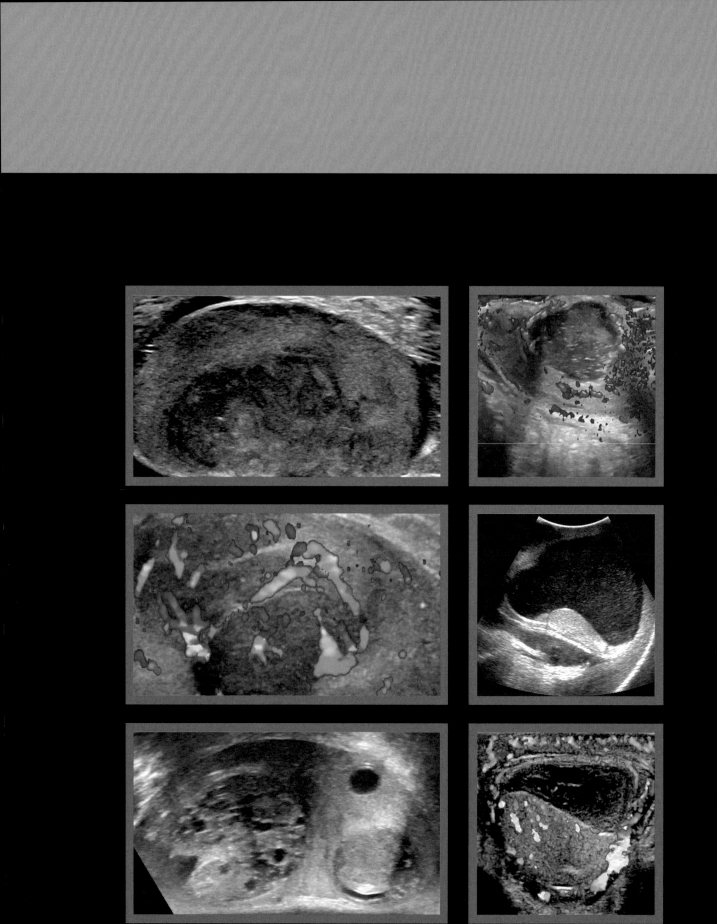

SECTION 20
Scrotum

Generic Imaging Patterns

Intratesticular Mass	604
Testicular Cystic Lesions	608
Extratesticular Cystic Mass	610
Extratesticular Solid Mass	612
Diffuse Testicular Enlargement	616
Decreased Testicular Size	618
Testicular Calcifications	620

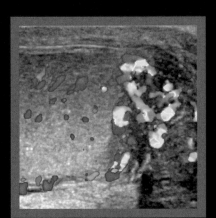

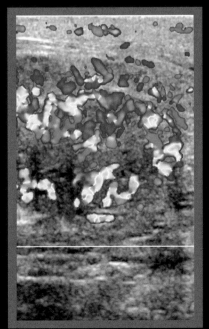

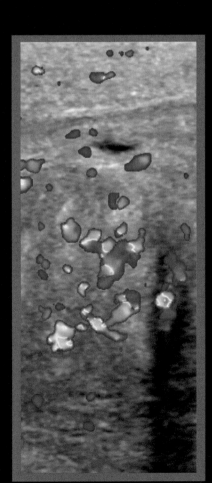

DIFFERENTIAL DIAGNOSIS

Common

- Testicular Carcinoma: Germ Cell Tumors
- Epididymitis/Orchitis
- Testicular Torsion/Infarction

Less Common

- Testicular Abscess
- Testicular Hematoma
- Testicular Lymphoma, Leukemia, and Metastases
- Gonadal Stromal Tumors, Testis
- Testicular Epidermoid Cyst

Rare but Important

- Granulomatous Orchitis
- Adrenal Rests
- Testicular Lipomatosis
- Leydig Cell Hyperplasia

ESSENTIAL INFORMATION

Key Differential Diagnosis Issues

- Age, clinical presentation, color Doppler exam
  - Trauma and avascular testicular mass: Consider hematoma
  - Young male patient, acute scrotal pain, ↑ color Doppler flow within epididymis and adjacent testis: Epididymoorchitis, abscess, segmental infarction
  - Acute scrotal pain, heterogeneous (or normal) testis with no or relatively ↓ Doppler flow: Testicular torsion
  - Young male patient with slowly growing, palpable, hypoechoic testicular mass: Seminoma or mixed germ cell tumor
  - Testicular mass and endocrinopathy: Gonadal stromal tumor
  - Older man or HIV(+) patient with bilateral hyperemic testicular masses: Lymphoma
- US findings are key (but overlap among various tumors)
  - Histopathologic correlation is needed
- CEUS and scrotal MR can be used to troubleshoot undifferentiated lesions

Helpful Clues for Common Diagnoses

- **Testicular Carcinoma: Germ Cell Tumors**
  - Most common neoplasm in males aged 15-34 years
  - Vast majority are seminomas (~ 50%) and nonseminomatous mixed germ cell tumors (~ 50%)
  - Seminoma: Typically solitary, homogeneous testicular mass
    - Sometimes large enough to replace/enlarge entire testis
    - Rare: Multifocal, bilateral or partially cystic/necrotic
  - Nonseminomatous germ cell tumors: Mixed tumors, teratoma, teratocarcinoma, embryonal cell carcinoma, yolk sac tumor, choriocarcinoma
    - Often mixed echogenicity, heterogeneous masses ± cystic components, calcification
    - Imaging overlap precludes imaging diagnosis
      - Same treatment regardless of tumor type (radical orchiectomy), so subtyping by imaging is unimportant

- Tumor markers and demographics (β-hCG, AFP, LDH) may suggest nonseminomatous component
- Occasionally, testicular carcinoma presents first as retroperitoneal lymphadenopathy
  - Important to evaluate scrotum with US in young to middle-aged man presenting with retroperitoneal mass
- Rarely, regressed/burnt-out germ cell tumor presents as vague, hypoechoic, scar-like mass or calcification

- **Epididymitis/Orchitis**
  - Most common cause for acute scrotal pain in adolescent boys and adults
  - Epididymis primarily involved: 20-40% with secondary orchitis due to contiguous spread of infection
  - Ill-defined, focal testicular echogenicity or diffusely enlarged, heterogeneous testis
    - No true mass
  - Relatively ↑ Doppler flow
    - Rare mimic: Torsion-detorsion
  - Primary mumps orchitis: Uni- or bilateral
    - Enlarged, heterogeneous, hyperemic testis; often spares epididymis

- **Testicular Torsion/Infarction**
  - Torsion: Grayscale US appearance depends upon time, course, and degree of infarction
    - Early presentation: Normal or mildly heterogeneous ± enlarged
    - Later presentation: Enlarged, heterogeneous, hypoechoic → may be confused for mass
    - Chronic: Small, atrophic testis with hypovascularity
  - Spiral twist of spermatic cord cranial to testis (whirlpool sign)
  - Color Doppler US critical for diagnosis
    - 80-90% sensitivity for acute torsion
  - Infarction
    - Complication of epididymoorchitis or may occur after surgery (retroperitoneal, inguinal hernia)
    - Segmental infarction: Wedge-shaped areas of abnormal echogenicity and absent flow
    - Can be differentiated from true mass by lack of round borders and flow
    - Rarely, global testicular infarction appears similar to torsion but no twist of cord

Helpful Clues for Less Common Diagnoses

- **Testicular Abscess**
  - Clinical history critical: Persistent/worsening symptoms on antibiotics or untreated epididymoorchitis
  - Avascular, intratesticular collection of variable echogenicity ± surrounding pyocele
  - CEUS or MR can be used to troubleshoot if concern for mass; abscess shows no central enhancement

- **Testicular Hematoma**
  - Typically focal, elongated, avascular intratesticular "mass" and history of trauma (a.k.a. testicular fracture containing blood)
  - Echogenicity depends upon hematoma age
    - Acute hematoma may be relatively echogenic
  - Critical additional findings on scrotal US
    - Tunica integrity and surrounding testicular viability (assessed by color Doppler)

– Viable testis may allow for tunica repair, hematocele evacuation of testicular salvage
- Small, contained intratesticular hematomas: US follow-up needed to ensure resolution (and to exclude underlying neoplasm)

- **Testicular Lymphoma, Leukemia, and Metastases**
  - Lymphoma
    - Most common testicular tumor in men > 60 years
      □ Multiple lesions; 50% of cases are bilateral
    - Often large in size at time of diagnosis; commonly occurs in association with disseminated disease
    - Ill-defined, predominantly hypoechoic lesions: ↑ flow on color Doppler US
  - Leukemia: Enlarged, homogeneous, hypoechoic vascular mass or multifocal nodules
  - Metastases are rare; most common sites of origin include prostate, lung, and GI tract

- **Gonadal Stromal Tumors, Testis**
  - Majority are benign but are indistinguishable from germ cell tumors
  - Clinical history (endocrinopathy secondary to ↑ estrogen or testosterone by tumor) may be suggestive
    - Children: Precocious puberty/gynecomastia
    - Adults: Impotence, ↓ libido

- **Testicular Epidermoid Cyst**
  - Benign tumor: Likely monodermal teratoma composed entirely of ectoderm
  - Sharply circumscribed, round, encapsulated lesion
    - Classic onion skin with concentric layers of keratin and desquamated squamous cells
    - No flow on color Doppler US
  - Classic appearance should prompt testis-sparing enucleation rather than radical orchiectomy

Helpful Clues for Rare Diagnoses

- **Granulomatous Orchitis**
  - Multiple ill-defined, hypoechoic masses: Mycobacterium infection, sarcoid or idiopathic
- **Adrenal Rests**

- Clinical history (congenital adrenal hyperplasia) suggests diagnosis
  - Aberrant adrenal rests trapped within developing gonad: Without stimulation, typically < 5 mm and not seen by imaging
  - If exposed to ↑ ACTH, enlarge and become palpable masses
  - May result in testicular structure damage, spermatogenesis disorder, infertility
- Bilateral, often hypoechoic testicular lesions centered about mediastinum testis

- **Testicular Lipomatosis**
  - Occurs often in Cowden syndrome (*PTEN* mutation)
  - Multiple subcentimeter hyperechoic foci without shadowing or abnormal Doppler

- **Leydig Cell Hyperplasia**
  - Associated with cryptorchidism, congenital adrenal hyperplasia, Kleinfelter syndrome, hCG-producing tumor or exogenous hCG
  - Multiple small (1-6 mm), hypoechoic nodules
  - Often not palpable and may be discovered incidentally

SELECTED REFERENCES

1. Sintim-Damoa A et al: Pearls and pitfalls of pediatric scrotal imaging. Semin Ultrasound CT MR. 43(1):115-29, 2022
2. Katabathina VS et al: Testicular germ cell tumors: classification, pathologic features, imaging findings, and management. Radiographics. 41(6):1698-716, 2021
3. Tsili AC et al: Ultrasonography of the scrotum: revisiting a classic technique. Eur J Radiol. 145:110000, 2021
4. Ramjit A et al: Complete testicular infarction secondary to epididymoorchitis and pyocele. Radiol Case Rep. 15(4):420-3, 2020
5. Saxon P et al: Segmental testicular infarction: report of seven new cases and literature review. Emerg Radiol. 19(3):217-23, 2012
6. Wasnik AP et al: Scrotal pearls and pitfalls: ultrasound findings of benign scrotal lesions. Ultrasound Q. 28(4):281-91, 2012
7. Venkatanarasimha N et al: Case 175: testicular lipomatosis in Cowden disease. Radiology. 261(2):654-8, 2011
8. Woodward PJ et al: From the archives of the AFIP: tumors and tumorlike lesions of the testis: radiologic-pathologic correlation. Radiographics. 22(1):189-216, 2002

Testicular Carcinoma: Germ Cell Tumors

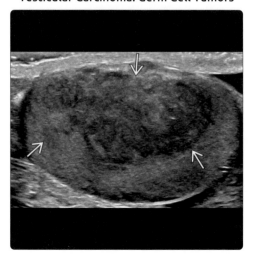

Testicular Carcinoma: Germ Cell Tumors

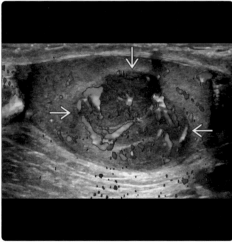

(**Left**) *Longitudinal US of the testis in a 32-year-old man shows a solid, hypoechoic, mildly heterogeneous mass ➡. Pathology revealed mixed germ cell tumor.* (**Right**) *Longitudinal color Doppler US of the testis in a 32-year-old man shows a hypoechoic, lobulated, homogeneous mass with strong color Doppler flow ➡. Pathology revealed pure seminoma. Differentiating between seminoma and nonseminomatous germ cell tumors is difficult and not necessary as the treatment is the same.*

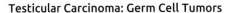

Testicular Carcinoma: Germ Cell Tumors

(Left) *Longitudinal US of the testis in a 20-year-old man with a palpable mass shows multiple masses ➡ in the testis, which are heterogeneous and partially cystic. Heterogeneous lesions are more likely to be mixed germ cell tumors, as in this case.* (Right) *Transverse color Doppler US shows enlarged, hypoechoic and hypervascular left testis ➡ compared to the right ➡. Also note the epididymal enlargement and hypervascularity ➡. Orchitis can rarely appear mass-like and focal, but clinical history usually is helpful.*

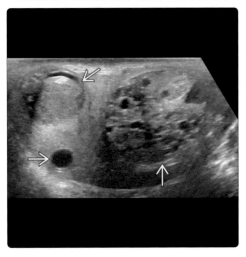

Epididymitis/Orchitis

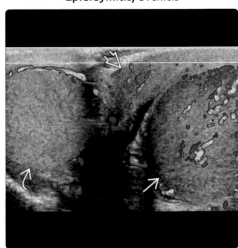

Testicular Torsion/Infarction

(Left) *Longitudinal US in a 15-year-old boy with 72 hours of scrotal pain shows an enlarged, heterogeneous testis with no color Doppler flow. This was a late presentation of torsion, and the testis was not salvageable.* (Right) *Transverse scrotal US in a 22-year-old man 3 days after football injury to the groin shows a heterogeneous cystic lesion ➡ in the testis, consistent with intratesticular hematoma. Note associated hematocele ➡ and irregular tunica ➡. Hematomas may appear different depending on the age of blood products.*

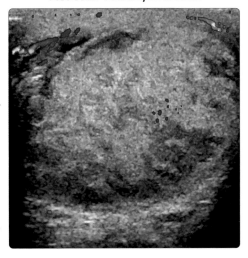

Testicular Hematoma

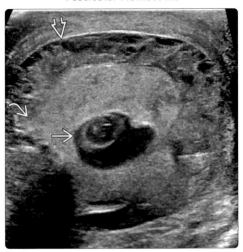

Testicular Abscess

(Left) *Color Doppler US in a patient with known epididymitis presenting with worsening symptoms shows 2 small, hypoechoic collections ➡ with rim vascularity, consistent with intratesticular abscesses. This patient was successfully managed with antibiotics.* (Right) *Longitudinal color Doppler US shows a large, mass-like, hypoechoic lesion ➡ in the testis. The lack of internal blood flow and the history of worsening pain on antibiotics for epididymitis makes abscess the most likely diagnosis.*

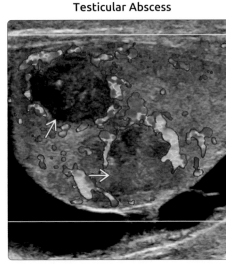

Testicular Abscess

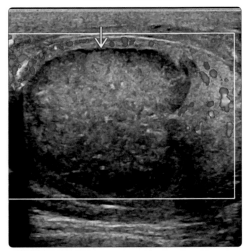

Testicular Lymphoma, Leukemia, and Metastases

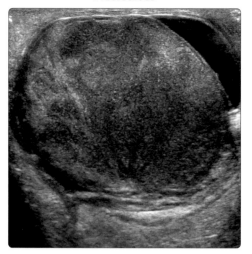

Gonadal Stromal Tumors, Testis

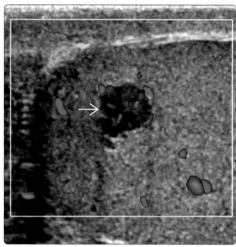

(Left) *US of an 83-year-old man with a scrotal mass shows an enlarged, heterogeneous testis. Retroperitoneal adenopathy was identified in the same setting. The age of the patient and US findings suggested lymphoma; B-cell lymphoma was identified at orchiectomy.* (Right) *Longitudinal color Doppler US in a 19-year-old man with elevated estrogen levels shows a small, hypoechoic mass ➡ with internal blood flow. Leydig cell tumor (the most common stromal tumor) was found at partial orchiectomy.*

Testicular Epidermoid Cyst

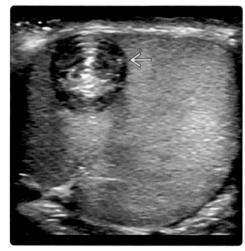

Adrenal Rests

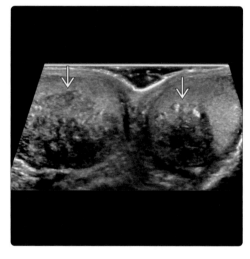

(Left) *US of a young male patient shows a well-circumscribed, hypoechoic testicular mass ➡. Its characteristic onion skin appearance is almost pathognomic of an epidermoid cyst, which was successfully enucleated.* (Right) *Transverse US of both testes in a 17-year-old boy with history of congenital adrenal hyperplasia and a palpable mass shows bilateral hypoechoic masses with echogenic foci and calcification ➡. These lesions were centered around the mediastinum testis.*

Testicular Lipomatosis

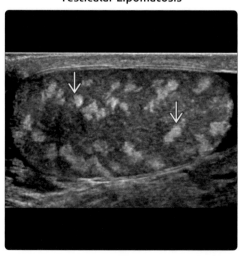

Leydig Cell Hyperplasia

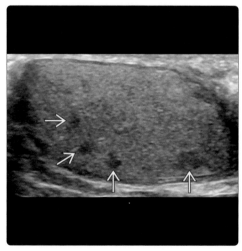

(Left) *Longitudinal US of the testis shows multiple irregular, nonshadowing, hyperechoic foci ➡. The contralateral testis had the same findings. Color Doppler US (not shown) was normal. This is typical of lipomatosis and is often seen in Cowden syndrome.* (Right) *Longitudinal US shows several very small, hypoechoic nodules ➡ in the testis. Biopsy revealed Leydig cell hyperplasia, which can occur in a variety of settings and often has this appearance.*

DIFFERENTIAL DIAGNOSIS

Common

- Nonseminomatous Germ Cell Tumor
- Tubular Ectasia of Rete Testis
- Tunica Albuginea Cyst

Less Common

- Intratesticular Cyst
- Testicular Abscess
- Posttraumatic Hematoma
- Epidermoid Cyst
- Intratesticular Varicocele

ESSENTIAL INFORMATION

Key Differential Diagnosis Issues

- Testicular cystic lesions commonly present as palpable mass and most are benign
- Most cystic neoplasms have complex features and solid components allowing easy differentiation
- Differentiation is largely based on location, size, and morphology; most cystic lesions have typical appearance

Helpful Clues for Common Diagnoses

- **Nonseminomatous Germ Cell Tumor**
  - Pure teratomas are usually well-defined, complex, predominantly cystic masses ± calcification and fat
    - Cysts may be anechoic or complex depending on cyst contents
    - Mixed tumors with germ cell component may have cystic foci
  - Cystic necrosis or hemorrhage is sometimes encountered in germ cell tumors (often yolk sac and choriocarcinoma) and may mimic cystic lesion
- **Tubular Ectasia of Rete Testis**
  - Variably sized tubular and cystic lesions at mediastinum testis
  - No flow on color Doppler US
  - Associated with spermatocele, male infertility, and vasectomy

- **Tunica Albuginea Cyst**
  - Common etiology for palpable mass
  - Along tunica, may indent testis slightly
  - Usually solitary, 2-7 mm in diameter, can be septate

Helpful Clues for Less Common Diagnoses

- **Intratesticular Cyst**
  - Generally simple cysts with no septation
  - Near mediastinum testis
- **Testicular Abscess**
  - Usually complication of epididymoorchitis; usually late presentation or worsening on antibiotics
  - Simple or complex heterogeneous cystic collection with rim Doppler vascularity
  - Lack of internal Doppler flow argues against tumor but may be difficult to distinguish
    - History is important; follow-up US may be needed
    - CEUS can be used to evaluate enhancement pattern and help differentiate
- **Posttraumatic Hematoma**
  - Less common manifestation of trauma is intratesticular hematoma
  - Variable appearance depends on age of blood products
- **Epidermoid Cyst**
  - Rarely anechoic; typically, layered keratin creates lamellated (onion skin), echogenic appearance
  - May have calcified capsule
  - Benign; important to recognize so that testis-sparing surgery can be performed rather than radical orchiectomy
- **Intratesticular Varicocele**
  - May mimic tubular ectasia though veins are usually much larger than ductules
  - Color Doppler US confirms venous flow
  - Often without extratesticular varicocele component

SELECTED REFERENCES

1. Katabathina VS et al: Testicular germ cell tumors: classification, pathologic features, imaging findings, and management. Radiographics. 41(6):1698-716, 2021

Nonseminomatous Germ Cell Tumor

Tubular Ectasia of Rete Testis

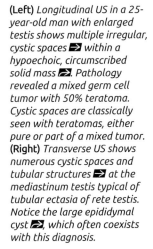
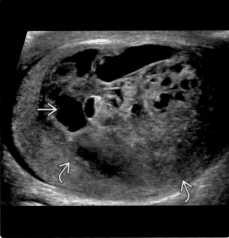
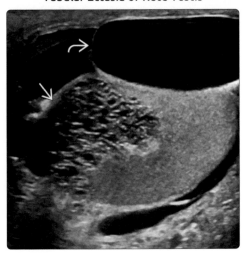

(Left) *Longitudinal US in a 25-year-old man with enlarged testis shows multiple irregular, cystic spaces ➡ within a hypoechoic, circumscribed solid mass ➔. Pathology revealed a mixed germ cell tumor with 50% teratoma. Cystic spaces are classically seen with teratomas, either pure or part of a mixed tumor.* **(Right)** *Transverse US shows numerous cystic spaces and tubular structures ➔ at the mediastinum testis typical of tubular ectasia of rete testis. Notice the large epididymal cyst ➔, which often coexists with this diagnosis.*

Testicular Cystic Lesions

Tunica Albuginea Cyst

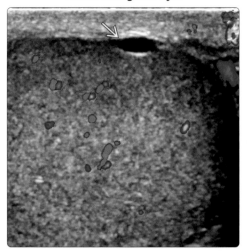

Intratesticular Cyst

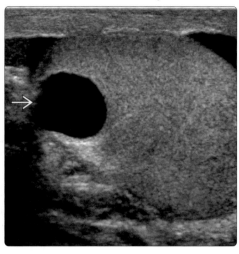

(Left) *Transverse US shows a small, oval simple cyst* ➡ *along the periphery of the testis. The location, size, and appearance is typical of a tunica albuginea cyst. These are common palpable complaints and are benign.* (Right) *Longitudinal US shows a simple cyst* ➡ *within the testicle. The lack of a soft tissue component distinguishes this from a cystic mass.*

Testicular Abscess

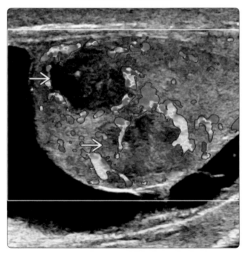

Posttraumatic Hematoma

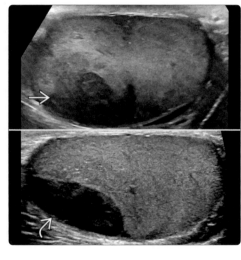

(Left) *Transverse color Doppler US shows 2 hypoechoic cystic lesions* ➡ *in the testis with increased peripheral Doppler flow. The patient had a history of epididymitis not responding to antibiotics, and these represent intratesticular abscesses.* (Right) *Longitudinal US of the testis performed immediately following trauma shows a vague, hypoechoic mass* ➡. *Follow-up 10 days later shows a complex cyst* ➡ *consistent with evolving hematoma. Appearance of hematomas will depend on the age of the blood products.*

Epidermoid Cyst

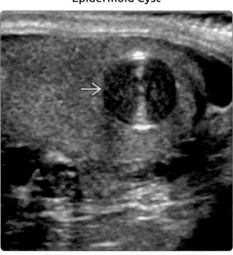

Intratesticular Varicocele

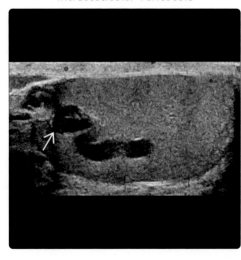

(Left) *Longitudinal US shows a circumscribed cystic mass* ➡ *with lamellated (onion skin) appearance. This is the classic appearance of an epidermoid cyst and should be recognized to avoid an unnecessary orchiectomy.* (Right) *Longitudinal US shows a cyst mimic with a dilated, tubular, hypoechoic structure* ➡ *near the mediastinum. Little Doppler flow is seen at rest, but increased flow was demonstrated with Valsalva maneuver, consistent with intratesticular varicocele.*

DIFFERENTIAL DIAGNOSIS

Common

- Hydrocele
- Spermatocele/Epididymal Cyst
- Varicocele (Mimic)

Less Common

- Hematocele
- Pyocele
- Scrotal Wall Fluid Collection

Rare but Important

- Epididymal Papillary Cystadenoma

ESSENTIAL INFORMATION

Helpful Clues for Common Diagnoses

- **Hydrocele**
  - Serous fluid contained within layers of tunica vaginalis
    - Congenital: Communicating hydrocele secondary to failure of processus vaginalis to close
    - Most idiopathic, some reactive to epididymitis, varicocelectomy, etc.
  - Surrounds testis except for "bare area" where tunica vaginalis is deficient
    - Displaces testis posteriorly
    - Differentiates from very large epididymal cyst
  - Chronic hydroceles contain low-level echoes (falling-snow sign)
- **Spermatocele/Epididymal Cyst**
  - Differentiated by contents (simple fluid within epididymal cyst, echogenic fluid containing spermatozoa within spermatocele) though makes little difference clinically
  - Epididymal cysts occur throughout epididymis
  - Associated with dilatation of rete testis
  - Large epididymal cysts may be confused for hydrocele; fluid does not surround testis as seen in hydrocele
- **Varicocele (Mimic)**
  - Multiple dilated, serpiginous veins of pampiniform plexus > 3 mm in diameter due to retrograde flow in gonadal vein
    - CDUS and morphology readily distinguishes varicocele from other extratesticular lesions
  - Enlarge and show increased velocity with Valsalva maneuver or upon standing

Helpful Clues for Less Common Diagnoses

- **Hematocele**
  - Blood within tunica vaginalis potential space
  - Post trauma (assess testicle CDUS carefully for absent flow and look for tunica rupture)
    - Occasionally post inguinal hernia repair
  - Echogenicity depends upon age of blood; acute clot may appear echogenic, subacute with many avascular strands similar to ovarian hemorrhagic cyst
- **Pyocele**
  - Complex fluid collection containing septations, low-level echoes within layers of tunica vaginalis
  - Generally complication of epididymoorchitis
  - Color Doppler US: Rim vascularity around collection and of scrotal wall and ↑ vascularity of epididymis ± testis
- **Scrotal Wall Fluid Collection**
  - Clinical context key (e.g., trauma → hematoma or fever, leukocytosis → abscess)
  - Fluid collection with gas → Fournier gangrene
  - Median raphe cyst: Midline cyst that occurs anywhere from penile meatus to perineum

Helpful Clues for Rare Diagnoses

- **Epididymal Papillary Cystadenoma**
  - Rare benign neoplasm, typically in young adult male patients
  - Associated with von Hippel-Lindau disease
  - Cystic or solid mass in epididymis

SELECTED REFERENCES

1. Srisajjakul S et al: Diagnostic clues, pitfalls, and imaging characteristics of '-celes' that arise in abdominal and pelvic structures. Abdom Radiol (NY). 45(11):3638-52, 2020

Hydrocele

Spermatocele/Epididymal Cyst

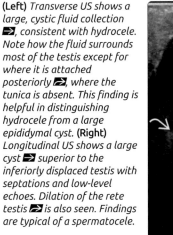

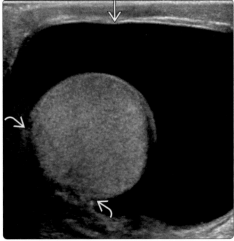

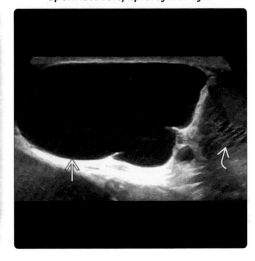

(Left) Transverse US shows a large, cystic fluid collection ➡, consistent with hydrocele. Note how the fluid surrounds most of the testis except for where it is attached posteriorly ➡, where the tunica is absent. This finding is helpful in distinguishing hydrocele from a large epididymal cyst. (Right) Longitudinal US shows a large cyst ➡ superior to the inferiorly displaced testis with septations and low-level echoes. Dilation of the rete testis ➡ is also seen. Findings are typical of a spermatocele.

Hydrocele

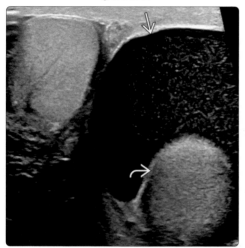

Varicocele (Mimic)

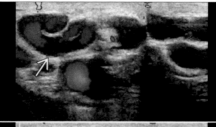
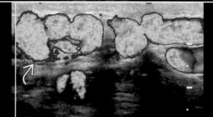

(Left) *Transverse US of both testis shows a large left complex hydrocele ➡ containing multiple punctate echoes. Echoes in the cyst fluid usually represent proteinaceous debris and are associated with chronicity. Note how the testis ➡ is displaced posteriorly, which is typical.* (Right) *Color Doppler US in a patient with a palpable mass shows a serpiginous, anechoic, cyst-like lesion ➡ with incomplete Doppler flow. With Valsalva, the Doppler flow increases ➡ in velocity due to reflux, consistent with varicocele.*

Hematocele

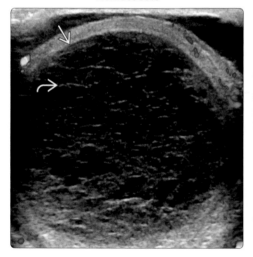

Pyocele

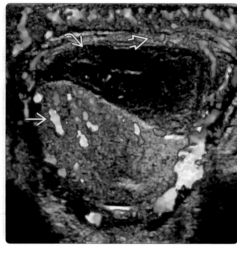

(Left) *Transverse US of the scrotum after surgery for epididymal cyst resection shows a complex cystic collection ➡ with fine strands ➡ showing no color Doppler flow. This is typical of a hematocele. Appearance will depend on the age of the blood products.* (Right) *Transverse color Doppler US in the setting of acute pain shows hyperemia of the left testis ➡, representing orchitis, as well as hyperemia of the tunica and scrotal skin ➡ around a complex septated fluid collection ➡, consistent with pyocele.*

Scrotal Wall Fluid Collection

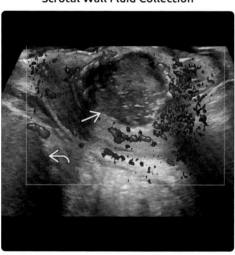

Epididymal Papillary Cystadenoma

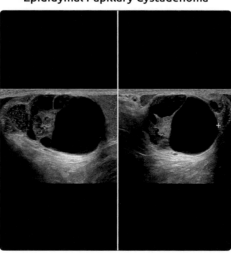

(Left) *Transverse US of the scrotum in a patient with pain and erythema shows a hypoechoic complex cyst ➡ with ↑ rim color Doppler vascularity. Note the superficial location at the skin surface, separate from the testis ➡, consistent with a scrotal wall abscess.* (Right) *Sagittal and transverse scrotal US shows a mixed cystic and solid epididymal head mass. Patient history of von Hippel-Lindau suggested epididymal papillary cystadenoma, a rare benign epididymal lesion. (Courtesy T. Desser, MD.)*

DIFFERENTIAL DIAGNOSIS

Common
- Epididymitis
- Inguinal Hernia
- Torsion of Testicular Appendage
- Scrotal Pearl
- Sperm Granuloma

Less Common
- Adenomatoid Tumor
- Mesenchymal Tumors, Scrotum
- Fibrous Pseudotumor
- Papillary Cystadenoma, Epididymis

Rare but Important
- Metastatic Disease
- Polyorchidism
- Mesothelioma of Tunica Vaginalis

ESSENTIAL INFORMATION

Key Differential Diagnosis Issues
- Clinical presentation + US findings key
- Painful lesions: Epididymitis, appendix testicular torsion, complicated hernia, occasionally sperm granuloma
- Neoplasms, on the other hand, are generally nonpainful and present as palpable masses or vague discomfort
- Most extratesticular masses are benign

Helpful Clues for Common Diagnoses
- **Epididymitis**
  - US: Increase or decrease in echogenicity depending upon acute or chronic stage
    - Echogenic tissues surrounding epididymis (edema)
  - Enlarged, hyperemic epididymis on color Doppler US
    - 20-40% present with concomitant orchitis → enlarged, heterogeneous and hyperemic testis
  - Epididymitis is usually diffuse, however, may be focal generally in tail as this is 1st site of ascending infection
    - Focal epididymitis in tail often presents as heterogeneous mass with increased Doppler flow
  - Epididymal abscess: Focal heterogeneous collection in epididymis with hypervascular Doppler rim
- **Inguinal Hernia**
  - Typically, indirect type may descend into scrotum and simulate extratesticular mass
    - Direct hernias, when large, can also descend into scrotum
  - Bowel or fat seen within scrotum or inguinal canal
    - Fat is identified by increased echogenicity, lack of peristalsis and should be able to be traced up to internal inguinal ring
    - Bowel is identified by typical alternating hyper- and hypoechoic layers as well as peristalsis and luminal contents on US
    - Important to identify vascularity, normal wall thickness, and peristalsis of bowel to exclude strangulation
  - Valsalva or standing US is important and may show dynamic nature of hernia
- **Torsion of Testicular Appendage**

- Most common cause of acute scrotal pain in child
- Mean age is 9 years, whereas testicular torsion occurs later at mean of 14 years
- US: Enlarged, round, hypoechoic, avascular nodule along testis or epididymis at site of patient pain + hyperemia of surrounding tissues
  - Size cutoff of 5.6 mm is specific for torsion
  - Reactive hydrocele
- **Scrotal Pearl**
  - Detached and calcified testicular appendages secondary to prior torsion or inflammation
  - Commonly seen incidentally on US and frequent palpable complaint
  - US: Small, round, echogenic, calcified nodule with shadowing
  - May be fixed or mobile
- **Sperm Granuloma**
  - Nonspecific appearance; clinical history of vasectomy or other causes of epididymal tubular obstruction (trauma, infection) can suggest diagnosis
  - US: Heterogeneous appearance often with hyperechoic wall and hypoechoic center
    - May contain punctate, hyperechoic foci
  - Often associated with postvasectomy appearance of epididymis: Enlarged with tubular ectasia

Helpful Clues for Less Common Diagnoses
- **Adenomatoid Tumor**
  - 2nd most common extratesticular tumor
    - 36% of all extratesticular neoplasms
  - Typically located in epididymal tail
  - US: Well-defined, solid mass with variable echogenicity from iso- to hyperechoic
    - Hypovascularity on color Doppler, may be peripheral
- **Mesenchymal Tumors, Scrotum**
  - Lipoma most common extratesticular benign neoplasm; may be difficult to distinguish from fat-containing hernia
    - Hernia tends to be anterior to spermatic cord; lipoma lateral or posterior
    - Hernia moves with Valsalva; lipoma static
    - US: Variable echogenicity; soft → deforms with transducer pressure
    - Sometimes lower echogenicity than surrounding fat tissue; may see fine septa/lobulations
    - MR: Fat signal, no enhancement or soft tissue
  - Leiomyoma: Variable echogenicity, edge shadowing, whorled, Doppler flow
  - Most common malignant tumors include rhabdomyosarcoma (child) and liposarcoma, leiomyosarcoma (adult)
    - Large, irregular, heterogeneous vascular mass originating or extending into inguinal canal
- **Fibrous Pseudotumor**
  - Reactive fibrous proliferation, usually associated with/attached to tunica
  - US: Generally hypoechoic with strong posterior shadowing
    - Absent flow on color Doppler US
  - MR: Very low-signal mass on T2 MR
    - Slow and low enhancement with gadolinium administration

- May be multifocal
- Reactive hydrocele
- Range in size from millimeters to 8 cm in diameter
- **Papillary Cystadenoma, Epididymis**
  - Epididymal component of von Hippel-Lindau syndrome (VHL)
    - Seen in 65% of patients with VHL
  - Often bilateral; found in young adults
  - Ill-defined, solid mass with scattered cysts

Helpful Clues for Rare Diagnoses

- **Metastatic Disease**
  - Typically GU, GI tumors
  - Usually multiple other metastatic sites
- **Polyorchidism**
  - Extremely rare congenital disorder
  - Extratesticular mass with similar echo pattern as adjacent testis: MR for confirmation
  - Classified based upon presence or absence of epididymis/vas deferens
  - Mimic: Splenogonadal fusion
- **Mesothelioma of Tunica Vaginalis**
  - Complex hydrocele with multiple nodules or masses arising from tunica

SELECTED REFERENCES

1. Karbasian N et al: Pathologic conditions at imaging of the spermatic cord. Radiographics. 42(3):741-75, 2022
2. Hannappel TD et al: Imaging appearance of cystic and solid mesothelioma of the tunica vaginalis. Radiol Case Rep. 15(7):809-11, 2020
3. Sharbidre KG et al: Imaging of scrotal masses. Abdom Radiol (NY). 45(7):2087-108, 2020
4. Mittal PK et al: Spectrum of extratesticular and testicular pathologic conditions at scrotal MR imaging. Radiographics. 38(3):806-30, 2018
5. Secil M et al: Imaging features of paratesticular masses. J Ultrasound Med. 36(7):1487-509, 2017
6. Bertolotto M et al: Imaging of mesothelioma of tunica vaginalis testis. Eur Radiol. 26(3):631-8, 2016
7. Mukherjee S et al: Clinico-radiological and pathological evaluation of extra testicular scrotal lesions. J Cytol. 30(1):27-32, 2013
8. Park SB et al: Imaging features of benign solid testicular and paratesticular lesions. Eur Radiol. 21(10):2226-34, 2011

Epididymitis

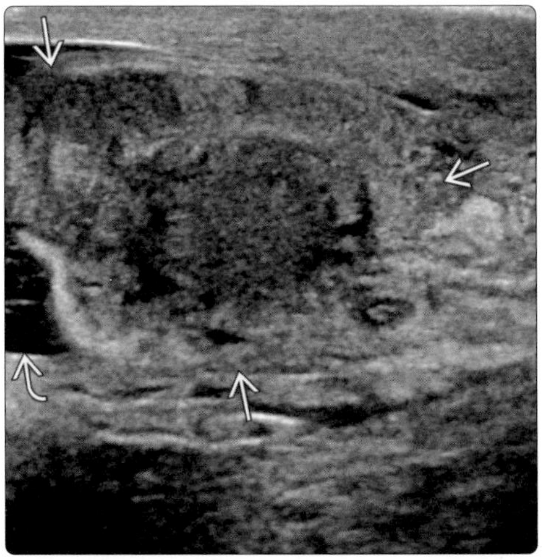

Epididymitis

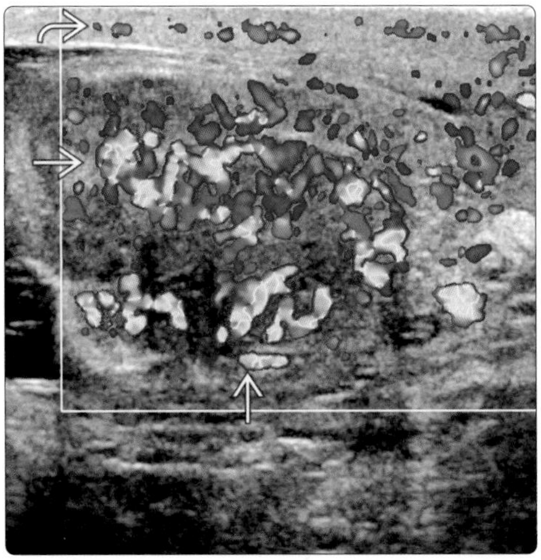

(Left) *Longitudinal US shows a heterogeneous, enlarged, mass-like area ➡ at the epididymal tail. Notice adjacent complex hydrocele with septations ↪.* **(Right)** *Color Doppler US in the same patient shows marked hyperemia of the mass ➡ and also of the overlying scrotal skin ↪. The patient had acute pain and dysuria. Findings are typical of epididymitis, which sometimes causes mass-like enlargement.*

Epididymitis

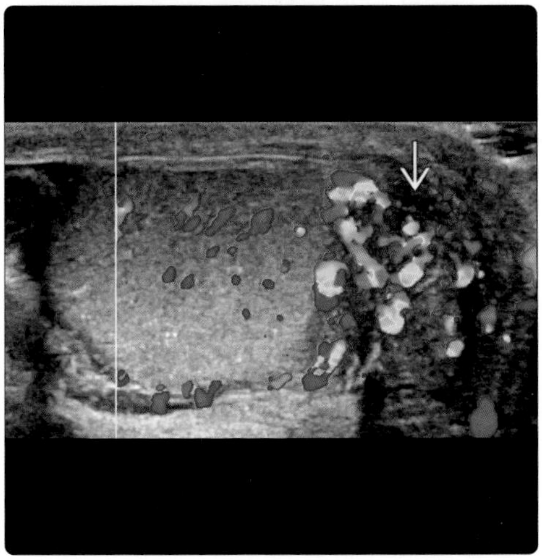

Epididymitis

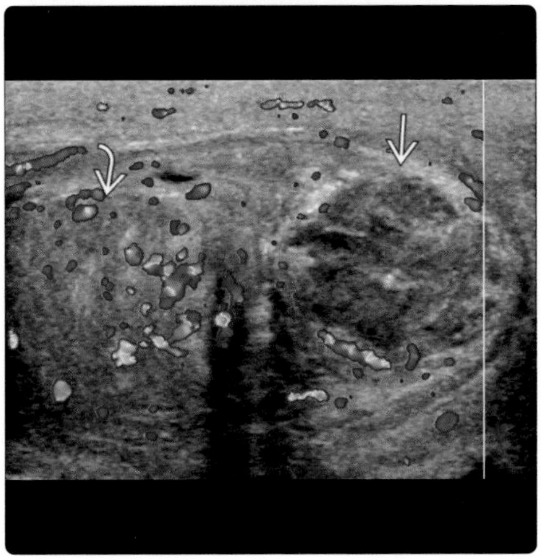

(Left) *Longitudinal color Doppler US in a patient with acute pain shows a markedly hypervascular mass ➡ at the epididymal tail. It is important to remember that epididymitis starts in the tail and spreads to the head and testis, so focal painful masses in the tail are often infection.* **(Right)** *Longitudinal color Doppler US shows a round, heterogeneous mass ➡ inferior to the testis ↪ with peripheral Doppler flow only. Note hyperemia of the testis as well. This represented an epididymal tail abscess in the setting of epididymoorchitis.*

Inguinal Hernia

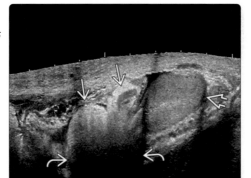

Inguinal Hernia

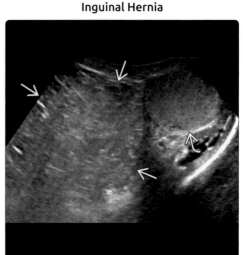

(Left) *Extended field-of-view US shows a large inguinal hernia that displaces the testis ➡. "Dirty" shadowing ➡ is shown posterior to the gas-containing bowel ➡. Peristalsis seen in real time is also useful to identify bowel.* (Right) *Longitudinal US shows a large, echogenic mass ➡ with scattered fine septa displacing the testis ➡ inferiorly, typical of a fat-containing hernia. Lack of bowel signature, gas, and peristalsis allows differentiation from a bowel-containing hernia.*

Torsion of Testicular Appendage

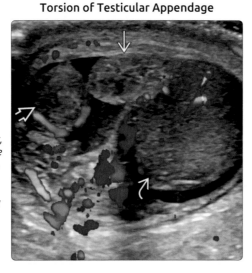

Sperm Granuloma

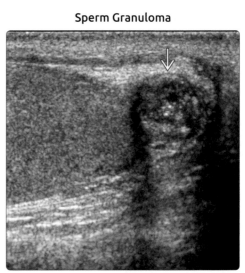

(Left) *Transverse color Doppler US of the right scrotum in an 8-year-old with acute pain shows a heterogeneous, avascular, oval mass ➡ adjacent to the testis ➡ and epididymis ➡. This is typical of appendage torsion.* (Right) *Longitudinal US shows a round, hypoechoic, heterogeneous mass ➡ at the epididymal tail with punctate, echogenic foci internally and peripheral flow (not shown). The patient reported a history of vasectomy.*

Adenomatoid Tumor

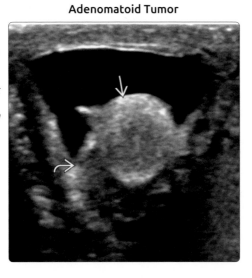

Adenomatoid Tumor

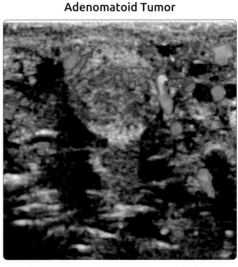

(Left) *Transverse US in a 56-year-old patient with a new, palpable scrotal mass shows a small, round, hyperechoic extratesticular mass ➡ in the inferior right scrotum adjacent to the tail of the epididymis ➡.* (Right) *Color Doppler US in the same patient shows mild vascularity within this mass. The patient went on to surgery and adenomatoid tumor was found. This is the typical US appearance.*

Mesenchymal Tumors, Scrotum

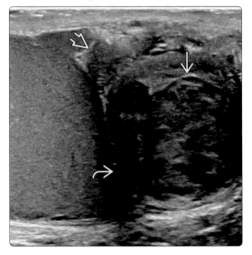

Mesenchymal Tumors, Scrotum

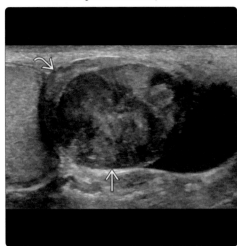

Mesenchymal Tumors, Scrotum

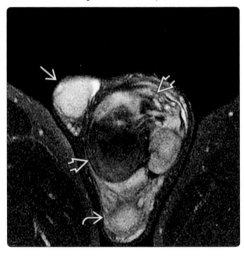

Fibrous Pseudotumor

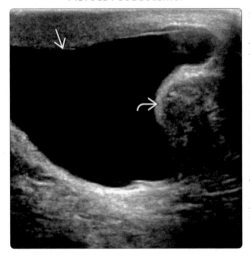

Papillary Cystadenoma, Epididymis

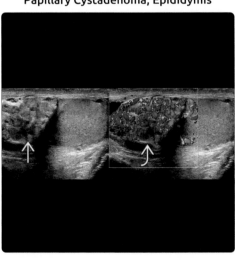

Polyorchidism

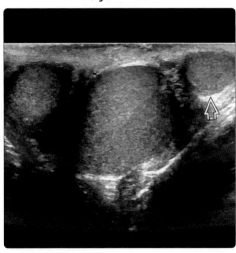

(Left) *Longitudinal US in a 60-year-old patient shows a large, heterogeneous, hypoechoic extratesticular mass* ➡ *near the tail of the epididymis* ➡. *Edge shadowing is seen* ➡. *Imaging is nonspecific in this case. Resection found a leiomyoma.* (Right) *Longitudinal US shows a round, hypoechoic mass* ➡ *at the epididymal tail* ➡. *Resection showed leiomyosarcoma. Distinguishing mesenchymal tumors can be difficult though malignant lesions tend to be large and heterogeneous, unlike this case.*

(Left) *Axial T2 MR of an older man performed to evaluate a growing extratesticular mass shows a mixed-signal mass* ➡, *which displaces right* ➡ *and left* ➡ *testes. A spermatic cord liposarcoma was resected. MR is particularly helpful for evaluating large, extratesticular masses.* (Right) *Longitudinal US shows a large hydrocele* ➡ *and a round, hypoechoic, shadowing mass* ➡ *along the tunica vaginalis. These lesions range in size from small and multifocal to solitary and large.*

(Left) *US of a young male patient with von Hippel-Lindau syndrome (VHL) to assess growing bilateral extratesticular lesions shows an enlarged, heterogeneous right epididymis* ➡, *which is hyperemic on color Doppler* ➡. *The left was similar-appearing. Papillary cystadenomas of epididymis are rare; benign lesions are strongly associated with VHL.* (Right) *US to evaluate a palpable scrotal mass shows a supernumerary testis* ➡.

DIFFERENTIAL DIAGNOSIS

Common

- Orchitis
- Testicular Torsion/Infarction
- Testicular Carcinoma
- Scrotal Trauma

Less Common

- Testicular Lymphoma/Leukemia
- Testicular Metastases
- Testicular Cyst

ESSENTIAL INFORMATION

Key Differential Diagnosis Issues

- Diagnosis depends, not on US appearance alone, but on combination of clinical and imaging features

Helpful Clues for Common Diagnoses

- **Orchitis**
  - Characterized by edema of testes contained within rigid tunica albuginea
  - Heterogeneous parenchymal echogenicity and septal accentuation seen as hypoechoic bands
  - Diffuse increase in testicular parenchymal vascularity on color Doppler US
  - Epididymitis almost always coexists in cases of bacterial infection
  - Isolated orchitis occurs typically in viral infection, such as mumps
- **Testicular Torsion/Infarction**
  - Testicular torsion
    - In early torsion, testis is typically normal in size and grayscale appearance
    - After 12 hours, enlargement and heterogeneity is seen, and testicle is often nonviable
    - Whirlpool sign or "torsion knot" at level of spermatic cord; dampened or absent vascularity in testis
  - Testicular infarction
    - Segmental infarction: Wedge-shaped, heterogeneous area with no flow; most commonly seen with epididymitis
    - Global infarction: Diffusely enlarged, hypoechoic testis similar to torsion
- **Testicular Carcinoma**
  - Discrete, hypoechoic or mixed echogenic testicular mass ± vascularity
  - May be large enough to completely replace entire tests with no normal tissue seen
- **Scrotal Trauma**
  - Generally, well-defined traumatic event is clue; handlebar, sports injuries common
  - Discrete, linear/irregular fracture plane within testis, tunica albuginea rupture with extrusion of tubules, hematocele
  - Intratesticular hematoma: Avascular, mass-like lesion; echogenicity of hematoma depends on its age

Helpful Clues for Less Common Diagnoses

- **Testicular Lymphoma/Leukemia**
  - Uni- or multifocal nodules or diffuse, infiltrative, hypoechoic lesions in man > 60 years
  - 20-35% of cases bilateral
  - Color Doppler US shows straight normal vessels coursing through lesion
- **Testicular Metastases**
  - Metastases are rare; most common sites include prostate, lung, and GI tract
    - Ill-defined, mostly hypoechoic lesions
    - Associated with disseminated disease
- **Testicular Cyst**
  - Intratesticular cysts are usually simple cysts located near mediastinum testis
  - May be associated with tubular ectasia of rete testis
  - Need to differentiate from cystic neoplasms
    - Search carefully for solid components and internal vascularity

(Left) *Transverse color Doppler US shows an enlarged, hypoechoic, hyperemic right testis* *compared to the left* ⮢ *with a complex hydrocele or developing pyocele* ⮢. **(Right)** *Sagittal grayscale US of the left testis demonstrates an enlarged, heterogeneous testis* ⇨ *with surrounding pyocele* ⮢ *and overlying skin thickening* ⮢, *suggestive of acute orchitis.*

Orchitis

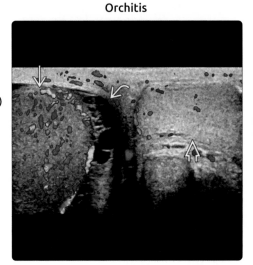

Orchitis

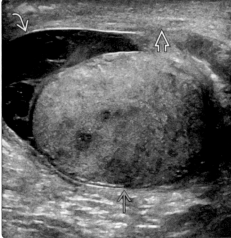

Testicular Torsion/Infarction

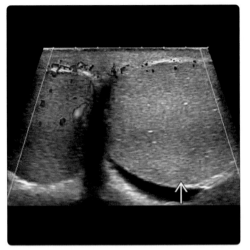

Testicular Carcinoma

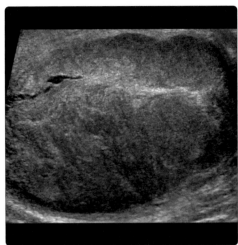

(Left) Transverse color Doppler US in an 11-year-old boy shows an enlarged, mildly hyperechoic left testis ➡ with no blood flow, consistent with torsion. The testis was viable and salvaged in the OR. (Right) Longitudinal US shows a large, hypoechoic, heterogeneous mass replacing the entire testis. Pathology showed pure embryonal carcinoma.

Testicular Carcinoma

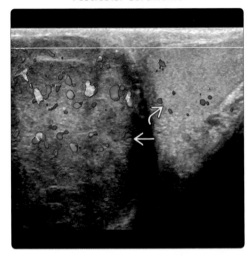

Scrotal Trauma

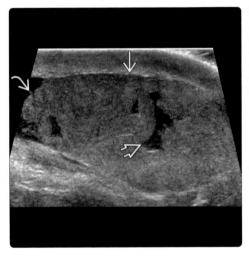

(Left) Transverse color Doppler US shows an enlarged, hyperemic right testicle ➡ compared to the left ➡. Notice the abnormal heterogeneous, hypoechoic parenchyma, consistent with a large mass replacing the entire testis. A seminoma was found at resection. (Right) Longitudinal US of the testis after a motorcycle crash shows an enlarged testis ➡ with internal fluid areas ➡. Notice the irregular surface ➡ and lack of distinct capsule, which represents rupture with extrusion of tubules.

Testicular Lymphoma/Leukemia

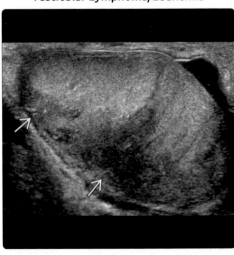

Testicular Cyst

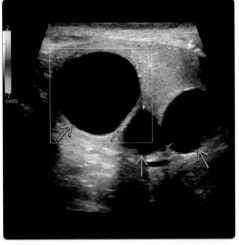

(Left) Longitudinal US in a 62-year-old man shows an enlarged testis with infiltrative, hypoechoic lesions ➡. Doppler US (not shown) showed normal vessels running through these areas. Diffuse large B-cell lymphoma was found, the most common lymphoma to involve the testis. (Right) Transverse color Doppler US demonstrates an enlarged left testis with multiple anechoic structures ➡ without internal blood flow or solid components, compatible with testicular cysts.

DIFFERENTIAL DIAGNOSIS

Common
- Testicular Infarction
- Scrotal Trauma
- Cryptorchidism
- Hypogonadism

Rare but Important
- Chronic Mass Effect
- Polyorchidism
- Mumps Orchitis

ESSENTIAL INFORMATION

Key Differential Diagnosis Issues
- Reduction in size considered significant if volume of affected testis reduced to 20% of unaffected testis
- Consider testicular atrophy if combined axis measurements of testes differ by ≥ 10 mm or if testicular size < 4 x 2 cm
- Atrophic testis is often decreased in echogenicity and shows decreased color Doppler flow
  - Sometimes shows striated appearance with linear bands of decreased echogenicity (tiger stripes); fibrosis interspersed with normal tissue
- Differentiation of causes is often based on age and history
- Atrophy important as it is associated with male subfertility or infertility

Helpful Clues for Common Diagnoses
- **Testicular Infarction**
  - Posttorsion atrophy: Variable success of testicular salvage, resulting in ischemia and atrophy
    - Particularly likely if long duration of pain (> 12 h) and heterogeneous grayscale US at time of torsion
  - Infarction is known complication of inguinal hernia surgery
  - Segmental or global infarction is rare complication of epididymoorchitis
  - Missed torsion: In utero cord torsion (45%) or may present later in life

- Uniformly hypoechoic or focal mixed echogenicity of testis (or striated appearance) with absence of flow are features of diffuse or focal infarction, respectively
  - Reduced echogenicity is sensitive marker of poor outcome compared to clinical parameters
- **Scrotal Trauma**
  - Hematoma, fracture, or rupture leads to nonviable parenchyma and may result in atrophy depending on severity of injury and management
- **Cryptorchidism**
  - Exhibits different degrees of atrophy with altered parenchymal echogenicity
    - Less echogenic and smaller than normally descended testis
- **Hypogonadism**
  - Androgen deprivation therapy for prostate cancer
  - Klinefelter syndrome: Most common cause of primary hypogonadism
    - Leydig cell hyperplasia: Hyperechoic lesions
  - Pituitary neoplasm, Kallmann syndrome, hypogonadotrophic hypogonadism, sickle cell disease
  - Transgender person (male to female) on estrogen therapy

Helpful Clues for Rare Diagnoses
- **Chronic Mass Effect**
  - Longstanding hernia or hydrocele may compromise testicular blood flow and result in atrophy
- **Polyorchidism**
  - Homogeneously echogenic oval structure with echogenicity identical to that of normal testis but smaller in size
- **Mumps Orchitis**
  - Occurs in 15-30% of postpubertal males and results in atrophy in 40-70%
  - During active infection, testis is enlarged and hypervascular; later, small and hypovascular

SELECTED REFERENCES

1. Yang DM et al: Small testes: clinical characteristics and ultrasonographic findings. Ultrasonography. 40(3):455-63, 2021

Testicular Infarction

Testicular Infarction

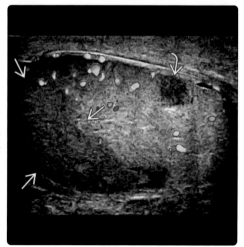

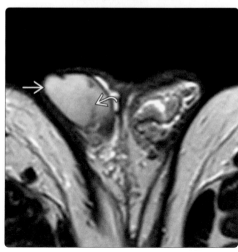

(Left) Longitudinal color Doppler US of the testis shows a large, hypoechoic, wedge-shaped area ➡ with absent color flow, consistent with segmental infarction. A similar, smaller area ➡ is also seen. This classically occurs in the setting of epididymitis and is often treated conservatively. (Right) Axial T2 MR in the same patient 2 years later shows an atrophic right testicle ➡ with T2-dark fibrotic band ➡.

Scrotal Trauma

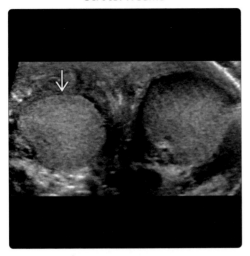

Cryptorchidism

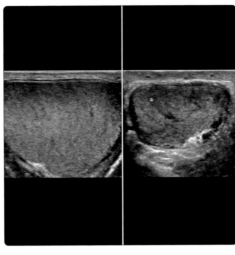

(Left) Transverse US shows an asymmetrically small right testis ⇨ compared to the left. The patient had sustained testicular rupture 6 months prior and underwent surgical repair. (Right) Transverse US of both testes in a 48-year-old man who had undergone orchiopexy as a child is shown. Notice the smaller, hypoechoic and heterogeneous left testicle compared to the right, consistent with atrophy. This should not be mistaken for a mass.

Hypogonadism

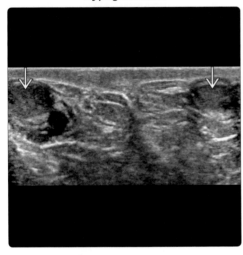

Hypogonadism

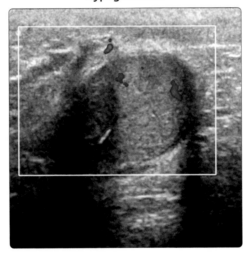

(Left) Transverse US in a 28-year-old man with Klinefelter syndrome shows markedly small testes ⇨, consistent with hypogonadism. (Right) Transverse color Doppler US in a transgender (male-to-female) patient shows a small, hypoechoic and hypovascular testis. This is due to hypogonadism from estradiol therapy.

Chronic Mass Effect

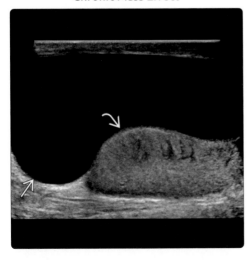

Mumps Orchitis

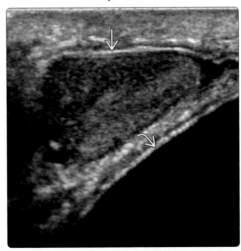

(Left) Longitudinal US shows a large fluid collection ⇨ partially surrounding the testis, consistent with a hydrocele. The testis ⇨ is small and hypoechoic with dark bands, consistent with atrophy and fibrosis. (Right) Longitudinal US of the right testis in a 68-year-old man shows a small, hypoechoic testis ⇨. A large left epididymal cyst ⇨ is partially seen. This patient had mumps orchitis as a child and developed atrophy after the infection.

DIFFERENTIAL DIAGNOSIS

Common
- Testicular Microlithiasis
- Scrotal Pearl (Mimic)
- Germ Cell Tumor

Less Common
- Scrotal Trauma
- Epidermoid Cyst
- Scrotal Tuberculosis

Rare but Important
- Large Cell Calcifying Sertoli Cell Tumor

ESSENTIAL INFORMATION

Key Differential Diagnosis Issues
- Correlation between clinical and US features essential
  - Incidental finding: Testicular microlithiasis, scrotal pearl
  - Mass with intrinsic calcification: Testicular tumors, epidermoid cyst
  - Associated with trauma: Testicular hematoma, hematocele

Helpful Clues for Common Diagnoses
- **Testicular Microlithiasis**
  - Multiple small (1-3 mm), discrete, nonshadowing, echogenic intratesticular foci; rarely large calcification
  - Unilateral or bilateral involvement
  - May be seen concurrently with tumor but common benign finding alone
- **Scrotal Pearl (Mimic)**
  - Calcification of detached testicular epididymal appendages due to previous inflammation or torsion of appendages
  - Solitary discrete, echogenic, shadowing focus in tunica vaginalis along margin of testis; not truly intratesticular
- **Germ Cell Tumor**
  - Solid testicular mass; calcification may be present in seminoma or nonseminomatous germ cell tumors

- Calcifications more common in tumors that contain teratomatous components
- Pure teratoma (postpubertal type) often has macrocalcification
- **Burnt-out germ cell tumor**: Regression of primary testis tumor that has already spread to lymph nodes or metastasized
  - Linear or nodular macrocalcification, scar-like hypoechoic area, atropic testis
  - Most common in teratoma and choriocarcinoma

Helpful Clues for Less Common Diagnoses
- **Scrotal Trauma**
  - Foci of calcification could be due to remote testis hematoma or fracture
    - No associated soft tissue mass
- **Epidermoid Cyst**
  - Lamellated appearance on US is classic
  - May have peripheral calcified rim or focal calcification
- **Scrotal Tuberculosis**
  - Epididymis most commonly involved
  - Orchitis may appear as diffuse, hypoechoic enlargement or multiple hypoechoic nodules or numerous miliary nodules
  - Tuberculous infections may calcify after treatment/healing and produce rim-like tunica calcification

Helpful Clues for Rare Diagnoses
- **Large Cell Calcifying Sertoli Cell Tumor**
  - ~ 40% occur in Peutz-Jeghers or Carney complex
  - Present at mean of 16 years of age
  - Calcified, round mass; may be multifocal and bilateral

SELECTED REFERENCES

1. Katabathina VS et al: Testicular germ cell tumors: classification, pathologic features, imaging findings, and management. Radiographics. 41(6):1698-716, 2021

(Left) *Longitudinal US shows numerous 1-mm calcifications* ➡ *without shadowing, consistent with microlithiasis. There is an association with malignancy; however, imaging follow-up is generally not recommended.* **(Right)** *Longitudinal US shows an oval, shadowing calcification* ➡ *at the margin of the testis. Transverse US shows that the calcification is within the tunica* ➡ *and extratesticular, typical of a scrotal pearl, which may present as a palpable complaint.*

Testicular Microlithiasis

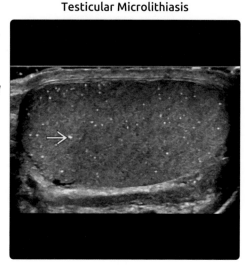

Scrotal Pearl (Mimic)

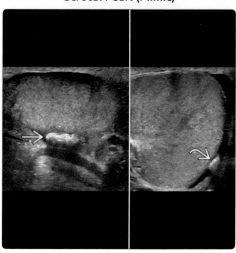

Germ Cell Tumor

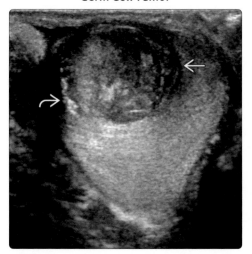

Germ Cell Tumor

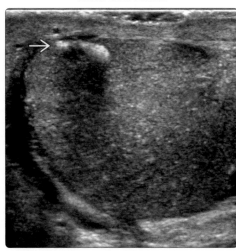

(Left) Transverse US in a 19-year-old shows a round, hyperechoic testicular mass ➡ with peripheral calcification ➡. Pathology showed a nonseminomatous mixed germ cell tumor. (Right) Transverse US in a 25-year-old with multiple enlarged retroperitoneal nodes shows a linear, calcified lesion ➡ in the testis without a mass. This represented a burnt-out germ cell tumor.

Germ Cell Tumor

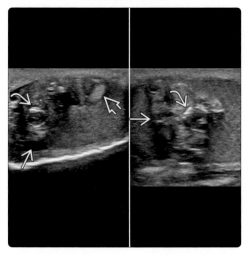

Scrotal Trauma

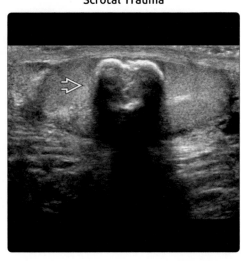

(Left) Transverse and longitudinal US in a 28-year-old shows a heterogeneous mass ➡ with multiple calcifications ➡ and echogenic foci ➡. Pathology showed postpubertal teratoma. (Right) Sagittal US of the right testis shows a densely calcified mass ➡. Pathology confirmed fibrosis with heterotopic ossification, likely secondary to prior traumatic injury.

Epidermoid Cyst

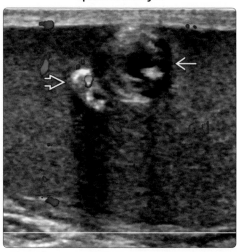

Large Cell Calcifying Sertoli Cell Tumor

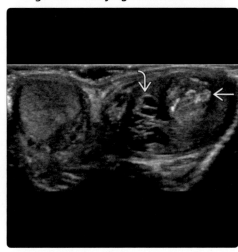

(Left) Longitudinal US shows a circumscribed, avascular mass ➡ with a somewhat lamellated appearance. A focus of peripheral calcification ➡ is seen with shadowing and twinkle artifact. Such an appearance should suggest epidermoid, and a partial orchiectomy may be appropriate. (Right) Transverse US of both testes in a 11-year-old shows a solid, partially calcified mass ➡ in the left testis. Dilated rete testis ➡ is seen adjacent. Pathology showed large cell calcifying Sertoli cell tumor.

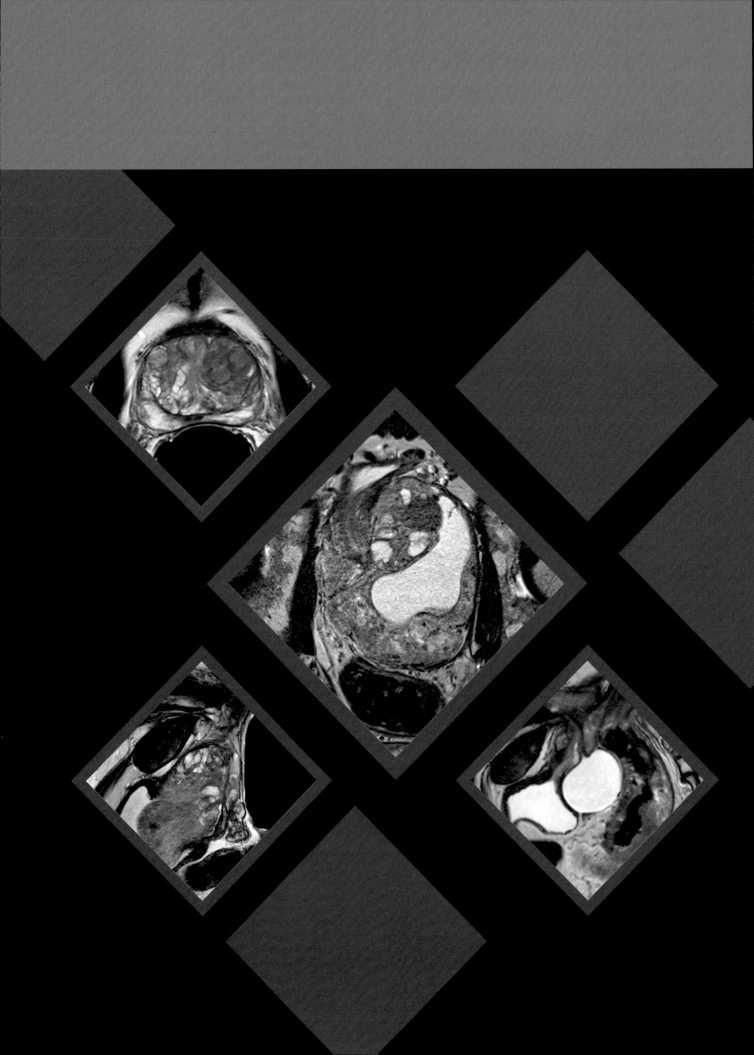

SECTION 21
Prostate and Seminal Vesicles

Generic Imaging Patterns

Focal Lesion in Prostate   624
Enlarged Prostate   630

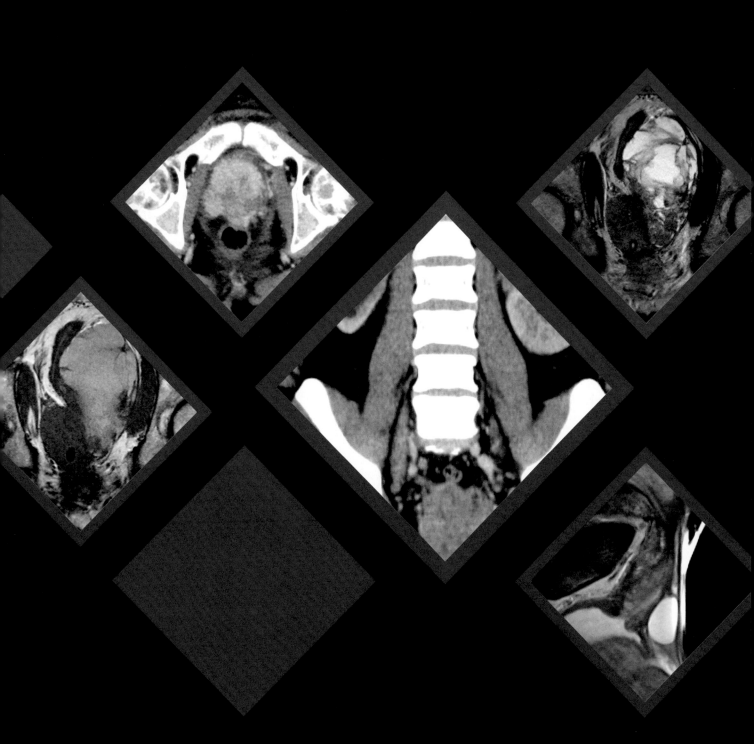

DIFFERENTIAL DIAGNOSIS

Common

- Benign Prostatic Hyperplasia Nodules
  - Typical Nodule
  - Atypical Nodule
  - Cystic or Hemorrhagic Nodule
  - Exophytic Nodule
- Prostatic Carcinoma
- Prostatitis
- Normal Central Zone (Mimic)
- Prostatic Calcification
- Prostatic Utricle Cyst
- Hemorrhage

Less Common

- Müllerian Duct Cyst
- Prostatic Abscess
- Ejaculatory Duct Cyst
- Granulomatous Prostatitis

Rare but Important

- Other Rare Prostatic Tumors

ESSENTIAL INFORMATION

Helpful Clues for Common Diagnoses

- **Benign Prostatic Hyperplasia Nodules**
  - T2 MR: Enlarged transition zone (TZ) with multiple nodules; signal of nodule depends on histologic composition
    - ↑ signal intensity: Proliferation of glandular elements
    - ↓ signal intensity: Proliferation of stromal elements
    - Sometimes referred to as "organized chaos" appearance → heterogeneous appearance of benign prostatic hyperplasia (BPH) organized into encapsulated nodular areas
  - Nodules may extend into bladder base → intravesical prostatic protrusion
  - **Typical BPH nodule**: Completely encapsulated nodule (PI-RADS T2 score 1)
    - Sometimes coronal and sagittal better show encapsulation
    - May show variable DWI but that does not change overall PI-RADS score of 1
  - **Atypical BPH nodule**: Mostly encapsulated or homogeneous, low-signal, circumscribed nodule without encapsulation
    - If marked DWI (score 4/5), upgraded to overall PI-RADS 3
    - Overall low chance of cancer in these nodules (~ 6%)
  - **Cystic BPH nodule**: Cystic degeneration of BPH nodule is most common cystic prostatic lesion
    - May contain ↑ T1 signal due to proteinaceous or hemorrhagic contents
  - **Exophytic (extruded) BPH nodule:** TZ nodule extends beyond pseudocapsule into peripheral zone (PZ)
    - May mimic PZ cancer with moderate to marked DWI
    - However, usually heterogeneous and encapsulated on T2 MR and abutting pseudocapsule, allowing for differentiation
- **Prostatic Carcinoma**
  - > 95% of tumors are adenocarcinoma
  - Location
    - 70-75% in PZ, 20-30% in TZ, and < 5% in central zone (CZ)
  - Multiparametric MR (mpMR)
    - T2
      - PZ: Focal, hypointense lesion with round/oval, lenticular, or subcapsular shape
      - TZ: Ill-defined, lenticular shape, ↓ signal intensity lesion ± invasion of anterior fibromuscular stroma
    - DWI: Marked ↑ signal intensity on high b-value image (b > 1,400 s/mm²) and marked ↓ signal intensity on ADC map
    - DCE: Early enhancement ± delayed washout
  - Differentiation of BPH nodule from cancer originating from TZ can be challenging and is mainly based on morphologic features
    - PI-RADS T2 score 4/5: Noncircumscribed, homogeneous, hypointense, often anterior location
    - PI-RADS T2 score 3: Heterogeneous with obscured margins
      - Upgrade to score 4 if DWI score is 5 (marked DWI and ADC signal ≥ 1.5 cm)
- **Prostatitis**
  - Clinical history is helpful for differential diagnosis, e.g., urinary symptoms; gland tender at palpation
  - mpMR
    - Can be diffuse or focal
    - Often asymptomatic and may be manifestation of chronic prostatitis &/or fibrosis
    - Best clue: Wedge shape or linear lesion in PZ with mild/moderate DWI/ADC
      - PI-RADS: PZ T2 score 2 and DWI score 2 → overall PI-RADS 2
    - DCE often shows enhancement, generally sustained and does not washout like tumor
    - Sometimes diffuse involving nearly entire PZ; DWI score 1-3 helps distinguish from tumor
    - Occasionally round and can mimic cancer (DWI score 3 and +DCE → overall PI-RADS 4)
- **Prostatic Calcification**
  - Common feature of chronic prostatitis and of no clinical significance
    - Caused by calcium precipitation inside acini whose ducts are obstructed by inflammation
  - mpMR: ↓ signal intensity on all sequences
  - CT: Hyperdense foci
- **Prostatic Utricle Cyst**
  - Cystic dilatation of prostatic utricle, acquired or congenital
    - Congenital associated with hypospadias, undescended testes, and unilateral renal agenesis
  - Intraprostatic, midline, arises from verumontanum, usually confined to prostate
  - Usually small, tubular, or pear-shaped
  - Often communicates with urethra
- **Hemorrhage**
  - Common after TRUS biopsy and usually appears in PZ and seminal vesicles
  - In general, hemorrhage is often mild and does not obscure cancer

– Rarely, it is severe and limits interpretation

○ Hemorrhage tends to involve benign tissue, and cancers are located elsewhere

○ Hemorrhage exclusion sign: Cancer foci in PZ show lack of ↑ T1 signal due to hemorrhage sparing cancer and filling normal glands

Helpful Clues for Less Common Diagnoses

- **Müllerian Duct Cyst**
  ○ Originates from remnant of müllerian duct
  ○ Usually large midline cyst extending above prostatic base
    – Differentiation from utricle cyst is difficult and generally clinically irrelevant
  ○ Oval/teardrop-shaped, rarely communicates with urethra

- **Prostatic Abscess**
  ○ Complication of acute prostatitis or seeding from hematogenous spread of infection
  ○ One or multiple prostatic rim-enhancing collections ± septa ± gas
  ○ More common in periphery of gland
    – May extend beyond prostate

- **Ejaculatory Duct Cyst**
  ○ Secondary to congenital or inflammatory obstruction of ejaculatory duct
  ○ Located along course of ejaculatory duct
    – Paramedian at base, midline at verumontanum
  ○ Can be associated with dilated, obstructed seminal vesicle
  ○ Intracystic calculi are common

- **Granulomatous Prostatitis**
  ○ Etiology: Idiopathic > prior BCG therapy for bladder cancer > TB
  ○ 3 patterns seen on T2 MR: Diffuse (most common), nodular, or cystic with mural nodule
    – Often located in PZ
    – When nodular, often has polygonal shape with notch along border
  ○ DWI: Typically shows marked restricted diffusion → PI-RADS 4/5

○ DCE: Avid enhancement

○ Diagnosis can be suspected in man with prior history of BCG therapy for bladder cancer
  – However, biopsy usually required given that it is **indistinguishable from cancer**

Helpful Clues for Rare Diagnoses

- **Other Rare Prostatic Tumors**
  ○ **Mucinous cystadenoma or cystadenocarcinoma**
    – Large, multiloculated cystic mass; variable high fluid signal intensity on both T1/T2 MR (similar to other mucinous tumors in body)
    – Little areas of diffusion restriction
    – Metastatic lymph nodes may contain mucin (cystic)
    – Patients typically present with obstructive voiding symptoms
  ○ **Stromal tumor of uncertain malignant potential (STUMP)**
    – Large, well-circumscribed mass with heterogeneous appearance on T2 MR (variable amounts of cystic and solid components)
    – Can appear similar to prostate sarcoma or BPH nodules
  ○ **Prostate sarcomas**
    – Predominantly solid, heterogeneous, vascular mass; high-grade tumors show tumor necrosis; occurs more often in younger men (35-60 years of age)
    – Typically large and locally advanced at diagnosis
    – Rhabdomyosarcoma: Most common tumor in children and adolescents
    – Postradiation sarcomas: Occur at median of 6 years after radiation, tend to be large and aggressive

SELECTED REFERENCES

1. Marcal LP et al: Mesenchymal neoplasms of the prostate and seminal vesicles: spectrum of disease with radiologic-pathologic correlation. Radiographics. 42(2):417-32, 2022
2. Turkbey B et al: Prostate Imaging Reporting and Data System Version 2.1: 2019 Update of Prostate Imaging Reporting and Data System Version 2. Eur Urol. 76(3):340-51, 2019

Typical Nodule

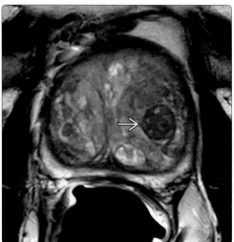

Typical Nodule

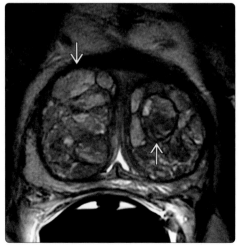

(Left) *Axial T2 MR shows benign prostatic hyperplasia (BPH) with typical heterogeneous but organized appearance. An encapsulated, heterogeneous nodule* ➔ *stands out from the background. PI-RADS T2 score is 1.* **(Right)** *Axial T2 MR of the prostate shows an enlarged transition zone with multiple encapsulated, heterogeneous nodules* ➔ *of varying signal intensity. These are typical BPH nodules. PI-RADS T2 score is 1.*

Atypical Nodule

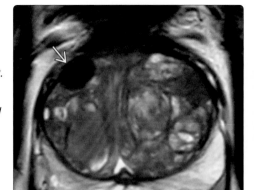

Atypical Nodule

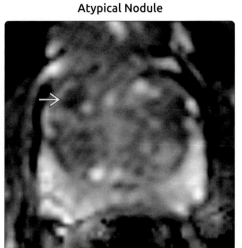

(Left) *Axial T2 MR shows an anterior transition zone T2 dark nodule ➡, which is sharply circumscribed and homogeneous without a capsule. PI-RADS T2 score is 2.* (Right) *Axial ADC map in the same patient shows mild ↓ signal ➡. Corresponding DWI MR showed no ↑ signal. DWI score is 3. Overall PI-RADS score is 2.*

Cystic or Hemorrhagic Nodule

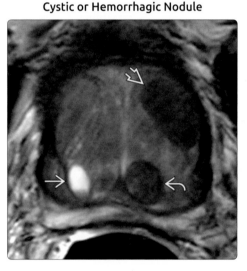

Cystic or Hemorrhagic Nodule

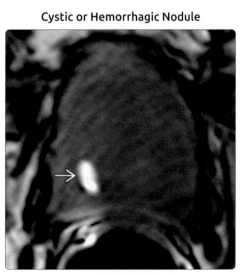

(Left) *Axial T2 MR shows a hyperintense cyst ➡ in within BPH, consistent with cystic BPH nodule. Typical ➡ and atypical ➡ nodules are also seen.* (Right) *Axial T1 MR in the same patient shows hyperintensity within the cystic nodule ➡, representing proteinaceous or hemorrhagic fluid.*

Exophytic Nodule

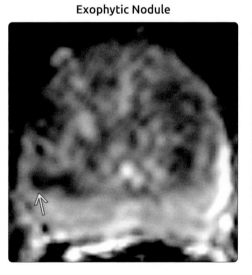

Exophytic Nodule

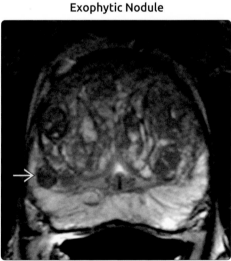

(Left) *Axial ADC map shows focal, marked ↓ signal ➡. Corresponding DWI MR showed marked ↑ signal in the right peripheral zone, and DWI was score 4.* (Right) *Axial T2 MR in the same patient shows a corresponding focal, round lesion ➡ in the right peripheral zone. Note that it abuts the pseudocapsule and shows a thin, dark capsule. This is a pitfall for peripheral zone cancer and should be scored as a transition zone lesion. PI-RADS score is 1.*

Prostatic Carcinoma

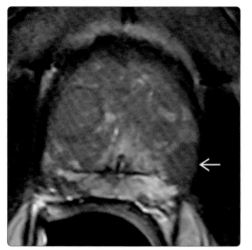

Prostatic Carcinoma

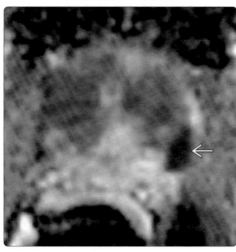

(Left) *Axial T2 MR shows a focal, oval, homogeneous, hypointense, circumscribed lesion ➡ in the left peripheral zone.* **(Right)** *Axial ADC map in the same patient shows marked ↓ signal ➡. Corresponding DWI MR showed marked ↑ signal. PI-RADS DWI score was 5. Overall PI-RADS score is 5. Biopsy showed Gleason 4+3 (grade group 3) cancer.*

Prostatic Carcinoma

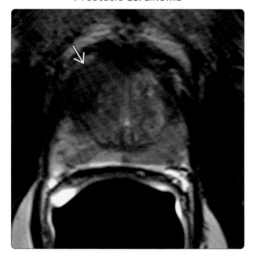

Prostatic Carcinoma

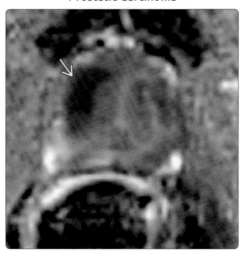

(Left) *Axial T2 MR shows a noncircumscribed, lenticular, homogeneous, hypointense lesion ➡ ≥ 1.5 cm in the right anterior transition zone. PI-RADS T2 score is 5.* **(Right)** *Axial ADC map in the same patient shows marked ↓ signal ➡. DWI score was 5. Overall PI-RADS score is 5. Targeted biopsy showed Gleason 3+4 (grade group 2) cancer.*

Prostatitis

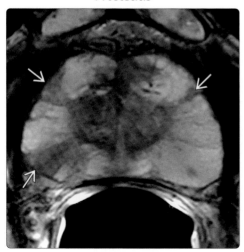

Prostatitis

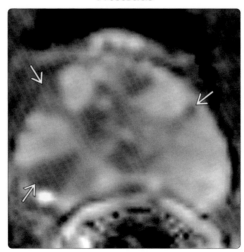

(Left) *Axial T2 MR shows multiple bilateral, wedge-shaped and streaky, hypointense lesions ➡ in the peripheral zone. PI-RADS T2 score is 2.* **(Right)** *Axial ADC map in the same patient shows mild hypointensity ➡ in wedge-shaped and linear lesions. PI-RADS DWI score was 2. Overall PI-RADS score is 2.*

Normal Central Zone (Mimic)

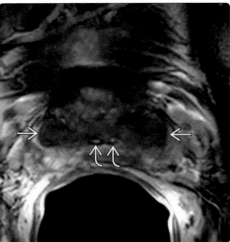

Normal Central Zone (Mimic)

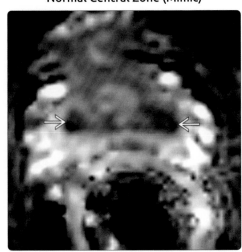

(Left) *Axial T2 MR shows round, T2 dark nodules at the base of the prostate, which at first glance appear to represent focal lesions ➡. However, note the symmetry and location adjacent to the ejaculatory ducts ➡. (Right) Axial ADC map in the same patient shows restricted diffusion ➡ in these areas. This is the typical location and appearance of the normal central zone and should not be confused with a tumor.*

Prostatic Calcification

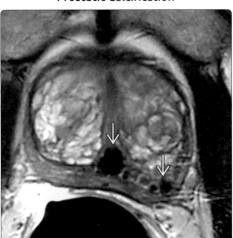

Prostatic Calcification

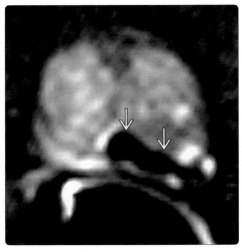

(Left) *Axial T2 MR shows multiple round, T2 dark foci ➡ in the left peripheral zone. (Right) Axial DWI MR in the same patient shows signal void ➡ in the left peripheral zone due to calcification.*

Prostatic Utricle Cyst

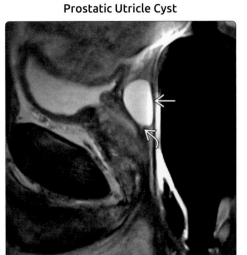

Hemorrhage

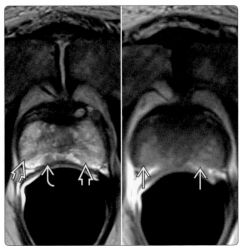

(Left) *Sagittal T2 MR shows a simple cyst ➡ in the midline base of the prostate. There is suggestion of communication with the urethra ➡. (Right) Axial MR shows moderate, diffuse T1 hyperintensity ➡ and patchy/linear T2 hypointensity ➡ throughout the peripheral zone due to postbiopsy hemorrhage. This however did not obscure a small, round PI-RADS 4 lesion ➡.*

Prostatic Abscess

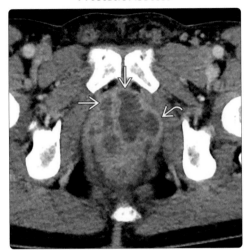

Ejaculatory Duct Cyst

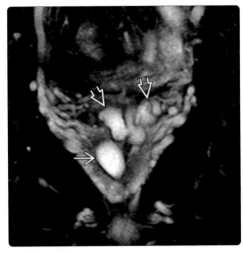

(Left) *Axial CECT in a patient with history of IV drug use shows large, lobulated, complex, rim-enhancing collections* ➔ *in the prostate extending into left periprostatic soft tissues* ➔. (Right) *Coronal T2 FS MR in man with low sperm count shows a right paramedian cyst* ➔ *along the course of the ejaculatory duct, consistent with ejaculatory duct cyst. Also note the dilated left seminal vesicle* ➔, *presumably due to obstruction of the left ejaculatory duct.*

Granulomatous Prostatitis

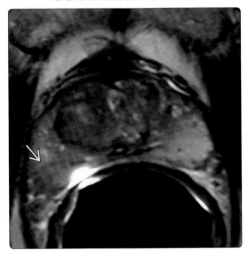

Granulomatous Prostatitis

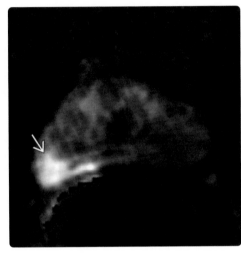

(Left) *Axial T2 MR in a 61-year-old with a PSA of 7 ng/mL and history of prior bladder cancer treated with BCG shows a focal, hypointense nodule* ➔ *in the right peripheral zone.* (Right) *Axial DWI MR shows marked hyperintensity of the lesion* ➔. *DWI score is 4, and overall PI-RADS score is 4. MR-guided prostate biopsy showed granulomatous prostatitis.*

Other Rare Prostatic Tumors

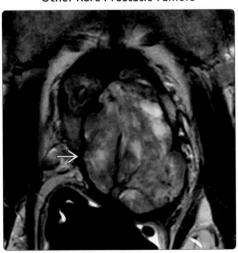

Other Rare Prostatic Tumors

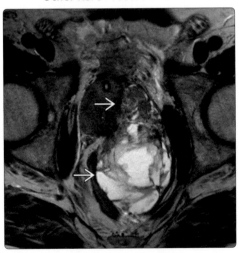

(Left) *Axial T2 MR shows a large, heterogeneous mass* ➔ *arising from the prostate and extending into the periprostatic space. Note the T2 dark capsule. Biopsy revealed STUMP.* (Right) *Axial T2 MR shows a large, heterogeneous, cystic and solid mass* ➔ *arising from the left prostate and extending into the perirectal space. Biopsy revealed mucinous adenocarcinoma.*

DIFFERENTIAL DIAGNOSIS

Common
- Benign Prostatic Hyperplasia

Less Common
- Prostatic Adenocarcinoma
- Prostatitis ± Abscess
- Prostatic Cyst
- Secondary Involvement of Periprostatic Tumors

Rare but Important
- Other Rare Prostatic Tumors
- IgG4-Related Disease

ESSENTIAL INFORMATION

Key Differential Diagnosis Issues
- Normal prostate typically 3 x 3 x 5 cm
- Prostate considered enlarged when > 25 mL

Helpful Clues for Common Diagnoses
- **Benign Prostatic Hyperplasia**
  - By far, most common cause of prostatomegaly (50% prevalence by 50-60 years of age)
  - Glandular and stromal hyperplasia in transition zone (TZ); peripheral zone compressed
  - Heterogeneously enlarged TZ compressing peripheral and central zones
  - May extend into bladder base → intravesical prostatic protrusion (previously called median lobe hypertrophy)

Helpful Clues for Less Common Diagnoses
- **Prostatic Adenocarcinoma**
  - Most cases of prostate cancer do not cause global enlargement
  - Locally advanced prostate cancer: Look for avid, homogeneous enhancement on CT with invasion of seminal vesicle or extracapsular extension
- **Prostatitis ± Abscess**
  - Prostatitis: Diffusely, mildly enlarged prostate (but may be normal in size), ↑ enhancement, periprostatic fat stranding
  - Prostatic abscess: Uni- or multilocular collection with thick walls/septa and rim enhancement
- **Prostatic Cyst**
  - Large utricle cyst (midline), ejaculatory duct cyst (paramedian), or müllerian duct cysts (midline, extending above base)
- **Secondary Involvement of Periprostatic Tumors**
  - Bladder and rectal cancers most common

Helpful Clues for Rare Diagnoses
- **Other Rare Prostatic Tumors**
  - **Mucinous cystadenoma or cystadenocarcinoma**
    - Large, multiloculated cystic mass; variable fluid signal intensity on T1/T2 MR
    - Patients typically present with obstructive voiding symptoms
  - **Stromal tumor of uncertain malignant potential (STUMP)**
    - Large, well-circumscribed mass with heterogeneous appearance on T2 MR (variable amounts of cystic and solid components)
    - Can appear similar to prostate sarcoma or BPH nodules
  - **Prostate sarcomas**
    - Predominantly solid, heterogeneous, vascular mass; high-grade tumors show tumor necrosis; occurs more often in younger men (ages 35-60)
- **IgG4-Related Disease**
  - Diffuse enlargement and infiltration or periprostatic infiltrating mass
  - Look for other organ involvement: Pancreas, bile ducts, kidneys, RPF

SELECTED REFERENCES

1. Marcal LP et al: Mesenchymal neoplasms of the prostate and seminal vesicles: spectrum of disease with radiologic-pathologic correlation. Radiographics. 42(2):417-32, 2022

Benign Prostatic Hyperplasia

Benign Prostatic Hyperplasia

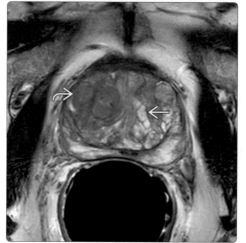

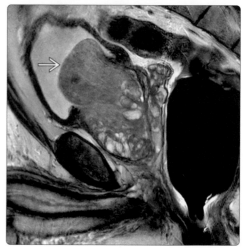

(Left) Axial T2 MR shows an enlarged transition zone of prostate due to benign prostatic hyperplasia (BPH). This is the typical appearance with multiple encapsulated nodules of various signal intensity. Higher intensity areas ➡ represent glandular hyperplasia, whereas lower intensity areas ➡ represent stromal hyperplasia. (Right) Sagittal T2 MR shows markedly enlarged prostate gland due to BPH of transition zone. Note extension into bladder base ➡, which is termed intravesical prostatic protrusion.

Prostatic Adenocarcinoma

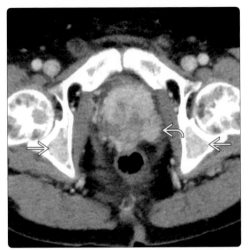

Prostatitis ± Abscess

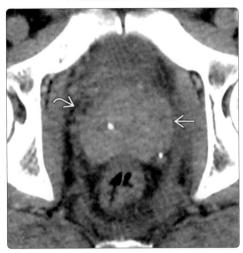

(Left) *Axial CECT in a patient with bone pain shows an enlarged prostate due to locally advanced prostate cancer. The hyperenhancement and extension beyond the capsule ➡ is typical. Bone metastases ➡ are also seen.* (Right) *Axial CECT in a patient with a UTI shows a mildly enlarged and hyperenhancing prostate ➡. Subtle periprostatic fat stranding ➡ is also seen. Findings are suggestive of prostatitis.*

Prostatitis ± Abscess

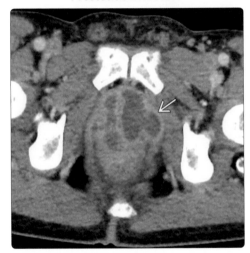

Prostatic Cyst

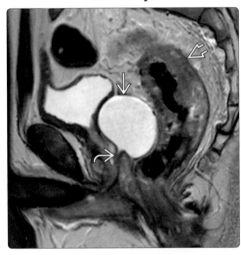

(Left) *Axial CECT shows an enlarged prostate due to multilocular, rim-enhancing fluid collections ➡, typical of prostatic abscess.* (Right) *Sagittal T2 MR shows an enlarged prostate due to a large midline cyst ➡, which communicates with the urethra ➡, consistent with a utricle cyst. Rectal cancer ➡ is also seen.*

Other Rare Prostatic Tumors

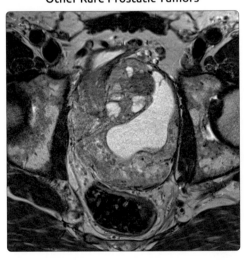

Other Rare Prostatic Tumors

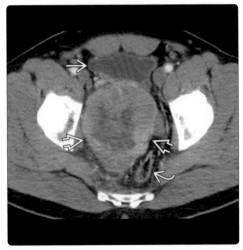

(Left) *Axial T2 MR shows massive enlargement of the process due to a heterogeneous cystic and solid mass. Biopsy showed STUMP, a rare smooth muscle tumor that is typically benign but can act aggressively.* (Right) *A centrally necrotic, enhancing pelvic mass ➡ arising from the prostate anteriorly displaces the bladder ➡. The rectum ➡ is separate. Surgical pathology from a surgical resection revealed prostate sarcoma, not otherwise specified.*

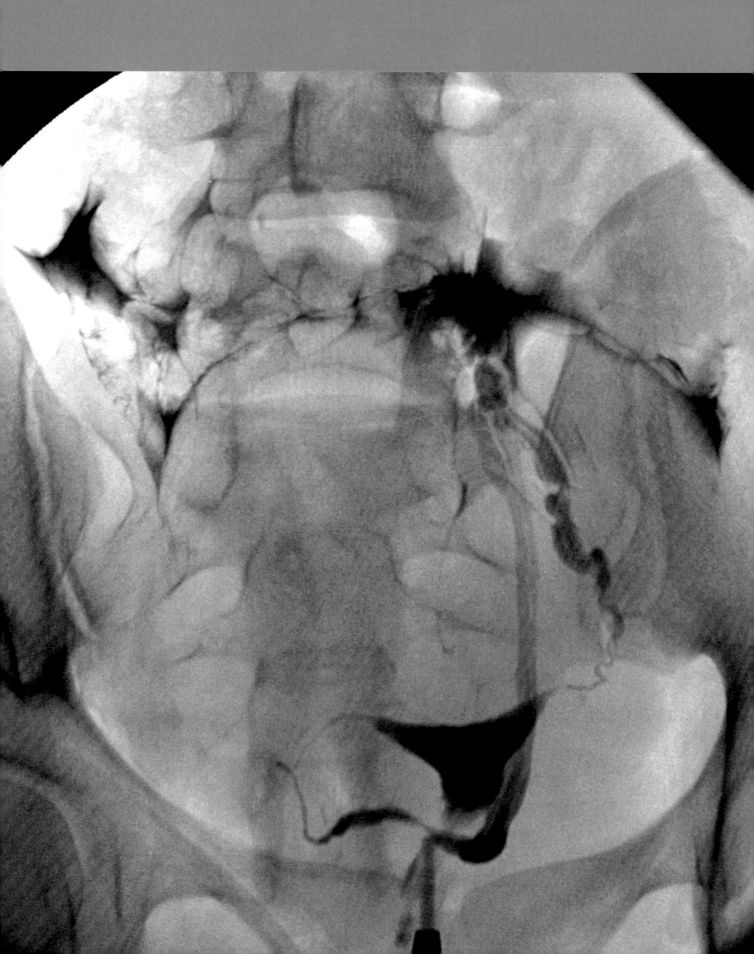

SECTION 22
Female Pelvis

Generic Imaging Patterns

Pelvic Fluid   634
Female Lower Genital Cysts   638
Extraovarian Adnexal Mass   644

Clinically Based Differentials

Acute Pelvic Pain in Nonpregnant Women   650

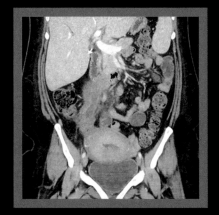
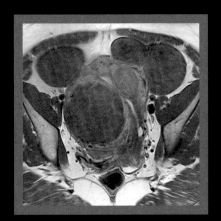
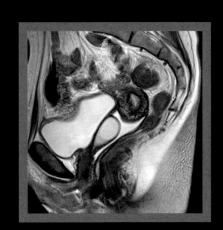

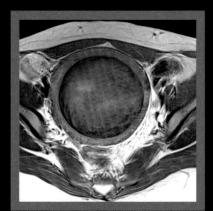
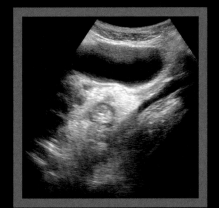
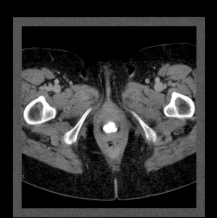

DIFFERENTIAL DIAGNOSIS

Common

- Physiologic Fluid
- Ruptured Hemorrhagic Cyst
- Pelvic Inflammatory Disease
- Ruptured Ectopic Pregnancy

Less Common

- Peritoneal Inclusion Cysts
- Pelvic Abscess due to Bowel Disease
  - Appendicitis
  - Other Bowel-Related Abscess
- Ascites
- Endometriosis

Rare but Important

- Ovarian Torsion
- Ovarian Carcinoma
- Ovarian Metastases
- Ovarian Hyperstimulation Syndrome
- Ruptured Endometrioma

ESSENTIAL INFORMATION

Key Differential Diagnosis Issues

- Simple fluid
  - Anechoic at US, fluid attenuation at CT, and fluid signal intensity at MR
  - Small amount of simple fluid in asymptomatic woman is likely physiologic
  - Large amount of simple fluid, likely ascites
  - If signs of metastatic disease, check ovaries
- Fluid with debris in cul-de-sac
  - Blood: Patient may be hemodynamically unstable
    - Ruptured hemorrhagic cyst
      - □ Variable amount of pelvic blood
      - □ Blood can extend along paracolic gutter and to subdiaphragmatic spaces
    - Ruptured ectopic pregnancy
    - Endometriosis
    - Ruptured endometrioma
  - Pus: Patient acutely ill with elevated WBC count and fever
    - Pelvic inflammatory disease
    - Pelvic abscess due to bowel disease
  - Cells: Ovarian carcinoma and metastatic disease
- Fluid with septations
  - Peritoneal inclusion cysts
  - Endometriosis
  - Loculated ascites

Helpful Clues for Common Diagnoses

- **Physiologic Fluid**
  - Small amount of simple fluid may be seen during all phases of menstrual cycle
    - Ruptured follicles
    - Retrograde menstruation
    - Increase in ovarian permeability under estrogen stimulation
  - Should not be seen in postmenopausal women

- **Ruptured Hemorrhagic Cyst**
  - Hematocrit may initially be normal if patient has not had time to hemodilute after rehydration
  - Check for fluid by kidneys and around liver in cases of massive hemoperitoneum
    - Sentinel clot sign
      - □ Blood closest to rupture site has more time to retract, forming higher attenuation clotted blood, and pinpoint origin of hemoperitoneum
  - Characteristic imaging appearance of hemorrhagic cyst
    - US: Different patterns may be seen
      - □ Echogenic, avascular, homogeneous, or heterogeneous nonshadowing in early stage
      - □ Retracted clot
      - □ Avascular, mass-like structure within anechoic cyst with characteristic concave contour
      - □ May jiggle with transducer ballottement
      - □ Reticular, lacy, fishnet, or spongy pattern
    - CT
      - □ Usually single unilocular cyst containing high-attenuation homogeneous fluid (around 50 HU) and partial or complete rim enhancement
    - MR
      - □ Usually single unilocular cyst
      - □ High signal intensity on T1WI, remains high on T1WI FS
      - □ High or low signal intensity on T2WI
      - □ No T2-dark spots
      - □ Pelvic blood usually has high signal intensity on T1WI

- **Pelvic Inflammatory Disease**
  - Adnexal cystic mass with irregular thick wall in case of tuboovarian abscess
  - Fluid-filled fallopian tubes in case of pyosalpinx
  - May be associated with peritoneal thickening because of associated peritonitis
  - Associated stranding of pelvic fat

- **Ruptured Ectopic Pregnancy**
  - Positive pregnancy test
  - Fluid is usually echogenic and may contain particulate matter
    - Pelvic hemorrhage is specific finding of ectopic pregnancy with 86-93% positive predictive value when β-hCG levels are abnormal
  - Adnexal mass separate from ovary may be seen
    - May see tubal ring ± yolk sac and embryonic pole
  - Hematocrit may initially be normal if patient has not had time to hemodilute after rehydration

Helpful Clues for Less Common Diagnoses

- **Peritoneal Inclusion Cysts**
  - History of prior surgery or pelvic inflammatory conditions (e.g., Crohn disease)
  - Fluid usually simple at imaging with angular margins
  - Multilocular cystic lesion surrounding normal ovary (usually at margin)
  - Loculi separated by thin septa
  - No mass effect on pelvic structures
    - Cyst insinuates itself between pelvic structures rather than displace them

- **Pelvic Abscess due to Bowel Disease**

- o Patient acutely tender in region of complex fluid collection
- o May see abnormal loop of bowel/appendix in region
- **Ascites**
  - o Many causes include liver cirrhosis, heart failure, hypoproteinemia, etc.
  - o Usually simple-appearing fluid
  - o Ascites may also be seen in Meigs syndrome
    - Triad of ascites, pleural effusion, and benign ovarian tumor (fibroma, Brenner tumor, and, occasionally, granulosa cell tumor)
- **Endometriosis**
  - o Women with endometriosis have larger than normal amount of peritoneal fluid volume
    - Usually small amount of fluid and difficult to distinguish from physiologic fluid
  - o Fluid may be simple or hemorrhagic
  - o Evidence of peritoneal adhesions with obliteration of cul-de-sac may be found
    - Negative sliding sign
      - □ Gentle pressure by transvaginal probe to assess whether rectum glides freely across posterior vaginal wall and whether rectosigmoid glides freely over uterus
    - Kissing ovaries
      - □ Ovaries are adherent to each other behind uterus due to pelvic adhesions
  - o Peritoneal endometriotic implants or areas of fibrosis may be seen on MR

Helpful Clues for Rare Diagnoses

- **Ovarian Torsion**
  - o Nausea and vomiting
  - o Ovarian edema
    - Asymmetric enlargement (largest diameter > 5 cm when no ovarian lesion is present)
    - Thicker than expected ovarian parenchyma surrounding lesion
    - Peripheralization of follicles (string of pearls sign)

- Small amount of fluid usually surrounds torsed ovary or within cul-de-sac
  - □ In up to 87% of cases
- Changes of parenchymal edema ± hemorrhage
  - □ Heterogeneity at US
  - □ Increased attenuation at NECT
  - □ Increased T1 signal intensity at MR
- o Twisted vascular pedicle
- o Strange situs, usually located in midline and superior to fundus of uterus
- o Vascular flow may be absent on Doppler US, but its presence does not exclude torsion
- **Ovarian Carcinoma**
  - o Pelvic ascites ± soft tissue nodules on surface of pelvic organs
  - o Large cystic and solid adnexal mass
- **Ovarian Metastases**
  - o Usually bilateral
  - o Known abdominal primary tumor, usually from gastrointestinal source
  - o Always check appendix for neoplasm, if no known primary tumor
- **Ovarian Hyperstimulation Syndrome**
  - o Enlarged ovaries containing numerous simple cysts
  - o Pelvic fluid in severe cases
- **Ruptured Endometrioma**
  - o Several key imaging features help to make confident preoperative diagnosis of ruptured endometrioma
    - Pericyst hemorrhagic fluid
    - Adnexal inflammation
    - Irregular cyst wall
    - Collapsed cyst
    - Diffuse peritonitis

SELECTED REFERENCES

1. Strachowski LM et al: Pearls and pitfalls in imaging of pelvic adnexal torsion: seven tips to tell it's twisted. Radiographics. 41(3):E97, 2021
2. Fonseca EKUN et al: Ruptured endometrioma: main imaging findings. Radiol Bras. 51(6):411-2, 2018

Physiologic Fluid

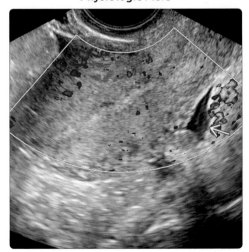

Ruptured Hemorrhagic Cyst

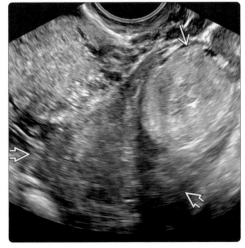

(Left) *Transvaginal color Doppler US shows a small amount of simple fluid ➡ posterior to the uterus within the cul-de-sac. A small amount of simple free fluid within the pelvis in a premenopausal woman is a common finding that may be seen in all phases of the menstrual cycle.* **(Right)** *Transvaginal US shows an echogenic left ovarian lesion ➡ representing hemorrhagic cyst with a large amount of echogenic pelvic fluid ➡.*

Ruptured Hemorrhagic Cyst

(Left) *Axial CECT in the same patient shows a large amount of high-attenuation fluid* ➡ *filling the pelvis. The CT appearance is concerning and can be confused with carcinomatosis.* (Right) *Coronal CECT in the same patient shows high-attenuation fluid* ➡ *filling the pelvis and extending along the paracolic gutters to the perihepatic region* ➡. *The fluid has high attenuation with the highest attenuation present around the left ovary (sentinel clot sign)* ➡. *A small area of active extravasation* ➡ *is also seen.*

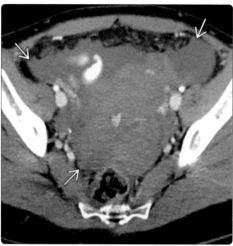

Ruptured Hemorrhagic Cyst

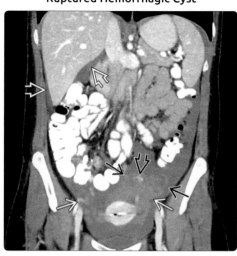

Pelvic Inflammatory Disease

(Left) *Axial CECT shows a small amount of pelvic fluid* ➡. *The peritoneum of the cul-de-sac is slightly thickened and enhancing* ➡. *There is stranding of the pelvic fat* ➡. *A high-attenuation right ovarian lesion* ➡ *is present and was found to represent an abscess.* (Right) *Coronal CECT in the same patient shows thickening and enhancement of the right fallopian tube* ➡.

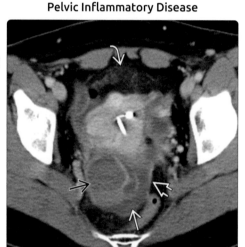

Pelvic Inflammatory Disease

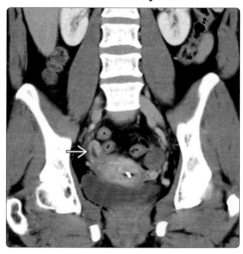

Ruptured Ectopic Pregnancy

(Left) *Transvaginal US shows large amount of echogenic fluid within the cul-de-sac* ➡ *with retracted clot* ➡ *due to hemoperitoneum.* (Right) *Transvaginal color Doppler US in the same patient shows an adnexal mass* ➡ *separate from the ovary* ➡ *and displaying peripheral ring of increased vascularity.*

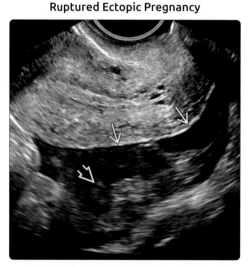

Ruptured Ectopic Pregnancy

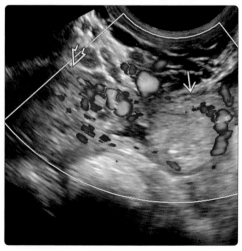

Peritoneal Inclusion Cysts

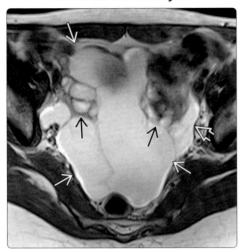

Peritoneal Inclusion Cysts

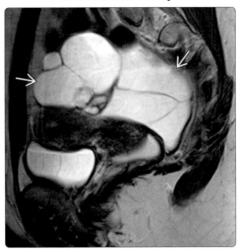

(Left) Axial T2 MR in a patient with a history of multiple pelvic surgeries shows a multilocular cystic lesion ➡ occupying much of the pelvic cavity. The lesion surrounds both ovaries ➡ and insinuates itself between pelvic structures ➡ without significant mass effect. (Right) Sagittal T2 MR in the same patient shows a multilocular cystic mass ➡ superior to the uterus. The mass is composed of multiple loculi separated by thin septa.

Endometriosis

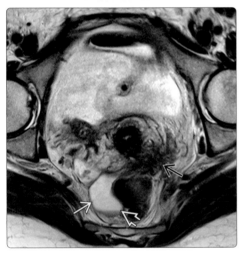

Ovarian Torsion

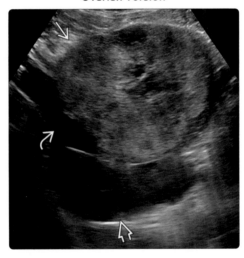

(Left) Axial oblique T2 MR shows free pelvic fluid ➡ with a fluid level ➡ and an ill-defined, infiltrative mass-like structure of low signal intensity ➡ obliterating the left side of the cul-de-sac, containing small foci of high signal intensity. (Right) Transabdominal pelvic US shows an enlarged ovary ➡ located anterior to the uterus ➡. A small amount of fluid is present around the enlarged ovary ➡.

Ovarian Torsion

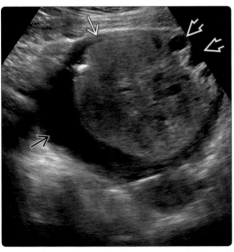

Ruptured Endometrioma

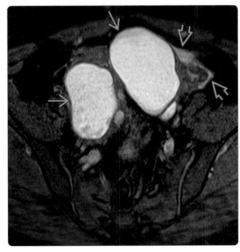

(Left) Transabdominal pelvic US in the same patient shows an enlarged ovary ➡ containing multiple peripheral follicles ➡ and surrounded by a small amount of fluid ➡. (Right) Axial T1 FS MR in a woman who presented with severe pelvic pain shows bilateral ovarian high signal intensity lesions ➡ representing known endometriomas. There is left adnexal high signal intensity hemorrhagic free fluid ➡, consistent with an endometrioma rupture.

DIFFERENTIAL DIAGNOSIS

Common

- Epidermal Inclusion Cyst
- Nabothian Cyst
- Skene Gland Cyst
- Bartholin Gland Cyst
- Gartner Duct Cyst
- Müllerian Duct Cysts
- Urethral Diverticulum
- Cystocele

Less Common

- Posthysterectomy Inclusion Cyst

Rare but Important

- Endometrioma of Rectovaginal Septum
- Subpubic Cartilaginous Cyst
- Endocervicosis

ESSENTIAL INFORMATION

Key Differential Diagnosis Issues

- Relation to level of perineal membrane and symphysis pubis
  - Above
    - Gartner duct cyst
    - Endometrioma of rectovaginal septum
    - Urethral diverticulum
    - Nabothian cyst
    - Endocervicosis
    - Müllerian duct cysts
    - Posthysterectomy inclusion cysts
  - Below
    - Skene gland cyst
    - Bartholin gland cyst
    - Epidermal inclusion cyst
    - Cystocele
    - Subpubic cartilaginous cyst

Helpful Clues for Common Diagnoses

- **Epidermal Inclusion Cyst**
  - Most common vaginal cyst; ≈ 23% of all vaginal cysts
  - Located at sites of prior trauma or surgery around vaginal introitus
    - Commonly at posterior or lateral vaginal walls
      - Episiotomy is common cause
    - May also affect clitoris
      - Usually in setting of female circumcision
  - US
    - Hypoechoic mass with variable echogenic foci without color Doppler signals
  - CT
    - Homogeneous, well-defined lesion with attenuation higher than simple fluid
      - Can be mistaken for solid mass
- **Nabothian Cyst**
  - Located within uterine cervix
    - Single cyst or multiple cysts in fibrous cervical stroma
  - Few millimeters in diameter but may reach 4 cm or more

- Intermediate or slightly high signal intensity on T1 and prominent high signal intensity on T2 MR
- Purely cystic without solid component
  - Distinguish nabothian cysts from malignant adenoma malignum
- **Skene Gland Cyst**
  - Rounded or ovoid cyst located lateral to external urethral orifice
  - Inferior to symphysis pubis and below level of perineal membrane
  - US
    - Anechoic or low-level echoes
  - CT
    - Fluid attenuation
  - MR
    - Variable T1 and T2 signal intensity depending on presence of hemorrhage &/or proteinaceous material
      - Usually hyperintense on T2 MR when uncomplicated
- **Bartholin Gland Cyst**
  - Located at posterolateral vaginal introitus
    - At or below level of symphysis pubis, inferior to perineal membrane
  - US
    - Anechoic or low-level echoes
  - CT
    - Fluid attenuation
  - MR
    - Variable T1 and T2 signal intensity depending on presence of hemorrhage &/or proteinaceous material
      - Usually hyperintense on T2 MR when uncomplicated
  - Thin wall without significant enhancement in absence of complication
    - Bartholin abscess will show thickened and irregular rim enhancement with adjacent inflammatory stranding
- **Gartner Duct Cyst**
  - Remnants of embryologic paired mesonephric (wolffian) duct
  - Classically located in anterolateral wall of upper vagina
    - Above level of perineal membrane and symphysis pubis
    - Commonly arising from upper vaginal wall (though may be located distally as well)
  - US
    - Anechoic or low-level echoes
  - CT
    - Fluid attenuation
  - MR
    - Variable T1 and T2 signal intensity depending on presence of hemorrhage &/or proteinaceous material
      - Usually hyperintense on T2 MR when uncomplicated
  - May be associated with other congenital urogenital abnormalities, such as ectopic ureteral insertion and unilateral renal agenesis/hypoplasia
- **Müllerian Duct Cysts**
  - Remnants of embryologic paramesonephric ducts
  - Usually single

- Typically located in anterolateral vaginal wall
  - May be located at posterior vaginal wall
- US
  - Anechoic or low-level echoes
- CT
  - Fluid attenuation
- MR
  - Variable T1 and T2 signal intensity depending on presence of hemorrhage &/or proteinaceous material
    - Usually hyperintense on T2 MR when uncomplicated
- **Urethral Diverticulum**
  - Round, oval, crescentic, horseshoe- or saddlebag-shaped, or circumferential periurethral cystic lesions
  - Located at posterolateral aspect of mid to distal urethra
    - Above level of perineal membrane and symphysis pubis
  - Direct urethral communication may be seen
    - High-resolution, fat-saturated, postcontrast T1 FSE MR can be useful in identification of diverticular neck
  - Anechoic on US, fluid attenuation on CT, and hyperintense on T2 MR when uncomplicated
  - Stones within diverticula may be seen (≈ 5-10% of cases)
- **Cystocele**
  - Defined as abnormal descent of bladder neck inferior to pubococcygeal line (PCL) on midline sagittal image, either at rest or upon stress
    - PCL is line drawn from inferior aspect of pubic bone to last coccygeal joint
  - Often associated with additional pelvic organ prolapse or pelvic floor laxity
  - Small cystocele may simulate pelvic floor cystic lesion on axial imaging
  - Diagnosis is made upon recognizing clear communication with bladder lumen

Helpful Clues for Less Common Diagnoses

- **Posthysterectomy Inclusion Cyst**
  - Occur at vaginal cuff as late complication of surgery
  - On images, these commonly appear as simple cysts

- May have variable T1 and T2 signal intensity depending on presence of hemorrhage &/or proteinaceous material

Helpful Clues for Rare Diagnoses

- **Endometrioma of Rectovaginal Septum**
  - Centered in rectovaginal region between rectum posteriorly and posterior vaginal wall anteriorly
  - Cyst with homogeneous low-level internal echoes on US
  - Homogeneous well-defined structure on CT with attenuation higher than simple fluid
    - ~ 40 HU
  - Hemorrhagic cyst with characteristic T1 hyperintensity and T2 shading on MR
- **Subpubic Cartilaginous Cyst**
  - Midline, rounded, cystic mass
  - Located anterosuperior to urethra and posteroinferior to pubic symphysis
  - Sclerotic &/or erosive changes may be seen in symphysis pubis on CT and plain radiography
  - Hypointense relative to muscle on T1 and heterogeneously hyperintense on T2 MR
  - Thin enhancing wall with no internal enhancement
  - MR may show direct communication between cyst and pubic symphysis
- **Endocervicosis**
  - Closely clustered cysts of various sizes surrounding proximal 1/3 of urethra and may extend into bladder
  - Usually low signal intensity on T1 and high signal intensity on T2 MR
  - No solid elements and no enhancement with gadolinium

SELECTED REFERENCES

1. Zulfiqar M et al: Imaging of the vagina: spectrum of disease with emphasis on MRI appearance. Radiographics. 41(5):1549-68, 2021
2. Tubay M et al: Resident and fellow education feature: what is that cyst? Common cystic lesions of the female lower genitourinary tract. Radiographics. 34(2):427-8, 2014
3. Eskridge MR et al: MRI of endocervicosis: an unusual cause of clustered periurethral cystic masses involving the bladder. AJR Am J Roentgenol. 188(2):W147-9, 2007

Epidermal Inclusion Cyst

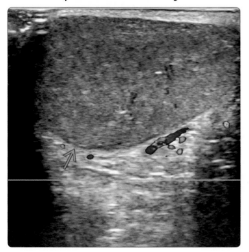

Epidermal Inclusion Cyst

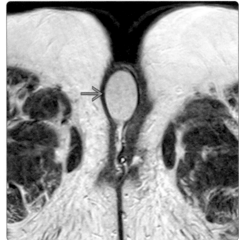

(Left) Transperineal US shows a right labia majora lesion ➡. The mass is hypoechoic with posterior acoustic enhancement. There is no blood flow within the mass, confirming its cystic nature despite its solid appearance. (Right) Axial T2 MR in the same patient shows a well-defined lesion ➡ within the right labia majora. The lesion demonstrates high T2 signal intensity.

Female Lower Genital Cysts

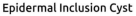

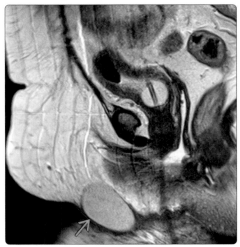

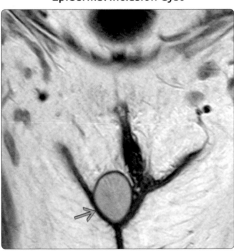

(Left) *Sagittal T2 MR in the same patient shows a well-defined lesion ⇨ within the right labia majora. The lesion demonstrates high T2 signal intensity and is located immediately under the skin.* (Right) *Coronal T2 MR in the same patient shows a well-defined lesion ⇨ within the right labia majora. The lesion demonstrates high T2 signal intensity.*

Nabothian Cyst

Nabothian Cyst

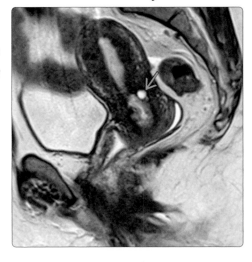

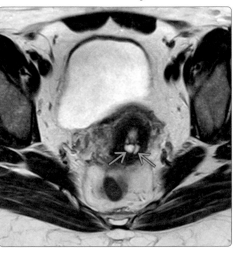

(Left) *Sagittal T2 MR shows a hyperintense cystic lesion ⇨ within the cervical dark stroma.* (Right) *Axial T2 MR in the same patient shows hyperintense cystic lesions ⇨ within the cervical dark stroma.*

Nabothian Cyst

Nabothian Cyst

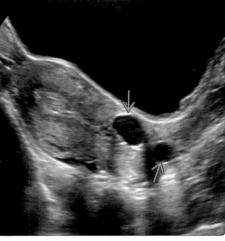

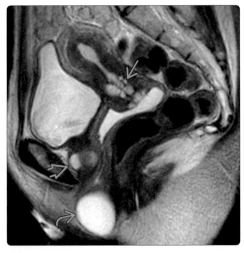

(Left) *Sagittal transabdominal pelvic US shows 2 simple-appearing cystic lesions ⇨ within the uterine cervix.* (Right) *Sagittal T2 MR shows multiple small cervical cysts ⇨ representing nabothian cysts. Note also the presence of urethral diverticulum ⇨ and a Bartholin gland cyst ⇨.*

Skene Gland Cyst

Skene Gland Cyst

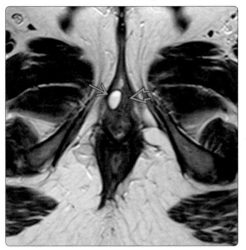

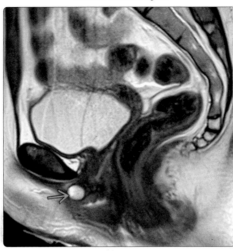

(Left) *Axial T2 MR shows a well-defined, oval, cystic structure* ⇨*, adjacent to the urethral meatus* ⇨*, demonstrating homogeneous high signal intensity.* (Right) *Sagittal T2 MR shows a well-defined, oval structure* ⇨ *demonstrating homogeneous high signal intensity adjacent to the urethral meatus. The cyst is located below the level of the symphysis pubis.*

Bartholin Gland Cyst

Bartholin Gland Cyst

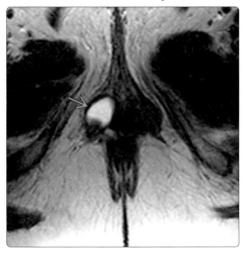

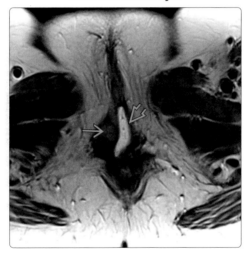

(Left) *Axial T2 MR shows an oval structure* ⇨ *at the right side of the vaginal introitus. The lesion shows high signal intensity, characteristic of uncomplicated cyst.* (Right) *Axial T2 MR in a patient who presented with vaginal pain shows an oval structure* ⇨ *at the right side of the vaginal introitus* ⇨*. The lesion shows signal intensity that is lower than gel within the vaginal introitus and slightly higher than signal intensity of pelvic muscles.*

Bartholin Gland Cyst

Bartholin Gland Cyst

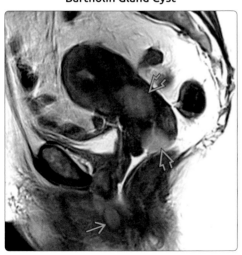

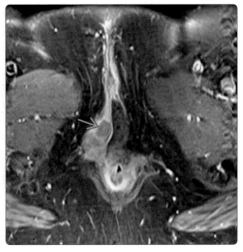

(Left) *Sagittal T2 MR in the same patient shows an oval structure* ⇨ *at the vaginal introitus, below the level of the symphysis pubis. The lesion shows intermediate signal intensity. Note also the presence of unrelated cervical masses* ⇨*.* (Right) *Axial T1 C+ FS MR in the same patient shows a structure* ⇨ *on the right side of the vaginal introitus. The lesion shows a thin enhancing wall and no enhancement of its content. Pus was aspirated from the cyst, consistent with Bartholin abscess.*

Gartner Duct Cyst

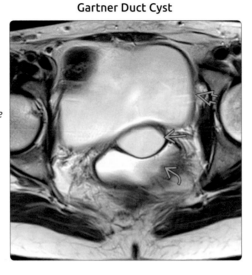

Gartner Duct Cyst

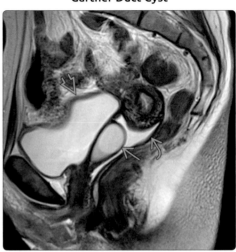

(Left) *Axial T2 MR shows a lesion ⇨ between the urinary bladder anteriorly ⇨ and the gel-filled vagina ⇨ posteriorly. The lesion shows homogeneous high signal intensity.* (Right) *Sagittal T2 shows a lesion ⇨ between the urinary bladder anteriorly ⇨ and the gel-filled vagina ⇨ posteriorly. The lesion shows homogeneous high signal intensity. An anterior wall vaginal cyst may be a Gartner duct cyst or a müllerian cyst, whereas a posterior wall cyst is likely a müllerian cyst.*

Urethral Diverticulum

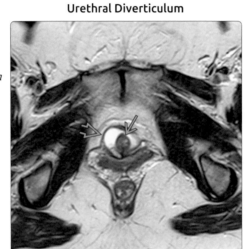

Urethral Diverticulum

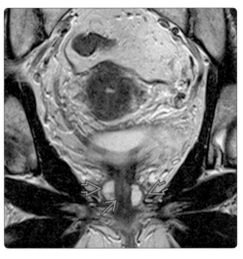

(Left) *Axial T2 MR shows a horseshoe-shaped T2 high signal intensity lesion ⇨ surrounding the urethra ⇨.* (Right) *Coronal T2 MR shows a lesion with T2 high signal intensity ⇨ on both sides of the urethra ⇨.*

Cystocele

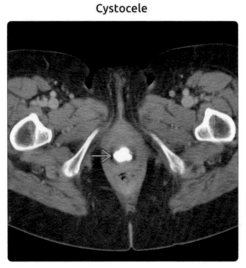

Cystocele

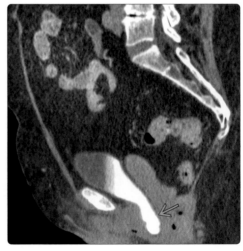

(Left) *Axial CECT shows a rounded lesion ⇨ at about the level of the vaginal introitus that is filled with contrast.* (Right) *Sagittal CECT shows downward extension of the urinary bladder ⇨ far below a line drawn from the lower border of the symphysis pubis to the last coccygeal joint.*

Endometrioma of Rectovaginal Septum

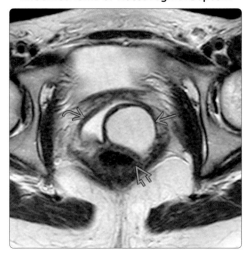

Endometrioma of Rectovaginal Septum

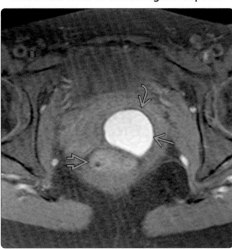

(Left) *Axial T2 MR shows a lesion* ⇨ *between the rectum* ⇨ *and the gel-filled vagina* ⇨. *The lesion shows homogeneous high signal intensity.* (Right) *Axial T1 FS MR shows a lesion* ⇨ *between the rectum* ⇨ *and the vagina* ⇨. *The lesion shows homogeneous high signal intensity. The high T1 signal intensity is due to blood products.*

Endocervicosis

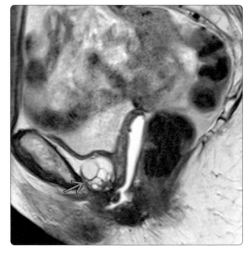

Endocervicosis

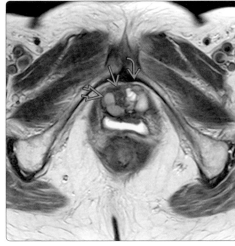

(Left) *Sagittal T2 MR shows a cluster of periurethral cysts* ⇨. (Right) *Axial T2 MR shows a cluster of periurethral cysts* ⇨ *surrounding the upper urethra* ⇨. *Some cysts* ⇨ *show signal intensity less than simple fluid, likely due to hemorrhage.*

Endocervicosis

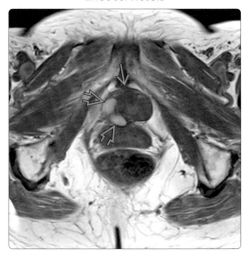

Endocervicosis

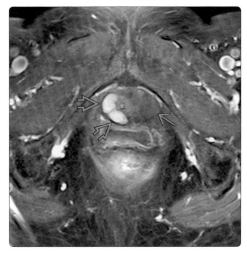

(Left) *Axial T1 MR shows a cluster of periurethral cysts* ⇨. *Some cysts* ⇨ *show high signal intensity, likely due to hemorrhage.* (Right) *Axial T1 C+ FS MR shows a cluster of periurethral cysts* ⇨. *Some cysts* ⇨ *show high signal intensity, likely due to hemorrhage. There was no enhancement following contrast injection.*

DIFFERENTIAL DIAGNOSIS

Common

- Tubal
  - Tubal Ectopic Pregnancy
  - Hydrosalpinx
  - Pyosalpinx
  - Hematosalpinx
  - Primary Fallopian Tube Carcinoma
  - Tubal Leiomyoma
  - Fimbrial Cyst
- Gynecologic (Not Tubal)
  - Endometriosis
    - Endometrioma
    - Endometrial Implant
  - Subserosal Leiomyoma
  - Paraovarian/Paratubal Cysts
  - Exophytic Ovarian Mass

Less Common

- Peritoneal Inclusion Cyst
- Lymphocele
- GI Related
  - Bowel Loop
  - Bowel Obstruction
  - Sigmoid Diverticulitis
  - Appendicitis
  - Appendiceal Mucocele
  - Meckel Diverticulitis
  - GI Duplication Cyst
- GU Related
  - Hydroureter
  - Bladder Diverticulum
  - Renal Ectopia (Pelvic Kidney)
- Tarlov Cyst
- Pelvic Varices

Rare but Important

- Wolffian Duct Remnant
- Particle Disease Related to Hip Prosthesis
- Tubal Torsion
- Heterotopic Pregnancy
- Tubal Carcinoma
- Nerve Sheath Tumor
- Sarcoma
  - Ovarian Vein Leiomyosarcoma
  - Extraperitoneal Sarcoma

ESSENTIAL INFORMATION

Key Differential Diagnosis Issues

- Is patient pregnant?
  - Ectopic pregnancy, tubal
  - Ectopic pregnancy, heterotopic
- Is patient febrile with elevated WBC count?
  - Pelvic inflammatory disease (salpingitis, pyosalpinx)
  - Appendicitis, diverticulitis, Meckel diverticulitis
- Is mass tubular?
  - Fallopian tube
  - GI (bowel obstruction, mucocele)

- GU (hydroureter)
- Vascular (varices, aneurysm, venous leiomyosarcoma)
- Is mass intimately associated with ovary?
  - If adherent to ovary, may be exophytic ovarian mass
  - Tubal lesions may compress ovary and appear to arise from ovary
  - Pelvic inflammatory disease (tuboovarian abscess)
- Is mass related to uterus?
  - Leiomyomas may show broad base of attachment to uterus
  - Leiomyomas may show blood flow from uterus (bridging vessels sign)

Helpful Clues for Common Diagnoses

- **Tubal**
  - **Tubal ectopic pregnancy**
    - Pain &/or bleeding in 1st trimester
    - Echogenic, vascular ring-like mass separate from ovary
    - May see yolk sac or embryo
    - Free fluid with debris is blood
  - **Hydrosalpinx**
    - Tubular, anechoic mass; incomplete septations
    - Separate from ovary
    - Prior pelvic inflammatory disease or endometriosis
  - **Pyosalpinx**
    - Tubular, hypoechoic mass; incomplete septations
    - Separate from ovary
    - Internal debris ± fluid level
    - Irregular margins, thick wall
    - Free fluid
    - Clinical findings of infection
      - Pain, fever, elevated WBC count
      - Vaginal discharge
      - Cervical motion tenderness
  - **Hematosalpinx**
    - Associated with tubal ectopic pregnancy or endometriosis
    - Distended fallopian tube with fluid and debris
    - Rarely due to fallopian tube carcinoma
- **Gynecologic (Not Tubal)**
  - **Endometriosis**
    - Endometrioma ("chocolate" cyst) with diffuse, homogeneous, low-level internal echoes
      - ± layering debris
      - Thick wall
      - May have punctate calcifications in wall of cyst
      - May have septations with blood flow
    - May also see endometrial implants and fibrotic plaques
    - Cyclic pelvic pain
  - **Subserosal leiomyoma**
    - Fibrous appearance with shadowing
    - Separate from ovary
    - Connection to uterus may be visualized
    - Blood flow from uterus may be present (bridging vessel sign)
    - MR helpful in establishing diagnosis
  - **Paraovarian/paratubal cysts**
    - Separate from ovary
    - Thin walled

– Anechoic
– Tend not to change in size over time
– Most commonly arise from peritoneal mesothelium of broad ligament or less commonly from fimbrial of fallopian tube

Helpful Clues for Less Common Diagnoses

- **Peritoneal Inclusion Cyst**
  o History of prior surgery
  o Cystic mass surrounding ovarian tissue
  o Conforms to shape of pelvic space as allowed by adjacent organs
  o Septations with blood flow can simulate malignancy
- **Lymphocele**
  o Septated cystic mass resulting from disrupting lymphatics following surgery
  o Not associated with ovaries or uterus
- **GI Related**
  o **Bowel loop**
    – Assess for peristalsis
    – Change in appearance over time
  o **Appendicitis**
    – Rebound tenderness to scanning in right lower quadrant
    – Dilated, tubular, blind-ending structure in region of patient's pain
    – Tubular structure noncompressible
    – ± adjacent fluid or appendicolith
    – Clinical signs of infection
- **GU Related**
  o **Renal ectopia (pelvic kidney)**
    – Reniform shape of mass
    – Collecting system
    – Absent kidney in ipsilateral renal fossa

Helpful Clues for Rare Diagnoses

- **Tubal Torsion**
  o Acute, colicky pain
  o Associated with tubal mass or paraovarian cyst
  o Elongated cystic mass that tapers near cornua

- **Heterotopic Pregnancy**
  o Intrauterine and extrauterine pregnancy
  o Common in patients undergoing assisted fertilization
  o Check for ovary separate from mass
- **Tubal Carcinoma**
  o Seen between and separate from uterus and ovary
  o Tube may be dilated: Hydrosalpinx with mural nodules
  o Tube may be enlarged with tubular solid mass
- **Sarcoma**
  o Leiomyosarcoma may begin in wall of ovarian vein and extend into inferior vena cava

Alternative Differential Approaches

- Acute pelvic pain, no signs of infection
  o Endometriosis
  o Bowel obstruction
  o Hydroureter
  o Tubal torsion
- Acute pelvic pain with signs of infection
  o Pelvic inflammatory disease (salpingitis, pyosalpinx, tuboovarian abscess)
  o Diverticulitis (sigmoid or Meckel)
  o Appendicitis
- Acute pelvic pain with positive pregnancy test
  o Ectopic pregnancy (tubal, heterotopic)
- Asymptomatic/incidental mass
  o Hydrosalpinx
  o Leiomyoma (tubal, subserosal uterine)
  o Cyst (paraovarian, paratubal, fimbrial, peritoneal inclusion cyst, GI duplication, bladder diverticulum, Tarlov)
  o Endometriosis
  o Appendiceal mucocele
  o Lymphocele
  o Malignancy (tubal, sarcoma, nerve sheath)
  o Wolffian duct remnant
  o Particle disease of hip prosthesis

Hydrosalpinx

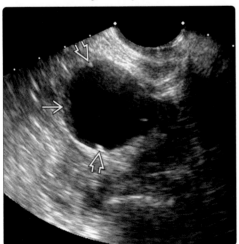

Hydrosalpinx

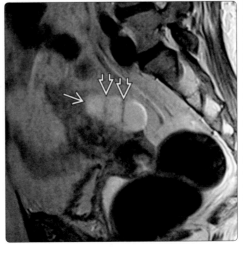

(Left) Transvaginal US shows a cystic adnexal mass ➡ with multiple tiny, echogenic mural nodules ➡. The structure is tubular and separate from the ovary (not shown). This is hydrosalpinx with "mural nodules" representing the longitudinal folds of the fallopian tube. (Right) Sagittal T2 MR shows a tubular adnexal mass ➡ separate from the ovary. Note the incomplete septations ➡. Signal is hyperintense on T2 MR and hypointense on T1 MR with no enhancement, consistent with hydrosalpinx.

Extraovarian Adnexal Mass

Pyosalpinx

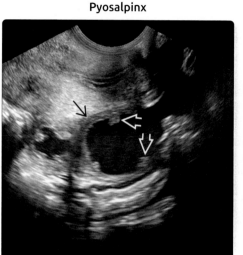

Pyosalpinx

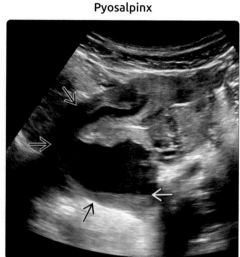

(Left) *Transvaginal US shows a complex cystic adnexal mass ⇨ separate from the ovary. The thickened wall and nodular projections ⇨ give the appearance of a cogwheel, consistent with pyosalpinx.* (Right) *Transabdominal US in the same patient shows the complex cystic adnexal mass ⇨ is tubular. Note the thickened wall and the fluid-debris level ➡. The ipsilateral ovary is separate.*

Hematosalpinx

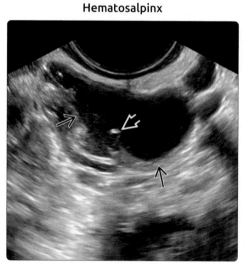

Hematosalpinx

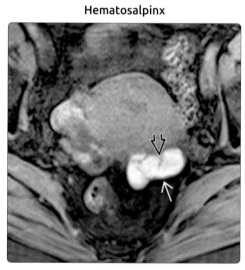

(Left) *Transvaginal US shows an adnexal mass ⇨ with low-level internal echoes, a thick wall, and incomplete septations ⇨. The ovary is not shown but separate. The tubular shape and incomplete septations suggest a fallopian tube. Internal echoes and thick wall can be seen with pyosalpinx or hematosalpinx.* (Right) *Axial T1 FS MR in the same patient shows a tubular, hyperintense left adnexal mass ➡ with incomplete septations ⇨ compatible with hematosalpinx. In this nonpregnant patient, this is consistent with endometriosis.*

Fimbrial Cyst

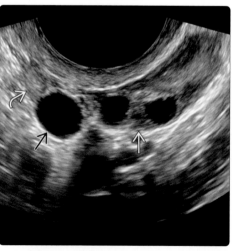

Fimbrial Cyst

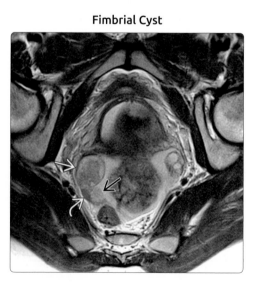

(Left) *Transvaginal US shows a simple cyst ⇨ adjacent to, but separate from, the ovary ➡. Tubular soft tissue ➡ extending to the cyst is better seen in real time.* (Right) *Axial oblique T2 MR in the same patient shows the right fallopian tube ➡ extending to a simple cyst ⇨, which is separate from the right ovary ➡. This is consistent with a fimbrial cyst.*

Endometrial Implant

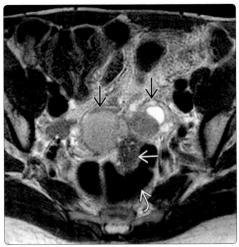

Endometrial Implant

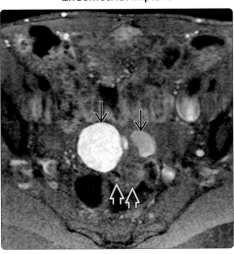

(Left) Axial T2 MR shows bilateral ovaries ➡ with endometriomas. There is an extraovarian adnexal mass ➡ adjacent to the ovaries and intimately associated with the sigmoid colon ➡. The ill-defined margins and T2-bright foci in the mass are compatible with endometrial implant. (Right) Axial T1 FS MR in the same patient shows the hyperintense endometriomas ➡. The endometrial implant contains hyperintense foci ➡, compatible with hemorrhagic glands.

Subserosal Leiomyoma

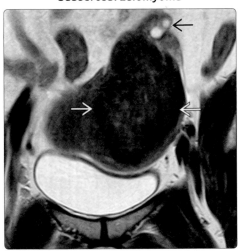

Subserosal Leiomyoma

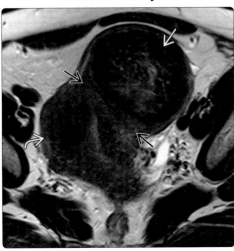

(Left) Coronal T2 MR shows the normal left ovary ➡ with an adjacent, circumscribed, hypointense mass ➡. (Right) Axial T2 MR in the same patient shows the hypointense mass ➡ has a broad-based attachment ➡ to the uterus ➡, consistent with subserosal leiomyoma. MR can be very helpful in localizing an adnexal mass due to its multiplanar capability and soft tissue contrast.

Paraovarian/Paratubal Cysts

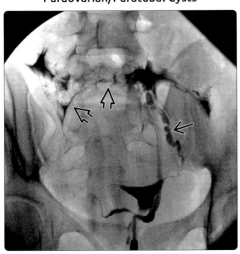

Paraovarian/Paratubal Cysts

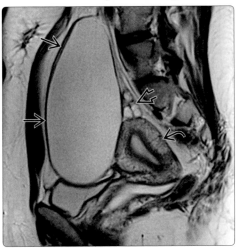

(Left) Hysterosalpingography shows peritoneal contrast ➡ being displaced by a large central pelvic mass. The left fallopian tube ➡ is also stretched around the mass. (Right) Sagittal T2 MR in the same patient shows a large simple cyst ➡ separate from the ovary ➡ and uterus ➡. This was a large paratubal cyst.

Peritoneal Inclusion Cyst

Peritoneal Inclusion Cyst

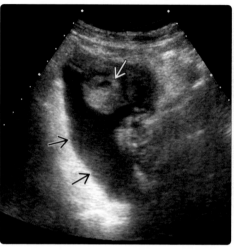

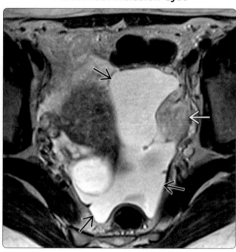

(Left) *Longitudinal US of the pelvis shows the left ovary* ➡ *with associated loculated fluid* ➡ *and posterior acoustic enhancement.* (Right) *Axial T2 MR in the same patient shows loculated fluid* ➡ *in the pelvic peritoneal cavity surrounding the left ovary* ➡. *There is no mass effect on adjacent structures; rather, the fluid fills the space provided. This is characteristic of peritoneal inclusion cyst.*

Lymphocele

Lymphocele

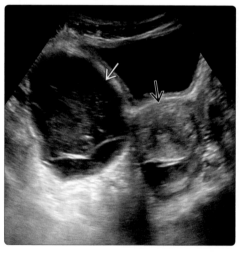

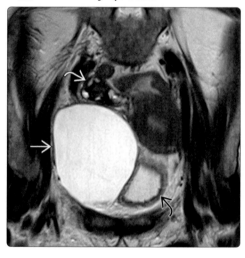

(Left) *Transverse US of the pelvis shows the uterus* ➡ *and a right adnexal hypoechoic mass* ➡ *with internal septations and posterior acoustic enhancement.* (Right) *Coronal oblique T2 MR in the same patient shows the cystic mass* ➡ *along the right pelvic sidewall displacing the urinary bladder* ➡. *The uterus and right ovary* ➡ *are separate and displaced superolaterally. This was a lymphocele related to renal transplant surgery. Note that the mass is not between the uterus and ovary as with most tubal pathologies.*

Sigmoid Diverticulitis

Sigmoid Diverticulitis

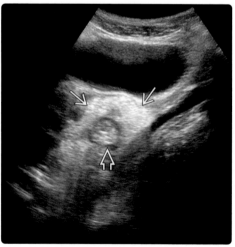

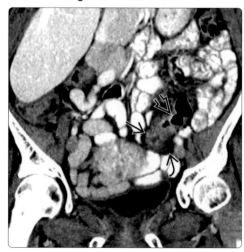

(Left) *Transabdominal US shows a bowel loop* ➡ *with surrounding echogenic inflammation* ➡. *This was separate from the ovary.* (Right) *Coronal CECT in the same patient shows focal fat stranding and inflammation* ➡ *surrounding a thick-walled diverticulum* ➡ *arising from the sigmoid colon* ➡.

Appendicitis

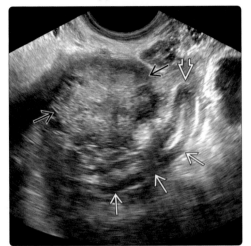

Appendicitis

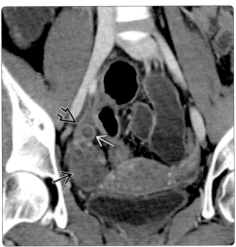

(Left) *Transvaginal US of the right ovary* ➡ *shows an adjacent, tubular* ➡, *blind-ending* ➡ *structure with bowel signature.* (Right) *Coronal CECT in the same patient confirms appendicitis with a dilated, hyperenhancing appendix* ➡ *adjacent to the right ovary* ➡. *Note the periappendiceal fluid and peritoneal enhancement* ➡.

Appendiceal Mucocele

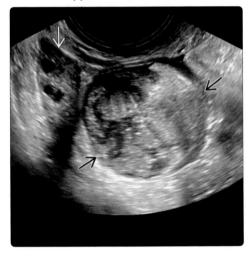

Appendiceal Mucocele

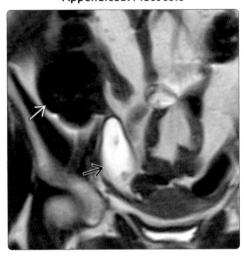

(Left) *Transvaginal US shows a normal right ovary* ➡ *and an adjacent, but separate, echogenic mass* ➡. *The mass was tubular (not evident on this image).* (Right) *Coronal T2 MR in the same patent shows the tubular cystic structure* ➡ *extending from the tip of the cecum* ➡, *consistent with a dilated appendix. There is no surrounding inflammation, consistent with appendiceal mucocele.*

Sarcoma

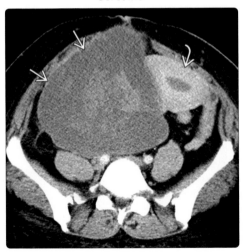

Sarcoma

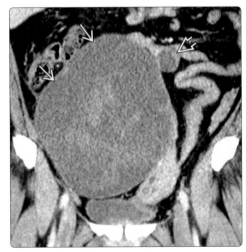

(Left) *Axial CECT shows a large, solid and cystic right adnexal mass* ➡ *displacing the uterus* ➡ *to the left.* (Right) *Coronal CECT in the same patient shows the right adnexal mass* ➡ *displacing the right ovary* ➡ *superiorly and the fallopian tube (not shown) stretched around the mass. Surgical resection revealed spindle cell sarcoma of the mesosalpinx.*

DIFFERENTIAL DIAGNOSIS

Common

- Ovarian Follicular Cyst
- Ovarian Corpus Luteum
- Ovarian Hemorrhagic Cyst
- Pelvic Inflammatory Disease

Less Common

- Endometrioma
- Ovarian Torsion
- Complicated Paraovarian Cyst
- Malpositioned Intrauterine Device

Rare but Important

- Complications of Uterine Leiomyoma
- Complications of Mature Cystic Teratoma
- Ovarian Vein Thrombosis/Thrombophlebitis
- Ovarian Hyperstimulation Syndrome
- Hematosalpinx
- Ovarian Abscess due to Diverticulitis
- Cervical Stenosis

ESSENTIAL INFORMATION

Key Differential Diagnosis Issues

- Ovarian abnormalities
  - Ovarian follicular cyst
  - Ovarian corpus luteum (CL)
  - Ovarian hemorrhagic cyst
  - Pelvic inflammatory disease (PID): Tuboovarian abscess (TOA)
  - Ovarian endometrioma
  - Ovarian torsion
  - Complications of mature cystic teratoma
  - Ovarian hyperstimulation syndrome
- Adnexal abnormalities
  - PID: Salpingitis/pyosalpinx
  - Complicated paraovarian cyst
  - Hematosalpinx
  - Ovarian vein thrombosis/thrombophlebitis
- Uterine abnormalities
  - PID: Endometritis
  - Complications of uterine leiomyomas
  - Malpositioned IUD
  - Cervical stenosis

Helpful Clues for Common Diagnoses

- **Ovarian Follicular Cyst**
  - Physiologic cysts seen only in premenopausal women
  - Painful cysts are often large, measuring 3-8 cm
  - Thin-walled simple cyst
  - ± curvilinear septations (i.e., cumulus oöphorus)
  - Resolve on follow-up examinations
- **Ovarian Corpus Luteum**
  - Postovulatory CL measures up to 3 cm
  - Collapsed, thick-walled cyst with crenulated margin
    - Doppler US demonstrates prominent peripheral blood flow with low-resistance waveform
    - Peripheral enhancement at CT and MR

- May appear completely solid on US with peripheral increased vascularity
- Presence of CL may lead to ovarian stromal edema → acute pelvic pain
  - Can mimic ovarian torsion on US
    - Enlarged ovaries and peripherally displaced follicles
- **Ovarian Hemorrhagic Cyst**
  - Various sonographic patterns depending on chronicity
    - Acute hemorrhage is echogenic, avascular, homogeneous, or heterogeneous nonshadowing
    - Diffuse pattern of low-level echoes
    - Retracted clot
      - Avascular, mass-like structure within anechoic cyst
      - Has characteristic concave contour
      - May jiggle with transducer ballottement
    - Reticular, lacy, fishnet, or spongy pattern
    - Doppler US shows peripheral vascularity with low-impedance flow on spectral Doppler imaging
  - MR demonstrates single unilocular cyst
    - High signal intensity on T1, remains high on T1 FS
    - May be hypointense on T2 (more commonly hyperintense)
    - No T2 shading or T2-dark spots
- **Pelvic Inflammatory Disease**
  - Pelvic pain, cervical motion tenderness, ↑ WBC
  - Swollen tubes with thickened endosalpingeal folds (cog-wheel sign)
  - Tubal obstruction and dilatation with complex fluid or fluid-pus level (pyosalpinx)
    - Waist sign: Best to discriminate fluid-filled tube from other adnexal masses
  - Endometrial thickening/fluid (endometritis)
  - Complex adnexal mass comprised of adhesed ovary and tube (TOA)
  - Echogenic fluid (pus) in cul-de-sac

Helpful Clues for Less Common Diagnoses

- **Endometrioma**
  - US
    - Unilocular cyst contains homogeneous, low-level echoes → characteristic ground-glass appearance
    - ± small, echogenic mural foci (35% of endometriomas)
  - MR
    - High signal intensity on T1, remains high on T1 FS
    - T2 shading
    - T2-dark spots
  - Rupture of endometrioma is rare, commonly occurs during pregnancy
    - Pericyst hemorrhagic fluid
    - Adnexal inflammation
    - Irregular cyst wall
    - Collapsed cyst
    - Diffuse peritonitis
- **Ovarian Torsion**
  - Pelvic pain localized to side of torsion
  - Ovarian edema
    - Asymmetric enlargement (largest diameter > 5 cm when no ovarian lesion is present)
    - Thicker than expected ovarian parenchyma surrounding lesion

- Peripheralization of follicles (string of pearls sign)
- Small amount of fluid surrounds torsed ovary or within cul-de-sac (87% of cases)
- Changes of parenchymal edema ± hemorrhage
- Twisted vascular pedicle
- Abnormal situs, usually located in midline and superior to fundus of uterus
- Vascular flow may be absent on Doppler US, but its presence does not exclude torsion

- **Complicated Paraovarian Cyst**
  o May cause pain due to rupture or torsion
  o Well-defined, unilocular, contain simple fluid and separate from ovary
- **Malpositioned Intrauterine Device**
  o IUD-associated complications of displacement, myometrial penetration, and perforation result in acute pelvic pain
  o US, particularly 3D US, best to detect IUD malposition

Helpful Clues for Rare Diagnoses

- **Complications of Uterine Leiomyoma**
  o Red degeneration (hemorrhagic necrosis)
    - Peripheral or diffuse high signal intensity on T1
    - Variable signal intensity on T2
  o Torsion and infarction
    - Change in location of pedunculated fibroid
    - May demonstrate twisted vascular pedicle
    - Hypoenhancement/nonenhancement due to infarction
- **Complications of Mature Cystic Teratoma**
  o May be lead point for torsion
  o Rupture is rare complication
    - Free-floating abdominal fat, fat-fluid level
    - Discontinuity of cyst wall
    - Inflammatory stranding of surrounding fat
- **Ovarian Vein Thrombosis/Thrombophlebitis**
  o Occurs primarily in postpartum setting
  o Involves right ovarian vein in 70-90% of cases
  o Presents clinically as pelvic pain and fever
  o US is often inconclusive

- o CT and MR are imaging modalities of choice
    - Intraluminal filling defect and enlargement of vein
- **Ovarian Hyperstimulation Syndrome**
  o History of ovulation induction therapy
  o Massively enlarged multicystic ovaries
  o ± ascites, pleural &/or pericardial effusions
- **Hematosalpinx**
  o May occur in setting of tubal endometriosis, ectopic pregnancy, tumor, and torsion
  o US demonstrates hypoechoic tubular adnexal structure + internal echoes, no blood flow on Doppler evaluation
  o Hyperattenuating tubular adnexal structure separate from ovary on CT
  o MR imaging shows hyperintense tubular adnexal structure on T1 FS and T2 ± T2 shading
- **Cervical Stenosis**
  o Commonly caused by endometrial atrophy in postmenopausal women
    - Also tumors, trauma, and instrumentation
  o Results in accumulation of fluid within endometrial cavity
  o At imaging, appears as distended uterine cavity filled with fluid (hydrometra) or blood (hematometra)

Other Diagnoses to Consider

- Ectopic pregnancy
  o Should always be considered in premenopausal woman with positive pregnancy test
- Nongynecologic causes of pelvic pain
  o GI causes
    - e.g., diverticulitis, appendicitis, Crohn disease, etc.
  o Urinary causes
    - e.g., urolithiasis, cystitis, etc.

SELECTED REFERENCES

1. Basta Nikolic M et al: Imaging of acute pelvic pain. Br J Radiol. 94(1127):20210281, 2021
2. Olpin JD et al: Imaging of acute pelvic pain: nonpregnant. Radiol Clin North Am. 58(2):329-45, 2020
3. Rogers D et al: Corpus luteum with ovarian stromal edema is associated with pelvic pain and confusion for ovarian torsion. Abdom Radiol (NY). 44(2):697-704, 2019

Ovarian Follicular Cyst

Ovarian Corpus Luteum

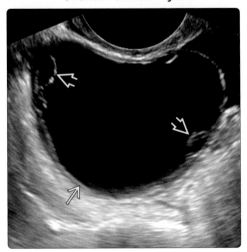
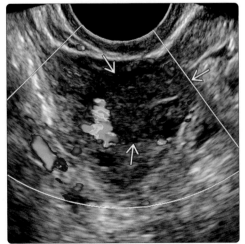

(Left) *Transvaginal US shows a unilocular ovarian cyst ➡ measuring ~ 8 cm with peripheral curvilinear septations ⧉ representing the cumulus oophorus. Follow-up 4 weeks later revealed complete resolution.* **(Right)** *Transvaginal color Doppler US shows a slightly hypoechoic, avascular ovarian structure ➡ with peripherally increased vascularity. Follow-up 4 weeks later revealed complete resolution.*

Ovarian Hemorrhagic Cyst

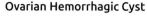

(Left) *Axial CECT shows a large amount of high-attenuation pelvic fluid ➡ surrounding the uterus ➡.* **(Right)** *Axial CECT in the same patient shows high-attenuation pelvic fluid ➡ and a right ovarian lesion ➡ that is predominantly cystic with a high-attenuation nodular structure ➡ representing a hemorrhagic cyst with retracted clot. Hemoperitoneum is the result of rupture of the hemorrhagic cyst.*

Ovarian Hemorrhagic Cyst

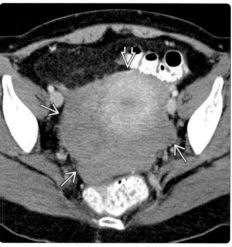
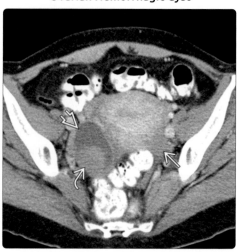

(Left) *Axial T2 MR shows a left adnexal fluid-filled lesion ➡ with a thick wall and fluid level. Note the inflammatory stranding of the fat surrounding the abscess ▣.* **(Right)** *Coronal T1 C+ FS MR in the same patient shows the left adnexal lesion ➡ with a thick, uniformly enhancing wall due to tuboovarian abscess.*

Pelvic Inflammatory Disease

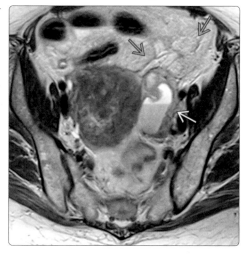
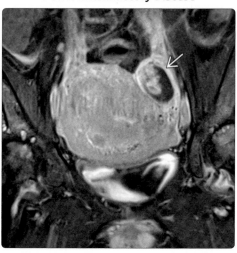

(Left) *Axial T2 MR shows bilateral adnexal masses ➡ with high signal intensity and areas of very low signal intensity ➡.* **(Right)** *Axial T1 FS MR in the same patient shows bilateral adnexal masses ➡ with high signal intensity. Adjacent to the left lesion, there is free fluid of high signal intensity ➡ due to hemoperitoneum resulting from rupture of endometrioma.*

Endometrioma

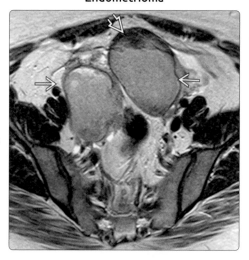
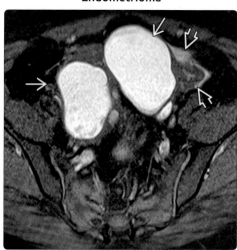

Ovarian Torsion

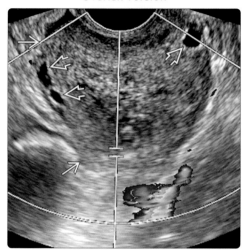

Ovarian Torsion

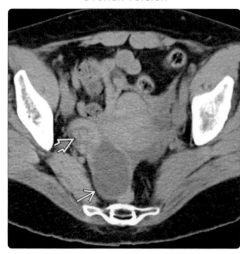

(Left) *Color Doppler US shows an enlarged right ovary ➡ (~ 6 cm) with absent flow. Small follicles ➡ are seen at the periphery (string of pearls sign).* **(Right)** *Axial NECT in the same patient shows an enlarged, nonenhancing ovary ➡ and twisting of the vascular pedicle ➡.*

Complications of Uterine Leiomyoma

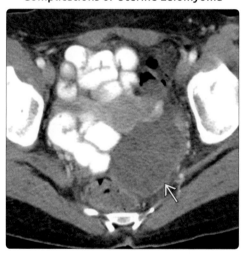

Complications of Uterine Leiomyoma

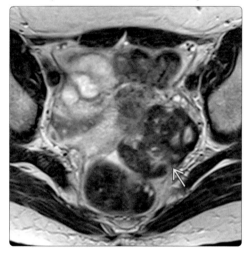

(Left) *Axial CECT shows a poorly enhancing left adnexal mass ➡.* **(Right)** *Axial T2 MR in the same patient shows a left adnexal mass ➡. The mass was separate from the ovary and showed low signal intensity with small areas of high signal intensity.*

Complications of Uterine Leiomyoma

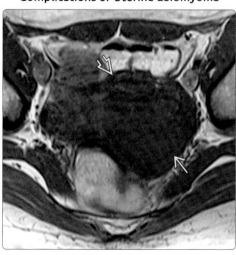

Complications of Uterine Leiomyoma

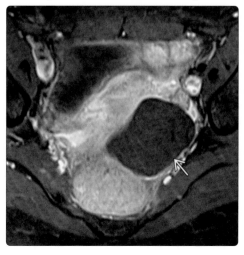

(Left) *Axial T1 MR in the same patient shows a left adnexal mass ➡ with intermediate signal intensity similar to that of the uterus ➡.* **(Right)** *Axial T1 C+ FS MR in the same patient shows a left adnexal mass ➡. The mass shows no enhancement following contrast administration. Comparison with prior imaging showed change in the location of the mass relative to the uterus. The imaging features are consistent with torsion of an exophytic uterine leiomyoma.*

Complications of Uterine Leiomyoma

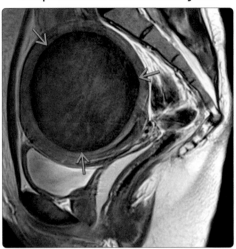

Complications of Uterine Leiomyoma

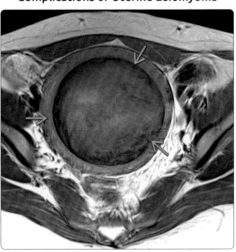

(Left) *Sagittal T2 MR in a young woman who presented with acute pelvic pain 2 weeks after delivery shows a low signal intensity rim at the periphery of an intramural leiomyoma ➡ due to abundant intracellular methemoglobin in the peripheral thrombosed vessels.* (Right) *Sagittal T2 MR in the same patient shows a low signal intensity rim at the periphery of the intramural leiomyoma ➡.*

Complications of Uterine Leiomyoma

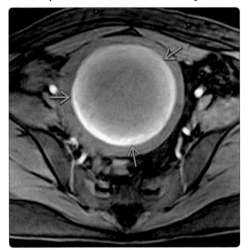

Complications of Uterine Leiomyoma

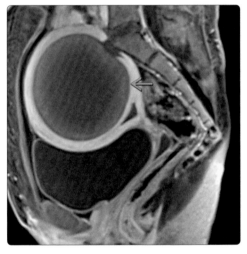

(Left) *Axial T1 MR in the same patient shows an intramural uterine leiomyoma with peripheral rim of high signal intensity ➡, likely secondary to the proteinaceous content of the blood or the T1-shortening effects of methemoglobin.* (Right) *Sagittal T1 C+ FS MR in the same patient shows absence of enhancement of the intramural leiomyoma ➡.*

Ovarian Vein Thrombosis/Thrombophlebitis

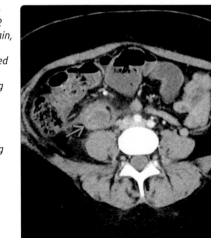

Ovarian Vein Thrombosis/Thrombophlebitis

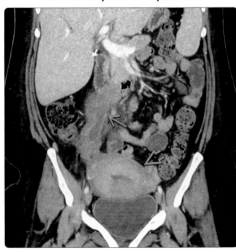

(Left) *Axial CECT in 25-year-old woman who presented 2 weeks after delivery with pain, fever, and elevated WBC shows a dilated, nonpacified right ovarian vein ➡ with stranding of the surrounding fat.* (Right) *Coronal CECT in the same patient shows a dilated, nonpacified right ovarian vein ➡ with stranding of the surrounding fat. Note the enlarged postpartum uterus ➡.*

Hematosalpinx

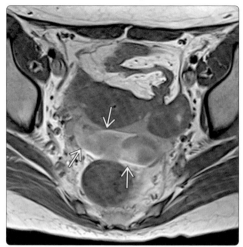

Hematosalpinx

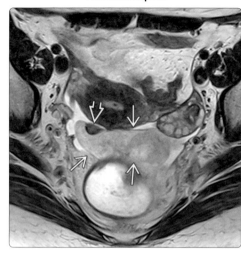

(Left) *Axial T1 MR shows a distended, tubular structure* ⇨ *posterior to the uterus with heterogeneous, predominantly high signal intensity.* (Right) *Axial T2 MR in the same patient shows a distended, tubular structure* ⇨ *with high signal intensity due to blood-filled fallopian tube (hematosalpinx) caused by endometrial implant* ⇨.

Ovarian Abscess due to Diverticulitis

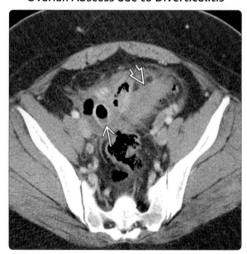

Ovarian Abscess due to Diverticulitis

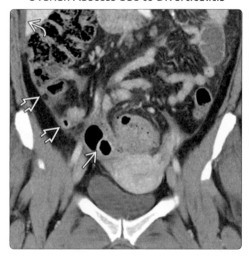

(Left) *Axial CECT shows a right air- and fluid-filled adnexal cavity* ⇨ *adjacent to an inflamed sigmoid colon* ⇨. (Right) *Coronal CECT shows a right air- and fluid-filled adnexal cavity* ⇨. *Note the extension of inflammatory changes along the right paracolic gutter* ⇨ *to the perihepatic region* ⇨.

Cervical Stenosis

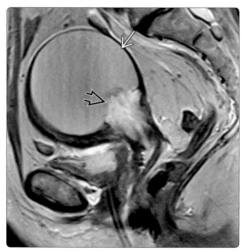

Cervical Stenosis

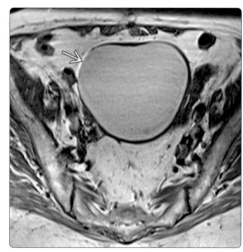

(Left) *Sagittal T2 MR shows a distended uterine cavity* ⇨ *filled with high signal intensity fluid due to an obstructing cervical mass* ⇨. (Right) *Axial T1 MR in the same patient shows distention of the uterine cavity* ⇨. *The cavity is filled with blood exhibiting high signal intensity (hematometra).*

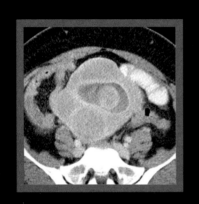
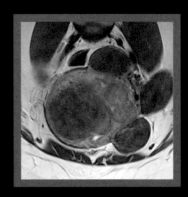
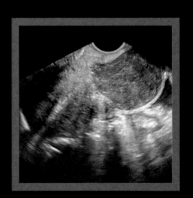
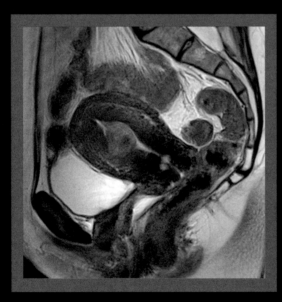
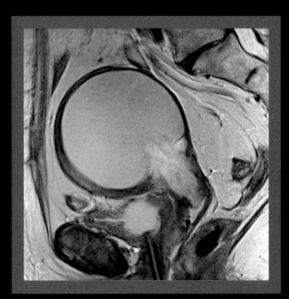
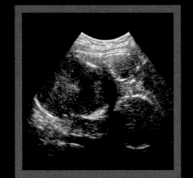
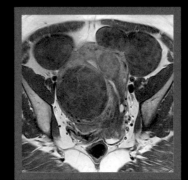
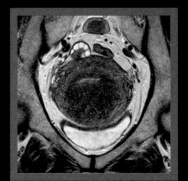

SECTION 23
Uterus

Generic Imaging Patterns

Enlarged Uterus   658
Thickened Endometrium   662

Clinically Based Differentials

Abnormal Uterine Bleeding   668

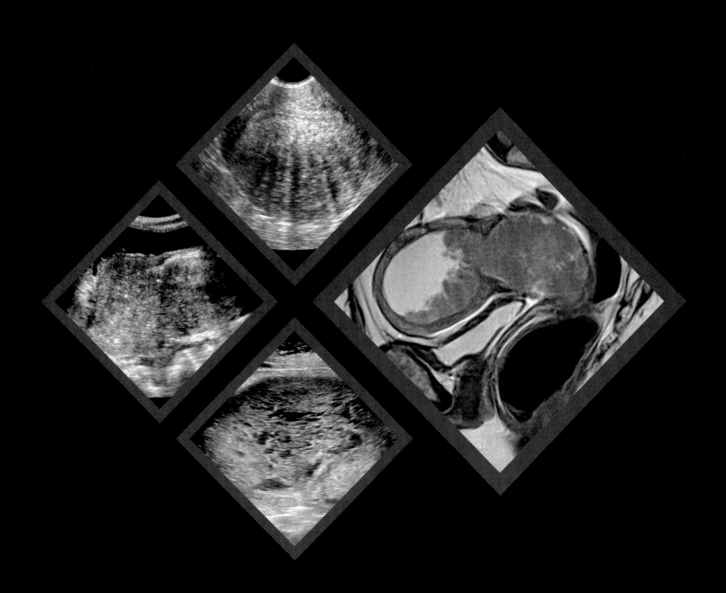

DIFFERENTIAL DIAGNOSIS

Common

- Leiomyoma
- Adenomyosis
- Post Partum
  - Normal Post Partum
  - Endometritis

Less Common

- Endometrial Cancer

Rare but Important

- Uterine Leiomyosarcoma
- Cervical Lesion
  - Cervical Cancer
  - Cervical Stenosis
  - Cervical Leiomyoma

ESSENTIAL INFORMATION

Key Differential Diagnosis Issues

- Enlarged uterus without focal mass
  - Diffuse adenomyosis
  - Postpartum uterus
  - Endometrial cancer
- Enlarged uterus with focal mass
  - Multiple round, well-defined masses
    - Intramural leiomyomas
  - Single ill-defined mass
    - Focal adenomyosis
    - Endometrial cancer
- Fluid in endometrial cavity causing uterine enlargement
  - Cervical stenosis
  - Cervical cancer
- Lesion centered in cervix
  - Cervical leiomyoma
  - Cervical cancer
- MR can differentiate various etiologies of enlarged uterus

Helpful Clues for Common Diagnoses

- **Leiomyoma**
  - Focal, well-defined masses
  - Lobulated external contour of uterus
  - MR is diagnostic
    - Well-defined, T2-hypointense masses
- **Adenomyosis**
  - Asymmetric myometrial thickening
  - Cystic spaces in myometrium
  - Alternating bands of increased through transmission and shadowing
  - Uterus may be tender during examination
  - MR is diagnostic
    - Thickened junctional zone (≥ 12 mm)
    - Myometrial hyperintense foci

Helpful Clues for Less Common Diagnoses

- **Endometrial Cancer**
  - Typically postmenopausal woman with bleeding
  - Diffuse uterine enlargement
  - Ill-defined endometrium

Helpful Clues for Rare Diagnoses

- **Cervical Lesion**
  - MR best modality for visualization and differentiation of cervical abnormalities
  - Cervical cancer
    - US: Hypoechoic, ill-defined lesion
    - MR: T2-hyperintense cervical mass
    - ± hydronephrosis
    - ± fluid in endometrial cavity
  - Cervical leiomyoma
    - US: Well-defined, shadowing, hypoechoic lesion
    - MR: Well-defined, T2-hypointense mass
    - Typically will not obstruct endocervical canal
  - Cervical stenosis
    - No identifiable mass
    - Fluid distention of endometrial cavity
    - Thin surrounding endometrium
    - History of curettage or childbearing

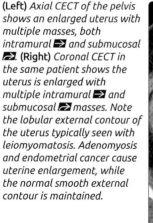

(Left) *Axial CECT of the pelvis shows an enlarged uterus with multiple masses, both intramural ➡ and submucosal ⬈. **(Right)** Coronal CECT in the same patient shows the uterus is enlarged with multiple intramural ➡ and submucosal ➡ masses. Note the lobular external contour of the uterus typically seen with leiomyomatosis. Adenomyosis and endometrial cancer cause uterine enlargement, while the normal smooth external contour is maintained.*

Leiomyoma

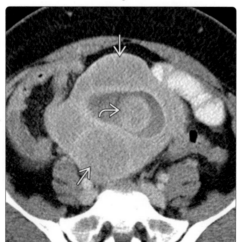

Leiomyoma

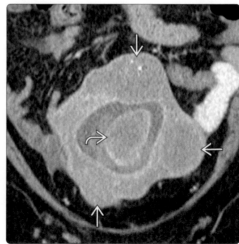

Leiomyoma

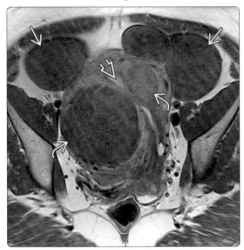

Leiomyoma

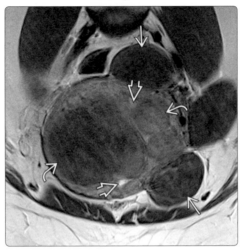

(Left) *Axial oblique T2 FSE MR shows enlargement of the uterus and distortion of the endometrial stripe* ⇒ *by well-defined, hypointense intramural* ⇉ *and subserosal* ⇒ *masses. MR is helpful for diagnosis and mapping of leiomyomas prior to treatment.* (Right) *Coronal oblique T2 FSE MR in the same patient shows marked distortion of the endometrial stripe* ⇒ *by multiple intramural leiomyomas* ⇉. *Note the lobular external uterine contour due to subserosal leiomyomas* ⇉.

Leiomyoma

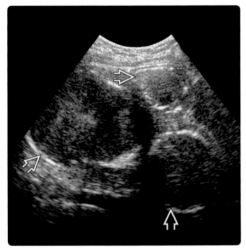

Uterine Leiomyosarcoma

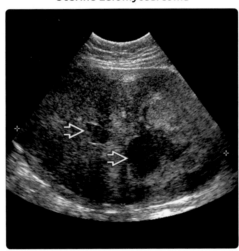

(Left) *Longitudinal US shows an enlarged uterus (> 20 cm in length) with multiple masses* ⇒ *surrounded by calcific rims, consistent with degenerated leiomyomas.* (Right) *Longitudinal US shows an enlarged uterus with a hypoechoic mass (calipers) with areas of necrosis* ⇒. *The uterus had rapidly increased in size since a study 3 months prior, raising the likelihood of malignancy.*

Adenomyosis

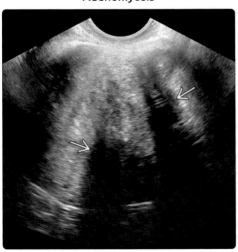

Adenomyosis

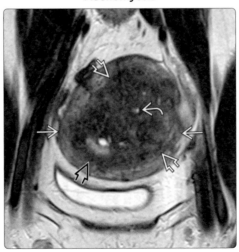

(Left) *Transverse transvaginal US of the pelvis shows an enlarged uterus with ill-defined, shadowy* ⇒, *hypoechoic areas.* (Right) *Coronal oblique T2 FSE MR in the same patient shows enlargement of the uterus* ⇒ *by focal, hypointense thickening* ⇒ *of the posterior junctional zone with foci of hyperintensity* ⇉. *Note the normal thin junctional zone anteriorly* ⇉. *Adenomyomas are typically contiguous with the junctional zone and may have functional endometrial glands, as in this case.*

Adenomyosis

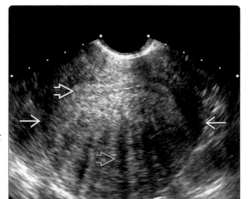

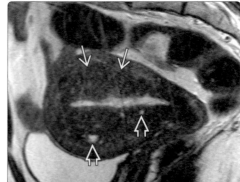

(Left) *Transverse transvaginal US shows an enlarged uterus ➡ with asymmetric thickening of the posterior wall and alternating echogenic and hypoechoic striations ➡ emanating from the junctional zone. Note the normal endometrial echo complex ➡. **(Right)** Sagittal T2 FSE MR shows enlargement of the uterus ➡ with diffuse thickening of the junctional zone. Hyperintense foci ➡ in the thickened junctional zone are typical of adenomyosis and represent endometrial glands. The external contour of the uterus is smooth.*

Endometritis

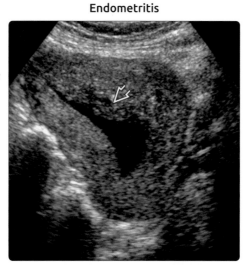

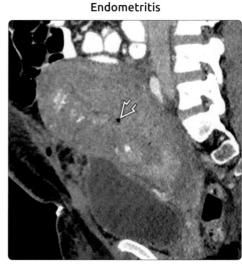

(Left) *Longitudinal US shows an enlarged uterus with endometrial fluid and a shaggy, irregular appearance to the endometrium anteriorly ➡. **(Right)** Sagittal CECT of the pelvis in a postpartum patient with fever shows enlargement of the uterus with foci of gas ➡ in the endometrial cavity. These can be normal postpartum findings, and the clinical history of fever and pain should be used to help make the diagnosis of endometritis, as in this case.*

Endometrial Cancer

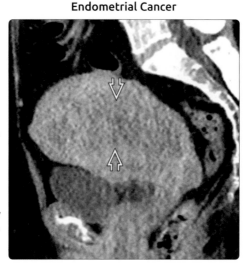

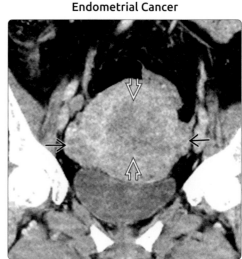

(Left) *Sagittal CECT of the pelvis shows an enlarged uterus with ill-defined central hypodensity ➡. The overall shape of the uterus is preserved with a smooth external contour. **(Right)** Coronal CECT in the same patient again shows the enlarged uterus with a normal external contour and central ill-defined hypodensity ➡. The ill-defined endometrial mass fills and distends the endometrial cavity, resulting in uterine enlargement. Biopsy confirmed endometrial cancer. Ovaries ➡ are noted.*

Cervical Cancer

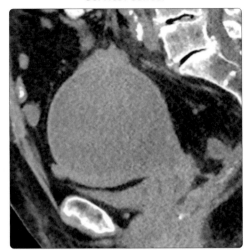

Cervical Cancer

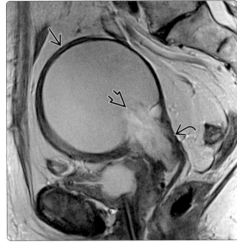

(Left) *Sagittal NECT of the pelvis shows an enlarged uterus. There is the suggestion of hypodense distention of the uterine cavity and thinning of the surrounding myometrium.* (Right) *Sagittal T2 FSE MR in the same patient shows the uterus ⟹ is enlarged due to fluid-filled distention of the uterine cavity. The cervical obstruction is due to a hyperintense mass ⟹. There is preservation of an outer rim of low-signal cervical stroma ⟹, confirming the absence of parametrial invasion. Biopsy confirmed adenocarcinoma.*

Cervical Cancer

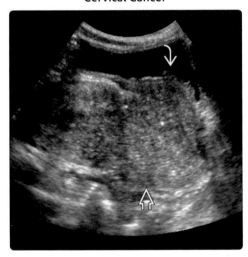

Cervical Stenosis

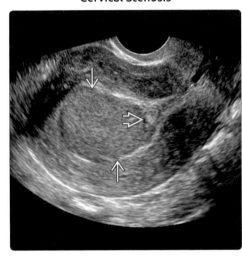

(Left) *Longitudinal US shows a large, irregular, hypoechoic mass in the region of the cervix ⟹. The mass invades the bladder ⟹.* (Right) *Longitudinal US after endometrial ablation shows that the endometrial cavity is filled with complex fluid ⟹ with some echogenic debris ⟹. The surrounding endometrium is thin.*

Cervical Leiomyoma

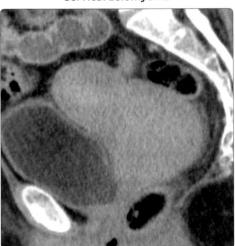

Cervical Leiomyoma

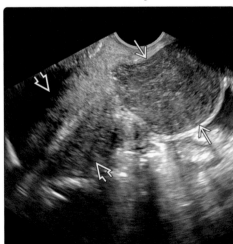

(Left) *Sagittal NECT shows enlargement of the cervix with homogeneous density and smooth external margins.* (Right) *Longitudinal transvaginal US in the same patient shows a well-defined, homogeneously hypoechoic mass ⟹ in the cervix. Note the normal uterine body ⟹ and lack of distention of the uterine cavity.*

DIFFERENTIAL DIAGNOSIS

Common

- Secretory-Phase Endometrium
- Endometrial Polyps
- Leiomyoma
- Diffuse Adenomyosis
- Early Pregnancy

Less Common

- Endometrial Hyperplasia
- Endometrial Cancer
- Tamoxifen-Induced Changes
- Retained Products of Conception
- Hematometra

Rare but Important

- Endometritis
- Molar Pregnancy
- Unopposed Estrogen
- Metastatic Disease

ESSENTIAL INFORMATION

Key Differential Diagnosis Issues

- Diffuse endometrial thickening
  - Normal secretory-phase endometrium
  - Endometrial hyperplasia
  - Endometrial cancer
  - Diffuse adenomyosis
  - Hematometra
  - Focal endometrial lesions can also mimic diffuse thickening
    - Techniques that may be helpful for identifying focal abnormality
      - □ Color Doppler US
      - □ 3D US
      - □ Phase of menstruation
- Focal endometrial thickening
  - Endometrial polyp
  - Endometrial cancer
  - Submucosal leiomyoma
- Postpartum patient
  - Endometritis
  - Retained products of conception
- Indistinct endometrial-myometrial interface
  - Endometrial cancer
  - Adenomyosis
  - Submucosal leiomyoma

Helpful Clues for Common Diagnoses

- **Secretory-Phase Endometrium**
  - In latter 1/2 of menstrual cycle, endometrium can be thick, heterogeneous, and echogenic
  - Follow-up early in subsequent menstrual cycle will show thin endometrium
- **Endometrial Polyps**
  - Focal endometrial lesion
  - Typically more echogenic than surrounding endometrium
  - May have cysts

- Stalk with flow
- May have broad base
- Frequently multiple
- Smooth margins
- May have surrounding thin endometrium

- **Leiomyoma**
  - Submucosal leiomyoma is > 50% within endometrium
  - Intramural leiomyoma can cause appearance of endometrial thickening
  - Iso- or hypoechoic lesion
  - Posterior acoustic shadowing
  - Can be confirmed with MR
    - Well-defined, T2-hypointense myometrial mass
- **Diffuse Adenomyosis**
  - Endometrial pseudowidening
  - Enlarged, globular uterus
  - Indistinct endometrial-myometrial interface
  - Subendometrial cysts
  - Can be confirmed with MR
    - Thickened junctional zone (JZ) ≥ 12 mm
    - High signal intensity foci in JZ on T1 and T2 MR
- **Early Pregnancy**
  - Positive urine/serum human chorionic gonadotropin
    - Normal early pregnancy
    - Miscarriage
    - Ectopic pregnancy
    - Hydatiform mole, complete mole
    - Hydatiform mole, partial mole

Helpful Clues for Less Common Diagnoses

- **Endometrial Hyperplasia**
  - Typically diffuse endometrial thickening but may be focal
  - ± cystic spaces
  - Well-defined endometrial-myometrial interface
  - Risk factors
    - Nulliparity
    - Obesity
    - Age > 70
    - Hypertension
    - Diabetes mellitus
    - Tamoxifen

- **Endometrial Cancer**
  - Irregular endometrial thickening ± mass
  - Heterogeneous endometrium with areas of hypoechogenicity
  - Ill-defined margins, indistinct endometrial-myometrial interface
  - Myometrial invasion is diagnostic
  - Typically postmenopausal woman with abnormal bleeding
  - Postmenopausal patients who present with vaginal bleeding should undergo transvaginal US
    - Abnormal thickness of endometrium > 5 mm, regardless of hormone replacement therapy
- **Tamoxifen-Induced Changes**
  - ↑ incidence with ↑ dose and time of treatment
  - Reactivation of foci of adenomyosis
  - Due to estrogenic effect in endometrium, can lead to polyps, hyperplasia, and carcinoma

- Endometrial cancer in patients taking tamoxifen is frequently in endometrial polyps
- **Retained Products of Conception**
  - Focal endometrial lesion
  - May have calcifications
  - May have blood flow, but lack of flow does not exclude diagnosis
- **Hematometra**
  - Echogenic fluid in endometrial cavity
    - Mobile debris
    - No flow on Doppler US
  - Look for underlying cause of obstruction
    - Uterine duplication anomaly
    - Leiomyoma
    - Endometrial cancer
    - Cervical cancer
    - If thin surrounding endometrium and no obstructing lesion, cervical stenosis is diagnosis of exclusion

Helpful Clues for Rare Diagnoses

- **Endometritis**
  - In postpartum patient, painful enlarged uterus
  - In nonpregnant patient, associated with pelvic inflammatory disease
  - Clinical diagnosis; imaging is nonspecific
  - Elevated white blood cell count
- **Molar Pregnancy**
  - Most common type of gestational trophoblastic disease
  - Hyperechoic early in pregnancy with classic grape-like appearance developing as pregnancy advances
- **Unopposed Estrogen**
  - Can result in endometrial polyps, hyperplasia, and carcinoma
  - Estrogen use without progesterone
  - Due to chronic anovulatory states (i.e., polycystic ovary syndrome), exogenous estrogen exposure, tamoxifen, obesity, estrogen-secreting ovarian tumors (i.e., thecoma, granulosa cell tumor)
- **Metastatic Disease**
  - Ovarian primary with metastasis to endometrium

- Cervical primary with direct extension to endometrium
  - MR helpful for cervical cancer staging, local extent of disease, and to differentiate cervical from endometrial primary when both are involved by tumor
- Distant primary with hematogenous metastasis to endometrium

Other Essential Information

- Use transvaginal US for best evaluation of endometrium
- Sonohysterography can differentiate focal and diffuse endometrial abnormalities to determine best sampling technique
  - Diffuse thickening can be sampled with blind biopsy
  - Focal mass best assessed with hysteroscopic biopsy
- Sonohysterography helpful if endometrium is not adequately visualized by transvaginal US in symptomatic patient
- In uterine duplication anomalies, must evaluate each endometrium separately
  - 3D US and MR can be helpful for further evaluation

Alternative Differential Approaches

- Solid or complex ovarian lesion in association with endometrial lesion
  - Estrogenic effect from granulosa cell tumor or thecoma produces endometrial abnormality
  - Concordant ovarian and endometrial carcinoma
  - Endometrioid tumor
  - Metastatic disease

SELECTED REFERENCES

1. Gupta A et al: Imaging of the endometrium: physiologic changes and diseases: women's imaging. Radiographics. 37(7):2206-7, 2017
2. Barwick TD et al: Imaging of endometrial adenocarcinoma. Clin Radiol. 61(7):545-55, 2006
3. Smith-Bindman R et al: How thick is too thick? When endometrial thickness should prompt biopsy in postmenopausal women without vaginal bleeding. Ultrasound Obstet Gynecol. 24(5):558-65, 2004
4. Davis PC et al: Sonohysterographic findings of endometrial and subendometrial conditions. Radiographics. 22:803-16, 2002

Secretory-Phase Endometrium

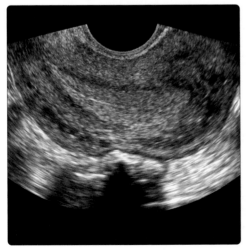

Endometrial Polyps

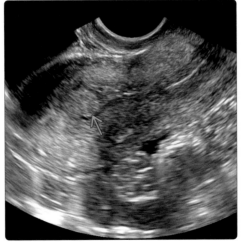

(Left) *Longitudinal transvaginal US of the uterus shows a homogeneous, symmetric endometrial echo complex that measures 11 mm, which is normal in the secretory phase of the menstrual cycle. There is no focal thickening, heterogeneity, or abnormal blood flow.* (Right) *Longitudinal transvaginal US of the uterus shows focal, echogenic thickening* ⇒ *of the fundal endometrium. Note the normal thin endometrium of the lower uterine segment.*

(Left) *Sagittal T2 FS MR of the uterus in the same patient shows focal endometrial ⇨ thickening and mild heterogeneity. Small endometrial polyps can be difficult to see on MR, and focal thickening of the stripe can be a clue, as in this case.* **(Right)** *Longitudinal color Doppler US of the uterus shows diffuse endometrial thickening. No focal abnormality could be identified on grayscale imaging, but Doppler shows focal flow ➡ extending into endometrium.*

Endometrial Polyps

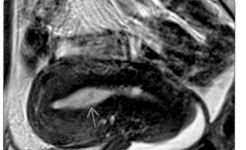

Endometrial Polyps

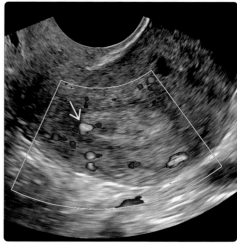

(Left) *Saline-infused sonohysterogram in the same patient shows a small, echogenic endometrial lesion ⇨. This was removed and confirmed to be an endometrial polyp. Doppler US can help indicate a focal lesion when grayscale imaging only shows diffuse endometrial thickening.* **(Right)** *Transvaginal color Doppler US of the uterus shows focal, hyperechoic thickening ⇨ of the endometrial echo complex with a focus of vascular flow ⇨.*

Endometrial Polyps

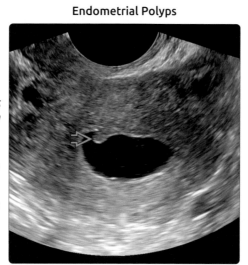

Endometrial Polyps

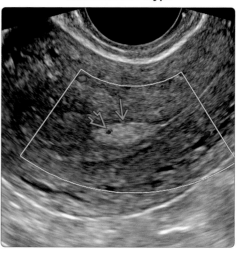

(Left) *Coronal 3D US of the uterus in the same patient shows an echogenic endometrial mass ➡, consistent with endometrial polyp. 3D US has been shown to be helpful in identifying focal endometrial abnormalities when the endometrium appears thick on 2D imaging.* **(Right)** *Longitudinal transvaginal US shows a hypoechoic mass ⇨ projecting into the endometrial cavity with the appearance of a thick endometrium (calipers).*

Endometrial Polyps

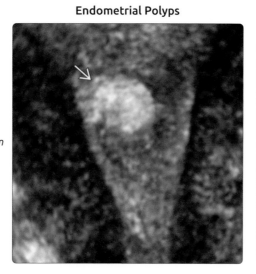

Leiomyoma

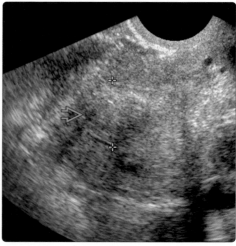

Leiomyoma

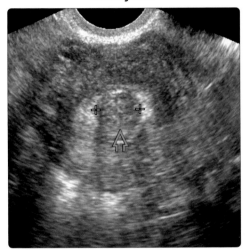

Leiomyoma

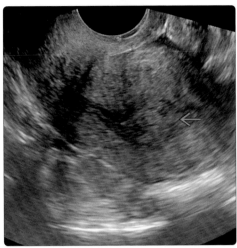

(Left) *Transverse transvaginal US in the same patient during secretory phase shows how the leiomyoma ⇉ (calipers) is now more apparent when surrounded by echogenic endometrium.* (Right) *Transvaginal US shows an isoechoic, shadowing mass ⇉ centrally in the uterus. The normal endometrial echo complex is obscured. The differential diagnosis for a mass in this location includes submucosal leiomyoma or endometrial cancer.*

Leiomyoma

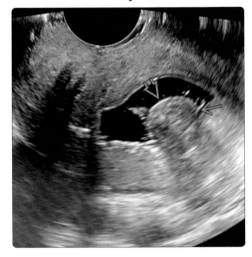

Leiomyoma

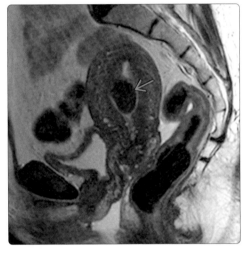

(Left) *Saline-infused US in the same patient shows the isoechoic, shadowing mass ⇉. The echogenic endometrial lining ⇉ overlying the lesion is thin and intact, confirming submucosal leiomyoma and not endometrial lesion.* (Right) *Sagittal T2 FSE MR shows a well-defined, homogeneously hypointense mass ⇉ projecting into the endometrial cavity, consistent with submucosal leiomyoma.*

Leiomyoma

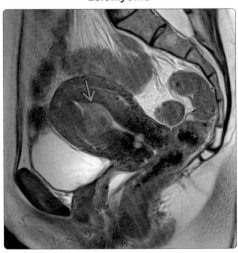

Diffuse Adenomyosis

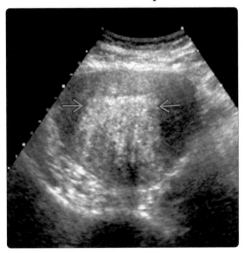

(Left) *Sagittal T2 FSE MR shows a well-defined, subendometrial, heterogeneous mass ⇉ projecting into endometrial cavity, consistent with submucosal leiomyoma.* (Right) *Transabdominal US shows ill-defined thickening of an endometrial echo complex ⇉. There is asymmetric thickening of the posterior uterine wall with echogenic and hypoechoic striations emanating from the endometrial-myometrial interface, indicating that endometrial thickening is due to diffuse adenomyosis.*

Early Pregnancy

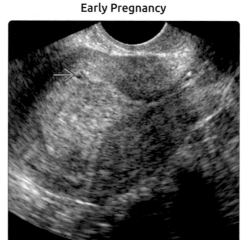

Endometrial Hyperplasia

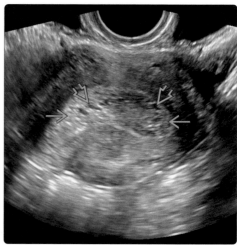

(Left) *Longitudinal transvaginal US in a woman with bleeding in the 1st trimester shows a heterogeneous endometrium with small cysts* ⮕*. Follow-up showed a normal early pregnancy.* (Right) *Transvaginal US of the uterus shows diffuse thickening of the endometrial echo complex* ⮕ *with foci of cystic change* ⮕*.*

Endometrial Cancer

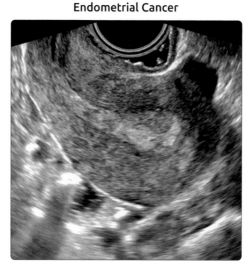

Endometrial Cancer

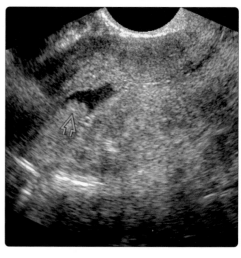

(Left) *Transvaginal US shows endometrial thickening and heterogeneous echogenicity. Although the differential is wide for this appearance, cancer should always be excluded, particularly in a postmenopausal woman with bleeding. This was confirmed to be endometrial cancer on biopsy and hysterectomy.* (Right) *Longitudinal transvaginal US shows fluid in the endometrial cavity with a focal area of endometrial thickening* ⮕ *in the fundal region.*

Tamoxifen-Induced Changes

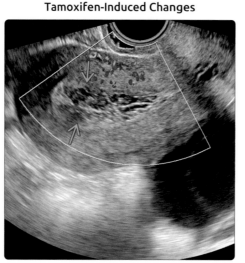

Retained Products of Conception

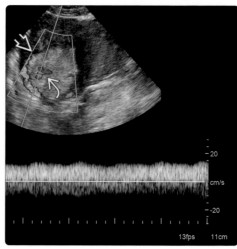

(Left) *Transvaginal Doppler US in a 35-year-old woman taking tamoxifen shows a thickened, heterogeneous endometrium* ⮕ *with multiple cysts.* (Right) *Color Doppler US in a patient who presented with postpartum bleeding following full-term vaginal delivery shows markedly echogenic endometrium* ⮕ *with large feeding vessels* ⮕*.*

Retained Products of Conception

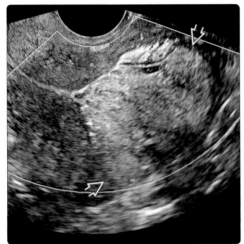

Molar Pregnancy

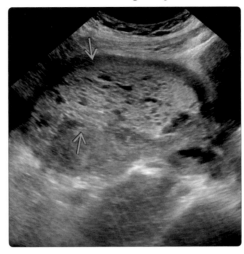

(Left) Color Doppler US in another patient who presented with postpartum bleeding following full-term vaginal delivery shows markedly echogenic endometrium ⬌ without significant vascularity. Retained products of conception can have variable vascularity. (Right) Transvaginal US of the uterus in a patient with markedly elevated β-hCG shows cystic thickening ⬌ of the endometrial echo complex.

Molar Pregnancy

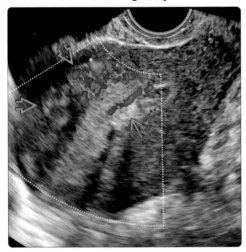

Unopposed Estrogen

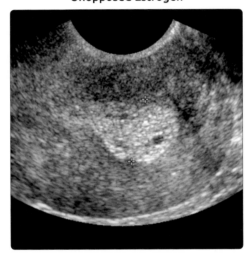

(Left) Color Doppler US in the same patient shows irregular thickening of the endometrial echo complex ⬌ with extension into the myometrium ⬌, consistent with persistent gestational trophoblastic disease. Abnormal tissue shows increased vascularity. (Right) Transvaginal US in a patient with granulosa cell tumor of the ovary shows a 15-mm endometrium (calipers) with cysts. In the setting of ovarian mass, endometrial abnormalities may be due to an estrogen secretion by the tumor.

Unopposed Estrogen

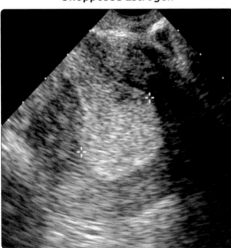

Metastatic Disease

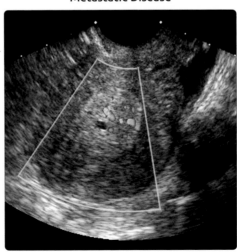

(Left) Transvaginal US in a patient with oligomenorrhea and PCOS shows a thickened, 23-mm endometrium (calipers). Chronic anovulation and unopposed estrogen result in stimulation of endometrium and an increased risk of endometrial hyperplasia or, rarely, cancer. (Right) Color Doppler US shows blood flow within the thickened, heterogeneous endometrium. In this patient with breast cancer, tamoxifen change and metastatic disease were thought to be most likely. Biopsy showed metastatic disease from breast primary.

DIFFERENTIAL DIAGNOSIS

Common
- Anovulatory Bleeding
- Endometrial Polyp
- Endometrial Atrophy
- Leiomyoma
- Pregnancy and Complications
  - Subchorionic Hematoma
  - Tubal Ectopic Pregnancy
  - Hydatiform Mole

Less Common
- Adenomyosis
- C-Section Defect
- Endometrial Hyperplasia
- Endometrial Cancer
- Cervical Cancer
- Endometritis
- Retained Products of Conception

Rare but Important
- Uterine Leiomyosarcoma
- Vulva Carcinoma
- Vaginal Carcinoma
- Intrauterine Device Perforation
- Estrogen-Producing Tumor of Ovary
  - Granulosa Cell Tumor
  - Fibrothecoma, Ovary
- Ovarian Carcinoma
- Bleeding From GI or GU Tract

ESSENTIAL INFORMATION

Key Differential Diagnosis Issues
- Is patient premenopausal?
  - Anovulatory bleeding (most common)
  - Pregnancy and complications
  - Endometrial polyp
  - Leiomyoma, submucosal
  - Endometrial hyperplasia
  - Malignancy (uterine, endometrial, cervical)
  - Nongynecologic sources of bleeding: GI or urinary tract
- Is patient postmenopausal?
  - Bleeding due to hormone use
    - Hormones can affect endometrial thickness
  - Endometrial atrophy (most common)
  - Endometrial polyp
  - Endometrial cancer
    - > 90% present with bleeding in postmenopausal woman; therefore, if endometrium is not adequately seen on US, further imaging with SIS or MR must be recommended
  - Leiomyoma
  - Malignancy (uterine, endometrial, cervical)
  - Nongynecologic sources of bleeding: GI or urinary tract
- Is there focal thickening of endometrium?
  - Endometrial polyps (most common)
  - Submucosal leiomyoma
  - Endometrial hyperplasia, rarely focal
  - Endometrial cancer
- Is endometrial-myometrial interface obscured?
  - Leiomyoma, submucosal
  - Endometrial cancer
  - Adenomyosis
- Is patient pregnant?
  - Normal pregnancy
  - Subchorionic hematoma
  - Tubal ectopic pregnancy
  - Hydatiform mole
- Is patient peripartum?
  - Retained products of conception
  - Endometritis

Helpful Clues for Common Diagnoses
- **Endometrial Polyp**
  - Focal endometrial lesion
  - Echogenic ± cystic change
  - Smooth margins
  - ± vascular stalk
- **Endometrial Atrophy**
  - 50-75% of postmenopausal bleeding attributed to atrophy
  - US appearance of thin endometrium with < 5-mm double-layer thickness
- **Leiomyoma**
  - Shadowing
  - Iso- or hypoechoic
  - Submucosal leiomyomas most likely associated with bleeding
  - If > 50%, leiomyoma projects into endometrial cavity, can be removed hysteroscopically
  - MR is diagnostic and helpful for treatment planning
    - Circumscribed, hypointense mass on T2 MR
- **Pregnancy and Complications**
  - Positive urine/serum human chorionic gonadotropin
  - If intrauterine pregnancy
    - Normal pregnancy
    - Normal or abnormal intrauterine pregnancy with subchorionic hematoma
    - Miscarriage
    - Hydatidiform mole
    - Consider heterotopic pregnancy with ectopic if fertility treatment
  - If no intrauterine pregnancy visualized
    - Ectopic pregnancy
    - Normal pregnancy, too early to visualize
    - Miscarriage

Helpful Clues for Less Common Diagnoses
- **Adenomyosis**
  - Diffuse or asymmetric myometrial thickening and heterogeneity
  - ± tender uterus
  - ± small myometrial cysts
- **C-Section Defect**
  - Triangular collection in anterior lower uterine segment
  - Acts as reservoir for blood products, leading to intermenstrual bleeding
- **Endometrial Hyperplasia**
  - Diffuse thickening most common, but also can be focal

- ○ ± cystic spaces
- **Endometrial Cancer**
  - ○ Poor definition of endometrium
  - ○ Irregular, thickened, heterogeneous endometrium
  - ○ Loss of endometrial-myometrial interface
  - ○ Most commonly presents with abnormal bleeding in postmenopausal woman
  - ○ Risk factors: Recurrent bleeding, estrogen hormone replacement therapy, obesity, polycystic ovary syndrome, chronic anovulation, hypertension, diabetes mellitus
- **Cervical Cancer**
  - ○ May be missed by US when small
  - ○ MR used for staging

Other Essential Information

- Use transvaginal US for best evaluation of endometrium
- Measure greatest double-layer endometrial thickness in sagittal plane
- Sonohysterography helpful to distinguish focal and diffuse endometrial abnormality
  - ○ Diffuse thickening can be sampled with blind biopsy
  - ○ Focal mass best assessed with hysteroscopic biopsy
- Sonohysterography helpful if endometrium is not adequately visualized with transvaginal US
- In uterine duplication anomalies, must evaluate each endometrium separately
- Tamoxifen use leads to polyps, hyperplasia, and carcinoma, as well as reactivation of foci of adenomyosis
  - ○ Number of endometrial lesions related to cumulative dose
  - ○ Endometrial cancer in patients taking tamoxifen frequently arises in endometrial polyps
- Postmenopausal patients with bleeding
  - ○ If endometrium is not visualized adequately in its entirety, must further evaluate with another imaging modality, biopsy, or direct visualization
  - ○ < 5 mm likely atrophy, no need to biopsy
  - ○ Society of Radiologists in Ultrasound consensus: Double-layer endometrial thickness > 5 mm is abnormal

- – 96% sensitivity for endometrial cancer
- ○ Recommend biopsy for diffuse thickening
- ○ Recommend biopsy for any focal abnormality
- ○ Use of HRT increases false-positive rate

Alternative Differential Approaches

- Enlarged uterus
  - ○ Leiomyoma
  - ○ Adenomyosis
  - ○ Cervical stenosis with uterus distended with debris
  - ○ Endometrial carcinoma
- Solid or complex ovarian lesion in association with endometrial lesion
  - ○ Estrogenic effect from granulosa cell tumor leading to endometrial lesion
  - ○ Estrogen secretion from thecoma leading to endometrial lesion
  - ○ Concordant ovarian and endometrial carcinoma
  - ○ Endometrioid tumor
  - ○ Metastatic disease

SELECTED REFERENCES

1. Keller CA et al: Color Doppler imaging of vascular abnormalities of the uterus. Ultrasound Q. 38(1):72-82, 2022
2. Gonzalo-Carballes M et al: A pictorial review of postpartum complications. Radiographics. 40(7):2117-41, 2020
3. Cunningham RK et al: Adenomyosis: a sonographic diagnosis. Radiographics. 38(5):1576-89, 2018
4. Goldstein SR: Sonography in postmenopausal bleeding. J Ultrasound Med. 31(2):333-6, 2012
5. American College of Obstetricians and Gynecologists: ACOG Committee Opinion No. 426: the role of transvaginal ultrasonography in the evaluation of postmenopausal bleeding. Obstet Gynecol. 113(2 Pt 1):462-4, 2009
6. Kazandi M et al: Transvaginal sonography combined with saline contrast sonohysterography to evaluate the uterine cavity in patients with abnormal uterine bleeding and postmenopausal endometrium more than 5 mm. Eur J Gynaecol Oncol. 24(2):185-90, 2003
7. Davis PC et al: Sonohysterographic findings of endometrial and subendometrial conditions. Radiographics. 22:803-16, 2002
8. Goldstein RB et al: Evaluation of the woman with postmenopausal bleeding: Society of Radiologists in Ultrasound-Sponsored Consensus Conference statement. J Ultrasound Med. 20(10):1025-36, 2001

Endometrial Polyp

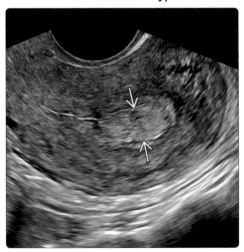

Endometrial Polyp

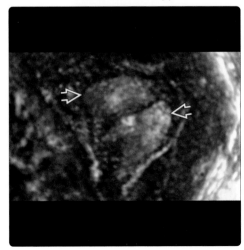

(Left) *Longitudinal transvaginal US of the uterus shows focal, hyperechoic thickening ➡ of the endometrial echo complex.* **(Right)** *3D US in the same patient shows to better advantage 2 endometrial polyps ➡ resulting in the focal endometrial thickening seen on 2D images. 3D US is helpful in clarifying focal abnormalities that may not be evident with 2D technique.*

Endometrial Polyp

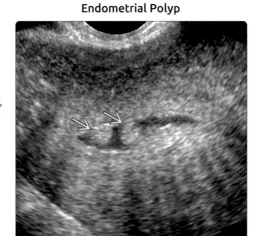

Endometrial Polyp

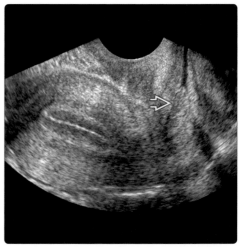

(Left) *Transverse hysterosonogram shows multiple small, echogenic masses ➡ arising from the endometrium.* **(Right)** *Longitudinal transvaginal US shows a well-defined, oblong, soft tissue echogenicity mass ➡ in the endocervical canal.*

Endometrial Polyp

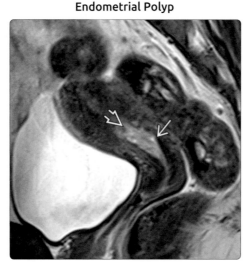

Endometrial Polyp

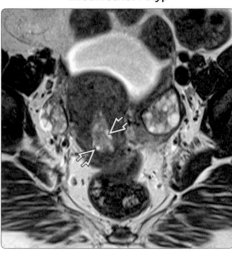

(Left) *Sagittal T2 MR shows focal endometrial thickening ➡ in the lower uterine segment extending through the internal cervical os ➡.* **(Right)** *Axial T2 MR in the same patient shows small cystic spaces ➡ in the focal endometrial thickening. This pedunculated polyp extends into the endocervical canal. Endometrial polyps tend to be isointense to normal endometrium and are seen on MR due to focal thickening and internal cystic spaces.*

Endometrial Atrophy

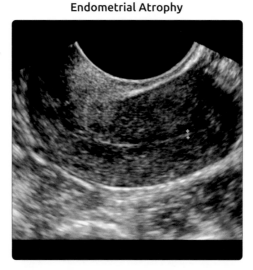

Leiomyoma

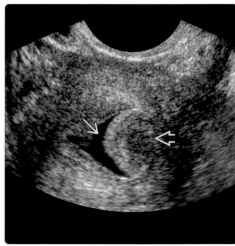

(Left) *Longitudinal transvaginal US shows a retroflexed uterus with a thin, atrophic endometrium (calipers).* **(Right)** *Oblique transvaginal US shows a hypoechoic mass ➡ projecting into the endometrial cavity with a small amount of endometrial fluid ➡. Note that > 50% of the leiomyoma projects into the endometrial cavity. This will allow for hysteroscopic removal of the leiomyoma.*

Abnormal Uterine Bleeding

Leiomyoma

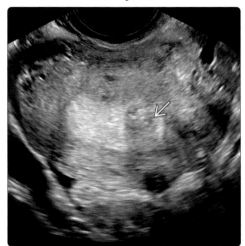

Leiomyoma

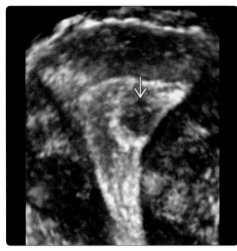

(Left) *Transverse transvaginal US of the uterus shows a hypoechoic, shadowing mass ➡ in the endometrium.* (Right) *Coronal 3D US in the same patient shows the hypoechoic mass ➡ projecting into the endometrium.*

Leiomyoma

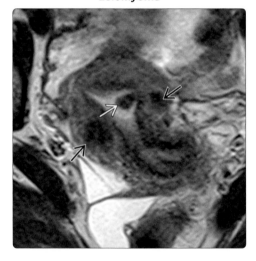

Leiomyoma

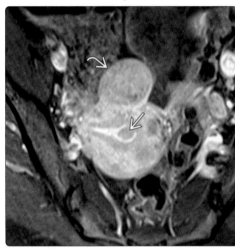

(Left) *Coronal oblique T2 MR in the same patient shows a pedunculated, circumscribed, hypoechoic mass ➡, consistent with submucosal leiomyoma. Note also the intramural leiomyomas ➡. MR is ideal for definitive diagnosis of leiomyomas.* (Right) *Axial T1 C+ FS MR in the same patient shows the pedunculated submucosal leiomyoma ➡. Despite its hypointensity relative to the surrounding endometrium, the leiomyoma is enhancing and is therefore viable. Note also the larger viable subserosal leiomyoma ➡ anteriorly.*

Pregnancy and Complications

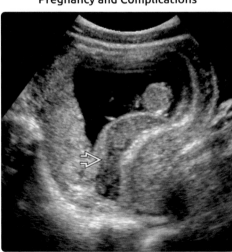

Pregnancy and Complications

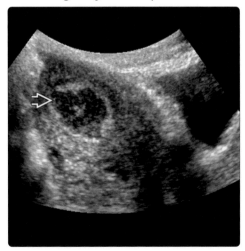

(Left) *Oblique US shows a marginal subchorionic hematoma ➡ in a patient 13 weeks pregnant with pain and bleeding.* (Right) *Longitudinal US shows a complex fluid collection ➡ in the endometrial cavity of a woman with an ectopic pregnancy. This finding is consistent with a pseudosac.*

Pregnancy and Complications

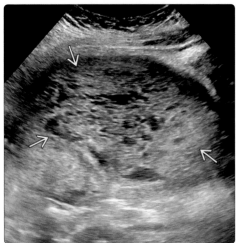

Endometrial Hyperplasia

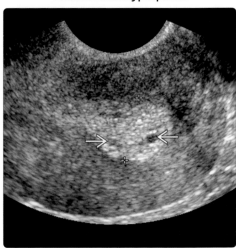

(Left) *Transverse US shows a typical complete hydatidiform mole with the uterus filled by a complex, hyperechoic mass with numerous small, cystic spaces ➡. (Right) Longitudinal transvaginal US in a patient with an ovarian granulosa cell tumor shows a thickened, heterogeneous endometrium measuring 15 mm (calipers) with multiple cysts ➡.*

Adenomyosis

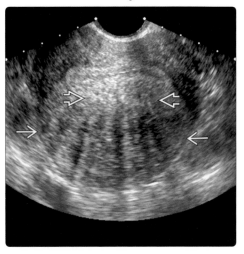

Adenomyosis

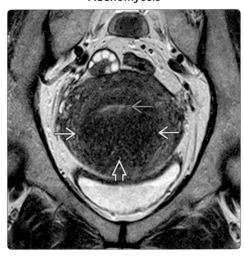

(Left) *Transverse transvaginal US of the uterus shows asymmetric thickening of the posterior uterine wall ➡ as well as echogenic and hypoechoic striations emanating from the ill-defined posterior endometrial-myometrial interface ➡. (Right) Coronal oblique T2 MR in the same patient shows thickening of junctional zone ➡ anteriorly with numerous punctate, hyperintense foci ➡. Cystic foci represent endometrial glands. Note the normal thickness of the endometrium ➡ and junctional zone posteriorly.*

C-Section Defect

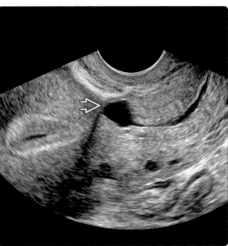

C-Section Defect

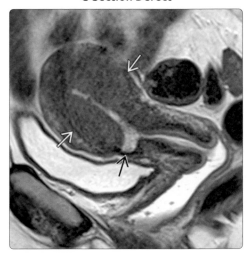

(Left) *Longitudinal transvaginal US shows focal myometrial thinning in the anterior lower uterine segment, consistent with C-section scar. There is a fluid collection ➡ in the scar. (Right) Sagittal T2 FSE FS MR in the same patient shows focal myometrial thinning in the anterior lower uterine segment at the site of prior C-section ➡. Blood products can collect in the defect, resulting in intermenstrual bleeding. Note also the diffuse thickening of the junctional zone ➡, consistent with diffuse adenomyosis.*

Endometrial Cancer

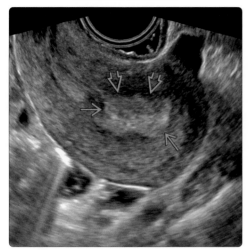

Endometrial Cancer

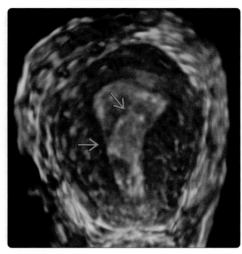

(Left) *Transvaginal US shows focal thickening and heterogeneity of the endometrial stripe ⇉ with irregular myometrial-endometrial interface ⇨.* (Right) *3D surface-rendered US of the uterus in the same patient confirms the focal mass on the left side of the endometrial cavity ⇨. Differential diagnosis for such a finding includes endometrial polyp, hyperplasia, and carcinoma. Biopsy was recommended and revealed endometrial carcinoma.*

Endometrial Cancer

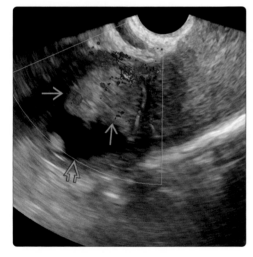

Endometrial Cancer

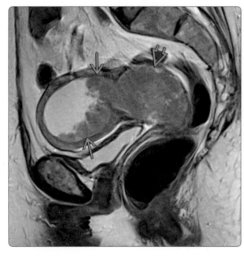

(Left) *Transvaginal US shows a polypoid, vascularized endometrial mass ⇉ and trapped intraluminal fluid ⇨. Evaluation of the cervix was difficult due to the inability to distinguish the cervical canal and mucosa.* (Right) *Axial T2 MR shows an eccentric, polypoid endometrial mass ⇨ with invasion of the cervical stroma ⇨. MR can be helpful for staging endometrial cancer due to the superior soft tissue contrast allowing visualization of tumor and its depth of invasion.*

Endometrial Cancer

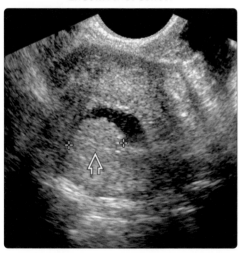

Cervical Cancer

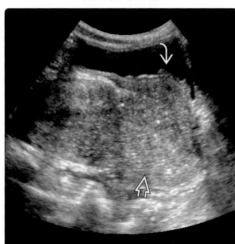

(Left) *Transverse transvaginal US shows fluid in the endometrial cavity with a focal, broad-based mass (calipers) in the posterior endometrium ⇨.* (Right) *Longitudinal US shows a large, irregular, hypoechoic mass in the region of the cervix ⇨. The mass invades the bladder ⇨.*

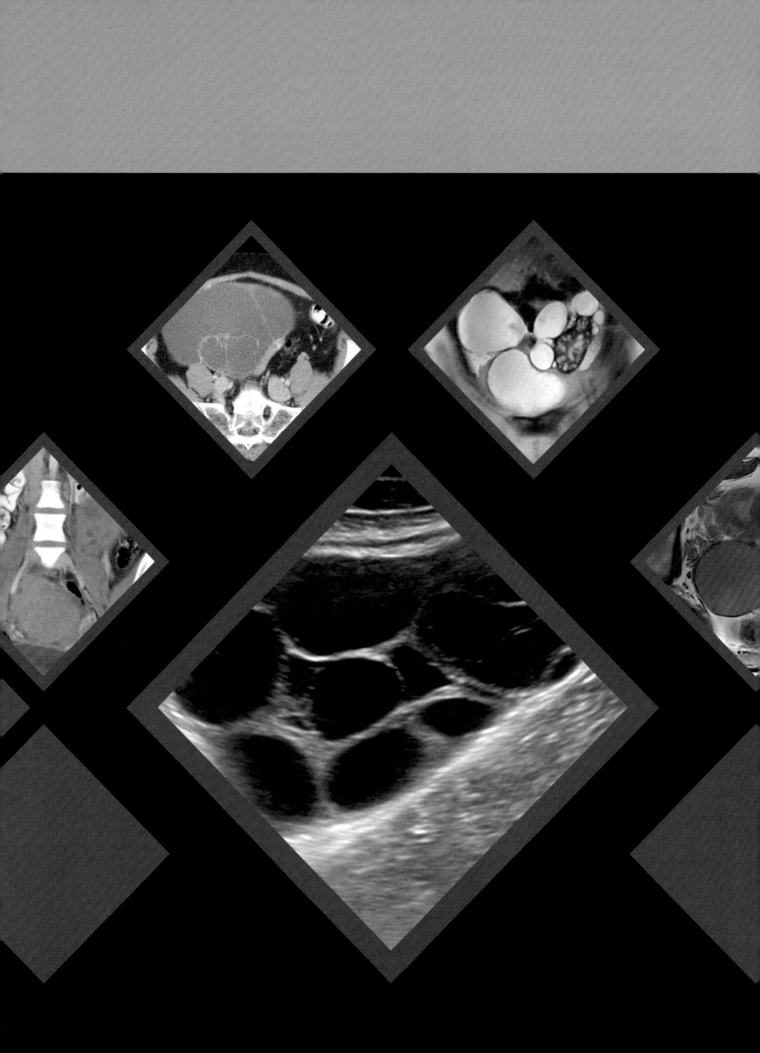

SECTION 24
Ovary

Generic Imaging Patterns

Multilocular Ovarian Cysts 676
Unilocular Ovarian Cysts 682
Solid Ovarian Masses 688
Calcified Ovarian Masses 692

Modality-Specific Imaging Findings

Magnetic Resonance Imaging

Ovarian Lesions With Low T2 Signal Intensity 696

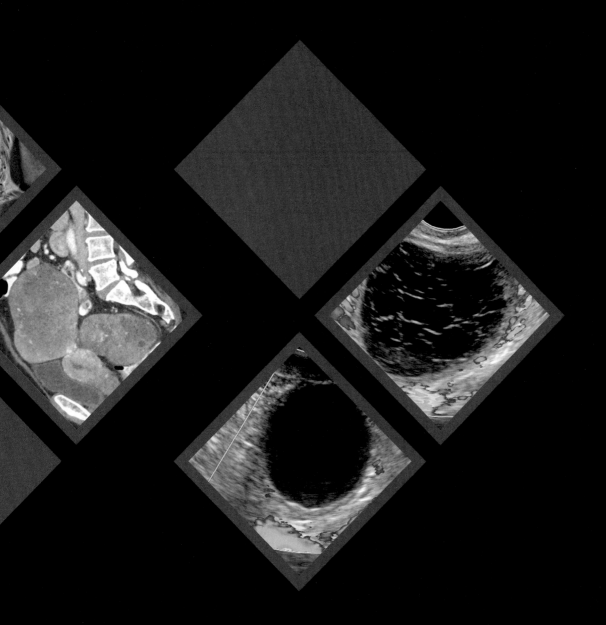

DIFFERENTIAL DIAGNOSIS

Common
- Mucinous Cystadenoma
- Serous Cystadenoma
- Polycystic Ovarian Syndrome
- Endometriomas
- Tuboovarian Abscess

Less Common
- Theca Lutein Cysts
- Cystadenofibroma
- Malignant Ovarian Epithelial Neoplasms
  - Serous Cystadenocarcinoma
  - Mucinous Cystadenocarcinoma
  - Endometrioid Carcinoma
  - Clear Cell Carcinoma
  - Transitional Cell Carcinoma
- Metastases

Rare but Important
- Brenner Tumor
- Struma Ovarii
- Ovarian Hyperstimulation Syndrome
- Granulosa Cell Tumor
- Yolk Sac Tumor

ESSENTIAL INFORMATION

Key Differential Diagnosis Issues
- Imaging pattern
  - Multilocular, cystic mass without solid component
    - Mucinous cystadenoma
    - Tuboovarian abscess
    - Borderline ovarian epithelial neoplasms
    - Serous cystadenoma
    - Granulosa cell tumor
  - Multilocular, cystic mass + solid component
    - Tuboovarian abscess
    - Serous cystadenoma
    - Mucinous cystadenoma
    - Cystadenofibroma
    - Brenner tumor
    - Malignant ovarian epithelial neoplasms
    - Struma ovarii
    - Yolk sac tumor
    - Granulosa cell tumor
  - Enlarged ovary with multiple cysts
    - Endometriomas
    - Polycystic ovarian syndrome
    - Ovarian hyperstimulation syndrome
    - Theca lutein cysts
- Ovarian cystic lesions associated with endometrial pathology
  - Endometrioid carcinoma
  - Granulosa cell tumor
  - Theca lutein cysts

Helpful Clues for Common Diagnoses
- **Mucinous Cystadenoma**
  - Almost always multilocular and may be quite large

- MR, CT, and ultrasound appearance of individual locules may vary as result of differences in degree of hemorrhage or protein content
    - Stained glass appearance on MR
- **Serous Cystadenoma**
  - Occasionally multilocular (more commonly unilocular)
  - Thin wall and thin septa
  - Usually anechoic on ultrasound, fluid attenuation on CT, and fluid signal intensity on MR
  - Occasionally contain small papillary projections
- **Polycystic Ovarian Syndrome**
  - Characterized clinically by menstrual irregularities, hirsutism, and obesity
  - Enlarged ovaries (volume > 10 cm³)
  - Numerous follicles 2-9 mm in size; criteria include
    - ≥ 25 follicles per ovary per 2013 Androgen Excess and PCOS Society Task Force
    - ≥ 20 follicles per ovary per 2018 ESHRE guidelines
  - Peripheral distribution of follicles → string of pearls appearance
- **Endometriomas**
  - Usually unilocular but presence of multiple endometriomas gives ovary multicystic appearance
  - Characteristic sonographic features include
    - Homogeneous low-level echoes
    - Echogenic mural foci
  - Characteristic MR features include
    - T2 shading
    - T2 dark spots
- **Tuboovarian Abscess**
  - Complex multilocular, cystic mass ± solid component
  - ± fluid-debris level
  - ± intracystic air
  - Surrounding inflammation, which may be seen as increased echogenicity of pelvic fat, or infiltration and enhancement of surrounding fat on CT and MR
  - Enhancement of wall and septa on CECT and MR
  - Thick-walled adnexal mass with low signal intensity contents on T1WI and high signal intensity on T2WI

Helpful Clues for Less Common Diagnoses
- **Theca Lutein Cysts**
  - Bilateral enlarged, multicystic ovaries, similar to ovarian hyperstimulation syndrome
  - Occurs in setting of gestational trophoblastic disease or multiple gestations
- **Cystadenofibroma**
  - Rims, plaques, or nodules of low signal intensity on T2WI
  - Locules show fluid characteristics on imaging in cases of serous cystadenofibroma
    - MR, CT, and ultrasound appearance of individual locules may vary as result of differences in degree of hemorrhage or protein content in cases of mucinous cystadenofibroma
- **Malignant Ovarian Epithelial Neoplasms**
  - Elevated CA 125
  - Mixed solid and cystic ovarian mass
  - Thick, irregular septa and large, vascular solid components
  - Invasion of surrounding structures

- Ascites, peritoneal caking, and nodal metastases in advanced disease
- **Metastases**
  - Commonly occur in setting of known gastrointestinal tract malignant tumor
  - Unilateral or bilateral
  - Mixed solid and cystic or solid with cystic areas due to necrosis

Helpful Clues for Rare Diagnoses

- **Brenner Tumor**
  - Solid component in multilocular, cystic mass may exhibit amorphous calcifications
  - Low signal intensity of solid component on T2WI
- **Struma Ovarii**
  - Multilocular, cystic mass with solid components (solid masses, thick wall, and septa)
  - Cyst fluid is anechoic or of low-level echogenicity on ultrasound
    - Cysts contain 1 or more vascularized, well-circumscribed, roundish echogenic structures with smooth contours (struma pearls)
  - Cystic spaces demonstrate high attenuation on CT
    - Due to presence of thyroglobulin
  - ± calcifications in solid component
  - Cystic spaces demonstrate locules of low intensity on T2WI and punctuate foci of high intensity on T1WI
  - May be associated with, or part of, mature cystic teratoma
    - Characteristic imaging features of mature cystic teratoma because of presence of fat
- **Ovarian Hyperstimulation Syndrome**
  - History of ovulation induction therapy
  - Massively enlarged ovaries, multicystic ovaries
  - Ascites as well as pleural or pericardial effusions in severe cases
  - Empty uterus
- **Granulosa Cell Tumor**
  - Multilocular ± solid component

- Cysts typically contain large numbers of small locules (> 10)
- Variable appearance of cyst content on imaging due to presence of hemorrhage
- Papillary projections may be found
- Most common estrogen-producing ovarian tumor
  - May be associated with endometrial hyperplasia, polyps, or carcinoma
- **Yolk Sac Tumor**
  - Elevated level of α-fetoprotein in young patient with pelvic mass
  - Mixed solid and cystic mass with hemorrhagic portion
  - Bright dot sign is common finding seen at contrast-enhanced CT and MR imaging as enhancing foci in wall or solid components
    - Due to dilated vessels in these highly vascular tumors
  - Capsular tears may be observed on imaging

SELECTED REFERENCES

1. Elsherif SB et al: Current update on malignant epithelial ovarian tumors. Abdom Radiol (NY). 46(6):2264-80, 2021
2. Marko J et al: Mucinous neoplasms of the ovary: radiologic-pathologic correlation. Radiographics. 39(4):982-97, 2019
3. Choi JI et al: Imaging features of complex solid and multicystic ovarian lesions: proposed algorithm for differential diagnosis. Clin Imaging. 40(1):46-56, 2016
4. Shaaban AM et al: Ovarian malignant germ cell tumors: cellular classification and clinical and imaging features. Radiographics. 34(3):777-801, 2014
5. Lujan ME et al: Updated ultrasound criteria for polycystic ovary syndrome: reliable thresholds for elevated follicle population and ovarian volume. Hum Reprod. 28(5):1361-8, 2013
6. Van Holsbeke C et al: Imaging of gynecological disease (3): clinical and ultrasound characteristics of granulosa cell tumors of the ovary. Ultrasound Obstet Gynecol. 31(4):450-6, 2008
7. Jung SE et al: CT and MR imaging of ovarian tumors with emphasis on differential diagnosis. Radiographics. 22(6):1305-25, 2002

Mucinous Cystadenoma

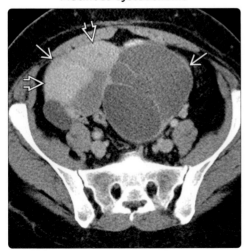

Serous Cystadenoma

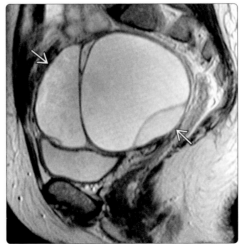

(Left) *Axial CECT shows bilateral, multilocular, cystic ovarian masses* ➡. *Some of the locules within the right ovarian lesion contain high-attenuation material* ➡ *due to hemorrhage or high protein content.* (Right) *Sagittal T2 MR shows a large, multilocular, cystic ovarian mass* ➡. *The lesion is composed of multiple locules separated by thin, smooth septa.*

Polycystic Ovarian Syndrome

Polycystic Ovarian Syndrome

(Left) *Transvaginal US shows an enlarged ovary* ➡️ *composed of numerous discrete, uniform, small ovarian cysts. Note the peripheral location of follicles, which results in a string of pearls appearance.* **(Right)** *Axial T2 MR shows enlarged ovaries* ➡️ *with numerous discrete, small ovarian cysts. Note the peripheral location of follicles, resulting in a string of pearls appearance.*

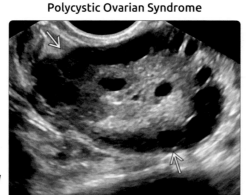

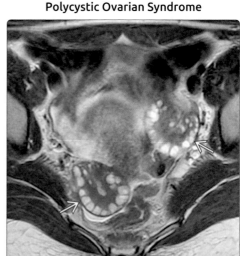

Endometriomas

Endometriomas

(Left) *Axial T2 MR shows bilateral, enlarged ovaries* ➡️*, each containing multiple discrete high-signal lesions. Some of the lesions show T2 shading* ➡️*. A left ovarian lesion shows a T2-dark spot* ➡️*.* **(Right)** *Axial T1 FS MR shows bilateral ovarian enlargement* ➡️*. Both ovaries contain multiple lesions displaying high signal intensity.*

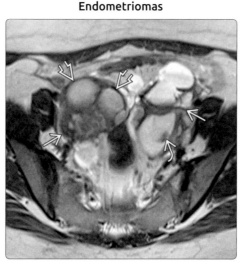

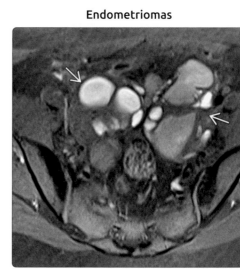

Tuboovarian Abscess

Tuboovarian Abscess

(Left) *Axial T2 MR shows a right ovarian mass* ➡️ *composed of multiple cystic loculi* ➡️ *and a thick rind of high signal intensity.* **(Right)** *Coronal T2 MR in the same patient shows a right ovarian mass* ➡️ *composed of multiple cystic loculi. Note the difference in signal intensity within various loculi.*

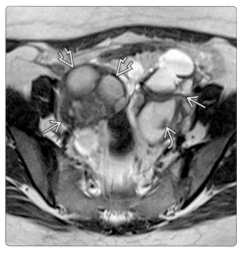

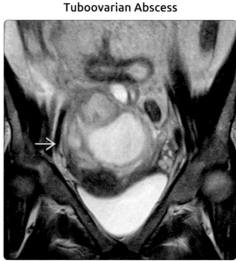

Multilocular Ovarian Cysts

Tuboovarian Abscess

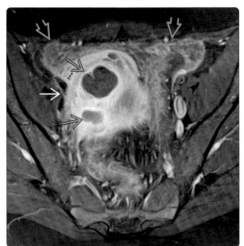

Tuboovarian Abscess

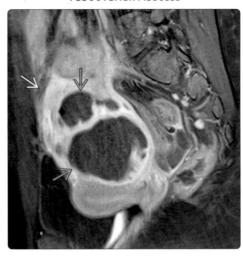

(Left) *Axial T1 C+ FS MR shows a right ovarian mass* ➡ *composed of multiple cystic loculi* ⬦ *and a thick, enhancing rind. Note enhancement of the pelvic fat* ⬦*.* (Right) *Sagittal T1 C+ FS MR shows a right ovarian mass* ➡ *composed of multiple cystic loculi* ⬦ *and a thick, enhancing rind. Individual loculi tend to be irregular in shape with irregular contour.*

Theca Lutein Cysts

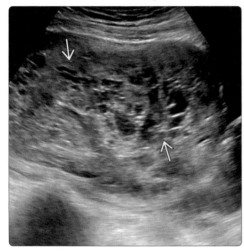

Theca Lutein Cysts

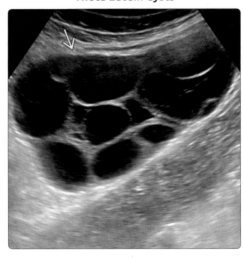

(Left) *Axial US in a patient with a high level of hCG shows a heterogeneous mass* ➡ *filling the uterine cavity due to hydatidiform mole.* (Right) *Transvaginal US in the same patient shows an enlarged ovary* ➡ *composed of numerous discrete cysts. The other ovary was similarly enlarged.*

Cystadenofibroma

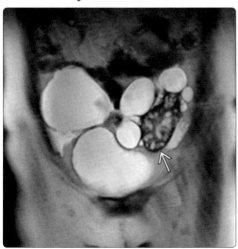

Malignant Ovarian Epithelial Neoplasms

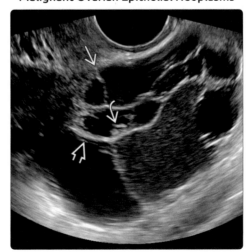

(Left) *Coronal T2 MR shows an enlarged left ovary* ➡ *with numerous intraovarian and exophytic cysts. Note the diffuse low signal intensity of the ovarian parenchyma in between the small parenchymal cysts.* (Right) *Transvaginal US shows a multilocular cystic mass* ➡ *composed of multiple locules displaying variable echogenicity. The septa are thick and irregular* ➡ *and show small papillary projections* ⤴*.*

(Left) *Axial T2 MR shows a multilocular cystic mass* ➡️ *with a peripheral solid component* ⮕. **(Right)** *Axial T1 C+ FS MR in the same patient shows a multilocular cystic mass* ➡️ *with an enhancing solid component* ⮕ *and a thick, enhancing wall* ⮕. *Pathologic examination revealed serous cystadenocarcinoma.*

Malignant Ovarian Epithelial Neoplasms

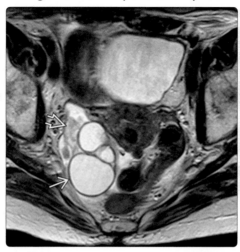

Malignant Ovarian Epithelial Neoplasms

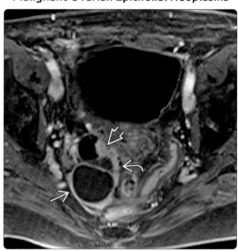

(Left) *Axial CECT shows a multilocular cystic mass* ➡️. *Pathologic examination revealed mucinous cystadenocarcinoma.* **(Right)** *Coronal CECT in a patient with history of colonic carcinoma shows bilateral enlarged, cystic ovaries* ➡️ *and a right lobe liver mass* ⮕ *due to metastatic disease.*

Malignant Ovarian Epithelial Neoplasms

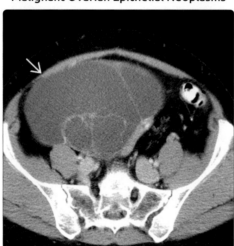

Metastases

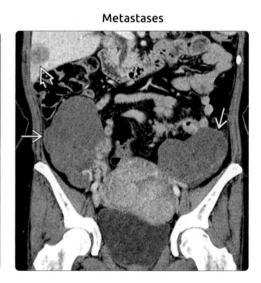

(Left) *Transvaginal US shows a multilocular cystic mass* ➡️ *containing multiple rounded, echogenic structures (strumal pearls)* ⮕. **(Right)** *Axial CECT shows a large pelvic mass* ➡️ *composed of large loculi separated by thin, enhancing septa. There is an intensely enhancing solid component* ⮕ *in the center of the mass.*

Struma Ovarii

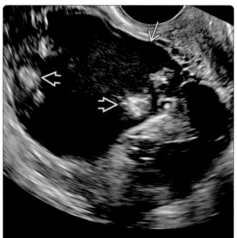

Struma Ovarii

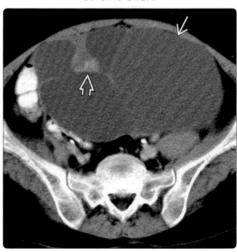

Struma Ovarii

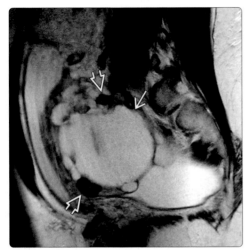

Ovarian Hyperstimulation Syndrome

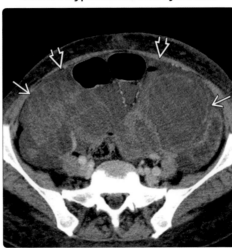

(Left) *Sagittal T2 MR shows a multilocular cystic mass ➡ composed of numerous locules filling the pelvic cavity. Note that some locules ⇒ demonstrate very low signal intensity, a characteristic feature of struma ovarii.* **(Right)** *Axial CECT in a patient receiving ovarian induction therapy for in vitro fertilization shows bilateral, enlarged, multicystic ovaries ➡ and small-volume ascites ⇒. Note also diffuse subcutaneous edema resulting from increased capillary permeability.*

Granulosa Cell Tumor

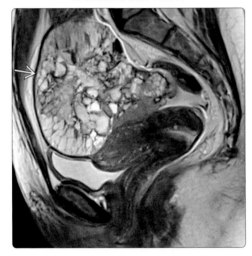

Granulosa Cell Tumor

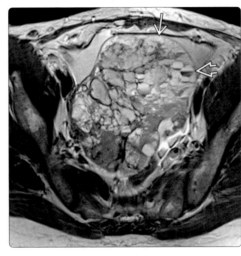

(Left) *Sagittal T2 MR shows a large, multilocular cystic mass ➡ composed of numerous small, cystic spaces.* **(Right)** *Axial T2 MR shows a large, multilocular cystic mass ➡ composed of numerous small cystic spaces. Some of the locules show fluid level ⇒ due to intracystic hemorrhage.*

Granulosa Cell Tumor

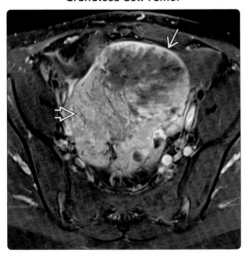

Yolk Sac Tumor

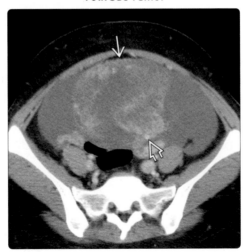

(Left) *Axial T1 C+ FS MR shows a large, multilocular cystic mass ➡ composed of numerous small cystic spaces, and enhancing solid component ⇒.* **(Right)** *Axial CECT shows a mixed solid and multilocular cystic mass ➡. The bright dot sign ⇒ represents aneurysmally dilated vascular structures and is commonly seen in yolk sac tumors due to its high vascularity.*

DIFFERENTIAL DIAGNOSIS

Common

- Physiologic Follicles
- Corpus Luteum
- Hemorrhagic Cyst
- Mature Cystic Teratoma
- Endometrioma
- Postmenopausal Cyst

Less Common

- Tuboovarian Abscess
- Serous Cystadenoma
- Mucinous Cystadenoma
- Serous Cystadenocarcinoma
- Mucinous Cystadenocarcinoma
- Cystadenofibroma

Rare but Important

- Granulosa Cell Tumor

ESSENTIAL INFORMATION

Key Differential Diagnosis Issues

- Complexity
  - Unilocular cyst: Cyst without septa and solid component
    - Simple cyst (round or oval with smooth, thin walls, no solid component or septation); anechoic with posterior acoustic enhancement on US, no internal flow at color Doppler US, fluid attenuation at CT, and homogeneous fluid signal intensity on MR
      - Physiologic follicles
      - Cystadenomas (serous and mucinous)
      - Cystadenofibroma
    - Complex cysts: Cyst containing any kind of nonviable components
      - Corpus luteum
      - Endometrioma
      - Hemorrhagic cyst
      - Dermoid cyst
      - Tuboovarian abscess
  - Unilocular solid cyst: Unilocular cyst with solid component
    - Dermoid cyst
    - Endometrioma
    - Cystadenoma (serous and mucinous)
    - Cystadenocarcinoma (serous and mucinous)
    - Cystadenofibroma
    - Granulosa cell tumor

Helpful Clues for Common Diagnoses

- **Physiologic Follicles**
  - Premenopausal woman
  - Thin-walled, round to oval, avascular simple cyst
    - May reach diameter up to 3 cm
    - When ovulation fails to occur → follicle continues to enlarge → follicular cyst
      - Remains simple in appearance
  - Curvilinear septation may be seen within dominant preovulatory follicle

- Represents oocyte and its supporting structures (i.e., cumulus oöphorus)

- **Corpus Luteum**
  - Postovulatory corpus luteum measures up to 3 cm
  - Thick-walled cyst with crenulated margin
  - Cyst can be collapsed and lack fluid, giving it relatively solid appearance
  - Doppler US demonstrates prominent peripheral blood flow with low-resistance waveform
  - CT/MR: Irregular, collapsed cyst with peripheral enhancement

- **Hemorrhagic Cyst**
  - Resolve on follow-up examinations
  - US: Different patterns may be seen
    - Echogenic, avascular, homogeneous, or heterogeneous nonshadowing in early stage
    - Retracted clot
      - Avascular mass-like structure within anechoic cyst with characteristic concave contour
      - May jiggle with transducer ballottement
    - Reticular, lacy, fishnet, or spongy pattern
  - MR
    - Usually single unilocular cyst
    - High signal intensity on T1 MR
      - Signal intensity remains high on T1 FS MR
    - Hyperintense or hypointense on T2 MR
    - No T2-dark spots

- **Mature Cystic Teratoma**
  - US
    - Focal, highly echogenic nodules
    - Heterogeneous internal echoes ± acoustic shadows
    - Multiple hyperechoic fine lines and dots
    - Atypical features include fluid-fluid level, anechoic cyst, and multiple floating globules
  - CT and MR
    - Presence of fat is characteristic
      - Fat attenuation on CT
      - High signal intensity on T1 and low signal intensity on T1 FS MR

- **Endometrioma**
  - US
    - Well-defined, smooth-walled cyst(s)
    - Contains homogeneous low-level echoes → characteristic ground-glass appearance
    - Small echogenic mural foci
    - Mural nodules (15%): Usually avascular (likely due to adherent mural clot or fibrin)
    - ± flow due to presence of endometrial tissue
  - MR
    - Single or multiple
    - High signal intensity on T1, remains high on T1 FS MR
      - To differentiate from fat-containing dermoid cyst
    - T2 shading (signal loss on T2 in cyst that appears hyperintense on T1 MR)
    - T2-dark spots (hypointense foci within cyst on T2 MR)

- **Postmenopausal Cyst**
  - Simple cyst in postmenopausal woman
  - Hemorrhagic cyst should not occur in late menopause
  - Normal CA 125

Helpful Clues for Less Common Diagnoses

- **Tuboovarian Abscess**
  - Occasionally presents as unilocular cystic mass ± irregular wall and mural vascularity
- **Serous and Mucinous Cystadenoma**
  - Simple cyst with thin wall
  - Persistent on follow-up examinations
  - Features suggestive of benignity include
    - Entirely cystic with diameter < 4 cm
      - □ ± small papillary projections
    - Thin wall < 3 mm
    - Lack of internal structure
    - Absence of both ascites and invasive features, such as peritoneal disease or adenopathy
- **Serous and Mucinous Cystadenocarcinoma**
  - Elevated CA 125
  - Features suggestive of malignancy include
    - Thick, irregular wall, thick septa, papillary projections, and large soft tissue component with necrosis
- **Cystadenofibroma**
  - Simple cyst with smooth wall of low T2 signal intensity
  - Wall is thicker than in simple functional cyst
  - May contain solid component with shadowing on US
  - Most demonstrate no or minimal color Doppler signals

Helpful Clues for Rare Diagnoses

- **Granulosa Cell Tumor**
  - Rare presentation
  - Hyperestrogenemia → endometrial pathology
  - Unilocular cyst with thick solid rind

SELECTED REFERENCES

1. Wang PS et al: Benign-appearing incidental adnexal cysts at US, CT, and MRI: putting the ACR, O-RADS, and SRU guidelines all together. Radiographics. 42(2):609-24, 2022
2. Taylor EC et al: Multimodality imaging approach to ovarian neoplasms with pathologic correlation. Radiographics. 41(1):289-315, 2021
3. Marko J et al: Mucinous neoplasms of the ovary: radiologic-pathologic correlation. Radiographics. 39(4):982-97, 2019
4. Jung SI: Ultrasonography of ovarian masses using a pattern recognition approach. Ultrasonography. 34(3):173-82, 2015

Physiologic Follicles

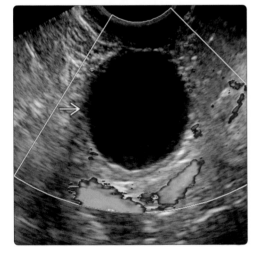

Physiologic Follicles

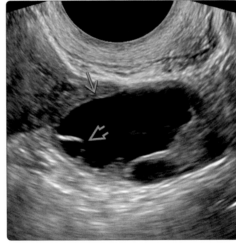

(**Left**) *Transvaginal color Doppler US in a 23-year-old woman shows a single, unilocular simple cyst measuring 28 mm ➡. The finding of such a cyst in a premenopausal woman woman does not require follow-up.* (**Right**) *Transvaginal US in a 28-year-old woman shows a single unilocular ➡ cyst measuring 25 mm. There is a curvilinear peripheral septation ➡, which indicates that the ovum is surrounded by a cumulus oöphorus within the mature follicle.*

Corpus Luteum

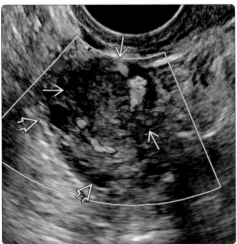

Hemorrhagic Cyst

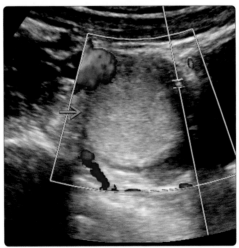

(**Left**) *Transvaginal color Doppler US shows an isoechoic ovarian lesion ➡ with peripheral vascularity surrounded by normal ovarian tissue ➡.* (**Right**) *Transabdominal US shows a hyperechoic avascular ovarian lesion ➡. Differential diagnosis includes an acute hemorrhagic cyst vs. dermoid cyst. This lesion resolved on follow-up imaging, confirming the diagnosis of a hemorrhagic cyst.*

Hemorrhagic Cyst

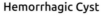

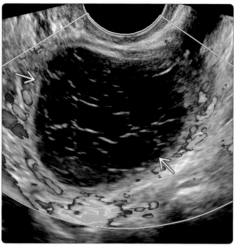

Mature Cystic Teratoma

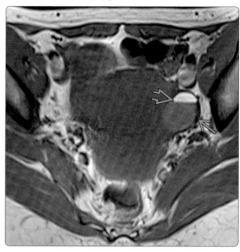

(Left) *Transvaginal color Doppler US shows a hypoechoic ovarian lesion* ➡ *with irregular internal avascular septa, giving the lesion a lacy or fishnet appearance.* **(Right)** *Axial T1 MR in the same patient shows a left ovarian lesion* ➡. *The lesion displays a fluid level* ➡. *The floating part has high signal intensity, similar to that of subcutaneous fat, while the dependent part has low signal intensity similar to that of simple fluid.*

Mature Cystic Teratoma

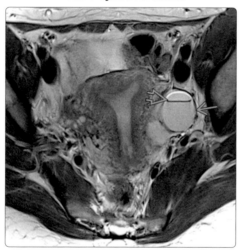

Mature Cystic Teratoma

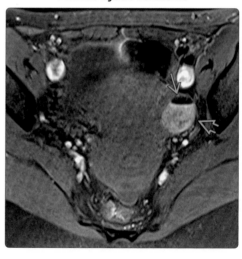

(Left) *Axial T2 MR in the same patient shows a left ovarian lesion* ➡. *The lesion displays high signal intensity with a fluid level* ➡. *The floating part has slightly higher signal intensity than the dependent part.* **(Right)** *Axial T1 FS MR in the same patient shows a left ovarian mass* ➡ *with suppression of the high signal intensity of the floating part* ➡ *(due to its fatty nature).*

Endometrioma

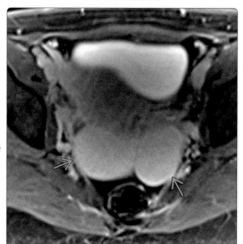

Endometrioma

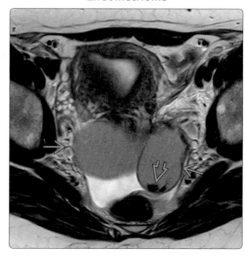

(Left) *Axial T1 C+ FS MR in the same patient shows bilateral ovarian endometriomas* ➡ *displaying high signal intensity without enhancement.* **(Right)** *Axial T2 MR in the same patient shows bilateral ovarian endometriomas* ➡ *displaying T2 shading (signal loss on T2 in a cyst that appears hyperintense on T1). Note also the T2-dark spots* ➡ *(hypointense foci within cyst).*

Endometrioma

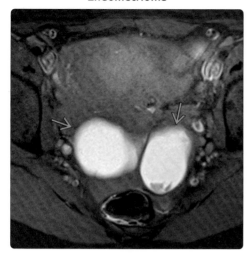

Endometrioma

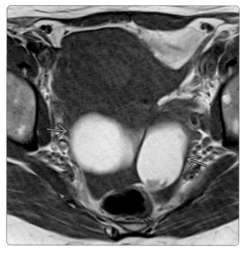

(Left) Axial T1 FS MR in the same patient shows bilateral ovarian endometriomas ➡ with high signal intensity. Persistent high signal intensity on T1 FS MR differentiates endometriomas, and hemorrhagic cysts, from dermoid cysts, which lose signal on this sequence. (Right) Axial T1 MR shows bilateral ovarian endometriomas ➡ with high signal intensity.

Endometrioma

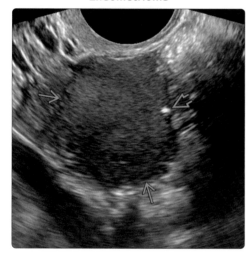

Endometrioma

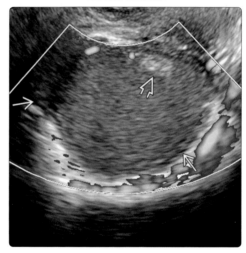

(Left) Transvaginal US shows a hypoechoic ovarian lesion ➡ with uniform low-level echoes and a mural echogenic focus ➡, a characteristic feature of endometriomas. (Right) Transvaginal color Doppler US shows an endometrioma ➡ with an avascular echogenic mural nodule ➡. The presence of a mural nodule does not necessarily mean malignant transformation, as nodules may develop as a result of retracted clot or nonmalignant changes of the endometrial tissue.

Postmenopausal Cyst

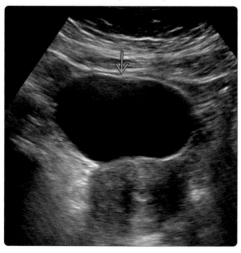

Tuboovarian Abscess

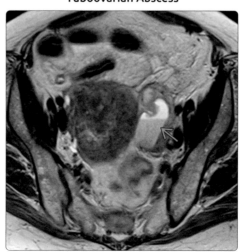

(Left) Transvaginal US in a 58-year-old woman shows a simple-appearing ovarian cyst ➡. CA 125 was normal, and the cyst has been stable for 3 years. (Right) Axial T2 MR shows a left ovarian lesion ➡ with fluid-fluid level. The dependent portion has lower signal intensity than simple fluid.

Tuboovarian Abscess

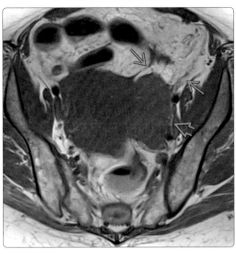

Tuboovarian Abscess

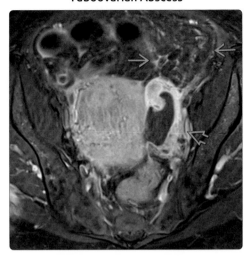

(Left) *Axial T1 MR in the same patient shows enlargement of the left ovary ➡. There is stranding of the fat surrounding the pelvis and left ovary ➡.* **(Right)** *Axial T1 C+ FS MR in the same patient shows a left ovarian lesion ➡ with an enhancing rind surrounding a unilocular, low-signal center. Note stranding of the pelvic fat ➡.*

Tuboovarian Abscess

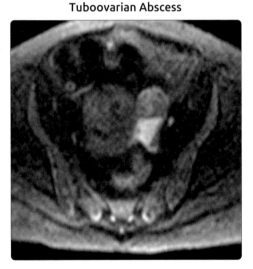

Serous Cystadenoma

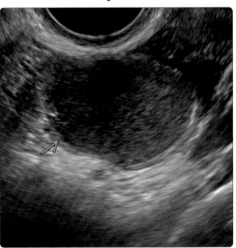

(Left) *Axial DWI MR in the same patient shows high signal intensity of the content of the lesion due to diffusion restriction.* **(Right)** *Transvaginal US shows a unilocular cyst ➡ containing homogeneous, low-level echoes, initially thought to represent an endometrioma.*

Serous Cystadenoma

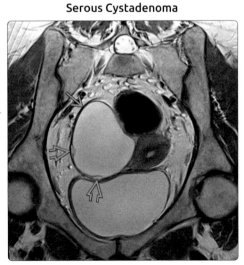

Serous Cystadenoma

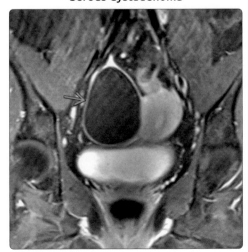

(Left) *Coronal T2 MR shows a right ovarian simple cystic lesion ➡ measuring 7 cm with homogeneous high signal. Ovarian follicles ➡ are seen stretched around the cyst.* **(Right)** *Coronal T1 C+ FS MR in the same patient shows a right ovarian low-signal lesion ➡ with a uniformly thin, enhancing wall. Pathologic examination revealed an ovarian serous cystadenoma.*

Mucinous Cystadenoma

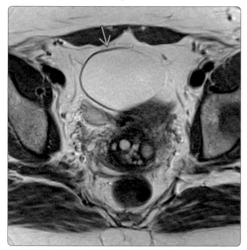

Mucinous Cystadenoma

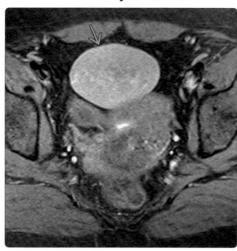

(Left) *Axial T2 MR shows a simple-appearing, unilocular ovarian lesion ⮕ with high signal intensity.* (Right) *Axial T1 FS MR in the same patient shows a unilocular ovarian lesion ⮕ with high signal intensity. Mucinous cystadenomas may show locules of high T1 signal due to mucin contents.*

Serous Cystadenocarcinoma

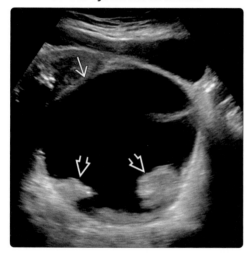

Cystadenofibroma

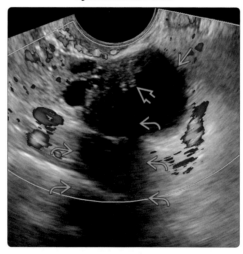

(Left) *Transabdominal US shows a unilocular cyst ⮕ with mural nodules ⮕. Pathologic examination revealed serous cystadenocarcinoma.* (Right) *Transvaginal US shows a unilocular ovarian cyst ⮕ containing an avascular solid component ⮕. There is significant shadowing ⮕ arising from the solid component, a characteristic feature of cystadenofibromas.*

Cystadenofibroma

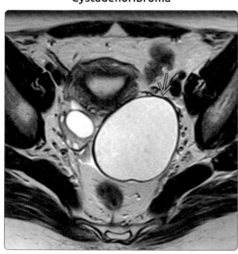

Granulosa Cell Tumor

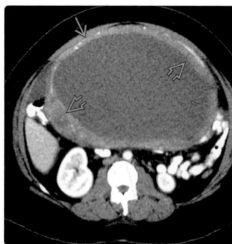

(Left) *Axial T2 MR shows a left ovarian cyst ⮕ with a smooth, fine low-signal wall.* (Right) *Axial CECT shows a large, predominantly unilocular cystic mass ⮕ with a thick rind of soft tissue attenuation ⮕. Pathologic evaluation revealed granulosa cell tumor.*

DIFFERENTIAL DIAGNOSIS

Common

- Malignant Epithelial Tumors
- Metastases
- Fibroma/Fibrothecoma/Thecoma
- Torsion and Massive Ovarian Edema

Less Common

- Brenner Tumor
- Granulosa Cell Tumor

Rare but Important

- Germ Cell Tumors
  - Dysgerminoma
  - Immature Teratoma
  - Yolk Sac Tumor
  - Choriocarcinoma
  - Carcinoid
- Sertoli-Leydig Cell Tumors
- Lymphoma
- Leukemia
- Hyperthecosis
- Fibromatosis
- Sarcoma
  - Chondrosarcomas
  - Fibrosarcomas
  - Endometrial Stromal Sarcomas
  - Angiosarcomas
  - Rhabdomyosarcomas
  - Leiomyosarcomas

ESSENTIAL INFORMATION

Key Differential Diagnosis Issues

- Hormone and tumor marker-producing tumors
  - Granulosa cell tumors → hyperestrogenism
  - Thecoma/fibrothecoma → hyperestrogenism
  - Carcinoid → carcinoid syndrome
  - Choriocarcinoma → β-hCG
  - Yolk sac tumor → α-fetoprotein
  - Sertoli-Leydig cell tumors → hyperandrogenism
  - Dysgerminoma → β-hCG (only 5% of cases)
  - Hyperthecosis → hyperandrogenism
- Calcifications
  - Malignant epithelial tumors
  - Brenner tumor
  - Dysgerminoma (speckled pattern)
  - Immature teratoma
- Low signal on T2 MR
  - Brenner tumor
  - Fibroma
  - Fibromatosis
  - Adenofibroma
- Bilateral
  - Malignant epithelial tumors
  - Metastases
  - Lymphoma
  - Dysgerminoma (6.5-10.0% of cases)
  - Hyperthecosis

- Preservation of normal follicles
  - Torsion and massive ovarian edema
  - Fibromatosis
  - Lymphoma
  - Leukemia (granulocytic sarcoma)

Helpful Clues for Common Diagnoses

- **Malignant Epithelial Tumors**
  - ↑ serum CA 125 level
  - Extensive peritoneal carcinomatosis ± calcifications
  - Tumor invasion of pelvic organs
  - Pelvic and retroperitoneal adenopathy
- **Metastases**
  - Term Krukenberg tumor is loosely used to describe any kind of ovarian metastases from any primary site
    - Should be reserved to metastases characterized histologically by signet-ring cell mucinous features
  - Bilateral in 60-80% of patients
  - Well-demarcated, intratumoral, cystic component is often identified
  - MR
    - Solid components appear to be T1 and T2 hypointense because of dense stromal reaction
    - Demonstrates diffusion restriction and enhancement on contrast-enhanced sequences
- **Fibroma/Fibrothecoma/Thecoma**
  - Fibrothecomas may manifest with hyperestrogenism
    - Endometrial polyps, hyperplasia, or carcinoma
  - US
    - Round, oval, or slightly lobulated tumors
    - Most are hypoechoic and solid with homogeneous internal echogenicity
    - Dramatic sound attenuation resulting in posterior acoustic shadowing, similar to uterine fibroids
    - Minimal to moderate vascularization on color Doppler
  - CT
    - Soft tissue attenuation ± calcifications
  - MR
    - Hypo- to isointense to pelvic muscles on T1 and low signal intensity on T2, similar to uterine fibroids
    - T1 C+: Mild enhancement
- **Torsion and Massive Ovarian Edema**
  - Diffuse ovarian enlargement with preserved shape
  - Edematous ovarian stroma with peripheral follicles
  - Variable vascular flow on Doppler studies
  - No or minimal enhancement with contrast-enhanced studies
  - Whirlpool sign: Twisted vascular pedicle
    - Highly sensitive (87%) and specific (88%)
  - Pelvic free fluid (nonspecific)
  - Displacement of adnexal structures/uterus

Helpful Clues for Less Common Diagnoses

- **Brenner Tumor**
  - US
    - Hypoechoic with posterior shadowing due to presence of calcifications
    - Minimal flow on color Doppler imaging
  - CT
    - Soft tissue attenuation ± calcifications (83% of cases)
  - MR

- Very low T2 signal intensity and low T1 signal intensity due to presence of fibrous elements
- At least moderate enhancement after contrast material administration

- **Granulosa Cell Tumor**
  - Hyperestrinism is common → endometrial hyperplasia, polyps, or carcinoma
  - US
    - Solid or mixed tumors with homogeneous or heterogeneous echogenicity
      - □ Heterogeneity results from intratumoral bleeding, infarcts, and fibrous degeneration
      - □ Swiss cheese pattern: Multiple small cysts in solid mass
    - ↑ vascularity is demonstrated on Doppler
  - CT and MR
    - Solid granulosa cell tumor has no specific features to suggest diagnosis

Helpful Clues for Rare Diagnoses

- **Dysgerminoma**
  - Most cases occur in adolescence and early adulthood
  - Tumor divided into component lobules by vascularized enhancing septa
    - Septa are usually hypo- or isointense on T2 and are difficult to appreciate on T1
- **Immature Teratoma**
  - Peak incidence 15-19 years of age; rarely seen in menopause
  - Predominantly solid mass with interspersed small foci of fatty elements, coarse irregular calcifications, and numerous cysts of variable sizes
- **Yolk Sac Tumor**
  - Most common in 2nd and 3rd decades; rare in women > 40 years old
  - Bright dot sign
    - Enhancing foci in wall or solid components attributed to dilated vessels
  - Capsular tears
  - Very rapid rate of growth

- **Choriocarcinoma**
  - ↑ β-hCG level
    - Presence of adnexal mass with ↑ β-hCG level → erroneous diagnosis of ectopic pregnancy
  - Solid or mixed solid and cystic adnexal mass
  - Strong enhancement of solid component
- **Carcinoid**
  - May be associated with carcinoid syndrome
    - Even in absence of metastases as ovarian veins drain directly into systemic circulation
- **Sertoli-Leydig Cell Tumors**
  - Hyperandrogenism
  - Small (almost always < 3 cm), unilateral, solid nodule
  - Hemorrhage, necrosis, and large size are suggestive of malignancy
  - Variable intensity on T2
  - Intense enhancement with contrast
- **Lymphoma**
  - Solid, homogeneous, large ovarian mass or bilateral ovarian involvement is seen in absence of ascites
  - Usually maintains normal ovarian structure and shows no invasion of surrounding structures
- **Hyperthecosis**
  - Hyperandrogenism
  - Bilateral symmetric ovarian enlargement
  - Mostly postmenopausal women
  - Homogeneous low echogenicity on ultrasound and low signal intensity on T2 with few, if any, follicles
- **Fibromatosis**
  - Marked T2-hypointense, thick rim of fibrous tissue surrounding ovary, referred to as black garland sign
  - Relative sparing of central ovarian parenchyma
  - Minimal or no enhancement in parenchymal phase following contrast administration

SELECTED REFERENCES

1. Cacioppa LM et al: Magnetic resonance imaging of pure ovarian dysgerminoma: a series of eight cases. Cancer Imaging. 21(1):58, 2021
2. Shaaban AM et al: Ovarian malignant germ cell tumors: cellular classification and clinical and imaging features. Radiographics. 34(3):777-801, 2014

Malignant Epithelial Tumors

Metastases

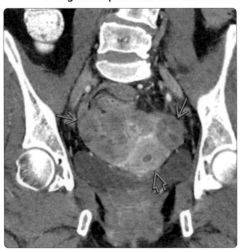

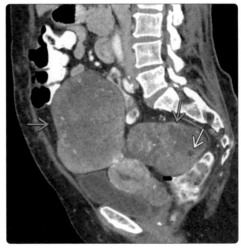

(Left) *Coronal CECT shows bilateral, predominantly solid masses* ⇨ *abutting the uterus* ⇨. *Both masses are solid with small, cystic areas.* **(Right)** *Sagittal CECT shows bilateral, solid ovarian masses* ⇨. *Well-demarcated cystic areas may be seen within the solid tumors* ⇨. *When bilateral, solid ovarian masses are found on imaging, the stomach, colon, appendix, pancreas, and biliary tract should be scrutinized for a mass as the source of primary tumor.*

Fibroma/Fibrothecoma/Thecoma

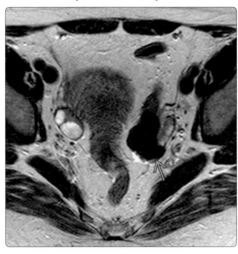

Fibroma/Fibrothecoma/Thecoma

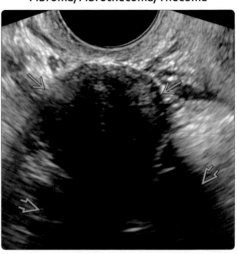

(Left) *Axial T2 MR shows a well-defined left ovarian mass ➡. The mass has homogeneous low signal intensity relative to pelvic muscles.* **(Right)** *Transvaginal US shows an ovarian mass ➡ with low echogenicity and dramatic sound attenuation, resulting in posterior acoustic shadowing ➡.*

Torsion and Massive Ovarian Edema

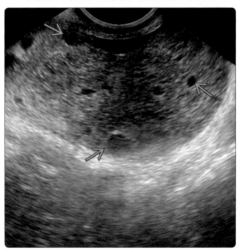

Torsion and Massive Ovarian Edema

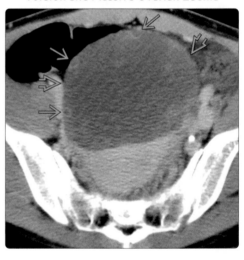

(Left) *Transvaginal US shows an enlarged ovary with heterogeneous echogenicity and scattered multiple follicles ➡.* **(Right)** *Axial CECT in a 23-year-old woman presenting with acute pelvic pain shows an enlarged left ovary ➡ with multiple preserved ovarian follicles ➡ that are predominantly at the periphery of the enlarged ovary.*

Brenner Tumor

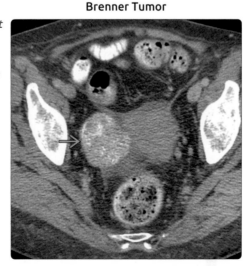

Granulosa Cell Tumor

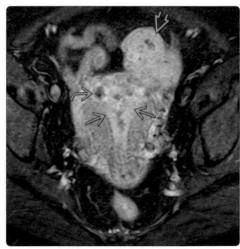

(Left) *Axial CECT shows a right ovarian mass ➡ with diffuse, amorphous calcifications.* **(Right)** *Axial T1 C+ FS MR shows an enhancing, solid left ovarian mass ➡ in a 45-year-old woman with vaginal bleeding. Note the thickened, enhancing endometrium ➡ with cystic changes ➡. Endometrial biopsy revealed endometrial hyperplasia.*

Dysgerminoma

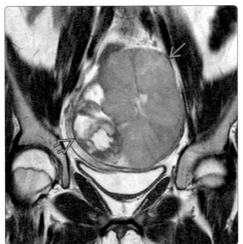

Immature Teratoma

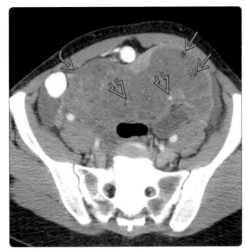

(Left) *Coronal T2 MR shows a multilobulated right ovarian mass ➡ that is hyperintense relative to muscle with hypointense septa separating it into multiple lobules. An associated mature cystic teratoma ➡ is also present.* (Right) *Axial CECT shows a large pelvic mass ➡ with heterogeneous attenuation with small foci of fat ➡ and calcifications ➡.*

Yolk Sac Tumor

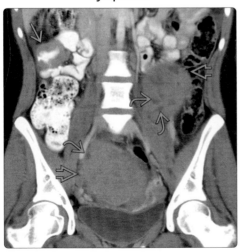

Sertoli-Leydig Cell Tumors

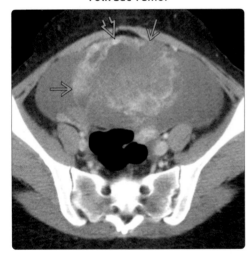

(Left) *Axial CECT shows a large abdominal mixed solid and cystic mass ➡ with small foci of enhancement ➡, a finding known as the bright dot sign, which indicates increased tumor vascularity.* (Right) *Axial T2 MR in a 17-year-old girl with virilism shows a right ovarian mass ➡ with high signal relative to pelvic muscles.*

Lymphoma

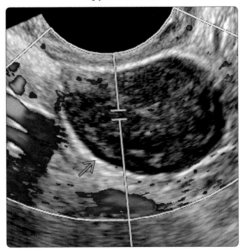

Hyperthecosis

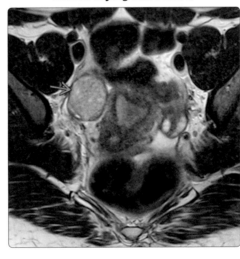

(Left) *Coronal CECT shows bilateral ovarian masses ➡ with preserved follicles ➡ within both the ovarian masses. Note also the circumferential thickening of the wall of the terminal ileum ➡ in this patient with Burkitt lymphoma.* (Right) *Transvaginal Doppler US in a 68-year-old woman with virilism shows an enlarged ovary ➡ with a volume of 12 cm³. The other ovary was similarly enlarged. Both ovaries showed homogeneous, low echogenicity without discernible masses.*

DIFFERENTIAL DIAGNOSIS

Common

- Mature Cystic Teratoma (Dermoid Cyst)
- Mucinous Ovarian Neoplasms
- Serous Ovarian Neoplasms
- Leiomyoma (Mimic)

Less Common

- Fibroma
- Brenner Tumor
- Cystadenofibroma

Rare but Important

- Immature Teratoma
- Dysgerminoma

ESSENTIAL INFORMATION

Key Differential Diagnosis Issues

- Associated with fat
  - Mature cystic teratoma (dermoid cyst)
  - Immature teratoma
- Not associated with fat
  - Mucinous ovarian neoplasms
  - Serous ovarian neoplasms
  - Fibroma
  - Cystadenofibroma
  - Brenner tumor
  - Dysgerminoma

Helpful Clues for Common Diagnoses

- **Mature Cystic Teratoma (Dermoid Cyst)**
  - Calcifications in form of tooth, coarse calcifications in Rokitansky nodule, or mural calcifications
  - Fat attenuation on CT
- **Mucinous Ovarian Neoplasms**
  - Calcifications in 34% of mucinous cystic tumors on CT
  - Patterns of calcifications
    - Fine, sand-like, intracystic calcifications located in necrotic material within cystic structures

    - More common in malignant tumors
  - Mural curvilinear calcification pattern
    - More common in benign tumors
- **Serous Ovarian Neoplasms**
  - Calcifications in 4.7% of serous cystic tumors on CT
  - Calcifications may be seen in peritoneal (sheet-like studding) and nodal metastases
  - Calcifications appear to be more common in low-grade serous carcinoma
- **Leiomyoma (Mimic)**
  - Calcified exophytic uterine leiomyoma can be mistaken for ovarian mass
  - Careful evaluation of relation of mass to uterus can establish its uterine origin
    - Bridging vascular sign

Helpful Clues for Less Common Diagnoses

- **Fibroma**
  - < 10% of fibromas calcify
  - Solid, T2-dark, hypoechoic mass with calcifications
- **Brenner Tumor**
  - Solid or mixed solid and cystic mass with calcifications in 83% of cases
  - Calcifications are frequently extensive and amorphous
- **Cystadenofibroma**
  - Calcifications may occur in solid component or even extend beyond mass into pelvis

Helpful Clues for Rare Diagnoses

- **Immature Teratoma**
  - Peak incidence 15-19 years of age
  - Solid mass with interspersed small foci of fat, calcifications, and numerous cysts of variable sizes
  - Coarse, irregular calcifications within solid component or mural calcifications in walls of cysts
- **Dysgerminoma**
  - Most cases occur in adolescence and early adulthood
  - Calcification may be present in speckled pattern
  - Multilobulated solid masses with prominent fibrovascular septa

---

Mature Cystic Teratoma (Dermoid Cyst)

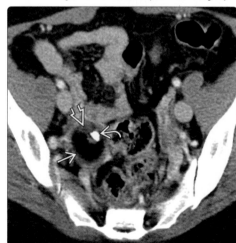

Mature Cystic Teratoma (Dermoid Cyst)

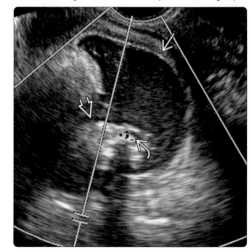

(Left) Axial CECT shows a right ovarian mass ➡ of predominantly fatty attenuation with a mural nodule of soft tissue attenuation (Rokitansky nodule) ➡ containing coarse calcifications ➡. (Right) Transvaginal color Doppler US shows a cystic ovarian lesion ➡ with echogenic mural nodule ➡ containing densely echogenic structure ➡ with posterior shadowing.

Mature Cystic Teratoma (Dermoid Cyst)

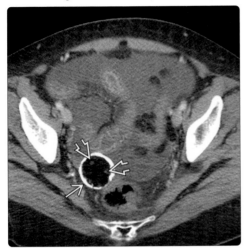

Mature Cystic Teratoma (Dermoid Cyst)

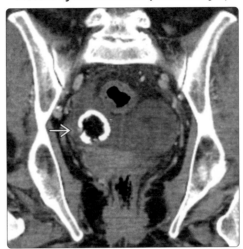

(Left) Axial CECT shows a fat-attenuation right ovarian lesion ➡ with a surrounding thick rim of irregular calcifications. Small foci of soft tissue attenuation ➡ are present within the fatty mass. (Right) Coronal CECT in the same patient shows a fat-attenuation right ovarian lesion ➡ with a surrounding thick, interrupted rim of irregular calcifications.

Mucinous Ovarian Neoplasms

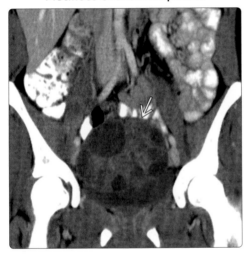

Mucinous Ovarian Neoplasms

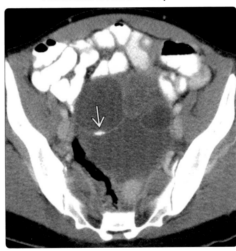

(Left) Coronal CECT shows a well-defined, predominantly solid pelvic mass ➡ with multiple well-defined, cystic spaces. (Right) Axial CECT in the same patient shows curvilinear calcifications ➡ in the wall of a cyst. Pathology revealed borderline mucinous tumor.

Serous Ovarian Neoplasms

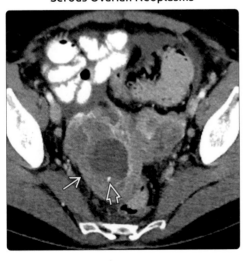

Serous Ovarian Neoplasms

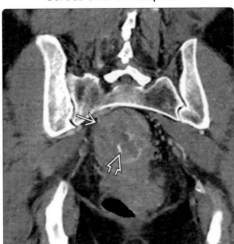

(Left) Axial CECT shows a mixed solid and cystic right ovarian mass ➡ with a small area of calcifications ➡. (Right) Coronal CECT in the same patient shows a right ovarian mass ➡ with a small area of calcifications ➡. Pathology revealed low-grade serous carcinoma.

Serous Ovarian Neoplasms

Serous Ovarian Neoplasms

(Left) *Axial CECT shows a cystic right ovarian mass* ➡ *with soft tissue attenuation mural nodules* ➡ *containing foci of calcifications* ➡. (Right) *Coronal CECT in the same patient shows extensive peritoneal metastases* ➡ *with a small, calcific focus* ➡ *within the peritoneal implants.*

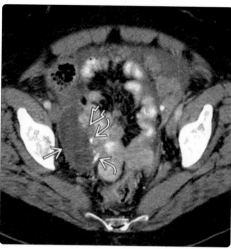

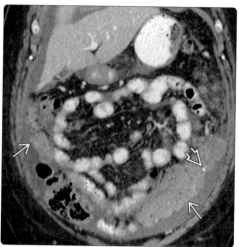

Leiomyoma (Mimic)

Leiomyoma (Mimic)

(Left) *Axial CECT shows a solid right adnexal mass* ➡ *with scattered foci of calcifications. Enhancing vessels* ➡ *are seen bridging from the uterus to the mass (bridging vascular sign), which help establish the uterine origin of the mass.* (Right) *Coronal CECT in the same patient shows the calcified right ovarian mass* ➡ *separate from the right ovary* ➡.

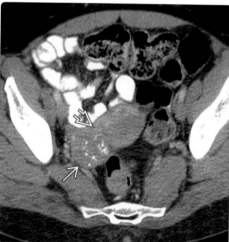

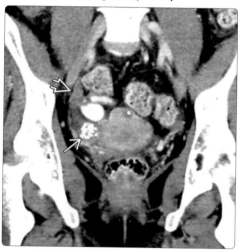

Fibroma

Fibroma

(Left) *Axial CECT shows a large pelvic mass* ➡ *with homogeneous attenuation, a large chunk of irregular calcifications* ➡, *and curvilinear calcifications of the wall* ➡. (Right) *Coronal CECT in the same patient shows a homogeneous soft tissue attenuation mass* ➡ *with peripheral curvilinear calcifications* ➡.

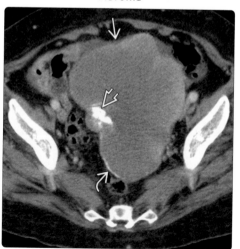

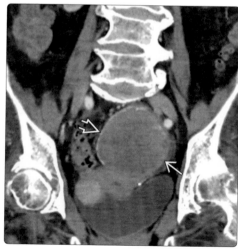

Brenner Tumor

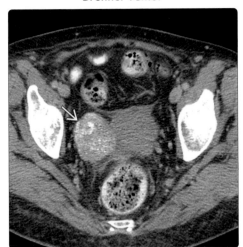

Brenner Tumor

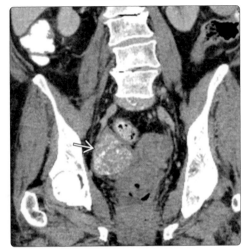

(Left) *Axial CECT shows a solid right ovarian mass ➡ with extensive amorphous calcifications.* (Right) *Coronal CECT in the same patient shows a solid right ovarian mass ➡ with extensive amorphous calcifications. Pathology revealed benign Brenner tumor.*

Cystadenofibroma

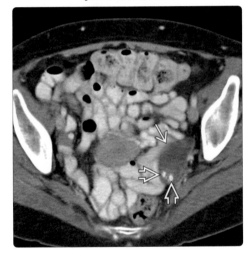

Cystadenofibroma

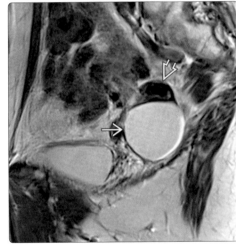

(Left) *Axial CECT shows a left ovarian mass ➡ with foci of coarse calcifications ➡.* (Right) *Sagittal T2 MR shows a left ovarian mass composed of cystic ➡ and solid ➡ components. The solid component has very low signal intensity due to fibrous tissue. Pathology revealed serous cystadenofibroma.*

Immature Teratoma

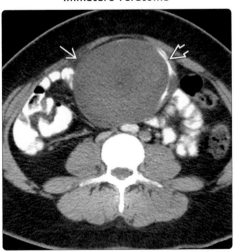

Immature Teratoma

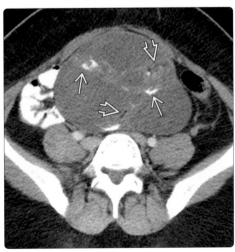

(Left) *Axial CECT shows a fluid-attenuation lesion ➡ with peripheral curvilinear calcifications ➡.* (Right) *Axial CECT in the same patient shows a multilobular mass with irregular, linear calcifications ➡ and small foci of fat attenuation ➡.*

DIFFERENTIAL DIAGNOSIS

Common

- Endometrioma
- Hemorrhagic Cyst
- Fibroma/Fibrothecoma

Less Common

- Krukenberg Tumor
- Mucinous Cystic Neoplasm
- Adenofibroma/Cystadenofibroma

Rare but Important

- Brenner Tumor
- Struma Ovarii
- Fibromatosis

ESSENTIAL INFORMATION

Key Differential Diagnosis Issues

- T2 signal intensity relative to pelvic muscles
  - T2 isointense relative to muscles
    - Endometrioma
    - Fibroma/fibrothecoma
    - Cystadenofibroma
    - Struma ovarii
  - T2 hyperintense relative to muscles
    - Hemorrhagic cyst
    - Krukenberg tumor
    - Mucinous cystic neoplasm
- Solid vs. cystic
  - Solid
    - Fibroma/fibrothecoma
    - Krukenberg tumor
    - Adenofibroma
  - Cystic
    - Endometrioma
    - Hemorrhagic cyst
    - Mucinous cystic neoplasm
  - Cystic and solid
    - Cystadenofibroma
    - Struma ovarii
    - Brenner tumor

Helpful Clues for Common Diagnoses

- **Endometrioma**
  - US
    - Well-defined, smooth-walled, uni- or multilocular cyst(s)
    - Contains homogeneous low-level echoes → characteristic ground-glass appearance
    - Small echogenic foci occur in 35% of endometrioma walls
      - ↑ likelihood that cystic mass is endometrioma
    - Atypical features that may be seen (15% of cases)
      - Mural nodules: Usually avascular (due to adherent mural clot or fibrin)
      - Flow due to presence of endometrial tissue
  - MR
    - Single or multiple, uni- or multilocular cyst
    - High signal intensity on T1 MR

- Signal intensity remains high on T1 FS MR (to differentiate from fat-containing mature cystic teratoma)
  - T2 shading (signal loss on T2 in ovarian cyst that appears hyperintense on T1 MR)
  - T2-dark spots (discrete, markedly hypointense foci within cyst on T2 MR ± T2 shading)

- **Hemorrhagic Cyst**
  - Physiologic cysts seen only in premenopausal women
  - Resolve on follow-up examinations
  - US: Different patterns may be seen
    - Echogenic, avascular, homogeneous, or heterogeneous nonshadowing in early stage
    - Retracted clot
      - Avascular mass-like structure within anechoic cyst
      - Has characteristic concave contour
      - May jiggle with transducer ballottement
    - Reticular, lacy, fishnet, or spongy pattern
      - Irregular fine lines that typically do not completely traverse cyst
  - MR
    - Usually single unilocular cyst
    - High signal intensity on T1 MR
      - Signal intensity remains high on T1 FS MR (to differentiate from fat-containing mature cystic teratoma)
    - May be hypointense on T2 MR (more commonly hyperintense)
      - No T2 shading
      - No T2-dark spots

- **Fibroma/Fibrothecoma**
  - Fibromas can be associated with ascites and pleural effusions in classic Meigs syndrome
  - Fibrothecomas may manifest with hyperestrogenism
    - Endometrial polyps, hyperplasia, or carcinoma
  - US
    - Round, oval, or slightly lobulated tumors often mistaken for exophytic fibroid
    - Most are hypoechoic and solid with regular or slightly irregular internal echogenicity
    - Dramatic sound attenuation resulting in posterior acoustic shadowing
    - Minimal to moderate vascularization on color Doppler images
  - MR
    - T1: Hypo- to isointense to pelvic muscles
    - T2: Low signal intensity
      - Allows differentiation from other solid ovarian masses
    - T1 C+: Mild enhancement

Helpful Clues for Less Common Diagnoses

- **Krukenberg Tumor**
  - Known primary tumors commonly originating from stomach (70% of cases), followed by breast, colon, and appendix
  - Bilateral in 60-80% of patients
  - MR
    - Heterogeneous solid and cystic masses with intratumoral cysts within solid component

– Variable hypointensity on T2 MR due to presence of metastatic mucin-filled signet-ring cells in ovarian stroma and abundant collagen formation
– Moderate to marked enhancement of solid component

- **Mucinous Cystic Neoplasm**
  o Usually large, multilocular cystic mass
  o Variable signal intensity in different loculi depending on mucin concentration
    – Some loculi can have low T2 signal intensity
- **Adenofibroma/Cystadenofibroma**
  o US
    – Primarily solid (adenofibromas)
      ▫ Resemble ovarian fibromas
    – Primarily cystic (cystadenofibromas)
      ▫ Predominantly cystic
      ▫ Irregular, thick wall or septa (possibly > 3 mm) in 30-67% of cases
      ▫ Solid component or papillary projections
  o MR
    – Uni- or multilocular cystic mass with solid fibrous component that demonstrates low signal intensity on T2 MR
    – Primarily solid (adenofibromas)
      ▫ Resemble ovarian fibromas with small foci of high-signal cystic spaces
    – Primarily cystic (cystadenofibromas)
      ▫ Solid, low-signal fibrous component may result in irregular wall or septal thickening (possibly > 3 mm)

Helpful Clues for Rare Diagnoses

- **Brenner Tumor**
  o US
    – Solid or mixed cystic and solid
    – Cystic content is anechoic or of low echogenicity
    – Minimal flow on color Doppler US
    – Calcifications in majority of cases (best seen on CUST)
  o MR
    – Very low T2 signal intensity and low T1 signal intensity due to presence of fibrous elements ± calcifications

  ▫ Imaging finding overlaps with those of fibrothecomas
  ▫ Solid component has low T2 signal intensity in mixed solid and cystic lesions
    – Typically demonstrates at least moderate enhancement after contrast material administration
    – Presence of calcification and coexisting epithelial neoplasms favors diagnosis of Brenner tumor over fibrothecoma
- **Struma Ovarii**
  o US
    – Solid and cystic appearance
    – May be associated with mature cystic teratoma
    – May show rounded or oval, echogenic nodules (stromal pearls)
  o MR
    – Hyperthyroidism in ~ 5% of patients
    – ± mature cystic teratoma with its characteristic appearance due to fat contents
    – Loculated cystic mass with variable signal characteristics
      ▫ Some locules may show marked hypointensity on T2 MR and intermediate signal intensity on T1 MR due to thick, gelatinous colloid
    – Strong enhancement of solid components on T1 C+ MR
- **Fibromatosis**
  o Enlarged ovary with preserved ovarian shape and follicles
  o Black garland sign: T2-hypointense rim surrounding ovary sparing central ovary
    – Distinguishes from solid ovarian masses

SELECTED REFERENCES

1. Avesani G et al: Pearls and potential pitfalls for correct diagnosis of ovarian cystadenofibroma in MRI: a pictorial essay. Korean J Radiol. 22(11):1809-21, 2021
2. Corwin MT et al: Differentiation of ovarian endometriomas from hemorrhagic cysts at MR imaging: utility of the T2 dark spot sign. Radiology. 271(1):126-32, 2014
3. Khashper A et al: T2-hypointense adnexal lesions: an imaging algorithm. Radiographics. 32(4):1047-64, 2012

Endometrioma

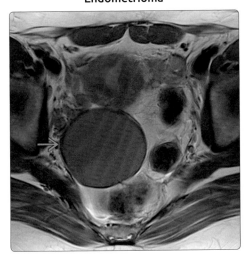

Endometrioma

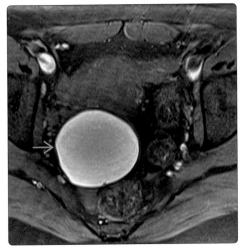

(Left) Axial T2 MR shows a right ovarian lesion ➔ with homogeneous signal intensity similar to that of pelvic muscles. (Right) Axial T1 MR shows a right ovarian mass ➔ with high signal intensity. This is an example of T2 shading (signal loss on T2 in an ovarian cyst that appears hyperintense on T1 MR).

Endometrioma

Endometrioma

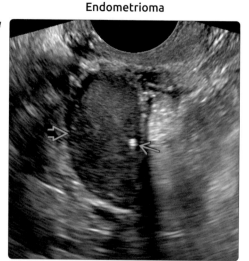

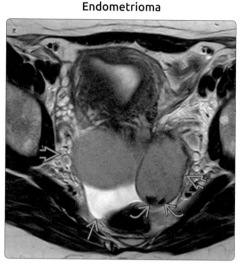

(Left) *Transvaginal US shows a hypoechoic ovarian lesion ➡ with homogeneous, low-level echoes and a small, echogenic mural focus ➡.* (Right) *Axial T2 MR shows 2 endometriomas ➡, both of which show signal intensity that is lower than that of simple fluid ➡. Multiple T2-dark spots ➡ are present within the left endometrioma.*

Hemorrhagic Cyst

Hemorrhagic Cyst

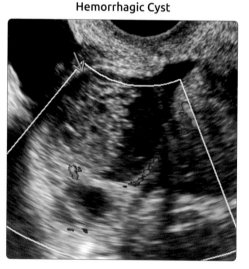

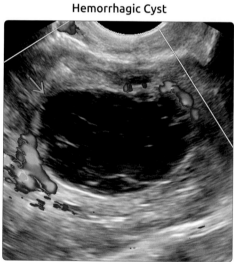

(Left) *Transvaginal color Doppler US shows an ovarian lesion ➡ with an avascular, heterogeneous, hyperechoic pattern.* (Right) *Transvaginal color Doppler US shows an ovarian lesion ➡ with irregular, fine lines that do not completely traverse the cyst, a pattern that has been described as cobweb, reticular, lacy, fishnet, or spongy.*

Hemorrhagic Cyst

Hemorrhagic Cyst

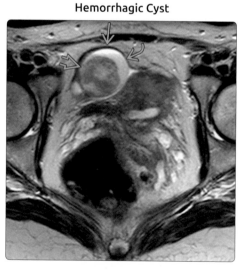

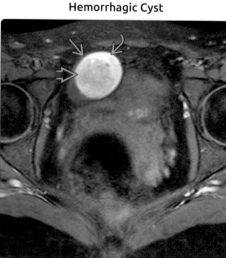

(Left) *Axial T2 MR shows a right ovarian hemorrhagic cyst ➡ with a retracted clot pattern. An eccentric low signal intensity blood clot ➡ is present within the high signal intensity component ➡.* (Right) *Axial T1 FS MR shows a right ovarian hemorrhagic cyst ➡ with a retracted clot pattern. An eccentric high signal intensity blood clot ➡ is present within the higher signal intensity component ➡.*

Fibroma/Fibrothecoma

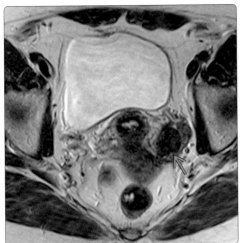

Fibroma/Fibrothecoma

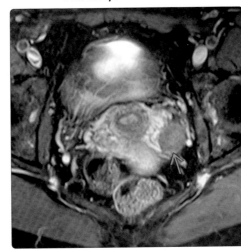

(Left) *Axial T2 MR shows a left ovarian mass ➡ with homogeneous low signal intensity.* (Right) *Axial T1 C+ FS MR shows poor enhancement of the left ovarian mass ➡.*

Fibroma/Fibrothecoma

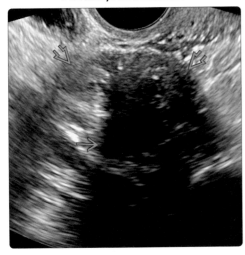

Fibroma/Fibrothecoma

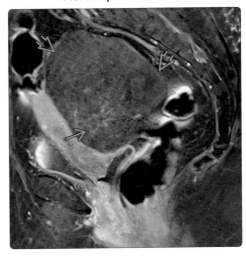

(Left) *Transvaginal US in the same patient shows a well-defined, hypoechoic ovarian lesion ➡ with marked attenuation of the sound waves, resulting in posterior acoustic shadowing ➡.* (Right) *Sagittal T1 C+ FS MR in the same patient shows a well-defined ovarian mass ➡ with minimal enhancement ➡.*

Krukenberg Tumor

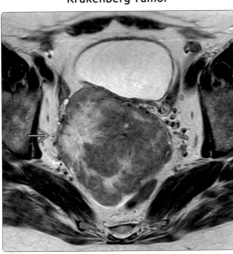

Krukenberg Tumor

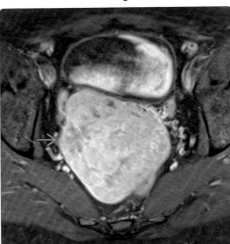

(Left) *Axial T2 MR in a patient with a history of gastric carcinoma shows a heterogeneous right ovarian mass ➡ with areas of low signal intensity similar to pelvic muscles.* (Right) *Axial T1 C+ FS MR in the same patient shows heterogeneous, intense enhancement of the right ovarian mass ➡.*

Mucinous Cystic Neoplasm

Mucinous Cystic Neoplasm

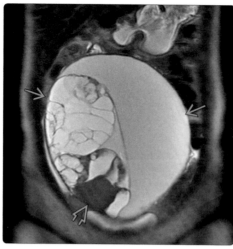

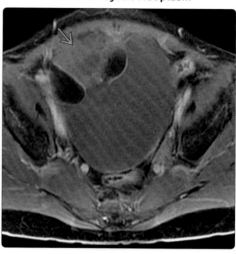

(Left) *Axial T2 MR shows a large, multilocular cystic ovarian mass ➡. Variable signal intensity of individual compartments with one of the compartments demonstrating very low signal intensity ➡.* (Right) *Axial T1 C+ FS MR in the same patient shows no enhancement of the compartment with low signal intensity ➡. Variable signal intensity in individual compartments results from variable mucin concentrations. Pathology revealed borderline mucinous neoplasm.*

Adenofibroma/Cystadenofibroma

Adenofibroma/Cystadenofibroma

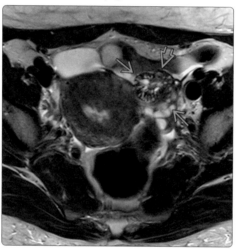

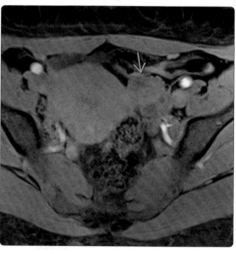

(Left) *Axial T2 MR shows a well-defined, predominantly solid left ovarian mass ➡. The solid component ➡ has low signal intensity with small foci of high signal intensity as a black sponge appearance.* (Right) *Axial T1 C+ FS in the same patient shows a well-defined, predominantly solid left ovarian mass ➡ with minimal homogeneous enhancement.*

Adenofibroma/Cystadenofibroma

Adenofibroma/Cystadenofibroma

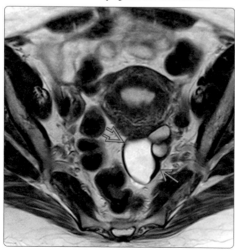

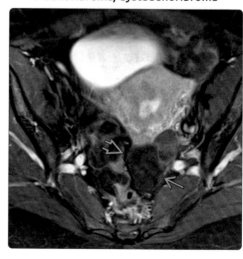

(Left) *Axial T2 MR shows a well-defined, multilocular left ovarian cystic mass ➡ with a relatively thick wall demonstrating low signal intensity ➡.* (Right) *Axial T1 C+ FS shows a well-defined, multilocular left ovarian cystic mass ➡ with minimal enhancement of the wall ➡.*

Ovarian Lesions With Low T2 Signal Intensity

Brenner Tumor

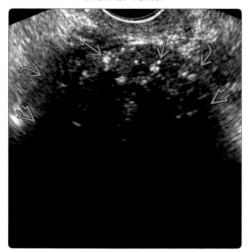

Brenner Tumor

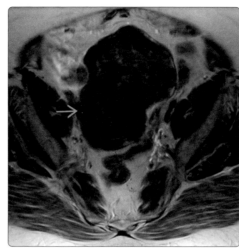

(Left) *Transvaginal US shows a solid ovarian mass ⇗ with foci of increased echogenicity and posterior shadowing ⇨ due to calcifications. There is marked attenuation of the sound waves resulting in posterior shadowing ⇨. The presence of calcifications favors Brenner tumor rather than fibroma.* **(Right)** *Axial T2 MR shows a pelvic mass ⇨ with relatively homogeneous low signal intensity. It is difficult to appreciate calcifications on MR.*

Struma Ovarii

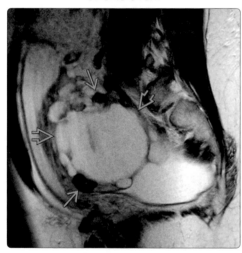

Struma Ovarii

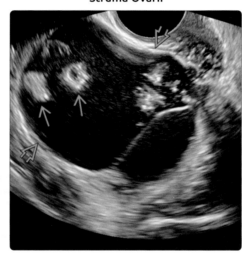

(Left) *Sagittal T2 MR in a 24-year-old woman shows a multilocular cystic mass ⇨. Most of the loculi demonstrate high signal intensity, while few demonstrate very low signal intensity ⇨.* **(Right)** *Transvaginal US shows a multilocular cystic ovarian mass ⇨ with multiple echogenic, rounded intracystic stroma pearls ⇨, a characteristic feature of struma ovarii.*

Fibromatosis

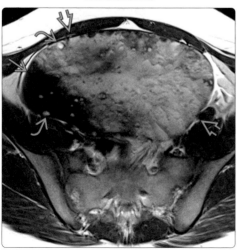

Fibromatosis

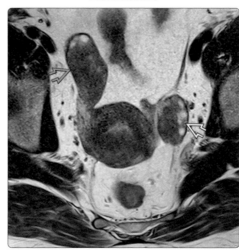

(Left) *Axial T2 MR in a 13-year-old girl with repeated episodes of severe pelvic pain shows a massively enlarged left ovary ⇨. The enlarged ovary has increased signal intensity except for a segmental area of very low signal ⇨ at the periphery. Note the preserved ovarian follicles ⇨ throughout the ovary.* **(Right)** *Axial T2 MR in a 46-year-old woman shows bilaterally enlarged ovaries ⇨ with preserved shape ⇨, low signal intensity, and preserved follicles.*

INDEX

A

Abdominal abscess
- acute left abdominal pain vs., **215**
- cystic mesenteric and omental mass vs., **10**
- elevated or deformed hemidiaphragm vs., **58**
- left upper quadrant mass vs., **124–125**
- pneumoperitoneum vs., **29**
- portal venous gas vs., **274–275**
- rectal or colonic fistula vs., **188, 189**
- stenosis, terminal ileum vs., **148**

Abdominal aortic aneurysm, ruptured, retroperitoneal hemorrhage vs., **476**

Abdominal calcifications, **22–27**
- differential diagnosis, **22**

Abdominal hernia, epigastric pain vs., **119**

Abdominal injection sites, calcifications in, abdominal calcifications vs., **23**

Abdominal manifestations, focal hypervascular liver lesion vs., **253**

Abdominal trauma, hemoperitoneum vs., **32**

Abdominal wall
- abscess, **48**
- calcifications, abdominal calcifications vs., **23**
- defect (hernia), **60–63**
    differential diagnosis, **60**
    left upper quadrant mass vs., **125**
- elevated or deformed hemidiaphragm, **58–59**
    differential diagnosis, **58**
- groin mass, **54–57**
- hematoma, left upper quadrant mass vs., **125**
- iliopsoas compartment mass, **52–53**
- mass, **48–51**
    differential diagnosis, **48**
    left upper quadrant mass vs., **125**
- subcutaneous mass, abdominal wall defect vs., **61**
- trauma, acute right lower quadrant pain vs., **209**
- traumatic hernia, abdominal wall defect vs., **61**

Abnormal bladder wall, **594–597**
- differential diagnosis, **594**

Abscess
- abdominal. *See* Abdominal abscess.
- amebic, anechoic liver lesion vs., **337**
- bilateral renal cysts vs., **508**
- hepatic. *See* Hepatic abscess.
- iliopsoas compartment mass vs., **52**
- inguinal, groin mass vs., **55**
- intrarenal, dilated renal pelvis vs., **557**
- pelvic, due to bowel disease, pelvic fluid vs., **634–635**
- prostatic
    enlarged prostate vs., **630**
    focal lesion in prostate vs., **624, 625**
- pyogenic hepatic, anechoic liver lesion vs., **336**
- renal, cystic renal mass vs., **504–505**
- splenic
    cystic splenic mass vs., **230**
    healed, multiple splenic calcifications vs., **226**
    solid splenic mass vs., **228**
- splenomegaly vs., **223**
- testicular
    intratesticular mass vs., **604**
    testicular cystic lesions vs., **608**
- tuboovarian
    acute pelvic pain vs., **650**
    multilocular ovarian cysts vs., **676**
    unilocular ovarian cysts vs., **682, 683**

Acalculous cholecystitis
- acute, diffuse gallbladder wall thickening vs., **374–375**
- distended gallbladder vs., **366**

Acanthosis, glycogenic, mucosal nodularity, esophagus vs., **76**

Acanthosis nigricans, mucosal nodularity, esophagus vs., **76**

Achalasia
- cricopharyngeal, lesion at pharyngoesophageal junction vs., **72**
- esophageal
    dilated esophagus vs., **80**
    esophageal dysmotility vs., **84**
    mimic, intrathoracic stomach vs., **102**

Acinar cell carcinoma
- hypervascular pancreatic mass vs., **422, 423**
- hypovascular pancreatic mass vs., **416, 417**

Acquired cystic kidney disease, bilateral renal cysts vs., **508**

Acute acalculous cholecystitis, diffuse gallbladder wall thickening vs., **374–375**

Acute appendicitis, stenosis, terminal ileum vs., **148**

Acute biliary inflammation, epigastric pain vs., **118**

Acute cortical necrosis
- enlarged kidney vs., **544, 545**
- hyperechoic kidney vs., **553**
- kidney transplant dysfunction vs., **497**
- small kidney vs., **549**

Acute esophageal inflammation, epigastric pain vs., **118**

Acute flank pain, **538–543**
- differential diagnosis, **538**
- musculoskeletal causes, **538**

Acute gastroduodenal inflammation, epigastric pain vs., **118**

Acute left abdominal pain, **214–219**
- differential diagnosis, **214**

INDEX

Acute pelvic pain, in nonpregnant women, **650–655**
- differential diagnosis, **650**

Acute rejection, kidney transplant dysfunction vs., **496**

Acute right lower quadrant pain, **208–213**
- differential diagnosis, **208**

Acute tubular injury
- delayed or persistent nephrogram vs., **530**
- enlarged kidney vs., **544**
- kidney transplant dysfunction vs., **496**
- wedge-shaped or striated nephrogram vs., **534**

Acute viral hepatitis, periportal lesion vs., **356**

Adenocarcinoma
- Cowper gland, urethral stricture vs., **600**
- primary, aneurysmal dilation of small bowel lumen vs., **146**
- prostatic, enlarged prostate vs., **630**

Adenofibroma, ovarian lesions with low T2 signal intensity vs., **696, 697**

Adenoma. *See also* Cystadenoma.
- adrenal
  - adrenal mass vs., **480**
  - mimic, cystic retroperitoneal mass vs., **460**
- hepatic
  - echogenic liver mass vs., **344–345**
  - focal hypervascular liver lesion vs., **252**
  - focal liver lesion with hemorrhage vs., **240**
  - hypoechoic liver mass vs., **341**
  - liver mass with central or eccentric scar vs., **236**
  - liver mass with mosaic enhancement vs., **258**
- metanephric, solid renal mass vs., **501**
- papillary, solid renal mass vs., **501**
- villous, solitary colonic filling defect vs., **172**

Adenomatoid tumor, extratesticular solid mass vs., **612**

Adenomatous polyp, gastric mass lesions vs., **90**

Adenomyomatosis
- diffuse gallbladder wall thickening vs., **374**
- hyperechoic gallbladder wall vs., **380**

Adenomyosis
- abnormal uterine bleeding vs., **668**
- diffuse, thickened endometrium vs., **662**
- enlarged uterus vs., **658**
- focal, enlarged uterus vs., **658**

Adhesions, small bowel obstruction vs., **164**

Adnexal mass, extraovarian, **644–649**
- differential diagnosis, **644**

Adnexal torsion, acute left abdominal pain vs., **214**

Adrenal adenoma
- adrenal mass vs., **480**
- mimic, cystic retroperitoneal mass vs., **460**

Adrenal calcifications, abdominal calcifications vs., **22–23**

Adrenal carcinoma, adrenal mass vs., **481**

Adrenal collision tumor, adrenal mass vs., **481**

Adrenal cortical carcinoma, left upper quadrant mass vs., **124**

Adrenal cyst
- adrenal mass vs., **480**
- cystic retroperitoneal mass vs., **460**
- left upper quadrant mass vs., **124**

Adrenal ganglioneuroma, adrenal mass vs., **481**

Adrenal hemorrhage
- acute flank pain vs., **539**
- adrenal mass vs., **480**
- retroperitoneal hemorrhage vs., **476**

Adrenal hyperplasia, adrenal mass vs., **481**

Adrenal infarction, acute flank pain vs., **539**

Adrenal mass, **480–485**
- abdominal calcifications vs., **23**
- differential diagnosis, **480**
- left upper quadrant mass vs., **124**

Adrenal metastases and lymphoma, left upper quadrant mass vs., **124**

Adrenal parenchymal calcifications, abdominal calcifications vs., **23**

Adrenal pheochromocytoma (mimic), hypervascular pancreatic mass vs., **422, 423**

Adrenal rest tumor, hepatic, hyperintense liver lesions (T1WI) vs., **299**

Adrenal rests, intratesticular mass vs., **604, 605**

Afferent loop syndrome
- cluster of dilated small bowel vs., **144**
- small bowel obstruction vs., **165**

AIDS
- cholangiopathy. *See* Cholangiopathy, AIDS.
- diffusely abnormal liver echogenicity vs., **334**
- hepatic involvement, diffuse hyperechoic liver vs., **328**
- mesenteric lymphadenopathy vs., **19**
- splenomegaly vs., **222**

Air (gas) bubbles
- gastric mass lesions vs., **90**
- multiple colonic filling defects vs., **174**

Alcohol-ablated liver tumors, mimic, fat-containing liver mass vs., **246**

Allograft nephropathy, chronic, small kidney vs., **548**

Alport syndrome, small kidney vs., **549**

Amebiasis, mass or inflammation of ileocecal area vs., **176**

Amebic abscess
- anechoic liver lesion vs., **337**
- hepatic
  - cystic hepatic mass vs., **248**
  - echogenic liver mass vs., **345**
  - epigastric pain vs., **119**
  - focal hepatic echogenic lesion vs., **323**
  - hypoechoic liver mass vs., **340**
  - liver lesion containing gas vs., **271**
  - liver lesion with capsule or halo on MR vs., **304**
  - multiple hypodense liver lesions vs., **309**
  - target lesions in liver vs., **348**

Ameboma, solitary colonic filling defect vs., **172**

Amiodarone therapy, diffuse increased attenuation, spleen vs., **232**

Ampullary carcinoma
- dilated pancreatic duct vs., **435**
- hypovascular pancreatic mass vs., **416–417**

Ampullary tumors
- dilated common bile duct vs., **398**
- duodenal mass vs., **131**
- gas in bile ducts or gallbladder vs., **369**

Amyloid
- abnormal bladder wall vs., **594, 595**
- urethral stricture vs., **600**

Amyloidosis
- diffusely abnormal liver echogenicity vs., **334**

- focal liver lesion with hemorrhage vs., **240**
- gastric dilation or outlet obstruction vs., **111**
- linitis plastica vs., **114, 115**
- renal, hyperechoic kidney vs., **553**
- splenomegaly vs., **223**
- thickened gastric folds vs., **105**
Anasarca, infiltration of peripancreatic fat planes vs., **438**
Anastomosis
- biliary-enteric
    high-attenuation (hyperdense) bile in gallbladder vs., **378**
- bowel-bowel, aneurysmal dilation of small bowel lumen vs., **146**
- surgical biliary-enteric, gas in bile ducts or gallbladder vs., **368**
Anechoic liver lesion, **336–339**
- differential diagnosis, **336**
Anemia, sickle cell, diffuse increased attenuation, spleen vs., **232**
Aneurysm
- aortic, extrinsic esophageal mass vs., **68**
- calcifications in wall of, abdominal calcifications vs., **23**
- calcifications within kidney vs., **488**
- groin, groin mass vs., **55**
- renal artery. *See* Renal artery, aneurysm.
- ruptured
    hemoperitoneum vs., **33**
    high-attenuation (hyperdense) ascites vs., **42**
Aneurysmal dilation, of small bowel lumen, **146–147**
- differential diagnosis, **146**
Angioedema, intestinal
- colonic wall thickening vs., **200, 201**
- segmental or diffuse small bowel wall thickening vs., **151**
Angiomyolipoma
- calcifications within kidney vs., **489**
- epithelioid
    calcifications within kidney vs., **489**
    fat-containing renal mass vs., **520–521**
    solid renal mass vs., **501**
- hepatic
    focal hepatic echogenic lesion vs., **323**
    focal hypervascular liver lesion vs., **253**
    hyperintense liver lesions (T1WI) vs., **299**
    multiple hypodense liver lesions vs., **309**
    multiple hypointense liver lesions (T2WI) vs., **295**
- renal
    fat-containing renal mass vs., **520**
    fat-containing retroperitoneal mass vs., **472**
    hyperechoic renal mass vs., **560**
    perirenal and subcapsular mass lesions vs., **516**
    retroperitoneal hemorrhage vs., **476**
    solid renal mass vs., **500**
- renal sinus lesion vs., **525**
Angiosarcoma
- hepatic
    focal hypervascular liver lesion vs., **253**
    liver mass with mosaic enhancement vs., **259**
Annular pancreas, duodenal mass vs., **130**
Anomalous blood supply, focal hyperperfusion abnormality vs., **282**

Anovulatory bleeding, abnormal uterine bleeding vs., **668**
Antral gastritis, linitis plastica vs., **114**
Aortic aneurysm, extrinsic esophageal mass vs., **68**
Aortic arch, extrinsic esophageal mass vs., **68**
Aortoenteric fistula, occult GI bleeding vs., **160**
Appendagitis, epiploic, fat-containing lesion of peritoneal cavity vs., **14**
Appendiceal mucocele
- abdominal calcifications vs., **23**
- extraovarian adnexal mass vs., **644**
Appendicitis
- acute, stenosis, terminal ileum vs., **148**
- acute flank pain vs., **539**
- acute left abdominal pain vs., **215**
- acute right lower quadrant pain vs., **208**
- extraovarian adnexal mass vs., **644, 645**
- mass or inflammation of ileocecal area vs., **176**
- pelvic fluid vs., **634**
- pneumoperitoneum vs., **29**
- portal venous gas vs., **274**
- right upper quadrant pain vs., **390, 391**
Appendix
- carcinoma
    acute right lower quadrant pain vs., **209**
    mass or inflammation of ileocecal area vs., **176**
- mucocele
    acute right lower quadrant pain vs., **209**
    mass or inflammation of ileocecal area vs., **177**
Arterial thrombosis, kidney transplant dysfunction vs., **497**
Arterioportal shunt
- cirrhosis, focal hyperperfusion abnormality vs., **282–283**
- focal hypervascular liver lesion vs., **252**
Arterioportal shunt, focal hypervascular liver lesion vs., **252**
Arteriovenous fistula, groin, groin mass vs., **54**
Arteriovenous malformation
- dilated renal pelvis vs., **557**
- hepatic, focal hyperperfusion abnormality vs., **283**
- renal, renal sinus lesion vs., **524**
Artery calcification, hepatic, periportal lesion vs., **357**
Ascariasis, **385**
Ascending cholangitis
- intrahepatic and extrahepatic duct dilatation vs., **388**
- periportal lesion vs., **356**
- right upper quadrant pain vs., **390**
Ascending urinary tract infection, right upper quadrant pain vs., **390**
Ascites
- exudative, high-attenuation (hyperdense) ascites vs., **42**
- free-flowing, **42**
- high-attenuation (hyperdense), **42–45**
    differential diagnosis, **42**
    hemoperitoneum vs., **33**
- lesser sac, mimic, cystic pancreatic mass vs., **426**
- loculated
    cystic mesenteric and omental mass vs., **10**
    left upper quadrant mass vs., **125**
- malignant, hemoperitoneum vs., **33**
- pelvic fluid vs., **634, 635**
- transudative, **42**
Asthma, pneumatosis of small intestine vs., **156**

INDEX

Asymmetric dilation, of intrahepatic bile ducts, **404–407**
- differential diagnosis, **404**
Asymmetric musculature, mimic, iliopsoas compartment mass vs., **52**
Atherosclerotic calcifications, abdominal calcifications vs., **23**
Atrial enlargement, left, extrinsic esophageal mass vs., **68**
Atrophy
- endometrial, abnormal uterine bleeding vs., **668**
- posttorsion, decreased testicular size vs., **618**
Atrophy or fatty replacement of pancreas, **432–433**
- differential diagnosis, **432**
Atypical hemangioma
- hepatic mass with central scar vs., **354**
- hypoechoic liver mass vs., **341**
Autoimmune disease, pneumatosis of small intestine vs., **156**
Autoimmune (IgG4) pancreatitis
- dilated pancreatic duct vs., **435**
- epigastric pain vs., **118–119**
Autosomal dominant polycystic disease
- bilateral renal cysts vs., **508**
- cystic pancreatic mass vs., **426, 427**
- enlarged kidney vs., **544–545**
- liver
  - cystic hepatic mass vs., **248**
  - focal liver lesion with hemorrhage vs., **240**
  - multiple hypodense liver lesions vs., **308**

B

Backwash ileitis, stenosis, terminal ileum vs., **148**
Bacterial cystitis, abnormal bladder wall vs., **594**
Barotrauma
- gas in or around kidney vs., **528**
- pneumatosis of small intestine vs., **156**
- pneumoperitoneum vs., **28**
Barrett esophagus
- esophageal strictures vs., **78, 78–79**
- mucosal nodularity, esophagus vs., **76**
Bartholin gland cyst, female lower genital cysts vs., **638**
Beak sign, small bowel obstruction, **164**
Behçet disease, esophageal ulceration vs., **74**
Benign hepatic cyst, hypoechoic liver mass vs., **340**
Benign prostatic hyperplasia
- enlarged prostate vs., **630**
- filling defect in urinary bladder vs., **584**
- nodules, focal lesion in prostate vs., **624**
Bezoar, gastric
- gastric dilation or outlet obstruction vs., **110**
- mimic, gastric mass lesions vs., **90**
Bilateral renal cysts, **508–511**
- differential diagnosis, **508**
Bile ducts
- abnormal, hypoechoic liver mass vs., **340**
- dilated, **398–403**
  - anechoic liver lesion vs., **337**
  - differential diagnosis, **398**

mimic, periportal lucency or edema vs., **288**
- gas in, **368–371**
  - differential diagnosis, **368**
  - liver lesion containing gas vs., **270**
Bile sump syndrome, gas in bile ducts or gallbladder vs., **369**
Biliary calculi, intrahepatic
- focal hepatic echogenic lesion vs., **322**
- hepatic calcifications vs., **266**
Biliary carcinoma, cystic hepatic mass vs., **248**
Biliary cholangitis, primary
- dysmorphic liver with abnormal bile ducts vs., **278**
- mosaic/patchy hepatogram vs., **262**
Biliary cystadenocarcinoma, anechoic liver lesion vs., **337**
Biliary cystadenoma
- anechoic liver lesion vs., **337**
- cystic hepatic mass vs., **248**
- hepatic calcifications vs., **267**
Biliary-enteric anastomosis, high-attenuation (hyperdense) bile in gallbladder vs., **378**
Biliary-enteric fistula, gas in bile ducts or gallbladder vs., **368**
Biliary hamartoma
- anechoic liver lesion vs., **337**
- cystic hepatic mass vs., **248**
- diffuse hyperechoic liver vs., **328**
- diffusely abnormal liver echogenicity vs., **334**
- dysmorphic liver with abnormal bile ducts vs., **279**
- echogenic liver mass vs., **345**
- focal hepatic echogenic lesion vs., **322**
- multiple hypo-, hyper- or anechoic liver lesions vs., **351**
- multiple hypodense liver lesions vs., **308**
Biliary infection, gas in bile ducts or gallbladder vs., **369**
Biliary inflammation, acute, epigastric pain vs., **118**
Biliary instrumentation, gas in bile ducts or gallbladder vs., **368**
Biliary intraductal papillary mucinous neoplasm
- asymmetric dilation of intrahepatic bile ducts vs., **404, 405**
- cystic hepatic mass vs., **248–249**
- dilated common bile duct vs., **398, 399**
- intrahepatic and extrahepatic duct dilatation vs., **388**
Biliary necrosis, posttransplant, periportal lucency or edema vs., **289**
Biliary parasites, hepatic calcifications vs., **267**
Biliary sphincterotomy, gas in bile ducts or gallbladder vs., **368**
Biliary stent
- high-attenuation (hyperdense) bile in gallbladder vs., **378**
- placement, gas in bile ducts or gallbladder vs., **368**
Biliary strictures, multiple, **408–411**
- differential diagnosis, **408**
Biliary tract
- biliary strictures in, multiple, **408–411**
- calcifications, abdominal calcifications vs., **22**
- dilated common bile duct, **398–403**
- hypointense lesion in biliary tree (MRCP), **412–413**
- intrahepatic bile ducts, asymmetric dilation of, **404–407**

INDEX

Biliary trauma
- dilated common bile duct vs., **398, 399**
- high-attenuation (hyperdense) bile in gallbladder vs., **378**

Biloma
- anechoic liver lesion vs., **336**
- cystic hepatic mass vs., **248**
- infected, hypoechoic liver mass vs., **341**
- liver lesion containing gas vs., **271**

Bladder, urinary
- abnormal wall, **594–597**
- distended, dilated renal calyces vs., **566**
- diverticulum
    extraovarian adnexal mass vs., **644**
    mimic, cystic dilation of distal ureter vs., **580**
    urinary bladder outpouching vs., **590**
- filling defect, **584–589**
- fistulas
    filling defect in urinary bladder vs., **584**
    gas within urinary bladder vs., **592**
    urinary bladder outpouching vs., **590**
- gas within, **592–593**
    differential diagnosis, **592**
- herniation, urinary bladder outpouching vs., **590**
- iatrogenic
    gas within urinary bladder vs., **592**
    urinary bladder outpouching vs., **590**
- neurogenic
    abnormal bladder wall vs., **594**
    urinary bladder outpouching vs., **590**
- outpouching, **590–591**
    differential diagnosis, **590**
- postoperative, urinary bladder outpouching vs., **590**
- schistosomiasis, abnormal bladder wall vs., **594, 595**
- underdistended, abnormal bladder wall vs., **594**

Bladder calculi, filling defect in urinary bladder vs., **584**

Bladder carcinoma
- abnormal bladder wall vs., **594**
- filling defect in urinary bladder vs., **584**
- rectal or colonic fistula vs., **188, 189**

Bladder instrumentation, rectal or colonic fistula vs., **188, 189**

Bladder stones, abdominal calcifications vs., **23**

Bladder trauma
- hemoperitoneum vs., **33**
- high-attenuation (hyperdense) ascites vs., **43**
- urinary bladder outpouching vs., **590**

Bladder tumor, cystic dilation of distal ureter vs., **580**

Bladder wall trauma, abnormal bladder wall vs., **594, 595**

Bland portal vein thrombosis, portal vein abnormality vs., **362**

Bleeding, from GI or GU tract, abnormal uterine bleeding vs., **668**

Blood clot
- delayed or persistent nephrogram vs., **530**
- echogenic material in gallbladder vs., **382**
- filling defect, renal pelvis vs., **570**
- filling defect in urinary bladder vs., **584**
- ureteral filling defect or stricture vs., **576**

Blood-filled renal pelvis, dilated renal calyces vs., **566, 567**

Bochdalek hernia, elevated or deformed hemidiaphragm vs., **58**

Boerhaave syndrome, esophageal outpouchings (diverticula), **82–83**

Bone tumor, groin mass vs., **55**

Bosniak I cysts, cystic renal mass vs., **504**

Bosniak II cysts, cystic renal mass vs., **504**

Bowel-bowel anastomosis, aneurysmal dilation of small bowel lumen vs., **146**

Bowel calcifications, abdominal calcifications vs., **23**

Bowel disease, pelvic abscess due to, pelvic fluid vs., **634–635**

Bowel inflammation, epigastric pain vs., **119**

Bowel loop, extraovarian adnexal mass vs., **644, 645**

Bowel obstruction
- epigastric pain vs., **119**
- extraovarian adnexal mass vs., **644**

Bowel perforation, pneumoperitoneum vs., **29**

Breast cancer, linitis plastica vs., **114**

Brenner tumor
- calcified ovarian masses vs., **692**
- multilocular ovarian cysts vs., **676, 677**
- ovarian lesions with low T2 signal intensity vs., **696, 697**
- solid ovarian masses vs., **688–689**

Bronchobiliary fistula, gas in bile ducts or gallbladder vs., **369**

Bronchogenic cyst
- cystic retroperitoneal mass vs., **461**
- extrinsic esophageal mass vs., **68**

Bronchus, left main, extrinsic esophageal mass vs., **68**

Brucellosis, multiple splenic calcifications vs., **226**

Brunner gland hyperplasia
- groove pancreatitis, duodenal mass vs., **130**
- thickened duodenal fold vs., **138**

Budd-Chiari syndrome
- dysmorphic liver with abnormal bile ducts vs., **278**
- focal hyperdense hepatic mass on nonenhanced CT vs., **315**
- hepatomegaly vs., **330**
- mosaic/patchy hepatogram vs., **262**
- widespread low attenuation within liver vs., **318**

C

C-section defect, abnormal uterine bleeding vs., **668**

Calcifications. *See also* Urolithiasis.
- abdominal, **22–27**
    differential diagnosis, **22**
- extrahepatic, hepatic calcifications vs., **267**
- hepatic artery
    focal hepatic echogenic lesion vs., **322**
    hepatic calcifications vs., **266**
    mimic, gas in bile ducts or gallbladder vs., **368**
- pancreatic, **444–447**
- within primary hepatic tumor, focal hyperdense hepatic mass on nonenhanced CT vs., **314–315**
- prostatic
    abdominal calcifications vs., **23**

focal lesion in prostate vs., **624**
- testicular, **620–621**
    differential diagnosis, **620**
Calcified granuloma
- liver
    focal hepatic echogenic lesion vs., **322**
    hepatic calcifications vs., **266**
- multiple hypointense liver lesions (T2WI) vs., **294**
Calcified lymph nodes, abdominal calcifications vs., **23**
Calcified metastasis, echogenic liver mass vs., **344**
Calcified ovarian masses, **692–695**
- differential diagnosis, **692**
Calcified rim, masses with, focal hepatic echogenic lesion vs., **323**
Calcified scar
- abdominal calcifications vs., **23**
- abdominal wall mass vs., **48**
Calcified scar, masses with, focal hepatic echogenic lesion vs., **323**
Calcineurin inhibitor toxicity, kidney transplant dysfunction vs., **496**
Calcinosis syndromes
- abdominal calcifications vs., **23**
- abdominal wall mass vs., **49**
Calcium bile, milk of, high-attenuation (hyperdense) bile in gallbladder vs., **378**
Calculi, bladder, filling defect in urinary bladder vs., **584**
Calculi parasites, intrahepatic, hepatic calcifications vs., **267**
Calculous cholecystitis, acute, diffuse gallbladder wall thickening vs., **374**
Calyceal diverticulum
- congenital renal anomalies vs., **493**
- dilated renal calyces vs., **566, 567**
Canal of Nuck hydrocele, groin mass vs., **55**
Cancer, small bowel obstruction vs., **164**
Candida esophagitis
- esophageal strictures vs., **78**
- esophageal ulceration vs., **74**
- intraluminal mass vs., **66**
- mucosal nodularity, esophagus vs., **76**
- odynophagia vs., **86**
Candidiasis, hepatic, cystic hepatic mass vs., **248**
Capsular retraction, liver "mass" with, **244–245**
Carcinoid tumor
- mass or inflammation of ileocecal area vs., **176**
- mimic, hypervascular pancreatic mass vs., **422, 423**
- misty (infiltrated) mesentery vs., **36**
- occult GI bleeding vs., **160**
- segmental or diffuse small bowel wall thickening vs., **151**
- small bowel obstruction vs., **165**
- solid mesenteric or omental mass vs., **5**
- solid ovarian masses vs., **688, 689**
- stenosis, terminal ileum vs., **148**
- of stomach, target (bull's-eye) lesions, stomach vs., **98–99**
Caroli disease
- anechoic liver lesion vs., **337**

- asymmetric dilation of intrahepatic bile ducts vs., **404, 405**
- cystic hepatic mass vs., **249**
- dysmorphic liver with abnormal bile ducts vs., **279**
- multiple biliary strictures vs., **408, 409**
- multiple hypo-, hyper- or anechoic liver lesions vs., **351**
- multiple hypodense liver lesions vs., **309**
- periportal lesion vs., **357**
Cartilaginous cyst, subpubic, female lower genital cysts vs., **638, 639**
Castleman disease
- mesenteric lymphadenopathy vs., **19**
- perirenal and subcapsular mass lesions vs., **517**
- renal sinus lesion vs., **525**
Cathartic abuse
- segmental colonic narrowing vs., **195**
- smooth ahaustral colon vs., **206**
Caustic esophagitis
- esophageal strictures vs., **78**
- esophageal ulceration vs., **74**
- odynophagia vs., **86**
Caustic gastritis, portal venous gas vs., **274**
Caustic gastroduodenal injury
- linitis plastica vs., **114–115**
- pneumatosis of small intestine vs., **157**
- thickened duodenal fold vs., **138**
- thickened gastric folds vs., **104**
Cavernous hemangioma
- focal hypervascular liver lesion vs., **252**
- hepatic
    echogenic liver mass vs., **344**
    focal hepatic echogenic lesion vs., **322**
    focal hyperdense hepatic mass on nonenhanced CT vs., **314**
    focal hyperperfusion abnormality vs., **282–283**
    liver "mass" with capsular retraction vs., **244**
    liver mass with central or eccentric scar vs., **236**
    multiple hypodense liver lesions vs., **308**
Cecal carcinoma, stenosis, terminal ileum vs., **148**
Cecal volvulus
- colonic ileus vs., **182**
- mass or inflammation of ileocecal area vs., **176**
Celiac-sprue disease
- dilated duodenum vs., **136**
- mesenteric lymphadenopathy vs., **19**
- pneumatosis of small intestine vs., **156**
- segmental or diffuse small bowel wall thickening vs., **150**
- thickened duodenal fold vs., **138**
Central scar, hepatic mass with, **354–355**
- differential diagnosis, **354**
Cervical cancer
- abnormal uterine bleeding vs., **668, 669**
- enlarged uterus vs., **658**
- ureteral filling defect or stricture vs., **576**
Cervical carcinoma
- dilated renal calyces vs., **566**
- filling defect in urinary bladder vs., **584**
- rectal or colonic fistula vs., **188–189**
Cervical leiomyoma, enlarged uterus vs., **658**
Cervical lesion, enlarged uterus vs., **658**

Cervical lymphadenopathy, lesion at pharyngoesophageal junction vs., **72**

Cervical osteophytes, lesion at pharyngoesophageal junction vs., **72**

Cervical stenosis
- acute pelvic pain vs., **650, 651**
- enlarged uterus vs., **658**

Chagas disease, dilated esophagus vs., **80**

Chemical proctocolitis
- colonic thumbprinting vs., **198**
- colonic wall thickening vs., **200, 201**

Chemoembolization, transarterial hepatic, gas in bile ducts or gallbladder vs., **369**

Chemotherapy
- cholangitis
      asymmetric dilation of intrahepatic bile ducts vs., **404, 405**
      dysmorphic liver with abnormal bile ducts vs., **278**
      multiple biliary strictures vs., **408, 409**
      periportal lucency or edema vs., **288, 288–289**
- post, small kidney vs., **549**

Chemotherapy-induced enteritis, segmental or diffuse small bowel wall thickening vs., **150**

Chemotherapy-induced gastritis, thickened gastric folds vs., **105**

Cholangiocarcinoma
- asymmetric dilation of intrahepatic bile ducts vs., **404**
- distal common bile duct, **398**
- echogenic liver mass vs., **344**
- focal hepatic echogenic lesion vs., **323**
- focal hypervascular liver lesion vs., **252, 253**
- hepatic calcifications vs., **266**
- hypovascular pancreatic mass vs., **416, 417**
- intrahepatic and extrahepatic duct dilatation vs., **388**
- intrahepatic/hilar, dysmorphic liver with abnormal bile ducts vs., **278**
- liver mass
      with capsular retraction vs., **244**
      with central or eccentric scar vs., **236**
      with mosaic enhancement vs., **258–259**
- multiple biliary strictures vs., **408**
- peripheral, multiple hypointense liver lesions (T2WI) vs., **294**
- periportal lucency or edema vs., **289**

Cholangiography, intraluminal contrast after, high-attenuation (hyperdense) bile in gallbladder vs., **378**

Cholangiopathy
- AIDS
      asymmetric dilation of intrahepatic bile ducts vs., **404**
      diffuse gallbladder wall thickening vs., **375**
      dilated common bile duct vs., **398, 399**
      dysmorphic liver with abnormal bile ducts vs., **278**
      multiple biliary strictures vs., **408**
- ischemic, multiple biliary strictures vs., **408**

Cholangitis
- AIDS-related, periportal lucency or edema vs., **288**
- ascending
      asymmetric dilation of intrahepatic bile ducts vs., **404**
      epigastric pain vs., **118**
      intrahepatic and extrahepatic duct dilatation vs., **388**
      multiple biliary strictures vs., **408**
      periportal lesion vs., **356**
      periportal lucency or edema vs., **288**
      right upper quadrant pain vs., **390**
- autoimmune (IgG4), multiple biliary strictures vs., **408, 409**
- chemotherapy
      asymmetric dilation of intrahepatic bile ducts vs., **404, 405**
      dysmorphic liver with abnormal bile ducts vs., **278**
      multiple biliary strictures vs., **408, 409**
      periportal lucency or edema vs., **288–289**
- IgG4-related sclerosing, asymmetric dilation of intrahepatic bile ducts vs., **404, 405**
- ischemic, asymmetric dilation of intrahepatic bile ducts vs., **404, 405**
- multiple hypo-, hyper- or anechoic liver lesions vs., **351**
- periportal lucency or edema vs., **288**
- primary sclerosing
      asymmetric dilation of intrahepatic bile ducts vs., **404**
      dilated common bile duct vs., **398, 399**
      dysmorphic liver with abnormal bile ducts vs., **278**
      focal hyperdense hepatic mass on nonenhanced CT vs., **315**
      liver "mass" with capsular retraction vs., **244**
      multiple biliary strictures vs., **408**
      periportal lucency or edema vs., **288**
      widened hepatic fissures vs., **276**
- recurrent pyogenic
      asymmetric dilation of intrahepatic bile ducts vs., **404–405**
      dilated common bile duct vs., **398, 399**
      intrahepatic and extrahepatic duct dilatation vs., **388**
      multiple biliary strictures vs., **408–409**
      periportal lucency or edema vs., **288**

Cholecystitis
- acalculous
      acute, dilated gallbladder vs., **384**
      distended gallbladder vs., **366**
- acute
      duodenal mass vs., **131**
      epigastric pain vs., **118**
      hemorrhagic, dilated gallbladder vs., **385**
      right upper quadrant pain vs., **390**
- acute acalculous, diffuse gallbladder wall thickening vs., **374–375**
- acute calculous
      diffuse gallbladder wall thickening vs., **374**
      dilated gallbladder vs., **384**
- acute flank pain vs., **539**
- acute right lower quadrant pain vs., **208**
- chronic, diffuse gallbladder wall thickening vs., **374**
- complicated, echogenic material in gallbladder vs., **382**
- emphysematous
      gas in bile ducts or gallbladder vs., **368**
      hyperechoic gallbladder wall vs., **380**
- focal hyperperfusion abnormality vs., **282**
- hemorrhagic, high-attenuation (hyperdense) bile in gallbladder vs., **378**
- infectious, dilated gallbladder vs., **385**

- other causes of, dilated gallbladder vs., **385**
- xanthogranulomatous, focal gallbladder wall thickening vs., **372**

Cholecystokinin secretion, decreased, distended gallbladder vs., **366**

Cholecystosis, hyperplastic
- diffuse gallbladder wall thickening vs., **374**
- focal gallbladder wall thickening vs., **372**
- hyperechoic gallbladder wall vs., **380**

Choledochal cyst
- dilated common bile duct vs., **398, 399**
- dilated gallbladder vs., **384**
- dysmorphic liver with abnormal bile ducts vs., **279**
- intrahepatic and extrahepatic duct dilatation vs., **388**
- mimic
    cystic pancreatic mass vs., **427**
    distended gallbladder vs., **366**

Choledochocele, duodenal mass vs., **130**

Choledocholithiasis
- dilated common bile duct vs., **398**
- dilated pancreatic duct vs., **435**
- epigastric pain vs., **118**
- gas in bile ducts or gallbladder vs., **368**
- hypointense lesion in biliary tree (MRCP) vs., **412**
- intrahepatic and extrahepatic duct dilatation vs., **388**
- mimic, pancreatic calcifications vs., **444**
- periportal lesion vs., **356**
- right upper quadrant pain vs., **390**

Cholelithiasis
- echogenic material in gallbladder vs., **382**
- right upper quadrant pain vs., **390**

Choriocarcinoma, solid ovarian masses vs., **688, 689**

Chronic bladder outlet obstruction, abnormal bladder wall vs., **594**

Chronic cholecystitis, diffuse gallbladder wall thickening vs., **374**

Chronic cystitis, abnormal bladder wall vs., **594**

Chronic hepatitis, diffusely abnormal liver echogenicity vs., **334**

Chronic kidney disease, hyperechoic kidney vs., **552**

Chronic mass effect, decreased testicular size vs., **618**

Chronic obstructive pulmonary disease, pneumatosis of small intestine vs., **156**

Chronic renal failure, thickened duodenal fold vs., **138**

Ciliated hepatic foregut cyst
- anechoic liver lesion vs., **337**
- cystic hepatic mass vs., **249**

Cirrhosis
- diffuse hyperechoic liver vs., **328**
- diffusely abnormal liver echogenicity vs., **334**
- dysmorphic liver with abnormal bile ducts vs., **278**
- fatty, hepatomegaly vs., **331**
- irregular hepatic surface vs., **360**
- mimic, multiple biliary strictures vs., **408**
- misty (infiltrated) mesentery vs., **36**
- mosaic/patchy hepatogram vs., **262**
- multiple hypointense liver lesions (T2WI) vs., **294**
- periportal lucency or edema vs., **289**
- portal hypertension with, splenomegaly vs., **222**

- regenerating nodules, multiple hypointense liver lesions (T2WI) vs., **294**
- with regenerative/dysplastic nodule
    multiple hypo-, hyper- or anechoic liver lesions vs., **350**
    multiple hypodense liver lesions vs., **309**
- widened hepatic fissures vs., **276**

Cirrhotic regenerating nodule, focal hyperdense hepatic mass on nonenhanced CT vs., **314**

Clear cell carcinoma, multilocular ovarian cysts vs., **676**

Closed loop small bowel obstruction, cluster of dilated small bowel vs., **144**

Coagulopathic hemorrhage
- filling defect, renal pelvis vs., **570**
- hemoperitoneum vs., **32**
- high-attenuation (hyperdense) ascites vs., **42**
- liver, focal liver lesion with hemorrhage vs., **240**
- retroperitoneal, **476**
    acute left abdominal pain vs., **215**
- spontaneous, perirenal and subcapsular mass lesions vs., **516**

Colitis
- acute
    acute left abdominal pain vs., **214**
    right upper quadrant pain vs., **390, 391**
- granulomatous
    segmental colonic narrowing vs., **194**
    smooth ahaustral colon vs., **206**
- infectious
    acute left abdominal pain vs., **214**
    acute right lower quadrant pain vs., **208**
    colonic thumbprinting vs., **198**
    colonic wall thickening vs., **200**
    rectal or colonic fistula vs., **188**
    segmental colonic narrowing vs., **194**
    toxic megacolon vs., **186**
- ischemic
    acute left abdominal pain vs., **214**
    acute right lower quadrant pain vs., **209**
    colonic ileus vs., **182**
    colonic thumbprinting vs., **198**
    colonic wall thickening vs., **200**
    segmental colonic narrowing vs., **194**
    smooth ahaustral colon vs., **206**
    toxic megacolon vs., **186**
- neutropenic
    acute right lower quadrant pain vs., **209**
    colonic thumbprinting vs., **198**
    colonic wall thickening vs., **200–201**
    segmental colonic narrowing vs., **195**
- pseudomembranous
    colonic thumbprinting vs., **198**
    colonic wall thickening vs., **200**
    diverticulitis, multiple colonic filling defects vs., **174**
- radiation
    segmental colonic narrowing vs., **195**
    smooth ahaustral colon vs., **206**
- stercoral
    acute left abdominal pain vs., **214**
    fecal impaction, colonic ileus vs., **182**

- ulcerative
  - acute left abdominal pain vs., **214**
  - colonic thumbprinting vs., **198**
  - colonic wall thickening vs., **200**
  - multiple colonic filling defects vs., **174**
  - segmental colonic narrowing vs., **194**
  - smooth ahaustral colon vs., **206**
  - toxic megacolon vs., **186**

Collagen vascular diseases, splenomegaly vs., **223**

Collateral vessels and varices, soft-tissue-density retroperitoneal mass vs., **466**

Collecting system
- dilated renal calyces, **566–569**
- filling defect, renal pelvis, **570–573**
- gas in, filling defect, renal pelvis vs., **570**

Colon
- acute left abdominal pain, **214–219**
- acute right lower quadrant pain, **208–213**
- carcinoma
  - acute left abdominal pain vs., **214**
  - acute right lower quadrant pain vs., **209**
  - colonic wall thickening vs., **200**
  - duodenal mass vs., **130**
  - mass or inflammation of ileocecal area vs., **176**
  - multiple colonic filling defects vs., **174**
  - rectal or colonic fistula vs., **188**
  - segmental colonic narrowing vs., **194**
  - solitary colonic filling defect vs., **172**
- fistula, **188–193**
- ileocecal area, mass or inflammation of, **176–181**
- ileus or dilation, **182–185**
  - differential diagnosis, **182**
- intramural hematoma, colonic thumbprinting vs., **198**
- mesenchymal tumor, multiple colonic filling defects vs., **174**
- multiple colonic filling defects, **174–175**
- parasites, multiple colonic filling defects vs., **174**
- pneumatosis of, colonic wall thickening vs., **200, 201**
- polyps
  - multiple colonic filling defects vs., **174**
  - solitary colonic filling defect vs., **172**
- segmental colonic narrowing, **194–197**
- solitary colonic filling defect, **172–173**
- spasm, segmental colonic narrowing vs., **194**
- thumbprinting, **198–199**
- toxic megacolon, **186–187**
- tuberculosis
  - mass or inflammation of ileocecal area vs., **176, 177**
  - segmental colonic narrowing vs., **194**
- urticaria, multiple colonic filling defects vs., **174**
- varices, multiple colonic filling defects vs., **174**
- wall thickening, **200–205**
  - differential diagnosis, **200**

Colon cancer, perforated or obstructed, acute flank pain vs., **539**

Colon mass, extrinsic, duodenal mass vs., **131**

Colonic ileus, toxic megacolon vs., **186**

Colonic interposition, mimic, pneumoperitoneum vs., **29**

Colorectal carcinoma, colonic ileus vs., **182**

Colorectal trauma, rectal or colonic fistula vs., **188, 189**

Colovesical fistula, gas within urinary bladder vs., **592**

Column of Bertin
- hyperechoic renal mass vs., **560**
- hypertrophied, congenital renal anomalies vs., **492**

Common bile duct
- dilated, **398–403**
  - differential diagnosis, **398**
- stone, distal, obstructing, pancreatic duct dilatation vs., **456**

Compartment syndrome, kidney transplant dysfunction vs., **497**

Compensatory renal hypertrophy, enlarged kidney vs., **544**

Conception, retained products of, thickened endometrium vs., **662, 663**

Concretions, **22**

Conduit wall calcifications, **22**

Congenital absence of hepatic segments, widened hepatic fissures vs., **276**

Congenital heart disease, mosaic/patchy hepatogram vs., **262**

Congenital hepatic fibrosis
- dysmorphic liver with abnormal bile ducts vs., **279**
- mosaic/patchy hepatogram vs., **262**
- widened hepatic fissures vs., **276**

Congenital midureteral stricture, ureteral filling defect or stricture vs., **576, 577**

Congenital renal anomalies, **492–495**
- differential diagnosis, **492**

Congestion, splenomegaly vs., **222**

Congestive heart failure
- diffuse gallbladder wall thickening vs., **374**
- hepatomegaly vs., **330**
- splenomegaly vs., **222**

Contracted gallbladder, with gallstones, hyperechoic gallbladder wall vs., **380**

Contrast-induced nephropathy, delayed or persistent nephrogram vs., **531**

Coronary artery disease, epigastric pain vs., **119**

Corpus luteum
- ovarian, acute pelvic pain vs., **650**
- ruptured, acute right lower quadrant pain vs., **208**
- unilocular ovarian cysts vs., **682**

Cortical necrosis, acute, kidney transplant dysfunction vs., **497**

Cortical nephrocalcinosis, calcifications within kidney vs., **488–489**

Cortical parenchymal defect, hyperechoic renal mass vs., **560**

Costal cartilage calcification, mimic, abdominal calcifications vs., **23**

Courvoisier sign, **384**

Cowden disease, mucosal nodularity, esophagus vs., **76**

Cowper gland adenocarcinoma, urethral stricture vs., **600**

Crohn colitis
- acute left abdominal pain vs., **214**
- colonic wall thickening vs., **200**
- segmental colonic narrowing vs., **194**

Crohn disease
- abnormal bladder wall vs., **594, 595**
- acute right lower quadrant pain vs., **208**
- epigastric pain vs., **119**

- esophageal strictures vs., **78**
- esophageal ulceration vs., **74**
- gastric dilation or outlet obstruction vs., **111**
- gastric ulceration without mass vs., **100**
- linitis plastica vs., **115**
- mass or inflammation of ileocecal area vs., **176**
- occult GI bleeding vs., **160**
- rectal or colonic fistula vs., **188**
- segmental or diffuse small bowel wall thickening vs., **150**
- small bowel obstruction vs., **164**
- smooth ahaustral colon vs., **206**
- stenosis, terminal ileum vs., **148**
- thickened duodenal fold vs., **138**
- thickened gastric folds vs., **105**
- toxic megacolon vs., **186**
Crossed renal ectopia, congenital renal anomalies vs., **492**
Cryptorchidism
- decreased testicular size vs., **618**
- groin mass vs., **54–55**
- mimic, abdominal wall defect vs., **60**
- primary or within, soft-tissue-density retroperitoneal mass vs., **467**
Cushing syndrome, atrophy or fatty replacement of pancreas vs., **432**
Cystadenocarcinoma
- enlarged prostate vs., **630**
- focal lesion in prostate vs., **624, 625**
- hepatic calcifications vs., **267**
- mucinous
    multilocular ovarian cysts vs., **676**
    unilocular ovarian cysts vs., **682, 683**
- serous
    multilocular ovarian cysts vs., **676**
    unilocular ovarian cysts vs., **682, 683**
Cystadenofibroma
- calcified ovarian masses vs., **692**
- multilocular ovarian cysts vs., **676**
- ovarian lesions with low T2 signal intensity vs., **696, 697**
- unilocular ovarian cysts vs., **682, 683**
Cystadenoma
- biliary, cystic hepatic mass vs., **248**
- mucinous
    enlarged prostate vs., **630**
    focal lesion in prostate vs., **624, 625**
    multilocular ovarian cysts vs., **676**
    unilocular ovarian cysts vs., **682, 683**
- papillary, extratesticular solid mass vs., **612, 613**
- serous
    cystic retroperitoneal mass vs., **460**
    left upper quadrant mass vs., **124**
    microcystic, cystic retroperitoneal mass vs., **461**
    multilocular ovarian cysts vs., **676**
    unilocular ovarian cysts vs., **682, 683**
Cystic calcification, abdominal, **22**
Cystic dilation of distal ureter, **580–581**
- differential diagnosis, **580**
Cystic duct insertion (mimic), hypointense lesion in biliary tree (MRCP) vs., **412**
Cystic duct remnant, periportal lesion vs., **357**

Cystic fibrosis
- cystic pancreatic mass vs., **427**
- pancreas
    atrophy or fatty replacement of pancreas vs., **432**
    fat-containing lesion of peritoneal cavity vs., **15**
    pancreatic calcifications vs., **445**
- pneumatosis of small intestine vs., **156**
- small bowel obstruction vs., **164**
Cystic hepatic mass, **248–251**
- differential diagnosis, **248**
Cystic kidney disease
- acquired, bilateral renal cysts vs., **508**
- medullary, bilateral renal cysts vs., **508, 509**
Cystic lesions
- periureteral, mimic, cystic dilation of distal ureter vs., **580**
- testicular, **608–609**
Cystic mass, extratesticular, **610–611**
Cystic metastases, cystic pancreatic lesion vs., **449**
Cystic neoplasm
- mimic, cystic mesenteric and omental mass vs., **10**
- mucinous, ovarian lesions with low T2 signal intensity vs., **696, 697**
Cystic ovarian neoplasm, cystic mesenteric and omental mass vs., **10**
Cystic pancreatic lesion, **448–451**
- differential diagnosis, **448**
Cystic pancreatic mass, **426–431**
- differential diagnosis, **426**
Cystic pancreatic neuroendocrine tumor, cystic pancreatic lesion vs., **449**
Cystic pheochromocytoma, cystic retroperitoneal mass vs., **460**
Cystic renal cell carcinoma, cystic renal mass vs., **504, 505**
Cystic renal mass, **504–507**
- differential diagnosis, **504**
Cystic splenic mass, **230–231**
- differential diagnosis, **230**
Cystic teratoma, mature
- calcified ovarian masses vs., **692**
- complications of, acute pelvic pain vs., **650, 651**
- cystic retroperitoneal mass vs., **461**
- unilocular ovarian cysts vs., **682**
Cystitis
- bacterial, abnormal bladder wall vs., **594**
- chronic, abnormal bladder wall vs., **594**
- emphysematous
    abnormal bladder wall vs., **594, 595**
    gas within urinary bladder vs., **592**
    rectal or colonic fistula vs., **188**
- eosinophilic, abnormal bladder wall vs., **594, 595**
- fungal, abnormal bladder wall vs., **594, 595**
- gas within urinary bladder vs., **592**
- rectal or colonic fistula vs., **188**
- tuberculous, abnormal bladder wall vs., **594, 595**
- viral, abnormal bladder wall vs., **594, 595**
Cystitis cystica et glandularis, filling defect in urinary bladder vs., **585**
Cystocele
- female lower genital cysts vs., **638, 639**
- urinary bladder outpouching vs., **590**

Cystoides intestinalis, pneumatosis, pneumoperitoneum vs., **29**

Cysts
- adrenal. *See* Adrenal cyst.
- Bartholin gland, female lower genital cysts vs., **638**
- Bosniak I/II, cystic renal mass vs., **504**
- bronchogenic, extrinsic esophageal mass vs., **68**
- choledochal, mimic, distended gallbladder vs., **366**
- complex, hyperechoic renal mass vs., **560**
- congenital, cystic pancreatic lesion vs., **449**
- dermoid
    calcified ovarian masses vs., **692**
    cystic mesenteric and omental mass vs., **11**
    fat-containing lesion of peritoneal cavity vs., **14**
- duplication. *See* Duplication cyst.
- ejaculatory duct, enlarged prostate vs., **630**
- epidermoid
    testicular, intratesticular mass vs., **604, 605**
    testicular calcifications vs., **620**
    testicular cystic lesions vs., **608**
- epididymal, extratesticular cystic mass vs., **610**
- fimbrial, extraovarian adnexal mass vs., **644**
- Gartner duct, female lower genital cysts vs., **638**
- gastric duplication, stomach intramural mass vs., **96**
- hemorrhagic
    ovarian, acute pelvic pain vs., **650**
    ovarian lesions with low T2 signal intensity vs., **696**
    ruptured, pelvic fluid vs., **634**
    unilocular ovarian cysts vs., **682**
- hepatic. *See* Hepatic cysts.
- hydatid. *See* Hydatid cyst.
- inclusion, posthysterectomy, female lower genital cysts vs., **638, 639**
- intratesticular, testicular cystic lesions vs., **608**
- milk of calcium, hyperechoic renal mass vs., **560**
- Müllerian duct
    enlarged prostate vs., **630**
    female lower genital cysts vs., **638–639**
    focal lesion in prostate vs., **624, 625**
- nabothian, female lower genital cysts vs., **638**
- paraovarian/paratubal, extraovarian adnexal mass vs., **644–645**
- parapelvic, dilated renal pelvis vs., **556**
- peripelvic
    bilateral renal cysts vs., **508**
    cystic renal mass vs., **504**
    dilated renal pelvis vs., **556**
- peritoneal inclusion, pelvic fluid vs., **634**
- postmenopausal, unilocular ovarian cysts vs., **682**
- pyelogenic, dilated renal pelvis vs., **557**
- Skene gland, female lower genital cysts vs., **638**
- Tarlov, extraovarian adnexal mass vs., **644**
- testicular, diffuse testicular enlargement vs., **616**
- tunica albuginea, testicular cystic lesions vs., **608**

D

Deep venous thrombosis, chronic, abdominal calcifications and, **23**

Dengue fever, diffuse gallbladder wall thickening vs., **375**

Dermatomyositis, pneumatosis of small intestine vs., **156**

Dermoid cyst
- calcified ovarian masses vs., **692**
- cystic mesenteric and omental mass vs., **11**
- fat-containing lesion of peritoneal cavity vs., **14**

Desmoid
- abdominal wall mass vs., **49**
- solid mesenteric or omental mass vs., **4**

Diabetes, colonic ileus vs., **182**

Diabetic nephropathy
- chronic, small kidney vs., **548**
- hyperechoic kidney vs., **552**

Diaphragm
- eventration of, elevated or deformed hemidiaphragm vs., **58**
- hernia, traumatic, elevated or deformed hemidiaphragm vs., **58**
- paralyzed, elevated or deformed hemidiaphragm vs., **58**

Diaphragmatic insertions, mimic, solid mesenteric or omental mass vs., **4**

Diffuse adenomyosis
- enlarged uterus vs., **658**
- thickened endometrium vs., **662**

Diffuse gallbladder wall thickening, **374–377**
- differential diagnosis, **374**

Diffuse increased attenuation, spleen, **232–233**

Diffuse neoplastic infiltration, hepatomegaly vs., **331**

Diffuse testicular enlargement, **616–617**
- differential diagnosis, **616**

Diffusely abnormal liver echogenicity, **334–335**
- differential diagnosis, **334**

Dilatation, senescent and postoperative, dilated common bile duct vs., **398**

Dilated duodenum, **136–137**
- differential diagnosis, **136**

Dilated gallbladder, **384–387**
- differential diagnosis, **384**

Dilated pancreatic duct, **434–437**
- differential diagnosis, **434**

Dilated renal calyces, **566–569**
- differential diagnosis, **566**

Dilated small bowel, cluster of, **144–145**
- differential diagnosis of, **144**

Direct hernias, **60**

Distended gallbladder, **366–367**
- differential diagnosis, **366**

Distended urinary bladder
- dilated renal calyces vs., **566**

Diverticula, small bowel
- aneurysmal dilation of small bowel lumen vs., **146**
- pneumoperitoneum vs., **29**

Diverticulitis
- acute flank pain vs., **539**

- acute left abdominal pain vs., **214**
- acute right lower quadrant pain vs., **208**
- cecal, mass or inflammation of ileocecal area vs., **176**
- colonic ileus vs., **182**
- colonic thumbprinting vs., **198**
- colonic wall thickening vs., **200**
- dysmorphic liver with abnormal bile ducts vs., **278**
- filling defect in urinary bladder vs., **584**
- gas within urinary bladder vs., **592**
- infiltration of peripancreatic fat planes vs., **439**
- Meckel
    acute right lower quadrant pain vs., **209**
    extraovarian adnexal mass vs., **644**
- ovarian abscess due to, acute pelvic pain vs., **650**
- pneumoperitoneum vs., **28**
- portal venous gas vs., **274**
- rectal or colonic fistula vs., **188**
- right upper quadrant pain vs., **390, 391**
- segmental colonic narrowing vs., **194**
- sigmoid
    colonic, abnormal bladder wall vs., **594, 595**
    extraovarian adnexal mass vs., **644**
- solitary colonic filling defect vs., **172**
Diverticulosis
- multiple colonic filling defects vs., **174**
- segmental colonic narrowing vs., **194**
Diverticulum
- bladder
    extraovarian adnexal mass vs., **644**
    mimic, cystic dilation of distal ureter vs., **580**
    urinary bladder outpouching vs., **590**
- calyceal
    dilated renal calyces vs., **566, 567**
    dilated renal pelvis vs., **557**
- duodenal, gas in bile ducts or gallbladder vs., **368**
- Killian-Jamieson, **82**
- pulsion, **82, 102**
- traction, **82**
- urethral, female lower genital cysts vs., **638, 639**
- Zenker, **82**
Dominant polycystic disease, autosomal, liver, focal liver lesion with hemorrhage vs., **240**
"Double duct" sign, pancreatic duct dilatation vs., **456**
Drainage catheter, echogenic material in gallbladder vs., **382**
Dromedary hump, congenital renal anomalies vs., **492**
Drug effects, dilated gallbladder vs., **384**
Drug-induced esophagitis
- epigastric pain vs., **118**
- esophageal strictures vs., **78**
- esophageal ulceration vs., **74**
- lesion at pharyngoesophageal junction vs., **72**
- odynophagia vs., **86**
Duct dilatation, intrahepatic and extrahepatic, **388–389**
- differential diagnosis, **388**
Duodenal diverticulum
- gas in bile ducts or gallbladder vs., **368**
- mimic
    cystic pancreatic mass vs., **426**
    hypovascular pancreatic mass vs., **416**
    pancreatic calcifications vs., **444**

Duodenal mass, **130–135**
- differential diagnosis, **130**
- gastric dilation or outlet obstruction vs., **111**
Duodenal varices, thickened duodenal fold vs., **138**
Duodenitis, thickened duodenal fold vs., **138**
Duodenum
- adenocarcinoma, dilated pancreatic duct vs., **435**
- carcinoma
    hypovascular pancreatic mass vs., **416, 417**
- carcinoma, duodenal mass vs., **130**
- dilated, **136–137**
    differential diagnosis, **136**
- diverticulitis, infiltration of peripancreatic fat planes vs., **439**
- hematoma
    duodenal mass vs., **130**
    thickened duodenal fold vs., **138**
- laceration, thickened duodenal fold vs., **138**
- polyps, duodenal mass vs., **130**
- stricture, gastric dilation or outlet obstruction vs., **111**
- ulcer
    epigastric pain vs., **118**
    gastric dilation or outlet obstruction vs., **110**
    infiltration of peripancreatic fat planes vs., **438**
    right upper quadrant pain vs., **390**
    thickened duodenal fold vs., **138**
Duplex collecting system, congenital renal anomalies vs., **493**
Duplication cyst
- duodenal, cystic pancreatic mass vs., **427**
- duodenal mass vs., **130**
- gastric, stomach intramural mass vs., **96**
- gastrointestinal
    aneurysmal dilation of small bowel lumen vs., **146**
    extraovarian adnexal mass vs., **644**
    gastric mass lesions vs., **91**
Dysgerminoma
- calcified ovarian masses vs., **692**
- solid ovarian masses vs., **688, 689**
Dysmotility, esophageal, **84–85**
- differential diagnosis, **84**
Dyspepsia, functional, epigastric pain vs., **118**
Dysplastic kidney, multicystic, small kidney vs., **548**
Dysplastic nodules
- cirrhosis with, multiple hypointense liver lesions (T2WI) vs., **294**
- hepatic, focal hyperdense hepatic mass on nonenhanced CT vs., **314**
- hyperintense liver lesions (T1WI) vs., **298**
Dystrophic calcification
- abdominal, **22**
- calcifications within kidney vs., **488**

E

Eccentric scar, liver mass with central or, **236–239**
Echinococcal cysts
- abdominal calcifications vs., **22**

- echogenic liver mass vs., **345**
- hepatic, hepatic mass with central scar vs., **354**
- hepatic, multiple hypo-, hyper- or anechoic liver lesions vs., **351**
- multiple splenic calcifications vs., **226**

Echogenic liver mass, **344–347**
- differential diagnosis, **344**

Echogenic material, in gallbladder, **382–383**
- differential diagnosis, **382**

Ectopic pancreatic tissue, target (bull's-eye) lesions, stomach vs., **98**

Ectopic pregnancy
- acute pelvic pain vs., **650, 651**
- ruptured
  acute right lower quadrant pain vs., **209**
  hemoperitoneum vs., **32**
  pelvic fluid vs., **634**
- tubal
  abnormal uterine bleeding vs., **668**
  extraovarian adnexal mass vs., **644**

Ectopic ureter, cystic dilation of distal ureter vs., **580**

Edema, misty (infiltrated) mesentery, **36**

Ejaculatory duct cyst
- enlarged prostate vs., **630**
- focal lesion in prostate vs., **624, 625**

Emphysematous cholecystitis
- gas in bile ducts or gallbladder vs., **368**
- hyperechoic gallbladder wall vs., **380**

Emphysematous cystitis
- abnormal bladder wall vs., **594, 595**
- gas within urinary bladder vs., **592**
- rectal or colonic fistula vs., **188**

Emphysematous pyelitis
- filling defect, renal pelvis vs., **570**
- gas in or around kidney vs., **528**

Emphysematous pyelonephritis, hyperechoic renal mass vs., **560–561**

Empyema, gallbladder, distended gallbladder vs., **366**

Endocervicosis, female lower genital cysts vs., **638, 639**

Endocrine disorders, colonic ileus vs., **182**

Endometrial atrophy, abnormal uterine bleeding vs., **668**

Endometrial cancer
- abnormal uterine bleeding vs., **668, 669**
- enlarged uterus vs., **658**
- thickened endometrium vs., **662**

Endometrial carcinoma
- dilated renal calyces vs., **566**
- rectal or colonic fistula vs., **188**

Endometrial hyperplasia
- abnormal uterine bleeding vs., **668–669**
- thickened endometrium vs., **662**

Endometrial implant, extraovarian adnexal mass vs., **644**

Endometrial polyps
- abnormal uterine bleeding vs., **668**
- thickened endometrium vs., **662**

Endometrioid carcinoma, multilocular ovarian cysts vs., **676**

Endometrioma
- extraovarian adnexal mass vs., **644**
- multilocular ovarian cysts vs., **676**
- ovarian, acute pelvic pain vs., **650**

- ovarian lesions with low T2 signal intensity vs., **696**
- rectovaginal septum, female lower genital cysts vs., **638, 639**
- ruptured, pelvic fluid vs., **634, 635**
- solitary colonic filling defect vs., **172**
- unilocular ovarian cysts vs., **682**

Endometriosis
- abdominal wall mass vs., **49**
- acute flank pain vs., **538**
- acute left abdominal pain vs., **214**
- acute right lower quadrant pain vs., **208, 209**
- colonic wall thickening vs., **200**
- cystic mesenteric and omental mass vs., **11**
- extraovarian adnexal mass vs., **644**
- filling defect in urinary bladder vs., **584**
- inguinal canal, groin mass vs., **55**
- mass or inflammation of ileocecal area vs., **176**
- multiple colonic filling defects vs., **174**
- pelvic fluid vs., **634, 635**
- segmental colonic narrowing vs., **194, 195**
- segmental or diffuse small bowel wall thickening vs., **151**
- ureteral filling defect or stricture vs., **576**

Endometritis
- acute pelvic pain vs., **650**
- enlarged uterus vs., **658**
- thickened endometrium vs., **662, 663**

Endometrium
- secretory-phase, thickened endometrium vs., **662**
- thickened, **662–667**
  differential diagnosis, **662**

Enlarged prostate, **630–631**
- differential diagnosis, **630**

Enteritis
- chemotherapy-induced, segmental or diffuse small bowel wall thickening vs., **150**
- infectious
  segmental or diffuse small bowel wall thickening vs., **150**
  stenosis, terminal ileum vs., **148**
- ischemic
  occult GI bleeding vs., **160**
  pneumatosis of small intestine vs., **156**
  segmental or diffuse small bowel wall thickening vs., **150**
  small bowel obstruction vs., **165**
- mesenteric
  acute right lower quadrant pain vs., **208**
  segmental or diffuse small bowel wall thickening vs., **150**
- portal, segmental or diffuse small bowel wall thickening vs., **150**
- radiation
  occult GI bleeding vs., **160**
  segmental or diffuse small bowel wall thickening vs., **151**
  small bowel obstruction vs., **165**
  stenosis, terminal ileum vs., **148**

Enterocolitis, necrotizing, pneumatosis of small intestine vs., **157**

Enterocutaneous fistula, mimics, abdominal wall defects vs., **61**

Enterovesical fistula, gas within urinary bladder vs., **592**

Eosinophilic cholangitis, multiple biliary strictures vs., **408, 409**

Eosinophilic cystitis, abnormal bladder wall vs., **594, 595**

Eosinophilic gastritis
- linitis plastica vs., **114**
- thickened gastric folds vs., **105**

Epidermal inclusion cyst, female lower genital cysts vs., **638**

Epidermoid cyst
- testicular, intratesticular mass vs., **604, 605**
- testicular calcifications vs., **620**
- testicular cystic lesions vs., **608**

Epidermolysis bullosa dystrophica and pemphigoid, esophageal ulceration vs., **74**

Epididymal cyst, extratesticular cystic mass vs., **610**

Epididymal papillary cystadenoma, extratesticular cystic mass vs., **610**

Epididymis
- extratesticular solid mass vs., **612, 613**
- testicular calcifications vs., **620**

Epididymitis
- extratesticular solid mass vs., **612**
- intratesticular mass vs., **604**

Epigastric hernia, abdominal wall defects vs., **60**

Epigastric pain, **118–123**
- differential diagnosis, **118**

Epiploic appendagitis
- acute flank pain vs., **539**
- acute left abdominal pain vs., **214**
- acute right lower quadrant pain vs., **208**
- fat-containing lesion of peritoneal cavity vs., **14**
- right upper quadrant pain vs., **390, 391**

Epithelial tumors, malignant, solid ovarian masses vs., **688**

Epithelioid angiomyolipoma
- calcifications within kidney vs., **489**
- fat-containing renal mass vs., **520–521**
- solid renal mass vs., **501**

Epithelioid hemangioendothelioma
- hepatic, echogenic liver mass vs., **345**
- hepatic calcifications vs., **267**
- liver "mass" with capsular retraction vs., **244**
- liver mass with central or eccentric scar vs., **236**
- multiple hypodense liver lesions vs., **309**

Erdheim-Chester disease
- perirenal and subcapsular mass lesions vs., **517**
- renal sinus lesion vs., **525**

Erosive gastritis, **104**
- linitis plastica vs., **114**

Erythematosus, systemic lupus, diffuse increased attenuation, spleen vs., **232**

Erythematosus, systemic lupus, multiple splenic calcifications vs., **226**

Esophageal carcinoma
- dilated esophagus vs., **80**
- epigastric pain vs., **119**
- esophageal strictures vs., **78**
- intraluminal mass vs., **66**
- lesion at pharyngoesophageal junction vs., **72**
- mimic, extrinsic esophageal mass vs., **68**
- mucosal nodularity, esophagus vs., **76**

Esophageal foreign body
- epigastric pain vs., **119**
- intraluminal mass vs., **66**
- odynophagia vs., **86**

Esophageal inflammation, acute, epigastric pain vs., **118**

Esophageal spasm, diffuse, esophageal dysmotility vs., **84**

Esophageal tumors, intramural (mesenchymal), extrinsic esophageal mass vs., **68**

Esophageal varices, extrinsic esophageal mass vs., **68**

Esophageal webs, lesion at pharyngoesophageal junction vs., **72**

Esophagitis. *See also Candida* esophagitis; Caustic esophagitis; Reflux esophagitis.
- drug-induced
  - epigastric pain vs., **118**
  - esophageal strictures vs., **78**
  - esophageal ulceration vs., **74**
  - lesion at pharyngoesophageal junction vs., **72**
  - odynophagia vs., **86**
- eosinophilic, **78**
- radiation, esophageal strictures vs., **78**
- viral
  - esophageal ulceration vs., **74**
  - intraluminal mass vs., **66**
  - mucosal nodularity, esophagus vs., **76**
  - odynophagia vs., **86**

Esophagus
- adenoma, **66**
- Barrett, mucosal nodularity, esophagus vs., **76**
- dilated, **80–81**
  - differential diagnosis, **80**
- dysmotility, **84–85**
  - differential diagnosis, **84**
- extrinsic mass, **68–71**
  - differential diagnosis, **68**
- intraluminal mass, **66–67**
  - differential diagnosis, **66**
- lesion at pharyngoesophageal junction, **72–73**
- metastases and lymphoma
  - dilated esophagus vs., **80**
  - esophageal strictures vs., **78**
  - extrinsic mass, **68**
  - intraluminal mass vs., **66**
- mucosal nodularity, esophagus vs., **76–77**
  - differential diagnosis, **76**
- odynophagia, **86–87**
  - differential diagnosis, **86**
- outpouchings (diverticula), **82–83**
- strictures, **78–79**
  - differential diagnosis, **78**
- tumors, intramural benign, intraluminal mass vs., **66**
- ulceration, **74–75**
  - differential diagnosis, **74**

Estrogen, unopposed, thickened endometrium vs., **662, 663**

Estrogen-producing tumor of ovary, abnormal uterine bleeding vs., **668**

Ethiodol-treated tumor, liver, hepatic calcifications vs., **266**

Everted ureterocele, urinary bladder outpouching vs., **590**

Excretion, vicarious, high-attenuation (hyperdense) ascites vs., **42**

Exophytic hepatic mass, gastric mass lesions vs., **90**

Exophytic ovarian mass, extraovarian adnexal mass vs., **644**

External hernias
- acute left abdominal pain vs., **215**
- cluster of dilated small bowel vs., **144**
- small bowel obstruction vs., **164**

Extraadrenal myelolipoma, fat-containing retroperitoneal mass vs., **472**

Extrahepatic calcifications, hepatic calcifications vs., **267**

Extramedullary hematopoiesis
- Fat-containing retroperitoneal mass vs., **472**
- perirenal and subcapsular mass lesions vs., **516, 517**
- soft-tissue-density retroperitoneal mass vs., **467**

Extraovarian adnexal mass, **644–649**
- differential diagnosis, **644**

Extraperitoneal sarcoma, extraovarian adnexal mass vs., **644**

Extrarenal pelvis
- dilated renal pelvis vs., **556**
- prominent (mimic), dilated renal calyces vs., **566**

Extrarenal sources, gas in or around kidney vs., **528**

Extratesticular cystic mass, **610–611**
- differential diagnosis, **610**

Extratesticular solid mass, **612–615**
- differential diagnosis, **612**

Extrinsic colon mass, duodenal mass vs., **131**

Extrinsic compression
- of liver, focal hyperperfusion abnormality vs., **283**
- mimic, esophageal strictures vs., **78**

Extrinsic gallbladder lesion, duodenal mass vs., **131**

Extrinsic hepatic mass, duodenal mass vs., **131**

Extrinsic pancreatic masses, duodenal mass vs., **130–131**

Extrinsic renal mass, duodenal mass vs., **131**

Exudative ascites, high-attenuation (hyperdense) ascites vs., **42**

F

Fallopian tube carcinoma, primary, extraovarian adnexal mass vs., **644**

Familial polyposis
- multiple colonic filling defects vs., **174**
- multiple masses or filling defects vs., **142**

Fat attenuation, lesions causing, and echogenic lesions, **560**

Fat-containing lesion, peritoneal cavity, **14–17**
- differential diagnosis, **14**

Fat-containing liver mass, **246–247**
- differential diagnosis, **246**
- focal hepatic echogenic lesion vs., **323**

Fat-containing renal mass, **520–523**
- differential diagnosis, **520**

Fat necrosis
- fat-containing lesion of peritoneal cavity vs., **14**
- solid mesenteric or omental mass vs., **5**

Fatty cirrhosis, hepatomegaly vs., **331**

Fatty infiltration
- asymmetric, normal variant, atrophy or fatty replacement of pancreas vs., **432**
- multifocal, multiple hypodense liver lesions vs., **308**

Fatty liver
- cystic hepatic mass vs., **248**
- diffusely abnormal liver echogenicity vs., **334**
- fat-containing liver mass vs., **246**
- focal sparing, focal hyperdense hepatic mass on nonenhanced CT vs., **314**
- hepatomegaly vs., **330**
- mass (mimic), focal hyperdense hepatic mass on nonenhanced CT vs., **314**
- right upper quadrant pain vs., **390**

Fatty sparing
- focal, hypoechoic liver mass vs., **340**
- liver, periportal lesion vs., **356**

Fecal impaction
- acute left abdominal pain vs., **214**
- stercoral colitis, colonic ileus vs., **182**

Fecalith, abdominal calcifications vs., **23**

Feces
- multiple colonic filling defects vs., **174**
- solitary colonic filling defect vs., **172**

Female genital tract, pneumoperitoneum from, **29**

Female pelvis
- acute pelvic pain in nonpregnant women, **650–655**
- extraovarian adnexal mass, **644–649**
- lower genital cysts, **638–643**
- pelvic fluid, **634–637**

Female reproductive organ calcification, abdominal calcifications vs., **23**

Femoral hernia
- abdominal wall defects vs., **60**
- groin mass vs., **54**
- small bowel obstruction vs., **164**

Fibroepithelial polyp
- acute flank pain vs., **538**
- ureteral, ureteral filling defect or stricture vs., **576, 577**

Fibrofatty mesenteric proliferation ("creeping fat") (mimic), fat-containing lesion of peritoneal cavity vs., **14**

Fibrolamellar carcinoma
- echogenic liver mass vs., **345**
- focal hepatic echogenic lesion vs., **323**
- focal hyperdense hepatic mass on nonenhanced CT vs., **314**
- hepatic mass with central scar vs., **354**

Fibrolamellar hepatocellular carcinoma
- focal hypervascular liver lesion vs., **253**
- hepatic calcifications vs., **266**
- liver mass with central or eccentric scar vs., **236**
- liver mass with mosaic enhancement vs., **258**
- multiple hypointense liver lesions (T2WI) vs., **294–295**

Fibroma
- calcified ovarian masses vs., **692**
- ovarian lesions with low T2 signal intensity vs., **696**
- solid ovarian masses vs., **688**

Fibromatosis
- ovarian lesions with low T2 signal intensity vs., **696, 697**
- solid ovarian masses vs., **688, 689**
Fibropolycystic liver diseases, dysmorphic liver with abnormal bile ducts vs., **279**
Fibrosis
- focal confluent, liver "mass" with capsular retraction vs., **244**
- retroperitoneal
    delayed or persistent nephrogram vs., **530**
    dilated renal calyces vs., **566**
    iliopsoas compartment mass vs., **52**
    perirenal and subcapsular mass lesions vs., **516, 517**
    ureteral filling defect or stricture vs., **576**
Fibrothecoma
- abnormal uterine bleeding vs., **668**
- ovarian lesions with low T2 signal intensity vs., **696**
- solid ovarian masses vs., **688**
Fibrous pseudotumor, extratesticular solid mass vs., **612–613**
Fibrovascular polyp, intraluminal mass vs., **66**
Filling defect
- renal pelvis, **570–573**
    differential diagnosis, **570**
- ureteral, **576–579**
    differential diagnosis, **576**
- in urinary bladder, **584–589**
    differential diagnosis, **584**
Fimbrial cyst, extraovarian adnexal mass vs., **644**
Fistula
- arteriovenous, renal sinus lesion vs., **524**
- biliary-enteric, high-attenuation (hyperdense) bile in gallbladder vs., **378**
- bladder
    filling defect in urinary bladder vs., **584**
    gas within urinary bladder vs., **592**
    urinary bladder outpouching vs., **590**
- colon, **188–193**
    differential diagnosis, **188**
- colovesical, gas within urinary bladder vs., **592**
- enterocutaneous, mimic, abdominal wall defects vs., **61**
- enterovesical, gas within urinary bladder vs., **592**
- gallbladder, hyperechoic gallbladder wall vs., **380**
- vesicocutaneous, gas within urinary bladder vs., **592**
- vesicovaginal, gas within urinary bladder vs., **592**
Flow artifact (mimic), hypointense lesion in biliary tree (MRCP) vs., **412**
Focal adenomyosis, enlarged uterus vs., **658**
Focal confluent fibrosis
- liver "mass" with capsular retraction vs., **244**
- widened hepatic fissures vs., **276**
Focal fatty sparing, hypoechoic liver mass vs., **340**
Focal gallbladder wall thickening, **372–373**
- differential diagnosis, **372**
Focal hepatic echogenic lesion, **322–327**
- differential diagnosis, **322**
Focal hydronephrosis, cystic renal mass vs., **504, 505**
Focal hyperdense hepatic mass, on nonenhanced CT, **314–317**
- differential diagnosis, **314**

Focal hyperperfusion abnormality (THAD or THID), **282–287**
- differential diagnosis, **282**
Focal hypervascular liver lesion, **252–257**
- differential diagnosis, **252**
Focal lesion, in prostate, **624–629**
- differential diagnosis, **624**
Focal liver lesion with hemorrhage, **240–243**
Focal nodular hyperplasia
- fat-containing liver mass vs., **246**
- focal hyperperfusion abnormality vs., **283**
- focal hypervascular liver lesion vs., **252**
- hepatic calcifications vs., **267**
- hepatic mass with central scar vs., **354**
- hyperintense liver lesions (T1WI) vs., **298–299**
- hypoechoic liver mass vs., **341**
- liver lesion with capsule or halo on MR vs., **304**
- liver mass with central or eccentric scar vs., **236**
Focal steatosis
- echogenic liver mass vs., **344**
- focal hepatic echogenic lesion vs., **322**
Follicular cyst, ovarian, acute pelvic pain vs., **650**
Food, multiple masses or filling defects vs., **142**
Foregut cyst, hepatic ciliated, cystic hepatic mass vs., **249**
Foreign body
- esophageal
    epigastric pain vs., **119**
    intraluminal mass vs., **66**
    odynophagia vs., **86**
- filling defect in urinary bladder vs., **585**
- perforation, acute right lower quadrant pain vs., **209**
- rectal or colonic fistula vs., **188, 189**
- retained, liver lesion containing gas vs., **270–271**
- solitary colonic filling defect vs., **172**
Free-flowing ascites, **42**
Functional dyspepsia, epigastric pain vs., **118**
Fundoplication complications
- dilated esophagus vs., **80**
- esophageal dysmotility vs., **84**
- gastric dilation or outlet obstruction vs., **110**
- mimic, esophageal diverticulum, **82**
Fungal cystitis, abnormal bladder wall vs., **594, 595**
Fungal hepatic abscess, target lesions in liver vs., **348**
Fungal infection, adrenal, adrenal mass vs., **481**
Fungus ball, filling defect, renal pelvis vs., **570**

G

Gallbladder
- carcinoma
    asymmetric dilation of intrahepatic bile ducts vs., **404**
    diffuse gallbladder wall thickening vs., **375**
    dilated common bile duct vs., **398, 399**
    dilated gallbladder vs., **384**
    duodenal mass vs., **131**
    focal gallbladder wall thickening vs., **372**
    high-attenuation (hyperdense) bile in gallbladder vs., **378**

- contracted, with gallstones, hyperechoic gallbladder wall vs., **380**
- dilated, **384–387**
- distended, **366–367**
    differential diagnosis, **366**
- echogenic material in, **382–383**
    differential diagnosis, **382**
- empyema, distended gallbladder vs., **366**
- fistula, hyperechoic gallbladder wall vs., **380**
- gas in, **368–371**
    differential diagnosis, **368**
    liver lesion containing gas vs., **270**
- hemorrhage, dilated gallbladder vs., **384–385**
- high-attenuation (hyperdense) bile in, **378–379**
    differential diagnosis, **378**
- hydrops, distended gallbladder vs., **366**
- hyperechoic wall, **380–381**
    differential diagnosis, **380**
    iatrogenic, **380**
- intrahepatic and extrahepatic duct dilatation of, **388–389**
- lesion, extrinsic, duodenal mass vs., **131**
- lymphoma, focal gallbladder wall thickening vs., **372**
- metastases
    diffuse gallbladder wall thickening vs., **375**
    focal gallbladder wall thickening vs., **372**
- porcelain, focal gallbladder wall thickening vs., **372**
- right upper quadrant pain, **390–395**
- sludge, high-attenuation (hyperdense) bile in gallbladder vs., **378**
- torsion/volvulus, dilated gallbladder vs., **385**
- varices, diffuse gallbladder wall thickening vs., **375**
- wall polyps, focal gallbladder wall thickening vs., **372**
- wall thickening
    diffuse, **374–377**
    focal, **372–373**
Gallstones
- abdominal calcifications vs., **22**
- adherent, hyperechoic gallbladder wall vs., **380**
- contracted gallbladder, hyperechoic gallbladder wall vs., **380**
- gas within, gas in bile ducts or gallbladder vs., **368**
- ileus, small bowel obstruction vs., **165**
- large, hyperechoic gallbladder wall vs., **380**
- layering of small, high-attenuation (hyperdense) bile in gallbladder vs., **378**
- right upper quadrant pain vs., **390**
Ganglioneuroma, soft-tissue-density retroperitoneal mass vs., **466**
Gardner syndrome
- gastric mass lesions vs., **90–91**
- multiple colonic filling defects vs., **174**
- multiple masses or filling defects vs., **142**
Gartner duct cyst, female lower genital cysts vs., **638**
Gas
- within gallbladder lumen, echogenic material in gallbladder vs., **382**
- within gallstones, gas in bile ducts or gallbladder vs., **368**
- in or around kidney, **528–529**

- within urinary bladder, **188, 592–593**
    differential diagnosis, **592**
- in wall of ileal conduit, pneumatosis of small intestine vs., **157**
Gas-containing masses, focal hepatic echogenic lesion vs., **323**
Gas-filled duodenal bulb, hyperechoic gallbladder wall vs., **380**
Gas granules, bubbles, undissolved, mucosal nodularity, esophagus vs., **76**
Gastric bezoar, gastric dilation or outlet obstruction vs., **110**
Gastric carcinoma
- dilated esophagus vs., **80**
- epigastric pain vs., **119**
- esophageal dysmotility vs., **84**
- extrinsic esophageal mass vs., **68**
- gastric dilation or outlet obstruction vs., **110**
- gastric mass lesions vs., **90**
- gastric ulceration without mass vs., **100**
- left upper quadrant mass vs., **124**
- linitis plastica vs., **114**
- target (bull's-eye) lesions, stomach vs., **98**
- thickened gastric folds vs., **104**
Gastric distention, left upper quadrant mass vs., **124**
Gastric diverticulum, mimic, adrenal mass vs., **481**
Gastric duplication cyst, stomach intramural mass vs., **96**
Gastric freezing, linitis plastica vs., **115**
Gastric ileus, gastric dilation or outlet obstruction vs., **110**
Gastric injury, linitis plastica vs., **114**
Gastric intramural hematoma, stomach intramural mass vs., **96**
Gastric mass lesion, **90–95**
- differential diagnosis, **90**
Gastric masses, left upper quadrant mass vs., **124**
Gastric metastases and lymphoma
- duodenal mass vs., **130**
- epigastric pain vs., **119**
- gastric dilation or outlet obstruction vs., **111**
- gastric mass lesions vs., **90**
- linitis plastica vs., **114**
- stomach intramural mass vs., **96**
- target (bull's-eye) lesions, stomach vs., **98**
- thickened gastric folds vs., **104**
Gastric polyps, gastric dilation or outlet obstruction vs., **111**
Gastric stromal tumors, target (bull's-eye) lesions, stomach vs., **98**
Gastric tumors, intramural
- gastric mass lesions vs., **90**
- stomach intramural mass vs., **96**
Gastric ulcer
- epigastric pain vs., **118**
- gastric dilation or outlet obstruction vs., **110**
- gastric ulceration without mass vs., **100**
- infiltration of peripancreatic fat planes vs., **438**
- thickened gastric folds vs., **104**
- without mass, **100–101**
    differential diagnosis, **100**

Gastric varices
- gastric mass lesions vs., **90**
- stomach intramural mass vs., **96**

Gastric volvulus, gastric dilation or outlet obstruction vs., **110**

Gastritis
- chemotherapy-induced, thickened gastric folds vs., **105**
- eosinophilic
  - linitis plastica vs., **114**
  - thickened gastric folds vs., **105**
- epigastric pain vs., **118**
- gastric ulceration without mass vs., **100**
- granulomatous, linitis plastica vs., **114**
- linitis plastica vs., **114**
- NSAID-induced, gastric ulceration without mass vs., **100**
- radiation, thickened gastric folds vs., **105**
- thickened gastric folds vs., **104**

Gastroduodenal inflammation, acute, epigastric pain vs., **118**

Gastroduodenal injury, caustic
- gastric ulceration without mass vs., **100**
- linitis plastica vs., **114–115**
- pneumatosis of small intestine vs., **157**
- thickened duodenal fold vs., **138**
- thickened gastric folds vs., **104**

Gastrointestinal bleeding
- occult, **160–163**
  - differential diagnosis, **160**
- overt, occult GI bleeding vs., **160**

Gastrointestinal stromal tumor
- aneurysmal dilation of small bowel lumen vs., **146**
- esophageal, intraluminal mass vs., **66**
- gastric mass lesions vs., **90**
- mimic
  - cystic pancreatic mass vs., **426, 427**
  - hypervascular pancreatic mass vs., **422, 423**
- occult GI bleeding vs., **160**
- segmental colonic narrowing vs., **195**
- solid mesenteric or omental mass vs., **5**
- stomach, epigastric pain vs., **119**

Gastrointestinal tract
- acute inflammatory conditions of, misty (infiltrated) mesentery vs., **36**
- perforation
  - hemoperitoneum vs., **33**
  - high-attenuation (hyperdense) ascites vs., **43**

Gastroparesis
- gastric dilation or outlet obstruction vs., **110**
- left upper quadrant mass vs., **124**

Genital cysts, female lower, **638–643**
- differential diagnosis, **638**

Genital tract, female, pneumoperitoneum from, **29**

Germ cell tumor
- burnt-out, testicular calcifications vs., **620**
- intratesticular mass vs., **604**
- nonseminomatous
  - intratesticular mass vs., **604**
  - testicular cystic lesions vs., **608**
- retroperitoneal, soft-tissue-density retroperitoneal mass vs., **467**
- testicular calcifications vs., **620**

Giant cell carcinoma, hypovascular pancreatic mass vs., **416, 417**

Glisson capsule, pseudolipoma, fat-containing lesion of peritoneal cavity vs., **15**

Glomerulocystic disease, bilateral renal cysts vs., **508, 509**

Glomerulonephritis
- acute, enlarged kidney vs., **544**
- chronic, small kidney vs., **548**
- hyperechoic kidney vs., **552**
- wedge-shaped or striated nephrogram vs., **534**

Glutaraldehyde-induced injury, **78**
- esophageal strictures vs., **78**

Glycogen storage disease
- diffusely abnormal liver echogenicity vs., **334**
- hepatomegaly vs., **331**
- splenomegaly vs., **223**

Glycogenic acanthosis, mucosal nodularity, esophagus vs., **76**

Gonadal stromal tumors, testicular, intratesticular mass vs., **604, 605**

Graft torsion, kidney transplant dysfunction vs., **497**

Graft-vs.-host disease
- esophageal strictures vs., **78**
- pneumatosis of small intestine vs., **157**
- segmental or diffuse small bowel wall thickening vs., **151**

Granuloma
- calcified
  - liver, focal hepatic echogenic lesion vs., **322**
  - multiple hypointense liver lesions (T2WI) vs., **294**
- splenic and hepatic, abdominal calcifications vs., **22**

Granulomatous colitis
- segmental colonic narrowing vs., **194**
- smooth ahaustral colon vs., **206**

Granulomatous gastritis, linitis plastica vs., **114**

Granulomatous infection, healed, multiple splenic calcifications vs., **226**

Granulomatous orchitis, intratesticular mass vs., **604, 605**

Granulomatous prostatitis, focal lesion in prostate vs., **624, 625**

Granulosa cell tumor
- abnormal uterine bleeding vs., **668**
- multilocular ovarian cysts vs., **676, 677**
- solid ovarian masses vs., **688, 689**
- unilocular ovarian cysts vs., **682, 683**

Groin aneurysm, groin mass vs., **55**

Groin arterial puncture site complication, retroperitoneal hemorrhage vs., **476**

Groin arteriovenous fistula, groin mass vs., **54**

Groin hematoma, groin mass vs., **54**

Groin mass, **54–57**

Groin pseudoaneurysm, groin mass vs., **54**

Groove pancreatitis, **434**
- hypovascular pancreatic mass vs., **416, 417**
- infiltration of peripancreatic fat planes vs., **439**
- pancreatic calcifications vs., **445**

Growing teratoma syndrome, fat-containing retroperitoneal mass vs., **472**

Gynecologic causes, acute flank pain, **539**

Gynecologic source, hemoperitoneum vs., **32**

H

Hamartoma, biliary. *See* Biliary hamartoma.
Hamartomatous polyposis syndromes
- gastric mass lesions vs., **91**
- multiple masses or filling defects vs., **142**
Healed granulomatous infection, multiple splenic calcifications vs., **226**
Healed splenic abscess, multiple splenic calcifications vs., **226**
Heart failure
- congestive
  hepatomegaly vs., **330**
  splenomegaly vs., **222**
- misty (infiltrated) mesentery vs., **36**
Helicobacter pylori gastritis, linitis plastica vs., **114**
HELLP syndrome
- focal hyperdense hepatic mass on nonenhanced CT vs., **315**
- focal liver lesion with hemorrhage vs., **240**
- hemoperitoneum vs., **32**
- hyperintense liver lesions (T1WI) vs., **298**
Hemangioendothelioma
- epithelioid
  hepatic calcifications vs., **267**
  liver "mass" with capsular retraction vs., **244**
  liver mass with central or eccentric scar vs., **236**
  multiple hypodense liver lesions vs., **309**
- focal hepatic echogenic lesion vs., **323**
Hemangioma
- adrenal, adrenal mass vs., **481**
- atypical
  hepatic mass with central scar vs., **354**
  hypoechoic liver mass vs., **341**
- focal hyperdense hepatic mass on nonenhanced CT vs., **315**
- hepatic, multiple hypo-, hyper- or anechoic liver lesions vs., **350**
- perirenal and subcapsular mass lesions vs., **516**
- renal sinus lesion vs., **525**
Hematocele, extratesticular cystic mass vs., **610**
Hematologic disorders, splenomegaly vs., **222**
Hematoma
- abdominal wall mass vs., **48**
- gastric
  gastric mass lesions vs., **91**
  intramural, stomach intramural mass vs., **96**
- groin, groin mass vs., **54**
- hepatic
  focal hyperdense hepatic mass on nonenhanced CT vs., **314**
  hypoechoic liver mass vs., **340**
  liver lesion with capsule or halo on MR vs., **304**
  multiple hypo-, hyper- or anechoic liver lesions vs., **351**
  multiple hypointense liver lesions (T2WI) vs., **295**
- iliopsoas, iliopsoas compartment mass vs., **52**
- intramural, gallbladder, focal gallbladder wall thickening vs., **372**
- liver, hyperintense liver lesions (T1WI) vs., **298**
- mesenteric, mimic, solid mesenteric or omental mass vs., **4**
- posttraumatic, testicular cystic lesions vs., **608**
- spherical, coagulopathic hemorrhage, liver, **240**
- splenic, multiple splenic calcifications vs., **226**
- subchorionic, abnormal uterine bleeding vs., **668**
- testicular, intratesticular mass vs., **604–605**
Hematometra, thickened endometrium vs., **662, 663**
Hematosalpinx
- acute pelvic pain vs., **650, 651**
- extraovarian adnexal mass vs., **644**
Hemidiaphragm, elevated or deformed, **58–59**
- differential diagnosis, **58**
Hemobilia, hypointense lesion in biliary tree (MRCP) vs., **412**
Hemochromatosis, secondary, diffuse increased attenuation, spleen vs., **232**
Hemolytic uremic syndrome, colonic wall thickening vs., **200, 201**
Hemonephrosis, dilated renal pelvis vs., **556**
Hemoperitoneum, **32–35**
- differential diagnosis, **32**
- nontraumatic causes of, high-attenuation (hyperdense) ascites vs., **42**
- traumatic, high-attenuation (hyperdense) ascites vs., **42**
Hemorrhage
- coagulopathic
  hemoperitoneum vs., **32**
  high-attenuation (hyperdense) ascites vs., **42**
  liver, focal liver lesion with hemorrhage vs., **240**
- focal lesion in prostate vs., **624–625**
- focal liver lesion with, **240–243**
- gallbladder, dilated gallbladder vs., **384–385**
- within hepatic tumor, focal hyperdense hepatic mass on nonenhanced CT vs., **314**
- intramural, segmental or diffuse small bowel wall thickening vs., **151**
- mesenteric, misty (infiltrated) mesentery vs., **37**
- misty (infiltrated) mesentery vs., **36**
- neoplastic, hemoperitoneum vs., **33**
- recent hepatic, anechoic liver lesion vs., **336**
- renal, acute flank pain vs., **538**
- retroperitoneal, **476–477**
  differential diagnosis, **476**
  soft-tissue-density retroperitoneal mass vs., **466**
Hemorrhagic cholecystitis, high-attenuation (hyperdense) bile in gallbladder vs., **378**
Hemorrhagic cyst
- ovarian, acute pelvic pain vs., **650**
- ovarian lesions with low T2 signal intensity vs., **696**
- ruptured, pelvic fluid vs., **634**
- unilocular ovarian cysts vs., **682**
Hemorrhagic pancreatitis, hemoperitoneum vs., **33**
Hemorrhoids, multiple colonic filling defects vs., **174**
Henoch-Schönlein purpura, dilated gallbladder vs., **385**

Hepatic abscess
- amebic
  - echogenic liver mass vs., **345**
  - epigastric pain vs., **119**
  - focal hepatic echogenic lesion vs., **323**
  - liver lesion containing gas vs., **271**
  - liver lesion with capsule or halo on MR vs., **304**
  - multiple hypodense liver lesions vs., **309**
  - target lesions in liver vs., **348**
- fungal, target lesions in liver vs., **348**
- hydatid, epigastric pain vs., **119**
- pyogenic
  - cystic hepatic mass vs., **248**
  - epigastric pain vs., **119**
  - focal hepatic echogenic lesion vs., **322**
  - focal hyperperfusion abnormality vs., **282**
  - hyperintense liver lesions (T1WI) vs., **298**
  - hypoechoic liver mass vs., **340**
  - liver lesion containing gas vs., **270**
  - liver lesion with capsule or halo on MR vs., **304**
  - multiple hypo-, hyper- or anechoic liver lesions vs., **350–351**
  - multiple hypodense liver lesions vs., **308**
  - right upper quadrant pain vs., **390, 391**
  - target lesions in liver vs., **348**
Hepatic adenoma
- echogenic liver mass vs., **344–345**
- focal hepatic echogenic lesion vs., **323**
- focal hyperdense hepatic mass on nonenhanced CT vs., **314–315**
- focal hypervascular liver lesion vs., **252**
- focal liver lesion with hemorrhage vs., **240**
- hepatic calcifications vs., **266**
- hepatic mass with central scar vs., **354**
- hyperintense liver lesions (T1WI) vs., **298**
- hypoechoic liver mass vs., **341**
- liver lesion with capsule or halo on MR vs., **304**
- liver mass with central or eccentric scar vs., **236**
- liver mass with mosaic enhancement vs., **258**
- multiple hypodense liver lesions vs., **309**
- multiple hypointense liver lesions (T2WI) vs., **294**
- target lesions in liver vs., **348**
Hepatic adrenal rest tumor, hyperintense liver lesions (T1WI) vs., **299**
Hepatic angiomyolipoma
- echogenic liver mass vs., **345**
- focal hypervascular liver lesion vs., **253**
- multiple hypointense liver lesions (T2WI) vs., **295**
Hepatic angiosarcoma, liver mass with mosaic enhancement vs., **259**
Hepatic artery calcifications
- focal hepatic echogenic lesion vs., **322**
- hepatic calcifications vs., **266**
- mimic, gas in bile ducts or gallbladder vs., **368**
- periportal lesion vs., **357**
Hepatic attenuation difference, transient, focal hypervascular liver lesion vs., **252**
Hepatic atypical hemangioma, target lesions in liver vs., **348**
Hepatic calcifications, **266–269**
- abdominal calcifications vs., **22**
- differential diagnosis, **266**
Hepatic cavernous hemangioma
- echogenic liver mass vs., **344**
- focal hepatic echogenic lesion vs., **322**
- focal hyperperfusion abnormality vs., **282–283**
- focal hypervascular liver lesion vs., **252**
- hepatic calcifications vs., **266**
- liver "mass" with capsular retraction vs., **244**
- liver mass with central or eccentric scar vs., **236**
- multiple hypodense liver lesions vs., **308**
Hepatic chemoembolization, transarterial, gas in bile ducts or gallbladder vs., **369**
Hepatic congestion, passive
- periportal lucency or edema vs., **288**
- right upper quadrant pain vs., **390, 391**
Hepatic cysts. *See also* Hydatid cyst.
- anechoic liver lesion vs., **336**
- cystic hepatic mass vs., **248**
- focal liver lesion with hemorrhage vs., **240**
- hemorrhagic, hyperintense liver lesions (T1WI) vs., **298**
- hepatic calcifications vs., **266**
- multiple hypo-, hyper- or anechoic liver lesions vs., **350**
- simple, multiple hypodense liver lesions vs., **308**
Hepatic echinococcal cyst
- anechoic liver lesion vs., **337**
- hepatic mass with central scar vs., **354**
- multiple hypo-, hyper- or anechoic liver lesions vs., **351**
Hepatic epithelioid hemangioendothelioma, echogenic liver mass vs., **345**
Hepatic fissures, widened, **276–277**
Hepatic granulomas, abdominal calcifications vs., **22**
Hepatic hemangioma, multiple hypo-, hyper- or anechoic liver lesions vs., **350**
Hepatic hematoma
- focal hyperdense hepatic mass on nonenhanced CT vs., **314**
- hypoechoic liver mass vs., **340**
- liver lesion with capsule or halo on MR vs., **304**
- multiple hypo-, hyper- or anechoic liver lesions vs., **351**
- multiple hypointense liver lesions (T2WI) vs., **295**
- target lesions in liver vs., **348**
Hepatic hemorrhage, recent, anechoic liver lesion vs., **336**
Hepatic infarction
- liver lesion containing gas vs., **270**
- portal venous gas vs., **274**
- widespread low attenuation within liver vs., **318**
Hepatic inflammation, epigastric pain vs., **119**
Hepatic inflammatory pseudotumor
- cystic hepatic mass vs., **249**
- periportal lucency or edema vs., **289**
Hepatic injury, toxic, widespread low attenuation within liver vs., **318**
Hepatic ligaments and fissures, echogenic liver mass vs., **344**
Hepatic lipoma, echogenic liver mass vs., **345**
Hepatic lymphoma
- anechoic liver lesion vs., **337**
- diffuse hyperechoic liver vs., **328**
- diffuse/infiltrative, periportal lesion vs., **356**
- diffusely abnormal liver echogenicity vs., **334**
- hypoechoic liver mass vs., **341**

- liver "mass" with capsular retraction vs., **244**
- mosaic/patchy hepatogram vs., **262**
- multiple hypo-, hyper- or anechoic liver lesions vs., **350**
- multiple hypodense liver lesions vs., **308**
- periportal lucency or edema vs., **289**
- target lesions in liver vs., **348**
- widespread low attenuation within liver vs., **318**

Hepatic mass
- with central scar, **354–355**
  - differential diagnosis, **354**
- extrinsic, duodenal mass vs., **131**
- left upper quadrant mass vs., **124**

Hepatic metastases
- anechoic liver lesion vs., **336**
- cystic hepatic mass vs., **248**
- diffuse hyperechoic liver vs., **328**
- duodenal mass vs., **130**
- echogenic liver mass vs., **344**
- epigastric pain vs., **119**
- fat-containing liver mass vs., **246**
- focal hepatic echogenic lesion vs., **322**
- focal hyperdense hepatic mass on nonenhanced CT vs., **314**
- focal hypervascular liver lesion vs., **252**
- focal liver lesion with hemorrhage vs., **240**
- hepatic calcifications vs., **266**
- hepatic mass with central scar vs., **354**
- hyperintense liver lesions (T1WI) vs., **298**
- hypoechoic liver mass vs., **340**
- irregular hepatic surface vs., **360**
- liver lesion with capsule or halo on MR vs., **304**
- liver "mass" with capsular retraction vs., **244**
- liver mass with central or eccentric scar vs., **236**
- mimic, multiple biliary strictures vs., **408, 409**
- mosaic/patchy hepatogram vs., **262**
- multiple hypo-, hyper- or anechoic liver lesions vs., **350**
- multiple hypodense liver lesions vs., **308, 309**
- multiple hypointense liver lesions (T2WI) vs., **294**
- periportal lucency or edema vs., **289**
- target lesions in liver vs., **348**
- widespread low attenuation within liver vs., **318**

Hepatic microabscesses, multiple hypo-, hyper- or anechoic liver lesions vs., **351**
Hepatic neoplasm, subcapsular, irregular hepatic surface vs., **360**
Hepatic opportunistic infection
- hepatic calcifications vs., **266–267**
- multiple hypodense liver lesions vs., **308–309**
- widespread low attenuation within liver vs., **318**

Hepatic pseudolipoma, hyperintense liver lesions (T1WI) vs., **299**
Hepatic pseudotumor, focal hyperdense hepatic mass on nonenhanced CT vs., **315**
Hepatic resection, postsurgical, irregular hepatic surface vs., **360**
Hepatic rupture, irregular hepatic surface vs., **360**
Hepatic sarcoidosis
- diffuse hyperechoic liver vs., **328**
- diffusely abnormal liver echogenicity vs., **334**
- mosaic/patchy hepatogram vs., **262**
- multiple hypointense liver lesions (T2WI) vs., **295**

- widespread low attenuation within liver vs., **318**

Hepatic sarcoma, undifferentiated
- cystic hepatic mass vs., **249**
- liver mass with mosaic enhancement vs., **259**

Hepatic schistosomiasis
- diffuse hyperechoic liver vs., **328**
- hepatic calcifications vs., **267**
- periportal lesion vs., **357**

Hepatic steatosis
- multiple hypo-, hyper- or anechoic liver lesions vs., **350**
- right upper quadrant pain vs., **390**

Hepatic surface, irregular, **360–361**
- differential diagnosis, **360**

Hepatic transplantation, liver lesion containing gas vs., **271**
Hepatic trauma
- focal hepatic echogenic lesion vs., **323**
- focal liver lesion with hemorrhage vs., **240**
- high-attenuation (hyperdense) bile in gallbladder vs., **378**
- periportal lesion vs., **356**
- periportal lucency or edema vs., **289**
- retroperitoneal hemorrhage vs., **476**

Hepatic tumor. *See also* Hepatic adenoma.
- epigastric pain vs., **119**
- hemorrhage within, focal hyperdense hepatic mass on nonenhanced CT vs., **314**
- liver lesion containing gas vs., **271**
- right upper quadrant pain vs., **390, 391**

Hepatic venous gas, liver lesion containing gas vs., **271**
Hepatitis
- acute
  - diffuse gallbladder wall thickening vs., **374**
  - diffusely abnormal liver echogenicity vs., **334**
  - hepatomegaly vs., **330**
  - right upper quadrant pain vs., **390**
- chronic, diffusely abnormal liver echogenicity vs., **334**
- diffuse hyperechoic liver vs., **328**
- mosaic/patchy hepatogram vs., **262**
- radiation, widespread low attenuation within liver vs., **318**
- viral and alcoholic, epigastric pain vs., **119**
- widespread low attenuation within liver vs., **318**

Hepatocellular carcinoma
- cystic hepatic mass vs., **249**
- diffuse hyperechoic liver vs., **328**
- diffusely abnormal liver echogenicity vs., **334**
- duodenal mass vs., **130**
- echogenic liver mass vs., **344**
- fat-containing liver mass vs., **246**
- fibrolamellar
  - focal hypervascular liver lesion vs., **253**
  - hepatic calcifications vs., **266**
  - liver mass with central or eccentric scar vs., **236**
  - liver mass with mosaic enhancement vs., **258**
  - multiple hypointense liver lesions (T2WI) vs., **294–295**
- focal hepatic echogenic lesion vs., **323**
- focal hyperdense hepatic mass on nonenhanced CT vs., **314**
- focal hyperperfusion abnormality vs., **282**
- focal hypervascular liver lesion vs., **252**
- focal liver lesion with hemorrhage vs., **240**

- hepatic calcifications vs., **266**
- hepatic mass with central scar vs., **354**
- hyperintense liver lesions (T1WI) vs., **298**
- hypoechoic liver mass vs., **340–341**
- infiltrative
    hepatomegaly vs., **331**
    irregular hepatic surface vs., **360**
- liver lesion with capsule or halo on MR vs., **304**
- liver "mass" with capsular retraction vs., **244**
- liver mass with central or eccentric scar vs., **236**
- liver mass with mosaic enhancement vs., **258**
- multiple hypo-, hyper- or anechoic liver lesions vs., **350**
- multiple hypodense liver lesions vs., **308**
- multiple hypointense liver lesions (T2WI) vs., **294**
- periportal lucency or edema vs., **289**
- target lesions in liver vs., **348**
- widespread low attenuation within liver vs., **318**
Hepatogram, mosaic/patchy, **262–263**
- differential diagnosis, **262**
Hepatolithiasis, asymmetric dilation of intrahepatic bile ducts vs., **404, 405**
Hepatomegaly, **330–333**
- differential diagnosis, **330**
- duodenal mass vs., **131**
- left upper quadrant mass vs., **124**
Hereditary hemorrhagic telangiectasia
- focal hyperperfusion abnormality vs., **283**
- focal hypervascular liver lesion vs., **252**
- mosaic/patchy hepatogram vs., **262**
- multiple hypointense liver lesions (T2WI) vs., **295**
Hernia
- Bochdalek, elevated or deformed hemidiaphragm vs., **58**
- diaphragmatic, traumatic, elevated or deformed hemidiaphragm vs., **58**
- external, cluster of dilated small bowel vs., **144**
- femoral
    abdominal wall defects vs., **60**
    abdominal wall mass vs., **48**
    groin mass vs., **54**
- hiatal
    dilated esophagus mimic, **80**
    elevated or deformed hemidiaphragm vs., **58**
    extrinsic esophageal mass vs., **68**
    intrathoracic stomach vs., **102**
    mimic, esophageal diverticulum, **82**
- incisional, abdominal wall defects vs., **60**
- inguinal
    abdominal wall defects vs., **60**
    abdominal wall mass vs., **48**
    extratesticular solid mass vs., **612**
    groin mass vs., **54**
- lumbar
    abdominal wall defects vs., **60**
    abdominal wall mass vs., **48**
- Morgagni, elevated or deformed hemidiaphragm vs., **58**
- obturator, abdominal wall defects vs., **61**
- paraduodenal, cluster of dilated small bowel vs., **144**
- perineal, abdominal wall defects vs., **61**
- sciatic, abdominal wall defects vs., **61**
- small bowel obstruction vs., **164**

- transmesenteric postoperative, cluster of dilated small bowel vs., **144**
- umbilical
    abdominal wall defects vs., **60–61**
    abdominal wall mass vs., **48**
- ventral
    abdominal wall defects vs., **60**
    abdominal wall mass vs., **48**
    acute left abdominal pain vs., **215**
    small bowel obstruction vs., **164**
Heterotopic pregnancy
- extraovarian adnexal mass vs., **644, 645**
Hiatal hernia
- dilated esophagus mimic, **80**
- elevated or deformed hemidiaphragm vs., **58**
- extrinsic esophageal mass vs., **68**
- intrathoracic stomach vs., **102**
- mimic, esophageal diverticulum, **82**
Hibernoma (brown fat), fat-containing retroperitoneal mass vs., **472**
High-attenuation (hyperdense) ascites, **42–45**
- differential diagnosis, **42**
- hemoperitoneum vs., **33**
High-attenuation (hyperdense) bile, in gallbladder, **378–379**
- differential diagnosis, **378**
Histiocytosis, Langerhans cell, xanthomatous lesions in, fat-containing liver mass vs., **246**
Histoplasmosis, multiple splenic calcifications vs., **226**
HIV, mesenteric lymphadenopathy vs., **19**
HIV-associated nephropathy
- chronic, small kidney vs., **548**
- enlarged kidney vs., **544, 545**
- hyperechoic kidney vs., **553**
Horseshoe kidney
- congenital renal anomalies vs., **492**
- enlarged kidney vs., **545**
Hydatid cyst
- cystic mesenteric and omental mass vs., **11**
- cystic pancreatic mass vs., **426, 427**
- hepatic
    asymmetric dilation of intrahepatic bile ducts vs., **404, 405**
    echogenic liver mass vs., **345**
    focal hepatic echogenic lesion vs., **323**
    hepatic calcifications vs., **266**
    liver lesion containing gas vs., **271**
- hepatic, cystic hepatic mass vs., **248**
Hydatid disease, hepatic, dysmorphic liver with abnormal bile ducts vs., **279**
Hydatiform mole, abnormal uterine bleeding vs., **668**
Hydrocele
- canal of Nuck, groin mass vs., **55**
- extratesticular cystic mass vs., **610**
Hydrometrocolpos, cystic mesenteric and omental mass vs., **11**
Hydronephrosis, enlarged kidney vs., **544**
Hydrops
- dilated gallbladder vs., **384**
- gallbladder, distended gallbladder vs., **366**

Hydrosalpinx, extraovarian adnexal mass vs., **644**

Hydroureter, extraovarian adnexal mass vs., **644**

Hyperechoic gallbladder wall, **380–381**
- differential diagnosis, **380**
- iatrogenic, **380**

Hyperechoic liver, diffuse, **328–329**
- differential diagnosis, **328**

Hyperechoic metastases, echogenic liver mass vs., **344**

Hyperechoic renal mass, **560–563**
- differential diagnosis, **560**

Hyperintense liver lesions (T1WI), **298–303**
- differential diagnosis, **298**

Hyperparathyroidism, pancreatic calcifications vs., **445**

Hyperperfusion abnormality, focal, **282–287**
- differential diagnosis, **282**

Hyperplastic cholecystosis
- diffuse gallbladder wall thickening vs., **374**
- focal gallbladder wall thickening vs., **372**
- hyperechoic gallbladder wall vs., **380**

Hyperplastic polyps, gastric mass lesions vs., **90**

Hyperstimulation syndrome, ovarian
- acute pelvic pain vs., **650, 651**
- multilocular ovarian cysts vs., **676, 677**
- pelvic fluid vs., **634, 635**

Hypertension, portal
- cirrhosis with, splenomegaly vs., **222**
- colonic wall thickening vs., **200**
- colopathy, colonic thumbprinting vs., **198**
- misty (infiltrated) mesentery vs., **36**
- portal vein abnormality vs., **362**

Hyperthecosis, solid ovarian masses vs., **688, 689**

Hypervascular pancreatic mass, **422–425**
- differential diagnosis, **422**

Hypervolemia, systemic, periportal lucency or edema vs., **288**

Hypoalbuminemia, diffuse gallbladder wall thickening vs., **374**

Hypodense liver lesions, multiple, **308–312**
- differential diagnosis, **308**

Hypoechoic liver mass, **340–343**
- differential diagnosis, **340**

Hypogonadism, decreased testicular size vs., **618**

Hypointense lesion in biliary tree (MRCP), **412–413**
- differential diagnosis, **412**

Hypointense liver lesions (T2WI), multiple, **294–297**
- differential diagnosis, **294**

Hypotension
- delayed or persistent nephrogram vs., **530**
- systemic, segmental or diffuse small bowel wall thickening vs., **150**

Hypothyroidism, colonic ileus vs., **182**

Hypovascular pancreatic mass, **416–421**
- differential diagnosis, **416**

I

Iatrogenic and postoperative stricture, ureteral filling defect or stricture vs., **576**

Iatrogenic injury
- hemoperitoneum vs., **32**
- pneumoperitoneum vs., **28**
- urethral stricture vs., **600**

Iatrogenic material, periportal lesion vs., **357**

Iatrogenic ureteral injury, acute flank pain vs., **538**

IgG4-related disease
- enlarged prostate vs., **630**
- ureteral filling defect or stricture vs., **576, 577**

IgG4-related kidney disease
- infiltrative renal lesions vs., **512, 513**
- solid renal mass vs., **501**
- wedge-shaped or striated nephrogram vs., **534, 535**

Ileal conduit, gas in wall of, pneumatosis of small intestine vs., **157**

Ileocecal area, mass or inflammation of, **176–181**
- differential diagnosis, **176**

Ileocecal valve
- lipoma of, mass or inflammation of ileocecal area vs., **176**
- lipomatous infiltration
  mass or inflammation of ileocecal area vs., **176**
  mimic, fat-containing lesion of peritoneal cavity vs., **15**
- prominent, mass or inflammation of ileocecal area vs., **176**

Ileocolitis, infectious, mass or inflammation of ileocecal area vs., **176**

Ileus
- colonic, **182–185**
  differential diagnosis, **182**
  toxic megacolon vs., **186**
- colonic ileus vs., **182**
- dilated duodenum vs., **136**
- gastric, gastric dilation or outlet obstruction vs., **110**
- small bowel obstruction vs., **164**

Iliopsoas bursitis, groin mass vs., **55**

Iliopsoas compartment mass, **52–53**
- differential diagnosis, **52**

Iliopsoas hematoma, iliopsoas compartment mass vs., **52**

Immature teratoma
- calcified ovarian masses vs., **692**
- solid ovarian masses vs., **688, 689**

Incisional hernia, abdominal wall defects vs., **60**

Inclusion cyst
- epidermal, female lower genital cysts vs., **638**
- peritoneal
  cystic mesenteric and omental mass vs., **11**
  extraovarian adnexal mass vs., **644, 645**
- posthysterectomy, female lower genital cysts vs., **638, 639**

Indirect hernia, **60**

Infarction
- acute pelvic pain vs., **651**

- hepatic
    liver lesion containing gas vs., **270**
    portal venous gas vs., **274**
    widespread low attenuation within liver vs., **318**
- renal
    acute flank pain vs., **539**
    acute left abdominal pain vs., **215**
    chronic, small kidney vs., **549**
    gas in or around kidney vs., **528**
    wedge-shaped or striated nephrogram vs., **534**
- splenic
    cystic splenic mass vs., **230**
    diffuse increased attenuation, spleen vs., **232**
    mimic, solid splenic mass vs., **228**
    multiple splenic calcifications vs., **226**
    splenomegaly vs., **223**
- testicular
    diffuse testicular enlargement vs., **616**
    intratesticular mass vs., **604**
Infected biloma, hypoechoic liver mass vs., **341**
Infection
- healed granulomatous, multiple splenic calcifications vs., **226**
- primary, iliopsoas compartment mass vs., **52**
- recurrent, small kidney vs., **548**
- secondary, iliopsoas compartment mass vs., **52**
Infectious cholecystitis, dilated gallbladder vs., **385**
Infectious colitis
- acute left abdominal pain vs., **214**
- acute right lower quadrant pain vs., **208**
- colonic thumbprinting vs., **198**
- colonic wall thickening vs., **200**
- duodenal mass vs., **130**
- portal venous gas vs., **274**
- rectal or colonic fistula vs., **188**
- segmental colonic narrowing vs., **194**
- toxic megacolon vs., **186**
Infectious enteritis
- segmental or diffuse small bowel wall thickening vs., **150**
- stenosis, terminal ileum vs., **148**
Infectious ileocolitis, mass or inflammation of ileocecal area vs., **176**
Infectious/inflammatory nodes, soft-tissue-density retroperitoneal mass vs., **466**
Infectious ureteritis, ureteral filling defect or stricture vs., **576**
Inferior vena cava, duplications and anomalies of, soft-tissue-density retroperitoneal mass vs., **466**
Infiltrating lesions, gastric dilation or outlet obstruction vs., **111**
Infiltration
- leukemic or lymphomatous, of peritoneum, misty (infiltrated) mesentery vs., **37**
- of peripancreatic fat planes, **438–443**
    differential diagnosis, **438**
- postsurgical mesenteric, misty (infiltrated) mesentery vs., **36**
Infiltrative diseases, splenomegaly vs., **222**
Infiltrative granulomatous diseases, linitis plastica vs., **115**

Infiltrative hepatocellular carcinoma
- hepatomegaly vs., **331**
- irregular hepatic surface vs., **360**
Infiltrative metastasis, diffusely abnormal liver echogenicity vs., **334**
Infiltrative renal lesions, **512–515**
- differential diagnosis, **512**
Infiltrative renal mass
- delayed or persistent nephrogram vs., **531**
- wedge-shaped or striated nephrogram vs., **535**
Inflammation
- by intrinsic or adjacent process, distended gallbladder vs., **366**
- misty (infiltrated) mesentery, **36**
- near ampulla, gas in bile ducts or gallbladder vs., **369**
Inflammatory bowel disease, pneumatosis of small intestine vs., **157**
Inflammatory diseases, urethral stricture vs., **600**
Inflammatory myofibroblastic pseudotumor, filling defect in urinary bladder vs., **585**
Inflammatory polyp, esophagus, intraluminal mass vs., **66**
Inflammatory pseudotumor
- hepatic, cystic hepatic mass vs., **249**
- liver "mass" with capsular retraction vs., **244**
Inguinal abscess, groin mass vs., **55**
Inguinal canal
- endometriosis, groin mass vs., **55**
- metastases to, groin mass vs., **55**
Inguinal hernia
- abdominal wall defects vs., **60**
- acute left abdominal pain vs., **215**
- extratesticular solid mass vs., **612**
- groin mass vs., **54**
- small bowel obstruction vs., **164**
Inguinal lymphadenopathy, groin mass vs., **54**
Injection site, abdominal wall mass vs., **48**
Instrumentation, gas in or around kidney vs., **528**
Intensity difference, focal hyperperfusion abnormality vs., **282**
Internal hernia, small bowel obstruction vs., **165**
Interparietal hernia, **60**
Interstitial fibrosis, kidney transplant dysfunction vs., **496**
Interstitial nephritis, acute, hyperechoic kidney vs., **552**
Intestinal lymphangiectasia, misty (infiltrated) mesentery vs., **37**
Intestinal scleroderma, dilated duodenum vs., **136**
Intestines. *See also* Colon; Diverticulum; Small intestine.
- lipoma, fat-containing lesion of peritoneal cavity vs., **15**
- lymphoma
    multiple masses or filling defects vs., **142**
    segmental or diffuse small bowel wall thickening vs., **151**
- metastases
    multiple masses or filling defects vs., **142**
    segmental or diffuse small bowel wall thickening vs., **151**
- parasitic disease
    multiple masses or filling defects vs., **142**
    small bowel obstruction vs., **165**

- trauma
    pneumatosis of small intestine vs., **157**
    pneumoperitoneum vs., **28**
    small bowel obstruction vs., **165**
- tumor, intramural benign
    multiple masses or filling defects vs., **142**
    occult GI bleeding vs., **160**
Intraductal papillary mucinous neoplasm
- cystic pancreatic lesion vs., **448**
- cystic pancreatic mass vs., **426**
- dilated pancreatic duct vs., **434–435**
- pancreatic calcifications vs., **445**
- pancreatic duct dilatation vs., **456**
Intraductal stones, asymmetric dilation of intrahepatic bile ducts vs., **404, 405**
Intrahepatic bile ducts, asymmetric dilation of, **404–407**
- differential diagnosis, **404**
Intrahepatic biliary calculi
- focal hepatic echogenic lesion vs., **322**
- hepatic calcifications vs., **266**
Intrahepatic calculi parasites, hepatic calcifications vs., **267**
Intrahepatic cholangiocarcinoma, liver mass with central or eccentric scar vs., **236**
Intrahepatic pseudocyst, cystic hepatic mass vs., **249**
Intraluminal duodenal lesions, duodenal mass vs., **130**
Intraluminal mass, esophagus, differential diagnosis, **66**
Intramural benign intestinal tumors
- multiple masses or filling defects vs., **142**
- occult GI bleeding vs., **160**
Intramural duodenal lesions, duodenal mass vs., **130**
Intramural gastric tumors, stomach intramural mass vs., **96**
Intramural hematoma
- colon, colonic thumbprinting vs., **198**
- gallbladder, focal gallbladder wall thickening vs., **372**
- solitary colonic filling defect vs., **172**
Intramural hemorrhage
- colonic wall thickening vs., **200, 201**
- segmental or diffuse small bowel wall thickening vs., **151**
Intramural leiomyomas, enlarged uterus vs., **658**
Intramural mass, **96–97**
- differential diagnosis, **96**
Intrapancreatic splenule, solid pancreatic lesion vs., **453**
Intrarenal abscess, dilated renal pelvis vs., **557**
Intrarenal varices, dilated renal pelvis vs., **557**
Intratesticular cyst, testicular cystic lesions vs., **608**
Intratesticular mass, **604–607**
- differential diagnosis, **604**
Intratesticular varicocele, testicular cystic lesions vs., **608**
Intrathoracic stomach, **102–103**
- differential diagnosis, **102**
Intrauterine device
- malpositioned, acute pelvic pain vs., **650, 651**
- perforation, abnormal uterine bleeding vs., **668**
Intussusception
- acute right lower quadrant pain vs., **209**
- mass or inflammation of ileocecal area vs., **177**
- mimic, fat-containing lesion of peritoneal cavity vs., **15**
- small bowel obstruction vs., **165**
Inverted appendical stump, solitary colonic filling defect vs., **172**

Inverted papilloma, filling defect in urinary bladder vs., **585**
Irregular hepatic surface, **360–361**
- differential diagnosis, **360**
Ischemic cholecystitis, dilated gallbladder vs., **385**
Ischemic colitis
- acute left abdominal pain vs., **214**
- acute right lower quadrant pain vs., **209**
- colonic ileus vs., **182**
- colonic thumbprinting vs., **198**
- colonic wall thickening vs., **200**
- mass or inflammation of ileocecal area vs., **176**
- pneumatosis of small intestine vs., **156**
- portal venous gas vs., **274**
- segmental colonic narrowing vs., **194**
- smooth ahaustral colon vs., **206**
- toxic megacolon vs., **186**
Ischemic enteritis
- acute right lower quadrant pain vs., **209**
- occult GI bleeding vs., **160**
- pneumatosis of small intestine vs., **156**
- portal venous gas vs., **274**
- segmental or diffuse small bowel wall thickening vs., **150**
- small bowel obstruction vs., **165**

J

Junctional parenchymal defect, fat-containing renal mass vs., **520**
Juxtaglomerular cell tumor, solid renal mass vs., **501**

K

Kaposi sarcoma
- abdominal wall mass vs., **49**
- target (bull's-eye) lesions, stomach vs., **98**
Keloid, abdominal wall mass vs., **48**
Kidney
- acute flank pain, **538–543**
- bilateral renal cysts, **508–511**
- calcifications within, **488–491**
    differential diagnosis, **488**
- congenital renal anomalies, **492–495**
    differential diagnosis, **492**
- cystic renal mass, **504–507**
- delayed or persistent nephrogram, **530–533**
- enlarged, **544–547**
    differential diagnosis, **544**
- fat-containing mass, **520–523**
- gas in or around, **528–529**
- horseshoe
    congenital renal anomalies vs., **492**
    enlarged kidney vs., **545**
- hyperechoic, **552–555**
    differential diagnosis, **552**

- infarction
    chronic, small kidney vs., **549**
    gas in or around kidney vs., **528**
    wedge-shaped or striated nephrogram vs., **534**
- infiltrative lesions, **512–515**
- instrumentation of, filling defect, renal pelvis vs., **570**
- lymphoma, dilated renal pelvis vs., **557**
- perirenal and subcapsular mass lesions, **516–519**
- prominent vessel, dilated renal pelvis vs., **556**
- renal scar, fat in, fat-containing renal mass vs., **520**
- renal sinus lesion, **524–527**
- small, **548–551**
    differential diagnosis, **548**
- solid mass, **500–503**
- solid renal mass, **500–503**
    differential diagnosis, **500**
- supernumerary, small kidney vs., **549**
- transplant dysfunction, **496–499**
    differential diagnosis, **496**
- transplant rejection, hyperechoic kidney vs., **552**
- trauma
    hyperechoic renal mass vs., **561**
    perirenal and subcapsular mass lesions vs., **516**
    retroperitoneal hemorrhage vs., **476**
    wedge-shaped or striated nephrogram vs., **534**
- tumors, primary, enlarged kidney vs., **544**
- wedge-shaped or striated nephrogram, **534–537**
Killian-Jamieson diverticulum, esophageal outpouchings
    (diverticula) vs., **82**
Krukenberg tumor, ovarian lesions with low T2 signal
    intensity vs., **696–697**
Kwashiorkor, pancreatic calcifications vs., **445**

L

Langerhans cell histiocytosis, xanthomatous lesions in, fat-
    containing liver mass vs., **246**
Large cell calcifying Sertoli cell tumor, testicular
    calcifications vs., **620**
Lead poisoning, chronic, small kidney vs., **549**
Left upper quadrant mass, **124–127**
  - differential diagnosis, **124**
Leiomyoma
  - abnormal uterine bleeding vs., **668**
  - cervical, enlarged uterus vs., **658**
  - enlarged uterus vs., **658**
  - extratesticular solid mass vs., **612**
  - intramural, enlarged uterus vs., **658**
  - intramural, thickened endometrium vs., **662**
  - mimic, calcified ovarian masses vs., **692**
  - perirenal and subcapsular mass lesions vs., **516**
  - renal sinus lesion vs., **525**
  - solid renal mass vs., **501**
  - submucosal, thickened endometrium vs., **662**
  - subserosal, extraovarian adnexal mass vs., **644**
  - thickened endometrium vs., **662**
  - tubal, extraovarian adnexal mass vs., **644**

Leiomyomatosis peritonealis disseminata, solid mesenteric
    or omental mass vs., **5**
Leiomyosarcoma
  - extratesticular solid mass vs., **612**
  - ovarian vein, extraovarian adnexal mass vs., **644, 645**
  - perirenal and subcapsular mass lesions vs., **517**
  - soft-tissue-density retroperitoneal mass vs., **466**
  - uterine
      abnormal uterine bleeding vs., **668**
      enlarged uterus vs., **658**
Lesser sac ascites (mimic), cystic pancreatic mass vs., **426**
Leukemia
  - abdominal wall mass vs., **49**
  - delayed or persistent nephrogram vs., **531**
  - renal, infiltrative renal lesions vs., **512**
  - solid mesenteric or omental mass vs., **5**
  - solid renal mass vs., **500**
  - testicular
      diffuse testicular enlargement vs., **616**
      intratesticular mass vs., **604, 605**
Leukoplakia, mucosal nodularity, esophagus vs., **76**
Leydig cell hyperplasia, intratesticular mass vs., **604, 605**
Lichen sclerosus, urethral stricture vs., **600**
Lipoma
  - abdominal wall mass vs., **48**
  - extratesticular solid mass vs., **612**
  - fat-containing renal mass vs., **520**
  - of ileocecal valve, mass or inflammation of ileocecal
      area vs., **176**
  - intestine, fat-containing lesion of peritoneal cavity vs.,
      15
  - liver, hyperintense liver lesions (T1WI) vs., **299**
  - retroperitoneal, fat-containing retroperitoneal mass,
      472
  - spermatic cord, groin mass vs., **54**
Lipomatosis
  - peritoneal, fat-containing lesion of peritoneal cavity vs.,
      15
  - renal replacement
      fat-containing renal mass vs., **520**
      renal sinus lesion vs., **524**
  - renal sinus, lucent, dilated renal pelvis vs., **557**
  - testicular, intratesticular mass vs., **604, 605**
Lipomatous infiltration, ileocecal valve, mimic, fat-
    containing lesion of peritoneal cavity vs., **15**
Lipomatous pseudohypertrophy
  - atrophy or fatty replacement of pancreas vs., **432**
  - pancreas, mimic, fat-containing lesion of peritoneal
      cavity vs., **15**
Lipomatous solitary fibrous tumor, fat-containing renal
    mass vs., **521**
Liposarcoma
  - abdominal wall defects vs., **61**
  - extratesticular solid mass vs., **612**
  - fat-containing lesion of peritoneal cavity vs., **15**
  - fat-containing liver mass vs., **246**
  - fat-containing renal mass vs., **520**
  - fat-containing retroperitoneal mass vs., **472**
  - groin mass vs., **55**
  - liver, hyperintense liver lesions (T1WI) vs., **299**

- metastatic, liver mass with mosaic enhancement vs., **258**
- misty (infiltrated) mesentery vs., **37**
- perirenal and subcapsular mass lesions vs., **516**
- primary or metastatic, liver mass with mosaic enhancement vs., **258**

Lithium nephropathy
- bilateral renal cysts vs., **508**
- hyperechoic kidney vs., **553**

Liver
- anechoic liver lesion, **336–339**
- biopsy/trauma, focal hyperperfusion abnormality vs., **282**
- congested, hepatomegaly vs., **330**
- cystic hepatic mass, **248–251**
- diffusely abnormal liver echogenicity, **334–335**
- dysmorphic, with abnormal bile ducts, **278–281**
    differential diagnosis, **278**
- dysplastic nodules, **298**
- echogenic liver mass, **344–347**
- fatty, hepatomegaly vs., **330**
- fatty sparing, periportal lesion vs., **356**
- focal hepatic echogenic lesion, **322–327**
- focal hyperdense hepatic mass on nonenhanced CT, **314–317**
- focal hyperperfusion abnormality, **282–287**
    differential diagnosis, **282**
- focal hypervascular lesion, **252–257**
- focal liver lesion with hemorrhage, **240–243**
- hematoma, hyperintense liver lesions (T1WI) vs., **298**
- hepatic calcifications, **266–269**
    differential diagnosis, **266**
- hepatic fissures, widened, **276–277**
    differential diagnosis, **276**
- hepatic mass with central scar, **354–355**
- hyperechoic, diffuse, **328–329**
    differential diagnosis, **328**
- hyperintense lesions (T1WI), **298–303**
    differential diagnosis, **298**
- hypodense lesions, multiple, **308–312**
- hypoechoic liver mass, **340–343**
- hypointense lesions, multiple (T2WI), **294–297**
- irregular hepatic surface, **360–361**
- lesion with capsule or halo on MR, **304–307**
    differential diagnosis, **304**
- metastases
    focal hyperperfusion abnormality vs., **282**
    widened hepatic fissures vs., **276**
- mosaic/patchy hepatogram, **262–263**
    differential diagnosis, **262**
- multiple hypo-, hyper- or anechoic liver lesions, **350–353**
- normal anatomic pitfalls, **322–323**
- periportal lesion, **356–359**
- periportal lucency or edema, **288–293**
    differential diagnosis, **288**
- portal vein abnormality, **362–363**
- portal venous gas, **274–275**
    differential diagnosis, **274**
- posttransplant, periportal lucency or edema vs., **289**
- regenerating (cirrhotic) nodules, **294**

- target lesions in, **348–349**
    differential diagnosis, **348**
- tumors
    alcohol-ablated, mimic, fat-containing liver mass vs., **246**
    asymmetric dilation of intrahepatic bile ducts vs., **404**
- widespread low attenuation, **318–321**

Liver disease, fibropolycystic, dysmorphic liver with abnormal bile ducts vs., **279**

Liver lesion
- with capsule or halo on MR, **304–307**
    differential diagnosis, **304**
- containing gas, **270–273**
    differential diagnosis, **270**

Liver mass
- with capsular retraction, **244–245**
- with central or eccentric scar, **236–239**
- fat-containing, **246–247**
- with mosaic enhancement, **258–261**

Localized cystic renal disease, cystic renal mass vs., **504, 505**

Loculated ascites, cystic mesenteric and omental mass vs., **10**

Loin pain hematuria syndrome, acute flank pain vs., **539**

Lumbar hernia
- abdominal wall defects vs., **60**
- abdominal wall mass vs., **48**

Lung volume, loss, unilateral, elevated or deformed hemidiaphragm vs., **58**

Lupus, pneumatosis of small intestine vs., **156**

Lupus nephritis, chronic, small kidney vs., **548**

Lymph nodes
- calcified, abdominal calcifications vs., **23**
- mediastinal, extrinsic esophageal mass vs., **68**

Lymphadenopathy
- cervical, lesion at pharyngoesophageal junction vs., **72**
- cystic mesenteric and omental mass vs., **11**
- inguinal, groin mass vs., **54**
- peripancreatic, mimic, hypovascular pancreatic mass vs., **416**
- periportal, asymmetric dilation of intrahepatic bile ducts vs., **404**
- porta hepatis, periportal lucency or edema vs., **289**
- postsurgical, mesenteric lymphadenopathy vs., **19**
- reactive
    due to localized abdominal inflammation, mesenteric lymphadenopathy vs., **18**
    due to systemic inflammation, mesenteric lymphadenopathy vs., **18**

Lymphangiectasia, intestinal
- misty (infiltrated) mesentery vs., **37**
- segmental or diffuse small bowel wall thickening vs., **151**

Lymphangioleiomyomatosis
- retroperitoneum, cystic retroperitoneal mass vs., **461**
- soft-tissue-density retroperitoneal mass vs., **467**

Lymphangioma
- abdominal calcifications vs., **23**
- cystic retroperitoneal mass vs., **461**
- perirenal and subcapsular mass lesions vs., **516–517**

Lymphangiomatosis, renal, dilated renal pelvis vs., **557**
Lymphocele
- cystic mesenteric and omental mass vs., **10**
- extraovarian adnexal mass vs., **644, 645**
- retroperitoneal, cystic retroperitoneal mass vs., **460–461**

Lymphoepithelial cyst
- cystic pancreatic lesion vs., **449**
- cystic pancreatic mass vs., **426, 427**

Lymphoid follicles
- multiple colonic filling defects vs., **174**
- small bowel, multiple masses or filling defects vs., **142**

Lymphoma
- abdominal wall mass vs., **49**
- adrenal, adrenal mass vs., **481**
- colonic
  colonic thumbprinting vs., **198**
  colonic wall thickening vs., **200, 201**
  multiple colonic filling defects vs., **174**
  segmental colonic narrowing vs., **194**
  solitary colonic filling defect vs., **172**
- cystic pancreatic mass vs., **426, 427**
- diffuse gallbladder wall thickening vs., **375**
- diffuse/infiltrative hepatic, periportal lesion vs., **356**
- esophageal strictures vs., **78**
- filling defect in urinary bladder vs., **585**
- gallbladder, focal gallbladder wall thickening vs., **372**
- gastric
  linitis plastica vs., **114**
  target (bull's-eye) lesions, stomach vs., **98**
- gastric mass lesions vs., **90**
- hepatic
  anechoic liver lesion vs., **337**
  diffuse hyperechoic liver vs., **328**
  diffusely abnormal liver echogenicity vs., **334**
  hypoechoic liver mass vs., **341**
  liver "mass" with capsular retraction vs., **244**
  mosaic/patchy hepatogram vs., **262**
  multiple hypo-, hyper- or anechoic liver lesions vs., **350**
  multiple hypodense liver lesions vs., **308**
  periportal lucency or edema vs., **289**
  target lesions in liver vs., **348**
  widespread low attenuation within liver vs., **318**
- hepatomegaly vs., **331**
- infiltration of peripancreatic fat planes vs., **439**
- intestinal
  mass or inflammation of ileocecal area vs., **176–177**
  multiple masses or filling defects vs., **142**
  occult GI bleeding vs., **160**
  segmental or diffuse small bowel wall thickening vs., **151**
  small bowel obstruction vs., **164–165**
- intraluminal mass vs., **66**
- mesenteric lymphadenopathy vs., **18**
- misty (infiltrated) mesentery vs., **36**
- perirenal and subcapsular mass lesions vs., **516**
- renal sinus lesion vs., **524–525**
- retroperitoneal, dilated renal pelvis vs., **557**
- small bowel, aneurysmal dilation of small bowel lumen vs., **146**
- soft-tissue-density retroperitoneal mass vs., **466**
- solid mesenteric or omental mass vs., **4**
- solid ovarian masses vs., **688, 689**
- solid pancreatic lesion vs., **453**
- solid renal mass vs., **500**
- solid splenic mass vs., **228**
- splenic
  cystic splenic mass vs., **230**
  splenomegaly vs., **222–223**
- testicular
  diffuse testicular enlargement vs., **616**
  intratesticular mass vs., **604, 605**

Lymphomatous infiltration, of peritoneum, misty (infiltrated) mesentery vs., **37**

M

Macrocystic serous cystadenoma, cystic pancreatic mass vs., **426**
Malakoplakia, ureteral filling defect or stricture vs., **576, 577**
Malaria
- infectious cholecystitis, **385**
- splenomegaly vs., **223**
Malignant ascites, hemoperitoneum vs., **33**
Malignant epithelial tumors, solid ovarian masses vs., **688**
Malignant ovarian epithelial neoplasms, multilocular ovarian cysts vs., **676–677**
Malpositioned intrauterine device, acute pelvic pain vs., **650, 651**
Malrotation, bands, small bowel obstruction vs., **164**
Mastocytosis
- mesenteric lymphadenopathy vs., **19**
- segmental or diffuse small bowel wall thickening vs., **151**
Mature cystic teratoma
- calcified ovarian masses vs., **692**
- complications of, acute pelvic pain vs., **650, 651**
- cystic retroperitoneal mass vs., **461**
- unilocular ovarian cysts vs., **682**
Meckel diverticulitis
- acute right lower quadrant pain vs., **209**
- extraovarian adnexal mass vs., **644**
Meckel diverticulum, small bowel obstruction vs., **165**
Medication-induced pneumatosis, pneumatosis of small intestine vs., **156**
Medullary cystic disease
- bilateral renal cysts vs., **508, 509**
- complex, small kidney vs., **549**
Medullary nephrocalcinosis
- calcifications within kidney vs., **488**
- hyperechoic renal mass vs., **560**
Megacalycosis, dilated renal calyces vs., **566, 567**
Megacolon, toxic, colonic ileus vs., **182**
Megaureter
- congenital, cystic dilation of distal ureter vs., **580**
- congenital renal anomalies vs., **493**
- dilated renal calyces vs., **566, 567**

Melanoma, abdominal wall mass vs., **49**

Ménétrier disease, thickened gastric folds vs., **104**

Mesenchymal neoplasms, filling defect in urinary bladder vs., **585**

Mesenchymal tumors
- benign, solid mesenteric or omental mass vs., **5**
- colon, multiple colonic filling defects vs., **174**
- duodenal mass vs., **130**
- gastric mass lesions vs., **90**
- scrotum, extratesticular solid mass vs., **612**
- solitary colonic filling defect vs., **172**
- target (bull's-eye) lesions, stomach vs., **98**

Mesenteric adenitis
- acute right lower quadrant pain vs., **208**
- mass or inflammation of ileocecal area vs., **176**
- mesenteric lymphadenopathy vs., **19**
- segmental or diffuse small bowel wall thickening vs., **150**

Mesenteric calcifications, abdominal calcifications vs., **23**

Mesenteric cyst, cystic mesenteric and omental mass vs., **10**

Mesenteric enteritis
- acute right lower quadrant pain vs., **208**
- segmental or diffuse small bowel wall thickening vs., **150**

Mesenteric hematoma, mimic, solid mesenteric or omental mass vs., **4**

Mesenteric hemorrhage, misty (infiltrated) mesentery vs., **37**

Mesenteric infiltration, postsurgical, misty (infiltrated) mesentery vs., **36**

Mesenteric lymphadenopathy, **18–21**
- differential diagnosis, **18**
- solid mesenteric or omental mass vs., **4**

Mesenteric mass
- cystic, differential diagnosis, **10**
- solid, **4–9**
    differential diagnosis, **4**

Mesenteric varices, occult GI bleeding vs., **160**

Mesenteritis, sclerosing
- abdominal calcifications vs., **23**
- fat-containing lesion of peritoneal cavity vs., **14**
- infiltration of peripancreatic fat planes vs., **439**
- mesenteric lymphadenopathy vs., **19**
- misty (infiltrated) mesentery vs., **36**
- solid mesenteric or omental mass vs., **4**

Mesh hernia repair, mimic, groin mass vs., **54**

Mesothelioma
- benign multicystic peritoneal, cystic mesenteric and omental mass vs., **11**
- cystic retroperitoneal, cystic retroperitoneal mass vs., **461**
- misty (infiltrated) mesentery vs., **37**
- solid mesenteric or omental mass vs., **4**
- of tunica vaginalis
    extratesticular solid mass vs., **612, 613**

Metabolic calcification, calcifications within kidney vs., **488**

Metanephric adenoma, solid renal mass vs., **501**

Metastases
- adrenal, adrenal mass vs., **480**

- colonic
    colonic thumbprinting vs., **198**
    colonic wall thickening vs., **200, 201**
    multiple colonic filling defects vs., **174**
    segmental colonic narrowing vs., **194**
    solitary colonic filling defect vs., **172**
- cystic pancreatic mass vs., **426, 427**
- filling defect in urinary bladder vs., **585**
- gallbladder
    diffuse gallbladder wall thickening vs., **375**
    focal gallbladder wall thickening vs., **372**
- gastric
    duodenal mass vs., **130**
    epigastric pain vs., **119**
    gastric dilation or outlet obstruction vs., **111**
    gastric mass lesions vs., **90**
    linitis plastica vs., **114**
    stomach intramural mass vs., **96**
    target (bull's-eye) lesions, stomach vs., **98**
    thickened gastric folds vs., **104**
- hepatic
    anechoic liver lesion vs., **336**
    cystic hepatic mass vs., **248**
    diffuse hyperechoic liver vs., **328**
    duodenal mass vs., **130**
    echogenic liver mass vs., **344**
    epigastric pain vs., **119**
    fat-containing liver mass vs., **246**
    focal hepatic echogenic lesion vs., **322**
    focal hyperdense hepatic mass on nonenhanced CT vs., **314**
    focal hypervascular liver lesion vs., **252**
    focal liver lesion with hemorrhage vs., **240**
    hepatic calcifications vs., **266**
    hepatic mass with central scar vs., **354**
    hyperintense liver lesions (T1WI) vs., **298**
    hypoechoic liver mass vs., **340**
    irregular hepatic surface vs., **360**
    liver lesion with capsule or halo on MR vs., **304**
    liver "mass" with capsular retraction vs., **244**
    liver mass with central or eccentric scar vs., **236**
    mimic, multiple biliary strictures vs., **408, 409**
    mosaic/patchy hepatogram vs., **262**
    multiple hypo-, hyper- or anechoic liver lesions vs., **350**
    multiple hypodense liver lesions vs., **308, 309**
    multiple hypointense liver lesions (T2WI) vs., **294**
    periportal lucency or edema vs., **289**
    target lesions in liver vs., **348**
    widespread low attenuation within liver vs., **318**
- hepatomegaly vs., **331**
- hyperechoic, echogenic liver mass vs., **344**
- infiltrative, diffusely abnormal liver echogenicity vs., **334**
- to inguinal canal, groin mass vs., **55**
- intestinal
    mass or inflammation of ileocecal area vs., **176–177**
    multiple masses or filling defects vs., **142**
    occult GI bleeding vs., **160**
    segmental or diffuse small bowel wall thickening vs., **151**

small bowel obstruction vs., **164–165**
- mesenteric lymphadenopathy vs., **18**
- multilocular ovarian cysts vs., **676, 677**
- ovarian, pelvic fluid vs., **634, 635**
- pancreatic
  hypervascular pancreatic mass vs., **422**
  and lymphoma, hypovascular pancreatic mass vs., **416, 417**
  pancreatic calcifications vs., **445**
- periportal lesion vs., **356**
- peritoneal
  cluster of dilated small bowel vs., **144**
  cystic mesenteric and omental mass vs., **10**
  linitis plastica vs., **115**
  mimic, liver "mass" with capsular retraction vs., **244**
  misty (infiltrated) mesentery vs., **37**
  small bowel obstruction vs., **164**
  solid mesenteric or omental mass vs., **4**
- periureteral, dilated renal calyces vs., **566**
- renal
  hyperechoic renal mass vs., **561**
  infiltrative renal lesions vs., **512–513**
- retroperitoneal
  delayed or persistent nephrogram vs., **530**
  fat-containing retroperitoneal mass, **475**
  ureteral filling defect or stricture vs., **576**
- small bowel, aneurysmal dilation of small bowel lumen vs., **146**
- soft tissue, abdominal wall mass vs., **49**
- soft-tissue-density retroperitoneal mass vs., **466**
- solid ovarian masses vs., **688**
- solid pancreatic lesion vs., **453**
- solid renal mass vs., **500–501**
- splenic
  cystic splenic mass vs., **230**
  solid splenic mass vs., **228**
- splenomegaly vs., **223**
- testicular
  diffuse testicular enlargement vs., **616**
  intratesticular mass vs., **604, 605**
Metastatic calcification, abdominal, **22**
Metastatic disease
- extratesticular solid mass vs., **612, 613**
- liver mass with mosaic enhancement vs., **258**
- thickened endometrium vs., **662, 663**
Metastatic liposarcoma, liver mass with mosaic enhancement vs., **258**
Metastatic malignant teratoma, fat-containing lesion of peritoneal cavity vs., **15**
Microcystic adenoma, cystic pancreatic mass vs., **426**
Microlithiasis, testicular, testicular calcifications vs., **620**
Miliary tuberculosis, diffuse hyperechoic liver vs., **328**
Milk of calcium
- bile, high-attenuation (hyperdense) bile in gallbladder vs., **378**
- calcifications within kidney vs., **488**
- cyst, hyperechoic renal mass vs., **560**
Mirizzi syndrome, asymmetric dilation of intrahepatic bile ducts vs., **404, 405**
Misty (infiltrated) mesentery, **36–41**
- differential diagnosis, **36**

Mixed epithelial and stromal tumor family
- cystic renal mass vs., **504, 505**
- renal sinus lesion vs., **525**
Molar pregnancy, thickened endometrium vs., **662, 663**
Mönckeberg calcifications, abdominal calcifications vs., **23**
Mononucleosis
- mesenteric lymphadenopathy vs., **19**
- splenomegaly vs., **222**
Morgagni hernia, elevated or deformed hemidiaphragm vs., **58**
Mosaic enhancement, liver mass with, **258–261**
Mosaic/patchy hepatogram, **262–263**
- differential diagnosis, **262**
Mucinous cystadenocarcinoma
- multilocular ovarian cysts vs., **676**
- unilocular ovarian cysts vs., **682, 683**
Mucinous cystadenoma
- enlarged prostate vs., **630**
- focal lesion in prostate vs., **624, 625**
- multilocular ovarian cysts vs., **676**
- unilocular ovarian cysts vs., **682, 683**
Mucinous cystic neoplasm
- cystic pancreatic lesion vs., **448**
- cystic pancreatic mass vs., **426**
- cystic retroperitoneal mass vs., **460**
- hypovascular pancreatic mass vs., **416**
- left upper quadrant mass vs., **124**
- ovarian lesions with low T2 signal intensity vs., **696, 697**
- of pancreas, solid pancreatic lesion vs., **453**
- pancreatic calcifications vs., **445**
Mucinous ovarian neoplasms, calcified ovarian masses vs., **692**
Mucinous pancreatic cystic tumors, dilated common bile duct vs., **398, 399**
Mucocele
- appendiceal
  abdominal calcifications vs., **23**
  acute right lower quadrant pain vs., **209**
  extraovarian adnexal mass vs., **644**
  mass or inflammation of ileocecal area vs., **176, 177**
- dilated gallbladder vs., **384**
Müllerian duct cysts
- enlarged prostate vs., **630**
- female lower genital cysts vs., **638–639**
- focal lesion in prostate vs., **624, 625**
Multicystic dysplastic kidney, small kidney vs., **548**
Multicystic peritoneal mesothelioma, benign, cystic mesenteric and omental mass vs., **11**
Multicystic renal dysplasia
- bilateral renal cysts vs., **508, 509**
- cystic renal mass vs., **504, 505**
- enlarged kidney vs., **545**
Multifocal fatty infiltration, multiple hypodense liver lesions vs., **308**
Multilocular cystic nephroma
- cystic retroperitoneal mass vs., **460**
- dilated renal pelvis vs., **557**
Multilocular ovarian cysts, **676–681**
- differential diagnosis, **676**
Multiloculated cystic renal neoplasm of low malignant potential, cystic renal mass vs., **504, 505**

Multiple colonic filling defects, **174–175**
- differential diagnosis, **174**

Multiple gastric masses, gastric mass lesions vs., **91**

Multiple hypo-, hyper- or anechoic liver lesions, **350–353**
- differential diagnosis, **350**

Multiple hypodense liver lesions, **308–312**
- differential diagnosis, **308**

Multiple hypointense liver lesions (T2WI), **294–297**
- differential diagnosis, **294**

Multiple masses or filling defects, small bowel, **142–143**
- differential diagnosis, **142**

Multiple myeloma
- delayed or persistent nephrogram vs., **531**
- wedge-shaped or striated nephrogram vs., **534, 535**

Multiple sclerosis, colonic ileus vs., **182**

Multiple splenic calcifications, **226–227**
- differential diagnosis, **226**

Mumps orchitis, decreased testicular size vs., **618**

Muscle asymmetry, mimic, abdominal wall mass vs., **48**

Muscular disorders, lesion at pharyngoesophageal junction vs., **72**

Myasthenia gravis, lesion at pharyngoesophageal junction vs., **72**

Myelolipoma, adrenal
- adrenal mass vs., **481**
- fat-containing retroperitoneal mass vs., **472**

N

Nabothian cyst, female lower genital cysts vs., **638**

Nasogastric intubation
- esophageal strictures vs., **78**
- esophageal ulceration vs., **74**

Neck hematoma, lesion at pharyngoesophageal junction vs., **72**

Neck mass, lesion at pharyngoesophageal junction vs., **72**

Necrosis
- biliary, posttransplant, periportal lucency or edema vs., **289**
- fat
  fat-containing lesion of peritoneal cavity vs., **14**
  solid mesenteric or omental mass vs., **5**

Necrotizing enterocolitis, pneumatosis of small intestine vs., **157**

Neoplasm
- primary, iliopsoas compartment mass vs., **52**
- secondary, iliopsoas compartment mass vs., **52**

Neoplastic hemorrhage, hemoperitoneum vs., **33**

Neoplastic infiltration, diffuse, hepatomegaly vs., **331**

Nephrectomy, partial, small kidney vs., **548**

Nephritis
- chronic, small kidney vs., **549**
- radiation, wedge-shaped or striated nephrogram vs., **534, 535**

Nephrocalcinosis
- cortical
  calcifications within kidney vs., **488–489**
  hyperechoic kidney vs., **552, 553**
- medullary
  calcifications within kidney vs., **488**
  hyperechoic kidney vs., **552**

Nephrogram
- delayed or persistent, **530–533**
  differential diagnosis, **530**
- wedge-shaped or striated, **534–537**
  differential diagnosis, **534**

Nephrolithiasis, right upper quadrant pain vs., **390**

Nephropathy
- chronic hypertensive, small kidney vs., **548**
- contrast-induced, delayed or persistent nephrogram vs., **531**
- radiation, chronic, small kidney vs., **549**

Nephrosclerosis, hypertensive, hyperechoic kidney vs., **552**

Nerve sheath tumor
- extraovarian adnexal mass vs., **644**
- malignant peripheral, soft-tissue-density retroperitoneal mass vs., **466–467**
- renal sinus lesion vs., **525**

Neuroendocrine tumors
- calcifications within kidney vs., **489**
- renal sinus lesion vs., **525**
- solid renal mass vs., **501**

Neurofibroma, soft-tissue-density retroperitoneal mass vs., **466**

Neurogenic bladder
- abnormal bladder wall vs., **594**
- urinary bladder outpouching vs., **590**

Neurogenic tumor
- cystic retroperitoneal mass vs., **460**
- of retroperitoneum, **524**
- soft-tissue-density retroperitoneal mass vs., **466–467**

Neuromuscular disorders
- colonic ileus vs., **182**
- esophageal dysmotility vs., **84**

Neutropenic colitis
- acute right lower quadrant pain vs., **209**
- colonic thumbprinting vs., **198**
- colonic wall thickening vs., **200–201**
- mass or inflammation of ileocecal area vs., **176, 177**
- segmental colonic narrowing vs., **195**

Nodular hyperplasia, focal
- fat-containing liver mass vs., **246**
- focal hyperperfusion abnormality vs., **283**
- focal hypervascular liver lesion vs., **252**
- hepatic calcifications vs., **267**
- hepatic mass with central scar vs., **354**
- hyperintense liver lesions (T1WI) vs., **298–299**
- hypoechoic liver mass vs., **341**
- liver lesion with capsule or halo on MR vs., **304**
- liver mass with central or eccentric scar vs., **236**

Nodular regenerative hyperplasia
- focal hypervascular liver lesion vs., **252–253**
- hyperintense liver lesions (T1WI) vs., **299**
- liver lesion with capsule or halo on MR vs., **304**
- liver mass with central or eccentric scar vs., **236**
- multiple hypointense liver lesions (T2WI) vs., **295**

Nonhemorrhagic adrenal infarction, acute flank pain vs., **539**

Nonneoplastic pancreatic cysts, cystic pancreatic mass vs., **426, 427**

Nonseminomatous germ cell tumor
- intratesticular mass vs., **604**
- testicular cystic lesions vs., **608**

Normal anatomic pitfalls, echogenic liver mass vs., **344**

Normal central zone, mimic, focal lesion in prostate vs., **624**

Normal postoperative pneumoperitoneum, pneumoperitoneum vs., **28**

Normal trigone, abnormal bladder wall vs., **594**

NSAID-induced gastritis, gastric ulceration without mass vs., **100**

Nutcracker syndrome, acute flank pain vs., **539**

O

Obesity
- atrophy or fatty replacement of pancreas vs., **432**
- colonic wall thickening vs., **200**

Obstetric source, hemoperitoneum vs., **32**

Obstructed flow, of bile, distended gallbladder vs., **366**

Obstructing urolithiasis, acute flank pain vs., **538**

Obturator hernia
- abdominal wall defects vs., **61**
- small bowel obstruction vs., **164**

Occult gastrointestinal bleeding, **160–163**
- differential diagnosis, **160**

Odynophagia, **86–87**
- differential diagnosis, **86**

Ogilvie syndrome, colonic ileus vs., **182**

Omental infarct
- acute flank pain vs., **539**
- acute left abdominal pain vs., **215**
- acute right lower quadrant pain vs., **208**
- fat-containing lesion of peritoneal cavity vs., **14**
- right upper quadrant pain vs., **390, 391**

Omental mass
- cystic, differential diagnosis, **10**
- solid, **4–9**
    differential diagnosis, **4**

Oncocytoma
- calcifications within kidney vs., **489**
- fat-containing renal mass vs., **521**
- renal
    hyperechoic renal mass vs., **561**
    solid renal mass vs., **500**

Opportunistic infection
- diffuse increased attenuation, spleen vs., **232**
- hepatic
    hepatic calcifications vs., **266–267**
    multiple hypodense liver lesions vs., **308–309**
    widespread low attenuation within liver vs., **318**
- intestinal
    segmental or diffuse small bowel wall thickening vs., **150**
    thickened duodenal fold vs., **138**

Orchitis
- diffuse testicular enlargement vs., **616**
- granulomatous, intratesticular mass vs., **604, 605**
- intratesticular mass vs., **604**
- mumps, decreased testicular size vs., **618**
- testicular calcifications vs., **620**

Ossification, **22**

Ossified scar, abdominal calcifications vs., **23**

Osteophytes, cervical, lesion at pharyngoesophageal junction vs., **72**

Osteosarcoma, calcifications within kidney vs., **489**

Outpouching, urinary bladder, **590–591**
- differential diagnosis, **590**

Ovarian abscess, due to diverticulitis, acute pelvic pain vs., **650**

Ovarian carcinoma
- abnormal uterine bleeding vs., **668**
- pelvic fluid vs., **634, 635**
- rectal or colonic fistula vs., **188**

Ovarian corpus luteum, acute pelvic pain vs., **650**

Ovarian cyst
- hemorrhagic
    acute pelvic pain vs., **650**
    acute right lower quadrant pain vs., **208–209**
- multilocular, **676–681**
    differential diagnosis, **676**
- ruptured, hemoperitoneum vs., **32**
- unilocular, **682–687**

Ovarian edema
- massive, solid ovarian masses vs., **688**
- pelvic fluid vs., **634, 635**

Ovarian endometrioma, acute pelvic pain vs., **650**

Ovarian follicular cyst, acute pelvic pain vs., **650**

Ovarian hyperstimulation syndrome
- acute pelvic pain vs., **650, 651**
- multilocular ovarian cysts vs., **676, 677**
- pelvic fluid vs., **634, 635**

Ovarian mass
- calcified, **692–695**
- exophytic, extraovarian adnexal mass vs., **644**
- solid, **688–691**
    differential diagnosis, **688**

Ovarian metastases, pelvic fluid vs., **634, 635**

Ovarian neoplasms
- mucinous, calcified ovarian masses vs., **692**
- serous, calcified ovarian masses vs., **692**

Ovarian vein leiomyosarcoma, extraovarian adnexal mass vs., **644, 645**

Ovarian vein thrombosis, acute pelvic pain vs., **650, 651**

Ovary
- calcified ovarian masses, **692–695**
- estrogen-producing tumor, abnormal uterine bleeding vs., **668**
- lesions with low T2 signal intensity, **696–701**
- multilocular ovarian cysts, **676–681**
- solid ovarian masses, **688–691**
- torsion
    acute pelvic pain vs., **650, 650–651**
    acute right lower quadrant pain vs., **208–209**
    pelvic fluid vs., **634, 635**
    solid ovarian masses vs., **688**

Overt GI bleeding, occult GI bleeding vs., **160**

P

Pain
- acute flank, **538–543**
    differential diagnosis, **538**
- acute right lower quadrant, **208–213**
- right upper quadrant, **390–395**
Pancake kidney, congenital renal anomalies vs., **493**
Pancreas
- atrophy or fatty replacement of, **432–433**
- calcifications, **444–447**
    differential diagnosis, **444**
- cystic fibrosis
    atrophy or fatty replacement of pancreas vs., **432**
    fat-containing lesion of peritoneal cavity vs., **15**
    pancreatic calcifications vs., **445**
- cystic mass, **426–431**
    cystic retroperitoneal mass vs., **460**
- dilated pancreatic duct, **434–437**
    differential diagnosis, **434**
- dorsal, agenesis of
    atrophy or fatty replacement of pancreas vs., **432**
    hypovascular pancreatic mass vs., **416, 417**
- hypervascular pancreatic mass, **422–425**
- hypovascular pancreatic mass, **416–421**
- infected necrotizing fluid collections, gas in or around
    kidney vs., **528**
- lesion
    cystic, **448–451**
    solid, **452–455**
- lipomatous pseudohypertrophy, mimic, fat-containing
    lesion of peritoneal cavity vs., **15**
- mucinous cystic neoplasm of, solid pancreatic lesion vs.,
    453
- normal anatomic variants of, mimic, hypovascular
    pancreatic mass vs., **416**
- pancreatic duct dilatation, **456–457**
    differential diagnosis, **456**
- peripancreatic fat planes of, infiltration of, **438–443**
- senescent change
    dilated pancreatic duct vs., **434**
    pancreatic calcifications vs., **444**
- serous cystadenoma
    cystic pancreatic lesion vs., **448**
    cystic pancreatic mass vs., **426**
    duodenal mass vs., **131**
    hypervascular pancreatic mass vs., **422**
    hypovascular pancreatic mass vs., **416**
    pancreatic calcifications vs., **444**
    solid pancreatic lesion vs., **452–453**
- shock, infiltration of peripancreatic fat planes vs.,
    438–439
Pancreatic calcifications, **444–447**
- abdominal calcifications vs., **22**
- differential diagnosis, **444**

Pancreatic cystic masses, cystic retroperitoneal mass vs.,
    460
Pancreatic divisum, dilated pancreatic duct vs., **435**
Pancreatic duct dilatation, **456–457**
- differential diagnosis, **456**
- isolated, pancreatic duct dilatation vs., **456**
Pancreatic ductal adenocarcinoma
- cystic pancreatic mass vs., **426, 427**
- dilated common bile duct vs., **398**
- dilated pancreatic duct vs., **434**
- hypovascular pancreatic mass vs., **416**
Pancreatic ductal carcinoma
- infiltration of peripancreatic fat planes vs., **438**
- intrahepatic and extrahepatic duct dilatation vs., **388**
- necrotic, cystic pancreatic lesion vs., **449**
- pancreatic duct dilatation vs., **456**
- solid pancreatic lesion vs., **452**
- stomach, epigastric pain vs., **119**
Pancreatic inflammation, epigastric pain vs., **118**
Pancreatic intraductal papillary mucinous neoplasm,
    duodenal mass vs., **131**
Pancreatic masses
- left upper quadrant mass vs., **124**
- other, dilated common bile duct vs., **398, 399**
Pancreatic metastases
- hypervascular pancreatic mass vs., **422**
- and lymphoma, hypovascular pancreatic mass vs., **416,
    417**
- pancreatic calcifications vs., **445**
Pancreatic neuroendocrine tumor
- cystic pancreatic lesion vs., **449**
- cystic pancreatic mass vs., **426, 427**
- dilated pancreatic duct vs., **435**
- duodenal mass vs., **131**
- hypervascular pancreatic mass vs., **422**
- hypovascular pancreatic mass vs., **416, 417**
- left upper quadrant mass vs., **124**
- pancreatic calcifications vs., **444**
- solid pancreatic lesion vs., **452**
Pancreatic panniculitis, abdominal wall mass vs., **49**
Pancreatic pseudocyst
- cystic mesenteric and omental mass vs., **10**
- cystic pancreatic lesion vs., **448**
- cystic pancreatic mass vs., **426**
- cystic retroperitoneal mass vs., **460**
- cystic splenic mass vs., **230**
- dilated common bile duct vs., **398, 399**
- duodenal mass vs., **130**
- left upper quadrant mass vs., **124**
- pancreatic calcifications vs., **445**
- stomach intramural mass vs., **96**
Pancreatic pseudopapillary neoplasm, hypervascular
    pancreatic mass vs., **422, 423**
Pancreatic solid neoplasm, hypervascular pancreatic mass
    vs., **422, 423**
Pancreatic tissue, ectopic
- gastric mass lesions vs., **90, 91**
- stomach intramural mass vs., **96**
- target (bull's-eye) lesions, stomach vs., **98**
Pancreaticobiliary parasites, dilated common bile duct vs.,
    398, 399

Pancreatitis
- acute
  - acute right lower quadrant pain vs., **209**
  - diffuse gallbladder wall thickening vs., **374**
  - dilated duodenum vs., **136**
  - epigastric pain vs., **118**
  - gastric dilation or outlet obstruction vs., **110**
  - hypovascular pancreatic mass vs., **416, 417**
  - infiltration of peripancreatic fat planes vs., **438**
  - misty (infiltrated) mesentery vs., **36**
  - portal venous gas vs., **274**
  - right upper quadrant pain vs., **390**
  - solid mesenteric or omental mass vs., **4**
  - thickened duodenal fold vs., **138**
  - thickened gastric folds vs., **104**
- acute flank pain vs., **539**
- autoimmune
  - hypovascular pancreatic mass vs., **416, 417**
  - infiltration of peripancreatic fat planes vs., **439**
- chronic
  - abdominal calcifications vs., **22**
  - atrophy or fatty replacement of pancreas vs., **432**
  - dilated common bile duct vs., **398**
  - dilated pancreatic duct vs., **434**
  - epigastric pain vs., **118**
  - gastric dilation or outlet obstruction vs., **110–111**
  - hypovascular pancreatic mass vs., **416**
  - pancreatic calcifications vs., **444**
  - pancreatic duct dilatation vs., **456**
  - solid pancreatic lesion vs., **452**
- focal acute, solid pancreatic lesion vs., **452**
- groove
  - hypovascular pancreatic mass vs., **416, 417**
  - infiltration of peripancreatic fat planes vs., **439**
- hemorrhagic, hemoperitoneum vs., **33**
- hereditary, pancreatic calcifications vs., **445**
- pseudocyst, thickened gastric folds vs., **104**
- segmental colonic narrowing vs., **194–195**
- traumatic, infiltration of peripancreatic fat planes vs., **438**
Pancreatitis-related collection, cystic retroperitoneal mass vs., **460**
Pancreatobiliary parasites
- asymmetric dilation of intrahepatic bile ducts vs., **404, 405**
- hepatic calcifications vs., **266**
- multiple biliary strictures vs., **408, 409**
Panniculitis
- acute left abdominal pain vs., **215**
- pancreatic, abdominal wall mass vs., **49**
Papillary adenoma, solid renal mass vs., **501**
Papillary cystadenoma
- epididymal, extratesticular cystic mass vs., **610**
- extratesticular solid mass vs., **612, 613**
Papillary necrosis, renal
- dilated renal calyces vs., **566, 567**
- filling defect, renal pelvis vs., **570**
Papillary serous carcinoma, primary, solid mesenteric or omental mass vs., **5**
Papilloma
- esophagus, intraluminal mass vs., **66**

- filling defect, renal pelvis vs., **570**
- inverted, filling defect in urinary bladder vs., **585**
- ureteral, ureteral filling defect or stricture vs., **576, 577**
Papillomatosis, esophageal, mucosal nodularity, esophagus vs., **76**
Paraduodenal hernia
- cluster of dilated small bowel vs., **144**
- small bowel obstruction vs., **165**
Paraganglioma, soft-tissue-density retroperitoneal mass vs., **466**
Paraovarian cyst
- complicated, acute pelvic pain vs., **650, 651**
- extraovarian adnexal mass vs., **644–645**
Parapelvic cyst, dilated renal pelvis vs., **556**
Pararenal fluid collections, dilated renal pelvis vs., **556**
Parasitic infestation, echogenic material in gallbladder vs., **382**
Parastomal hernias, **60**
Paratubal cysts, extraovarian adnexal mass vs., **644–645**
Paraumbilical varices, abdominal wall mass vs., **48**
Parenchymal calcifications, adrenal, abdominal calcifications vs., **23**
Parkinson disease, colonic ileus vs., **182**
Particle disease, related to hip prosthesis, extraovarian adnexal mass vs., **644**
Passive hepatic congestion
- mosaic/patchy hepatogram vs., **262**
- periportal lucency or edema vs., **288**
- widespread low attenuation within liver vs., **318**
Patchy steatosis, mimic, fat-containing liver mass vs., **246**
Peliosis, splenic, solid splenic mass vs., **228**
Peliosis hepatis
- focal hypervascular liver lesion vs., **253**
- hyperintense liver lesions (T1WI) vs., **299**
- multiple hypointense liver lesions (T2WI) vs., **295**
Pelvic abscess
- due to bowel disease, pelvic fluid vs., **634–635**
- rectal or colonic fistula vs., **188, 189**
Pelvic cancer, locally advanced, ureteral filling defect or stricture vs., **576**
Pelvic fluid, **634–637**
- differential diagnosis, **634**
Pelvic fractures, urethral stricture vs., **600**
Pelvic infection, reaction to, abnormal bladder wall vs., **594–595**
Pelvic inflammatory disease
- acute pelvic pain vs., **650**
- acute right lower quadrant pain vs., **208**
- pelvic fluid vs., **634**
Pelvic malignancies
- delayed or persistent nephrogram vs., **530**
- rectal or colonic fistula vs., **188**
Pelvic mass, extravesical, filling defect in urinary bladder vs., **584**
Pelvic neoplasm, invasion by, abnormal bladder wall vs., **594**
Pelvic pain, nongynecologic causes, **650, 651**
Pelvic trauma, retroperitoneal hemorrhage vs., **476**
Pelvic varices, extraovarian adnexal mass vs., **644**
Penile fracture, urethral stricture vs., **600**

Peptic ulcer, perforated, diffuse gallbladder wall thickening vs., **375**

Perforated ulcer, pneumoperitoneum vs., **28**

Perforation, bowel, pneumoperitoneum vs., **29**

Perfusion artifact, mimic, solid splenic mass vs., **228**

Periampullary duodenal adenocarcinoma, dilated common bile duct vs., **398**

Periampullary tumors, gas in bile ducts or gallbladder vs., **369**

Peribiliary cysts
- anechoic liver lesion vs., **337**
- dysmorphic liver with abnormal bile ducts vs., **278**
- periportal lesion vs., **357**
- periportal lucency or edema vs., **289**

Pericaval fat deposition, fat-containing liver mass vs., **246**

Perigastric mass (mimic), gastric mass lesions vs., **90**

Perineal hernia, abdominal wall defects vs., **61**

Peripancreatic fat planes, infiltration of, **438–443**
- differential diagnosis, **438**

Peripancreatic lymphadenopathy, mimic, hypovascular pancreatic mass vs., **416**

Peripancreatic vascular abnormalities, hypervascular pancreatic mass vs., **422, 423**

Peripancreatic vascular lesions (mimic), pancreatic calcifications vs., **444**

Peripelvic cysts
- bilateral renal cysts vs., **508**
- cystic renal mass vs., **504**
- dilated renal pelvis vs., **556**

Peripheral cholangiocarcinoma
- liver lesion with capsule or halo on MR vs., **304**
- liver mass with central or eccentric scar vs., **236**

Periportal lesion, **356–359**
- differential diagnosis, **356**

Periportal lucency or edema, **288–293**
- differential diagnosis, **288**

Periportal lymphadenopathy, asymmetric dilation of intrahepatic bile ducts vs., **404**

Periprostatic tumors, secondary involvement of, enlarged prostate vs., **630**

Perirenal abscess, perirenal and subcapsular mass lesions vs., **516**

Perirenal and subcapsular mass lesions, **516–519**
- differential diagnosis, **516**

Perirenal hemorrhage, **516**
- retroperitoneal hemorrhage vs., **476**

Peristalsis, segmental colonic narrowing vs., **194**

Peritoneal calcifications, abdominal calcifications vs., **23**

Peritoneal inclusion cyst
- cystic mesenteric and omental mass vs., **11**
- extraovarian adnexal mass vs., **644, 645**
- pelvic fluid vs., **634**

Peritoneal lipomatosis, fat-containing lesion of peritoneal cavity vs., **15**

Peritoneal metastases
- cluster of dilated small bowel vs., **144**
- cystic mesenteric and omental mass vs., **10**
- mimic, liver "mass" with capsular retraction vs., **244**
- misty (infiltrated) mesentery vs., **37**
- small bowel obstruction vs., **164**
- solid mesenteric or omental mass vs., **4**

Peritonealis disseminata, leiomyomatosis, solid mesenteric or omental mass vs., **5**

Peritoneum and mesentery
- abdominal calcifications, **22–27**
- fat-containing lesion, peritoneal cavity, **14–17**
- hemoperitoneum, **32–35**
- high-attenuation (hyperdense) ascites, **42–45**
- mesenteric and omental mass, cystic, **10–13**
- mesenteric lymphadenopathy, **18–21**
- misty (infiltrated) mesentery, **36–41**
- pneumoperitoneum, **28–31**
- solid mesenteric or omental mass, **4–9**

Peritonitis
- acute left abdominal pain vs., **215**
- hemoperitoneum vs., **33**
- misty (infiltrated) mesentery vs., **36**
- pneumoperitoneum vs., **29**
- sclerosing, abdominal calcifications vs., **23**
- tuberculous, solid mesenteric or omental mass vs., **4**

Peritransplant collection, kidney transplant dysfunction vs., **496**

Periureteral cystic lesions, mimic, cystic dilation of distal ureter vs., **580**

Periureteral metastases, dilated renal calyces vs., **566**

Persistent fetal lobulation, congenital renal anomalies vs., **492**

Pharyngitis, odynophagia vs., **86**

Pharyngoesophageal junction lesion, differential diagnosis, **72**

Pheochromocytoma
- adrenal mass vs., **480**
- cystic, cystic retroperitoneal mass vs., **460**
- left upper quadrant mass vs., **124**

Phleboliths, abdominal calcifications vs., **23**

Physiologic dilatation, dilated gallbladder vs., **384**

Physiologic fluid, pelvic fluid vs., **634**

Physiologic follicles, unilocular ovarian cysts vs., **682**

Pills, multiple masses or filling defects vs., **142**

Plasma cell neoplasms, perirenal and subcapsular mass lesions vs., **517**

Pleural effusion, subpulmonic (mimic), elevated or deformed hemidiaphragm vs., **58**

Pneumatosis
- of colon, colonic wall thickening vs., **200, 201**
- colonic thumbprinting vs., **198**
- cystoides intestinalis
    pneumatosis of small intestine vs., **157**
    pneumoperitoneum vs., **29**
- of intestine, portal venous gas vs., **274**
- medication-induced, pneumatosis of small intestine vs., **156**
- multiple colonic filling defects vs., **174**
- small intestine, **156–159**
    differential diagnosis of, **156**

Pneumobilia
- focal hepatic echogenic lesion vs., **322**
- hypointense lesion in biliary tree (MRCP) vs., **412**
- multiple hypointense liver lesions (T2WI) vs., **294**
- periportal lesion vs., **356**

- portal venous gas vs., **274**

Pneumocystis carinii, multiple splenic calcifications vs., **226**

Pneumoperitoneum, **28–31**
- differential diagnosis, **28**

Polyarteritis nodosa, pneumatosis of small intestine vs., **156**

Polycystic disease, autosomal dominant
- liver, cystic hepatic mass vs., **248**
- liver, focal liver lesion with hemorrhage vs., **240**
- multiple hypodense liver lesions vs., **308**

Polycystic kidney disease, autosomal dominant
- bilateral renal cysts vs., **508**
- enlarged kidney vs., **544–545**

Polycystic liver disease, anechoic liver lesion vs., **336**

Polycystic ovarian syndrome, multilocular ovarian cysts vs., **676**

Polymyositis, pneumatosis of small intestine vs., **156**

Polyorchidism
- decreased testicular size vs., **618**
- extratesticular solid mass vs., **612, 613**

Polyps
- endometrial
    abnormal uterine bleeding vs., **668**
    thickened endometrium vs., **662**
- fibrovascular, intraluminal mass vs., **66**
- hyperplastic, gastric mass lesions vs., **90**

Porcelain gallbladder
- abdominal calcifications vs., **22**
- focal gallbladder wall thickening vs., **372**
- high-attenuation (hyperdense) bile in gallbladder vs., **378**
- hyperechoic gallbladder wall vs., **380**

Porta hepatis lymphadenopathy, periportal lucency or edema vs., **289**

Portal biliopathy, multiple biliary strictures vs., **408, 409**

Portal collaterals, hepatic, multiple hypointense liver lesions (T2WI) vs., **295**

Portal enteritis, segmental or diffuse small bowel wall thickening vs., **150**

Portal hypertension
- cirrhosis with, splenomegaly vs., **222**
- colonic wall thickening vs., **200**
- colopathy, colonic thumbprinting vs., **198**
- infiltration of peripancreatic fat planes vs., **438**
- misty (infiltrated) mesentery vs., **36**
- portal vein abnormality vs., **362**
- varices, thickened gastric folds vs., **104**

Portal vein
- abnormality, **362–363**
    differential diagnosis, **362**
- aneurysm (mimic), cystic pancreatic mass vs., **426, 427**
- bland, thrombosis, portal vein abnormality vs., **362**
- calcification, hepatic calcifications vs., **267**
- cavernous transformation of, periportal lesion vs., **356**
- occlusion, focal hyperperfusion abnormality vs., **283**
- pulsatile, portal vein abnormality vs., **362**
- thrombophlebitis, dysmorphic liver with abnormal bile ducts vs., **278**
- thrombosis, periportal lucency or edema vs., **289**
- tumor thrombus, portal vein abnormality vs., **362**

Portal vein gas
- focal hepatic echogenic lesion vs., **322**
- liver lesion containing gas vs., **270**
- mimic, gas in bile ducts or gallbladder vs., **368**
- mimic, hypointense lesion in biliary tree (MRCP) vs., **412**
- multiple hypointense liver lesions (T2WI) vs., **295**
- portal vein abnormality vs., **362**

Portal venous gas, **274–275**
- differential diagnosis, **274**
- liver lesion containing gas vs., **270**

Portomesenteric venous thrombosis, misty (infiltrated) mesentery vs., **37**

Portosystemic collaterals
- periportal lesion vs., **356**
- portal vein abnormality vs., **362**

Post ablative therapy, small kidney vs., **548**

Post endoscopy, pneumatosis of small intestine vs., **156**

Post surgery, small kidney vs., **548**

Post vagotomy, dilated gallbladder vs., **384**

Post Whipple procedure, gastric dilation or outlet obstruction vs., **110**

Postcholecystectomy dilatation, of common bile duct, **398**

Post esophagectomy
- intrathoracic stomach vs., **102**
- mimic
    dilated esophagus vs., **80**
    esophageal outpouchings (diverticula) vs., **82**

Posthysterectomy inclusion cyst, female lower genital cysts vs., **638, 639**

Postmenopausal cyst, unilocular ovarian cysts vs., **682**

Postoperative bladder, urinary bladder outpouching vs., **590**

Postoperative packing material, hyperintense liver lesions (T1WI) and, **298**

Postoperative state
- bowel
    pneumatosis of small intestine vs., **156**
    rectal or colonic fistula vs., **188**
- filling defect in urinary bladder vs., **585**
- focal hepatic echogenic lesion and, **323**
- kidney, gas in or around kidney vs., **528**
- stomach, fluid collection, intrathoracic stomach vs., **102**

Postoperative stricture, segmental colonic narrowing vs., **195**

Postpartum uterus, enlarged uterus vs., **658**

Postradiation sarcomas, focal lesion in prostate vs., **624, 625**

Postradiation therapy, for neck malignancy, lesion at pharyngoesophageal junction vs., **72**

Postsurgical fat necrosis, fat-containing retroperitoneal mass vs., **472**

Postsurgical hepatic fissures, widened hepatic fissures vs., **276**

Postsurgical hepatic resection, irregular hepatic surface vs., **360**

Postsurgical lymphadenopathy, mesenteric lymphadenopathy vs., **19**

Postsurgical mesenteric infiltration, misty (infiltrated) mesentery vs., **36**

Posttorsion atrophy, decreased testicular size vs., **618**

Posttransplant liver
- multiple biliary strictures vs., **408**
- periportal lucency or edema, **289**

Posttraumatic hematoma, testicular cystic lesions vs., **608**

Postvagotomy state
- dilated duodenum vs., **136**
- dilated esophagus vs., **80**
- esophageal dysmotility vs., **84**

Pregnancy
- complications, abnormal uterine bleeding vs., **668**
- early, thickened endometrium vs., **662**
- heterotopic, extraovarian adnexal mass vs., **644, 645**
- molar, thickened endometrium vs., **662, 663**
- ureterectasis of, dilated renal calyces vs., **566**

Presbyesophagus, esophageal dysmotility vs., **84**

Primary adenocarcinoma, aneurysmal dilation of small bowel lumen vs., **146**

Primary biliary cholangitis
- dysmorphic liver with abnormal bile ducts vs., **278**
- multiple hypointense liver lesions (T2WI) vs., **295**

Primary hepatic tumor, calcification within, focal hyperdense hepatic mass on nonenhanced CT vs., **314–315**

Primary pelvic malignancy, dilated renal calyces vs., **566**

Primary retroperitoneal mucinous cystadenoma, cystic retroperitoneal mass vs., **461**

Prominent duodenal ampulla mimicking mass, duodenal mass vs., **130**

Prominent ileocecal valve, mass or inflammation of ileocecal area vs., **176**

Prostate
- abscess, focal lesion in prostate vs., **624, 625**
- adenocarcinoma, enlarged prostate vs., **630**
- calcifications
    abdominal calcifications vs., **23**
    focal lesion in prostate vs., **624**
- carcinoma
    dilated renal calyces vs., **566**
    filling defect in urinary bladder vs., **584**
    focal lesion in prostate vs., **624**
    rectal or colonic fistula vs., **188**
- cyst, enlarged prostate vs., **630**
- enlarged, **630–631**
- focal lesion, **624–629**
- sarcomas
    enlarged prostate vs., **630**
    focal lesion in prostate vs., **624, 625**
- tumors
    enlarged prostate vs., **630**
    focal lesion in prostate vs., **624, 625**
- utricle cyst, focal lesion in prostate vs., **624**

Prostatitis
- enlarged prostate vs., **630**
- focal lesion in prostate vs., **624**
- granulomatous, focal lesion in prostate vs., **624, 625**

Pseudoaneurysm
- filling defect, renal pelvis vs., **570**
- mimic, cystic pancreatic mass vs., **426, 427**
- renal artery, renal sinus lesion vs., **524**

Pseudoaneurysm, groin, groin mass vs., **54**

Pseudocyst
- intrahepatic, cystic hepatic mass vs., **249**
- pancreatic
    cystic mesenteric and omental mass vs., **10**
    cystic splenic mass vs., **230**

Pseudodiverticulosis, intramural, esophageal outpouchings (diverticula) vs., **82**

Pseudolipoma
- Glisson capsule, fat-containing lesion of peritoneal cavity vs., **15**
- hepatic, hyperintense liver lesions (T1WI) vs., **299**

Pseudomembranous colitis
- colonic thumbprinting vs., **198**
- colonic wall thickening vs., **200**
- diverticulitis, multiple colonic filling defects vs., **174**

Pseudomyxoma peritonei
- abdominal calcifications vs., **23**
- cystic mesenteric and omental mass vs., **10**
- high-attenuation (hyperdense) ascites vs., **42, 43**
- left upper quadrant mass vs., **125**

Pseudomyxoma retroperitonei, cystic retroperitoneal mass vs., **461**

Pseudopneumatosis, pneumatosis of small intestine vs., **156**

Pseudotumor
- fibrous, extratesticular solid mass vs., **612–613**
- hepatic, focal hyperdense hepatic mass on nonenhanced CT vs., **315**
- inflammatory, liver, liver "mass" with capsular retraction vs., **244**

Ptotic kidney, congenital renal anomalies vs., **492**

Pulmonary disease, pneumatosis of small intestine vs., **156**

Pulmonary fibrosis, pneumatosis of small intestine vs., **156**

Pulsatile portal vein, portal vein abnormality vs., **362**

Pulsatile vascular compression (mimic), hypointense lesion in biliary tree (MRCP) vs., **412**

Pulsion diverticulum, esophageal outpouchings (diverticula) vs., **82**

Pyelitis, renal sinus lesion vs., **524**

Pyelogenic cyst, dilated renal pelvis vs., **557**

Pyelonephritis
- acute
    acute left abdominal pain vs., **215**
    enlarged kidney vs., **544**
    hyperechoic kidney vs., **552**
    hyperechoic renal mass vs., **561**
    infiltrative renal lesions vs., **512**
    wedge-shaped or striated nephrogram vs., **534**
- acute flank pain vs., **538**
- acute right lower quadrant pain vs., **208**
- delayed or persistent nephrogram vs., **530**
- emphysematous
    gas in or around kidney vs., **528**
    hyperechoic kidney vs., **553**
    hyperechoic renal mass vs., **560–561**
- filling defect, renal pelvis vs., **570**
- kidney transplant dysfunction vs., **496**
- right upper quadrant pain vs., **390, 391**
- xanthogranulomatous
    dilated renal calyces vs., **566, 567**

enlarged kidney vs., **545**

gas in or around kidney vs., **528**

hyperechoic renal mass vs., **561**

infiltrative renal lesions vs., **512, 513**

perirenal and subcapsular mass lesions vs., **516, 517**

Pyocele, extratesticular cystic mass vs., **610**

Pyogenic abscess, hepatic
- anechoic liver lesion vs., **336**
- cystic hepatic mass vs., **248**
- echogenic liver mass vs., **344**
- focal hepatic echogenic lesion vs., **322**
- hyperintense liver lesions (T1WI) vs., **298**
- hypoechoic liver mass vs., **340**
- liver lesion with capsule or halo on MR vs., **304**
- multiple hypo-, hyper- or anechoic liver lesions vs., **350–351**
- multiple hypodense liver lesions vs., **308**
- target lesions in liver vs., **348**

Pyogenic cholangitis, recurrent
- asymmetric dilation of intrahepatic bile ducts vs., **404–405**
- dysmorphic liver with abnormal bile ducts vs., **279**
- intrahepatic and extrahepatic duct dilatation vs., **388**
- multiple biliary strictures vs., **408–409**
- periportal lesion vs., **357**

Pyonephrosis
- acute flank pain vs., **538–539**
- dilated renal calyces vs., **566**
- dilated renal pelvis vs., **556**
- gas in or around kidney vs., **528**

Pyosalpinx
- acute pelvic pain vs., **650**
- extraovarian adnexal mass vs., **644**

Q

Quadrant mass, left upper, **124–127**
- differential diagnosis, **124**

R

Radiation colitis
- segmental colonic narrowing vs., **195**
- smooth ahaustral colon vs., **206**

Radiation enteritis
- occult GI bleeding vs., **160**
- segmental or diffuse small bowel wall thickening vs., **151**
- small bowel obstruction vs., **165**
- stenosis, terminal ileum vs., **148**

Radiation hepatitis, widespread low attenuation within liver vs., **318**

Radiation nephritis, wedge-shaped or striated nephrogram vs., **534, 535**

Radiation therapy
- infiltrative renal lesions, **512, 513**
- misty (infiltrated) mesentery, **37**
- multiple biliary strictures vs., **408, 409**

Reactive lymphadenopathy
- due to localized abdominal inflammation, mesenteric lymphadenopathy vs., **18**
- due to systemic inflammation, mesenteric lymphadenopathy vs., **18**

Rectal carcinoma
- dilated renal calyces vs., **566**
- filling defect in urinary bladder vs., **584**
- rectal or colonic fistula vs., **188**
- solitary colonic filling defect vs., **172**

Rectal mucosal prolapse, segmental colonic narrowing vs., **195**

Rectovaginal septum, endometrioma, female lower genital cysts vs., **638, 639**

Red degeneration, acute pelvic pain vs., **651**

Reflux, into dilated renal pelvis, dilated renal pelvis vs., **556**

Reflux esophagitis
- dilated esophagus vs., **80**
- epigastric pain vs., **118**
- esophageal dysmotility vs., **84**
- esophageal strictures vs., **78**
- esophageal ulceration vs., **74**
- mucosal nodularity, esophagus vs., **76**
- odynophagia vs., **86**

Reflux nephropathy, chronic, small kidney vs., **548**

Refractile artifact, echogenic liver mass vs., **344**

Regenerating nodules, cirrhotic
- focal hyperdense hepatic mass on nonenhanced CT vs., **314**
- multiple hypointense liver lesions (T2WI) vs., **295**

Regenerative hyperplasia, nodular
- focal hypervascular liver lesion vs., **252–253**
- hyperintense liver lesions (T1WI) vs., **299**
- liver lesion with capsule or halo on MR vs., **304**
- liver mass with central or eccentric scar vs., **236**
- multiple hypointense liver lesions (T2WI) vs., **295**

Renal abscess
- cystic renal mass vs., **504–505**
- gas in or around kidney vs., **528**

Renal agenesis, congenital renal anomalies vs., **492–493**

Renal angiomyolipoma
- duodenal mass vs., **130**
- fat-containing renal mass vs., **520**
- left upper quadrant mass vs., **125**

Renal anomalies, congenital, **492–495**
- differential diagnosis, **492**

Renal artery
- aneurysm
  dilated renal pelvis vs., **557**
  renal sinus lesion vs., **524**
- stenosis
  chronic, small kidney vs., **549**
  delayed or persistent nephrogram vs., **530, 531**
  transplant, kidney transplant dysfunction vs., **497**

Renal atrophy
- postobstructive, small kidney vs., **548**

- posttraumatic, small kidney vs., **549**
Renal calculi
- acute right lower quadrant pain vs., **208**
- calcifications within kidney vs., **488**
- hyperechoic renal mass vs., **560**
Renal cell carcinoma
- acute flank pain vs., **539**
- acute left abdominal pain vs., **215**
- calcifications within kidney vs., **488**
- cystic
    cystic renal mass vs., **504, 505**
    cystic retroperitoneal mass vs., **460**
- delayed or persistent nephrogram vs., **531**
- enlarged kidney vs., **544**
- fat-containing renal mass vs., **520**
- filling defect, renal pelvis vs., **570**
- gastric mass lesions vs., **90**
- hyperechoic renal mass vs., **560**
- infiltrative renal lesions vs., **512**
- left upper quadrant mass vs., **125**
- mimic
    adrenal mass vs., **481**
    hypervascular pancreatic mass vs., **422, 423**
- perirenal and subcapsular mass lesions vs., **516**
- renal sinus lesion vs., **524**
- retroperitoneal hemorrhage vs., **476**
- solid renal mass vs., **500**
Renal cystic dysplasia, small kidney vs., **549**
Renal cysts
- abdominal calcifications vs., **23**
- bilateral, **508–511**
- cystic retroperitoneal mass vs., **460**
- simple, bilateral renal cysts vs., **508**
Renal dysplasia, multicystic
- bilateral renal cysts vs., **508, 509**
- cystic renal mass vs., **504, 505**
- enlarged kidney vs., **545**
Renal ectopia
- crossed fused
    congenital renal anomalies vs., **492**
    enlarged kidney vs., **545**
- extraovarian adnexal mass vs., **644, 645**
- simple, congenital renal anomalies vs., **492**
Renal failure
- chronic, thickened duodenal fold vs., **138**
- diffuse gallbladder wall thickening vs., **374**
- misty (infiltrated) mesentery vs., **36**
Renal hemorrhage
- acute flank pain vs., **538**
- acute left abdominal pain vs., **215**
Renal hypoplasia, small kidney vs., **549**
Renal infarction
- acute flank pain vs., **539**
- acute left abdominal pain vs., **215**
- chronic, small kidney vs., **549**
- gas in or around kidney vs., **528**
Renal junctional line, hyperechoic renal mass vs., **560**
Renal leukemia, infiltrative renal lesions vs., **512**
Renal lymphoma, infiltrative renal lesions vs., **512**
Renal malrotation, congenital renal anomalies vs., **492**

Renal mass
- extrinsic, duodenal mass vs., **131**
- left upper quadrant mass vs., **125**
- solid, **500–503**
    differential diagnosis, **500**
Renal medullary carcinoma
- infiltrative renal lesions vs., **512**
- solid renal mass vs., **500**
Renal metastases
- hyperechoic renal mass vs., **561**
- infiltrative renal lesions vs., **512–513**
Renal oncocytoma, hyperechoic renal mass vs., **561**
Renal papillary necrosis
- delayed or persistent nephrogram vs., **530**
- dilated renal calyces vs., **566, 567**
- filling defect, renal pelvis vs., **570**
- hyperechoic renal mass vs., **560**
Renal pelvis
- blood-filled, dilated renal calyces vs., **566, 567**
- dilated, **556–559**
    differential diagnosis, **556**
- filling defect, **570–573**
    differential diagnosis, **570**
- obstructed, dilated renal pelvis vs., **556**
- physiologic distention of, dilated renal pelvis vs., **556**
Renal plasmacytoma, infiltrative renal lesions vs., **512, 513**
Renal ptosis, acute flank pain vs., **539**
Renal replacement lipomatosis
- fat-containing renal mass vs., **520**
- renal sinus lesion vs., **524**
Renal sarcoidosis, infiltrative renal lesions vs., **512, 513**
Renal sarcoma, infiltrative renal lesions vs., **512, 513**
Renal scar, fat in, hyperechoic renal mass vs., **560**
Renal sinus cysts, mimic, dilated renal calyces vs., **566**
Renal sinus hemorrhage, dilated renal pelvis vs., **556**
Renal sinus lesion, **524–527**
- differential diagnosis, **524**
Renal tuberculosis
- abdominal calcifications vs., **23**
- dilated renal calyces vs., **566, 567**
Renal tumors, primary, infiltrative, enlarged kidney vs., **544**
Renal vein stenosis, delayed or persistent nephrogram vs., **530, 531**
Renal vein thrombosis
- acute
    dilated renal pelvis vs., **557**
    enlarged kidney vs., **544, 545**
- delayed or persistent nephrogram vs., **530, 531**
- wedge-shaped or striated nephrogram vs., **534, 535**
Renomedullary interstitial cell tumor, solid renal mass vs., **501**
Respiratory motion artifact (mimic), hypointense lesion in biliary tree (MRCP) vs., **412**
Retained foreign body, liver lesion containing gas vs., **270–271**
Retained products of conception, thickened endometrium vs., **662, 663**
Rete testis, tubular ectasia, testicular cystic lesions vs., **608**

Retroperitoneal abscess, cystic retroperitoneal mass vs., **461**

Retroperitoneal fibrosis
- acute flank pain vs., **539**
- dilated renal calyces vs., **566**
- iliopsoas compartment mass vs., **52**
- renal sinus lesion vs., **525**
- soft-tissue-density retroperitoneal mass vs., **466**
- ureteral filling defect or stricture vs., **576**

Retroperitoneal germ cell tumor, soft-tissue-density retroperitoneal mass vs., **467**

Retroperitoneal hemorrhage, **476–477**
- acute flank pain vs., **538**
- differential diagnosis, **476**

Retroperitoneal mass
- cystic, **460–465**
    differential diagnosis, **460**
- fat-containing, **472–475**
    differential diagnosis, **472**
- soft-tissue-density, **466–471**
    differential diagnosis, **466**

Retroperitoneal metastasis, ureteral filling defect or stricture vs., **576**

Retroperitoneal paraganglioma (mimic), hypervascular pancreatic mass vs., **422, 423**

Retroperitoneal sarcoma
- left upper quadrant mass vs., **125**
- mimic, cystic retroperitoneal mass vs., **460**

Retroperitoneal teratoma, cystic pancreatic mass vs., **426, 427**

Retroperitoneum
- cystic retroperitoneal mass, **460–465**
    differential diagnosis, **460**
- fibrosis
    delayed or persistent nephrogram vs., **530**
    perirenal and subcapsular mass lesions vs., **516, 517**
- lymphangioleiomyomatosis, cystic retroperitoneal mass vs., **461**
- metastases and lymphoma
    delayed or persistent nephrogram vs., **530**
    dilated renal pelvis vs., **557**
    fat-containing retroperitoneal mass, **475**
- retroperitoneal hemorrhage, **476–477**
    differential diagnosis, **476**
- retroperitoneal mass, fat-containing, **472–475**
    differential diagnosis, **472**
- solid mesenteric or omental mass vs., **5**
- varices or vessels (mimic), adrenal mass vs., **480**

Rhabdomyolysis
- abdominal wall mass vs., **49**
- delayed or persistent nephrogram vs., **531**
- wedge-shaped or striated nephrogram vs., **534, 535**

Rhabdomyosarcoma, extratesticular solid mass vs., **612**

Richter hernia, **60**

Right upper quadrant pain, **390–395**
- differential diagnosis, **390**

Rosai-Dorfman disease
- perirenal and subcapsular mass lesions vs., **517**
- renal sinus lesion vs., **525**

S

Salpingitis, acute pelvic pain vs., **650**

Sarcoidosis
- gastric dilation or outlet obstruction vs., **111**
- hepatic
    diffuse hyperechoic liver vs., **328**
    diffusely abnormal liver echogenicity vs., **334**
    mosaic/patchy hepatogram vs., **262**
    multiple hypointense liver lesions (T2WI) vs., **295**
    widespread low attenuation within liver vs., **318**
- hepatomegaly vs., **331**
- linitis plastica vs., **114, 115**
- mesenteric lymphadenopathy vs., **19**
- multiple biliary strictures vs., **408, 409**
- multiple splenic calcifications vs., **226**
- solid splenic mass vs., **228**
- splenomegaly vs., **223**
- thickened gastric folds vs., **105**

Sarcoma
- abdominal wall mass vs., **49**
- extraovarian adnexal mass vs., **644, 645**
- extraperitoneal, extraovarian adnexal mass vs., **644**
- Kaposi
    abdominal wall mass vs., **49**
    target (bull's-eye) lesions, stomach vs., **98**
- prostate
    enlarged prostate vs., **630**
    focal lesion in prostate vs., **624, 625**
- renal, infiltrative renal lesions vs., **512, 513**
- renal sinus lesion vs., **525**
- retroperitoneal, mimic, cystic retroperitoneal mass vs., **460, 461**
- soft-tissue-density retroperitoneal mass vs., **466**
- solid renal mass vs., **500**

Scar, calcified, abdominal wall mass vs., **48**

Schistosomiasis
- bladder, abnormal bladder wall vs., **594, 595**
- diffusely abnormal liver echogenicity vs., **334**
- hepatic
    diffuse hyperechoic liver vs., **328**
    hepatic calcifications vs., **267**
    periportal lesion vs., **357**
- irregular hepatic surface vs., **360**
- widened hepatic fissures vs., **276**

Schwannoma
- hypovascular pancreatic mass vs., **416, 417**
- pancreatic, hypervascular pancreatic mass vs., **422, 423**
- target (bull's-eye) lesions, stomach vs., **98**

Sciatic hernia, abdominal wall defects vs., **61**

Scleroderma
- esophageal
    dilated esophagus vs., **80**
    esophageal dysmotility vs., **84**
- esophageal strictures vs., **78**
- intestinal, dilated duodenum vs., **136**
- pneumatosis of small intestine vs., **157**

Sclerosing cholangitis
- intrahepatic and extrahepatic duct dilatation vs., **388**
- primary, liver "mass" with capsular retraction vs., **244**
Sclerosing mesenteritis
- abdominal calcifications vs., **23**
- acute left abdominal pain vs., **215**
- fat-containing lesion of peritoneal cavity vs., **14**
- mesenteric lymphadenopathy vs., **19**
- misty (infiltrated) mesentery vs., **36**
- solid mesenteric or omental mass vs., **4**
Sclerosing peritonitis
- abdominal calcifications vs., **23**
- cluster of dilated small bowel vs., **144**
Scrotal pearl
- extratesticular solid mass vs., **612**
- mimic, testicular calcifications vs., **620**
Scrotum
- decreased testicular size, **618–619**
- diffuse testicular enlargement, **616–617**
- extratesticular cystic mass, **610–611**
- extratesticular solid mass, **612–615**
- intratesticular mass, **604–607**
- testicular calcifications, **620–621**
- testicular cystic lesions, **608–609**
- trauma
    decreased testicular size vs., **618**
    diffuse testicular enlargement, **616**
    testicular calcifications vs., **620**
- tuberculosis, testicular calcifications vs., **620**
- wall fluid collection, extratesticular cystic mass vs., **610**
Sebaceous cyst, abdominal wall mass vs., **48**
Secretory-phase endometrium, thickened endometrium vs., **662**
Segmental colonic narrowing, **194–197**
- differential diagnosis, **194**
Seminoma, intratesticular mass vs., **604**
Senescent change
- atrophy or fatty replacement of pancreas vs., **432**
- colon, smooth ahaustral colon vs., **206**
- pancreas
    dilated pancreatic duct vs., **434**
    pancreatic calcifications vs., **444**
- widened hepatic fissures vs., **276**
Seroma
- adrenal (liquefied hematoma), cystic retroperitoneal mass vs., **461**
- cystic hepatic mass vs., **248**
- retroperitoneal (liquefied hematoma), cystic retroperitoneal mass vs., **461**
Serous cystadenocarcinoma
- multilocular ovarian cysts vs., **676**
- unilocular ovarian cysts vs., **682, 683**
Serous cystadenoma
- cystic retroperitoneal mass vs., **460**
- left upper quadrant mass vs., **124**
- microcystic, cystic retroperitoneal mass vs., **461**
- multilocular ovarian cysts vs., **676**
- pancreatic
    cystic pancreatic lesion vs., **448**
    cystic pancreatic mass vs., **426**
    duodenal mass vs., **131**

hypervascular pancreatic mass vs., **422**
hypovascular pancreatic mass vs., **416**
pancreatic calcifications vs., **444**
solid pancreatic lesion vs., **452–453**
- unilocular ovarian cysts vs., **682, 683**
Serous ovarian neoplasms, calcified ovarian masses vs., **692**
Sertoli cell tumor, large cell calcifying, testicular calcifications vs., **620**
Sertoli-Leydig cell tumors, solid ovarian masses vs., **688, 689**
Shock bowel, segmental or diffuse small bowel wall thickening vs., **150**
Shock pancreas, infiltration of peripancreatic fat planes vs., **438–439**
Shwachman-Diamond syndrome
- atrophy or fatty replacement of pancreas vs., **432**
- pancreatic calcifications vs., **445**
Sickle cell anemia, diffuse increased attenuation, spleen vs., **232**
Sigmoid colonic diverticulitis, abnormal bladder wall vs., **594, 595**
Sigmoid diverticulitis, extraovarian adnexal mass vs., **644**
Sigmoid volvulus
- acute left abdominal pain vs., **214, 215**
- colonic ileus vs., **182**
Simple hepatic cysts, multiple hypodense liver lesions vs., **308**
Simple renal ectopia, congenital renal anomalies vs., **492**
Simple small bowel obstruction, cluster of dilated small bowel vs., **144**
Skene gland cyst, female lower genital cysts vs., **638**
Sloughed papilla, ureteral filling defect or stricture vs., **576**
Sludge/sludge ball/echogenic bile, echogenic material in gallbladder vs., **382**
Small intestine
- aneurysmal dilation of, lumen, **146–147**
- carcinoma
    occult GI bleeding vs., **160**
    small bowel obstruction vs., **165**
    stenosis, terminal ileum vs., **148–149**
- dilated small bowel, cluster of, **144–145**
- diverticula
    aneurysmal dilation of small bowel lumen vs., **146**
    pneumoperitoneum vs., **29**
- intubation, iatrogenic, small bowel obstruction vs., **165**
- lymphoma, aneurysmal dilation of small bowel lumen vs., **146**
- metastases, aneurysmal dilation of small bowel lumen vs., **146**
- multiple masses or filling defects, **142–143**
    differential diagnosis, **142**
- obstruction, **164–169**
    aneurysmal dilation of small bowel lumen vs., **146**
    differential diagnosis, **164**
    dilated common bile duct vs., **398, 399**
    dilated duodenum vs., **136**
    epigastric pain vs., **119**
    pneumatosis of small intestine vs., **156–157**
    portal venous gas vs., **274**

- occult GI bleeding, **160–163**
  - differential diagnosis, **160**
- pneumatosis of, **156–159**
  - differential diagnosis of, **156**
- stenosis, terminal ileum, **148–149**
- transplantation
  - cluster of dilated small bowel vs., **144**
  - misty (infiltrated) mesentery vs., **37**
  - pneumatosis of small intestine vs., **157**
- vasculitis
  - misty (infiltrated) mesentery vs., **37**
  - occult GI bleeding vs., **160**
  - segmental or diffuse small bowel wall thickening vs., **151**
- wall thickening, segmental or diffuse, **150–155**
  - differential diagnosis, **150**
Smooth ahaustral colon, **206–207**
- differential diagnosis, **206**
Soft tissue calcifications, abdominal calcifications vs., **23**
Soft tissue metastases, abdominal wall mass vs., **49**
Solid mass
- extratesticular, **612–615**
- focal hepatic echogenic lesion vs., **323**
Solid mass calcification, abdominal, **22**
Solid ovarian masses, **688–691**
- differential diagnosis, **688**
Solid pancreatic lesion, **452–455**
- differential diagnosis, **452**
Solid pseudopapillary neoplasm
- cystic pancreatic lesion vs., **449**
- cystic pancreatic mass vs., **426–427**
- hypovascular pancreatic mass vs., **416, 417**
- pancreatic calcifications vs., **445**
- solid pancreatic lesion vs., **453**
Solid renal mass, **500–503**
- differential diagnosis, **500**
"Solid" serous adenoma, cystic pancreatic mass vs., **426**
Solid splenic mass, **228–229**
- differential diagnosis, **228**
Solitary colonic filling defect, **172–173**
- differential diagnosis, **172**
Solitary fibrous tumor
- hypervascular pancreatic mass vs., **422, 423**
- lipomatous, fat-containing renal mass vs., **521**
- liver mass with mosaic enhancement vs., **259**
- soft-tissue-density retroperitoneal mass vs., **467**
Solitary rectal ulcer syndrome, solitary colonic filling defect vs., **172**
Space-occupying masses, splenomegaly vs., **222**
Sperm granuloma, extratesticular solid mass vs., **612**
Spermatic cord lipoma
- abdominal wall defects vs., **61**
- groin mass vs., **54**
Spermatocele, extratesticular cystic mass vs., **610**
Spherical hematoma, coagulopathic hemorrhage, liver, **240**
Sphincter of Oddi
- contraction of (mimic), hypointense lesion in biliary tree (MRCP) vs., **412**
- dysfunction, epigastric pain vs., **118**
- patulous, gas in bile ducts or gallbladder vs., **368**

Sphincterotomy, biliary, gas in bile ducts or gallbladder vs., **368**
Spigelian hernia
- abdominal wall defects vs., **60**
- abdominal wall mass vs., **48**
- acute left abdominal pain vs., **215**
Spinal cord injury, colonic ileus vs., **182**
Spleen
- abscess
  - cystic splenic mass vs., **230**
  - healed, multiple splenic calcifications vs., **226**
  - solid splenic mass vs., **228**
- accessory
  - mimic, hypervascular pancreatic mass vs., **422, 422–423**
  - perirenal and subcapsular mass lesions vs., **516, 517**
  - stomach intramural mass vs., **96**
- calcifications, abdominal calcifications vs., **22**
- cyst
  - abdominal calcifications vs., **22**
  - cystic splenic mass vs., **230**
  - multiple splenic calcifications vs., **226**
- cystic splenic mass, **230–231**
- diffuse increased attenuation, **232–233**
- granulomas, abdominal calcifications vs., **22**
- hematoma, multiple splenic calcifications vs., **226**
- infarction
  - cystic splenic mass vs., **230**
  - diffuse increased attenuation, spleen vs., **232**
  - mimic, solid splenic mass vs., **228**
  - multiple splenic calcifications vs., **226**
  - splenomegaly vs., **223**
- infection
  - cystic splenic mass vs., **230**
  - solid splenic mass vs., **228**
- lymphoma
  - cystic splenic mass vs., **230**
  - splenomegaly vs., **222–223**
- metastases
  - cystic splenic mass vs., **230**
  - solid splenic mass vs., **228**
- multiple splenic calcifications, **226–227**
- neoplasms, primary, multiple splenic calcifications vs., **226**
- ruptured
  - hemoperitoneum vs., **33**
  - high-attenuation (hyperdense) ascites vs., **42**
- solid splenic mass, **228–229**
- splenomegaly, **222–225**
- trauma
  - cystic splenic mass vs., **230**
  - mimic, solid splenic mass vs., **228**
  - splenomegaly vs., **223**
- tumors
  - cystic splenic mass vs., **230**
  - mimic, hypervascular pancreatic mass vs., **422, 423**
  - primary, solid splenic mass vs., **228**
  - primary, splenomegaly vs., **223**
Splenic mass
- cystic, **230–231**
  - differential diagnosis, **230**

INDEX

- left upper quadrant mass vs., **124**
- solid, **228–229**
    differential diagnosis, **228**
Splenic peliosis, solid splenic mass vs., **228**
Splenic vein occlusion, splenomegaly vs., **223**
Splenomegaly, **222–225**
- differential diagnosis, **222**
- gastric mass lesions vs., **90**
- left upper quadrant mass vs., **124**
Splenosis
- gastric mass lesions vs., **90**
- solid mesenteric or omental mass vs., **5**
- stomach intramural mass vs., **96**
Squamous cell carcinoma, infiltrative renal lesions vs., **512, 513**
Steatohepatitis
- epigastric pain vs., **119**
- hepatomegaly vs., **330–331**
Steatosis
- diffuse hyperechoic liver vs., **328**
- diffusely abnormal liver echogenicity vs., **334**
- epigastric pain vs., **119**
- focal
    echogenic liver mass vs., **344**
    focal hepatic echogenic lesion vs., **322**
- hepatic
    multiple hypo-, hyper- or anechoic liver lesions vs., **350**
    right upper quadrant pain vs., **390**
- hyperintense liver lesions (T1WI) vs., **298**
- mimic, cystic hepatic mass vs., **248**
- mosaic/patchy hepatogram vs., **262**
- patchy, mimic, fat-containing liver mass vs., **246**
- periportal lucency or edema vs., **289**
- widespread low attenuation within liver vs., **318**
Stenosis, terminal ileum, **148–149**
Stercoral colitis
- acute left abdominal pain vs., **214**
- fecal impaction, colonic ileus vs., **182**
Steroid medications, atrophy or fatty replacement of pancreas, **432**
Stomach
- apposed walls of, gastric mass lesions vs., **90**
- dilation or outlet obstruction, **110–113**
    differential diagnosis, **110**
- gastric mass lesion, **90–95**
    differential diagnosis, **90**
- gastric ulceration without mass, **100–101**
    differential diagnosis, **100**
- intramural mass, **96–97**
    differential diagnosis, **96**
- intrathoracic, **102–103**
    differential diagnosis, **102**
- linitis plastica (limited distensibility), **114–117**
    differential diagnosis, **114**
- target (bull's-eye) lesions, stomach, **98, 98–99**
    differential diagnosis, **98**
- thickened gastric folds, **104–109**
    differential diagnosis, **104**
Storage diseases, splenomegaly vs., **223**
Straddle injuries, urethral stricture vs., **600**

Stricture
- esophageal, **78–79**
- urethral, **600–601**
    differential diagnosis, **600**
    idiopathic, urethral stricture vs., **600**
    infectious, urethral stricture vs., **600**
Stromal tumor of uncertain malignant potential (STUMP)
- enlarged prostate vs., **630**
- focal lesion in prostate vs., **624, 625**
Strongyloides, dilated duodenum vs., **136**
Struma ovarii
- multilocular ovarian cysts vs., **676, 677**
- ovarian lesions with low T2 signal intensity vs., **696, 697**
Subcapsular collection, delayed or persistent nephrogram vs., **530–531**
Subcapsular fluid collections, enlarged kidney vs., **544**
Subcapsular hemorrhage, **516**
Subcapsular hepatic neoplasm, irregular hepatic surface vs., **360**
Subchorionic hematoma, abnormal uterine bleeding vs., **668**
Subclavian artery, aberrant, extrinsic esophageal mass vs., **68**
Subdiaphragmatic mass, elevated or deformed hemidiaphragm vs., **58**
Submucosal leiomyoma, thickened endometrium vs., **662**
Subphrenic fat, mimic, pneumoperitoneum vs., **29**
Subpubic cartilaginous cyst, female lower genital cysts vs., **638, 639**
Subserosal leiomyoma, extraovarian adnexal mass vs., **644**
Superior mesenteric artery syndrome, dilated duodenum vs., **136**
Superior vena cava obstruction
- abdominal manifestations, focal hyperperfusion abnormality vs., **283**
- focal hypervascular liver lesion vs., **253**
Supernumerary kidney, congenital renal anomalies vs., **493**
Surgical biliary-enteric anastomosis, gas in bile ducts or gallbladder vs., **368**
Surgical complications, esophageal dysmotility, **84**
Surgical devices, focal hepatic echogenic lesion and, **322**
Susceptibility artifact (mimic), hypointense lesion in biliary tree (MRCP) vs., **412**
Syphilis
- gastric dilation or outlet obstruction vs., **111**
- linitis plastica vs., **114, 115**
Syringocele, urethral stricture vs., **600**
Systemic diseases
- solid mesenteric or omental mass vs., **5**
- wall thickening due to, diffuse gallbladder wall thickening vs., **374**
Systemic hypervolemia
- mosaic/patchy hepatogram vs., **262**
- periportal lucency or edema vs., **288**
Systemic hypotension, segmental or diffuse small bowel wall thickening vs., **150**
Systemic infection, splenomegaly vs., **223**
Systemic lupus erythematosus
- diffuse increased attenuation, spleen vs., **232**
- dilated gallbladder vs., **385**

- multiple splenic calcifications vs., **226**

T

Tailgut cyst, cystic retroperitoneal mass vs., **461**
Tamoxifen-induced changes, thickened endometrium vs., **662–663**
Target lesions, stomach, **98**
- differential diagnosis, **98**
Tarlov cyst, extraovarian adnexal mass vs., **644**
Technical artifact (mimic)
- diffuse hyperechoic liver and, **328**
- diffusely abnormal liver echogenicity vs., **334**
Telangiectasia, hereditary hemorrhagic
- focal hypervascular liver lesion vs., **252**
- mosaic/patchy hepatogram vs., **262**
- multiple hypointense liver lesions (T2WI) vs., **295**
Teratoma
- fat-containing liver mass vs., **246**
- immature
   calcified ovarian masses vs., **692**
   solid ovarian masses vs., **688, 689**
- liver, hyperintense liver lesions (T1WI) vs., **299**
- mature
   cystic mesenteric and omental mass vs., **11**
   fat-containing lesion of peritoneal cavity vs., **14**
- retroperitoneal, fat-containing retroperitoneal mass, **472**
- testicular cystic lesions vs., **608**
Testicular appendage, torsion of, extratesticular solid mass vs., **612**
Testis
- abscess
   intratesticular mass vs., **604**
   testicular cystic lesions vs., **608**
- calcifications, **620–621**
   differential diagnosis, **620**
- carcinoma
   diffuse testicular enlargement vs., **616**
   intratesticular mass vs., **604**
- cyst, diffuse testicular enlargement vs., **616**
- cystic lesions, **608–609**
   differential diagnosis, **608**
- decreased size, **618–619**
- diffuse enlargement, **616–617**
- epidermoid cyst, intratesticular mass vs., **604, 605**
- gonadal stromal tumors, intratesticular mass vs., **604, 605**
- hematoma, intratesticular mass vs., **604–605**
- infarction
   decreased testicular size vs., **618**
   diffuse testicular enlargement vs., **616**
- leukemia
   diffuse testicular enlargement vs., **616**
   intratesticular mass vs., **604, 605**
- lipomatosis, intratesticular mass vs., **604, 605**
- lymphoma
   diffuse testicular enlargement vs., **616**

intratesticular mass vs., **604, 605**
- metastases
   diffuse testicular enlargement vs., **616**
   intratesticular mass vs., **604, 605**
- microlithiasis, testicular calcifications vs., **620**
- torsion
   diffuse testicular enlargement vs., **616**
   intratesticular mass vs., **604**
Theca lutein cysts, multilocular ovarian cysts vs., **676**
Thecoma, solid ovarian masses vs., **688**
Thickened duodenal fold, **138–139**
- differential diagnosis, **138**
Thickened endometrium, **662–667**
- differential diagnosis, **662**
Thickened gastric folds, **104–109**
- differential diagnosis, **104**
Thoracic infection or inflammation, right upper quadrant pain vs., **390, 391**
Thoracic processes, mimics, pneumoperitoneum vs., **29**
Thorotrast, diffuse increased attenuation, spleen vs., **232**
Thrombophlebitis, acute pelvic pain vs., **650, 651**
Thrombosed esophageal varix, intraluminal mass vs., **66**
Thrombosis
- chronic deep venous, abdominal calcifications and, **23**
- portomesenteric venous, misty (infiltrated) mesentery vs., **37**
Thumbprinting, colonic, **198–199**
- differential diagnosis, **198**
Thyroid, enlarged, extrinsic esophageal mass vs., **68**
Torsion
- acute pelvic pain vs., **651**
- ovarian
   acute pelvic pain vs., **650**
   solid ovarian masses vs., **688**
- testicular
   diffuse testicular enlargement vs., **616**
   intratesticular mass vs., **604**
- testicular appendage, extratesticular solid mass vs., **612**
- tubal, extraovarian adnexal mass vs., **644, 645**
Toxic hepatic injury, widespread low attenuation within liver vs., **318**
Toxic megacolon, **186–187**
- colonic ileus vs., **182**
- differential diagnosis, **186**
- smooth ahaustral colon vs., **206**
Traction diverticulum, esophageal outpouchings (diverticula) vs., **82**
Transarterial hepatic chemoembolization, gas in bile ducts or gallbladder vs., **369**
Transient hepatic attenuation difference
- focal hyperperfusion abnormality vs., **282**
- focal hypervascular liver lesion vs., **252**
Transitional cell carcinoma, multilocular ovarian cysts vs., **676**
Transmesenteric internal hernia
- epigastric pain vs., **118**
- small bowel obstruction vs., **165**
Transmesenteric postoperative hernia, cluster of dilated small bowel vs., **144**

INDEX

Transplant dysfunction, kidney, **496–499**
- differential diagnosis, **496**
Transplant renal artery stenosis, kidney transplant dysfunction vs., **497**
Transplantation
- renal, chronic allograft rejection, small kidney vs., **548**
- small bowel, misty (infiltrated) mesentery vs., **37**
- small intestine, cluster of dilated small bowel vs., **144**
Transudative ascites, **42**
Trauma
- abdominal, hemoperitoneum vs., **32**
- bladder
    hemoperitoneum vs., **33**
    high-attenuation (hyperdense) ascites vs., **43**
    urinary bladder outpouching vs., **590**
- bladder wall, abnormal bladder wall vs., **594, 595**
- colorectal or vaginal, rectal or colonic fistula vs., **188, 189**
- filling defect, renal pelvis vs., **570**
- hepatic
    focal hepatic echogenic lesion vs., **323**
    focal liver lesion with hemorrhage vs., **240**
    high-attenuation (hyperdense) bile in gallbladder vs., **378**
    periportal lesion vs., **356**
    periportal lucency or edema vs., **289**
    retroperitoneal hemorrhage vs., **476**
- intestinal
    pneumatosis of small intestine vs., **157**
    pneumoperitoneum vs., **28**
    small bowel obstruction vs., **165**
- pelvic, retroperitoneal hemorrhage vs., **476**
- renal
    cystic renal mass vs., **504, 505**
    hyperechoic renal mass vs., **561**
    perirenal and subcapsular mass lesions vs., **516**
    retroperitoneal hemorrhage vs., **476**
    wedge-shaped or striated nephrogram vs., **534**
- scrotal
    decreased testicular size vs., **618**
    diffuse testicular enlargement, **616**
    testicular calcifications vs., **620**
- splenic
    cystic splenic mass vs., **230**
    mimic, solid splenic mass vs., **228**
    splenomegaly vs., **223**
Traumatic hemoperitoneum, high-attenuation (hyperdense) ascites vs., **42**
Trigone, normal, abnormal bladder wall vs., **594**
Tubal carcinoma, extraovarian adnexal mass vs., **644, 645**
Tubal ectopic pregnancy
- abnormal uterine bleeding vs., **668**
- extraovarian adnexal mass vs., **644**
Tubal leiomyoma, extraovarian adnexal mass vs., **644**
Tubal torsion, extraovarian adnexal mass vs., **644, 645**
Tuberculoma, solitary colonic filling defect vs., **172**
Tuberculosis
- adrenal, adrenal mass vs., **481**
- calcifications within kidney vs., **489**
- colon
    mass or inflammation of ileocecal area vs., **176, 177**

    segmental colonic narrowing vs., **194**
- gastric dilation or outlet obstruction vs., **111**
- linitis plastica vs., **114, 115**
- mesenteric lymphadenopathy vs., **19**
- miliary, diffuse hyperechoic liver vs., **328**
- multiple splenic calcifications vs., **226**
- renal
    abdominal calcifications vs., **23**
    dilated renal calyces vs., **566, 567**
    enlarged kidney vs., **545**
    hyperechoic kidney vs., **553**
- scrotal, testicular calcifications vs., **620**
- stenosis, terminal ileum vs., **148**
- thickened gastric folds vs., **105**
- of urinary tract, hyperechoic renal mass vs., **561**
- wedge-shaped or striated nephrogram vs., **534, 535**
Tuberculous autonephrectomy, small kidney vs., **549**
Tuberculous cystitis, abnormal bladder wall vs., **594, 595**
Tuberculous peritonitis, solid mesenteric or omental mass vs., **4**
Tuberous sclerosis, bilateral renal cysts vs., **508**
Tuboovarian abscess
- acute left abdominal pain vs., **214**
- acute pelvic pain vs., **650**
- multilocular ovarian cysts vs., **676**
- unilocular ovarian cysts vs., **682, 683**
Tubular atrophy, kidney transplant dysfunction vs., **496**
Tubular ectasia of rete testis, testicular cystic lesions vs., **608**
Tubular injury, acute, kidney transplant dysfunction vs., **496**
Tubular necrosis, acute
- hyperechoic kidney vs., **552**
- small kidney vs., **549**
Tumor
- echogenic material in gallbladder vs., **382**
- filling defect, renal pelvis vs., **570**
- thrombus, portal vein, portal vein abnormality vs., **362**
Tunica albuginea cyst, testicular cystic lesions vs., **608**
Tunica vaginalis, mesothelioma of, extratesticular solid mass vs., **612, 613**
Twinkling artifacts, **560**
Typhlitis
- acute right lower quadrant pain vs., **209**
- colonic thumbprinting vs., **198**
- colonic wall thickening vs., **200–201**
- mass or inflammation of ileocecal area vs., **176, 177**
- segmental colonic narrowing vs., **195**

U

Ulcer
- duodenal
    epigastric pain vs., **118**
    gastric dilation or outlet obstruction vs., **110**
    infiltration of peripancreatic fat planes vs., **438**
    right upper quadrant pain vs., **390**
    thickened duodenal fold vs., **138**

- perforated, pneumoperitoneum vs., **28**

Ulcerative colitis
- acute left abdominal pain vs., **214**
- colonic thumbprinting vs., **198**
- colonic wall thickening vs., **200**
- multiple colonic filling defects vs., **174**
- portal venous gas vs., **274**
- segmental colonic narrowing vs., **194**
- smooth ahaustral colon vs., **206**
- stenosis, terminal ileum vs., **148**
- toxic megacolon vs., **186**

Umbilical hernia
- abdominal wall defects vs., **60–61**
- abdominal wall mass vs., **48**

Underdistended bladder, abnormal bladder wall vs., **594**

Undifferentiated hepatic sarcoma
- cystic hepatic mass vs., **249**
- liver mass with mosaic enhancement vs., **259**

Undifferentiated pleomorphic sarcoma, perirenal and subcapsular mass lesions vs., **516**

Unilocular ovarian cysts, **682–687**
- differential diagnosis, **682**

Unopacified bowel (mimic), hypovascular pancreatic mass vs., **416**

Urachal carcinoma, filling defect in urinary bladder vs., **585**

Urachal remnant
- cystic mesenteric and omental mass vs., **11**
- urinary bladder outpouching vs., **590**

Ureter
- calculus, obstructing, delayed or persistent nephrogram vs., **530**
- distal, cystic dilation of, **580–581**
- duplication, dilated renal calyces vs., **566**
- ectopic, cystic dilation of distal ureter vs., **580**
- fibroepithelial polyp, ureteral filling defect or stricture vs., **576, 577**
- filling defect or stricture, **576–579**
    differential diagnosis, **576**
- obstruction
    acute, wedge-shaped or striated nephrogram vs., **534**
    cystic dilation of distal ureter vs., **580**
    dilated renal calyces vs., **566**
- stone, dilated renal calyces vs., **566**
- stricture
    acute flank pain vs., **538**
    delayed or persistent nephrogram vs., **530**
- tumor, cystic dilation of distal ureter vs., **580**

Ureteral papilloma, ureteral filling defect or stricture vs., **576, 577**

Ureterectasis of pregnancy, dilated renal calyces vs., **566**

Ureteritis, infectious, ureteral filling defect or stricture vs., **576**

Ureteritis cystica, ureteral filling defect or stricture vs., **576–577**

Ureterocele
- congenital renal anomalies vs., **493**
- cystic dilation of distal ureter vs., **580**
- everted, urinary bladder outpouching vs., **590**
- filling defect in urinary bladder vs., **584**

Ureteropelvic junction obstruction
- acute flank pain vs., **538**
- congenital renal anomalies vs., **493**
- dilated renal calyces vs., **566**

Urethra
- carcinoma, urethral stricture vs., **600**
- diverticulum, female lower genital cysts vs., **638–639**
- stricture, **600–601**
    differential diagnosis, **600**
    idiopathic, urethral stricture vs., **600**
    infectious, urethral stricture vs., **600**
- trauma, urethral stricture vs., **600**

Urinary bladder. *See* Bladder, urinary.

Urinary obstruction
- delayed or persistent nephrogram vs., **530**
- kidney transplant dysfunction vs., **497**

Urinary retention, acute flank pain vs., **538**

Urinary tract
- calcifications, abdominal calcifications vs., **22–23**
- tuberculosis, hyperechoic renal mass vs., **561**

Urinoma
- cystic retroperitoneal mass vs., **460**
- perirenal and subcapsular mass lesions vs., **516, 517**

Urolithiasis
- acute left abdominal pain vs., **214–215**
- acute right lower quadrant pain vs., **208**
- cystic dilation of distal ureter vs., **580**
- filling defect, renal pelvis vs., **570**
- obstructing, acute flank pain vs., **538**
- renal sinus lesion vs., **524**
- ureteral filling defect or stricture vs., **576**

Urothelial carcinoma
- acute flank pain vs., **538**
- delayed or persistent nephrogram vs., **530**
- dilated renal calyces vs., **566**
- dilated renal pelvis vs., **556**
- enlarged kidney vs., **544**
- filling defect, renal pelvis vs., **570**
- infiltrative renal lesions vs., **512**
- renal sinus lesion vs., **524**
- solid renal mass vs., **500**
- ureteral filling defect or stricture vs., **576**

Urticaria, colon, multiple colonic filling defects vs., **174**

Uterine bleeding, abnormal, **668–673**
- differential diagnosis, **668**

Uterine carcinoma, rectal or colonic fistula vs., **188–189**

Uterine fibroids
- acute left abdominal pain vs., **214**
- acute right lower quadrant pain vs., **208**
- segmental colonic narrowing vs., **194**

Uterine leiomyoma, complications of, acute pelvic pain vs., **650, 651**

Uterine leiomyosarcoma
- abnormal uterine bleeding vs., **668**
- enlarged uterus vs., **658**

Uterus
- abnormal uterine bleeding, **668–673**
- enlarged, **658–661**
    abnormal uterine bleeding vs., **668, 669**
    differential diagnosis, **658**
- postpartum, enlarged uterus vs., **658**

- thickened endometrium, **662–667**
Utricle cyst
- enlarged prostate vs., **630**
- prostatic, focal lesion in prostate vs., **624**

V

Vagal stimulation, decreased, distended gallbladder vs., **366**
Vaginal carcinoma, abnormal uterine bleeding vs., **668**
Vaginal trauma, rectal or colonic fistula vs., **188, 189**
Varices, paraumbilical, abdominal wall mass vs., **48**
Varicocele
- groin mass vs., **54**
- intratesticular, testicular cystic lesions vs., **608**
- mimic, extratesticular cystic mass vs., **610**
Varix, hemorrhoidal, solitary colonic filling defect vs., **172**
Vas deferens calcifications, abdominal calcifications vs., **23**
Vascular abnormalities, mimic, multiple splenic calcifications vs., **226**
Vascular calcifications
- abdominal calcifications vs., **23**
- calcifications within kidney vs., **488**
Vascular compression, ureteral filling defect or stricture vs., **576, 577**
Vascular diseases, collagen, splenomegaly vs., **223**
Vascular ectasia, intestinal, occult GI bleeding vs., **160**
Vascular injury, chronic, small kidney vs., **549**
Vascular lesions, renal sinus lesion vs., **524**
Vascular masses
- echogenic liver mass vs., **344**
- focal hepatic echogenic lesion vs., **323**
Vascular metastases, echogenic liver mass vs., **344**
Vasculitis
- hyperechoic kidney vs., **552**
- perirenal and subcapsular mass lesions vs., **516**
- small bowel, misty (infiltrated) mesentery vs., **37**
- small bowel obstruction vs., **165**
- small intestine
    occult GI bleeding vs., **160**
    segmental or diffuse small bowel wall thickening vs., **151**
- ureteral filling defect or stricture vs., **576, 577**
- wedge-shaped or striated nephrogram vs., **534–535**
Venoocclusive disease
- diffusely abnormal liver echogenicity vs., **334**
- hepatomegaly vs., **331**
Venous collaterals, hepatic, multiple hypointense liver lesions (T2WI) vs., **295**
Venous thrombosis, kidney transplant dysfunction vs., **497**
Ventral hernia
- abdominal wall defects vs., **60**
- abdominal wall mass vs., **48**
- acute left abdominal pain vs., **215**
- small bowel obstruction vs., **164**
Vesicocutaneous fistula, gas within urinary bladder vs., **592**
Vesicoureteral reflux, dilated renal calyces vs., **566**

Vesicovaginal fistula, gas within urinary bladder vs., **592**
Vessels
- abnormal, hypoechoic liver mass vs., **340**
- anechoic liver lesion vs., **336–337**
- multiple hypo-, hyper- or anechoic liver lesions vs., **351**
Vicarious excretion
- hemoperitoneum vs., **33**
- high-attenuation (hyperdense) ascites vs., **42**
- high-attenuation (hyperdense) bile in gallbladder vs., **378**
Villous adenoma, solitary colonic filling defect vs., **172**
Viral cystitis, abnormal bladder wall vs., **594, 595**
Viral hepatitis, acute, periportal lesion vs., **356**
Visceral organ cysts, cystic mesenteric and omental mass vs., **10**
Von Hippel-Lindau disease
- bilateral renal cysts vs., **508–509**
- cystic pancreatic mass vs., **426, 427**
Vulva carcinoma, abnormal uterine bleeding vs., **668**

W

Whipple disease
- mesenteric lymphadenopathy vs., **19**
- segmental or diffuse small bowel wall thickening vs., **151**
Whirl sign, small bowel obstruction, **164**
Widespread low attenuation, within liver, **318–321**
- differential diagnosis, **318**
Wilson disease
- diffusely abnormal liver echogenicity vs., **334**
- widespread low attenuation within liver vs., **318**
Wolffian duct remnant, extraovarian adnexal mass vs., **644**
Wunderlich syndrome, acute flank pain vs., **538**

X

Xanthogranulomatous cholecystitis
- diffuse gallbladder wall thickening vs., **375**
- focal gallbladder wall thickening vs., **372**
Xanthogranulomatous pyelonephritis
- acute flank pain vs., **539**
- calcifications within kidney vs., **488**
- dilated renal calyces vs., **566, 567**
- enlarged kidney vs., **545**
- gas in or around kidney vs., **528**
- hyperechoic renal mass vs., **561**
- infiltrative renal lesions vs., **512, 513**
- perirenal and subcapsular mass lesions vs., **516, 517**
- renal sinus lesion vs., **524**
Xanthoma, liver, hyperintense liver lesions (T1WI) vs., **299**
Xanthomatous lesions, in Langerhans cell histiocytosis, fat-containing liver mass vs., **246**

INDEX

Y

Yolk sac tumor
- multilocular ovarian cysts vs., **676, 677**
- solid ovarian masses vs., **688, 689**

Z

Zenker diverticulum, esophageal outpouchings
    (diverticula), **82**
Zollinger-Ellison syndrome
- dilated duodenum vs., **136**
- gastric ulceration without mass vs., **100**
- thickened duodenal fold vs., **138**
- thickened gastric folds vs., **104**